Psychiatric Dictionary

Psychiatric Dictionary
SIXTH EDITION

ROBERT JEAN CAMPBELL, M.D.

New York   Oxford
OXFORD UNIVERSITY PRESS
1989

Oxford University Press

Oxford New York Toronto
Delhi Bombay Calcutta Madras Karachi
Petaling Jaya Singapore Hong Kong Tokyo
Nairobi Dar es Salaam Cape Town
Melbourne Auckland

and associated companies in
Berlin Ibadan

Published by Oxford University Press, Inc.,
200 Madison Avenue, New York, New York 10016

Oxford is a registered trademark of Oxford University Press

Library of Congress Cataloging-in-Publication Data

Campbell, Robert Jean, 1926–
Psychiatric dictionary/Robert Jean Campbell.—6th ed.
p. cm.
Bibliography: p.
ISBN 0-19-505293-5
1. Psychiatry—Dictionaries. I. Title.
[DNLM: 1. Psychiatry—dictionaries. WM 13 H665p]
RC437.H5 1989
616.89'003'21—dc 19
DNLM/DLC
for Library of Congress   88-12579 CIP

2 4 6 8 9 7 5 3

Printed in the United States of America
on acid-free paper

Preface to the Sixth Edition

Since the fifth edition of this dictionary was published in 1981, psychiatry has continued to battle the stigmatization and discrimination its patients suffer and to confront the misconceptions that many hold about its substance and its methods. At the same time, it has had to respond to externally directed forces that try to define its boundaries, regulate its application, and limit its extension. It has had to develop ways of communicating effectively with the rest of medicine, with legislators and public officials, with the courts, with the media, and with the public. In many instances, this has meant a more precise description of its treatments, its theories, and its research strategies. It has also meant an accommodation to the different and sometimes conflicting viewpoints of other scientific disciplines and of other sectors of society.

All these interchanges have required a familiarity with the languages of those sectors, and nowadays even the lone practitioner in a private office must have more knowledge of official nomenclature, treatment options, informed consent, drug–drug interactions, and duty to warn—to cite but a few examples—than would have been considered even relevant a decade ago. In this new edition of the dictionary, the editor has tried to include as much of such new knowledge as is necessary, without losing sight of the work's primary function, to define *psychiatric* terms.

Like the rest of medicine, the way in which psychiatry is practiced has been changing. Entrepreneurial medicine, developed in response to an imposed philosophy of marketplace competition among "health care providers," has fostered the development of managed care systems. Within such systems, the psychiatrist must be familiar with alternative levels of care, with different systems such as the HMO and the PPO, with such concepts as adverse selection, offset, moral hazard, outliers, skimming, cost shifting, and case mix index. None of these terms is psychiatric, or even medical, yet they are defined because of the practitioner's need to know.

The situation is similar in areas of science whose influence on psychiatry has become more significant than it was in the past. With the many advances in chemical neuroanatomy, neuropsychology, and neurometrics have come a host of terms with which the reader must be familiar in order to understand the current psychiatric literature. Such terms are defined in this dictionary for those whose training antedated these developments.

Coincident with the knowledge explosion in the neurological sciences has been a dramatic expansion of knowledge in particular areas of clinical psychiatry: the sleep and eating disorders, agoraphobia and panic disorder, depression, speech disorders, disorders in cognitive functioning, and others. Equally important have been treatment advances and outcome studies in different treatment approaches. Some of the artificial boundaries between different therapies have been breached, and treatments that lie far outside the realm of "orthodox" therapy have been tested. Every new finding demands a description and requires that some kind of hypothesis be adduced to explain it. A specialized dictionary such as this should include all these descriptions and speculations and indicate, if possible, how they might fit with earlier descriptions. At the same time, outdated terms should be avoided to make way for new entries. In meeting the demands of a printing schedule, the editor must, of course, decide on a cutoff point, after which no new entries can be accommodated and no outmoded ones expunged. In consequence, any such compilation is certain to fall short of perfection; some entries will at best be seen as needless variants, others will be thought to have been banished before they outlived their usefulness, and still others will have been denied the early recognition they deserve. As Samuel Johnson noted, dictionaries are like watches: the worst is better than none, and the best cannot be expected to go quite right.

The last edition of this dictionary incorporated the new language of DSM-III. This edition incorporates the terms of its official revision, DSM-III-R, as well as some of the more controversial terms that were suggested for inclusion in that revision but were ultimately rejected. As in previous editions, inclusion of the official terminology did not lead automatically to the exclusion of older, more familiar terms. Many of those, in fact, are given preference because they are more familiar, and because they continue to be more widely used.

The edition continues the tradition of giving encyclopedic treatment to many terms, and through the liberal use of cross-references it tries to relate entries to associated terms and to put them in perspective within a broader category. It is hoped that such an approach makes the dictionary more readable, and more useful to a broader range of readers.

By definition, a dictionary is derivative and reflective of the work of others. Just as no attempt is made within the text itself to cite the originator of each term, so no listing of people who helped in the preparation of this edition can claim to include them all. To some, however, my indebtedness is so great that they cannot go unnamed: Jeffrey W. House and Marion Osmun, and their associates at Oxford University Press, particularly Carole Schwager, for their unstinting editorial help; Susan Heffner at the American Psychiatric Association's Library for her biographical research; Cynthia and Richard Zirinsky for fashioning the milieu in which this work could proceed; and Cesare L. Santeramo for deftly protecting that milieu against intrusion.

New York, New York   R. J. C.
June 1988

Preface to the First Edition

As the title of this dictionary implies its material has been drawn mainly from the words and concepts current in the field of psychiatry—with definitions and illustrative quotations that aim to give these terms vital, clinical meaning. Though brevity was the ideal, in many instances, where needed, the articles are more or less encyclopedic in character.

The framework of the dictionary is made up of psychiatric terms, but considerable attention has been devoted to terms in allied fields—clinical neurology, constitutional medicine, genetics and eugenics, mental deficiency, forensic psychiatry, social service, nursing, and occupational therapy.

A liberal use of cross-references, including the familiar *q.v.* and *see also,* and double registration of compound expressions under the main idea and under the modifying part, should make the book more serviceable and the search for desired information easier and more efficient. For instance, the impulse to buy is registered as *oniomania* and as *buy, impulse to;* excessive hunger is registered as *bulimia* and as *hunger, excessive.* Thus a technical or scientific term that has escaped one's memory for the moment may usually be found under its popular English equivalent: *automatic action* is listed as such and as *paraphonic state* and as *action, automatic.*

This psychiatric dictionary comprises all important terms and concepts used during the span of time approximately since Hippocrates up to our own day. Terms no longer in use are marked *obs.* (obsolete); those which are losing currency have been designated as *obst.* (obsolescent). Accordingly, it is possible for the reader to gain an appreciation of the historical development of psychiatric nomenclature and to grasp more clearly the meaning of old and new scientific achievements in the field.

This volume contains approximately 7500 title-entries, including personal names most eminent in the field of psychiatric science. Each entry registers a phonetic transcription of its pronunciation (see Key to Pronunciation used in the transliteration) and the philosophical derivation of the term.

Preface to the First Edition

Dr. Leland E. Hinsie is responsible for the definition of terms used in descriptive psychiatry, psychoanalysis, analytical psychology, psychobiology, forensic psychiatry, mental deficiency, sexology, nursing, and social work.

The philological part of the dictionary was done by Dr. Jacob Shatzky. The entire manuscript was prepared for the press by Mr. Judah A. Joffe, to whom the authors and their collaborators are sincerely grateful.

Miss Margaret Neubart did all the secretarial work connected with this volume, and has earned our deepest thanks for her efficiency and capability.

We wish to express our appreciation to the collaborators; to the many authors and publishers who permitted us to quote from their works; and last, but not least, we appreciate with deep gratification the close and cordial cooperation of the staff of the Oxford University Press.

September 1940   L.E.H.

J.S.

Key to Pronunciation

ā (bāke), e (thēme), í (fīne), ō (slōpe), ū (tūbe)
a (back), e (them), i (fin), o (slop), u (tub)

â—shâre, fâir, beâr
ä—fäther
a͏̇—a͏̇sk, bra͏̇nch, ba͏̇th
aw—saw, caught, thought
ē—plantar, her, first, motor,
  purpose, voyeur; folie de persecution
ô—ôften, lông, dôg, sôft
oi—toil, boy, void
o͞o—so͞on, move (mo͞ov), rule (ro͞ol)
oo—foot, bush (boosh), wood, would
  (wood), wool
ou—out, now, bough
b—as in back, bell, cupboard, raspberry
ch—as in church, itch, question (kwes'-
  chun), nature, virtuous
d—as in do, bidden
f—as in for, effort, phonetic, cough
g—as in go, league, ghastly
gz—as in examine, example
h—as in how, h(a)emophilia, cajal
hw—as in what, nowhere
j—as in just, judge (juj), gist, gestation
k—as in cake, (kāk), tick, eunuch, choir
  (kwīr)
K—as in Loch Lomond, Bach (bäK)
ks—as in complex, experimental
kw—as in equal, quite, choir (kwīr)
l—as in let, lost, doll, Lloyd
m—as in made, more, immediate, trimmed,
  dumb, tomb, solemn
n—as in no, never, innumerable, sinned
  (sind), benign (bē-nīn'), knee

ñ—as in cañon
N—as in F. bon (bôN)
ng—as in sing-song, tongue, language
  (lang'gwij), slink (slingk), finger
  (fing'gēr), puncture (pungk'chēr)
p—as in put, place, spot, stop, stopped
  (stopt)
r—as in red, root, berry, rheumatism, logo-
  rrh(o)ea
s—as in say, paste, miss, cent, concept,
  patience, scissors, sciatica, schizm,
  psyche
sh—as in shall, fashion, rash, chagrin,
  machine, brioche, crustacea, pernicious,
  physician, schist, conscience, nausea,
  tension, sugar, remission, tissue,
  intention, differential
t—as in tin, but, mitt, doubt, looked,
  stripped, thyme, ptotic
th—as in thick, bath, health, litho-
TH—as in their, father, bathe
u—as in F. menu (mē-nü'), G. Wüllner
v—as in vase, reverse, save, of (ov)
w—as in will, question (kwes'chun), suave,
  choir (kwīr)
y—as in year, million, pinion
z—as in zygote, gauze, raise, Times,
  positive, possess, scissors (siz'ērz),
  xenophobia
zh—as in seizure, glazier, abrasion,
  division, measure, garbage
'—as in chasm (kàz'm), principle (prin'sip'l)

Abbreviated Book References

Abraham, K. (*SP*) *Selected Papers*, tr. by Bryan, D. and Strachey, A., 1927

Bleuler, E. (*TP*) *Textbook of Psychiatry*, tr. by Brill, A. A., 1930

Brain, W. R. (*DNS*) *Diseases of the Nervous System*, 4th ed., 1951

Fenichel, O. (*PTN*) *The Psychoanalytic Theory of Neurosis*, 1945

Ferenczi, S. (*FCT*) *Further Contributions to the Theory and Technique of Psycho-Analysis*, tr. by Suttie, J. I., 1926

Fitch, J. A. (*SWYB*) in *Social Work Year Book 1939*, ed. by Kurtz, R. H., 1939

Freud, S. (*BW*) *The Basic Writings of Sigmund Freud*, tr. by Brill, A. A., 1938

    (*CP*) *Collected Papers*, Vols. 1–4, tr. by Riverie, J., 1924–25

    (*ID*) *The Interpretation of Dreams*, 3rd ed., tr. by Brill, A. A., 1933

Healy, W., Bronner, A. F., and Bowers, A. M. (*SMP*) *The Structure and Meaning of Psychoanalysis*, 1930

Hinsie, L. E. (*UP*) *Understandable Psychiatry*, 1948

Hunt, J. McV. (*PBD*) *Personality and the Behavior Disorders*, 1944

Janet, P. (*PH*) *Psychological Healing*, Vols. 1–2, tr. by Paul, E. and C., 1925

Jelliffe, S. E. and White, W. A. (*DNS*) *Diseases of the Nervous System*, 6th ed., 1935

Jung, C. G. (*CAP*) *Contributions to Analytical Psychology*, tr. by Baynes, H. G. and C. F., 1928

    (*PT*) *Psychological Types*, tr. by Baynes, H. G., 1923

Kempf, E. J. (*PP*) *Psychopathology*, 1921

Kraepelin, E. (*DP*) *Dementia Praecox*, tr. by Barclay, R. M., 1919

Kretschmer, E. (*HS*) *Hysteria*, tr. by Boltz, O., 1926

Slavson, S. R. (*IGT*) *An Introduction to Group Therapy*, 1943

Stekel, W. (*CD*) *Compulsion and Doubt*, 1949

    (*ID*) *The Interpretation of Dreams*, 1943

Tredgold, A. F. (*TMD*) *A Text-Book of Mental Deficiency*, 6th ed., 1937

Tuke, D. H. (*DPM*) *A Dictionary of Psychological Healing*, Vols. 1–2, 1892

Abbreviations

AA	Alcoholics Anonymous; Achievement Age
AANB	Alpha-amino-n-butyric acid
AAS	Ascending activating system (reticular activating system)
ACh	Acetylcholine
AChE	Acetylcholinesterase
ACT	Adaptive Control of Thought; atropine coma therapy
AD	Alzheimer's disease; average deviation
ADAMHA	Alcohol, Drug Abuse, and Mental Health Administration
ADD	Attention deficit disorder
ADDH	Attention deficit disorder with hyperactivity
ADH	Alcohol dehydrogenase
ADIS	Anxiety Disorders Interview Schedule
ADL	Activities of daily living
ADS	Alternative delivery system
AEP	Auditory evoked potential
AFP	Alpha-fetoprotein
AHP	Allied health professional
AI	Artificial intelligence
AIDS	Acquired immune deficiency syndrome
AIP	Attention and information processing
ALC	Alternate level of care
ALDH	Aldehyde dehydrogenase
AMPT	Alpha-methyl-paratyrosine
ARCOS	Automation of [controlled drug] Reports and Consolidated Orders System
ASDC	Association of Sleep Disorders Centers
ATC	Alcoholism Treatment Center
AVT	Arginine vasotocin
AZT	Azidothymidine

Abbreviations

BAL	Blood alcohol level; British anti-Lewisite
BCAA	Branched-chain amino acids
BDI	Beck Depression Inventory
BEAM	Brain electrical activity mapping
BEP	Brief and emergency psychotherapy
BLS	Buccal-lingual-masticatory syndrome
BWAM	Brain wave activity measurement
BWS	Battered wife syndrome
C-L	Consultation-liaison
CA	Catecholamine; chronological age
CABG	Coronary artery bypass grafting
CAMP	$3',5'$-cyclic adenosine monophosphate
CARE	Comprehensive Assessment and Referral Evaluation
CAT	Computerized axial tomography; choline acetyltransferase
CBA	Cost/benefit analysis
CBZ	Carbamazepine (Tegretol)
CCHP	Consumer choice health plan
CDI	Continuing disability investigation
CEA	Cost-effectiveness analysis
CET	Cerebral electrotherapy; computer electroencephalographic tomography
CHAMPUS	Civilian Health and Medical Program, Uniformed Services
CLAMS	Clinical Linguistic and Auditory Milestone Scale
CMCHS	Civilian-Military Contingency Hospital System
CMI	Case-mix index
CMP	Chronic mental patient; competitive medical plan(s)
CNV	Contingent negative variation
COLA	Cost of living adjustment
COMT	Catechol-O-methyl-transferase
CPR	Cardiopulmonary resuscitation
CSM	Chronic symptomatic maladjustment (= neuroses)
CT	Computerized tomography; conduction time
CTS	Carpal tunnel syndrome
CVS	Chorionic villus sampling
DA	Dopamine
DAT	Dementia of the Alzheimer type
DAWN	Drug Abuse Warning Network
DBH	Dopamine-beta-hydroxylase
DHHS	Department of Health and Human Services

DIB	Diagnostic Interview for Borderlines
DIMS	Disorders of initiating and maintaining sleep
DIS	Diagnostic Interview Schedule
DMPEA	3,4-dimethoxyphenethylamine; pink spot
DNA	Deoxyribonucleic acid
DO	Directive-organic (orientation or therapist)
DoD	Department of Defense
DOES	Disorders of excessive somnolence
DRG	Diagnosis-related group
DSD	Depressive spectrum disorder; depression *sine* depression
DSH	Deliberate self-harm
DSIP	Delta sleep-inducing peptide
DSPS	Delayed sleep phase syndrome
DST	Dexamethasone suppression test
DTs	Delirium tremens
DWI	Driving while intoxicated
EAP	Employee assistance program
ECT	Electroconvulsive therapy
EOG	Electro-oculograph
EP	Evoked potential
EPS	Extrapyramidal symptoms or syndrome
ERP	Event-related potential
ESL	English is (the subject's) second language
ESN	Educationally subnormal
ESP	Extrasensory perception
EST	Electroshock therapy
est	Erhard seminar training
EUCD	Emotionally unstable character disorder
FAST	Functional assessment stages
FD	Fluphenazine decanoate
FDA	Food and Drug Administration
FEHBP	Federal employees' health benefit program
FI	Fiscal intermediary
FPDD	Familial pure depressive disease
GABA	Gamma-aminobutyric acid
GAD	Generalized anxiety disorder
GDS	Global Deterioration Scale

Abbreviations

GGTP	Gamma-glutamyl transpeptidase
GHAA	Group Health Association of America
HACS	Hyperactive child syndrome
HBO	Health benefits organization(s)
HCA	Heterocyclic antidepressant drug
HCFA	Health Care Financing Administration of DHHS
HD	Huntington's disease
HEW	Health, Education and Welfare (Department of)
HGPRT	Hypoxanthine guanine phosphoribosyl transferase
HHS	Health and Human Services (Department of)
HI	Hyperglycemic index
HIAA	Hydroxyindoleacetic acid
HIF	Higher intellectual function
HIV	Human immunodeficiency virus
HMO	Health maintenance organization
HPA	Hypothalamic-pituitary-adrenocortical axis
HR	High risk
HSA	Health systems agency
HSV	Herpes simplex virus
HTLV-III	Human T-cell leukemia virus, type III
5HT	5-hydroxytryptamine (serotonin)
I-R	Individual-response (specificity)
IBTA	Individualized Behavior Therapy for Alcoholics
ICSS	Intracranial self-stimulation
IPT	Interpersonal psychotherapy
IQ	Intelligence quotient
IS	Ischemic scale; index of sexuality
ISD	Inhibited sexual desire
IRM	Inherited releasing mechanism
JCAH	Joint Commission on the Accreditation of Hospitals
KIPS	Knowledge information processing systems
KS	Kaposi sarcoma
L-K	Linguistic-kinesic
LAAM	L-alpha-acetylmethadol
LIPS	Logical inferences per second
LPU	Least publishable unit

LSD	Lysergic acid diethylamide
LTM	Long-term memory
LUMPS	Large urban medical practices
MAC	Maximum allowable cost
MAOI	Monoamine oxidase inhibitor
MBD	Minimal brain dysfunction
MCAT	Medical College Admission Test
MCR	Mother-child relationship
MDD	Major depressive disorder
MDI	Manic-depressive illness; major depressive illness
MeSH	**Me**dical **S**taff–**H**ospital joint business venture
MF	Multifactoral (model of inheritance)
MHP	Mental health professional
MHPG	3-Methoxy-4-hydroxy-phenyl-glycol
MIS	Medical Improvement Standard
MLD	Metachromatic leukodystrophy
MMECT	Multiple monitored electroconvulsive therapy
MMT	Multimodal therapy
MN	Metanephrine
MPD	Multiple personality disorder
MPI	Maudsley Personality Inventory
MPPS	Massive parallel processing system
MRI	Magnetic resonance imaging
MS	Multiple sclerosis
MSER	Mental Status Examination Report
MSIS	Multi-State Information System
MSRPP	Multidimensional Scale for Rating Psychiatric Patients (Lorr scale)
MSUD	Maple syrup urine disease
MVP	Mitral valve prolapse
MZ	Monozygote, monozygotic
MZA	Monzygotic twins reared apart
MZT	Monozygotic twins reared together
N	Cranial nerve
n	Number of subjects, size of sample
NAMH	National Association for Mental Health
NAPPH	National Association of Private Psychiatric Hospitals
NDATUS	National Drug and Alcoholism Treatment Utilization Survey
NE	Norepinephrine

Abbreviations

NFD	Neurofibrillary degeneration
NFT	Neurofibrillary tangle
NFTT	Nonorganic failure to thrive
NGI,NGRI	Not guilty by reason of insanity
NIAAA	National Institute on Alcohol Abuse and Alcoholism
NIH	National Institutes of Health
NIMH	National Institute of Mental Health
NMN	Normetanephrine
NMR	Nuclear magnetic resonance
NMS	Neuroleptic malignant syndrome
NPT	Nocturnal penile tumescence
NTD	Neural tube defect
OBS	Organic brain syndrome; obstetrics; obsolete
OD	Daily; right eye
OFD	Orofacial dyskinesia
OIT	Organic integrity test
OT	Occupational therapy
OTA	Office of Technology Assessment (U. S. Congress)
PA	Physician's assistant; public affairs; psychoanalysis
PAC	Professional advisory committee
PAD	Primary affective disorder
PCP	Pneumocystis carinii pneumonia; phencyclidine
PD	Panic disorder
PDA	Prescription drug abuse
PDD	Primary degenerative dementia
PDI	Primary depressive illness
PE	Pneumoencephalogram
PHF	Paired helical filaments (of the neurofibrillary tangle)
PHS	Public Health Service (DHHS)
PI	Paradoxical intention
PMI	Patient medication instruction
PML	Progressive multifocal leukoencephalopathy
PO	Postoperative; by mouth
POMS	Profile of Mood States
POW	Prisoner of war
PPA	Preferred provider arrangement
PPO	Preferred provider organization

PPS	Prospective payment system
PrL	Prolactin
PRO	Peer review organization
ProPAC	Prospective Payment Assessment Commission
PSA	Proportion of survivors affected
PSE	Present State Examination
PSG	Polysomnography
PSR	Physicians for Social Responsibility
PSRO	Professional standards review organization
PT	Physical therapy; physiotherapy; patient
PTA	Post-traumatic amnesia; parent-teachers' association
PTSD	Post-traumatic stress disorder
PUD	Peptic ulcer disease
QB	Quantitative Electrophysiological Battery
QD	Daily
QID	Four times a day
QNS	Quantity not sufficient
RBD	REM behavior disorder
rCBF	Regional cerebral blood flow
RCT	Randomized clinical trial
RDC	Research Diagnostic Criteria
REM	Rapid eye movement (sleep)
RFLP	Restriction fragment length polymorphism
RIF	Reduction in force
RNA	Ribonucleic acid
RPMD	Rheumatic pain modulation disorder
S	Subject
SAD	Seasonal affective disorder
SADS	Schedule for Affective Disorders and Schizophrenia
SAHS	Sleep apnea hypersomnolence syndrome
SCID	Structured Clinical Interview for DSM-III
SCN	Suprachiasmatic nucleus of the anterior hypothalamus
SCOPE	Systematic, complete, objective, practical, and empirical set of diagnostic procedures
SCOR	Skin conductance orienting response
SDAT	Senile dementia, Alzheimer type
SDD	Sporadic depressive disease

Abbreviations

SET	Self-instructional training
SHG	Self-help group(s)
SIP	Special internal predisposition
SMA	Sequential multichannel autoanalyzer
SMR	Sensory motor rhythm
SNF	Skilled nursing facility
SOD	Sexual orientation disturbance
SOP	Standard operating procedure
SPECT	Single photon emission computed tomography
SPEM	Smooth pursuit eye movements
SSA	Social Services Administration
SSDI	Social service disability insurance
SST	Social skills training; Self-Statement Training
STAPP	Short-term anxiety-provoking psychotherapy
STD	Sexually transmitted disease
STM	Short-Term memory
STR	Scientific-technical revolution
SWS	Slow wave sleep
TAT	Thematic apperception test
TCA	Tricyclic antidepressant
TCP	Terminal Care Project
TD	Tardive dyskinesia
TIA	Transient ischemic attack
TID	Three times a day
TLC	Tender loving care
TLE	Temporal lobe epilepsy
TLP	Time-limited psychotherapy
TPE	Therapeutic plasma exchange
TPN	Total parenteral nutrition
TRH	Thyroid-releasing hormone (protirelin)
TSH	Thyroid-stimulating hormone
T_3RU	T_3 resin uptake
T_4	Thyroxin
UFC	Urinary free cortisol
VA	Veterans Administration
VBR	Ventricle-to-brain ratio
VD	Venereal disease

VEP	Visual evoked potential
VLSIC	Very large scale integrated circuit(s)
VMA	3-Methoxy-4-hydroxymandelic acid
VNA	Visiting Nurse Association
WFMH	World Federation for Mental Health
WHO	World Health Organization
WPA	World Psychiatric Association
YAVIS	Young, attractive, verbal, intelligent, and successful

Psychiatric Dictionary

A

a In Rorschach scoring, animal response, increasing percentage of which indicates lack of imagination.

A-P psychiatrist Analytic-psychological psychiatrist; Hollingshead and Redlich so designated that group of psychiatrists whose approach is essentially nondirective and utilizes a psychodynamic orientation with acceptance of such basic psychoanalytic concepts as unconscious mental activity, conflict, respression, and transference. See *D-O psychiatrist*.

A type behavior See *type A*

A$_{obj}$ Rorschach scoring symbol for a response derived from or connected with the body of an animal; such a response is more commonly scored as *a* (q.v.).

AA Abbreviation for (1) *achievement age* (q.v.); (2) *Alcoholics Anonymous* (q.v.).

Abadie's sign (à-bà-dez') (Jean Marie Abadie, French ophthalmologist, 1842–1932) An early sign in *tabes* (q.v.) in which there is loss of deep pain from pressure on the testes or Achilles tendon.

abalienation *Obs.* Loss or failing of the senses or mental faculties.

abandonment Discontinuation of treatment by the physician before he has been dismissed by the patient, obtained the consent of the patient to withdraw, or furnished another doctor to continue treatment.

abasia (à-bā'z(h)ē-à) Inability to walk. See *astasia-abasia*.

abderite *Obs.* Stupid person. Abdera was a town in Thrace, the birthplace of Democritus; its inhabitants were said to be more stupid than other people.

ABEPP American Board of Examiners in Professional Psychology.

Aberdeen system See *system, Aberdeen*.

aberration, mental Any morbid deviation from normal activity; when used today the term ordinarily does not relate to deviations in intelligence, and it often implies a temporary condition.

abient See *avoidant*.

abilities, primary mental See *test, PMA*.

ability Power to perform, whether physical, mental, moral, or legal, with the connotation that the act can be performed now, without further education or training. *Aptitude* refers to the level of competence to which a person can be brought by a specified level of training.

ability, volitional See *volition*.

abiotrophy (ab-i-ot'-rō-fē) Premature loss of vitality of cells or tissues. The longevity of the heart, for instance, may be appreciably shorter than that of other organs of the body, leading to early disturbance in function which upsets homeostasis or organ-equilibrium. Lewis has shown that in schizophrenia the heart is hypoplastic and hence functionally inadequate. He believes that the shut-in type of personality, so often found in patients with schizophrenia, is a secondary result of cardiovascular inadequacy.

The concept of abiotrophy was used by Gowers as a possible explanation of dementia: precocious aging of the central nervous system was due to limited viability of the nerve cells concerned. Such an explanation, however, exaggerates the similarities and overlooks the very marked differences between the different members of the organic dementia group.

ablation Removal or interruption of function of a bodily part or organ, especially by surgical means. See *lobotomy, prefrontal*.

ablemo- Combining form meaning feeble, weak, less than normal, inadequate.

ablutomania Morbid impulse to wash or bathe, or incessant preoccupation with thoughts of washing or bathing; seen often in *obsessive-compulsive psychoneurosis* (q.v.).

abnormal psychology That division of psychology devoted to the study of mental disorders and psychopathology.

abnormality Variant, disorder, *disease* (q.v.); any state or condition that is outside the usual statistical range. Such a state may be a result of disease in some cases, but in others it is no more than the expression of variability. As noted by Culver and Gert (*Philosophy of Medicine,* 1982), there has been a tendency in medicine to define a normal range for trait x and thereby to have discovered two new diseases—hyper-x and hypo-x.

aboiement (à-bwà-mäN′) *Obs.* Involuntary production of abnormal sounds. It is often observed in schizophrenics who may make many animalistic sounds. See *syndrome, Gilles de la Tourette.*

abortion, therapeutic Interruption of pregnancy for medical reasons. In 1969 and 1970, efforts to reform or repeal abortion laws had been mounted in a majority of states. In 1973, the United States Supreme Court stipulated that the only legal restriction to be imposed on first-trimester abortions was that the procedure be performed by, or under the direction of, a licensed physician. Since then, the abortion mortality rate has fallen faster than the maternal mortality rate. For the three years 1972 to 1974, for example, the death-to-case rate for legal abortion in the United States was 3.9/100,000—approximately one-ninth the mortality rate for pregnancy and childbirth. (Willard Gates et al., *Journal of the American Medical Association 237,* 1977)

Since the Supreme Court decriminalization of medically conducted abortion (in *Roe v. Wade* and *Doe v. Bolton*), controversy has focused on whether to make abortion services more widely available or to limit their availability. Different states (and also different countries) define the indications for medical abortion along a range of considerations, the major ones being: (1) risk to the pregnant woman's life, physical health or mental health; (2) risk to the physical or mental integrity of the child if born (the eugenic consideration); (3) rape or incest (the juridical consideration); and (4) effects on the existing family (the socioeconomic consideration).

aboulia *Abulia* (q.v.).

above and below When Adler uses this term, he implies the unconscious notion existing in every psyche, male or female, of femaleness as a degradation and maleness as an ideal. In other words, there is the conception of man as *above* and woman as *below*, femininity being a position of inferiority to be avoided while masculinity is a goal of superiority to be striven for.

ABPN American Board of Psychiatry and Neurology, Inc., established in 1934 as the official agency to examine and certify physicians as specialists (*diplomates*) in psychiatry, child psychiatry, neurology, and neurology with special competence in child neurology.

Abraham, Karl (1877–1925) First psychoanalyst in Germany; manic-depressive psychosis, pregenital stages, character types, symbolism.

abreaction The process of bringing to consciousness and thus to adequate expression, of material that has been unconscious (usually because of repression). Abreaction refers to the two aspects of a "complex"—the intellectual representation and the accompanying affect—and includes not only the recollection of forgotten memories and experiences but their reliving with appropriate emotional display and discharge of affect. The method used to bring the repressed material into consciousness is called *catharsis* (q.v.); the term abreaction technically refers to the end-result.

The term *abreaction of emotion* refers to the discharge of emotion in the course of psychotherapy. This process is usually facilitated by the patient's gaining awareness of the causal relationship between the previously undischarged emotion and the symptoms. When such a discharge of emotion occurs during psychotherapy, it is often possible for the patient to see the link between his current irrational behavior and his demands toward his therapist, as well as the forgotten earlier counterpart from which the emotional attitude originated. The patient is thereby enabled to modify his anachronistic, immature, incongruous, and unreal emotional demands in favor of more adequate and appropriate behavior.

abreaction, motor The living-out of an unconscious impulse through muscular or motor expression.

abscess, brain Abscess of the brain (purulent encephalitis, encephalopyosis) is an inflammatory condition due to the invasion of pyogenic microorganisms resulting in a circumscribed collection of pus in any part of the brain.

absence 1. Loss of consciousness in a hysterical attack. 2. Petit mal. See *epilepsy*.

absent state The vacant, transfixed, dreamlike state characteristic of the patient with a temporal lobe seizure. Also characteristic of such seizures are hallucinations of smell or taste (the uncinate seizure; see *fit, uncinate*), a feeling of dreamlike detachment, and the experience of *panoramic memory*, in which the patient may feel that he is rapidly reenacting long periods of his life.

absentmindedness A tendency to be occupied with one's own thoughts to such degree that only inadequate attention is given to events that occur in external reality; consequently, memory may seem to be faulty, especially for routine and relatively insignificant happenings. Absentmindedness, then, is habitual inattention, but without the implication of severe pathology such as is associated with autism and withdrawal.

absorption Engrossment with one object or idea with inattention to others.

abstinence Self-denial; forgoing the indulgence of one's appetite, craving, or desire. In the case of *alcoholism* and *addiction (qq.v.)*, abstinence refers to the habitual avoidance or denial of the substance in question.

The term is used with a slightly different meaning in relation to psychoanalytic treatment. Freud advocated that in certain conditions (anxiety hysteria and obsessional neurosis) analytic treatment be carried out in a state of abstinence. By this, he did not refer only to sexual abstinence, nor did he imply that the patient was to be denied any and every satisfaction. Rather, abstinence rules were directed at substitutions for symptoms and were aimed at preserving a level of frustration that was optimal for treatment response. The analyst was enjoined to oppose those activities, interests, pleasures, and habits of the patient that drained off anxiety that was better handled during treatment sessions.

abstinence syndrome Withdrawal syndrome. See *addiction*.

abstract attitude Categorical attitude. Goldstein noted that one characteristic of the patient with an *organic mental disorder* is a relative inability to assume the abstract attitude or to shift readily from the abstract to the *concrete* (where thinking is determined by and cannot proceed beyond some immediate experience) or vice versa. The *abstract* attitude includes the following abilities: assuming a mental set voluntarily; shifting voluntarily from one aspect of a situation to another; keeping in mind simultaneously various aspects of a situation; grasping the essentials of a whole, breaking the whole into its parts, and isolating these voluntarily; abstracting common properties; planning ahead ideationally; assuming an attitude to the merely possible; thinking or performing symbolically; and detaching the ego from the outer world. See *syndrome, organic*.

abstracting disabilities Difficulties in organizing and understanding the inputs once information has been recorded in the brain.

abstraction "The drawing out or isolation of a content (e.g. a meaning or general character, etc.) from a connection, containing other elements, whose combination as a totality is something unique or individual, and therefore inaccessible to comparison." (Jung, *PT*) Abstraction is an activity that belongs to psychological functions in general, and Jung differentiates among abstracting thinking, abstracting feeling, abstracting sensation, and abstracting intuition.

abstractionism, systematic See *dissociation, semantic*.

absurdity In psychoanalysis, anything that is contradictory or incoherent or meaningless in a train of thought or a constellation of ideas.

abulia Absence of willpower or wishpower; the term implies that the subject has a desire to do something but the desire is without power or energy. Abulia itself is rare and with few exceptions occurs only in the schizophrenias. The more frequent disturbance in the will is a reduction or impairment (*hypobulia*) rather than a complete absence. Bleuler included abulia and hypobulia among the fundamental symptoms of the schizophrenias.

Social abulia means inactivity, focal or diffuse, of a person toward the environment, due to inability to settle on a plan of action. There may be a desire to contact the environment, but the desire has no power of action.

abulic-akinetic syndrome See *syndrome, akinetic-abulic.*

abuse, alcohol See *alcoholism.*

abuse, child See *syndrome, battered child.*

academic underachievement disorder A pattern of failing grades or inadequate school performance despite adequate (or even superior) intellectual potential and a supportive environment.

academic (work) inhibition A form of performance anxiety concerning school or occupational tasks, manifested as examination anxiety, inability to write reports, or difficulty in concentration despite adequate intellectual or performance ability as demonstrated by previously adequate functioning.

acalculia (à-kal-kū′lē-a) A type of *aphasia* (q.v.) characterized by inability to perform arithmetic operations, seen most commonly with parietal lobe (retrolandic) lesions. Various groups of acalculia are recognized: (1) *dyscalculia* of the spatial type in which disturbance of spatial organization of numbers predominates and is often associated with spatial dyslexia, spatial agnosia, sensorikinetic apraxia, somatospatial apractognosia, and directional and vestibular oculomotor disorders; (2) predominance of alexia or agraphia for numbers and figures, and (3) anarithmia, in which disturbances in the performance of arithmetic operations predominate. The second and third groups are often associated with speech disturbances and alterations in the process of verbalization.

acanthesthesia (à-kan-thes-thē′zhē-à) A type of paresthesia in which the patient experiences a sensation of pinpricks.

acarophobia A morbid dread of mites. The meaning of the term has been extended to include a wide variety of small things, animate (e.g. worms) or inanimate (e.g. pins, needles). The fear may be associated with the idea that insects or worms are crawling beneath the skin, as may occur in patients suffering from alcoholism or drug addiction. It may be associated with Lilliputian ideas.

acatalepsia Impairment of the reasoning faculty; abnormal inability to comprehend.

acatalepsy *Obs.* Formerly used synonymously with *dementia.*

acatamathesia *Obs.* Inability to understand language. This is the perceptive (sensory) aspect of aphasia. See *speech disorders.*

acataphasia A form of disordered speech in which "the patients either do not find the expression appropriate to their thoughts, but only produce something with a similar sound ('displacement paralogia'), or they let their speech fall into quite another channel ('derailment paralogia'). A patient said he was 'wholly without head on the date' for 'he did not know the date'; another complained he 'lived under protected police' instead of 'under the protection of police.' " (Kraepelin, *DP*) See *speech disorders.*

acathexis (à-kà-thek′sis) Lack of emotional charge or psychic energy with which an object would ordinarily be invested. Certain things, objective or subjective, hold no feelings or emotions for a person; they are not infused with emotions; they are not charged or cathected. This idea has received special consideration in the field of psychoanalysis, with reference to the attachment of affects to ideas or thoughts. Some patients have an unusual capacity for separating affect from an idea that is highly significant to them. The affect may be transferred to an indifferent or inconsequential idea or it may attach itself to some unconscious material. Thus one may express an idea or a series of ideas that seem to have no meaning or feeling for him. At times an entire complex may be utterly devoid of affect when it comes into consciousness.

acathisia (à-kath-i′zē-à) Also termed acathisia paraesthetica, acathisia psychasthenica, acathisia spastica. Inability to sit down because of the intense anxiety provoked by the thought of doing so. In acathisia spastica, the thought or act of sitting provokes hysterical convulsions.

Haase first applied the term (1955) to the inability to sit still and to other irritative, hyperkinetic symptoms that are sometimes seen as a complication of neuroleptic therapy. See *akatizia.*

acceleration, developmental Precocious growth in any area—motor, perceptual, langauge, or social. An uneven growth pattern is often found in schizophrenia, with unusual sequences of retardation and acceleration especially in postural development. This has been interpreted by some as a disorder of timing and integration of neurological maturation. (Fish, B. *Archives of Neurology 2*, 1960)

accentuation, interface See *network*.

acceptance See *tolerance, social*.

accessibility Receptivity to external influences. Inaccessibility is characteristic of *withdrawal* (q.v.).

accessory Additional, contributory, or secondary as opposed to fundamental or primary. In psychiatry, the term is chiefly used in reference to the symptomatology of the schizophrenias, whose symptoms were divided by Bleuler into (1) fundamental or primary symptoms and (2) accessory or secondary symptoms.

accident, cerebrovascular Apoplexy; stroke; often abbreviated to CVA. Cerebrovascular accidents include those conditions in which gross cerebral damage, hemorrhage, or softening follows a group of acute vascular disorders—cerebral thrombosis (82%), cerebral hemorrhage (15%), and cerebral embolism (3%).

Cerebral thrombosis is commonly a manifestation of cerebral arteriosclerosis and occurs in old age, although children with an acute infectious disease, young adults with cerebral syphilis, and young and middle-aged alcoholics may also develop cerebral thrombosis. See *arteriosclerosis, cerebral; multi-infarct dementia*.

Often the patient awakens in the morning completely paralyzed on one side of the body, monoplegic or aphasic. Thrombosis may also occur during the daytime, especially when the patient is inactive. Most cases recover with gradual recession of the pathologic change.

Cerebral hemorrhage may occur suddenly, without warning, as a true "stroke." It occurs most commonly as a result of arteriosclerosis or hypertension or as a complication of alcoholism, in the middle and older age groups.

Children and young adults with congenital abnormalities of the cerebral vasculature, such as aneurysms, may likewise be afflicted. Since hypertension of the essential type is so frequently familial, death from cerebral hemorrhage correspondingly runs in families. The exciting causes are such acts as straining at stool, coughing, retching, coitus, violent emotion, or heavy eating, all of which elevate the blood pressure. Thus hemorrhage frequently occurs in the daytime during periods of activity. Unconsciousness occurs suddenly, and the patient topples over or falls to the ground. Coma may gradually deepen and the patient may die in a few hours. More common is a coma of several days' duration during which the patient may rouse a little and then lapse back into deep coma. Some patients gradually recover consciousness and survive the attack.

Cerebral embolism creates the same clinical picture as cerebral thrombosis, but emboli are usually multiple and the syndrome may be more bizarre. The commonest causes of emboli are (1) diseases of the heart—as with auricular fibrillation and coronary occlusion with mural thrombi, which may break off and become embolic to the brain; or as in bacterial endocarditis, with valvular vegetations, which may become dislodged and flow to the brain; and (2) pulmonary diseases, with septic emboli lodging in a cerebral vessel, damaging the wall of the vessel and producing one or more brain abscesses and sometimes meningitis. Cerebral embolism comes on suddenly, without warning, and severe general symptoms appear as in hemorrhages. There may be convulsions and coma. Death may occur in a few hours when the embolus has lodged in vital area. The embolism may produce only softening, but most frequently hemorrhage also. It is the most frequent cause of sudden hemiplegia in childhood.

accident, intentional Huddleson stresses the consideration that accidents may be psychologically determined. "If an outraged employee with no other means of retaliation is so preoccupied, worried, or angry that he 'accidentally' thrusts his hand between gears and thus gains many weeks of compensation and care in lieu of employment and chagrin following the threat of imminent discharge, sociologic sympathy with his predicament ought not to obscure a psychologic estimate of his injury as virtually self-inflicted." (Huddleson, J.H. *Accidents, Neuroses and Compensation*, 1932)

accident proneness See *proneness, accident.*

accident, purposeful See *proneness, accident.*

accidental In psychoanalysis, accidental refers to that which is adventitious or of external origin, in contradistinction to that which is endowed or of inherent origin. Accidental experiences are of two kinds: dispositional, when they occur early in life and strongly influence character development; and definitive, when they occur later and act as precipitating or provocative agents.

accommodation Adjustment, especially of the eye for various distances.

1. Absolute accommodation is the accommodation of either eye separately; binocular accommodation is like accommodation in both eyes in coordination with convergence (the accommodation reflex). Accommodation occurs on shift of far to near vision, which is followed by thickening of the lens, convergence of the eyes, and constriction of the pupils. The most widely accepted theory of the mechanism of accommodation is that of Helmholtz: contraction of the ciliary muscle reduces the tension of the zonular muscle, thus permitting the elastic capsule of the lens to shape the lens and to increase its convexity. Convergence is produced by the action of both internal rectus muscles (innervated by N III); pupillary constriction is produced by the action of the sphincter muscle of the iris (innervated by the short ciliary nerves, the parasympathetic outflow from the Edinger-Westphal nucleus to the ciliary ganglion).

2. Nerve accommodation is the rise in threshold during the passage of a constant, direct electric current because of which only the make and break of the current stimulate the nerve.

3. Social accommodation refers to the functional changes in habits and customs occurring in persons and groups in response to other persons and groups and in response to the common environment. Such accommodation is typically made for the sake of social harmony. The concept of accommodation is used in analyzing attitudes in situations of superordination and subordination, as those of slavery, caste, class, status, and leadership. The social heritage, culture, and social organization are accommodations which are transmitted from generation to generation.

accountability In group psychotherapy, the participant's responsibility for his behavior within the therapy group and for reporting the reasons for that behavior.

accreditation Certification as being of a prescribed or desirable standard; credentialling; often a voluntary process in which a program or facility is reviewed by a professional organization responsible for setting standards of quality or competence. See *certification.*

accretion Growth by simple addition of parts or coherence of elements. Used particularly in learning psychology to refer to the learning of responses through frequency of association rather than through any inherent relatedness.

acculturation Originally, a term of social anthropology—the transfer of one ethnic group's culture to another. By extension, the implanting in children of the customs, beliefs, and ideals held to be important by adults of the culture group: a process of cultural indoctrination of children, much of which is carried out by educators without a formal plan, as an unconscious attempt at disseminating their own beliefs.

accumulation See *soteria.*

accuracy compulsion A term used in Rorschach interpretation to refer to the tendency of the subject to be overly accurate in his responses to the cards; he makes many corrections and indicates dissatisfaction with his responses but is unable to improve them.

acedia (á-sē'dē-á) *Obs.* A syndrome characterized by carelessness, listlessness, apathy, and melancholia.

acenesthesia (á-sen-es-thē'zhē-á) Absence of the feeling of physical existence, a common symptom in many psychiatric states.

acerophobia Fear of sourness.

acetylcholine (ACh) A reversible acetic acid ester which is synthesized from choline by the action of the enzyme choline acetyltransferase (CAT) and degraded enzymatically by acetylcholinesterase (AChE), which catalyzes the hydrolysis of acetylcholine. Acetylcholine is a neurotransmitter of the biogenic amine class that is active in both the peripheral and the central nervous system; approximately 5% of central neurons use it as a neurotransmitter.

There are two types of cholinergic (acetylcholine) receptors, nicotinic and muscarinic. Nicotinic receptors are mimicked by nicotine and blocked by α-bungarotoxin; the effect of their activation is excitatory. Muscarinic synapses, the predominant type in the central nervous system, are both inhibitory and excitatory; they are mimicked by muscarine and blocked by atropine.

There is evidence that central cholinergic neurons play a critical role in memory, in sleep, and in the regulation of mood.

ACh *Acetylcholine* (q.v.).

acheiria, achiria (à-kī'rē-à) Lacking hands; also, loss of sensation, total anesthesia, or a feeling of absence of the hands, sometimes a hysterical symptom.

achievement age (AA) The relationship between the chronological age and the age of achievement as established by standard achievement tests. The latter comprise a series of educational tests as distinguished from intelligence tests. Achievement age is synonymous with educational age and one speaks of educational or achievement quotient. When the latter is divided by the mental age (IQ) the result is expressed as *accomplishment quotient* (AQ).

Achilles reflex Ankle jerk. Tapping the Achilles tendon results in plantar flexion at the ankle due to contraction of the soleus and gastrocnemius muscles; the tibial nerve is both afferent and efferent for this reflex, and its center is S_{1-2}.

achluophobia Fear of darkness.

achromatic color response A Rorschach scoring term for a response of black, gray, white, or mention of lack of color; also designated *C'*. See *ShR*.

achromatic response A Rorschach scoring term for a response of texture or of anything that is described as achromatic.

achromatopsia (à-krō-mà-top'sē-à) Total color blindness.

Ackerman, Nathan W. (1908–71) Russian-born American psychoanalyst; child and family therapy.

acme In psychoanalysis the highest point of pleasure in sexual intercourse.

acmesthesia (ak-mes-thē'zhē-à) Perception of sharp points by touch rather than by pain, acuesthesia.

acoasm *Akoasm* (q.v.).

acolasia *Obs.* Morbid intemperance or lust.

aconuresis (à-kon-ū-rē'sis) See *enuresis*.

acoria (à-kō'rē-à) *Obs.* To Hippocrates it meant moderation in eating; but in Aretaeus it is used in regard to drink in the sense of insatiable desire. See *bulimia*. (Tuke, *DPM*)

acousma (à-kooz'mà) See *akoasm*.

acousticophobia Fear of sounds.

acquired immune deficiency syndrome See *syndrome, acquired immune deficicency*.

acquisitiveness *Hoarding* (q.v.). See *soteria*.

acrai (ä'krī) *Obs.* An Arabian term, synonymous with nymphomania and satyriasis.

acrasia, acrasy (à-krā'zē-à, ak'rà-sē) Morbid intemperance in anything; at one time it was synonymous with *acratia,* debility, impotence, inefficiency.

acrescentism, emotional Emotional deprivation.

acro- (ak'rō) Combining form meaning pertaining to extremity or tip, from Gr. ákros, highest, topmost.

acrocinesia, acrocinesis Excessive movements, such as those observed in the manic phase of manic-depressive psychosis.

acrocyanosis Blueness of the extremities, extending usually to the wrists and ankles; in psychiatric subjects, it is seen most frequently among schizophrenics, perhaps because in persons with an asthenic habitus the venous bed typically preponderates over the arterial.

acrodynia (-din'ē-à) *Pink disease;* erythredema polyneuropathy. A form of chronic mercury poisoning that occurs in infants and young children, mainly in the winter. It is characterized by irritability, purplish cold edema of the skin of the hands and feet, albuminuria, hematuria, and, in advanced cases, peripheral neuropathy and signs of cerebral and cerebellar involvement. Mortality is 5%, and neurologic involvement indicates a poor prognosis for complete recovery. Treatment is cystine, penicillamine, BAL (British anti-Lewisite, dimercaprol), or other sources of sulfhydryl compounds.

acroesthesia (-es-thē'zhē-à) Increased sensitivity to pain in the extremities.

acrohypothermy Abnormal coldness of the extremities, seen often in patients with schizophrenia, in whom it is commonly associated with *acrocyanosis* (q.v.).

acromania *Obs.* Chronic incurable insanity.

acromegaly, acromegalia Hyperpituitarism produced usually by an acidophilic adenoma of the anterior lobe (epithelial portion) of the hypophysis; acromegaly is sometimes seen in subjects with no adenoma whose hypophysis shows an increase in number of eosinophilic cells in an otherwise normal gland. The disorder was first clearly defined by Pierre Marie in 1886 and hence is sometimes called *Marie's disease.* Acromegaly occurs in adults after the epiphysial lines have closed; acidophilic adenomas arising prior to closure of the epiphysial lines in adolescence produce gigantism. Acromegaly consists of a localized increase in size of various structures (head, hands, feet, lips, jaw) resulting in a peculiar bodily configuration seen in no other disorder. Associated with this is profuse, offensive perspiration; bitemporal or frontal headache, excessive growth of hair, impotence, sterility, increase in basal metabolic rate, and glycosuria are also seen frequently. Bitemporal hemianopia develops with progression of the disorder.

Schizophrenic and manic-depressive psychoses are said to be rare in acromegaly, although it is regularly accompanied by striking alterations of personality: impulsiveness (about 90% of cases), moodiness and mood swings (60%), anger outbursts (50%), and often periodic or constant somnolence.

acromicria (-mik′rē-à) Term used in constitutional medicine, especially by Kretschmer and Pende, for the physical condition characterized by selective smallness and shortness of one or more extremities.

Benda proposed the term *congenital acromicria* to replace *mongolism* (q.v.), which he viewed as a form of pituitary hypofunction that to some extent is the opposite of acromegaly. See *syndrome, Down.*

acroparesthesia (-pār-es-thē′zē-a) Numbness, tingling, and/or other abnormal sensations of the extremities; seen frequently in organic disorders, especially peripheral nerve lesions, but by some the term is used only to refer to such unpleasant sensations occurring without demonstrable organic basis. Still less commonly, the term refers to an extreme degree of paresthesia.

acrophobia Fear of high places.

ACT Atropine coma therapy. See *therapy, atropine coma;* also adaptive control of thought in cognitive restructuring. See *therapy, behavior; therapy, cognitive.*

act, completion of See *ending, act.*

act ending See *ending, act.*

act-habit Any personality trait, habitual mode of response, etc., that is an outgrowth of cultural-environmental attitudes, such as minimal attention, scientific rearing, oversolicitousness, overwarmth, or overprotectiveness.

act, intervening In law, an act of the patient's own will; a voluntary act.

act, symptomatic Mistake, error; intending to do one thing but doing something else, which is usually in basic conflict with the intended action. Often called *Freudian slip* because of the assumption that it is based on unconscious wishes that the subject would consciously reject. According to Freud, symptomatic acts must fulfill three conditions: (1) they must fall within normal limits (i.e. they must not be morbid acts); (2) they must be temporary manifestations, subject to easy correction; and (3) if unrecognized by the individual committing them, they must be ascribed to inattention or accident when the subject's attention is called to them.

Symptomatic acts constitute some of the peculiarities of everyday life. They are expressed as mannerisms, slips of the tongue (*lapsus linguae*) or of memory (*lapsus memoriae*) or of the pen (*lapsus calami*), misprints, fake visual recognition, mislaying of objects, etc.

ACT system Adaptive Control of Thought system, a general model of the architecture of cognition developed by Anderson in his work in artificial intelligence.

act, unintentional See *act, symptomatic.*

ACTH Adrenocorticotropic hormone; one of the anterior pituitary hormones. See *syndrome, general adaptation.*

ACTH is also a *neuromodulator* (q.v.) in the central nervous system, and there is evidence that some ACTH analogues may improve selective attention, motivation, or mood. ACTH appears to be related to at least some neuropeptides.

acting in A type of *acting out* (q.v.) that occurs during therapy sessions; the patient discharges drive tension through action rather than through words.

acting out The partial discharge of drive tension that is achieved by responding to the present situation as if it were the situation that originally gave rise to the drive demand. Acting out is a displacement of behavioral response from one situation to another. See *alloplasticity*. Transference is a type of acting out in which the attitude or behavior is in response to certain definite persons.

Acting out is more than a single thought, expression, or movement; it is a real acting. Accordingly, compulsive acts and other symptoms that may involve a degree of acting are not considered to be acting out, for they are limited in extent and experienced as ego-alien.

In psychoanalysis, the patient may act out memories, instead of recalling them. A young woman, for example, imagined herself pregnant from a much older man during the course of her analysis. It later became apparent that the woman was acting out her infantile incestuous desires for her father, desires which, in the beginning, she was unable to verbalize under analysis. See *actualization*.

But acting out does not occur only in psychoanalysis. The character structure of a person, for example, is a chronic and habitual pattern of reaction that develops as the result of conflict between instinctual demands and the frustrating outer world. Although such a behavior pattern originates in the family situation, it is preserved throughout life as a typical method of reacting to any frustration. This displacement also constitutes acting out.

action, automatic In discussing *suggested action*, P. Janet writes: "These characteristics of the performance of suggested actions have often received specific names. Delboeuf proposed to speak of the state in which they were performed as a 'paraphonic state.' I myself have generally used the expression 'automatic' actions or beliefs. These tendencies, these dispositions to the performance of an aggregate of coordinated movements, may remain in 'latent condition,' or may be 'activated' more or less completely by passing through the stages of 'erection,' 'desire,' and 'effort,' in order to reach at length the stage of 'completed action,' or the stage of 'triumph.' " (*PH*)

action, chance See *chance action*.

action current Action potential; the basic unit of information transmittal within the nervous system, consisting of a regular sequence of small electrical deflections accompanying physiological activity of muscle or nerve. Such changes in electrical potential are commonly measured by the cathode ray oscillograph.

action, faulty See *act, symptomatic*.

Action for Mental Health See *Joint Commission on Mental Illness and Health*.

action guide *Principle* or *rule* (qq.v.).

action, ludic See *activity, ludic*.

action pattern See *instinct*.

action potential *Action current* (q.v.).

action potential, specific See *instinct*.

action, psychomotor Action resulting directly from an idea or perception.

action research See *research, action*.

action, social "The term 'social action' in its broadest sense implies any concerted movement by organized groups toward the achievement of desired objectives." (Fitch, *SWYB*) See *psychiatry, community*.

action, subconscious See *activity, ludic*.

action, symbolic Purposeless or symptomatic act. See *act, symptomatic*.

activated sleep See *dream*.

activating RNA See *chromosome*.

activation Stimulation of one organ system by another; the term stimulation is generally reserved for external influences only. Activation also is used to indicate the readout aspect of *memory* (q.v.).

activation pattern Desynchronization and suppression of the alpha waves of the EEG, with a shift to low-voltage rapid activity characteristic of sensory stimulation, attention, and mental activity. See *alpha wave training; electroencephalogram*.

active When applied to homosexual behavior in males, referring to insertion of the penis in anal intercourse or in fellatio; the one who inserts is termed active, the one who receives is termed passive. In some societies where male homosexuality per se was acceptable or tolerated, the passive role was considered unseemly, immoral, pathologic, or even punishable when adopted by adult males. By the first century A.D. terms came into being that differentiated between roles taken in homosexual behavior. Males who took the active role were called *exoleti, drauci,* *paedicatores,* and *glabri;* males who took the passive role were termed *calamiti, cinaedi, pathici, pueri.* (Boswell, J. *Christianity, Social Tolerance, and Homosexuality,* 1908.)

active technique When applied to psychotherapy, refers to anything that is not the classical *expectant technique* of psychoanalysis (i.e. maintaining neutrality throughout the analysis without recourse at any time to suggestion, exhortation, positive injunctions, or negative prohibitions); any more extensive interference on the part of the analyst than is usual in orthodox or classical psychoanalytic technique. Active techniques are associated particularly with the name of Ferenczi. Among the maneuvers utilized in active forms of therapy are injunctions or prohibitions aimed at habits, phobias, obsessions, psychosexual habits, etc. A major objection to the use of active techniques is that they encourage reenactment rather than memory work. See *psychotherapy; psychotherapy, brief.*

activities, graded In occupational therapy, those occupations and handicrafts that have been classified according to the degree of mental and physical effort required for accomplishment. By means of this classification it is possible to increase the complexity of the work as the capacity of the patient increases.

activity In occupational therapy, any occupation or interest wherein participation requires exertion of energy. See *passivity.*

activity, concealed antisocial The antisocial nature of certain types of behavior is sometimes concealed by the fact of its arising out of socially approved motivation. A. Kardiner refers to this as *concealed antisocial activity.* For example, he writes: "Competitiveness must be regarded in our society as a normal manifestation of self-assertion, when it is governed by the super-ego system. But there are neurotic and criminal forms of self-assertion. A neurotic self-assertion is an attempt to deny by force a deep feeling of inferiority or insecurity. There are some types of self-assertion that are injurious in intent, but that escape being criminal by a technicality. A good trader may misrepresent by omission, but not by commission. If he misrepresents by omitting damaging details, he is merely a sharp trader and is

both condemned and applauded; if he deliberately misrepresents, he is lying and is therefore only condemned. It is by this route that much concealed antisocial activity passes for normal." (*The Psychological Frontiers of Society,* 1945)

activity, group In occupational therapy, an activity in which several patients participate. Its chief value is its socializing effect on the mentally ill who are asocial.

activity, immobilizing Slavson suggests this term in relation to activity group psychotherapy as a form of *libido-binding* activities. By this he means activities that tie one down to a specific interest or occupation; to attain this he has devised a special environment for group psychotherapy, which is in contrast to *stimulating* or libido-activating activities. (*IGT*) See *psychotherapy, group.*

activity, libido-binding See *activity, immobilizing.*

activity, ludic Higher animals have a quantity of energy left after performing all the movements required by their physiological life processes. This excess energy must be expended (without purpose) in some way, most usually in play activity, called *ludic activity.*

activity quotient The ratio of the total number of verbs in a subject's speech or writing to the total number of adjectives; the activity quotient is said to be a measure of the subject's emotionality.

activity, socializing In therapy groups, this term denotes the activity that brings one member into interaction with other members of the group.

activity, stimulating The opposite of immobilizing activity. See *activity, immobilizing.*

activity theory of aging See *disengagement.*

actograph An apparatus designed to record the movements of a sleeper, usually by means of connection with the spring mattress.

actual neurosis See *neurosis, actual.*

actual self See *self.*

actualization 1. Fulfilling or realizing one's potential, the goal of many self-help groups. 2. *Acting out* (q.v.). Actualization of the transference refers to acting out within the context of the therapeutic relationship, ususally manifested as early, intense reactions of an erotic, hostile, or contemptuously devaluating nature.

actuarial Relating to the calculation of insurance premiums or risks. Actuarial factors that affect the costs of health care include age, sex, place of residence, previous episodes of illness, exposure to risk.

acuesthesia See *acmesthesia.*

aculalia (à-kū-lā'lē-à) Nonsensical or jargon speech, such as is seen with Wernicke's type of aphasia associated with lesions of the left angular gyrus (and usually also the base of the first and second temporal convolutions) in right-handed persons. The affected subject shows marked intellectual impairment, an inability to comprehend spoken or written language, and although the patient can speak he is likely to talk nonsense. This corresponds to Head's *syntactical aphasia.*

-acusia (-àkū'z[h]ē-à) Combining form meaning hearing.

acute affective reflex Kretschmer's term for the earliest indications of emotional discharge (usually, tremors) in response to great stress.

acute brain disorders In *DSM-I* (q.v.), various psychiatric syndromes due to temporary, reversible, diffuse impairment of brain tissue function. These disorders are part of the group formerly designated *organic psychoses;* the term acute, as used in the revised nomenclature, refers primarily to the reversibility of the process, and an acute brain disorder is one from which the patient will ordinarily recover. See *brain disorder; organic mental disorders; symptomatic; syndrome, organic.*

acute confusional state See *confusional state, acute.*

acute delusional psychoses See *psychosis, reactive.*

AD *Alzheimer's disease* (q.v.).

adaptability, cultural According to Freud, a person's capacity to transform egoistic impulses into social drives.

adaptability, heterogeneous See *adaptability, homogeneous.*

adaptability, homogeneous The capacity to adapt that is uniformly possessed by all members of the species, such as the adaptation to intensity of light entering the eye by means of the pupillary reflex. Homogeneous adaptability is differentiated from heterogeneous adaptability, which refers to genetic variability within the species or within a population (i.e. differences between individuals) in the capacity to adapt.

adaptation Fitting or conforming to the environment, usually with the implication that advantageous change has taken place. Adaptation is typically achieved through a combination of alloplastic maneuvers (which involve alteration of the external environment) and autoplastic maneuvers (which involve a change in the self). The end result of successful adaptation is *adjustment;* unsuccessful attempts at adaptation are termed *maladjustment.*

In occupational therapy, modification or alteration of an occupation to suit the specific need or disability of a patient.

In neurophysiology, the diminished rate of discharge shown by an end-organ subjected over a period of time to a constant stimulus. Adaptation in this sense is comparable to the term tolerance when the latter is used in reference to a drug.

adaptation, alloplastic See *psychodynamics, adaptational.*

adaptation, autoplastic See *psychodynamics, adaptational.*

adaptation, ontogenetic See *psychodynamics, adaptational.*

adaptation syndrome See *syndrome, general adaptation.*

adapted child In transactional analysis, that part of the child ego state that is subservient to parental influence: the constrained, compliant, dependent, inhibited, procrastinating, and withdrawing elements.

adaptedness The state that results from appropriate adjustments to conditions, as distinguished from adaptation, which strictly speaking refers only to the process whereby the adjustments are brought about. In common usage, the term adaptation has both meanings.

adaptiveness, social "From the point of view of mental deficiency, the most important group is that concerned with social adaptation, and in view of the ambiguity and various meanings attached to the term 'intelligence,' it might perhaps be advisable to apply the term 'common sense' to the quality which is characteristic of this group. In any case, whether we call it social adaptiveness, social intelligence, common sense, *nous,* or the more popular 'gumption,' the ability is clearly a composite one and made up of many different processes, such as comprehension, discrimination, reasoning, prevision and planning. . . . It is seen . . . that the psychological basis of mental deficiency consists essentially in the imperfect, and often irregular, development of that group of intellectual factors of mind which combine to form what we may designate *social adaptiveness.*" (Tredgold, *TMD*)

ADD *Attention deficit disorder* (q.v.); formerly called HACS (hyperactive child syndrome), hyperkinetic impulse disorder, or MBD (minimal brain dysfunction).

ADDH Attention deficit disorder with hyperactivity. See *attention deficit disorder.*

addict, object A term used to describe the behavior of certain schizophrenics who, to prove that they maintain some contact with the objective world, seek out and cling to objects and ideas and on the basis of this develop obsessions, monomania, elaborate inventions, etc.

addiction Strong dependence, both physiologic and emotional, on alcohol or some other drug. True addiction is characterized by the appearance of an *abstinence syndrome* of organic origin when the drug is withdrawn. It appears that in the addicted person the presence in the body of the addicting drug becomes necessary to maintain normal cellular functions, and when the drug is withdrawn, distortion of physiological processes ensues and abstinence symptoms are provoked. An addict, in other words, is a person who, whatever the apparent reason, has become physically and emotionally dependent on a drug, substance, or compound, so that he must maintain a certain level of intake of that substance. Often, in addition, the craving for the substance has a compulsive, overpowering quality, and there is often the tendency to use the substance in ever-increasing amounts. See *habituation.*

Addiction is considered to be a state of periodic or chronic intoxication, detrimental to the user and to society, produced by the repeated consumption of a natural or synthetic drug. The user has lost the power of self-control, at least in relation to the drug, and his behavior comes to be determined to a considerable extent by the use of chemical agents.

Because addiction usually implies physical dependence, it is gradually being replaced by the term drug dependency. See *alcoholism; dependency, drug; psychoactive substance dependence.*

addiction, cyclic A syndrome originally described by Wulff that occurs most commonly in women and consists of periods of depression, feelings of ugliness, and overeating or overdrinking alternating with periods of normal or elated mood, feelings of beauty, and ascetic behavior. By psychoanalytical definition these patients show a preoedipal mother conflict with unconscious hatred of the mother and of feminity. Their urge to eat is an attempt to incorporate something to counteract feminity—milk, penis, child and/or narcissistic supplies which soothe anxieties. See *dysphoria, hysteroid.*

addiction, enema The frequent and habitual taking of enemas to gratify deep, hidden, unconscious character needs, but usually rationalized "for health." See *anal eroticism.*

addiction, polysurgical Sometimes a manifestation of *factitious disorder,* at other times of *somatization disorder* or *hypochondriasis* (qq.v.); patients with polysurgical addiction solicit or, through multiple symptoms, obtain many operations even though no organic pathology is uncovered that would have warranted the surgical procedures. See *syndrome, Munchhausen.*

Addisonian syndrome See *syndrome, Addisonian.*

additive W A Rorschach scoring term for a response in which the subject reports details but finally combines these into a whole response.

ademonia Agitated depression.

ademosyne (à-dē-mos'i-nē) *Obs.* Nostalgia.

adenoid See *type, adenoid.*

adenoma, basophil(e) Tumor of the anterior lobe of the pituitary gland, characterized by a pluriglandular symptom complex *(Cushing's syndrome).* The symptoms are adiposity of the body and face but sparing the limbs, amenorrhea and hypertrichosis in women, acrocyanosis with cutis marmorata, hypertension, purple striae distensae, at times polycythemia and peculiar softening of bones, and frequently hyperglycemia.

Young adults are more commonly affected and duration of life is about five years following appearance of symptoms.

Psychoses develop in approximately 25% of cases; they are commonly of the manic, melancholic, or anxious-agitated variety. In another 35% of cases, there are marked personality changes, usually in the direction of apathy.

adenyl cyclase An enzyme believed to be responsible for the first step in a series of metabolic changes that constitutes the response to neurotransmitter-receptor interaction by some neurons. The interaction activates adenyl cyclase, which converts adenosine triphosphate to cyclic adenosine monophosphate (cAMP). In the second step (sometimes called the *second messenger system,*) cAMP catalyzes the phoshorylation of membrane proteins by protein kinase, resulting in alteration of the permeability of the postsynaptic membrane.

adephagia, addephagia *Obs.* A morbidly voracious appetite. See *bulimia.*

adiadochokinesis (à-dī-ad-ō-kō-ki-nē′sis) Loss of power to perform rapid alternating movements. This symptom is indicative of disorder of the cerebellum or its tracts.

adient Positively oriented or moving toward. The adient drive or behavior or response is a situation that results in behavior acting toward the stimulus, increasing and perpetuating its action; it is the opposite of the avoidant drive.

Adie's syndrome See *syndrome, Adie's.*

adiposogenital dystrophia See *Fröhlich's syndrome; syndrome. Laurence-Moon-Biedl.*

adjustment See *adaptation.*

adjustment disorders A group of maladaptive reactions to life stresses or crises, such as business reversals, divorce or family discord, physical illness, and the diffiiculties inherent in the move to a different developmental level (leaving home, marrying, becoming a parent, retiring, etc.). Symptoms and behavior are beyond the expected, normal range of reaction to such stressors and interfere with social or occupational functioning. Manifestations include any of the following, singly or in combination: depressed or anxious mood, conduct disturbances, work or academic inhibition, withdrawal, or physical complaints. The adjustment disorders typically remit when the stressor ceases, or when a new level of adaptation is reached. See *transient situational disturbances.*

adjustment reaction In the 1952 revision of psychiatric nomenclature (DSM-I), this term was used to refer to certain *transient situational disturbances* (q.v.) occurring in various periods of life.

adjustment, social Adaptation of the person to his social environment. Adjustment may take place by adapting one's self to the environment or by changing the environment.

Adler, Alfred (1870–1937) Austrian psychiatrist, founder of the school of Individual Psychology; inferiority complex; overcompensation.

admission certification See *review.*

admission, first A person admitted for the first time to an institution of a given class (e.g. mental hospital or institution for the retarded).

adolescence The state or period of growth from puberty to maturity. In normal subjects its beginning is marked by the appearance of secondary sexual characteristics, commonly at about age 12; its termination is at about age 20. Adolescence is the period in which sexual maturity is achieved in that for the first time both the sexual and reproductive instincts attain full maturity and unite into a single striving; it can further be considered the age of final establishment of a dominant positive ego identity, the age in which "tu-ism" replaces narcissism, the age in which sexual development dovetails into the development of object relationships leading to the mature, adult stage of impersonal object love (alloerotism) and unhampered orgastic sexuality.

According to Piaget, thinking changes in adolescence from the state of *concrete operations* to formal operational thinking, characterized by the ability to think abstractly, to construct hypotheses, and to use deductive reasoning.

adoptees, control See *cross-fostering.*

adoptees, index See *cross-fostering.*

adoption studies Investigations of adopted children as a way to estimate the degree of heritability of a given trait or disorder; the Danish studies of adoption and rearing of the offspring of schizophrenic parents by Seymour Kety and David Rosenthal and their coworkers (1968) are now classic.

Several techniques have been used:

1. *Adoptees' family method*—the investigator selects as an index case a person who,

adopted in childhood, by adulthood had been hospitalized with a diagnosis of schizophrenia; adoptees without psychiatric disorder serve as controls; the incidence of mental disorder in adoptive and biological parents, siblings and half-siblings is compared in index cases and controls.

2. *Adoptees study method*—biological parents of adoptees are divided into those with psychiatric disorder (index cases) and those without (controls); the adopted offspring are then studied for incidence of mental disorder.

3. *Adoptive parents method*—schizophrenics who have been adopted are compared with schizophrenics who have been reared by their biological parents and the incidence of mental disorder in adoptive and biological parents is compared.

4. *Cross-fostering*—the offspring of parents who are not schizophrenic are reared by adoptive parents who are schizophrenic; the adopted offspring are then studied for incidence of schizophrenia.

Adrenalin A proprietary brand of *epinephrine* (q.v.).

adrenergic Referring to neural excitation by catecholamines (e.g. dopamine, epinephrine, norepinephrine).

adrenergic circulatory state See *circulatory state, hyperdynamic β-adrenergic.*

adrenochrome See *psychotomimetic.*

adrenocortical insufficiency See *syndrome, Addisonian.*

adrenocorticotropic hormone (ACTH) One of the anterior pituitary hormones. See *syndrome, general adaptation.*

Adult ego state See *transactional analysis.*

adulthood Maturity. See *developmental levels.*

adultomorphism *Enelicomorphism;* interpretation of the behavior of children in terms of adult behavior. See *anthropomorph.*

advantage by illness See *illness, advantage by.*

adventitious motor overflow *Synkinesia* (q.v.).

adventurousness The condition characterizing the child in the preschool period in which there is an urge to rough-and-tumble freedom and curiosity. This involves the need of using the larger muscles rather than the smaller ones. Activities such as climbing, running, tricycle riding, ball playing, the use of big toys, the need to touch and handle everything within reach, and wandering away in search of

new adventures characterize this period. The short span of attention required produces a rapid shifting from one activity to another. See *wanderlust.*

adverse selection See *selection, adverse.*

advertising See *media.*

advocacy The act of pleading, defending, or interceding on behalf of another. A child advocacy system was recommended in the Report of the Joint Commission on Mental Health of Children (1969), largely in recognition of the fact that the organizational complexity of mental health services was of such degree that few parents had the ability effectively to engage the family and child with the system. Perhaps to a lesser degree, the same complexities render almost all human services relatively inaccessible to the people who need them most. See *expediter; psychiatry, community.*

Legal advocacy refers to efforts to establish and enforce legal rights; in psychiatry (as in the rest of medicine), it includes consumer-oriented efforts to improve the quality and quantity of services (*consumerism*) and civil-rights-oriented efforts to protect the freedoms and fundamental rights of patients. See *consumerism.*

Adx A Rorschach scoring symbol for a response of a part or a detail of an animal where most subjects would see the whole animal; also known as an oligophrenic response. See *Do.*

adynamia (ad-i-nā′mē-à) Weakness; asthenia; lack of energy.

aedoeomania *Obs.* Nymphomania.

aelurophobia *Ailurophobia* (q.v.).

AEP Average evoked potential. See *potential, evoked.*

aero- (ā-ēr-ō-) Combining form meaning air, from Gr. *aér.*

aero-acrophobia Fear of open, high spaces—the morbid dread of being at a great height such as occurs when one is in an airplane. This malady should not be confused with airsickness, which is a disturbance of vertigo-type.

aeroasthenia See *aeroneurosis.*

aeroneurosis A form of psychoneurosis, perhaps an actual neurosis, which is said to occur among aviators; the symptoms are anxiety, restlessness, and various physical phenomena.

aerophagia Swallowing of air, usually in such quantity as to produce abdominal distention and symptoms of hyperventilation (see *syndrome, hyperventilation*). The symptom is often based on unconscious wishes or conflicts, such as pregnancy wishes or cannibalistic impulses.

aerophobia Morbid dread of air, often ascribed to allegedly deleterious airborne influences; sometimes it also includes fear of one's own body odors.

aerumma (ē-room′nà) *Obs.* Melancholia associated with a physical ailment.

aeschromythesis (es-krō-mi-thē′sis) *Obs.* Obscene language, as in telephone scatologia. See *psychosexual*.

affect (ä′fekt) The feeling tone accompaniment of an idea or mental representation. The affects are the most direct psychic derivatives of the instincts and are psychic representatives of the various bodily changes by means of which the drives manifest themselves. The affects regularly attach themselves to ideas and other psychic formations to which they did not originally belong, and as a result their origin and meaning remain hidden from consciousness. If an affect is completely suppressed, it may appear not as an emotion but rather as physical changes of innervations, such as perspiration, tachycardia, or paresthesia. In other cases, especially in catatonic and manic states, the affects may appear without disguise.

Both "mood" and "affect" are abstractions, referring to a person's disposition to react emotionally in certain specific ways. Inferences about mood stem from present observations and past events, whereas inferences about affect usually stem from present observations only. Thus what is said about affect will also apply to mood, although what is said about mood (since it includes the past) may not apply to affect. Affect is the "feeling tone," the fluctuating, subjective aspect of emotion. See *mood*.

affect block See *block, affect*.

affect, blunted See *affectivity, disturbances of*.

affect, charge of "That part of the instinct which has become detached from the idea, and finds proportionate expression, according to its quantity, in processes which become observable to perception as affects." (Freud, *CP*) See *cathexis*.

affect, cooling of See *affectivity, disturbances of*.

affect, detached This is a term used by Freud to explain the psychological theory of obsessions and phobias. An idea that is unbearable to the ego may have its associated affect separated from it, and this affect persists in the psychical sphere. The unbearable idea is thus weakened and remains present in consciousness, detached from all associations. Its affect, now freed from the unbearable idea, attaches itself to other ideas, which are not in themselves unbearable, but which through this "false connection" grow to be obsessions. The detachment of its affect from an unbearable idea is undertaken as a defense against this idea.

affect, discharge of An energetic reaction to an affective experience that includes the whole range of voluntary and involuntary reflexes, by which, according to experience, the emotions—from weeping up to a clear act of revenge—are habitually worked off.

affect, dislocated See *affect, transposition of*.

affect, displacement of See *affect, transposition of*.

affect energy The energy that comes from the excitement engendered by applying a psychic stimulus to the whole human organism, with all its individual systems. Also called *affective energy*.

affect hunger See *hunger, affect*.

affect, inversion of *Counter-affect; reversal of affect;* transformation of an affect into its opposite. "If I am conversing with a person to whom I must show consideration while I should like to address him as an enemy, it is almost more important that I should conceal the expression of my affect from him than that I should modify the verbal expression of my thoughts." (Freud, *ID*)

affect-laden paranoia See *paranoia, affect-laden*.

affect, organ, localization of An affect, especially anxiety, can be felt in any organ of the body, but particularly in the organs that are directly supplied by the autonomic nervous system, such as the heart, lungs, stomach, intestines.

affect phantasy Jung's term for any phantasy that is strongly imbued with feelings.

affect, retention of See *affect, strangulated*.

affect, strangulated An affect that is repressed along with its attached mental content; it is retained in the unconscious and together with its psychic component produces morbid symptoms.

affect, transformation of in dreams In psychoanalytic interpretation it is often found that the feelings that one may really have masquerade in dreams as their exact opposites. The emotion of joy turns up as sorrow. Love is found disguised as the feeling of hatred. Sobs are discovered to be concealed by laughter. This process, usually referred to as the *transformation of an affect (feeling) into its opposite,* is one of the many processes by which the dream obscures its true meaning. If the psychic material out of which the dream is constructed contains an affect that has been repressed, this affect can gain representation in the dream by inversion into an opposite affect.

affect, transposition of Displacement of the affective component of an unconscious idea onto an unrelated and harmless idea, seen typically in obsessive-compulsive and depressive patients.

affectability *Obs.* The state of being able to express emotion or feeling. The expression is seldom employed in psychiatry, although inquiry is frequently made into the emotional susceptibility of the individual.

affectate *Obs.* To arouse feeling or emotion.

affectation Artificiality of manner or behavior. Affectation is a form of simulation in that there is a crudely disguised effort to act as someone else, usually for purposes of gaining esteem.

affected, germinally This genetic term (equivalent to the German *keimkrank*) qualifies an individual (1) as being heterozygous for some *recessive* morbid character and thus carrying the predisposition for this trait in its genotype without manifesting it phenotypically, or (2) as a homozygote for any kind of hereditary character with *inhibited* manifestation.

affectio hypochondriaca *Obs.* Hypochondriasis.

affection A general term, implying feeling and emotion, as distinguished from cognition and volition. Also used to refer to love or positive feelings for another that are not sexual.

affection, masked Stekel's term for the kind actions and tender behavior adopted by one person to disquise his feelings of hatred for another, as if wearing a mask of love to cover a face of hate. See *reaction formation.*

affection, partial Suggested by Hirschfield as a synonym for *fetishism.* See *fetish.*

affective Pertaining to affect.

affective cathexis See *cathexis.*

affective disorder, seasonal A depression that occurs regularly in the winter, or any episode of mania or depression that occurs as part of a regular pattern related to a particular time of year. It has been reported that sufferers from winter depression may be helped by exposure to bright (greater that 2500 Lux) artificial light (typically for two to three hours in the morning and again in the evening).

affective disorders A group of disorders characterized by a primary disturbance of mood, such as depression or elation; in DSM-III, the following are included:

1. Major affective disorders (see *depression; depression, unipolar; mania; psychosis, manic-depressive*): (a) bipolar disorder—mixed, manic, depressed; (b) major depression—single episode or recurrent.

2. Other specific affective disorders—cyclothymic disorder (see *cycloid; cyclothymia*); dysthymic disorder (depressive neurosis; see *depression, psychoneurotic*).

3. Atypical affective disorders—bipolar disorder, depression.

affective sensation See *feeling sensation.*

affective slumber See *Alzheimer's disease.*

affectivity Susceptibility to affective stimuli. Bleuler says that "every psychism can be divided into two parts, an intellectual and an affective." He then adds that "under the term affectivity we comprise the affects, the emotions and the feelings of pleasure and pain." (*TP*)

affectivity, disturbances of One of Bleuler's fundamental symptoms of the schizophrenias. Typical disturbances include indifference, blunted affect, shallowness, flatness, and constriction of the affects. Early in the course of the disorder there may be oversensitivity, overlability, or sanguineness. Mood is often inconsistent or exaggerated, with a lack of adaptability and of capacity for appropriate modulation of mood tone. Parathymia, paramimia, disharmony of mood, dissociation of affect and intellect, and contradictoriness of emotional expression are also among the schizophrenic disturbances of affectivity.

It is probably the incongruity between the affect displayed and the verbal productions of the patient that is more characteristic of schizophrenia than any other change in affect; lability of affect is seen in many organic brain disorders, and blunting or cooling of affect is particularly frequent in the presenile and senile mental disorders.

affectomotor Characterized by intense mental excitement and muscular movements. The combination, seldom seen alone, is usually found in conjunction with other symptoms and is a part of many psychiatric conditions. The term has been used loosely to refer to the manic phase of manic-depressive disorder, much in the same way that the expression *affective psychosis* has been employed.

affectosymbolic Burrow's term for the type of behavior that is distorted by emotional bias, associated with the undue attachment of man's feeling processes to symbolic constructs. Contrasted with organismic, orthopathic. A synonym is partitive.

affectualizing In transactional analysis, pseudoemotionality or play-acting of feelings as contrasted with authenic feelings that are basic to intimacy.

affectus animi *Obs.* (L. "disposition of mind") A general term for any type of mental disorder.

Affenliebe See *love, monkey.*

afferent (af'er-ent) Moving toward; in neurophysiology, concerned with transmission of nerve impulse into the central nervous system, in contrast to *efferent,* concerned with transmission of nerve impulse away from the central nervous system. See *reflex.*

affinal (a-fī'nal) Related by marriage.

affinity A marriage partner's relationship contracted with the other partner's (blood)-kindred, by the act of marrying. See *kinship.*

affinity hypothesis See *hypothesis, antagonism.*

affliction See *disease.*

AFP Alpha-fetoprotein. See *neural tube defect.*

after-contraction An involuntary movement occurring as a continuation of an original willed, voluntary movement; often utilized as a demonstration of suggestibility in the preinduction period of hypnosis by directing a subject to abduct his arm against a wall and after a few seconds telling him to step away from the wall. In many subjects, the previously abducted arm will then float upward involuntarily; this is termed after-contraction.

after-discharge Continuation of nerve impulse after cessation of the stimulus.

after-expulsion Secondary repression. See *repression.*

after-sensation Continuation of sense impression after stimulation of the sense organ has ceased; afterimage.

aftercare Continuing treatment and rehabilitation services provided to a patient within the community to which he has gone following inpatient hospitalization.

agapaxia Emotional hypersensitivity and hyperactivity to stimuli, as is seen particularly in persons of above-average intelligence.

agapism The doctrine exalting the value of love, especially in its general, nonsexual sense.

agastroneuria Neurasthenia of the stomach.

AGCT Army General Classification Test of intelligence, used during World War II and after. It is designed for use with literate adults.

age, basal In psychometrics, the highest age level of testing at which the subject passes all the subjects. See *scattering.*

âge critique (F. "critical age") The menopausal or climacteric period. See *developmental levels.*

âge de retour (F. "age of return") The period of old age or senility, when vital powers begin to be or are diminished. See *developmental levels.*

ageism Stereotyping of elderly people, on the basis of their age alone, in such a way as to create negative expectations of them, discriminate against them, and avoid dealing with their social and physiologic problems. At least in part, ageism may be based on primitive fears of aging and death, but the specific recognized pathologic fear of old age and/or of aging is termed *gerontophobia.*

agency-centered consultation See *consultant.*

agenesis, agenisia See *aplasia.*

agenetic Showing defective or absent development of some part or parts of the body.

agent, catalytic In group psychotherapy, a patient who activates catharsis in other patients.

agent provocateur (à-zhäN' prô-vô-kà-tēr') (F. "instigating agent") Precipitating cause.

ager naturae (à'ger nä-tōō'rī) (L. "the field of nature") The uterus.

agerasia (aj-ē-rā′sē-ȧ) A youthful appearance in an old person.

ageusia, ageustia (ȧ-gū′sē-ȧ, ȧ-gūs′tē-ȧ) Absence or impairment of the sense of taste; it may be due to disorder in the gustatory apparatus (i.e. the taste buds). It is also seen in psychiatric conditions, particularly in depressed patients who complain that food is tasteless. Ageusia is sometimes a part of depersonalization syndromes, such as occur in hysteria and the schizophrenias.

agglutination Condensation of more than one word-root or word into a single word. See *contamination; neologism.*

agglutinations, image Kretschmer says that in dreams and twilight states mental activity appears in the form of sensory images, which sometimes appear as scenes but more often as "fragments of pictures which apparently go on without rules or regulations, and, under the influence of affects, again conglomerate into peculiar image groups, the *image agglutinations.* The faces of several persons, several objects of similar emotional value, in the dreams are seen as one, and are conglomerated into unity; this we call, with Freud, *'condensation.'* " (HS)

aggregation Summation; integration; synthesis. Bernard subdivided evolution into five periods, each of which is a result of aggregation such as occurred when unicellular organisms first colonized to produce multicellular organisms (physical aggregation). In the fifth period, in which humans emerge, the aggregation is psychical, occurring through the instinct of gregariousness and leading to the emergence of a "supermind."

aggression, aggressiveness, aggressivity In psychiatry, the term refers to different concepts: (1) destrudo, the energy of the death drive or death instinct, as contrasted with libido; see *instinct, death;* (2) ideas and/or behavior which are angry, hateful, or destructive; (3) activity or action, especially when carried out in a forceful way. While the terms "rage" and "hate" are often used interchangeably to describe manifestations of the aggressive drive, some would differentiate between them, using "rage" to describe a primitive reaction that occurs before the formation of stable object representations, and "hate" or "hatred" to describe a type of object-directed representation of aggression. See *violence.*

Writers often fail to indicate which of the more than 200 definitions of aggression are included in their use of the term. Most agree, however, that an essential element is the intention to harm another, either physically or psychologically, and aggression is thereby differentiated from assertiveness, mastery, etc. Some authors also differentiate between *hostile aggression* and *instrumental aggression.* Hostile aggression is a response to an aversive stimulus such as an insult, mistreatment, or what is perceived as deliberate provocation; it is also known as aversively stimulated aggression. Instrumental aggression, on the other hand, refers to aggressive behavior that is needed to achieve some other reward (e.g. money, social acceptance, or fame).

The high level of violence characteristic of many television programs has been of concern to parents, educators, and physicians. The evidence so far available suggests that, far from providing a beneficial catharsis for pent-up feelings, fight scenes and similar aggressive presentations on the screen tend in both children and adults to activate ideas and feelings conducive to aggressive behavior.

aggression, animal The following types of aggressive behavior have been distinguished in animals:

1. *Predatory*—evoked by the presence of an object of prey; many workers do not consider this to be true aggression.

2. *Antipredatory*—defense of a territory against an intruder.

3. *Dominance*—evoked by a challenge to the animal's rank or desire for an object.

4. *Maternal*—evoked by the proximity of some threatening agent to the young of the particular female.

5. *Weaning*—evoked by the increased independence of the young when the parents will threaten or even gently attack their offspring.

6. *Parental disciplinary*—evoked by a variety of stimuli such as unwelcome suckling, rough or overextended play, wandering.

7. *Sexual*—evoked in males by females for the purpose of mating or the establishment of a prolonged union.

8. *Sex-related*—evoked by the same stimuli that produce sexual behavior.

9. *Inter-male*—evoked by the presence of a male competitor of the same species.

10. *Fear-induced*—evoked by confinement or cornering and inability to escape, or by the presence of some threatening agent.

11. *Irritable*—evoked by the presence of an attackable organism or object.

12. *Instrumental*—any changes in environment in consequence of the above types of aggression which increase the probability that aggressive behavior will occur in similar situations.

aggression panic See *homosexual panic.*

aggressive conduct disorder See *conduct disorders.*

aggressive instinct See *instinct, death.*

aging The process of gradual and cumulative decremental physical changes that usually develop with the passage of time and finally end with death.*Senescence,* or *primary aging,* is intrinsic to the organism and determined by inherent or hereditary factors. *Senility,* or *secondary aging,* refers to defects and disability secondary to environmental factors such as trauma and disease.

aging, cybernetic theory Aging is related to neuronal loss as reflected in increasing difficulty in handling information-transfer functions from environmental inputs.

aging, theories of Numerous theories of aging have been proposed, but at best each of them explains only some of the phenomena of aging. Among the major hypotheses are:

1. *Genetic redundancy*—life span is determined by the amount of DNA reserve within the genome that can be called upon to initiate and maintain vital functions.

2. *Watchspring theory*—the organism contains a fixed store of energy and when it is expended life ends.

3. *Free radical theory*—free radicals are molecular entities that have an unpaired electron, and they have their highest concentration in the mitochondria. Some believe they may be destructive intermediate by-products and that aging is due to loss of ability to destroy them or otherwise defend against them. Others have suggested that free radicals themselves defend the body against invading microorganisms and that aging brings about a loss of their defensive activity.

4. *Accumulation of deleterious material*—such as lipofuscin (an autooxidation product secondary to the increased degeneration of mitochondria that has been observed in brains of patients with Alzheimer's disease).

5. *Biologic programming*—the normal cell contains the memory and capability of ending the life of the cell, and after a determined number of doublings it stops reproducing itself.

6. *Immune system failure*—with aging, immune competence decreases and loss of control leads to the production of self-destructive autoantibodies.

7. *Cross-linkage* or *eversion theory*—the ester bonds that hold each interstitial collagen molecule together switch from within the molecule to between molecules of collagen. As the molecules of collagen become bound together connective tissue loses elasticity and can no longer maintain the structural integrity of tisse and organs.

8. *Aging clock theory*—the hypothalamus is the site of an aging clock, and loss of critical cells in the hypothalamus, whether genetically determined or due to trauma or disease, renders it unable to maintain homeostasis, for it can no longer respond appropriately to changes in the rest of the body.

For theories of the psychosocial aspects of aging see *continuity theory of aging; disengagement.*

agitation A tension state in which anxiety is manifested in the psychomotor area with hyperactivity (such as handwringing or pacing) and general perturbation. Severe agitation is sometimes termed jactation or jactitation.

agitolalia *Agitophasia; klazomania (qq.v.).*

agitophasia Cluttered speech due to excessive rapidity under stress of excitement.

agnomenatio See *homonym.*

agnosia (ag-nō′sē-à) Loss of ability to comprehend the meaning or to recognize the importance of various types of stimulation. The term agnosia is usually confined to loss of recognition of symbols in the nonlanguage field, for auditory and visual agnosias in the language field are essentially aphasias. The most common agnosias are: astereognosis (tactile agnosia; loss of power to perceive the shape and nature of an object and inability to identify it by superficial contact alone); anosognosia (ignorance of the existence of disease, especially hemiplegia or depersonalization in regard to paralyzed parts of the body); autotopagnosia or somatotopagnosia (impairment in ability to identify or orient the body or the relation of its individual parts); ideational or sensory apraxia is also essentially an agnosia. Finger agnosia, the inability to tell which finger has been touched by the examiner, has been reported to occur in many childhood schizophrenics and in children with minimal brain dysfunction.

agnosia, pain See *dwarfism, psychosocial.*

agnosia, social Reich's term for the inability of the psychopath to achieve satisfaction in living.

agnosia, tactile Inability to recognize objects, such as paper, glass, soap, cotton, metals, etc. by touching them. See *tactile sensation, double simultaneous.*

agnosia, visual-spatial A syndrome described by Paterson and Zangwill consisting of failure to analyze spatial relationships and inability to perform simple constructional tasks under visual control. This syndrome is usually associated with lesions of the posterior portions (occipitoparietal) of the right cerebral hemisphere in right-handed patients.

agonic social cohesion See *hedonism.*

agonist, inverse An active antagonist that in addition to occupying or blocking a receptor site exerts intrinsic activity.

agoraphobia Literally a dread of the marketplace, a morbid fear of open spaces. The term is currently applied to the severest form of *phobia* (q.v.), which usually is accompanied by panic attacks.

The central feature is a fear of leaving the security of home that develops, usually in the late teens or early twenties, after a preliminary phase of panic attacks, which lead to anticipatory dread that panic and a feeling of helplessness or humiliation (*catagelophobia*) will return in certain settings or situations such as crowds, stores, elevators, buses, subways, airplanes, theaters, tunnels—any place from which there is no easy escape or access to help.

Often the fears spread in time—as from the initial fear of being in a crowded department store, to a fear of taking the bus or crossing the bridge that would get one there, to going into the street in front of one's building, to entering the elevator in the building. The sufferer may finally become completely *homebound,* afraid even to leave the bedroom to go into other rooms of her house or apartment. (Between 65 and 95% of reported sufferers are women.)

It is sometimes easier for the agoraphobic if a specific person (the *phobic companion*) accompanies her; typically, such companionship becomes obligatory for the sufferer, whose demands are so insistent, unreasonable, and exacting that they provoke resentment and avoidance rather that the indulgent succoring that is sought. See *junctim.*

The most effective treatment appears to be a combination of antidepressant (e.g. imipramine or monoamine oxidase inhibitor) with behavior therapy (e.g. desensitization, flooding, or in vivo exposure). The antidepressant drug often controls or eliminates the spontaneous panic attacks, but directive or persuasive psychotherapy is usually required in addition to overcome the phobic-avoidant behavior. See *panic disorder.*

Many agoraphobics have been noted to be unusually sensitive to separation, often demonstrated from an early age as in school phobia. Some authorities believe agoraphobia to be a type of separation anxiety disorder. A pathologically lowered threshold for release of separation anxiety is posited by some to be based on a biological predisposition. Others emphasize unconscious conflicts over sexual or aggressive wishes (projected onto the proscribed territory), hostile-dependent conflicts as reenacted in the relationships between the agoraphobic and the phobic companion, object relation experiences with the childhood attachment-autonomy conflict, or pathologic family interactions.

agrammaphasia Ungrammatical, incoherent speech.

agrammatism Ungrammatical speech; a form of *aphasia* (q.v.), in which the patient forms words into a sentence without regard for grammatical rules of declension, conjugation, comparison of adjectives and adverbs, auxiliary verbs, prepositions, conjunctions, articles, etc. Agrammatism is seen most frequently in *Alzheimer's disease* and in *Pick's disease* (qq.v.). With some authors, the term is synonymous with *syntactic aphasia*. See *speech disorders*.

agraphia Loss of the power, or the inability, to communicate (ideas) in *writing,* and thus a subdivision of *aphasia* (q.v.). This is the motor (or expressive) aspect of the ailment of which the sensory (or perceptive) counterpart is *alexia* (q.v.). The inability may involve individual letters or syllables, words, or phrases, as in varieties of aphasia, and is usually attributed to cerebral disorders.

When agraphia is not a physiological ailment, but due to psychic or emotional factors and is merely voluntary, it is the graphic counterpart of *mutism* (q.v.). A patient who acknowledged organic ability to write was entirely unable to write a letter or a word, lest, as she thought, it would result in serious harm; she possessed excellent intelligence and manual dexterity. Patients with involutional melancholia are often inhibited emotionally from writing, but the inhibition in this respect is only representative of more or less categorical inhibition. See *acalculia; speech disorders.*

agraphia, acquired Loss of a previous ability to write resulting from brain injury or brain disease.

agraphia, congenital Failure to acquire any writing ability. Total failure is rare, although varying degrees of difficulty (dysgraphia) may accompany other developmental disorders of language or reading.

agraphognosia Inability to identify numbers or letters traced on the palm (or other parts of the body surface).

agriothymia (ag-rē-ō-thim'ē-à) Insane ferocity. *Obs.* "Maniacal furor"; at one time synonymous with "homicidal insanity."

agriothymia ambitiosa *Obs.* The desire to destroy nations; *Alexanderism.*

agriothymia hydrophobica Irresistible impulse to bite.

agriothymia religiosa *Obs.* The irrepressible desire to uproot and destroy other religions and those cultivating them. (Tuke, *DPM*)

agromania Morbid impulse to live in the open country or in solitude, sometimes a symptom of schizophrenia.

agrypnia *Obs.* Insomnia.

agrypnocoma (à-grip-nō-kō'mà) *Coma vigil* (q.v.).

agrypnotic (ag-rip-not'ik) Inducing wakefulness; somnifugous; relating to or characterized by insomnia.

ague, leaping (ā'gū) Dancing mania. See *choreomania.*

agyiophobia Fear of streets. See *agoraphobia.*

aha, ah-hah A term used to refer to a type of experience in which there is sudden insight into or solution of a problem; at a particular moment, the features of the problem suddenly fit together in a unitary pattern. See *brainstorm.*

ahypnia (ā-hip'nē-à) Insomnia.

AI Artificial intelligence. See *intelligence, artificial.*

aichmophobia (āk-mō-fō'bē-à) Fear or dread of pointed objects, such as knives, usually associated with the thought of using the feared object as an offensive weapon against someone, even though there is no conscious reason for doing so. The symptom often leads to peculiar eating habits, such as eating alone and without silverware, or to the selection of occupations in which dangerous implements or their symbolic equivalents are not likely to be encountered.

AID Abbreviation for *acute infectious diseases* (usually of childhood); also, more recently, acronym for *artificial insemination by donor,* or for *autoimmune diseases.* See *autoimmunity.*

aidoiomania *Erotomania* (q.v.).

AIDS See *syndrome, acquired immune deficiency.*

ailment, functional A mild transitory episodic symptom, usually the result of disturbed physiological functioning (pathophysiology). Such disturbed functionings are the visceral components of emotion, or the visceral expression of emotion or emotional conflicts. See *neurosis, vegetative.*

ailurophobia (ī-lū-rō-fō'bē-à) Fear of cats; also called *galeophobia* or *gatophobia.* The fear of cats has the same physical significance as the fear of animals in general. It is a fear of being injured by them; usually, upon careful inquiry, it is found that there is a dread of injury to a particular part of the body, typically the genital area or its psychical equivalent.

aim The activity in which an impulse or drive manifests itself and, more specifically, the activity by which the drive or impulse achieves gratification or discharge.

"What distinguishes the instincts from one another and furnishes them with specific attributes is their relation to their somatic *sources* and to their *aims*. The source of the instinct is an exciting process in an organ, and the immediate aim of the impulse lies in the release of this organ stimulus." (Freud, *BW*)

The modes of pleasure during the so-termed infancy period, that is, up to the latency period, chiefly center around the several erotogenic zones (oral, anal, dermal, muscular, etc.). During the latency period much of the energy and pleasure formerly identified with these zones is deflected into sublimations. The relinquishment of energy from the pregenital areas is called "*aim*-inhibited." At puberty there is reanimation to a greater or lesser extent of the aim-inhibited tendencies and their somatic manifestations.

aim inhibited See *aim.*

aim transference The transfer of a person's objectives from one life situation to another. The development of aim transference is encouraged particularly in short-term psychotherapy, when conditions do not permit the development and subsequent solution of the transference neurosis, as defined by psychoanalysts. Aim transference is illustrated by the case of an 18-year-old schizophrenic male whose mother allowed him no independence. She had dressed and fed the patient throughout his life. The patient himself desired to be independent and in fact wanted to become strong and dominant, like his father. These aims were encouraged in therapy and by the strong male personality of the psychiatrist, who arranged special situations that enabled the patient to become the active leader of a small group. This transfer of early aims to the therapeutic situation constitutes the aim transference. In the situation described, aim transference was reinforced by aim experience, when the therapist maneuvered the environment so that the patient was able to achieve his goals.

AIP 1. Acute intermittent porphyria. See *porphyria, acute intermittent.* 2. *Attention and information processing* (q.v.).

air pollution See *syndrome, air pollution.*

akataphasia (à-kat-à-fā′zhē-à) See *acataphasia.*

akatizia (à-ke-tē′zhē-à) *Acathisia* (q.v.); motor restlessness and, specifically, a feeling of muscular quivering; one of the possible complications of treatment with neuroleptics. Often, the symptom is of such intensity that it becomes impossible for the patients to sit still day or night, and it is described by them as more difficult to endure than any of the symptoms for which they had originally been treated. It may persist for a considerable time after the drug has been withdrawn, and it is sometimes mistaken for an agitated depression and wrongly treated.

Akerfeldt test See *ceruloplasmin.*

akinesia, akinesis Absence or diminution of voluntary motion; when seen as a part of psychiatric syndromes, it may range from moderate inactivity to almost complete immobility. Ordinarily, akinesia or hypokinesia is accompanied by a parallel reduction in mental activity. In the stuporous phase of catatonic schizophrenia, for example, there is almost complete physical and mental immobility.

Akinesia may be circumscribed in the sense that the patient becomes immobile only in a given setting or while under the influence of a particular trend of thought; this is sometimes termed *selective akinesia.*

akinesia algera A clinical syndrome characterized by general painfulness associated with any kind of movements. Moebius restricted the use of the term to those conditions arising on a psychogenic basis; to him it was a manifestation of hysteria.

akinetic-abulic syndrome See *syndrome, akinetic-abulic.*

akinetic epilepsy A type of petit mal epilepsy. See *epilepsy.*

akoasm (ak′ō-az′m) An elementary auditory hallucination. "Such would be simple sounds, as buzzing, crackling, ringing, and the like. The more complicated hallucinations which are conceived by the patient to be 'voices'—verbal auditory hallucinations—are known as *phonemes.*" (White, W.A. *Outlines of Psychiatry,* 1929)

akoluthia (à-ko-lū′thē-à) Semon's term for a phase of engraphy corresponding to what others have termed *primary memory* or *memory in the making.*

Al-Anon A self-help group fellowship of spouses, children, and relatives of alcoholics who are usually part of an AA group.

Al-Anon was developed as a parallel but separate movement to *Alcoholics Anonymous* (q.v.) in the late 1940s. Since then, *Alateen* has developed as a similar network of voluntary support groups composed of the teenaged children of alcholics.

alalia Speechlessness; loss of ability to talk. It was used in the 18th and into the 19th century for what is now generally denoted by *aphasia*. At present the *-lalia* frequently used in constructions like *echolalia* and *bradylalia*, connotes *talking* rather than *speaking—saying*, i.e. the exercise of the power of talking as contrasted with the faculty for significant or meaningful speech. See *speech disorders*.

alarm reaction See *reaction, alarm*.

Alateen See *Al-Anon; Alcoholics Anonymous*.

Albright's disease A syndrome consisting of multiple pseudocysts in the skeleton, segmental pigment disorders of the skin, and *pubertas praecox* (q.v.); the disease is due to hypothalamic-hypophysial dysfunction.

ALC Alternate level of care; services provided by a hospital to a patient even though services at an inpatient level are not necessary. Most patients receiving such services are suitable for skilled nursing or health-related services, but they are retained in hospital because the other services are not locally available.

alcohol-Antabuse reaction See *Antabuse*.

alcohol-sensitizing drug A compound that produces adverse reactions in the subject when he consumes alcohol. The most commonly used drug of this category in the United States is disulfiram (Antabuse).

alcoholic paranoid state A chronic condition, presumed to be primarily of organic origin, consisting of persisting infidelity or jealousy delusions, that appears mainly in male alcoholics. The condition is very rare, and many doubt that it exists at all.

alcoholic psychoses See *alcoholism*.

Alcoholics Anonymous (AA) An organization formed in 1935 by an Akron physician and a New York broker, both former alcoholics, for the purpose of rehabilitating alcoholics. Since its founding, Alcoholics Anonymous has expanded into an international movement. Its principles include (1) a belief in God or natural law, (2) frank self-appraisal, (3) a willingness to admit and correct wrongs done to others, (4) a trust in mankind, and (5)

dedication to the rescue of those who sincerely desire to conquer alcoholism by making them members of the organization as successful abstainers.

alcoholism *Alcohol dependence* (currently the preferred term); *alcohol addiction*. The terms refer to a variety of disorders associated with the repetitive ingestion of alcohol, usually over a long period of time, in amounts that the drinker is unable to handle physiologically, emotionally, or socially. In addition, the drinker typically is unable or unwilling to recognize that alcohol is the major factor in his disabilities, and so he continues to drink. His inability to control his intake—*loss of control*—is sometimes expressed as a compulsive craving, at other times as an inability to limit the amount of alcohol ingested once the initial drink has been taken. The alcoholic uses alcohol too much, and too often, and the results of his drinking are related to physiologic dependence on the depressant drug alcohol combined with a pattern of recurrent bouts of acute intoxication that are superimposed on the addiction. Alcoholism by definition is a chronic, and usually progressive disorder; the phrase "chronic alcoholism," although in common use, is tautologic.

Most investigators feel that alcoholism is a group of disorders. It is a genus with many species, according to Jellinek, who differentiated various forms:

1. *Alpha*—a psychological dependency on alcohol, which is used to relieve bodily or emotional pain; there is no loss of control, nor are there signs of progression to physiological dependence. Drinking is undisciplined, however, in regard to time, occasion, locale, amount, and behavioral effects. This type of alcoholism is sometimes called *problem drinking, escape drinking, symptomatic* or *reactive alcoholism, dyssocial drinking* (if effects are manifested chiefly in the family, social, or vocational sphere), or *thymogenic drinking* (if alcohol is used in a conscious effort to overcome social discomfort or to relieve emotional pain).

2. *Beta*—although no physical or psychological dependence is demonstrable, drinking leads to physical complications, such as in the gut, liver, pancreas, heart, vascular system, kidney, lungs, striate mus-

cle, brain, mechanisms of resistance and defense (manifested in proneness to infections and high incidence of certain types of malignancy), and complications of other coexisting illnesses. This type of alcoholism is sometimes called *somatopathic drinking;* some would include herein the French category *alcoolisation,* the regular (usually daily) consumption of relatively large amounts of alcohol that results in a general undermining of health and a shortened life span, but no specific complications and no physical or psychological dependence.

3. *Gamma*—the usual type of alcoholism seen in the United States, Canada, and other Anglo-Saxon and hard-liquor-drinking countries, characterized by increased *tolerance* (q.v.), cellular adaption to the repeated ingestion of the depressant substance, precipitation of a *withdrawal* or *abstinence* syndrome ("shakes," compulsive craving, convulsions, hallucinations, delirium; see *delirium tremens*) when alcohol intake is halted, and loss of control as defined above. This type of alcoholism is also known as *essential, addictive, regressive, malignant,* or *idiopathic.*

4. *Delta*—the usual type of alcoholism seen in France and other wine-drinking countries, characterized by increased tolerance, adaptive cell metabolism, and withdrawal symptoms, but rather than typical loss of control the delta alcoholic is unable to go on the "water wagon" for even one or two days without withdrawal symptoms. This type of alcoholism is also known as *inveterate drinking.*

5. *Epsilon*—a pattern of paroxysmal drinking bouts, during which the alcoholic drinks for days or weeks on end until he collapses; following recovery from one episode, he may stay dry for weeks or months until the next bout. Epsilon alcoholism is also known as *dipsomania* or *paroxysmal* or *periodic drinking.*

In DSM-III, *alcohol abuse* (305.0x) was used for persons whose drinking history suggests alcohol dependency even though confirmatory evidence is lacking; such a diagnosis required symptoms in at least two of the following groupings: legal (arrests, traffic accidents), vocational (absenteeism, suspension, or termination), serious interpersonal difficulties (fighting,

spouse or child abuse, etc.), and abnormal or deviant drinking patterns (which may include frequent *blackouts*—amnesia about periods of heavy drinking even though there was no loss of consciousness). Many writers avoid the word abuse on the grounds that it implies that the drinker could stop "if he really wanted to" and/or that it has the same pejorative implications as child abuse and self-abuse. As a result, *problem drinking* is sometimes used as an equivalent for alcohol abuse (see alpha alcoholism, above).

Because there are varieties of alcoholism, many theories of origin of the different varieties, and many ways in which those variants can affect the drinker and/or society, there is no agreed-upon, fixed terminology. The difficulty is compounded by the fact that alcohol ingestion, per se, is not generally considered to be deviant or abnormal behavior. The lines between "normal" social drinking, heavy drinking, problem drinking, and alcohol dependence are far from clear, and most workers in the field have been forced to construct ad hoc definitions of terms according to the focus of their investigations of *drinking behaviors* (q.v.).

It is generally agreed, nonetheless, that in the United States somewhere between 5 nd 10% of persons who consume alcohol will come to be recognized as alcohol dependent in time (although it may require as long as 20 years for the drinker to progress to that stage). Epidemiologic studies indicate that about 30% of the United States population are abstinent; 45% are infrequent or light drinkers (who consume one or two drinks at a time, at least once a month); 13% are moderate (who drink several times a month, but not more than four drinks per occasion); and the remaining 12% are heavy drinkers (they drink nearly every day, with 5 or more drinks per occasion at least once in a while). It is assumed that it is from the last group that most of those who qualify for the diagnosis of alcohol dependence are drawn. It is estimated that in the United States there are between 10 million and 13 million people with alcoholism, and although the disease strikes people in all walks of life, at every level of the social, educational, and economic scale, it occurs at excessively high rates in certain groups—in large city populations, in the economically deprived, the disenfranchised, the disadvantaged and in nonwhites. (See *Jellinek's formula.*) The American Indian has an incidence twice that of the general population, and high-consequence drinking is three times more prevalent in the lowest social class than in the upper-middle and highest classes. Alcoholism is three times more frequent in men than in women, and although its recognition is concentrated in those between 35 and 55 years of age, it is becoming increasingly recognized as a significant problem in the old as well as the young. Furthermore, once the alcoholic has been identified and diagnosed as such, inquiry reveals that he has been a heavy drinker and a problem drinker for many years before the diagnosis was made. On the basis of history alone, the male alcoholic is typically found to have begun drinking in his early twenties, the female alcoholic in her early thirties; but both sexes tend to be diagnosed, hospitalized, or otherwise to require intervention in their forties. This suggests that the disease has a more rapid course in the female, and there are indications that the female alcoholic may differ in other ways from her male counterpart.

Theories of the etiology of alcoholism abound. Psychodynamic explanations have been generally unsatisfactory, even though they have provided insight into many of the factors that precipitate or aggravate alcoholic consumption, and have delineated the factors that throw the alcoholic into conflict with various social units. Early psychoanalytic studies implicated a specific oral craving in the genesis of alcoholism— too severe frustration by an overindulgent mother, combined with an inconsistent or absent father, enforces a retreat to the earlier megalomaniacal phase of passive gratification through the oral route. A dearth of oral supplies produces chronic disappointment, which leads to rage that must be turned inward against the self in the form of tense depression. The latter, in turn, produces guilt, masochistic maneuvers, a giving up of the disappointing mother and a turning to the father in a passive, longing, dependent way.

In the United States, the family constel- lation of indulgent mother with inconsistent or absent father is considerably more common than alcoholism; no study has demonstrated that a particular personality type or a particular neurosis is characteristic of alcoholic persons. The psychologic factors adduced are not specific enough to indicate why alcoholism rather than some other disorder is their result or why particular social, racial, or economic groups are so susceptible to their influence. Epidemiologic, sociologic, clinical, and, more recently, genetic studies suggest that at least for some types of alcoholism, susceptibility may be based on a genetic predisposition.

Various organic mental disorders may be associated with or result from alcohol ingestion and alcoholism; they are described under separate listings, as follows:

alcohol amnestic syndrome (see *syndrome, Wernicke-Korsakoff*)

alcohol dementia

alcohol intoxication (see *intoxication, alcoholic*)

alcoholic withdrawal (see gamma alcoholism, above)

idiosyncratic or pathologic intoxication (see *intoxication, alcoholic*)

withdrawal delirium (see *delirium tremens*)

withdrawal hallucinosis

alcoholophilia, -mania *Rare.* Morbid craving for alcohol.

aldosteronism (al-dàs'têr-ō-nis'm) *Conn's syndrome;* consisting of severe metabolic and electrolytic changes due to hyperplasia or tumor of the adrenal cortex. Symptoms and signs include headache, muscular weakness, polydipsia, polyuria, low serum potassium, high serum sodium, and alkalosis.

alector A person who is unable to sleep.

alerting system See *formation, reticular.*

Alexander, Franz (1891–1964) Hungarian psychoanalyst; trained with Sachs and Abraham in Berlin; in 1929 appointed the first Professor of Psychoanalysis at the University of Chicago; chief contributions are in the area of brief analytic therapy and psychosomatic medicine.

Alexanderism *Obs.* (From Alexander the Great) *Agriothymia ambitiosa* (q.v.).

alexia Loss of the power to grasp the meaning of written or printed words; word-blindness; visual aphasia. See *acalculia;*

lobe, occipital; reading, disabilities of; speech disorders; syndrome, Potzl's.

alexia, acquired Loss of a previous skill in reading that follows disease or damage to the brain.

alexia, congenital Failure to acquire any reading ability; a rare disorder, usually associated with profound mental retardation. See developmental disorders, specific; dyslexia.

alexithymia Difficulty in describing or recognizing one's emotions; suggested by P. Sifneos to describe those persons who define emotions only in terms of somatic sensations or of behavioral reaction rather than relating them to accompanying thoughts. "They . . . give the impression they do not understand the meaning of the word 'feeling.' " (Short-Term Psychotherapy and Emotional Crisis, 1972) Their emotional functioning in general appears constricted and their phantasy life is limited and lackluster.

Some believe alexithymia reflects an absence of the ego functions that subserve affect and phantasy, but most writers explain it as due to primitive ego defenses that hide and distort the conscious experiences of affect and phantasy.

alexithymic deficit model See deficit model.

algedonic (al-jē-don'ik) Characterized by or relating to pleasure and pain, or the agreeable and the disagreeable.

-algesia (-al-jē'zē-à) Combining element meaning pain, from Gr. álgésis, sense of pain.

algesimeter (al-je-sim'ē-tēr) Same as algometer (q.v.).

algolagnia Any psychosexual disorder in which physical or mental pain is an essential part; algolagnia may be active (sadism) or passive (masochism).

algometer (al-gom'ē-tēr) An instrument that purports to measure sensitiveness to pain in terms of amount of pressure exerted on the skin by a blunt instrument. It is sometimes called algesimeter.

algophily (al-gof'i-lē) Rare. A term coined by Féré (L'Instinct Sexuel), synonymous with masochism.

algophobia Morbid fear of pain.

algopsychalia (al-gō-sī-kā'lē-à) See psychalgia.

algorithm, clinical Flow chart or decision tree; a graphic presentation of the sequential steps to be taken in making decisions about the diagnosis and treatment of a clinical problem.

Alice in Wonderland effect Metamorphosia (q.v.).

alienatio mentis (L. "alienation of the mind") Insanity.

alienation 1. A general term, now largely restricted to forensic psychiatry, indicating mental or psychiatric illness or insanity; when used in this way, alienation is ordinarily qualified by the adjective mental. 2. The repression, inhibition, blocking, or dissociation of one's own feelings so that they no longer seem effective, familiar, or convincing to the patient. Such alienation of one's own feelings is characteristic of obsessive-compulsive psychoneurosis. It may also be seen in the schizophrenias, but in the latter certain organs, body areas, or even the whole body are often perceived as if they did not belong to the person or as if they were different from the usual. The result is estrangement and depersonalization. 3. A mode of experience in which the person feels out of touch with himself; the syndrome often includes uncertainty about what role is expected of the person, doubt about his own decisions, loss of selfhood, dehumanization, and feelings of helplessness and futility. See identity crisis.

alienist Obs. Just as the term alienation in a psychiatric sense has been gradually restricted to the field of medical jurisprudence, so also the expression alienist refers to the specialist in psychiatry from the standpoint of law.

alienus (à-lē-ā'noos) Obs. Delirious, maniacal.

alimentary orgasm See orgasm, alimentary.

alimentation, forced Forced feeding; feeding in opposition to the will of the person being fed, as is frequently done in the treatment of patients with anorexia nervosa, persons who try to commit suicide through starvation, and prisoners on hunger strike. All such cases raise ethical questions about the rights of the person involved to refuse treatment and about the responsibility of the treater to override that person's autonomy.

all-or-none The principle that, regardless of the intensity of the stimulus, a single neuron reacts either with maximal intensity or not at all.

allachesthesia (à-làk-es-thē'zhē-à) Referral of a tactile sensation to a point remote from the point of stimulation; allesthesia. Usually, the displacement of sensation is symmetrical; it suggests a temporal lobe lesion.

allachesthesia, visual A rare phenomenon, indicative of parietal lobe lesion, consisting of referral or transposition of visual images to an opposite point in space.

Allan Dent disease *Arginosuccinic aciduria* (q.v.).

allele, allelomorph One of two or more genes that occupy the same locus on homologous chromosomes. If the individual has the same gene on a pair of homologous chromosomes, he is *homozygous* for that locus; if the homologous chromosomes differ he is *heterozygous* for that locus.

If a trait depends on a gene at a given locus, one allele may be dominant over the other (and the other is recessive to the first).

Three or more genes occupying the same locus in homologous chromosomes in a species are called *multiple alleles*. The best known instance of multiple alleles in man is in the blood groups.

allelic, allelomorphic Pertaining to or having the nature of an *allele* or *allelomorph*.

allesthesia See *allachesthesia; neglect, sensory*.

alliance and splitting In a weak or ineffective parental coalition, the assumption of the dominant role by one (typically the mother), who forms a coalition with the children, thereby consigning the other parent to a marginal, split-off and noninvolved role.

allo- Combining form meaning different, other.

alloch(e)iria (al-ō-kī′rē-à) A condition, apparently of neural origin, in which the location of touch or pain sensations is transferred to a corresponding place on the part of the body opposite to that stimulated.

allocortex Rhinencephalon; a part of the olfactory and allied systems of the cerebral cortex. The term is used primarily in speaking of the cytoarchitecture, or microscopic structure, of the cortex, in which case the allocortex is contrasted to the isocortex (or neocortex).

alloerotism, alloeroticism The final phase in the development of object relationships, marked by a stable integration or fusion of the drives and their deflection into appropriate channels; also known as the phase of impersonal socialization, adult sexuality, and mature genitality. It includes not only the ability to discharge libidinal impulses on a heterosexual object (as was achieved in the heteroerotic phase), but it also includes the ability to enter into a love relationship with the sexual object, a loving of the object more than a being loved by the object. See *ontogeny, psychic; stage, postambivalent*.

alloesthesia *Allachesthesia* (q.v.).

allolalia Any unusual or abnormal state of speech or utterance.

allometry In comparative biology, similarity based on physical accident rather than a common functioning background. See *analogy; homology*.

allophasis (al-of′à-zis) *Obs.* Incoherent speech.

alloplasticity *Acting out* (q.v.), often an expression of depression in children and adolescents.

alloplasty Adaptation by means of altering the external environment; contrasted with *autoplasty* (q.v.).

"Catalepsy and mimicry therefore would be regressions to a much earlier primitive method of adaptation of the organism, an autoplastic adaptation (adaptation by means of alteration in the organism itself), while flight and defense aim at an alteration in the environment (alloplastic adaptation)." (Ferenczi, *FCT*)

allopsyche The mind or psyche of another.

allotriogeustia, -geusia (a-lot-rē-ō-gūs′tē-à) 1. Perversion of the sense of taste. 2. Abnormal appetite.

allotriophagy (a-lot-rē-of′a-jē) Morbid impulse to eat unnatural foodstuffs; *pica* (q.v.).

allotriorhexia Compulsive plucking out of threads of clothes; usually the threads are then swallowed (*allotriophagia*).

allotropy (a-lot′rō-pē) Adolf Meyer's term for *allopsyche*.

Allport, Gordon Willard (1897–1967) U.S. psychologist and educator; developed a holistic psychology of human behavior, the core concepts of which are the *proprium* (the nuclear self or self-concept, consisting of those habits, attitudes, and values that are deeply ego-involved) and the *personal disposition* (the hierarchy of perceptual-motivational-behavioral unities that characterize a person). "Allport would certainly agree that, in many individuals, the Freudian framework labels for us the propriate strivings and the central dispositions. But he would equally assert that many therapeutic failures occur because the therapist keeps doggedly probing for infantile motivations in a personality where the propriate dispositions are organized around roles and conflicts of the adult situations." (Stagner, R. in *Handbook of Clinical Psychology*, ed. B.B. Wolman, 1965)

allusive thinking *Loosening* (q.v.) of associations; ideas are transmitted by inference and suggestion rather than directly, concepts seem diffuse and amorphous, and argument is often by analogy that seems irrelevant to the matter at hand.

alogia (à-lō′jē-à) Speechlessness usually due to intellectual deficiency or confusion. See *speech disorders*.

alogous (al′ō-gus) *Obs.* Unreasonable, irrational.

aloneness, autistic Kanner's term for the lack of desire for human contact that is a leading symptom of early infantile autism. See *autism, early infantile*.

Alpers's disease See *poliodystrophy, progressive infantile cerebral*.

alpha alcoholism See *alcoholism*.

alpha arc Refers to the sequence of a stimulus leading to motor behavior via a simple sensorimotor path. Beta arc refers to arousal of higher cortical paths by the functioning of an alpha arc (thus leading to a "sensation" rather than simple "awareness"), and not by an outside stimulus directly. The term alpha arc is approximately equivalent to *immediate response* in Watson's behavioristic psychology, while the term beta arc is roughly equivalent to Watson's *delayed response* or *implicit behavior*.

alpha EEG activity See *sleep*.

alpha index An index devised by Piotrowski for the diagnosis of schizophrenia on the basis of response to the Rorschach test. The index consists of the following criteria: the number of whole responses is no greater than 6; the sum of light shading responses is greater than the sum of the color responses; the presence of "dark shock"; a fall in sharply conceived forms below 70%. Accuracy of diagnosis is said to be 83–91%.

alpha rhythm, alpha wave See *electroencephalogram*.

alpha sleep A *sleep disorder* (q.v.) of the DIMS class with atypical polysomnographic features, consisting of the superimposition of alpha (high voltage) waves on the sleep EEG. In normal *sleep* (q.v.), alpha activity is decreased, but in alpha sleep there is *riddling* of the NREM sleep EEG. REM sleep is usually spared. The patient complains of interrupted and nonrestorative sleep. Alpha sleep may be idiopathic, or it may occur for a long period following withdrawal from drugs or alcohol.

alpha wave training A type of *biofeedback* (q.v.). Alpha brain waves (7.5–13.5 cps) are characteristic of relaxed and peaceful wakefulness (the *alpha state*). In alpha biofeedback training, the subject receives information on his EEG as a means of achieving a state of relaxation. In one technique, a tone sounds in the absence of alpha waves and disappears when the subject produces alpha waves.

alpinism A nonspecific term referring to neuropsychiatric syndromes appearing in relation to low atmospheric pressure, such as the asthenia syndrome of persons living in high altitudes.

ALS Amyotrophic lateral sclerosis. See *sclerosis, amyotrophic lateral*.

alter The other; the person in any social interaction with whom one interacts. See *ego*.

alter-egoism An altruistic feeling for only those who are in the same situation as oneself.

altered mind/body perception See *perception, altered mind/body*.

alternate care See *ALC*.

alternating psychosis The circular form of manic-depressive psychosis. See *psychosis, manic-depressive*.

alternative group session A regularly scheduled meeting of a therapy group that is held in the absence of the therapist. Alternate sessions are often scheduled at weekly intervals and may be held in the therapist's office or at the home of one of the group's members.

alternative psychologies Nontraditional approaches to an understanding of human behavior with emphasis on practical application, consciousness raising, achievement of potential, and self-determination. They are based on a variety of doctrines and philosophies, including (1) elements from well-established psychodynamic schemes such as Jung's analytical psychology, Reich's orgone theories, Gestalt theory; (2) data from neurophysiological studies such as altered states of consciousness, brain wave patterning, and biofeedback; (3) mystical or oriental philosophies such as yoga, zen buddhism, Taoism, astrology, the occult, parapsychology, psychical research; (4) popular movements such as est and sensitivity training.

altrigenderism (al-tri-jen'dēr-iz'm) The state of being attracted to the other gender. Beginning in the late infantile period the child takes an interest, to a greater or lesser extent, in members of the other *gender*, i.e. of the opposite sex. This term *altrigenderism* is suggested for socially approved unsexual activities between members of the two genders. When the interests become amorous, though not overtly sexual, *heteroerotism* is the proper term. When the sexual element (without sexual congress) enters into these relations, the condition is called *heterosexuality*, while *heterogenitality* as a term is limited to sexual intercourse.

altruism Regard for the interests and needs of others; a term coined by the French philosopher Auguste Comte (1798–1857), who maintained that the chief problem of existence is "vivre pour autrui" (to live for the sake of others). In psychiatric literature altruism and morality seem to be closely related, if not identical. Bleuler equates altruism with ethics.

"Freud says that the development from egotism and altruism is brought about through the formation of libidinal ties which inevitably limit narcism. This, according to him, is the only basis for the development of community interest." (Healy et al., *SMP*)

altruistic suicide See *anomie*.

alucinatio *Obs.* Hallucination.

alusia *Obs.* Insanity; hallucination.

alusia hypochondriaca *Obs.* Hypochondriasis.

alysm, alysmus *Obs.* Restlessness exhibited by a sick person.

alysosis (à-lē-sō'sis) Boredom, sometimes appearing as a central phenomenon in the simple form of schizophrenia. It is also known as *otiumosis*.

Alzheimer's disease (Alois Alzheimer, German neurologist, 1864–1915) Although formerly described as one of the presenile dementias, Alzheimer's disease now includes *primary degenerative dementia (PDD)* of both senile and presenile onset. It is also called *senile dementia, Alzheimer type (SDAT)*; *dementia, Alzheimer type (DAT)*; and *simple senile deterioration.*

Alzheimer's disease is a progressive, age-related, chronic cognitive dysfunction. The average course from onset to death is five years, with a range of one to ten years.

Alzheimer's disease is the predominant cause of dementia in late life and ranks fourth or fifth as the cause of death in the United States, accounting for about 100,000 deaths a year. Estimates of the prevalence rate range from 0.38 to 18.2%. In the United States, approximately 1 million people have severe dementia, and another 3 million have mild to moderate dementia. The likelihood of a first-degree relative developing SDAT is four times greater than in the general population, where the risk is well below 1%.

Symptoms and signs progress through two phases, the early confusional or forgetfullness phase and the later phase of severe dementia. Characteristic of the early phase is the *malignant amnestic syndrome,* consisting of shortened retention time, inability to recall events of the recent past, and inability to recall not only relatively unimportant facts associated with an experience but even the experience itself. Also impaired early are language and visuospatial skills. The language disturbances progress from simple word-finding difficulties and empty speech early in the illness to aphasia and even mutism late in its progression. Visuospatial abnormalities are manifested by disturbances of environmental orientation and difficulties in reproducing drawn figures (circle, square, cube).

In the second stage, apparent within a year or two after onset, disorientation is complete, rigidity of muscles becomes permanent (spastic contractures), and the patient shows purposeless hyperactivity in the emotional setting of perplexity and agitation. Aphasia, alexia, agraphia, apraxia, and agnosia are marked, speech is disrupted, and words or sentences are repeated senselessly (as *echolalia,* the echoing of phrases; *palilalia,* the reiteration of the last words of a sentence; or as *logoclonia,* the reiterative utterance of parts of words). The patient appears dull and apathetic, and both his attention and his emotions are difficult to arouse (*affective slumber*). Parkinsonism and convulsions may occur, and when the dementia is well advanced the patient may show the *signe du miroir*—he will sit for long periods in front of the mirror talking to his own reflection.

In the terminal stage, dementia is profound and the patient declines to a vegetative existence. Extreme emaciation may develop despite a ravenous appetite.

The pathology consists of generalized brain atrophy, with Alzheimer's neurofibrillary whorls (*agryrophilic dystrophy*), senile plaques, and granulovacuolar degeneration in the hippocampal pyramidal neurons. Etiology is unknown; there is evidence that some cases may be due to viral infection (perhaps a slow-growing virus) or autoimmune reactions. A genetically determined molecular defect leading to faulty handling of environmental aluminum has also been suggested by some researchers. The most consistent neurotransmitter abnormality is decrease in brain choline acetyltransferase, the enzyme necessary for the synthesis of acetylcholine. Almost all studies, however, have found multiple abnormalities and treatment approaches based on acetylcholine replacement have not been notably successful.

Esquirol first used the term *demence senile* in 1838. In 1907 Alzheimer described a type of presenile dementia accompanied by senile plaques and neurofibrillary tangles occurring in persons under 65. Arnold Pick had described Pick's presenile dementia in 1902. Until the 1960s, senile dementia was believed to be due to arteriosclerotic disease, but that is now recognized to be a relatively infrequent cause of senile or presenile dementia and is classified as a separate disorder, *multi-infarct dementia* (*MID*).

amathophobia Fear of dust.

amaurosis (am-aw-rō′sis) Complete blindness.

amaurotic family idiocy See *Tay-Sachs disease.*

amaxophobia Fear of being in a vehicle.

ambi- Combining form meaning both.

ambilevous (am-bi-le′vus) Poor in manual dexterity with both hands; "doubly left-handed," clumsy.

ambisexuality Ferenczi proposed that, from the standpoint of the psyche, the term ambisexuality be used instead of bisexuality. In their earliest manifestations emotions should not be regarded as masculine or feminine; rather they are qualities that have the capacity for association with masculinity, femininity, or both.

ambit, partial Burrow's term for the sphere of the organism's partial, false, conditioned *mergents* (q.v.). It represents a system of reflexly conditioned habituations that unites or separates clusters of individuals on a partitive or symbolic basis. Contrasted with total ambit.

ambit, total Burrow's term for the sphere of the organism's total or true *mergents* (q.v.). It embodies such reaction patterns as are expressive of an inherent principle of phyloorganismic equilibrium. Contrasted with partial ambit.

ambitendency Although some authors use the term ambitendency in the same sense that they use ambivalency, others seem to imply that an ambitendency is ambivalency in action. Bleuler equates ambivalence of the will with ambitendency. See *ambivalence.*

ambition Psychodynamically, ambition represents a fight against *shame* (q.v.) by proving that there is no need to be ashamed any more.

ambition, negative Reik's term used to describe the behavior of the masochist who evades every possibility of achieving his goal: he seems to follow the line of greatest resistance against himself, instead of that of greatest advantage for himself. The negative ambition is a grim reversal of an originally strong and positive ambition, in such a way that every opportunity is missed, every chance of success is turned into failure, every competition is avoided.

ambivalence, ambivalency Bipolarity; the coexistence of antithetic emotions, attitudes, ideas, or wishes toward a given object or situation. The term was coined by Bleuler, who differentiated among affective or emotional ambivalence, intellectual ambivalence, and ambivalence of the will. In current usage, the term ambivalence without further qualification ordinarily refers to affective ambivalence.

Ambivalence is characteristic of the unconscious and of children. Its overt appearance in the adult implies the presence of definite pathology, such as obsessive-compulsive psychoneurosis, manic-depressive psychosis, or schizophrenia.

Ambivalence is one of the fundamental symptoms of schizophrenia (Bleuler), and here it may appear in any one or more of its three forms. In affective ambivalence, the very same concept is accompanied simultaneously by pleasant and unpleasant feelings; thus a patient suffers the most intense anxiety that "they" will shoot her and yet constantly begs the doctor to shoot her. Another patient professes great love for her nurse and seems, in fact, to be very positively disposed toward the nurse, but in almost the same breath she asks how she can kill her. In ambivalence of the will, the desire to do a certain thing is accompanied by a desire not to do that thing. Thus a patient wants to eat and does not want to eat; or he demands work only to become furious when something is given him to do. In ambivalence of the intellect, an idea appears simultaneously with the counter-idea. One schizophrenic patient, for example, complained that he had no face and yet asked for a razor to shave the beard off his face; another answered "Definitely not" when asked directly if he heard voices and when then asked what they said replied, "Oh, all sorts of things." Ambivalence of the will and intellect are often at the basis of what is considered to be obsessive doubting in schizophrenic patients.

Affective ambivalence was noted by Abraham to be characteristic also of manic-depressive psychosis, and he described these patients as having a "constitutional ambivalence of the object cathexis." Among the psychoneuroses, the obsessive-compulsive group most characteristically shows ambivalence of severe degree. The ambivalence seen in the schizophrenias is often distinguishable from that seen in the manic-depressive and in the obsessive-compulsive groups in that schizophrenic ambivalence tends to be of severer degree, more widespread throughout all the object relationships of the patient, more overtly expressed and often fully conscious to the patient.

Ambivalence persists normally to some degree throughout life, but even in late childhood it is markedly reduced in comparison to the age period of 2 to 5 years, and in the adult it typically appears in one part in consciousness while the antithetic feeling or idea or goal remains unconscious. Ambivalence first makes its appearance in the oral sadistic stage, when introjection and incorporation are the important methods of forming object relationships. The object relationships of this stage represent the earliest and most extreme form of ambivalence, from which are later derived love and hate.

ambivalent Relating to the coexistence of antithetic emotions.

ambiversion The balance of the two traits, introversion and extraversion.

amblynoia simplex et catatonica (am-blē-noi′à) Dementia praecox (the schizophrenias).

amblyopia (am-blē-ō′pē-à) Dimness or partial loss of vision without discoverable lesion in eye structures or optic nerve; often it appears to develop as a result of intoxication with drugs, including tobacco.

ambulatory insulin treatment See *treatment, ambulatory insulin.*

ambulatory schizophrenia See *schizophrenia, ambulatory.*

amelectic (am-ē-lek′tik) *Rare.* Indifferent, careless, apathetic.

ameleia (am-el′ē-yà) Indifference.

amenomania A term introduced by B. Rush to denote a form of monomania, the equivalent of the manic phase of manic-depressive psychosis.

amentia *Obs.* Mental retardation; intellectual inadequacy. Amentia implies that the diminished intellectual capacity has been present from birth; in contrast, *dementia* (q.v.) implies that intellectual capacities were once intact but have since been dissipated, injured, or destroyed.

Different degrees of amentia were often specified by those who used the terms *idiocy* for what would currently be labeled profound retardation (Wechsler IQ below 25), *imbecility* for severe to moderate retardation (IQ 25–54), and *feeblemindedness* for mild retardation (IQ 55–69). Sometimes *moron* was used to refer to a mental retardate of mild degree. See *retardation, mental.*

amentia, deprivative Mental retardation (amentia) due to the lack of some constituent of the complete development of the brain. Among the several deprivative factors, three are well recognized. First, involvement of the endocrine glands, particularly the thyroid, associated with cretinism; second, malnutrition (*nutritional amentia*); third, lack of sensory stimuli (*amentia due to sense deprivation, isolation amentia*).

amentia, developmental Mental retardation that appears to be occasioned in part by germinal and in part by environmental factors, and particularly retardation with psychosocial (environmental) deprivation.

amentia, eclampsic *Obs.* Formerly applied to cases of mental retardation who manifested epileptiform convulsions for a short period only, in early infancy.

amentia, subcultural Tredgold says that "from the psychological aspect, many defectives appear to differ quantitatively rather than qualitatively from their nondefective fellows; indeed, they are often regarded as merely the tail end of a normal variation, and have been termed *subcultural* defectives by Dr. Lewis." (*TMD*)

amethystic Antiintoxicant; sobering; protecting from drunkenness. Used particularly in relation to alcohol in the sense of a "sobering-up" drug. No such agent has yet been discovered.

ametropia (à-me-trō′pē-à) Any error of refraction as a result of which parallel rays are focused not on the retina itself but in front of it (*myopia*) or behind it (*hyperopia*).

amimia (à-mim′ē-à) A disorder of language, characterized by the inability to use gestures appropriately to conform with the idea to be expressed. The person with amimia may also be unable to imitate or reproduce by motion the facial expressions and gestures of others. He may likewise make the inappropriate or wrong gestures in endeavoring to convey his thoughts or feelings, e.g. shaking his head sideways when saying yes, and nodding his head when saying no. This is the motor (or expressive) aspect of amimia. Its counterpart is sensory (or perceptive) amimia when the patient does not understand or assigns a wrong meaning to another's gesture, taking a sidewise shake of the head to mean consent, and a nod to mean disapproval.

amine An organic substance containing the radical group NH_2. Of particular interest are the *biogenic amines* because of their role in brain functioning. The biogenic amines are subdivided into the *catecholamines* (among which are epinephrine, mescaline, amphetamine, dopamine, and DMPEA) and the *indoles* (among which are tryptophan, serotonin, hydroxy-indolacetic acid, and bufotenine). See *epinephrine; ergotropic; neurotransmitter; serotonin.*

amine oxidase *Monoamine oxidase* (q.v.).

amixia Restriction of marriage to one race, caste, etc., to prevent miscegenation.

amnemonic (am-nē-mon′ik) Relating to loss of memory.

amnesia Inability to recall past experiences; loss of memory. *Anterograde amnesia* refers to inability to form new memories, either because of failure to consolidate what is perceived into permanent memory storage, or because of inability to retrieve memory from storage. *Retrograde amnesia* refers to loss of memory for events that occurred prior to the event or condition (toxin, trauma, vitamin deficiency, etc.) that is presumed to have caused the memory disturbance in the first place. See *amnestic syndrome; memory.*

amnesia, anterograde See *amnesia, retrograde.*

amnesia, autohypnotic *Repression* (q.v.), as opposed to normal forgetting.

amnesia, catathymic (kat-à-thī′mik) Circumscribed loss of memory that is limited to a single experience. For example, a patient with clear memory for all other events had no memory for circumstances connected with her pregnancy.

amnesia, circumscribed See *amnesia, retrograde.*

amnesia, continuous Anterograde amnesia.

amnesia, episodic Loss of memory for a specific happening without anterograde or retrograde extension, considered to be on the basis of repression and not primarily organic in nature.

amnesia, epochal "In the epochal type of amnesia a person, perhaps after a shock, suddenly loses all memory for lost *epochs;* it may be for days and even for years of his preceding life. In the classical case of Mr. Hanna, studied by Boris Sidis, the amnesia was for his whole previous life, so that the subject was like a new-born child." (Prince, M. *The Unconscious,* 1916)

amnesia, infantile Amnesia for the period of infancy and early childhood, i.e. from birth to the end of the fifth year of life. Memory for this period is practically nil and even those few isolated fragments that some people believe they can remember as "clearly as though it were yesterday" are seldom wholly accurate. See *memory, affect.*

amnesia, negativistic The delusion that memory and orientation are lost.

amnesia, posthypnotic Loss of memory for events transpiring during the hypnotic stage.

amnesia, retrograde Amnesia extending backward, to include material antedating the onset of amnesia proper; also called *circumscribed amnesia.* When the amnesia encompasses material subsequent to the onset of amnesia it is termed *anterograde amnesia* or *continuous amnesia.* See *dementia.*

amnesia, transient global (TGA) Abrupt onset of disorientation due to loss of ability to encode recent memories plus retrograde amnesia of variable duration, with retention of a remarkable degree of alertness and responsiveness and capacity for fairly complicated mental performances. The episode, which is almost never repeated, lasts for a few hours, when the patient regains his ability to encode recent memories despite amnesia for events that occurred during the acute phase. TGA is presumed to be due to transient ischemia of the hippocampus-fornix-hypothalamic system, although there is no direct proof of the theory. It is to be differentiated from hysterical amnesia and from the amnesia of temporal lobe epilepsy.

amnesia visualis verbalis *Obs.* Witmer's term (1907) for a type of *reading disability* (q.v.).

amnesic syndrome Profound loss of distant memory in a subject whose intelligence and recent memory are otherwise intact; related to bilateral lesions of the hippocampus and mammillary bodies. See *amnestic syndrome.*

amnestia *Obs.* Amnesia (q.v.).

amnestic aphasia See *aphasia, amnestic.*

amnestic apraxia See *apraxia, amnestic.*

amnestic syndrome One of the forms of *organic mental disorders* (q.v.), consisting of

impairment of *short-term memory* (i.e. unable to recall items 25 minutes after their presentation) but not of *immediate memory* (i.e. patient has a normal digit-span). Because of short-term memory impairment, memories are not consolidated and stored, or cannot be retrieved from storage; as a result, new memories cannot be formed (anterograde amnesia). Almost always there is some degree of retrograde amnesia, disorientation, apathy, inertia and emotional blandness. *Confabulation* (q.v.) may occur. The amnestic syndrome is rare and usually occurs in association with alcoholism. See *syndrome, Wernicke-Korsakoff.*

amniotic Equivalent of *intrauterine.*

amok See *amuck.*

amor lesbicus Sapphism. See *homosexuality, female.*

amoralia *Obs.* Moral imbecility; *psychopathic personality* (q.v.).

amorous paranoia See *jealousy, morbid.*

amorphosynthesis Faulty perception of the form of objects; one type of amorphosynthesis is *metamorphopsia* (q.v.).

amorphous communications See *communication, disordered.*

amotivational See *syndrome, amotivational.*

amphetamine Benzedrine; phenylisopropylamine; a sympathomimetic amine similar to ephedrine but with a greater ability to stimulate the higher centers, particularly the cortex. See *Benzedrine dependency; dependency, drug.*

amphetamines A generic name for a group of drugs including the substituted phenylethylamines (e.g. amphetamine, dextroamphetamine, methamphetamine) and other drugs with amphetaminelike actions, such as methylphenidate (Ritalin) and appetite suppressants. Sometimes all are called *speed,* although usually speed is used to refer to methamphetamine only.

All the drugs in this group are associated with abuse and dependence, and all can produce one or more organic mental disorders: intoxication, delirium, delusional syndrome, or withdrawal syndrome. See *Benzedrine dependency; dependency, drug.*

amphierotism (am-fē-er'ō-tiz'm) A term coined by Ferenczi to indicate the condition in which a person is able to conceive of him self as a male or female or both simultaneously.

amphigenesis (am-fi-jen'ē-sis) A form of sexual inversion in which a person, predominantly homosexual, is able also to have sexual relations with members of the opposite sex. Thus one speaks of amphigenic inversion in contradistinction to absolute inversion, in which sexuality is restricted to the members of the same sex only. See *swinging*.

amphimixis (am-fi-mik'sis) 1. A term used to indicate the fact that both parents contribute to the inheritance of their offspring. 2. Ferenczi's term for the union and integration of the component instincts (oral, anal, and urethral) into the genital function. The genitals attain their specific importance only when the earlier phases have been more or less surmounted and the genitals become the leading sexual zone and the central organ for discharging the entire libido. After puberty, the residues of the earlier developmental phases find expression in preparatory activities (forepleasure) and serve merely to stimulate the genital strivings.

amplifying somatic style A term suggested by Arthur J. Barsky and Gerald L. Klerman (*American Journal of Psychiatry 140*, 1983) as a replacement for *hypochondriasis* (q.v.). The phrase describes one particular mode of perceiving, evaluating, and expressing bodily sensations and is free from clinical assumptions and etiologic theories inherent in the older term.

Amsterdam retardation See *syndrome, de Lange*.

amuck A culture-specific syndrome of the Malaysian Peninsula consisting of an outburst of homicidal fury, vented indiscriminately against anyone who happens to cross the subject's path. Kraepelin suggested that amuck (amok) might be an epileptic variant similar to cursive epilepsy or episodic dyscontrol. Others, noting that the person who *runs amok* is often a male who has experienced rejection by the family of his prospective bride, have interpreted the syndrome as a culturally patterned response to a major threat to self-esteem.

amurakh A culture-specific syndrome occurring in Siberian women; because the major symptom is echopraxia, the syndrome is sometimes called *copying mania*.

amusia (a-mū'zē-a) Musical inability, whether for perception or (re-)production of vocal or instrumental sounds.

amychophobia (a-mi-kò-) Morbid fear of being scratched.

amygdala, amygdaloid nucleus (a-mig'da-là) A part of the basal ganglion complex; the amygdala is a small, discrete, nuclear mass situated on the roof of the temporal horn of the lateral ventricle at the inferior end of the caudate nucleus. It projects directly to the hypothalamus, and interruption of these connections gives rise to sham rage. See *rage, sham; rhinencephalon*.

amygdaloidectomy, amygdolectomy Ablation of the amygdaloid nucleus; this psychosurgical procedure has been used particularly in hallucinating patients, in the belief that the amygdaloid nucleus is a mechanism for transforming thought processes into temporally patterned motor movements, either of the vocal musculature as in subjective auditory experiences, or of the still vaguer projections or representations experienced through vision, taste, or smell. Bilateral amygdaloidecitomy in man has been reported to produce hypersexuality and other gross expressions of biological needs, hyperaggressivity, bulimia, polydipsia, and loss of social controls over behavior. See *syndrome, Klüver-Bucy*.

amyostasia (a-mi-ō-sta'zhē-a) Muscle tremor.

amyosthenia See *aphoria*.

amyotony (a-mī-ot'ō-nē) See *aphoria*.

amyotrophic lateral sclerosis See *sclerosis, amyotrophic lateral*.

Amytal interview (am'i-tal) See *narcotherapy*.

An Rorschach scoring symbol for anatomy response.

anabolic 1. Relating to the process of assimilating nutrients and converting them into protoplasm; the constructive side of metabolism. 2. *Obs.* In constitutional medicine, the anabolic biotype includes the *brachymorphic, megalosplanchnic, parasympathicotonic,* and *pyknic* types. See *type, pyknic*.

anabolism Biochemical changes by which food is converted into living materials within a cell or the combination of cells forming an organism.

anachoresis See *atelesis*.

anaclinic See *anaclitic*.

anaclisis (a-nàk'li-sis) A state of reclining. The infant is dependent on its mother or a substitute for its well-being and sustenance. Some people continue throughout life to depend on others for physical and emotional support and are termed anaclitic. An example is the passive, effeminate husband whose feelings, actions, and thoughts are largely regulated by a dominant wife.

According to Jones, anaclisis is the process of a sexual drive becoming attached to and exploiting various nonsexual self-preservative trends such as eating and defecation.

anaclitic, anaclinic Relating to or characterized by anaclisis or dependence on another or others; characterized by dependence of libido on another instinct, e.g. hunger. See *depression, anaclitic.*

"If we could speak of 'object choice' in this early stage of infancy, we would say that the first object choice is an anaclitic one, in which the individual leans on another object for gratification of hunger, bodily needs, for protection, and the like." (Nunberg, H. *Principles of Psychoanalysis,* 1955)

anacusia (à-nà-kū'sē-à) Total deafness.

anaesthesia See *anesthesia.*

anagogy, anagoge (an-a-gō'jē) Psychic material that is expressive of ideals. Some believe that dreams are susceptible of two different interpretations. One of the interpretations is that usually ascribed by psychoanalysts, namely, infantile sexual interpretation. The other is related to the spiritual, idealistic, nonsexual forces of the unconscious; hence the expression anagogic interpretation. The latter is of the kind stressed by Jung in his understanding of deep forces in the unconscious.

anal eroticism A psychoanalytic term for localization or concentration of libido in the anal zone. In psychoanalytic theory, the earliest concentration of libido is in the oral zone; with further development, most of it shifts to the anal region and, later, to the phallic area.

Part of the libido originally connected with the anal zone becomes attached to the habits and discipines identified with anal training (regularity of stool, control, cleanliness, etc.); the latter become incorporated into the personality as anal traits. Other portions of the original anal libido are invested in similar fashion in the results or products of anal activity. "Thus the interest in feces is carried on partly as interest in money, partly as a wish for a child, in which latter an anal-erotic and a genital impulse ('penis-envy') coincide."

(Freud, *CP*) See *character, anal; defense, character; envy, penis.*

anal sadism See *sadism, anal.*

anal sadistic Relating to anal sadism or the aggressive instinctual quality identified with the anal region and its functions. See *sadism, anal.*

anal triad See *triad, anal.*

analeptic A stimulating or restorative drug, such as caffeine or amphetamine. More specific antidepressant drugs (e.g. monoamine oxidase inhibitors and tricyclic compounds such as imipramine) are generally termed *psychoanaleptics.*

analfabetia partialis *Obs.* Wolff's term (1916) for a type of *reading disability* (q.v.).

analgesia, analgia Loss or absence of the sense of pain. Analgesia may be of somatic or psychic origin; the psychiatric conditions in which it is most frequently seen are schizophrenia, conversion hysteria, and hypnotic states.

anality A general term referring to the anal components of sexuality, to manifestations of instinctual conflict centering about the anal stage of sexual development, to manifestations of anal erogeneity which indicate fixation at the anal stage of development. Anality is prominent in obsessive-compulsive neurosis, hypochondriasis, and masochism. See *anal eroticism; phase, anal.*

analogous See *homologous.*

analogue, libido This is an expression introduced by Jung (analytical psychology) to refer to "the symbol which converts energy." He adds that "by this I define a representation that is suited to express the libido equivalent, by virtue of which the libido is led over into a form different from the original one. Mythology offers innumerable images of this sort, ranging from sacred objects like *churingas,* fetishes, etc., up to figures of gods. The rites with which the sacred objects are surrounded often disclose very plainly their character as transformers of energy. Thus, for example, the primitive rubs his *churinga* rhythmically and thereby takes into himself the magic power of the fetish, at the same time imparting a fresh 'charge' to the fetish." (Jung, *CAP*)

analogy In comparative biology, similarity based on common function. See *allometry; homology.*

analysand (à-nal'i-zand) The one who is being analyzed.

analysis *Psychoanalysis* (q.v.).

analysis, active A method of dream interpretation used in a technique in which the analyst does not confine himself to the mere passive elucidation of the subject's free associations but intervenes directly and actively, making revelations and giving advice suggested to him mainly by the manifest content of the dream. This method, introduced by Stekel, is also called "active analytical psychotherapy." (Stekel, *ID*) See *analysis, direct.*

analysis, anamnestic Jung's term for his method of psychoanalytic investigation and treatment. The term emphasizes the importance of tracing the historical development of the patient's disorder and the desirability of supplementing the subject's own account with material gleaned from family members and associates.

analysis, behavioral A way of examining patterned behavior at the micro level based on operant theory and social learning models of transactions. The basic assumption is that the most important determinants of behavior are in the external environment, and that analysis of events that vary together with behavior makes it possible to predict future behavior. Focus is on the presence and effects of reinforcers and punishers.

analysis, blind In Rorschach interpretation and percept analysis, inferring personality traits solely from the responses to the inkblots without knowledge of the subject, his symptoms, or his history other than age and sex.

analysis, character Psychoanalytic treatment of a character disorder. See *defense, character.*

analysis, child Psychoanalytic treatment of children that requires major modifications of the classical analytic technique. More activity is required of the analyst, for one thing, and play therapy must often substitute for free associations as a way to elicit the significant psychodynamic factors. See *technique, play; therapy, play.*

analysis, cohort See *cohort.*

analysis, content Interpretation of a subject's production on the basis of what is said, rather than on the basis of how it is said. The interpretation of symbols in a patient's dream, for example, is content analysis.

analysis, control Psychoanalytic treatment of a patient by a trainee in analysis whose therapeutic methods are under the close supervision of (i.e. are being "controlled" by) an experienced analyst.

analysis, cost/benefit (CBA) Comparison of the costs of a program or technology to resulting benefits, with both costs and benefits expressed by the same measure (usually monetary).

analysis, cost-effectiveness (CEA) Comparison of the costs of a program or alternative programs to the resultant benefits or effectiveness expressed in different measures. Costs are usually expressed in money, while benefits are expressed in such measures as number of lives saved or disabilities avoided or other objectives deemed worthwhile.

analysis, didactic See *analysis, orthodox; analysis, tuitional.*

analysis, direct A form of psychoanalytically oriented psychotherapy, advocated by John Rosen for treatment of schizophrenics, in which the therapist enters into the patient's delusional system and confronts him with interpretations of the meaning of his symptoms and behavior. Because such interpretations are based on the therapist's guesses about the patient's unconscious, the method is often referred to as *wild analysis.*

analysis, directed See *analysis, focused.*

analysis, discontinuous Interrupted or staggered analysis, especially a reduction in the frequency of sessions as part of gradual and planned termination of psychoanalytic treatment.

analysis, distributive In objective psychobiology, the analysis of information gained about the patient "is distributed by the physician along the various lines which are indicated by the patient's complaints and symptoms, by the problems which the physician himself can recognize, by the patient's imaginations concerning the present and the past as well as by actual situations, attitude to the future and outstanding features of his personality." (Diethelm, O. *Treatment in Psychiatry*, 1936)

analysis, ego In psychoanalytic treatment, the uncovering and interpreting of the ego's (and superego's) defenses against impulses. Libido analysis and ego analysis go hand in hand in treatment: libido analysis, for example, discovers *what* it is that has been repressed, while ego analysis discovers *why* the infantile ego found it necessary to repress the impulse in the first place.

analysis, existential See *existentialism*.

analysis, expectant See *analysis, focused*.

analysis, focused Selective analysis; directed analysis; a modification of the orthodox psychoanalytic technique (which is termed by Glover *expectant analysis* because the analyst waits and follows the spontaneous unfolding of the patient's psyche with leisurely, free-floating, analytical attention). In the focused or selective analysis, interpretations are purposively geared to a particular aspect of the patient's pathology— particular defenses, particular shades of transference, particular types of conflict, and particular stages of instinctual needs that seem to be of paramount importance.

analysis, fractional A technique employed by Alexander as one of his brief therapy methods. In fractional analysis, psychotherapy is suspended for calculated intervals, while the patient works through insights already attained and prepares himself for gaining more.

analysis, group Psychoanalytic group psychotherapy; resolution of individual conflict in a social network, where the symptom is reactivated and is translatable into communicative processes. Malcolm Pines (Tavistock Clinic), a pioneer in the application of psychoanalytic principles to the setting of group therapy, follows the proposition of Foulkes, one of the leading exponents of group therapy in England. The essence of the person is social, and neurosis and psychologic disturbances generally arise in disordered social relationships that develop from the unconscious forces of love and hate. The highly individualistic neurotic position is essentially group disruptive. The individual's inner world is actualized in the group setting. As each group member represents a deviation from the norm of the community to which all belong, together the group members are the norm from which each deviates. See *psychotherapy, group*.

analysis, minor A psychotherapeutic method in which the analysis of psychic material attempts neither an exhaustive study of (as does Freudian analysis in general) nor deeper delving into subconscious conflicts, but confines itself only to the elucidation of the salient details considered of primary importance in relation to the neurosis. Minor analysis is of shorter duration than orthodox, or Freudian, psychoanalysis. Through the interpretation of the most conspicuous of the psychic materials the analyst arrives at conclusions, makes revelations, and gives suggestions with the aim of enabling the patient to gain quick insight. (Stekel, *ID*)

analysis, orthodox Freudian analysis, better known as psychoanalysis, which uses primarily the technique of free association, interpretation of dreams, and elucidation of everyday mistakes in order to unmask the patient's unconscious motivations. The psychic material obtained in this manner is then made available to the patient, in order to prompt the emotional acceptance rather than mere intellectual knowledge of conflicts.

analysis, passive Stekel uses this expression to describe the feature of Freudian psychoanalysis that calls on the psychiatrist to wait patiently for the production of free associations by the subject and subsequently to interpret them without active intervention.

analysis, Schicksal Szondian depth analysis, an eclectic system that borrows heavily from Freudian and Jungian psychology and strongly emphasizes the "familial unconscious," or hereditary tendencies. See *test, Szondi*.

analysis, selective Pseudopsychoanalytic treatment in which the material (e.g. defense mechanisms, levels of development) chosen for interpretation is a function of the interests (and problems) of the therapist rather than a reflection of the psychic structure and function of the patient. To some extent, such selection is operative in all types of psychotherapy, including psychoanalysis, and is probably responsible at least in part for the effects the actual character and personality of the therapist have on his techniques and results. See *analysis, focused*.

analysis, structural A type of psychotherapy described by E. Berne (1957), based on the belief that psychiatric disorders arise from pathological relationships between the various ego states: exteropsychic (Parent), neopsychic (Adult), and archaeopsychic (Child). Structural analysis aims at strengthening the boundaries between these states so that the Adult can become the effective executive of a healthy way of living.

analysis, training See *analysis, tuitional.*

analysis, tuitional Didactic or training analysis; a term used by Ferenczi to refer to character analysis carried out for purposes of training in the concepts and problems of psychoanalysis (Freudian) through personal analysis of the analysand; who is in the position of a student who pays tuition for his instruction. See *analysis, orthodox.*

analysis, vector Alexander's term for the process of determining the degree of participation of the organism's basic tendencies—reception, elimination, and retention—in the genesis and development of neurosis.

analyst One who analyzes, that is, resolves a whole into its parts. While the term psychoanalyst has its generic meaning, it is usually understood today to refer to those who adhere to the formulations of the psychoanalysis of Freud. Analysts who follow Jung's concepts are called analytical psychologists; those who use the concepts of Meyer are psychobiologists; those following Adler are individual psychologists.

analyst, lay See *psychiatrist.*

analytic group psychotherapy See *psychotherapy, group.*

analytic psychology Jung's system of psychology, some of whose major elements are:

1. A personal unconscious as well as the *collective unconscious* (q.v.), containing prototypical or archetypal material and able to generate images prior to and independent of conscious experience. The archetypes are the themes with which humans have struggled throughout their history: Anima and Animus (the hidden opposite side of the male and female, respectively), Wise Old Man and Great Mother (the authority and power figures), etc.; see *archetype.*

2. Within consciousness, the ego (the center of the conscious field, the experiencing "me") surrounded by the *persona* (q.v.), or mask, which is the face the subject presents to the world.

3. A 16-category personality typology derived from the various combinations of *attitudes* and psychological *functions*—the attitudes (introversion and extraversion) influence the direction of energy in the psyche, while the paired functions (the rational pair is thinking and feeling, the perceptual pair is sensation and intuition) describe the ways in which the subject relates to the world, perceives it, and evaluates it; see *type, feeling; type, intuitive; type, rational; type, sensational; type, thinking.* During development, one of the attitudes and one of the functions become dominant and characterize the operation of that particular person; and one of the pair of functions orthogonal to the dominant function becomes the auxiliary function. Any personality is therefore described in terms of dominant attitude, first function, and auxiliary function.

4. The first half of life (to approximately 40 years of age) is concerned with establishing one's position in the world, through the operation of the dominant attitude and the first function. Then there is a shift from finding one's way in the world to finding one's way out, and in the ultimate confrontation with mortality the previously neglected and less conscious portions of the personality, the opposite attitude and the fourth function (the polar opposite of the first function), are given expression.

5. Life proceeds toward an ultimate outcome, consisting of the achievement of selfhood, making the potential actual, reconciling opposites, and making all the functions and the nondominant attitude conscious and thus available for use. The process of achieving that outcome is *individuation* (q.v.).

analytical Relating to analysis or to the separation of something into its parts.

analyzer Pavlov's term for the functional neural unit that provides the basis for differential sensitivity; the analyzer consists of receptor, afferent nerves, and their central connections.

anamnesia *Rare.* The recollection of phenomena which immediately precede an illness.

anamnesis The term literally means recollection. In medicine it commonly refers to the historical account of a patient's illness antedating the period of illness. It is distinguished from catamnesis, which refers to the history of the patient following an illness.

anamnesis, associative A type of psychiatric history-taking developed by Deutsch (1939) that attempts to elicit the causal relationship between the patient's somatic symptoms and his psychic structure. Of consequence in the anamnesis are not only the factual details but how they are said and when they are said in the interview. The patient is stimulated to give information by having him describe his organic complaints without making him aware of a psychological background. He is allowed to give a detailed account of his complaints and his ideas about the illness. Then he stops and waits to be questioned by the interviewer. When it is clear that the patient will not continue spontaneously, the examiner repeats one of the points of the patient's last sentence in interrogative form, using the same words the patient used insofar as possible. The patient then gives new information about his symptoms and is stimulated to further associations. Reference to others in his environment, present or past, then appear. The person who appears first in the case history is usually the relevant person from a psychosomatic point of view. Somatic and emotional symptoms with reference to this person are used as word stimuli for further associations. Then the patient himself usually correlates his organic illness with his emotional life. During the associative anamnesis, the examiner is on the lookout for three essential points in establishing the psychosomatic unity of the patient's complaints: the old conflict, the recent conflict, and the time factors involved. The associative anamnesis is used to greatest advantage with psychosomatic disorders. The anamnesis is taken in one sitting, which lasts from one to two hours.

anancasm (à-nang'kaz'm) Any form of repetitious, recurrent, orderly, stereotyped behavior or thinking which if left unperformed will lead to an increase in anxiety and tension. Though including obsessive and compulsive traits, the term does not apply to repeated fulfillment of recurrent physiologically determined needs such as

sleep and sex. H. Richter believes that phobias are also anancasms, because they may drive the subject to seek protection through compulsions or obsessions. (*American Journal of Psychiatry 96*, 1939–40)

anancastia (à-nang-kas'tē-à) Term for the compulsive, obsessive type of personality. See *defense, character; personality.*

anandria (an-an'drē-à) Absence of masculinity.

anaphase (an'à-fāz) The third state of the division of a cell by mitosis, characterized by polar migration of the chromosomes.

anaphia (an-à'fē-à) Absence of sense of touch; commonly used to refer to a relative rather than an absolute loss of tactile sensibility.

anaphrodisia *Obs.* Absence of sexual feeling.

anaphylaxis, psychic Reactivation of earlier symptoms by an event similar to the one that initially produced the symptoms. As in physical anaphylaxis, the initial event may be called the sensitizing agent, the later event the activating agent. A patient with severe asthma demonstrated psychic anaphylaxis; through psychoanalysis his symptoms were discovered to be derived from an early childhood experience of near-drowning. The asthma itself was an anxiety equivalent related to his fear of loss of love and his mother's scream for help. The sensitizing agent in this case was the early trauma of near-drowning; the activating agent was his fear of loss of love when his wife threatened to leave him. It is noteworthy that in psychic anaphylaxis, at least, the reaction is specific and is a response to the sensitizing agent rather than to the activating agent.

anarithmia A type of *acalculia* (q.v.).

anarthria (an-är'thrē-à) *Obs.* Complete inarticulateness; *aphasia* (q.v.). See *speech disorders.*

anasarca hystericum *Obs.* A transient swelling, generally of the abdominal parietes, in a hysterical person; phantom tumor; hysterical edema.

anathymiasis (à-na-thim-ī'à-sis) *Obs.* An old term for hysterical flatus or "the vapors," originally used by ancient Greek philosophers to describe the soul; an exhalation.

anaudia (an-aw'dē-à) *Aphonia* (q.v.).

anchoring symptoms Kernberg's term for the cardinal or key symptoms of psychopathology that suggest a specific diagnosis;

neurotic symptoms alone, for example, suggest a diagnosis of symtomatic neurosis, while defective reality testing indicates the presence of a borderline condition or functional psychosis and the dysmnesic syndrome points to the probability of an organic mental disorder.

ancillary Auxiliary, subordinate. In insurance terminology, ancillary costs or services are those related to diagnosis and treatment of the patient but not covered in the basic charge for the hospital bed or room, such as operating room, laboratory, and X-ray.

androgyneity, androgynism, androgyny Female pseudohermaphroditism, in which the subject is genetically female and has ovaries but manifests secondary characteristics of both sexes.

The term has been more loosely applied in psychoanalysis, anthropology, and general literature to refer to bisexuality or to the capacity to develop characteristics of either sex. Such usage has not always kept pace with recent advances in knowledge about human sexuality, so the sense in which any author is using the term can only be inferred from the context of the total production. The term may mean any of the following: (1) hermaphroditism, with physical features of both sexes; (2) confusion or uncertainty about one's *gender identity* (q.v.); (3) confusion or uncertainty about one's gender role, presenting a mixture of behaviors that will be labeled socially as both *masculine* and *feminine* (qq.v.). In this sense, the term is most commonly used to characterize a male as effeminate, often with the added implication that in sexual activity he prefers a partner of the same sex.

andromania *Nymphomania* (q.v.).

andromonoecism See *hermaphroditism.*

androphobia Morbid fear of men.

androphonia *Obs.* Homicide.

androphonomania *Obs.* Homicidal insanity.

anemia, cerebral An inexact, descriptive term for reduced blood flow to the brain. The diminished blood supply may be in the brain as a whole (generalized cerebral anemia) or it may be limited to one or more specific areas of the brain (local cerebral anemia). Generalized cerebral anemia may be acute, as in cardiac failure or in psychological or physiological shock, or it may be chronic, as in pernicious anemia, leukemia, other blood dyscrasias, repeated blood loss, cerebral arteriosclerosis, or cachexia. Symptoms of acute cerebral anemia include roaring in the ears, spots before the eyes, swaying, weakness, apathy, somnolence, unconsciousness, profuse sweating, and cold, pale skin. Symptoms of chronic cerebral anemia include headaches, feeling of pressure in the head, roaring in the ears, dizziness, insomnia, or drowsiness, and in many cases progression to an organic reaction with memory disturbances, delusions, and hallucinations.

Local cerebral anemia is seen in cerebral arteriosclerosis, intracranial tumor, vasospasm, hypertensive encephalopathy, etc. Symptoms include fleeting pareses, transient aphasias, temporary sensory disturbances, hemianopsia, and focal convulsive twitches.

anemic anoxia See *anoxia, cerebral.*

anemophobia Fear of wind.

aneos (a'nē-os) *Obs.* Struck with the loss of voice and reason.

anergasia (an-ēr-gas'ē-à) Loss of functional activity. When a clinical psychiatric syndrome is associated with structural pathology of the brain, it is classified by Adolf Meyer as an anergasia. The organic psychoses are called anergastic reaction types.

anergia, anergy (an-ēr'ji-à, an'ēr-jē) Lack of energy; passivity.

anerotism (an-er'ō-tiz'm) See *negativism, sexual.*

anesthesia, anaesthesia Absence of sensation.

anesthesia, glove A disorder in the sensory field in which the patient has no sense of feeling in an area roughly corresponding to that covered by a glove; this anesthesia is usually psychogenic (hysterical).

anesthesia, sexual *Frigidity, sexual* (q.v.).

anesthesia, spiritual Amorality; lack of moral or ethical standards. Apparent moral irresponsibility may be based on fear of making painful decisions.

anethopath (à-neth'ō-path) An ethically or morally uninhibited person.

anethopathy, anetopathy (an-eth-op'à-thē) Absence of moral inhibitions; unethicalness; Karpman's term (1949) for primary, essential, genuine, idiopathic psychopathy or *psychopathic personality* (q.v.). This is the group from which so-called habitual criminals come. In such cases, usually no deep-seated psychic motivations can be elicited, and patients appear to be "disease fast"—no matter what is done for them in terms of psychotherapy, their patterns of reaction continue unchanged. The conspicuous trait in their mental makeup is complete egocentricity, which is also reflected in their narcissistic sexual behavior.

aneuploidy (an'ū-ploi-dē) Cytogenetical anomaly; existence of an abnormal number of chromosomes not an exact multiple of the haploid number and/or the occurrence of abnormal chromosomes; karyotype abnormality. Among the best known examples of aneuploidy are D trisomy, E trisomy, G trisomy or Down's syndrome, XXX (superfemale), XXY (Klinefelter's syndrome), XO (Turner's syndrome), XYY, and XXYY. See *chromosome.*

aneuthanasia Painful death.

angel dust *Phencyclidine* (q.v.).

anginophobia Fear of choking.

angiogram (an'jē-ō-gram) An X-ray of the blood vessels of an area following injection of an artery supplying the area with a suitable contrast medium (usually Diodrast). In neurology, internal carotid angiography is used to study the arterial vessels of the cerebral hemispheres; vertebral angiography (arteriography) is used to study the circulation of the posterior fossa and the posterior portions of the cerebral hemispheres. Angiography is useful in demonstrating intracranial aneurysms, vascular malformations, and tumors.

angiomatosis, trigeminal cerebral *Sturge-Weber-Dimitri's disease;* hemangioma over the meninges of the parietal and occipital lobes and underlying maldevelopment of the brain resulting in mental retardation.

angular gyrus See *lobe, parietal; syndrome, angular gyrus.*

anhedonia (an-hē-dō'nē-à) Absence of pleasure in acts that are normally pleasurable. It is seen often in schizophrenics and may be one of the earliest signs in the pseudoneurotic variety described by Hoch and Polatin.

In behavioral terms, anhedonia is a state in which the reward value of usually reinforcing stimuli is blocked. As thus defined, anhedonia may be a side-effect of neuroleptic agents, but whether this effect results from direct interference with the reward system or because of the interference with response patterns is not yet clear.

anhidrosis (an-hi-drō'sis) Deficiency or absence of perspiration.

aniconia (à-ne-kō'nē-à) Absence of mental imagery.

anile To be in one's dotage; imbecilic.

anilingus Stimulation of the anal zone by the tongue and lips, usually as a part of sexual foreplay.

anima In Jung's terminology, the soul, that part of the psyche that is directed inward and is in touch with the unconscious; the anima is contrasted with the *persona* (q.v.), which is the outer attitude or outer character. Because the outer attitude is often the opposite of the inner, Jung also uses *anima* to refer to the feminine soul of a very masculine man and *animus* to refer to the masculine soul of a very feminine woman. Everyone, male or female, has both animus and anima, and Jung's description of personality types reflects the balance that is struck between the two. See *analytic psychology.*

animastic (an-i-mas'tik) Of or pertaining to the soul; psychic.

animatism (an'i-mà-tiz'm) The ascription of psychic qualities to inanimate as well as animate objects is called animatism; synonymous with *mentalism* (q.v.). The condition is vividly exemplified, for example, in schizophrenic subjects, who often personify the whole of the inanimate world, as if the latter possessed the same mental qualities as human beings do.

animi agitatio Mental agitation.

animism (an'imiz'm) The theory that all things in nature, both animate and inanimate, contain the so-called spirit or soul. See *animatism.*

animism, social The schizophrenic's selective interpretation of outer reality so as to conform to the emotion that possesses him at the moment. He feels inferior, unwanted, and unloved, sees every grouping of people in the street as a purposeful exclusion of him, and hears any question put to him as an affirmation of his worthlessness.

animus See *anima.*

anisocoria (an-ī-sō-kō'rē-à) Inequality of the pupils in size.

anisophrenia Depression.

ankle-jerk *Achilles reflex* (q.v.).

Anlage (án′là-gē) A particular genetic factor predisposing to a given trait or the entire *genotypical* structure of an individual. The term is an abbreviation of *Erbanlage,* or *hereditary predisposition,* and this is the sense in which it is used in American genetics. See *predisposition.*

Anna O A patient described by Freud, originally referred to Breuer at the age of 21 for a nervous cough and other symptoms that had appeared following the death of her father. Breuer discovered that one of her symptoms disappeared entirely after she had been able to recount the details of its first appearance. This was the origin of the "talking cure."

Anna O had numerous conversion symptoms, among them hysterical pregnancy (which covered the phantasy that she was pregnant by Breuer) and paralysis of her arm (related to her father's death, at which time she was sitting at his bedside with her arm pressed against the chair at the side of his bed).

annihilation, Milligan method See *Milligan annihilation method.*

anniversary hypothesis This hypothesis asserts the following: if a person has lost a parent by death in childhood, and that person subsequently marries and has children, and is later hospitalized for the first time for mental illness, the first hospitalization is likely to occur when the eldest child of that person is within one year of his own age when his parent died.

anniversary reaction Behavior, symptoms, dreams, etc. that occur on an anniversary of a significant experience; their time-specific relationship to the original experience is rarely recognized by the subject and they appear to be a type of *acting-out,* i.e. an attempt to master through reliving rather than through remembering. See *neurosis, Sunday.*

annulment A mental mechanism by which the patient annuls, i.e. renders nonexistent, certain specific events or ideas that are painful or disagreeable to him. In certain respects, this mechanism resembles repression, but it is basically of an entirely different nature. "The fundamental difference lies in the fact that in annulment painful experiences are shifted into daydreams, while in repression painful experi-

ences may be eliminated from consciousness and pushed into the unconscious, after which they may reappear in dreams or symptoms." (Stekel, *CD*)

annulment, marriage See *marriage, psychiatric aspects of.*

annulus fibrosus See *disk, herniated lumbar intervertebral.*

anoesia (an-ō-ē′sē-á) *Obs.* Mental retardation.

anoesis Absence of cognition or knowledge; a state of sheer feeling, having no reference to objects; noncognitive consciousness.

anoia (á-noi′á) *Obs.* Insanity; roughly comparable to *vesania* (q.v.).

anomalous Relating to deviations from the average, but excluding the deviations due to disease processes.

anomaly A deviation from the average. In medicine anomalies are distinguished from disease processes, although the clinical signs and symptoms may be similar in both. For example, an underdeveloped heart may be anomalous; it may be too small, organically and functionally, for the body in which it is located. The anomaly may be relative or absolute.

Personality may also be anomalous. The so-called *character neuroses* are of that order, in that the personalities are in the periphery of the normal or average personality circle. Schizoidism and cycloidism are also regarded as anomalies.

anomaly, constitutional See *inadequacy, constitutional.*

anomia *Obs.* Rush's term for congenital defect of the moral sense. In neurology, anomia is a type of aphasia with a disturbed capacity to name objects.

anomie Emile Durkheim (1858–1917) used this term to refer to lack of social control. He based his classification of suicide on the hypothesis of a relationship between suicide and social conditions. *Egotistic suicide* occurred in subjects who had lost their feelings of integration within their social group and were no longer subject to its controls. *Altruistic suicide* referred to sacrifice of one's life for the good of the social group. *Anomic suicide* occurs in a society that lacks "collective order" because it is in the midst of major social change; as a result, absence of regulation and control has permitted desires to grow beyond all hope of satisfaction.

anorexia Loss of appetite.

anorexia, elective Conscious restriction of the quantity of food eaten to the extent of incurring a morbid reaction to foodstuffs.

anorexia, mental *Obs. Anorexia nervosa* (q.v.).

anorexia nervosa An *eating disorder,* first described by Sir William Gull (1868) as *apepsia hysterica;* Gull proposed the term anorexia nervosa in 1874. The chief symptoms are deliberate restriction of food intake, weight loss, and, in women, amenorrhea. Other characteristic features include faulty perception of body image, considerable increase in bodily activity, an intense fear of gaining weight, an accompanying mood change of depression and unusual eating habits. It is noteworthy that although the syndrome is named anorexia, there need not be a loss of appetite; the important feature is that, for some reason, food is not taken in. Patients offer various rationalizations for this, ranging from disgust reactions to specific foods to fear of choking on food or fear of vomiting after eating. Secondary weight loss is pronounced and usually exceeds 25% of original body weight.

Anorexia nervosa occur typically in females between the ages of 12 and 21; it has been reported also, however, in older women and men (in which case impotence seems to be a cardinal feature). Anorexia nervosa is not a specific disorder and there is no neurosis or psychosis which is specific to this syndrome. Many authors stress the frequent occurrence of schizophrenia in such cases; others have grouped it with the obsessive-compulsive or hysterical disorders.

Differentiation should be made between anorexia nervosa, as described above, and pituitary cachexia (Simmonds' disease, panhypopituitarism). The latter tends to occur in middle age, is usually precipitated by physical illness, and weight loss occurs later in the course of the illness. In Simmonds' disease, amenorrhea is seen only in approximately 50% of cases, despite such other indications of endocrine dysfunction as premature aging, wrinkling of the skin, loss of sexual desire, and atrophy of the sexual organs. Lassitude and weakness are conspicuous in Simmonds' disease but are surprisingly infrequent in anorexia nervosa despite severe weight loss. The 17-ketosteroids are reduced in Simmonds' disease but normal in anorexia nervosa.

anorexia, primary mental See *anorexia, secondary mental.*

anorexia, secondary mental Loss of appetite secondary to voluntary restriction of food intake in order to relieve digestive symptoms. Appetite tends to be lost whenever hunger goes unrelieved for a long time, no matter what the reason for the initial deprivation of food.

anorexia, social Destruction of the appetite for food by starvation or severe malnutrition, as seen in the poor, who cannot afford adequate nourishment.

anorgasmy (à-nawr′gaz-mē) Lack of sexual pleasure.

anorthosis Sexual impotence.

anosmia (an-oz′mē-à) Absence of sense of smell.

anosognosia (à-nos-ō-gnō′zhē-à) Unawareness of physical illness. In persons with organic brain syndrome (first described by Anton in 1899), there is a tendency to suppress all knowledge of the disability. This is a protective mechanism that is particularly likely to occur when the incapacitation is total and so severe that the patient is unable to use the disturbed capacity at all. See *neglect, sensory; nonrecognition; syndrome, organic.*

anosphresia (an-os-phrē′sē-à) *Anosmia* (q.v.).

anoxia, cerebral Inadequate supply of oxygen to the brain, generally divided into four types: *anoxic anoxia,* as in respiratory failure, asphyxia, or altitude sickness; *anemic anoxia,* as in severe anemia, blood loss, and carbon monoxide poisoning; *stagnant anoxia,* as in circulatory or cardiac failure, cardiac arrhythmias, cardiac arrest, and cerebral vascular disease; and *metabolic anoxia,* as in hypoglycemia or cyanide poisoning.

ANS *Autonomic nervous system* (q.v.).

answers, syndrome of approximate A subject's tendency to answer questions with relevance to the general topic, but with glaring disregard for details—the so-called syndrome of approximate answers, also known in psychiatric literature as the *Ganser syndrome* (q.v.), the condition having been first described by him. See *syndrome, Ganser.*

For instance, when shown a 25-cent piece the patient calls it a dollar or a dime.

He writes three when asked to write two, raises the left arm when asked to raise the right, calls a match a cigarette; a comb is a brush or something to use for the hair. This syndrome usually occurs in persons facing criminal responsibility and may be an attempt to avoid trial and punishment. (Hinsie, *UP*)

Antabuse Trade name of a drug used in the treatment of alcoholism; chemically known as disulfiram and tetraethylthiuram disulfide. It appears that Antabuse interferes with the enzyme systems that normally break down alcohol in the organism. As a result, when alcohol is ingested by a subject with an adequate blood level of Antabuse, there occurs within a few minutes a characteristic response, the *alcohol-Antabuse* reaction. This consists of flushing, injection of the conjunctivae, sweating, a sensation of warmth, and tachycardia; in 20 to 30 minutes, additional symptoms may appear— headache, dizziness, chest pain, palpitation, dyspnea, pallor, and nausea. With more severe reactions, vomiting, hypotension, vasomotor collapse, and sometimes convulsions may occur. Alcoholics who sincerely wish to stop drinking are kept on a maintenance dose of Antabuse as an aid to control while other more specific therapeutic measures are utilized. Antabuse treatment is a form of deconditioning and as such is to be considered adjunctive therapy; used alone, it is ineffectual in curing alcoholism.

antagonism hypothesis See *hypothesis, antagonism.*

antagonist In pharmacology, a drug that reduces or blocks the action of another drug. Naloxone, for example, blocks the action of morphine by competing with it for receptor sites in the brain and other tissues. By occupying those sites Naloxone prevents morphine from binding to the receptors and exerting its effect.

antagonist, narcotic A substance with ability to block the euphorigenic and dependence-producing properties of opiates by competing with them for occupation of the same receptor sites.

anthropo- Combining form meaning human being.

anthropocentrism The doctrine or belief that humans are the center of the universe to which all else has reference.

anthropology The science of mankind in the widest sense; the history of human society. This term designates the extensive branch of natural science that studies the developmental aspects of humans as a species, using archaeology as one of its main methods.

Although anthropological research covers the history of human society regardless of time and space, it is primarily related to early times and primitive people, as it deals not only with the question of the earliest appearance of people and their rise from lower forms, but also with all the problems concerning the differential development of human races, languages, and cultural forms. Individuals have little, if any, significance in these studies and are bound to disappear in the cultural or racial groups to which they belong, since there exists no record of individual activity for prehistoric times.

Anthropology is usually subdivided into (1) zoological anthropology, investigating the evolutionary conditions of humanity; (2) descriptive anthropology, or ethnology, describing the division of mankind into races and studying the origin, distribution, and relations of these racial groups; (3) general anthropology, dealing with the evolution of mankind as a human society.

The last division is anthropology proper and, according to Franz Boas (*General Anthropology*, 1938), includes the following three main problems: (1) the reconstruction of human history; (2) the determination of types of historical phenomena and their sequences; (3) the dynamics of change.

anthropology, psychological The branch of anthropology that deals with the psychology of different civilizations and cultures and studies especially folklore, myths, and other expressions of the mentality of the people. Through comparisons the psychological investigations throw light on many observations made in children or in mentally sick persons in the culture. See *ethnology.*

anthropometry The scientific method pre-eminently applied in the field of *anthropology* (q.v.), which uses the measurement of the human body for the description of the typical anatomical variability of a population. In anthropology, more attention must be given to the bony structure than to any other part of the body, since a comparison between present and past conditions can usually be based only on comparisons of skeletons.

anthropomorph An expression used by some authors to designate a member of the group of psychologists and philosophers who in the past century studied the mental activities of animals and interpreted them in terms of human adult logic.

anthroponomy W. Hunter's term for behavioristic psychology.

anthropophobia Fear of humans in general.

anthropos Primal man; one of Jung's archetypes. See *archetype; archetype, mother.*

anthroposcopy (an'thrō-pos'kō-pē) *Obs.* Various debatable procedures of character-reading from the features or other parts of the human body.

anthrotype *Biotype* (q.v.); this term is used in some systems of constitutional medicine to classify various constellations of all the morphological, physiological, immunological, and psychological characteristics making up the human individual. It is usually interpreted in terms as general as those of biotypology, that is, in the sense of including the entire phenotypical makeup of human organisms.

anti-instinctual force See *anticathexis; countercathexis.*

antibody-barrier system See *barrier, blood-brain.*

anticathexis *Counterinvestment;* the energy that must be expended by the ego to maintain repression or otherwise block the entrance of id derivatives into consciousness.

anticholinergic syndrome See *syndrome, central anticholinergic.*

anticipation The act of dealing with, doing, foreseeing, or experiencing beforehand. Anticipation of the future is characteristic of the ego and is necessary for judgment and planning of suitable later action. Anticipation is dependent on reality testing, by trying in an active manner and in small dosage what might happen to one passively and in unknown dosage. With the development of speech, name symbols can be substituted for things, and thus anticipation can take place in the imagination in the model world of words. This affords the possibility of judging reality and is an important factor in development of the ability to tolerate tensions.

anticipatory maturation See *maturation, anticipatory, principle of.*

antidepressant Thymoleptic; referring to a drug used to treat depressive syndromes. The three major groups of antidepressants are (1) stimulants—including the amphetamines, methylphenidate, and similar sympathomimetics; because of their high potential for abuse, such drugs are not generally used as the primary or sole treatment for depression, but they may be useful adjuvants to other pharmacologic agents; (2) tricyclics (*TCA*), tetracyclics, etc.—including (a) tertiary amines: amitriptyline, doxepin, imipramine, (b) secondary amines: nortriptyline, protriptyline, desipramine; (3) monoamine oxidase inhibitors (MAOI)—including isocarboxazid, phenelzine, tranylcypromine.

antiexpectation technique See *therapy, paradoxical.*

antifetishism Hirschfeld's term for aversions that many latent homosexuals develop as a protection against conscious recognition of their homosexuality.

"One man dislikes women with large feet, another is repelled by women with hair on their bodies. Such a woman causes him to have a distinct nausea.... His search is endless because he is truly, though secretly, attracted by the male. His sexual goal is man." (Stekel, W. *Bi-Sexual Love,* 1922)

antikinesis *Obs.* All forms of nervous response; those recurring regularly and in a definite manner in response to stimulation are termed *reflexes,* while all the volitional responses in which there is a variable factor due to the greater complexity and elaboration in the physiological mechanism are called *antiklises.*

antiklisis (an-ti-klī'sis) See *antikinesis.*

antinodal behavior See *behavior, nodal.*

antipsychotics See *neuroleptic; psychotropics.*

antirisk factor See *risk factor.*

antisocial activity, concealed See *activity, concealed antisocial.*

antisocial personality *Psychopathic personality* (q.v.) or constitutional psychopathic state.

antisocial spectrum disorder A range of behaviors that have been interpreted as different manifestations of the same biological factors that predispose to conduct disorders and antisocial personality. Included are *alcoholism* and *somatization disorder,* based on the findings that the incidence of alcoholism is significantly above normal in the families of antisocial males and females, and that the incidence of somatization disorder is significantly above normal in the female relatives of antisocial subjects.

antitechnology bias See *Frankenstein factor.*

antithesis, neurotic Opposition, contrast. Adler uses this term to indicate that the neurotic measures a thing, a force, or an event, by an opposite which is fitted to it.

"Among these I have regularly found the following: (1) Above-beneath, (2) masculine-feminine. One furthermore always finds an arrangement of memories, feelings and actions according to this type of *antithesis* in the sense the patient takes them (not always in the generally accepted sense), i.e., inferior—beneath, feminine; powerful—above, masculine." (Adler, A. *The Neurotic Constitution,* 1917)

antlophobia Fear of floods.

anus Termination of the alimentary canal. See *anal erotism; anality.*

anxietas praesenilis (prī-se-nē′lis) Farrar describes three main forms of *involutional melancholia.* First, melancholia vera, characterized essentially by a clinical syndrome resembling manic-depressive psychosis; second, anxietas praesenilis, in which there is extreme anxiety with feelings of unreality; third, depressio apathetica, the central symptom of which is apathy.

anxietas tibiarum (tē-bē-ä′room) A nervous agitation, continually impelling the patient to change the position of his legs. See *akatizia; tachyathetosis.*

anxiety An affect that differs from other affects in its specific unpleasurable characteristics. Anxiety consists of a somatic, physiological side (disturbed breathing, increased heart activity, vasomotor changes, musculoskeletal disturbances such as trembling or paralysis, increased sweating, etc.) and of a psychological side. The latter includes "a specific conscious inner attitude and a peculiar feeling state characterized (1) by a physically as well as mentally painful awareness of being powerless to do anything about a personal matter; (2) by presentiment of an impending and almost inevitable danger; (3) by a tense and physi-

cally exhausting alertness as if facing an emergency; (4) by an apprehensive self-absorption which interferes with an effective and advantageous solution of reality-problems; and (5) by an irresolvable doubt concerning the nature of the threatening evil, concerning the probability of the actual appearance of the threat, concerning the best objective means of reducing or removing the evil, and concerning one's subjective capacity for making effective use of those means if and when the emergency arises." (Piotrowski, Z. *Perceptanalysis,* 1957) Anxiety is to be differentiated from fear, which lacks characteristics (4) and (5). Fear is a reaction to a real or threatened danger, whereas anxiety is more typically a reaction to an unreal or imagined danger.

Freud's earlier view was that anxiety arises by transformation of libido which cannot otherwise be discharged. He later abandoned this view and came to believe that anxiety arises automatically whenever the psyche is overwhelmed by an influx of stimuli too great to be mastered or discharged. Such *automatic anxiety* may arise in response to stimuli either of external or of internal origin, but most frequently it arises from the id, that is, from the drives (*id anxiety*). When anxiety develops automatically according to this pattern, the situation is called a traumatic one. Automatic anxiety is characteristic of infancy, when the ego is weak and immature, and of so-called actual anxiety neurosis of adult life.

There is a second type of anxiety, characteristic of the psychoneuroses, which Freud called *signal anxiety.* In the course of development the child learns to anticipate the advent of a traumatic situation and reacts to this possibility with anxiety before the situation becomes traumatic. The unpleasure arising from this threat of a danger situation automatically sets into operation the pleasure principle. The latter acts by enabling the ego to check or inhibit whatever id impulses might be giving rise to the danger situation. There is a series of typical danger situations that occur in sequence in the child's life; these persist to some degree throughout life in the unconscious, and it is one or another of these dangers that the psychoneurotic patient unconsciously fears. The first of these dangers, characteristic of ego development up to about 1½ years, is separation (known also as loss of the love object and as primal anxiety); the second, seen at 1 to 2 years, is loss of love; the third, seen at 2½ to 3 years, is castration or other genital injury; and the fourth, which is seen after the age of 5 or 6 years, when the superego has been formed, is guilt (disapproval and punishment by the superego).

Some differentiate between *state anxiety* (anxiety felt at a moment in time) and *trait anxiety* (a habitual, and perhaps in part a genetically determined tendency to be anxious in general).

anxiety, anal castration Fear of castration displaced, through regressive distortion, onto the anal area. Thus many "toilet phobias," such as fear of falling into the bowl or a fear that some monster will emerge from the toilet and crawl into one's anus, reveal themselves in analysis to refer to castration anxiety.

anxiety attack, equivalent of The physical symptoms often associated with manifest anxiety may alone constitute the anxiety-attack. These *equivalents* (physical symptoms) take on a variety of forms; e.g. attacks of sudden diarrhea or attacks of sweating, often nocturnal.

anxiety, automatic See *anxiety.*

anxiety, basic Horney's term for a feeling of loneliness and helplessness toward a potentially hostile world. This concept is more comprehensive than Freud's "real" anxiety. (*The Neurotic Personality of Our Time,* 1937)

anxiety, castration Fear of genital loss or injury. See *anxiety.*

The castration complex has its foundation laid down in the pregenital stage of development. Alexander, for example, refers to the many deprivations and losses suffered by the infant from the time of birth. He says that the child loses its mother's body and its fetal membrane at birth. A pleasure-giving organ is replaced by a painful condition. The next important loss is the pleasure-giving nipple (Staercke's oral primal castration); then the pleasure-giving stool is lost (Freud's anal primal castration); finally there is fear of the loss of the penis.

These early losses, first expressed or-

ganically, are indelibly imprinted on the psyche and appear later in the form of character traits, depending on the way they were solved or resolved in the early years.

anxiety, death A form of depression in which fear of death, poverty, etc., is the most prominent complaint.

anxiety depersonalization neurosis See *depersonalization.*

anxiety depression Reactive depression. See *depression; depression, psychoneurotic; depression, reactive.*

anxiety, depressive The specific anxiety observed in a person afflicted with depression. "The preservation of the good internalized objects with whom the ego is identified as a whole. In the latter case—which is the case of the depressive—the anxiety and feelings of suffering are of a much more complex nature. The anxiety lest the good objects and, with them, the ego should be destroyed, or that they are in a state of disintegration, is interwoven with continuous and desperate efforts to save the good objects both internalized and external." (Klein, M. *Contributions to Psycho-analysis 1921–45,* 1948)

anxiety, discharge of The process by which unconscious anxiety (tension) is chronically, repetitively, and more or less constantly nullified through action and deed in the integral activity of everyday life. These reality activities are utilized for the gratification of unconscious drives and urges. If this gratification did not occur more or less constantly and repetitively, these urges would succumb to repression and thus form the nidus for symptomatic anxiety and symptom formation. The trend toward the excessive utilization of this method of nullifying anxiety in contrast to such other common methods as the suppression of feeling or the guarding over thinking has been called "the flight into reality."

Sexual activity, with orgastic discharge, is a specific activity frequently employed as a method of discharging anxiety of unconscious origin.

anxiety disorders A group of disorders in which anxiety is the most prominent feature or in which anxiety appears when the affected person tries to resist his symptoms (e.g. phobias or compulsions). Included within this group are panic disorder, agoraphobia, social phobia, simple phobia, obsessive compulsive disorder, post-traumatic stress disorder, and generalized anxiety disorder. See *anxiety hysteria; anxiety neurosis; obsessive-compulsive psychoneurosis; panic disorder; phobia; post-traumatic stress disorder.*

anxiety disorders of childhood A group of disorders in which anxiety is the central feature, including (1) *separation anxiety disorder*—excessive anxiety about separation from significant others, such as worries that harm will befall attachment figures or the subject if separated, school phobia, and nightmares involving separation themes; (2) *avoidant disorder*—pathologic shyness that interferes with peer functioning, persistent shrinking from contact with strangers; (3) *overanxious disorder*—generalized persistent worrying about what the future holds or what humiliations the past contains, excessive need for reassurance, multiple unfounded somatic complaints.

anxiety, ego The threat of internal dangers to the ego in contrast to fear, which refers to the threat of external dangers to the ego. See *anxiety.*

anxiety elation psychosis See *cycloid psychosis.*

anxiety, elemental See *panic, primordial.*

anxiety, endogenous A general term that includes anxiety hysteria and agoraphobia with panic attacks. Characteristic are sudden, spontaneous panic attacks accompanied by multiple autonomic symptoms, overwhelming fear, a flight response, and polyphobic behavior. Psychotherapy, behavior therapy, and tranquilizers have been of limited benefit, but antidepressants such as phenelzine or imipramine have achieved good results in many cases.

anxiety, erotized A paradoxical reaction to anxiety in which, instead of flight from the source of anxiety, the tendency is to head directly toward the source and enjoy it.

anxiety, examination Freudian term for the anxiety attendant on examinations intensified by experiences of the past, usually unconscious, that had to do with "the punishments we suffered as children for misdeeds we had committed."

anxiety, free-floating Anxiety that is neither attached to ideational content nor otherwise channeled into substitutive symptoms; it is characteristic of *anxiety neurosis* (q.v.).

anxiety hysteria Phobic neurosis; a primitive reaction type and the most frequent neurosis of childhood. The main symptom is a specific fear (see listings under *fear of*) that has usually arisen from the binding of primary diffuse anxiety to a specific content. The thing that is feared may be feared because it represents a temptation (especially a situation that would ordinarily call forth an aggressive or a sexual response), or it may be feared because it represents the punishment for the forbidden impulse either directly or indirectly through symbolism, or it may be feared because of a combination of these factors. Further, the phobia may be a fear that the anxiety will return; this is seen in some agoraphobics whose initial attacks occurred in the street. The phobia may not represent castration and punishment directly, but may be concerned mainly with a fear of loss of love. See *agoraphobia; phobia.*

The defense in anxiety hysteria is (1) through anxiety itself, which gives warning to the ego so that the situation can be avoided; (2) repression of the impulse by development of substitutes for the real fear; (3) by projection of an internal instinctual danger onto an external perceptional danger (this is the most frequent type of displacement in anxiety hysteria); (4) by regression to childhood in order to ward off the wishes of the genital oedipal complex.

The two most famous cases of phobia in psychoanalytic literature are those of little Hans (Freud 1902) and the Wolf-Man (Freud 1918).

anxiety, ictal See *emotions, ictal.*

anxiety, id See *anxiety.*

anxiety, instinctual A term used by Freud interchangeably with the term *neurotic anxiety.* In discussing the meaning and significance of anxiety, Freud distinguishes between true anxiety and neurotic anxiety: true anxiety is anxiety in regard to a known real danger threatening from some external object; neurotic anxiety is anxiety in regard to an unknown danger. Upon investigation, this latter danger is found to be an instinctual danger. Accordingly, the term instinctual anxiety is used to refer to neurotic anxiety. But there are some cases in which neurotic anxiety is intermingled with true anxiety. In these cases the danger is known and real, but the anxiety in regard to it is disproportionately great.

anxiety neurosis In 1894, Freud detached the particular syndrome of anxiety neurosis from neurasthenia and described the clinical characteristics of anxiety neurosis as: general irritability, anxious expectation and pangs of conscience, the anxiety attack, and phobias. In anxious expectation there is a quantum of anxiety in a free-floating condition that is ever ready to attach itself to any suitable ideational content. Thus common physiological dangers, such as snakes or vermin, are exaggeratedly feared; and the affect of anxiety is also commonly attached to locomotion, as in agoraphobia. But this is not a true hysterical channeling, for it does not originate in a repressed idea. The anxiety attack includes cardiac disturbances, respiratory disturbances, sweating, tremor and shuddering, ravenous hunger often with giddiness, diarrhea, vertigo, congestion and vasomotor neurasthenia, paresthesiae, awakening in fright (the pavor nocturnus of adults), urinary frequency, seminal emissions, blurring of vision, tinnitus, general fatiguability, etc.; in other words, the somatic symptoms may involve any or all of the bodily systems.

Anxiety neurosis is very uncommon in its pure form. Freud considered that the etiology of the anxiety neurosis was a current or contemporary one, in which forced abstinence, frustrated sexual excitement, incomplete or interrupted coitus, sexual efforts that exceed the psychical capacity, etc., all unite in disturbing the equilibrium of psychical and somatic functions in sexual activity and in hindering the psychical cooperation necessary to relieve the nervous economy from sexual tension. He found that it appeared in females in the following cases: as virginal anxiety or anxiety in adolescents, provoked by their first meeting with libidinal strivings that had been largely unconscious throughout the latency period; as anxiety in women whose husbands suffer from ejaculatio praecox or from impaired potency; and as anxiety in women whose husbands practice coitus interruptus or reservatus; as anxiety in widows and voluntarily abstinent persons, when it is often combined with obsessional ideas; as anxiety in the climacteric during the last great increase in sexual need. Anxiety neurosis appears in men in the following cases: in the voluntarily abstinent, in prolonged sexual frustration as in a long courtship without intercourse, in men who practice coitus interruptus, and in aging men.

Freud considered the basis of anxiety neurosis to be a deflection of somatic sexual excitation from the psychical field, and the symptoms to be substitutes for the specific activity that should follow upon sexual excitation, should such activity be allowed. Neurasthenia, on the other hand, he considered to result from a deflection of methods of sexual gratification from more to less satisfactory means. Anxiety neurosis would thus be the somatic counterpart of hysteria; the excitation is from the soma and chemically mediated, and it cannot be mastered by the psyche and so is deflected into somatic channels. In hysteria, the excitation results from intrapsychic (rather than somatic) conflict that cannot be mastered and so is deflected into somatic channels.

anxiety, neurotic Freud distinguishes between objective anxiety and neurotic anxiety. He says that the latter is encountered in three forms. "First, we have free-floating, general apprehensiveness, ready to attach itself for the time being to any new possibility that may arise in the form of what we call expectant dread, as happens, for instance, in the typical anxiety-neurosis. Secondly, we find it firmly attached to certain ideas, in what are known as *phobias*, in which we can still recognize a connection with external danger, but cannot help regarding the anxiety felt toward it as enormously exaggerated. Thirdly and finally, we have anxiety as it occurs in hysteria and in other severe neuroses; this anxiety either accompanies symptoms or manifests itself independently, whether as an attack or as a condition which persists for some time, but always without having any visible justification in an external danger." (Freud, S. *New Introductory Lectures on Psycho-Analysis*, 1933)

anxiety object The displacement of anxiety to an object that is a symbolic representation of the individual who originally caused the anxiety. For example, a child fears a horse. The horse elicits marked anxiety in the child because the horse is a symbolic representation of the father, who was the original focus for anxiety. See *anxiety hysteria*.

anxiety, objective See *anxiety preparedness*.

anxiety, oral Anxiety occurring at the primary or oral stage of libidinal (personality) development (see *libido, displaceability of; phase, oral incorporative*). It is assumed that such massive expressions of infantile rage and fear are associated with or stem from phantasy images within the infant, of an immense internal object in countless small pieces. This image, theoretically an analytic reconstruction, has its origin in the ideas of swallowing, incorporating, and chewing up a dangerous or loved object, i.e. the parent, a body organ, or part thereof.

E.F. Sharpe states: "There must be some correlation between the excessive anxiety in oral stages, which is associated with the phantasy of a huge image of pieces inside; and the fact that at this time there is as little coordination of the bodily as of the psychical ego." (*Collected Papers on Psycho-analysis*, 1950)

anxiety, organic The anxiety that is associated with organic pain and that can be markedly attenuated in the dream state by the process of denial, transformation, and displacement; these mechanisms represent attempts at cure through wish-fulfillment.

anxiety, performance Anxiety related to the execution of a task; used particularly in sex therapy, to refer to persons whose sexual dysfunction is related to their concern about whether or not they perform well. Such performance anxiety tends to be incompatible with pleasure, so that the worrier ends up being unable to perform at all.

anxiety preparedness The increased sensory attention and motor tension that accompany anxiety and fear.

anxiety, primal See *anxiety*.

anxiety reaction In the 1952 nomenclature, the term for anxiety state or *anxiety neurosis* (q.v.).

anxiety, real Anxiety produced by actual danger in the external world of reality. Freud calls it *Realangst* (real anxiety).

anxiety resolution The therapeutic process through which the unconscious roots of anxiety are brought into consciousness and there mastered. The key to the resolution of anxiety is the recovery, in consciousness, by the subject, of repressed, albeit "forgotten" infantile, instinctual, conflict-ridden experiences, which have been mastered or overcome, and which remain fixation and regression focal points in the pseudo-adult character. Full ego maturity, in the neurotic, cannot be achieved except through this arduous path. All the forces of defense and resistance combine and conspire to defeat this process.

anxiety, separation The reaction seen in a child who is isolated or separated from its mother, consisting usually of tearfulness, irritability, and other signs of distress. This is considered by most to be an indication that the child is attempting to adjust to the changes imposed on him and therefore presumptive evidence of good emotional reactivity. Although these symptoms of protest may culminate in an acute physical upset and in temporary or even prolonged refusal to adjust, the separation symptoms are not in themselves thought to be evidence of personality defect or unbearable trauma. For a discussion of more pathologic reactions to separation, see *depression, anaclitic*.

anxiety, signal See *anxiety*.

anxiety state, prerelease The anxiety phenomena which some inmates of penal institutions develop through fear of being set free and having to face the world again.

anxiety, superego Anxiety caused by the unconscious functioning of the superego, which itself can become a source of continual danger because of inexorable demands for atonement. See *guilt*.

anxiety syndrome, organic See *organic anxiety syndrome*.

anxiety, true See *anxiety, basic*.

anxiety typology Description of different forms of the manifestations of anxiety. Most such typologies have been developed on an ad hoc basis and therefore have not been standardized on adequate population samples. Some consultation-liaison psychiatrists group surgical patients on the basis of preoperative anxiety into low-anxiety and high-anxiety groups. Low-anxiety patients have been called *repressors, avoiders,* or *deniers;* they typically have an external locus of control and see themselves as passive participants in their treatment. High-anxiety patients have been called *sensitizers* or *vigilant;* they typically have an internal locus of control and show more anticipatory anxiety. They ask more questions of the medical staff, demand more medication, report more pain, and have long hospital stays even after minor procedures.

anxiety, urethral Tension, anxiety, fear, and inhibition associated with urination.

anxiety, virginal Anxiety provoked by the first sexual experience. See *anxiety neurosis.*

anxiolytic See *psychotropics.*

anypnia (à-nip′nē-à) *Obs.* Sleeplessness.

aochlesia (ā-ō-klē′sē-à) *Obs.* Catalepsy.

APA American Psychiatric Association; founded as the Association of Medical Superintendents of American Institutions for the Insane in 1844, its name was changed to American Medico-Psychological Association in 1891, and to American Psychiatric Association in 1921. In 1986, approximately 31,000 members were recognized by the Association. Also American Psychological Association.

apallic Akinetic. See *syndrome, apallic.*

apandria (à-pan′drē-à) Aversion to men.

apanthropia, apanthropy *Obs.* Aversion to human society.

apastia (à-pas′tē-à) Abstinence from food as a symptom of a psychiatric disorder. See *anorexia nervosa.*

apathetic Without feeling; listless; hebetudinous.

apathy Want of feeling; absence of affect. The term refers to absence of feeling from the psychical, not from the somatic or physical point of view. It is observed in vivid form as a symptom in deep, stuporous states of depression and in certain schizophrenic syndromes.

apathy, emotional *Hebetude* (q.v.).

apathy, euphoric An expression used by Jung to refer to happy indifference, analogous to the "belle indifference" of the hysterical subject.

apeirophobia Fear of infinity. See *neurosis, infinity.*

apepsia hysterica *Obs. Anorexia nervosa* (q.v.).

aphalgesia, haphalgesia *Obs.* A rare type of psychogenic pain disorder; pain appears on contact with a substance that has some special significance for the subject, such as certain metals, liquids, or textures. For one subject, the mere thought of touching

a peach skin produced a throbbing pain in his right forearm. See *somatoform disorders.*

aphanisis (à-fan′i-sis) *Obs.* "Extinction of sexuality. The concept of 'castration' should be reserved, as Freud pointed out, for the penis alone, and should not be confounded with that of 'extinction of sexuality' for which the term 'aphanisis' is proposed." (Jones, E. *Papers on Psycho-Analysis,* 1938)

aphasia (à-fā′zhē-à) More properly, *dysphasia,* any disturbance in the comprehension or expression of language due to brain lesion and not the result of faulty innervation of the speech muscles or disorders of articulation or mental retardation. The word *language,* as used in this definition, refers not only to the expression or communication of thought by word, writing, and gesture, but also to the reception and interpretation of such acts when carried out by others and also to the retention, recall, and visualization of the symbols involved. Thus aphasia would technically include the agnosias and the apraxias.

Head aptly termed the present state of opinion on the aphasias as chaos. There are many systems of classification, some primarily anatomical (e.g. Bastian, Broadbent, Wernicke), others primarily functional or physiologic (e.g. Jackson, Marie, Goldstein, Head). Anatomical classifications have subdivided the aphasias into the motor type, with lesions in the lower precentral region, and the sensory type, with lesions in the superior temporal, the angular, or the supramarginal gyri. The sensory type is further divided into the cortical, subcortical, and transcortical groups.

Bannister (*Brain's Clinical Neurology,* 1985) classifies the dysphasias as follows:

1. *Broca's aphasia (expressive aphasia, motor aphasia, nonfluent aphasia)*—severely disordered expression in both speech and writing, with full understanding of both spoken and written language. Consonants are slurred and smaller words indicating relationships are omitted, producing *telegram speech.* In severe cases, repeated grunts may be the only utterances.

2. *Wernicke's aphasia (receptive aphasia, central aphasia, sensory aphasia)*—disordered comprehension and expression in both speech and writing. Speech has many errors in syntax and grammar and is sprinkled with wrong or nonexistent words. The

subject is unaware that he is speaking non-sense (*jargon aphasia*), and meaning, if any, can be conveyed only in a roundabout way through phonetic or verbal paraphasias. See *fluent aphasia*.

3. *Conduction aphasia*—so-called because the lesion is in the arcuate fasciculus, which connects Broca's area to Wernicke's area. Comprehension is normal, but speech is semantically abnormal and there is marked disturbance of repetition and difficulty in reading aloud.

4. *Angular gyrus lesions*—difficulty in comprehending spoken and written language; fluent speech may show echolalia and difficulty in naming objects (*nominal* or *amnesic aphasia*). Writing may demonstrate similar deficits.

5. *Global aphasia*—a combination of motor aphasia with a comprehension defect.

aphasia, amnestic (amnesic) Nominal aphasia; a difficulty in finding the right name for an object, even though the subject usually insists that he knows what the object is. In its mildest form, nominal or amnestic aphasia is a common disturbance and is seen following anxiety, fatigue, intoxication, or senility. When due to a focal cerebral lesion, amnestic aphasia usually indicates a lesion between the angular gyrus and the posterior part of the first temporal gyrus on the left side.

aphasia, auditory Word-deafness. "In pure or subcortical word-deafness the patient distinguishes words from other sounds but does not understand them, so that his own language sounds to him like a foreign tongue. Sometimes he recognizes the meaning of an individual word, but not of a whole sentence. Owing to this defect he cannot repeat words or write to dictation, but there is no other change in speaking, reading or spontaneous writing. . . . The lesion is thought to be in the subcortical white matter beneath the posterior part of the left first temporal convolution." (Brain, *DNS*)

aphasia, central Syntactical aphasia. "In central aphasia, the difficulty in understanding spoken speech is associated with gross disorder of thought and expression. Spoken speech is fluent, in marked contrast to the speech of the patient with expressive aphasia, but it is disordered by verbal and grammatical confusions—para-grammatism—difficulty in evoking words as names for objects, actions, and qualities, and the utterance of nonexistent or incorrect words—paraphasia (the syntactical aphasia of Head). The comprehension of spoken speech is impaired, but reading is less affected, and the patient can usually understand what he reads silently, though if he reads aloud he may be confused by the inaccuracies in his verbal expression of what he sees. Writing is usually less affected than articulate speech. Defective comprehension of spoken speech prevents the patient from noticing his own errors in speaking, and in severe cases he pours forth a stream of unintelligible jargon (jargon aphasia). The lesion responsible for central aphasia is situated in the left temporo-parietal region." (Brain, *DNS*)

aphasia, congenital A more or less general term used in the fields of neurology and neuropsychiatry. It refers to the inborn or constitutionally determined clinical symptomatic appearance of varied types of verbal or symbol-handling difficulty. The specific disability may appear in the fields of speaking, reading, writing, spelling, arithmetic, and even musical appreciation. The reading disability (*dyslexia*, or congenital word-blindness) has received the most intensive study.

Specific reading, writing, and spelling difficulty is often found connected with a tendency to reverse letters and words in reading and writing. This condition has been named *strephosymbolia*.

Congenital word-deafness, a rare form of congenital aphasia, is characterized by the inability of otherwise intelligent children to comprehend the meaning of words heard. Deafness, in the ordinary sense, is not present.

Certain forms of congenital aphasia, like stuttering, seem connected with the whole question of handedness, eyedness, footedness, laterality, or the predominance, physiologically, of one cerebral hemisphere over the other in motor function. (Hunt, *PBD*)

aphasia, expressive See *aphasia, motor*.

aphasia, fluent Wernicke type of aphasia, in contrast with nonfluent or Broca type of aphasia. Fluent aphasia is most commonly associated with posterior lesions in the part of the brain supplied by the left middle cerebral artery. Anterior lesions tend to produce nonfluent aphasia, often with associated spastic hemiparesis, apraxia, acalculia, or difficulties with constructions. See *aphasia, Wernicke's.*

aphasia, global Total aphasia, which results from massive destruction of the fronto-temporal region of the left hemisphere.

aphasia, jargon Loosely, any faulty, paraphasic speech or semantic disintegration. Some workers differentiate between neologistic and semantic types. See *aphasia; aphasia, central.*

Neologistic jargon refers to copious, unintelligible speech that consists in part of neologistic words resembling language. English phonemes are used with appropriate inflection by the patient, who is markedly fluent despite a severe comprehension defect. He often fails to perceive the nonsense he creates so copiously and may even deny completely that there is any difficulty. So striking a separation of auditory comprehension from speech production and the uncontrolled conglomeration of phonemes suggests a disconnection between the two major assumed physiological processes in speech, word building and its feedback control. In this type of disturbance, phonemic or literal paraphasias distort the original word into a neologism.

Semantic jargon refers to verbal paraphasias consisting of substituted, but in themselves understandable, words; included in this category are circumlocutory speech and recurrent utterances of jargon syllables.

aphasia, motor Expressive aphasia; verbal aphasia; word-dumbness. "In this form of aphasia the expressive aspect of speech suffers severely. In severe cases the patient may be completely speechless or able to say only 'yes' or 'no,' and even these words may be inappropriately used and cannot be repeated to order. He may be limited to the same phrase constantly repeated—a recurring utterance. Emotional speech suffers less than 'propositional,' and an otherwise almost speechless individual may be able to swear or utter other emotional ejaculations. . . . When the patient cannot think of the right word himself he will recognize it when it is offered to him." (Brain, *DNS*) The lesion responsible for

motor aphasia is usually on the posterior part of the third frontal convolution (Broca's area) and the lower part of the precentral convolution.

Brain also differentiates a type of aphasia called pure word-dumbness or subcortical motor aphasia in which uttered speech is disturbed in the same way as above but in which there are no associated disturbances in inner speech, comprehension, or writing. The lesion here is thought to be deep in the white matter in Broca's area.

aphasia, nominal See *aphasia, amnestic.*

aphasia, semantic The inability to grasp the meaning of words or speech. The patient may be able to utter words but does not understand their significance. He perceives the words, but does not apperceive them.

aphasia, sensory Receptive aphasia; inability to perceive speech by the senses, regardless of the retention of the power of using speech, which is usually meaningless and confined to parrotlike utterances. Sensory aphasia may combine visual aphasia and auditory aphasia.

aphasia, syntactical See *aphasia, central.*

aphasia, total Global aphasia; a combination of motor and sensory aphasia. See *aphasia, global.*

aphasia, transcortical Language disturbance produced by lesions which, although extensive, leave the Broca and Wernicke areas intact but isolated from the rest of the brain. In consequence, the patient may repeat spoken words even though he is unable to understand speech or produce it on his own.

aphasia, verbal See *aphasia, motor.*

aphasia, visual Word-blindness. In pure (subcortical) form, the patient can visualize colors but cannot recognize words, letters, or colors; he can write spontaneously but cannot copy. The lesion is in the lingual gyrus.

Visual aphasia is more often combined with agraphia; this is known as visual asymbolia or cortical word-blindness and is produced by a lesion of the left angular gyrus. Inability to read is termed *alexia.*

aphasia, Wernicke's *Receptive, central,* or *sensory* aphasia, due to a lesion in or near Wernicke's area of the brain (the posterior part of the superior temporal gyrus), characterized by speech in which the syntax appears normal but the content is meaning-less (*driveling*, or *jargon aphasia*), paraphasic utterances, loss of word complexity, and impaired comprehension of the speech of others.

aphelxia (af-elk′sē-à) See *ecphronia*.

aphemia *Obs*. Speechlessness; loss of power of speech; *aphasia* (q.v.).

aphemia pathematica *Obs*. Loss of speech due to fright.

aphemia plastica *Obs*. Voluntary *mutism* (q.v.).

aphephobia Haptephobia; haphephobia; fear of being touched.

aphonia, aphony (à-fō′nē-à, af′ō-ni) Voice-lessness; muteness. Aphony may be due to organic or psychic causes, though the term is generally used today with organic etiol-ogy in mind. Aphony conveys the idea that the patient is unable to use his voice owing to structural or organic changes.

aphoria *Obs. Amyotony;* asthenia and, particu-larly, the inability to increase energy or muscle tone through exercise (*amyos-thenia*). Janet thought it characteristic of neurotics.

aphoristic multiple sclerosis A type of multi-ple sclerosis characterized by pyramidal signs in both lower extremities, with subjec-tive symptoms limited to one extremity. See *sclerosis, multiple*.

aphrasia Inability to utter or understand words connected in the form of phrases. A subdivision of *aphasia* (q.v.) that involves only the order of words in the phrase and goes a stage beyond individual words: the patient's power (1) *expressive* (motor), i.e. to utter, or (2) *perceptive* (sensory), i.e. to understand, *single words* may be unim-paired, whereas *groups* of words forming phrases may baffle him completely as far as using or understanding them is con-cerned. See *speech disorders*.

aphrasia paranoica *Obs*. The clinical syn-drome characterized by stupor followed by talkativeness.

aphrenia *Obs*. Dementia. At one time aphre-nia was used synonymously with apoplexy, but that usage is now obsolete.

aphrenous (a-frē′nus) An early term for *insane*.

aphrodisia The state of sexual excitation.

aphrodisia phrenitica An early term for a psychiatric state thought to have sexual causes.

aphrodisiac Characterized by sexual excita-tion; also, any agent (e.g. odor) that stimu-lates sexual activity; entatic.

aphrodisiomania The state of excessive sex-ual excitement; morbid desire for venery; erotomania.

aphronesia (af-rō-nē-zē-à) *Obs*. Dementia.

aphthongia (áf-thông′ē-à, af-thông′jē-à) A form of motor aphasia characterized by spasm of the speech muscles.

apiphobia Morbid dread of bees.

apistiatria Loss of faith in the physician.

aplasia Complete or partial failure of tissue to grow or develop; arrested develop-ment; agenesis. It is to be distinguished from atrophy, which refers to the loss or diminution of structure which once had normal or average development. When tissue growth is partial, the term *hypoplasia* is used; when above average, *hyperplasia*.

aplastic Without power to grow toward nor-mal, healthy tissue.

aplestia (ap-les′tē-à) Greediness.

apnea, central Cessation of breathing due to neurologic disturbances of ventilatoy drive and frequency (in contrast to the more usual obstructive apnea, which is due to abnormalities of the nasal, pharyn-geal, or laryngeal passage). *Sleep apnea* and sleep hypopnea, the interruption of sleep by respiratory disturbances, may present only as complaints of sleepiness during the day, for the subject's breathing may be normal during waking hours and he does not remember the frequent awak-enings that have occurred during the night because of the respiratory abnormal-ity. See *sleep disorders*.

apocarteresis (ap-ō-kär-tē-rē′sis) Suicide by hunger or starvation.

apoclesis (ap-ō-klē′sis) Aversion to, or ab-sence of desire for, food.

apomathema (ap-ō-math′ē-mà) *Obs*. Loss of memory.

apoplectic See *habitus apoplecticus*.

apoplexy Stroke. See *accident, cerebrovascular*.

apopnixis *Globus hystericus* (q.v.).

apositia (à-pō-si′shē-a) *Obs*. Loathing of food.

apostle of the idiots The title generally applied to Edouard Séguin (1812–80), a French psychiatrist whose lifework was the care and welfare of the mentally retarded.

apparatus, autonomic "All the vital organs, including the ductless secretory glands, unstriped muscles and the ganglionic nervous systems that have to do with the *assimilation, conservation, distribution* and *expenditure* of energy-giving metabolic products and the *elimination* of the waste products. This includes the entire digestive, circulatory, respiratory and urinary systems, sex organs, glands of internal secretion, glands of external secretion and the autonomic nervous system." (Kempf, *PP*)

apparatus, autonomic affective "The various systems of the body, if grouped according to their functions, form two great divisions, the *autonomic apparatus* and its *projicient apparatus*. The sensory streams flowing from the periphery of different segments of the autonomic apparatus constitute the affective cravings or feelings, and the sensory streams flowing from the projicient apparatus, as it is compelled to work by the affective stream, constitutes the kinesthetic stream." (Kempf, *PP*)

apparatus, lie detector See *detector, lie.*

apparatus, projicient (prō-jish′ent) "The striped muscle apparatus and the cerebrospinal nervous system proper constitute the *projicient apparatus* which has been developed by the autonomic apparatus in order to master the environment." (Kempf, *PP*)

apparition *Rare.* Visual hallucination or visual illusion, particularly when such phenomena occur as part of an organic delirium. Such visual illusions result from the visual distortion of an object and the interpretation of the object in terms of the (usually unconscious and morbid) impulses of the patient. In alcoholic delirium, for instance, any object may be regarded as a person who is about to kill the patient.

apperception Conscious realization; awareness of the significance of a percept and particularly interpretation of what is apprehended by relating it to similar, already existing knowledge. See *distortion, apperceptive.*

apperception, scheme of By this term Adler indicates that the individual perceives what he wishes to perceive and selects from his whole experience what is useful in view of his directive fiction, forgetting or rejecting the rest of reality.

apperceptions, gestalt See *intelligence.*

appersonification, appersonation The act of embodiment or impersonation of another, typically on the basis of unconscious identification with another in part or in whole. While the phenomenon occurs in many psychiatric conditions, it may be overtly expressed in schizophrenics. One is thoroughly convinced that he is Christ; another says that he is the person who died in the next bed; a third affirms that she has the cancer her husband had. See *depersonifcation; personality, multiplication of.*

application groups See *Conferences, A.K. Rice Group Relations.*

applied ethics See *ethics, applied.*

apprehensio *Obs.* Catalepsy.

apprehension The simple or elementary intellectual act or process of becoming aware of some object or fact. *Misapprehension* is failure to understand or perceive correctly. Apprehension has also been used to refer to anxiety related to fear of some future event, but many prefer to call such anxiety *apprehensiveness.*

apprehension, irresistible Kraepelin's term for what is now termed *compulsive-obsessive psychoneurosis.*

apprehensiveness See *apprehension.*

approach Orientation, hypothesis, theory.

approach, environmental From the standpoint of the psychiatric social worker, "The *personal approach* is through the interview as it is employed to explore emotional reactions, interpret conflicts, suggest new points of view and stimulate interest in new lines of action. The *environmental approach* covers essentially manipulation of the material situations presented by physical illness, financial difficulty, employment, neighborhood conditions, etc.; this manipulation of the environment is exercised to relieve undue external pressure and call forth new and better attitudes in the client toward his responsibilities so that ultimately he may carry them unassisted." (*Proceedings of the American Association of Hospital Social Workers,* 1926) See *treatment, psychiatric social.*

approval Condonement; to be differentiated from social tolerance, in that what a society tolerates is not necessarily what a majority of its members personally approve of. See *tolerance, social.*

approximations, successive *Shaping* (q.v.).

apraxia "A disorder in the execution of learned skilled movement that cannot be explained by lack of comprehension or by inattention, sensory loss, weakness, ataxia, or basal ganglia disorder." (Watson, R.T., and Heilman, K.M. *Brain 106,* 1983)

apraxia, akinetic A condition in which the ability to carry out spontaneous movements is lost.

apraxia, amnestic Inability to carry out a movement on command, owing to inability to remember a command—though there is the ability to perform that movement.

apraxia, constructional or **constructive** A type of apraxia in which the patient, when asked to reproduce simple geometric patterns with matches, for example, is unable to connect the separate parts correctly; the end result is disorder and chaos. The defect is not related to intelligence and the patient with this kind of apraxia often recognizes his errors. See *syndrome, Gerstmann.*

apraxia, dressing A type of apraxia in which the patient is unable to don his clothes properly, putting his jacket on upside down, for example. Dressing apraxia is seen most commonly in parietal lobe lesions, such as occur in Pick's disease.

apraxia, dynamic Impaired ability to perform continuous movements, suggestive of pathology of the premotor cortex.

apraxia, ideational Sensory apraxia; loss of the conceptional process. The patient does not know the use of objects; he may fumble with a toothbrush, pen, or cigarette but will not know what to do with them.

apraxia, magnetic See *utilization behavior.*

apraxia, motor Along with ability to understand and name objects, the inability to carry out purposive movement with them.

apraxia, sensory See *apraxia, ideational.*

aprosexia Inability to maintain attention. This condition is common in organic states that affect the brain and psychiatric conditions in which (1) there are present overwhelming emotions that constantly interfere with thought processes; (2) ideas are sparse, as in states of pronounced depression; (3) ideas are so abundant that the patient cannot fix attention on external objects, as in productive mania; (4) fixed ideas of the patient compel his constant attention. The patient may show excellent attentive capacity when his special interests are involved, that is, aprosexia may be selective for certain matters.

aprosodia Inability to understand affect expressed by others, a type of fluent aphasia associated with a posterior lesion in the nondominant hemisphere; also, inappropriate emotional expression or lack of affective accompaniments of speech resulting in a bland, colorless, or blunted quality of the subject's communications. *Motor aprosodia,* the inability to express emotion in speech, is an expression of nondominant frontal lobe disease, while inappropriate emotional expression suggests nondominant temporal lobe involvement.

apsithyria, apsithuria *Obs.* Aphonia.

apsychia *Obs.* Loss of consciousness.

apsychognosia (à-sī-kog-nō′zē-à) Lack of awareness of one's own personality or mental state; used particularly to refer to the alcoholic's typical lack of awareness of the outside world's reaction to his drinking.

apsychosis *Rare.* In F.M. Barnes's terminology, absence of mental functioning and particularly of thinking, as in stupor. Barnes also speaks of *hyperpsychosis* (exaggeration of mental functioning), *hypopsychosis* (diminution of function), and *parapsychosis* (perversion of function). (*An Introduction to the Study of Mental Disorders,* 1923)

aptitude In occupational therapy, the ability and natural skill of a patient in certain lines of endeavor. See *test, aptitude.*

aquaphobia A special morbid fear of water, i.e. of going (for bathing or swimming purposes) into a *body* of water where one may drown.

arachnephobia Fear of spiders.

arachnoid (a-räk′noid) See *meninges.*

arachnoiditis See *pseudotumor cerebri.*

arc de cercle (F. "arc or segment of a circle") A pathological posture characterized by pronounced bending of the body, anteriorly or posteriorly.

arc, psychic reflex Ferenczi's term for that primitive onto- and phylogenetic stage of development in which adaptation is not achieved by a modification of the outer world, but instead by modifications of the organism itself, and particularly by simple motor discharge. Freud called this the *autoplastic* stage of development.

archaeology The science of antiquities. This term denotes the science that studies the history, use, and meaning of prehistoric objects in different countries, in order to throw light on the remote past of mankind (see *anthropology*).

"Under unusually favorable conditions

archaeological data give us information on the gradual changes of material culture and allow also inferences regarding a few aspects of the inner life of the people." (Boas, F. *General Anthropology*, 1938)

archaic Antiquated; stemming from a primitive or prehistoric age. Archaic modes of thinking and expression are seen most frequently in the schizophrenias. See *paleologic*.

archaism From the standpoint of analytical psychology (Jung), archaism means "the *ancient* character of psychic contents and functions. By this I do not mean archaistic, i.e., imitated antiquity, as exhibited or the nineteenth century 'Gothic,' but qualities which have the character of *survival*. All those psychological traits can be so described which essentially correspond with the qualities of primitive mentality. It is clear that archaism primarily clings to the phantasies of the unconscious, i.e., to such products of unconscious phantasy-activity as reach consciousness. The quality of the image is archaic when it poses unmistakable mythological parallels." (Jung, *PT*)

archeopsychism See *archaism*.

archetype In Jungian theory, an inherited idea or mode of thought, derived from the experience of the race, and present in the unconscious of the individual, controlling his ways of perceiving the world. An understanding of Jung's concept of these archetypes, especially with regard to his application of them in therapy, is basic for an understanding of Jung's system of psychology. See *analytic psychology*.

The unconscious part of the mind is separated by Jung into two subdivisions, termed by him the personal unconscious and the collective unconscious. The *personal unconscious* lies directly beneath consciousness and contains psychic material that is not in consciousness, yet is subject to conscious recall. Because it has to do with the person's life-experience this material can be made conscious, at least theoretically, since we are dealing with the actual person whom it concerns. Thus the term personal unconscious is particularly apt.

Constituting by far the largest area of the mind, and situated beneath the personal unconscious, is the *collective unconscious*. The material contained in this area is *not* derived from the life-experience of the person, but from the life-experience of the person's progenitors, *all of them*, and therefore of the entire human race. The whole history of human psychic functioning, the collective experience of humanity, is the inheritance of each individual psyche. The record of this history and experience contains ideas, modes of thought, patterns of reaction that are fundamental and typical in all humanity: the archetypes are their representations in the collective unconscious.

Jung believed that the collective unconscious represented the wisdom of the ages and, in consequence, contained tendencies superior to the individual's. This conception "had a significant influence on his therapeutic approach. A part of the process of self-development consisted in bringing a person into contact with his collective unconscious. This was done to a great extent through the interpretation of dreams. Jung saw the dream as having meanings on several levels. There was the personal meaning relating to the immediate life of the patient. If one pushed associations beyond that, one finally reached the collective unconscious meaning. Thus a dream about the father would finally come to a conception of all fatherhood, the father archetype. At this level supposedly the knowledge acquired by mankind through the centuries becomes available to the patient." (Thompson, C. *Psychoanalysis: Evolution and Development*, 1950)

"In the language of the unconscious, which is a picture-language, the archetypes appear in personified or symbolized picture form. Their number is relatively limited, for it corresponds to the 'possibilities of typical fundamental experiences,' such as human beings have had since the beginning of time. Their significance for us lies precisely in that 'primal experience' which they represent and mediate. The motives of the archetypal images are the same in all cultures. We find them repeated in all mythologies, fairy tales, religious traditions, and mysteries. What else is the myth of the night sea-voyage, of the wandering hero, or of the sea monster than our timeless knowledge, transformed into a picture of the sun's setting and rebirth? Prometheus, the stealer of fire, Hercules, the slayer of dragons, the numerous myths of creation, the fall from Paradise, the sacrificial mysteries, the virgin birth, the treacherous betrayal of the hero, the dismembering of Osiris, and many other myths and tales portray psychic processes in symbolic-imaginary form. Likewise the forms of the snake, the fish, the sphinx, the helpful animals, the World Tree, the Great Mother, and otherwise the enchanted prince, the *puer aeternus*, the Magi, the Wise Man, Paradise, etc., stand for certain figures and contents of the collective unconscious. The sum of the archetypes signifies thus for Jung the sum of all the latent potentialities of the human psyche—an enormous, inexhaustible store of ancient knowledge concerning the most profound relations between God, man, and the cosmos." (Jacobi, J. *The Psychology of C.G. Jung*, 1942)

archetype, mother "The archetype 'Mother' is pre-existent and superordinate to every form of manifestation of the 'motherly.' It is a constant core of meaning, which can take on all aspects and symbols of the 'motherly.' The primordial image of the mother and the characteristics of the 'Great Mother' with all paradoxical traits are the same in the soul of present-day man as in mythological times." (Jacobi, J. *The Psychology of C. G. Jung*, 1942) See *Magna Mater; individuation.*

archi-sleep See *dream.*

area, catchment See *psychiatry, community.*

area, delinquency A neighborhood or community with a disproportionately high rate of juvenile delinquents.

area striata See *lobe, occipital.*

arecoline A parasympathomimetic drug which has been noted on occasion to produce short-lived intervals of lucidity in schizophrenic subjects.

argininosuccinic aciduria (ar-jin-ēn-ō-suk-sin'Mik as-id-ūr'ē-à) A metabolic defect characterized by a high quantity of argininosuccinic acid in the cerebrospinal fluid and urine; associated with this are epilepsy, EEG dysrhythmia, and mental retardation. Known also as Allan-Dent disease.

Argyll Robertson pupil (Argyll Robertson, Scottish physician, 1837–1909) A pupil, usually miotic, that responds to accommodation but does not respond to light and reacts slowly to mydriatics. It is usually found in patients with neurosyphilis, al-

though it may appear in other conditions (traumatic brain injury, brain tumor, infectious diseases of the brain, multiple sclerosis, etc.).

aristogenic *Obs.* Best endowed eugenically. A term describing the individuals whose parenthood is to be encouraged through positive eugenic measures. See *eugenics.*

arithmetic disorder See *developmental disorders, specific.*

arithmomania A morbid impulse to count. The condition may be observed in a variety of psychiatric disorders, but most commonly in obsessive-compulsive neurosis.

"Case 6. Obsession of arithmomania. A woman became obliged to count the boards in the floor, the steps in the staircase, etc.—acts which she performed in a state of ridiculous distress.

"*Reinstatement.* She had begun the counting in order to turn her mind from obsessive ideas of temptation. She had succeeded in so doing, but the impulse to count had replaced the original obsession." (Freud, *CP*)

Arnold-Chiari malformation (Friedrich Arnold, German anatomist, 1803–90, and Hans Chiari; German physician, 1851–1916) A congenital abnormality of the central nervous system characterized by protrusion of the medulla and cerebellum into the spinal column. Hydrocephalus is usually present and, commonly, there is an associated meningomyelocele and lumbosacral spina bifida.

arousal Cortical vigilance or readiness; activation of the nervous system, alertness, wakefulness, usually with the implication that the subject is attentive and able to process information. See *formation, reticular.*

Sexual arousal refers to excitation or responsivity to erotic stimulation.

arrangement, neurotic The construction and marshaling of erroneous ideas on the part of a neurotic patient in order to justify his neurosis with apparently logical reasons, by rearranging the events of his life to suit his neurosis. These patients have an ingenious way of accounting for their failures; for instance, a man asserted that he had a "historic mission" to accomplish in life, yet did nothing in that direction and justified his hidden inferiority by saying to himself: "If you had sound nerves, if you did not suffer from night terrors, you would have gone far." This type of neurotic arrangement does not confine itself to the simple construction of erroneous ideas but may also be present in the somatic sphere: the patient magnifies an existing organ inferiority or creates one if it does not exist. (Stekel, *ID*)

arreptio (a-rep'shō) *Obs.* Insanity; mental disorder.

arrhostia (a-rōs'tē-à) *Obs.* Imbecillitas; mental retardation.

arrhythmokinesis Inability to maintain a desired or requested rhythmicity in the performance of an act.

arson See *pyromania.*

arsphenamine hemorrhagic encephalitis (ärs-fen'à-mēn hem-o-raj'ik en-sef-à-lī'tis) A toxic and probably idiosyncratic reaction (hence more correctly termed an encephalopathy) to the intravenous administration of arsphenamine. This is a rare complication and usually occurs one to two days after injection. Vomiting and headache are rapidly followed by restlessness and delirium, passing into coma with stertorous respiration and often generalized convulsions. In fatal cases, there is edema of the brain, capillary engorgement, and perivascular hemorrhage as well as nonhemorrhagic perivascular areas of necrosis and demyelination.

art The study of artistic productions has thrown much light on questions of psychology and psychopathology. Like dreams and phantasies, art is regarded as representing factors or themes of the psyche. From the psychiatric standpoint art is analyzed in much the same way that dreams and phantasies are. Freud applies his methods of investigation also to the problem of artistic creativeness, its nature and sources. "The artist is originally a man who turns from reality because he cannot come to terms with the demand for the renunciation of instinctual satisfaction as it is first made, and who then in phantasy-life allows full play to his erotic and ambitious wishes." (Freud, *CP*)

Jung says: "Art, like every other human activity, proceeds from psychic motives." Speaking of poetic art, he quotes Gerhart Hauptmann: "Poetry means the distant echo of the primitive world behind our veil of words." Jung expresses a similar idea when he asks "to what primordial image of the collective unconscious can we trace the image we see developed in the work of art?" He adds that "the shaping of the primordial image is, as it were, a translation into the language of the present which makes it possible for every man to find again the deepest spring of life which would otherwise be closed to him." (Jung, *CAP*)

arterenol (ar-te-rē'nol) Norepinephrine. See *epinephrine.*

arteriogram *Angiogram* (q.v.).

arteriosclerosis, cerebral Hardening of the arteries of the brain, the most common causes of which are primary degeneration of the intima of the cerebral vessels, degeneration secondary to hypertension, endarteritis (usually syphilitic), thromboangiitis, polyarteritis nodosa or periarteritis nodosa, and temporal arteritis. In DSM-III, this group of disorders is more limited in definition and is termed *multi-infarct dementia* (q.v.). Pathological changes are of two types—hyperplastic or hypoplastic degeneration of the internal elastic membrane. Hyperplastic degeneration produces focal parenchymatous lesions and mainly neurological symptoms (convulsions, aphasia, agnosia, apraxia, paralysis of the upper motor neuron type, tremor, chorea, athetosis, Parkinsonism); mental changes appear late in the course of the disorder.

Hypoplastic degeneration, on the other hand, produces gross hemorrhagic softenings and mainly mental symptoms: signs of frontal lobe damage such as *Witzelsucht* (q.v.), callousness, and euphoria; basal ganglia signs such as impulsiveness and whining; temporal lobe signs such as depression and visual hallucinations; and with parietal lobe involvement often hypochondriacal trends. In addition, there are general intellectual dulling with memory defects, emotional lability, hostility to all change, paranoid trends, loosely constructed delusions, confusion, and finally profound dementia.

arthritis Inflammation of a joint, usually manifested by pain and stiffness in the joint. Arthritis is commonly subdivided into *inflammatory* types, with exudative or proliferative changes or both, and *degenerative* types (also known as *osteoarthritis*), characterized by failure of the articular cartilage to repair itself adequately or normally. Of most interest to psychiatry is *rheumatoid (atrophic) arthritis,* consisting of chronic proliferative inflammation of the synovial membrane, involving multiple joints but with a predilection for the smaller ones, and characterized by wide variations in severity and a tendency to inexplicable remissions and exacerbations. Etiology is unknown, but because recurrences in many instances appear at least temporally to be related to emotional crisis, some authorities have considered rheumatoid arthritis to be primarily a psychophysiologic or psychosomatic disturbance. Alexander, for instance, believed that the specific dynamic pattern is the repression of all hostile, competitive tendencies. If the aggressive attack is inhibited at the stage of psychological preparation, a migraine attack develops; if it is inhibited at the stage of vegetative preparation, essential hypertension develops; while if it is inhibited at a neuromuscular phase, an inclination toward arthritic symptoms may develop. See *hypertension, essential.*

Current theories about arthritis implicate autoimmunity or disordered immune responses as significant factors in the production or precipitation of the tissue injury characteristic of rheumatoid arthritis.

arthritism See *diathesis, arthritic.*

arthritism, infantile In constitutional medicine this refers to the arthritic diathesis or arthritism that manifests itself in young children. See *diathesis, arthritic.*

arthro-, arthr- Combining form meaning joint, articulation.

arthropathy (är-throp'-a-thē) Joint disease, especially neuroarthropathy or trophoneurosis of the joint. Tabetic arthropathy, or Charcot's joint, consists of edema and effusions within the joints, associated usually with painless swellings; proliferation and destruction of the cartilage, capsule, and bone surface may occur with formation of new bone, fragments of which may be free within the joint ("joint mice").

articulation disorders See *developmental disorders, specific; speech disorders.*

artificial neurosis See *neurosis, experimental.*

artificialism Piaget's term for the child's tendency to believe that natural phenomena are caused by some human agency.

arugamama See *psychotherapy, Morita.*

"as if" This term, borrowed from the philosopher Vaihinger, is used by Adler to indicate the fictitious and imaginary goal of complete superiority that some persons set for themselves. "This goal introduces into our life a hostile and fighting tendency . . . whoever takes this goal of godlikeness seriously or literally, will soon be compelled to flee from real life and compromise, by seeking a life within life; if fortunate,—in art, but more generally,—in pietism, neurosis or crime." (Adler, A. *The Practice and Theory of Individual Psychology,* 1924) "As if" also is used to refer to a personality type seen typically in schizophrenics before or between acute episodes. See *personality, "as if."*

as-if performances Sullivan's term for those dramatizations in which a person ordinarily assumes various roles in order to avoid punishment or get tenderness; also included are those preoccupations in which a child loses himself in order to combat anxiety.

"as-if," pseudo See *"pseudo as-if."*

asaphia *Obs.* Indistinctness of voice.

asapholalia (à-sà-fō-lā'lē-à) Indistinct or *mumbling* speech (q.v.).

ascendance, ascendancy Dominance; used especially to refer to character traits and interpersonal or group relationships. See *submissiveness.*

asceticism See *character, ascetic.*

Aschner ocular phenomenon (Bernhardt Aschner, Viennese physician, 1883–1960) Pressure exerted over the eyeball produces a slowing of the pulse; also known as the oculocardiac reflex.

Aschner treatment of schizophrenia *Obs.* A method of "constitutional" therapy employed by the Viennese physician Bernhardt Aschner in the treatment of schizophrenia; the method includes the use of cold baths, sweats, drastic purgatives, emmenagogues, emetics, blisters, and periodic bloodletting.

ASDC Association of Sleep Disorders Centers; their nosology of sleep disorders is generally recognized as the "official" one.

asemasia (as-ē-mā'zē-à) *Asemia* (q.v.).

asemia (à-sē'mē-à) Loss of the ability, previously possessed, to make or understand any sign or token of communication, whether of organic or emotional origin. See *speech disorders.*

As in all speech disorders the perceptive and the expressive (or sensory and motor) aspects may manifest themselves singly or both combined, when the disability may be called total. The subdivisions of asemia are: amimia, alexia, agraphia. It includes the trainman's or switchman's inability to grasp the meaning of signs by semaphore or colored lights, the bellhop's irresponsiveness to the various buzzes or bell combinations, the telegrapher's inability to convey or "read" messages on the ticker, the student's blindness to letters, figures, and mathematical signs and symbols, the pianist's blank stare at a page of formerly familiar music, though he may still be able to play the piece from memory, the soldier's "disregard" of bugle calls.

asitia (a-sish'ē-a) Anorexia.

asocial Not social; indifferent to social values; without social meaning or significance.

asomatognosia See *somatognosia.*

asoticamania Self-destructive prodigality or squandering of money; profligate spending, which may constitute the outstanding behavioral feature of *mania* (q.v.).

Asperger's syndrome (Hans Asperger, Austrian physician, 1844–1954) See *psychopathy, autistic.*

aspermia, psychogenic (a-sper'mē-a) See *impotence, psychic.*

assembly, cell *Engram* (q.v.); any group of neurons that has come to function as a unit by reason of repeated stimulation.

assessment Diagnosis; evaluation. See *nosology.*

assimilation In analytical psychology (Jung), "the absorption or joining up of a new conscious content to already prepared subjective material, whereby the similarity of the new content with the waiting subjective material is specially emphasized, even to the prejudice of the independent quality of the new content. Fundamentally, assimilation is a process of apperception . . . which, however, is distinguished from pure apperception by this element of adjustment to the subjective material." (Jung, *PT*)

Jung maintains that *dissimilation* "represents the adjustment of subject to object, and a consequent estrangement of the subject from himself in favour of the object, whether it be an external object or a 'psychological' or inner object, as for instance an idea." (Ibid.)

In Fromm's theory of character, assimilation is one of two ways of relating to the world (the other is socialization). Assimilation types relate to material things rather than to people, and Fromm distinguishes five subtypes: (1) *receiving*—the person feels that the only way to get what he wants is to receive it passively from some outside source; (2) *exploiting*—the person feels that he can get what he wants only by stealing it or by using some artful, cunning scheme; (3) *hoarding*—the person doubts that he can ever get what he wants, so whatever he has must be saved and hoarded (similar to the anal character in other classifications); (4) *marketing*—the person values himself only in terms of salability to others and is dependent upon personal acceptance by them; such a person becomes alienated and estranged from his actions and his own life forces, an automaton who is ruled by the institutions of industrial society; (5) *working*—the only productive type in this group, characterized by the ability to reason objectively, to love unselfishly, and to work productively.

assimilation, social The process or processes by which peoples of diverse social origins and different cultural heritages, occupying a common territory, achieve a cultural solidarity.

Assimilation is generally considered in terms of the fusion of immigrants or of members of a minority group into the national culture, but it applies equally to the nature and degree of participation of a newcomer in a group, institution, or neighborhood.

association Relationship. In psychiatry, association refers particularly to the relationship between the conscious and the unconscious, ideas in the former being connected to the latter.

Associations may be free or induced. When a person without prompting is allowed to raise and to expand upon an idea or ideas, the process is known as "free" association. This is one of the methods used by psychoanalysts in tracing the origin and development of ideas or groups of ideas.

Induced associations involve the giving of stimulus words; "The experimenter calls out a word to the test-person, and the test-person immediately replies with the next association that comes into his mind." (Jung, *CAP*)

Originally the test was employed as a means by which complexes were revealed. It is still used by some for that purpose. As a rule, however, for practical, therapeutic purposes, the free association method is used, not alone for uncovering complexes, but principally for gaining information on the organization and development of the contents of the mind.

Freud "maintains that, when a subject is asked to make free associations from a given theme to which he is attending, and wholly to suspend the active-selective criticism that under such circumstances is instinctively exercised towards the incoming thoughts, the associations must be directly or indirectly related, in a causative manner to the initial theme." (Jones, E. *Papers on Psycho-Analysis*, 1938)

Jung uses the term *association method* to mean the procedure; the tests are called *association experiments*.

association, clang An association based on similarity of sound, without regard for differences in meaning; most frequently observed in the manic phase of manic-depressive disorder and in the schizophrenias. See *homonym*.

association disturbances See *associations, disturbances of*.

association-experiment See *association*.

association, false Stekel's term for the dreamer's various identifications simultaneously with several persons who nevertheless represent the same love object, these associations (given by the dreamer) being only partly valid, inasmuch as they correspond to incomplete situations and typically to two different situations reported by the patient as being only one.

This type of association may lead the analyst to details concerning one of the persons with whom the dreamer identifies his love object, when in reality this association pertains to another person, also a partial substitute for the real love object. (Stekel, *ID*)

association fibers See *commissure*.

association, free The trends of thought or chains of ideas that spontaneously arise when restraint and censorship upon logical thinking are removed and the subject orally reports everything that passes

through his mind. This fundamental technique of modern psychoanalysis assumes that when relieved of the necessity of logical thinking and reporting verbally everything going through his mind, the analysand will bring forward basic psychic material and thus make it available to analytical interpretation. This method was originally introduced by Freud after he had been disillusioned with the results of hypnosis. In trying to overcome the posthypnotic amnesia, Freud found out that, when urged to make an effort, the hypnotized subject was able to recall almost everything that had been said to him, although he could not remember anything that had happened during the hypnotic trance.

Freud applied the same technique to patients he could not hypnotize. He urged them to tell him everything that came to their minds, to leave out nothing, regardless of whether they considered it relevant. As he developed this method, he found that it was not as simple as he had thought, that these so-called free associations were really not free, but were determined by unconscious material which had to be analyzed and interpreted. He therefore designated this new technique psychoanalysis.

The methodological principle of free association is a common basis for the classical Freudian analysis and the Jungian type of analysis. (Freud, *BW;* Schilder, P. *Psychotherapy*, 1938)

association, induced See *association*.

association method See *association*.

association, psychosis of A form of psychosis in which certain of the mental symptoms of one patient (the principal) appear in similar or identical form in one or more other people (the associates) who are closely associated with the first. This association is typically intrafamilial, as in two siblings, or in parent and child, or in husband and wife; but it has also been reported among pairs of patients on a psychiatric ward and in pairs of friends who have been in intimate social contact over a period of time. When the number of people involved is two, the condition is sometimes called *folie à deux* (q.v.); there may be three (*folie à trois*), four (*folie à quatre*), or many (*folie à beaucoup*) involved. Other names by which this condition has been known are infectious insanity (Ideler, 1838); psychic infection (Hoffbauer, 1846); familial mental infection (Séguin, 1879); reciprocal insanity (Parsons, 1883); collective insanity (Ireland, 1886); double insanity (Tuke, 1887); influenced psychosis (Gordon, 1925); mystic paranoia (Pike, 1933); shared paranoid disorder (DSM-III). See *paranoia.*

Most writers agree that psychosis of association is limited to paranoid and depressive forms of psychosis, and in the case reports in the literature even purely depressive forms are a relative rarity. Four types of psychosis of association are recognized: (1) imposed (described by Laseque and Falret, 1877), in which the associate accepts the delusions of the principal with little elaboration, and separation of the patients typically results in disappearance of the delusions in the associate; (2) simultaneous (described by Regis, 1880), in which there is simultaneous appearance of identical symptoms in more than one subject, and these symptoms are typically depression and/or persecutory ideas; (3) communicated (described by Marandon de Montyel, 1881), in which the associate takes over the delusions of the principal and works them into his own system, often with elaboration, and these delusions are usually maintained even after separation of the two; and (4) induced (described by Lehmann, 1885), wherein a second receptive patient adds the principal's delusions to his own symptoms.

association test See *association.*

associationism That school of psychology that holds that mental development consists mainly of combinations and recombinations of basic, irreducible, mental elements. See *contextualism; reductionism.*

associations, contiguity of An internal connection which is still undisclosed will announce its presence by means of a temporal proximity of associations; just as in writing, if "a" and "b" are put side by side, it means that the syllable "ab" is to be formed out of them. (Freud, *CP*)

As an example, Freud refers to the case of Dora (Analysis of a Case of Hysteria) in which Dora recognizes that Frau K would always fall ill whenever Herr K returned from one of his long journeys, to be able to escape the conjugal duties that she so much detested. At this point Dora referred to her own alternations between good and bad health during the first years of her girlhood. Freud then suspected that her states of health depended on something else, in the same way as Frau K's.

associations, disturbances of One of Bleuler's fundamental symptoms of the schizophrenias. The associations are the innumerable related threads which guide thinking, and in the schizophrenias the associations are interrupted and lose their contiguity. As a result, thinking becomes haphazard, seemingly purposeless, illogical, confused, incorrect, abrupt, and bizarre. Among the many possible association disturbances are clang associations, indirect associations, stereotypy in speech, dearth of ideas to the point of monoideism, *thought deprivation* (blocking), *naming* (echopraxia) or *touching*, pressure of thoughts, inappropriate application of cliches, Klebedenken, impoverishment of thought, replacement of thinking proper by a senseless compulsion to associate.

associations, indirect One of the disturbances of associations seen often in the schizophrenias. With indirect associations, *A* may be connected to *B* and *B* may be connected to *C,* but the connecting link *B* is unexpressed so that the listener finds the statement incomprehensible, illogical, or bizarre.

associative thinking See *thinking, associative.*

assortative See *mating, assortative.*

assumptions, group See *group, basic assumptions*

assurance, quality See *quality assurance.*

astasia (à-stā′zē-à) The inability to stand, when there is no organic reason for the disability. See *astasia-abasia.*

astasia-abasia A form of hysterical ataxia with bizarre incoordination and inability to stand or walk, even though all leg movements can be performed normally while sitting or lying down.

astereognosis (às-ter-ē-og-nō′sis) Loss of power to perceive the shape and nature of an object and inability to identify it by superficial contact alone, in the absence of any demonstrable sensory defect; sometimes called tactile agnosia, although in astereognosis there is a defect in the higher correlation of proprioceptive sensations as well. Some use astereognosis for minor defects in which the patient cannot recognize form and tactile agnosia for more profound defects in which there is inability to identify objects. Astereognosis follows lesions of the parietal lobe, especially in the posterior portions.

asterixis A lapse of posture consisting of momentary loss of a fixed position of the hands or arms followed by a jerking recovery movement that restores the limb to its original position; also known as *flapping tremor,* it usually occurs in association with tremulousness in patients with some degree of central nervous system dysfunction secondary to metabolic disorders such as liver disease and uremia. It has also been reported as a side-effect of diphenylhydantoin.

asthenia Want or loss of strength, debility, diminution of the vital forces. In the field of constitutional medicine it does not imply the specific meaning conveyed by the adjective *asthenic.* See *type, asthenic.*

asthenia, mental Diminution of the capacity for mental work, usually related to hypoboulia and/or difficulty in concentration.

asthenia, neurocirculatory A clinical syndrome, also called *effort syndrome,* characterized by palpitation, shortness of breath, labored breathing, subjective complaints of effort and discomfort, all following slight exertion; other symptoms may be dizziness, tremulousness, sweating, insomnia. Neurocirculatory asthenia is most typically seen as a form of *anxiety neurosis* (q.v.), or of hyperventilation syndrome. See *syndrome, hyperventilation.*

asthenic See *type, asthenic.*

asthenic personality A *personality disorder* characterized by low energy level, easy fatigability, incapacity for enjoyment and lack of enthusiasm, and oversensitivity to physical and emotional stress. See *neurasthenia.*

asthenology The doctrine of diseases or anomalies, structural or functional, associated with weakness or debility. In psychiatry the term has special, though not exclusive, reference to matters pertaining to constitutional medicine, including such concepts as constitutional inadequacies, early structural or functional wearing out of organs or systems of organs, and imbalance of organic systems. For example, it is believed that among certain psychiatric patients, particularly the schizophrenic, the cardiovascular system retains puerile structure and function, as a consequence of which adult parts of the body have to get along with puerile parts. Such anomalies often lead to debility of a greater or lesser order. Asthenology includes studies of such disability or debility.

asthenophobia Fear of weakness.

asthenopia Weakness of vision or sight.

asthma, bronchial A respiratory disorder characterized by recurrent attacks of bronchiolar spasm, which traps air in the lungs and results in paralysis of the expiratory muscles, assumption of the inspiratory position, and use of all the accessory muscles of respiration. Asthma may be an anaphylactic reaction, or primarily hereditary, or a combination of extrinsic factors such as allergy with any number of intrinsic factors, including emotional and psychologic elements. In some asthmatics, the asthmatic attack may be an anxiety equivalent related to threat of separation from the protecting, encompassing mother and a cry for help. Maternal rejection is a recurrent motif in the history of such asthmatics, who are often of the obsessive-compulsive personality type with an anal-sadistic orientation.

asthma, sexual The asthmatic condition induced by the act of coitus.

astraphobia, astrapophobia Morbid fear of thunder and lightning.

astrocyte See *neuroglia.*

astrology The study of planets, particularly their influence on the destiny of the universe including human beings, their actions, personality, body, and health. The medicine of the Middle Ages was strikingly dominated by demonology, witchcraft, sorcery, and astrology, and statements that assumed there existed no infirmity or disease not due to the influence of some planet or planets were not uncommon. Saturn was assumed to govern the spleen; Jupiter ruled over the lungs, liver, and semen; Mars controlled the kidneys; Venus, the uterus, breasts, and genitals of the female; Mercury stood for the mental processes; and the Sun ruled the brain and the nerves, the right half of the body, and the left eye of the woman. Paracelsus expanded this school of medicinal thought considerably: among other things he believed that with a magnet he was able to shift the diseases of the body into the earth. (Hinsie, *UP*)

astyphia (à-stif′ē-à) Sexual impotence.

astysia (à-stis′ē-à) Sexual impotence.

asyllabia A form of aphasia (agraphia or alexia); inability to combine individual letters (or sounds) into syllables. See *speech disorders.*

asylum Originally defined as a place safe from violence or pillage. The ancients set apart certain places of refuge where the vilest criminals were protected, and the name later came to be applied specially to an institution that afforded a place of refuge or safety for the infirm or mentally ill.

asymbolia (as-im-bō′lē-à) Inability to make or understand symbols or signs.

A term proposed by F.C. Finkelburg in 1870 for what is now denoted by the more generally accepted term *asemia* (q.v.). Adolf Kussmaul argued that asymbolia is less comprehensive, because back of *symbol* stands an *idea* and thus it is narrower than *sign* or *token,* which frequently has merely a *feeling* back of it. See *speech disorders.*

asymbolia, pain A type of disordered recognition of the body, as is seen in parietal lobe lesions, in which the patient, although able to perceive painful stimuli, "shows a morbid poverty of emotional reaction to them. In every case described the lesion has been found in the left hemisphere but the whole body shows the abnormal response to pain." (Mayer-Gross, W., et al. *Clinical Psychiatry,* 1960)

asymbolia, visual See *aphasia, visual.*

asymmetry, mental The disparity in form and the unbalanced relationship between two opposite mental processes. In this regard, one may assert that a very frequent symptom in compulsion neurosis is the patient's tendency to compare various parts of his body with one another: some patients spend hours in front of a mirror comparing the two sides of their faces and even may often assert that they are of different form (asymmetric). This is but an expression of their mental disparity and unbalance and their conclusions are drawn merely with reference to their own egos. The patient compares not only different parts of his own body but also "compares himself with his father, with his brothers and sisters, and with other people." He compares also various achievements in his life, especially homosexual and heterosexual trends. (Stekel, *CD*)

asymptotic See *wish-fulfillment, asymptotic.*

asyndesis (às-in-dē′sis) A language disorder seen most commonly in the schizophrenias and to a lesser extent in other organic brain syndromes in which there is juxtaposition of elements without adequate linkage between them. Images and meanings that are connected in the mind of the patient are superimposed on each other in a sentence without explanation as to what the connecting links are; to the listener, the language then seems disjointed and disconnected. "One of our patients, for example, when asked what caused the wind to blow, said it was 'due to velocity, due to loss of air, evaporation of water . . . the contact of trees, of air in the trees.' " (Cameron, N. in *Language and Thought in Schizophrenia* ed. J.S. Kasansin, 1944) See *thinking-aside.*

asynergia (às-i-nēr′jē-à) See *ataxia.*

asynergia of Babinski, major Incoordination in standing and walking as a result of involvement of the cerebellum.

asynergia of Babinski, minor As a consequence of involvement of the cerebellum, there results a decomposition of movements giving rise to a "breaking up" of simple acts; when the patient attempts to carry out such acts as kneeling on a chair, elevating the leg while in a supine position, or sitting up from a recumbent position, the movements are disjointed and awkward.

asynesia (às-in-ē′zē-à) Profound mental dullness; stupidity.

asynesis (à-sin′ē-sis) *Obs.* Aphasia.

asynetous (à-sin′ē-tus) *Obs.* Stupid, foolish.

asynodia Failure of sexual partners to attain simultaneous orgasm; less commonly, sexual impotence.

At In Rorschach scoring, anatomy response, i.e. any response containing the image of a part of a human or animal organism that is not visible without cutting the body open. The *At* responses indicate attempts to compensate for a feeling of intellectual inferiority.

ataque A culture-specific syndrome found in Puerto Ricans, consisting of a convulsivelike episode that is believed to be a conversion defense against aggressive impulses.

ataraxy (a′tar-ak-sē) Absence of anxiety or confusion; untroubled calmness. The ataractic drugs are commonly called *tranquilizers*. See *psychotropics*.

atavism (at'à-viz'm) When mental or physical traits, dormant for one or more generations, reappear in the offspring, the condition is known as atavism. The term is commonly used in biology and less frequently in psychiatry. There are no clear-cut examples of atavism, strictly speaking, in psychology or psychiatry, although it is not unlikely that the many components of the sphere of the unconscious that constitute the *collective unconscious* of Jung may be regarded as atavistic, particularly when they are expressed overtly in the daily life of the person (as in schizophrenia).

ataxia Absence or lack of order; incoordination. In this general sense it may refer to the absence of order of any bodily function or system, physical or mental. It is most commonly used in the field of neurology to designate a loss of power of muscular coordination. The condition may be due to disorder in the brain or spinal cord. There is a form called autonomic or vasomotor ataxia, resulting from imbalance of the sympathetic and parasympathetic nervous systems.

The term ataxia is used also in conjunction with certain psychic functions. Stransky coined the expression *intrapsychic ataxia,* regarding it as a cardinal symptom of schizophrenia; it refers to lack of coordination between thoughts and feelings. A schizophrenic may laugh heartily while he believes that his body is being cut into millions of pieces. Intrapsychic ataxia is most vividly expressed in schizophrenia; it is not uncommon in hysteria; it may appear in other psychiatric and nonpsychiatric states.

ataxia, Friedreich's Familial, hereditary, and slowly progressive disorder consisting of degeneration of the posterior columns and spinocerebellar tracts of the spinal cord, mainly in its lower portion, and of the pyramidal tracts. Onset is between 5 and 15 years of age, with ataxia, loss of deep reflexes, nystagmus, dysarthria, intention tremor, and, because of early degeneration of the pyramidal tracts, development of pes cavus. (When accompanied by peroneal atrophy, the condition is termed *Roussy Levy syndrome.*) The Babinski and Romberg reflexes are usually posi-

tive and there is often a mild dementia. Death usually occurs within 20 years from first appearance of symptoms.

ataxia, hysterical See *astasia-abasia.*

ataxia, intrapsychic Stransky introduced this term in an effort to describe the condition of the emotions in schizophrenia. He stressed that patients with that disorder seemed not to show destruction of the feelings, but rather a separation of them from other mental phenomena; he spoke of *ataxic feelings.*

ataxia, locomotor See *tabes.*

ataxia, Marie's hereditary cerebellar (Pierre Marie, French physician, 1853–1940) A familial, hereditary disorder consisting of cerebellar and pyramidal tract degeneration and, in some cases, optic atrophy. Onset is during or after adolescence. Symptoms include ataxia, nystagmus, dysarthria, and intention tremor; in contrast to Friedreich's ataxia, reflexes are normal, pes cavus is not seen, and the Babinski and Romberg reflexes are negative. It would appear that this is a mixed group rather than a pure clinical or pathological entity.

ataxia, mental Intrapsychic ataxia. "In dementia praecox there is marked ataxia between the emotions and the intellectual and volitional powers of the mind. The dementia praecox patient may be depressed and have apparent reason to be so, yet his conduct at the time of apparent depression is in absolute opposition to the content of his consciousness. He cries when he should laugh, and vice versa." (Bowers, P.E. *Manual of Psychiatry,* 1924)

ataxia spirituum *Obs.* Nervous diathesis.

ataxia telangectasia A familial syndrome consisting of progressive cerebellar ataxia, oculocutaneous telangectases, and recurrent pulmonary infections; also known as *Louis-Bar's syndrome.*

ataxophemia Impaired coordination of words; incoherence.

atelesis Absence of integration or successful completion. The term has been used to refer to the three major dysjunctions prominent in schizophrenic psychopathology: dysjunction of inner world and environment (autism), dysjunction of ego and the contents of consciousness (*splitting* or *ego anachoresis*), and dysjunction of experience contents and the elementary forms of mental perception (*destruction of categories*).

atelia (á-tē′lē-á) The doctrine of incomplete development.

ateliosis (á-tē-lē-ō′sis) Dwarfism; incomplete development; the term may refer to psychic infantilism or puerilism, to mental retardation, and/or to physical dwarfism (microsomia).

atephobia Fear of ruin.

ater succus (ä′ter sook′koos) (L. "black juice or sap") *Obs.* Melancholia.

athetosis (ath-ē-tō′sis) Irregular, slow, objectively purposeless movement with some apparent pattern, occurring mainly in the toes and fingers, in the form of extension and flexion and spreading of the digits.

Athetosis results from a lesion in the extrapyramidal pathways, usually the corpus striatum, or from other lesions that interrupt the circuit of the suppressor reaction between cortical areas 4s and 4.

athletic See *type, athletic.*

athymia 1. Apathy, emotional indifference, or unresponsiveness. 2. Unconsciousness. 3. Mental retardation. 4. Melancholia. 5. Absence of the thymus gland.

atom, social "The social atom consists of the psychological relations of one individual to those other individuals to whom he is attracted or repelled, and their relation to him. It is the smallest social structure in a community. Developing from the time of birth, it first contains mother and child. As time goes on, the child adds from the persons who come into his orbit such persons as are unpleasant or pleasant to him, and, vice versa, those to whom he is unpleasant or pleasant. Persons who do not leave any impression, positive or negative, remain outside of the social atom as mere acquaintances. The feeling which correlates two or more individuals is called tele. The social atom is, therefore, a compound of the tele relationships of an individual. As positively or negatively charged persons may leave the individual's social atom and others may enter it, the social atom has a more or less everchanging constellation." (Moreno, J.L. *Who Shall Survive?* 1934)

atomism See *psychology, atomistic.*

atonic Relating to or characterized by atonia, i.e. by lack of tone or vital energy. It refers to the whole body, to a particular system of the body or to single organs, especially to contractile organs.

In the system of constitutional types described by Pende the term is used in a more specialized sense to indicate a subgroup of the *megalosplanchnic* (q.v.) hypervegetative constitution and also a subgroup of the *microsplanchnic* (q.v.) hypovegetative constitution. "We can understand the importance of our division of the great megalosplanchnic group into two subgroups, one of which we designate as the atonic and flaccid, and the other as the hypertonic and hypersthenic. The first includes individuals morphologically hypoevolute in almost all their organs, with a dominant parasympathicotonia and a torpid orientation of the nervous system and psyche; with slow metabolism; and with lymphatic plethora, a deficiency in the development of the arterial portion of the heart as compared with the venous, and of the blood as compared with the lymph." (Pende, N. *Constitutional Inadequacies,* 1928)

Similarly there is a distinction between the atonic and hyposthenic subgroup and the hypersthenic and hypertonic subgroup of the microsplanchnic hypovegetative constitution. In the former subgroup we have the slender type with small skeleton and muscles and also with hypoevolutism of the cardiovascular system and the endocrine glands.

The concept of an *atonic constitution* is further used in the system of Rostan, in which it refers to a type characterized by atonia of all systems, corresponding to the *lymphatic* type of classical antiquity and also in the system of Stiler, in which it is identical with the *ptotic habitus.* See *habitus, ptotic; type, lymphatic.*

atrabiliary, atrabilious *Obs.* Depressed or melancholic.

atrophy, optic A degenerative process involving the optic nerve fibers. The condition is primary or secondary. Primary optic atrophy may occur in tabes, multiple sclerosis, or may be due to poisons such as methyl alcohol, tryparsamide, lead, atoxyl, quinine, carbon bisulfide, and nitrobenzol. Occasionally the condition may occur following severe hemorrhage and in malaria. Ophthalmoscopically, the disk is grayish white in color, with some "cupping," the margins being sharply outlined. See *disease, Leber's.*

Secondary optic atrophy may occur as a

result of optic neuritis and choked disk. Here the fundus, disk, and vessels usually manifest residual signs of the previous condition.

Tumors of the pituitary gland, of the optic chiasm, and in some cases of the frontal lobe frequently give rise to optic atrophy—usually unilateral for a time.

atrophy, peroneal muscular Charcot-Marie-Tooth's disease; neural progressive muscular atrophy. A hereditary disorder, transmitted as a Mendelian dominant, more often affecting males, beginning between the ages of 5 and 10 years, with wasting of the small muscles in the peripheral limbs secondary to degeneration of the peripheral nerves and spinal cord. The muscular wasting results in a steppage gait, "fat bottle" calf when the lower part of the calf is wasted, and "inverted champagne bottle" limb when the lower third of the thigh is wasted. The disease runs a slow course and may become arrested at any stage; it does not shorten life, and there are no associated intellectual changes.

atrophy, progressive muscular See *sclerosis, amyotrophic lateral.*

atropine syndrome See *syndrome, central anticholinergic; therapy, atropine coma.*

attachment Bond, link, and in particular the affective tie between infant and caregiver. The mother is often the primary attachment figure, but the child can bond with many other responsive persons, including other children.

Bowlby interpreted smiling, clinging, vocal signals, and other communications as ways of maintaining attachment to the person(s) who provided protection against predators and comfort in distress. Attachment theory emphasizes the significance of the formation, disruption, and renewal of affective attachment bonds in the most intense human emotions, and Bowlby showed that disruption of those bonds heightens vulnerability to depression or despair. See *bonding.*

attachment disorder of infancy Also reactive attachment disorder of infancy and early childhood; characterized by marked disturbance in social relatedness that begins before the age of 5 years; also sometimes *failure to thrive.* The care of such children has been grossly deficient, either because of persistant disregard for the child's basic emotional needs (for comfort, stimulation, affection, etc.) or physical needs (food, housing, protection from physical abuse or sexual assault, etc.) or because of repeated changing of the primary caregiver so that stable attachments are not made.

attachment, liquidation of Janet uses this term to mean freedom from painful situations. "In this connexion, our first aim must be to put an end to the unceasing efforts occasioned by 'attachments.' We must 'disattach' the patients, we must unravel, as far as may be, the complicated situations in which they find themselves, and in which they have become enmeshed." (*PH*)

attack, first An illness occurring for the first time, whether or not it results in hospitalization, is a first attack.

attack, obsessive Rado's term for the major symptoms (as distinguished from obsessive character traits) of the *obsessive-compulsive psychoneurosis* (q.v.): (1) spells of doubting and brooding, (2) bouts of ritual making, and (3) fits of horrific temptation. According to Rado, obsessive attacks are derived from the temper (rage) tantrums of childhood, but the discharge of rage is slow and incomplete since it is always opposed by guilty fear. He terms this an interference pattern of discharge, i.e. a mechanism for the alternating discharge of opposite tensions. In the motor sphere, alternating discharge is expressed as bouts of ritual making; in the thinking sphere, as brooding spells.

attack, psychomotor A term sometimes used interchangeably with the term *psychic equivalent* of epilepsy. See *equivalent, epileptic.*

attention Conscious and willful focusing of mental energy on one object or one component of a complex experience and at the same time excluding other emotional or thought content; the act of heeding or taking notice or concentrating. Attention depends on consciousness and is thus a part of what is meant by the more general term *sensorium* (q.v.). *Attention span* (also known as *perceptual span*) is the number of briefly presented objects that can be recalled immediately; it is used as a test of immediate *memory* (q.v.).

Kenneth Nakdimen (*Bulletin of the Men-*

ninger Clinic 42, 1978) differentiates between alloplastic and autoplastic attention. He suggests that *alloplastic attention* is mainly a function of the left hemisphere: it is analytic-conceptualizing-abstracting and thus object-altering; it is characterized by maintenance of ego boundaries; and it includes that form of attention to attention that is commonly called *reflection. Autoplastic attention,* on the other hand, is a function of the right hemisphere; it is gestalt-imaging-concretizing attention that is synesthetic and self-altering; it is characterized by diffusion of ego boundaries; and it includes that form of attention called *imagination.*

attention and information processing (AIP) The basic neural steps that prepare the subject for response to a stimulus. The brain is constructed to receive and respond to significant stimuli, and information received through the sensory channels is sorted into relevant categories and distributed to various parts of the brain, which analyze and process the information.

Attention involves extensive areas of the brain (i.e. there is no one "attention center"), but it appears to be more dependent on the reticular formation (concerned with alertness and vigilance) and the right hemisphere than on other areas. Once the stimulus is received, inputs are sent to the cerebellum, reticular formation, and thalamus. Stimuli that eventually become conscious go to special neurons of the thalamus and thence to the cortex. Each kind of sensation goes to a primary sensory area of the cortex, next to the secondary sensory area, then to the association areas (which elaborate sensory information and join the various kinds of input to make a meaningful whole), and finally to the motor areas.

A lesion on one side of the brain may produce an attentional defect ("neglect") of the other side. A woman may apply makeup to only one side of her face, for example, or a man may shave only one side of his face.

attention, blocking of See *blocking.*

attention deficit disorder (ADD) Also attention deficit hyperactivity disorder; attention deficit disorder with hyperactivity (ADDH). A syndrome consisting of inattention, excessive motor activity, and impulsivity. Hyperactivity is manifested in restlessness and poorly organized excess activity that is haphazard, inconsistent, and lacking in clear goal orientation. The child fidgets, is always "on the go" or "running like a motor," and has difficulty sitting still. He frequently disrupts others at play and at work.

Other symptoms include specific learning deficits such as dyslexia; perceptual-motor deficits; defective coordination; lack of response to discipline and antisocial behavior, especialy in adolescence; interpersonal relationships marred by obstinacy, stubbornness, negativism, bullying; emotional lability, low frustration tolerance; temper outburst. In addition, neurologic examination of such children often uncovers "equivocal" abnormalities, or *soft signs,* such as transient strabismus, mixed and confused laterality, speech defects, or borderline EEG record. See *handicap, emotional.*

Etiology is unknown. Some believe it may be due to diencephalic dysfunction.

The syndrome appears early in life (in infancy or by the age of 2 or 3 years), is more common in boys (perhaps by as much as ten times the incidence in girls), and may occur in as many as 3% of prepubertal children. There is a family pattern, manifested in an increased frequency of the disorder in siblings and in the childhood history of parents (especially fathers).

Attention deficit disorder without hyperactivity is similar, but because of the wide variability in maturation of attention the diagnosis should not be made before the age of 4 years; less is known about this group than the hyperkinetic form.

It is recognized that the syndromes are heterogeneous and almost certainly encompass several distinct subgroups. It has been suggested that in at least one of those subgroups there is a strong genetic component, which may account for the frequently observed familial relationship between the hyperactive child syndrome and alcoholism, sociopathy, and hysteria. It has also been hypothesized that the latter disorders represent the persistence and symptomatic transformations of the childhood syndrome into adult life.

The syndromes described have been

given different names, including brain damage behavior syndrome, central nervous system deviation, minimal brain dysfunction (MBD), postencephalitic behavior disorder, choreatiform syndrome, hyperactive child syndrome (HACS), Strauss syndrome, and infantile hyperkinetic syndrome. Because of the heterogeneity of the group to which any of the foregoing labels apply, some workers advocate the abolishment of all of them and call for more intensive efforts to describe discrete subgroups and identify their etiologic mechanisms.

Follow-up studies indicate that the full syndrome persists in about a third of cases, and that a small subgroup (about 5%) have the residual type of ADDH, with attention deficit and impulsivity only. Some studies have also found a significant excess of antisocial personality disorders in adults who were hyperactive children.

Psychostimulants such as amphetamines or methylphenidate are generally effective in reducing hyperactivity and disruptive behavior, and some reports indicate that such drugs also improve academic performance. At the present time, between 1 and 2% of North American children receive psychostimulants as treatment for hyperactivity. Monoamine oxidase inhibitors have also been used successfully with such children; the mechanism of action appears not to be the same as that mediating their antidepressant effects.

attention, deterioration of Bleuler lists this as one of the fundamental symptoms of the schizophrenias, where often there is seen an impairment in the ability to heed, observe, and concentrate on external reality. This fundamental symptom appears to be related to deterioration of affectivity (another fundamental symptom) and the patient's loss of interest in many things about him. The impairment of attention is inconstant and shifting, for attention may appear normal when it is directed to something the patient wants to do. Inability to concentrate is seen also in other psychiatric disorders, but in this latter case it is almost always secondary, i.e. a result of emotional pressure, whereas in the schizophrenias it appears to be primary.

attention-getting Any means of gaining attention and recognition when the ego is

starved for them, as observed most often in a child who feels unloved. At first the child will attempt to do whatever he feels the parents like and will gain their attention. If this is not successful, the child will develop temper tantrums or other behavior disorders, preferring a display of displeasure or even a harsh disciplinary measure to no attention at all.

attention junkie A person who is pathologically dependent on applause, acclaim, approval, or other signs of acceptance by others; often applied to the hysteroid dysphoric. See *dysphoria, hysteroid.*

attentional dysfunction Defective selective or sustained attention, one of the most consistently reported abnormalities in adult schizophrenics. Reaction time measures selective attention; continuous performance tests measure sustained attention. It has been suggested that impaired ability to focus attention interferes with the acquisition of cognitive and social competence skills, and that the appearance of such dysfunction in children may identify specific subgroups who may be at increased risk of schizophrenia.

attitude "A readiness of the psyche to act or react in a certain direction. . . . To have a certain attitude means to be ready for something definite, even though this definite something is unconscious, since having an attitude is synonymous with an *a priori* direction toward a definite thing, whether this be present in consciousness or not." (Jung, *PT*) See *analytic psychology.*

Attempts have been made to measure attitudes but they have been criticized as measuring opinions rather than attitudes.

attitude, abstract See *abstract attitude.*

attitude, captative The early ego's appraisal of the external world solely in terms of the self. See *narcissism.*

attitude, catatonoid A type of behavior that resembles catatonia. According to Fenichel, it may be found in individuals who "are on the verge of becoming psychotic." Apparently, this phrase refers to a certain lack of the expected emotional response in personal or social situations: instead, there is found a stereotyped response, which never varies from situation to situation. For example, if the same vacant smile adorns an individual's countenance when he hears his friend's story of a recent personal tragedy or is told an uproarious anecdote, the individual demonstrates a catatonoid attitude. These stereotyped responses on the part of "schizoid characters," which occur when the individual becomes psychotic, would be easily recognized as catatonic symptoms. (Fenichel, *PTN*)

attitude, collective An *attitude* (q.v.) that is peculiar "not to one individual, but to many, at the same time, i.e. either to a society, a people, or to mankind in general." (Jung, *PT*)

attitude, concretizing The tendency of many schizophrenic patients to transform abstract parts of their life into concrete representations. Thus the patient who feels that his wife poisons his life may express feelings concretely by developing the delusion that she poisons his food.

attitude, fear An expression used by L. Kanner to designate a fear reaction observed in some children "who are literally *always afraid of everything.*" (*Child Psychiatry*, 1935)

attitude, inner Soul, according to Jung's point of view. See *anima*.

attitude, listening The expectation that one is about to hear something. S. Arieti emphasizes that such an attitude typically precedes hallucinations in schizophrenics: "If the patient learns to catch himself in the act of putting himself into the listening attitude. he, after some training, can prevent himself from doing so." (*Archives of General Psychiatry 6*, 1962)

attitude, masculine, in female neurotics. See *masculine attitude in female neurotics*.

attitude, mummy D.K. Henderson and R.D. Gillespie use this expression to denote the inactive, immobilized patient in the state of catatonic stupor.

"Then a state of dull stupor develops, with mutism, refusal of food, and with such a diminution of all activities that the patient may sit idly in one position, with the hands stretched out on the knees, and the head bowed between the shoulders, the whole aspect being that of a mummy." (*A Text-Book of Psychiatry*, 1936)

attitude passionelles See *hysteria*.

attitude, preadaptive The initial reaction to a stimulus or experience, before the subject has become accustomed to it. P. Steckler (*Archives of Neurology and Psychiatry 80*, 1958) notes that the preadaptive

attitude of schizophrenics to hallucinations or feelings of estrangement is of a fairly consistent pattern: anxiety, fear, search for reassurance, doubts as to sanity, search for a rational explanation, and, finally, autonomic and muscular system reactions.

attitude, referential An attitude of expectancy seen in some schizophrenic patients who, feeling themselves to be victims of hostility from others, search for references that will justify the underlying mood. See *attitude, listening*.

attitude therapy See *therapy, attitude*.

attitude tic See *tic, attitude*.

attitude type See *function type*.

attonity (at-on'i-tē) Attonity is a clinical state of stupor with complete or almost complete immobility. Bleuler believes that the condition occurs most frequently in the catatonic form of schizophrenia, though it is also observed in states of depression; it is then known as melancholia attonita. Other authorities consider that the latter designation refers also to the catatonic type of schizophrenia.

attributable risk See *risk factor*.

attribution Assignment of credit or responsibility. An *attribution error* is incorrect assignment of etiological significance, as in overestimating the influence of psychological factors (*dispositional attribution*) or environmental factors (*situational attribution*) in attempting to explain behavior.

atypical childhood psychosis A pervasive development disorder, with onset between 30 months and 12 years of age, consisting of grossly impaired emotional relationships, labile or flattened or inappropriate affect, catastrophic reactions to ordinary stress, resistance to change with ritualistic and repetitive behavior, motility disturbances, self-mutilation, etc. Other terms that have been applied to this disorder are atypical development, symbiotic psychosis, and childhood schizophrenia. See *autism, early infantile; developmental disorders, pervasive*.

atypical development See *development, atypical*.

atypical paranoid disorder See *paranoia*.

atypical polysomnograph disorder See *alpha sleep*.

atypical psychoses See *psychosis, reactive*.

audible thoughts See *symptoms, first-rank*.

audile (aw'dīl) Ear-minded; i.e. understanding better by hearing than by seeing.

audiogenic seizure See *seizure, audiogenic.*

audit Evaluation; *review* (q.v.). Medical audit is also known as *medical care evaluation (MCE);* when the care under review has been provided by nonphysicians the process is termed *patient care audit.*

Medical care evaluation studies are retrospective assessments of the quality of care or the nature of its utilization; they include investigation of suspected problems, analysis of the problems identified, and a plan for corrective action.

Claims review is also a retrospective assessment of the appropriateness of a claim for payment for a service rendered; it includes a determination that the claimant is eligible for reimbursement for the services provided, that charges are consistent with customary fees or published institutional rates, and that the service provided was necessary.

audition, thought A form of auditory hallucination in which everything the patient thinks or speaks is repeated by the voices; also known as *thought echoing* or *echo des pensées.*

auditory feedback See *feedback.*

auditory nerve See *nerve, acoustic.*

Aufgabe See *set.*

aulophobia Fear of seeing, handling, or playing a flute or similar wind instrument, which can be a phallic symbol.

aura A premonitory symptom that warns of some approaching physical or mental disorder. It is a symptom of a special nature in that it is not regarded as an essential part of the disease or disorder, because it disappears or loses its force after it has performed its function of warning.

The term is usually restricted to certain symptoms that appear in genuine epilepsy before the major symptoms set in. Bleuler says: "The attack is often preceded by prodromata which last a few hours, more rarely days; most frequently they are represented by 'moods,' but also by any ill-feeling, more rarely hallucinations and twilight states. In most instances these prodromata disappear in a trice with the attack." (Bleuler, *TP*)

In the grand mal type of epilepsy, an aura precedes loss of consciousness in about 60% of cases (the others are known as the "thunderclap" variety). The aura localizes the epileptogenic focus in the brain and thus appears in many forms, depending upon the specific location of the lesion: (1) *psychic aurae*—complex mental states such as feeling of unreality, or feeling of familiarity and déjà vu and déjà fait, disembodied feeling, intense but inexplicable fear; (2) *sensory aurae*—olfactory and gustatory hallucinations, visual hallucinations with complex scenes or simple flashes of light or balls of fire, auditory hallucinations of words, phrases, or merely crude sounds, and various paresthesiae; (3) *visceral aurae*—vertigo, epigastric discomfort; (4) *motor aurae*—as in cursive epilepsy.

aura cursoria A condition, usually associated with epilepsy, occurring immediately before a seizure and characterized by aimless running.

aurae, auditory (aw're) A form of epilepsy described as sensory seizures in which buzzing noises may occur suddenly, last a short period of time, and then disappear without the patient's having a grand mal attack. This would indicate a focus in the temporal lobe. In grand mal attacks, the patient occasionally may have an auditory aura just prior to the grand mal seizures, as a warning that a convulsive seizure is about to occur.

aurae, visual A form of epilepsy described as sensory seizures in which flashes of light may occur suddenly, last a short period of time, and then disappear without the patient's having a grand mal attack. This would indicate a focus in the temporooccipital area. In grand mal attacks, the patient occasionally may have a visual aura just before the grand mal seizure, as a warning that a convulsive attack is about to occur.

auroraphobia Fear of northern lights.

autarchy (aw'tär-kē) Supreme, autocratic power, absolute sovereignty; used in psychiatry in reference to the early infantile period, when no demands are made on the child and, insofar as possible, his instinctual demands are satisfied immediately. During this period the child is indeed absolute ruler—his slightest cry brings instinctual gratification, there is no need to deny himself pleasure, and there need be no deferral of pleasure.

autemesia Idiopathic vomiting, usually psychogenic in origin.

authoritarianism See *authority, irrational.*

authoritative imperative See *imperative, authoritative.*

authority, irrational Power or command over others that, contrary to reason and logic, is based on neurotic craving for power and has no justification in competence; authority imposed on o'hers through sheer will power, without their consent. Fromm distinguishes this from rational authority, which is based on genuine ability and competence and is exemplified by the teacher imparting knowledge to a pupil. The person who resorts to irrational authority for security may find power by being a *magic helper* (see *helper, magic*) or from various forms of intimidation; he may also find power through identification with the authoritarian force, be it a person, a group, or an idea. Hence Fromm considers Freud's superego a manifestation of authoritarian power.

The classical legend based on a vivid account by Pliny the Elder (*Historia Naturalis XXXV*) that gave rise to a widespread saying is a striking illustration of the gulf between rational and irrational authority. The great Greek painter Apelles (fl. 330 B.C.), who, valuing the opinion of the common folk, was in the habit of showing a new canvas in his studio and, hiding behind a painting, would listen to their observations. A passing shoemaker found fault with one sandal-loop being smaller than the other. The artist redrew it later in the day. The next morning the same shoemaker, emboldened by the artist's compliance, began to jeer about the leg. Emerging from his hiding place, Apelles squelched the glib critic with the crushing: "A cobbler should not judge above the sandal." ("Shoemaker, stick to your last.")

authypnobatesis (awth-hip-nō-bȧ-tē′sis) *Obs.* Spontaneous somnambulism.

autism A form of thinking, more or less genuinely of a subjective character; if objective material enters, it is given subjective meaning and emphasis. Autism generally implies that the material is derived from the subject himself, appearing in the nature of daydreams, phantasies, delusions, hallucinations, etc. The content of thought, in other words, is largely endogenous. In classical instances of autistic thinking, such as occurs in schizophrenia, the unconscious sphere makes the largest contribution to autism.

Autism, dereism, and introversion are closely allied to one another. Some authorities speak of the autistic temperament, meaning by it the introverted, retiring type that shrinks from all contact with life.

Autism, when it is a pervasive and generalized dereistic life-approach, is one of the fundamental symptoms of the schizophrenias (Bleuler).

In the autistic life-approach, the "Me" predominates, often to the exclusion of the "Not-Me," external reality gradually loses more and more of its significance, and the patient is attuned to and guided only by the inner workings of his being. He is totally selfish, in the most literal (and yet nonpejorative) sense of the term, for he is unable to turn his energies onto objects outside himself. He exaggerates the importance of inner physical sensations as well as his own ideas and emotions. He becomes involved in pseudo-philosophical speculations and has no time for mixing with his peers. He feels different from others, complains that he has never realized his potentialities, and is concerned with establishing an identity for himself.

autism, early infantile A syndrome described by Kanner consisting of (1) primary symptoms, including (a) withdrawal and (b) anxious, obsessive desire to maintain the status quo; and (2) secondary symptoms, including (a) exceptional object relationships, (b) intelligent, pensive facies despite low intelligence and, often, auditory impairment, (c) language disturbances, (d) monotonously repetitive motor behavior, and (e) fear of moving objects and loud noise.

Symptoms appear early in life or are present from the beginning: self-absorption, inaccessibility, aloneness, inability to relate, highly repetitive play and rage reactions if interrupted; predilection for rhythmical movements such as rolling, jumping, rocking and whirling; and many language disturbances such as pronominal reversals, inability to accept synonyms, and echolalia.

Incidence of autism has been estimated as 4.5 per 100,000. A genetic cause of the disorder is suggested by the following findings: (1) significant incidence of autism in identical twins and in the sibs of autistic children; (2) high male to female ratio (approximately 3.3 to 1); (3) association with other genetic and neurologic conditions, such as congential rubella, phenylketonuria, trisomy 21, and Schilder's disease. Contrary to earlier suggestions, there is little evidence of any association between autism and fragile X chromosome.

In DSM-III-R, autism is classified as one of the pervasive developmental disorders with onset in infancy (before 36 months of age) or childhood. Major deficits are qualitative impairment in both reciprocal social interaction and communication, and a restricted repertoire of activities, interests, and imaginative development. Manifestations include lack of awareness of the existence or feelings of others (e.g. breaks into a private meeting and does not realize he has intruded); preference for solitary play activities; failure to observe the conventions of social interaction appropriate for his age (e.g. invites playmates to come home with him and then shuts himself in his room without explanation); inadequate or abnormal nonverbal communication (e.g. does not smile when approaching another person socially, body stance is stiff and rigid); stereotyped and repetitive speech mannerisms and idiosyncratic use of words or phrases; abnormal volume, pitch, stress, or rhythm of speech; stereotypies of movement such as rocking or head banging; preoccupation with parts of objects or unusual objects (e.g. endlessly spins the wheels of a toy car or stares for hours in fascination at the spinning of the drier in the laundromat); insistence on routines and sameness; restricted patterns of interest; absence of developmentally appropriate imaginative activity.

autisme pauvre (aw-tēsm′ pōvr′) Literally, impoverished autism; term for the schizophrenic's withdrawal and detachment from reality that is not a deliberate retreat into phantasy life but is instead a product of will and affect disturbances which cut him off from meaningful contact with his environment.

autismus infantum Early infantile autism. See *autism, early infantile*.

autistic (aw-tis′tik) Mental activity that is more or less subjective and removed from reality.

Infancy research has demonstrated that the infant engages actively with the environment and, at least for short periods, regulates incoming stimulation even during the first months of life. Such data cast doubt on the classical theory of a stimulus barrier and a normal autistic phase, if that is defined as disinterest in or failure to register and respond to external stimuli. It seems more likely that the infant's social nature is intrinsically determined and begins to unfold from the earliest days of life.

autistic fantasy In DSM-III-R, a defense mechanism consisting of excessive daydreaming as a substitute for human relationships or more direct and effective action in dealing with conflicts or stressors.

autistic psychopathy See *psychopathy, autistic*.

autistic psychosis See *psychosis, symbiotic infantile*.

autoaggression See *syndrome, deliberate self-harm*.

autocastration, anticipatory A symbolic self-castration appearing as either a symptom or a personality trait, to forestall castration that under the circumstances is unconsciously perceived by the patient as an unavoidable threat. This anticipatory autocastration may be the unconscious reason for "feminine" behavior in boys: if the boy "castrates himself" by acting like a girl, he can no longer be threatened with actual castration.

Fenichel explains this behavior as a manifestation of primitive thinking. If the threatened individual punishes himself, he will be protected by the threatening force, which is the father or superego in unconscious terms. This thinking is clearly seen in prayer or in sacrifices to the gods, where the individual ingratiates himself with the gods by a self-inflicted lesser or symbolic punishment and thus wards off a more severe punishment.

Actual autocastration, however, takes place in some cases and apparently a "passive-submissive merging" with the omnipotent person is obtained thereby: by abandoning all activity the individual shares the omnipotence. By these means religious fanatics endeavor to obtain a union with God. (Fenichel, *PTN*)

autocatharsis Self-expression, especially as a form of therapy wherein the patient is encouraged to write down his experiences, thoughts, and feelings in order to rid himself of disturbing emotions.

autocentric Self-centered.

autochiria *Obs.* Suicide.

autochthonous (aw-tok′thō-nus) Aboriginal to the site of appearance, brought about by the independent activity of the structure in which the activity appears. See *delusion, autochthonous.*

autochthony The state of originating in an organ itself, independent of any essential influences outside of the organ in question. Many organs of the body act in part by virtue of forces inherent in the organs and in part because of forces or factors coming from distant sources. The heart, for instance, continues to beat for a time after it has been removed from the body. It is then said to function autochthonously. The same principle of independent action may be applied to the psyche, in the sense that the psyche can and does originate many of the forces found in it. The expression *psychogenic* carries this implication, for it means "born in the psyche." It is believed, for example, that dreams are products of the psyche; they are autochthonous to the psyche; they are psychogenic.

autoctonia (aw-tok-tō′nē-à) *Obs.* Suicide.

autodysosmophobia An obsessive fear or delusion that the person himself has a vile or repugnant odor; often combined with *automysophobia* (q.v.).

autoecholalia *Verbigeration* (q.v.).

autoechopraxia That form of stereotypy in which the patient, usually schizophrenic, constantly repeats an action which he had formerly experienced. The patient echoes, so to speak, his own motions. When he echoes that of another person, one speaks of echopraxia. Kraepelin says that "the patients stand or kneel for hours, days, or still longer, on the same spot, lie in the most uncomfortable positions in bed, fold their hands spasmodically, even till pressure-sores appear, take up the position of fencing." (*DP*)

autoeroticism, autoerotism Havelock Ellis invented the term "autoerotism" to mean "the phenomena of spontaneous sexual emotion generated in the absence of an external stimulus proceeding, directly or indirectly, from another person." (*Studies in the Psychology of Sex*, 1919)

Common usage has made autoerotism synonymous with masturbation. The latter, however, is a special subdivision of autoerotism. The term onanism has likewise been diverted to mean masturbation or autoerotism, though, as Ellis says, "Onan's device was not auto-erotic, but was an early example of withdrawal before emission, or *coitus interruptus*." (ibid.)

Autoeroticism is also a phase in the development of object relationships (see *ontogeny, psychic*). The drives are present from the beginning of life and at first are amorphous energy potentials in the undifferentiated psyche. Since there are no object relationships at birth, these energies are, perforce, directed to the infant himself. This is the period of autoeroticism, when no distinction is made between the self and the non-self, when little if any heed is paid to the external environment.

In psychoanalytic psychology, autoerotism is considered to be the most primitive form of relationship to the environment; it is followed by the narcissistic stage out of which objects develop. Freud appears to have held concurrently three contradictory views on the nature of the earliest relationship to the environment; in one view autoerotism was considered primary, in another, narcissism, and in still another, the most primitive relationship was considered to be primary object love. See *narcissism, primary.*

According to Abraham, the autoerotic stage first becomes manifest during the oral sucking period. It is the opinion of some (Rickman) that autoerotism is distinguished from narcissism in that the former is objectless, while in narcissism the "I" is recognizable. When the infant takes his own body as the love object, the condition is known as narcissism.

autoeroticism, secondary Self-pleasure indirectly connected with the erogenous zones. For example, the pleasure associated, not with the act of urination, but with the urine itself, is called secondary autoeroticism. A patient in the manic phase of manic-depressive psychosis drank her own urine.

autofellatio Putting one's own penis into one's mouth. "A considerable portion of the population does record attempts at self-fellation, at least in early adolescence. Only two or three males in a thousand are able to achieve the objective, but there are three or four histories of males who had depended upon self-fellation as a masturbatory technique for some appreciable period of time—in the case of one thirty-year-old-male, for most of his life." (Kinsey, A.C., et al. *Sexual Behavior in the Human Male*, 1948)

autofetishism Hirschfeld's term for the state of loving a material object (e.g. article of clothing) of one's own possession. The object acts as a sexual excitant.

autoflagellation Hirschfeld's term for the act of whipping oneself as a sexual excitant.

autogenic training A technique used to elicit the *relaxation response* (q.v.), consisting of six exercises: (1) focus on feelings of heaviness in the limbs; (2) cultivate a sense of warmth in the limbs; (3) concentrate on heart rate, (4) breathing, (5) warmth of the upper abdomen, and (6) coolness in the forehead.

autogeny, autogenic See *endogenous; endogeny.*

autognosis (aw-tog-nō'sis) Knowledge of oneself.

autohypnosis Self-hypnosis. In one of Freud's early communications (*Physical Mechanism of Hysterical Phenomena,* 1893), he emphasized the need on the part of the patient not only to remember the painful experience, but to live out its affect at the same time. He called this abreaction. Some patients are able to abreact on occasion when under the influence of autohypnosis.

autoimmunity An immunologic aberration in which antibody or sensitized lymphocyte reacts with the organism's own tissue. Whether the autoantibody causes, results from, or is merely coincident to human disease is unknown, even though it is a common belief that autoantibody attacks tissue and thereby causes autoimmune disease (*AID*)—among which are warm- and cold-antibody acquired hemolytic anemia, lupus erythematosus, chronic membranous glomerulonephritis, Hashimoto's thyroiditis, rheumatoid arthritis, mysasthenia gravis, scleroderma, and perhaps ulcerative colitis and some types of rheumatic heart disease. An alternative hypothesis is equally tenable—that autoimmunity may be due to genetically determined immunologic deficiencies which render the organism unable to respond immunologically to antigens (e.g. bacterium, virus, myoplasm, or other microorganism) that a normal immune system would readily eliminate. According to such a hypothesis, autoantibodies may be a secondary mechanism designed to eliminate the tissue killed or damaged by the antigen and/or designed to protect the attacked organ from further damage.

Human leukocyte antigens (HLAs) are the distinguishing markers of tissue types. There are more than 80 marker substances and hence thousands of possible combinations that are crucial to the regulation of the body's natural immune defense system. The gene complex of HLA is located on the short arm of chromosome 6. In many autoimmune diseases (including juvenile diabetes, myasthenia gravis, rheumatoid arthritis, systemic lupus, and perhaps narcolepsy) particular HLA types are found much more frequently than in the general population. The strongest association between an HLA substance and human disease was reported in 1971 by Paul Terasaki: HLA-B27, which is found in fewer than 6% of Americans, is present in more than 90% of persons who develop ankylosing spondylitis. HLA profiles are associated with disease susceptibility to a greater extent than any other known genetic marker in humans.

autoinfection, mental *Obs.* With this term Kornfeld in 1897 denoted a psychotic state in which the person believes himself wronged and brings every misfortune and unpleasant event into relation with his delusion.

autointoxication *Obs.* A term denoting toxicity allegedly due to the absorption of the waste products of metabolism or of the products of intestinal decomposition.

autokinesis Self-movement; frequently used in a specific way to designate the phenomenon of seeing and tracing the "movement" of a stationary pinpoint of light in a dark room. Persons with high autokinetic perception are said to demonstrate greater ego autonomy and more independent, nonconforming attitudes.

autolibido See *libido.*

autology Study of the self; self-analysis.

automagnetization Autosuggestion.

automasochism A term used by Hirschfeld synonymously with Freud's conception of *masochism* (q.v.).

automatic seizures A type of psychomotor epilepsy. See *epilepsy*.

automatism A condition in which activity is carried out without conscious knowledge on the part of the subject. Automatic actions and speech are seen in clear form in the catatonic form of schizophrenia in which incessant repetition may prevail without the patient's awareness. Automatisms are common also in other clinical states, particularly in those associated with a *fugue* (q.v.).

"Automatic actions are not directly noticed by the patient himself; he neither feels that he wishes to accomplish the action, nor that he executes it. If the action lasts for some time, he takes notice of it like a third person, by observing and listening." (Bleuler, *TP*) See *obedience, automatic*.

automatism, ambulatory A rhythmic form of automatic activity.

automatism, ambulatory comitial (kō-mish′ al) Tuke's term to denote automatic acts often observed in epileptic patients.

automatism, command A patient who strictly obeys a command, without the exercise of any critical judgment, is said to show command automatism. The condition may be induced through hypnosis. It is not uncommon during the stage of hypersuggestibility in the catatonic form of schizophrenia; the patient may "automatically" follow orders that lead to dangerous results.

automatism, postictal See *epilepsy*.

automatism, primary ictal A type of psychomotor epilepsy. See *epilepsy*.

automatization The process whereby an action becomes routine and automatic, without conscious effort or direction. While discussing the probable fundamental reason for the development of a neurosis, Waelder defines a neurosis as "the automatization of anxiety reaction," the individuals "remaining perpetually infantile in an important part of their being." A neurotic subject is therefore regarded as an automaton, acting at the mercy of his infantile impulses. The schizophrenic, whose life is built around concepts of infancy, succumbs completely to the deeply lying forces of his unconscious. The compulsive neurotic must give automatic obedience to his symptoms.

automonosexualism *Rare. Narcissism* (q.v.).

automysophobia Morbid dread that the person himself is filthy or smells bad—not infrequently a symptom of psychoneurosis.

autonomasia A variety of amnesic aphasia, characterized by an inability to recall names or substantives.

autonomic-affective law See *law, autonomic-affective*.

autonomic nervous system Vegetative nervous system. "The autonomic nervous system consists of a series of cerebrospinal nuclei and nerves with widely distributed ganglia and plexuses which subserve the vegetative functions of the body. In its peripheral ramifications the system is characterized by a series of synaptic junctions which are situated outside the central nervous system. From anatomic and physiologic points of view there are two primary divisions: (1) the parasympathetic, or craniosacral, and (2) the sympathetic, orthosympathetic or thoracicolumbar. This subdivision is based upon the point of outflow from the central nervous system, the distribution of peripheral ganglia, the general antagonism in physiologic effects on visceral tissues most of which receive innervation from both divisions, and the response to pharmacologic agents. Each peripheral division of the autonomic nervous system is characterized by a two-neuron chain and consists of two histologic elements, the preganglionic neuron which terminates in a peripheral ganglion, whence the postganglionic neuron of the second order carries impulses to their destinations on the viscera. No impulse goes directly to an organ of termination. Anatomically the two divisions are designated the craniosacral and the thoracicolumbar portions, or outflows, but clinically the favored terms are either parasympathetic and sympathetic systems or parasympathetic and sympathetic divisions." (DeJong, R.N. *The Neurologic Examination*, 1950)

The autonomic nervous system is under control of higher centers, the most important of which is the hypothalamus. The hypothalamus appears to be the chief subcortical center for the regulation of both sympathetic and parasympathetic activities and for the integration of these. The anterior and medial nuclei of the hypothalamus are chiefly concerned with parasympathetic functions, while the lateral and posterior hypothalamic nuclei are chiefly concerned with sympathetic regulation.

autonomous ego functions Basic psychological capacities that form the basis for the development of the *ego* (q.v.), such as attention, arousal, social relatedness (typically manifested in the infant as pleasure or smiling when held), and motivation.

autonomy The quality or state of being self-governing. The living organism does not represent merely an inactive element but is, to a large extent, a self-governing entity. The biological process therefore is not entirely a result of external forces, but is in part governed by specific biological forces which are endogenous. The organism possesses a certain degree of freedom in the sense of Spinoza: it acts according to its own inherent nature, which is based on intrinsic forces, and not under the compulsion of outside influences.

autonomy-heteronomy The autonomy of the organism is not absolute: the self-determination is restricted by outside influences that are heteronomous with relation to the organism. Every organismic process is always a resultant of two components, autonomy and heteronomy (endogenous and exogenous factors). In living beings of different species we find marked variations in the importance of autonomous and heteronomous determinants in their lives. Autonomy essentially means self-government; heteronomy means government from the outside. The expression autonomy-heteronomy is also used on the symbolic level, for instance, in relation to self-awareness. There is no absolute separation between the biological subject and the environment and therefore there is no sharp boundary between the experience of the self and the outside world. There are only degrees of ego proximity and ego distance. The degrees of ego proximity and ego distance are the symbolic expressions of the gradient of autonomy-heteronomy.

autonomy, sense of Erickson's phrase for that aspect of the ego that allows it to maintain its identity and to continue its integrative work even during the regressive pull of the middle game transference. Like the similar *cohesive self* (Kohut) and *object constancy* (Kernberg), the sense of autonomy is a measure of ego strength. See *game, middle*.

autonomy vs. doubt One of Erikson's eight stages of man. See *ontogeny, psychic*.

autonyctobatesis (aw-tō-nik-tō-bȧ-tē′sis) *Obs.* Somnambulism.

autopathic *Obs.* Feeling that has been distorted by self-consciousness and bias. Contrasted with *orthopathic* (q.v.).

autopathy (aw-top′ȧ-thē) Disease or disorder without apparent cause.

autophagy (aw-tof′ȧ-jē) Biting or eating one's own flesh.

autophilia Self-love; narcissism.

autophobia Morbid fear of being alone; fear of self.

autophonia *Obs.* Suicide.

autophonomania *Obs.* Suicidal insanity.

autoplasty The process of adapting by changing one's self, rather than by altering the external environment. Autoplastic adaptation may be normal and healthy (the patient's change in the course of psychoanalytic treatment, for example, which results from an autoplastic identification with the analyst), or they may be neurotic (as in symptom formation). See *alloplasty*.

autopsy negative death See *Bell's mania*.

autopsyche The mind of one's self.

autopsychosis, moral *Obs. Moral insanity*, i.e. psychopathic behavior traits, based on schizophrenia.

autoreceptor A receptor that controls the synthesis and release of neurotransmitters within the neuron on which it is located; sometimes called the presynaptic receptor to distinquish it from the postsynaptic receptor that is part of the feedback loop mechanism that mediates neurotransmitters originating from the antecedent neuron. Autoreceptor is the preferred term, however, because such receptors are located on the cell body and dendrites as well as in the presynaptic position on the nerve terminal.

autosadism *Masochism* (q.v.). "The first stage of sadism is thus aggression linked with activity against an outside object. The second stage, which may appear as a form of defense, consists of a turning against the subject which is identical with a change of object (auto-sadism). If the object is entirely absorbed by the ego, then the sadism is transformed into secondary masochism, which then grafts itself upon the primary masochism preceding the sadism, and strengthens it." (Nunberg. H. *Principles of Psychoanalysis*, 1955)

autoscopy Seeing one's "self" or "double" usually as the face and bust that imitate the movement and facial expressions of the original. The double typically appears misty, hazy, or semitransparent, and associated auditory, kinesthetic, and emotional perceptions are frequent. The commonest emotional reactions are sadness and bewilderment. Two forms of autoscopy are recognized: (1) symptomatic autoscopy, on an organic basis (such as irritative lesions in the temporoparietal lobes); and (2) idiopathic autoscopy, presumably a wish-fulfilling mechanism.

autosomal recessive See *recessiveness*.

autosome Ordinary chromosome that has no relation to sex and is distinguishable from the heterosome or sex chromosome. See *chromosome; sex determination*.

autosomnambulism Somnambulism occasioned by *self-hypnosis*.

autosuggestibility The state of influencing oneself; self-suggestibility.

autosuggestion When suggestion comes from the subject it is called autosuggestion, in contradistinction to heterosuggestion, that which emanates from another.

autosymbolism Hallucinations that represent, in symbolic form, what is thought or felt at a given instant. Autosymbolism is a phenomenon of the hypnagogic state, when neither full sleep nor full waking is predominant. It consists, essentially, of translation of thoughts into pictures and to this extent is identical with dream formation, differing from the latter only in that the other factors in dreamwork are absent.

autosynnoia (aw-tō-sin-oi'à) *Obs.* Complete or almost complete self-centeredness.

autotelik Pertaining to behavior and traits that express the central aims of the person, such as self-preservation.

autotomia In zoology this term refers to the severance of a part of the body; according to Ferenczi, this phenomenon appears to have its analogue in human activity. Some patients mutilate or cut off parts of the body that offend them. "A similar tendency for freeing oneself from a part of the body which causes pain is demonstrated in the normal 'scratch-reflex,' where the desire to scratch away the stimulated part is clearly indicated, in the ten-

dencies to self-mutilation in catatonia and in the like tendencies symbolically represented in the automatic actions of many tic patients." (*FCT*)

autotopagnosia (aw-tō-top-ag-nō'sē-à) Inability to identify or orient the body or the relation of its individual parts, i.e. a defect in appreciation of the body scheme. This type of agnosia occurs in lesions of the thalamoparietal pathways of the cortex in the region of the angular gyrus. The patient with such a lesion behaves as if he had no arm or leg on that side, even though he may feel stimuli on that side if his attention is called to the limb.

avalanche, law of See *conduction, avalanche; law of avalanche*.

Avellis' syndrome (George Avellis, German laryngologist, 1864–1916) A bulbar syndrome due to involvement of the vagus nerve and the bulbar portion of the spinal accessory nerve. Symptoms are homolateral paralysis of the soft palate, pharynx, and larynx and contralateral dissociate hemianesthesia, with loss of sensations of pain and temperature but not of touch and pressure.

aversion, partial *Antifetishism* (q.v.).

aversion therapy *Deterrent therapy;* treatment of alcoholism and alcohol abuse in which the ingestion of alcohol following classical conditioning is paired with an aversive stimulus (such as vomiting, electrical shock, or thoughts of undesirable consequences) so that the ingestion of alcohol in itself comes to evoke aversive thoughts or responses. Techniques include the use of chemical agents such as emetine to produce vomiting (*chemical aversion therapy*) and electroshock (*electrical aversion therapy*).

aviophobia Fear of flying.

avoidance A defense mechanism, akin to *denial* (q.v.), consisting of refusal to encounter situations, objects, or activities because they represent unconscious sexual or aggressive impulses and/or punishments for those impulses. Avoidance is a major defense in *phobia* and *anxiety hysteria* (qq.v.).

avoidant Negatively oriented or moving away from; an avoidant drive or behavior or response is a situation that results in behavior drawing away from the stimulus. Withdrawal behavior and defense reactions are types of avoidant behavior. Also known as abient behavior.

avoidant disorder See *anxiety disorders of childhood.*

avoided relationship See *group tension, common.*

avoiders See *anxiety typology.*

AVT Arginine vasotocin; a nonapeptide found in the pineal gland which may be involved in the regulation of sleep.

awakening, delayed See *paralysis, sleep.*

Awl, William M. (1799–1876) American psychiatrist; one of the "original thirteen" founders of the Association of Medical Superintendents of America (the forerunner of The American Psychiatric Association).

axial hyperkinesia See *hyperkinesia, axial.*

axon, axone See *neuron.*

aypnia (a-ip′nē-à) Insomnia, sleeplessness.

B

B type behavior See *type A*.

babbling A form of speech preceding articulate speech, characterized by sound combinations devoid of meaning.

Babcock sentence(s) Any of the statements suggested by Babcock (1930) to test a subject's ability to learn new information and reproduce it immediately. One that is frequently used is: One thing a nation must have to become rich and great is a large secure supply of wood.

Babinski-Nageotte's syndrome (Joseph François Felix Babinski, Paris physician 1857–1932, and Jean Nageotte, Paris histologist, 1866–1948) A bulbar syndrome produced by scattered lesions of the glossopharyngeal, vagus, spinal accessory (bulbar portion), and trigeminal nerves. Symptoms are homolateral paralysis of the tongue, pharynx, and larynx; homolateral loss of taste in posterior tongue; homolateral Horner's syndrome; homolateral loss of pain and temperature sense in the face; homolateral asynergia and ataxia with a tendency to fall to the side of the lesion; contralateral hemiplegia, and contralateral dissociate hemianesthesia with loss of pain and temperature sense but preservation of touch and pressure.

Babinski's reflex Described by Babinski in 1898 and 1903, as extension of the toes instead of flexion when stimulating the sole of the foot. It "consists in the comparatively slow dorsal extension of the great toe when the plantar reflex is tested and at the same time there is a slight spreading apart of the toes." (Jelliffe & White, *DNS*) The same phenomenon (great toe extension) may be produced by other tests—under *reflex* see *Chaddock, Gordon, Oppenheim*.

baby talk A form of speech characterized by defective articulation of certain conso-

nants; it is rapidly outgrown unless adults in the environment contribute to its maintenance by using it themselves in conversing with the child. In severe behavior disorders and schizophrenia, the patient may revert to this type of speech.

bacillophobia Morbid fear of bacilli or of microorganisms in general.

background *Ground* (q.v.).

backlash A type of *feedback* (q.v.), referring to the effect of its own overt responses upon the organism.

backwardness Educational retardation due not to intrinsic, but to extrinsic causes. "When these causes can be removed the arrears are usually made up, although in some cases this may not entirely take place. They compose about one-third of all retarded children. The causes of extrinsic backwardness are numerous, but may be grouped under the heading of (1) environmental or social; (2) physical." (Tredgold, *TMD*)

bacteriophage See *recombinant DNA*.

bad object See *object, bad*.

bad self See *self, bad*.

β-adrenergic circulatory state See *circulatory state, hyperdynamic β-adrenergic*.

bag lady See *street people*.

Bailey, Percival (1892–1973) Neurologist, neurosurgeon, neuropsychiatrist; best known for *Classification of the Tumors of the Glioma Group* and for his books on cytoarchitecture of primate and human brains.

Baillarger, Jules (bà-yär-zhä′) (1809–90) French psychiatrist; investigated manic-depressive insanity as *folie à double forme* (1853–54) and *cretinism* (1873).

BAL Blood alcohol level; also British anti-Lewisite—a chelating agent used as an antidote for poisoning by ingestion of particles of heavy metals such as antimony, arsenic, bismuth, chromium, gold, lead, mercury, and nickel.

balance, group The result of grouping patients in accordance with clinical and personal criteria in order to prevent intensification of a specific problem or set of problems.

balanced placebo design A research technique that allows for the effect of the subject's belief about what treatment he has received, by giving the experimental drug to one group of subjects who believe they have been given a placebo and giving a placebo to a second group who believe they have received the experimental drug.

balbutiate (bal-bū'shē-āt) *Rare.* To stammer.

balbuties (bal-boo'tē-ēz) *Stammering* or *stuttering* (qq.v.). Some authorities differentiate among *balbuties praecox* (starting before the age of 3 years), *balbuties vulgaris* (onset between the ages of 3 and 7), and *balbuties tarda* (onset after the age of 7).

ballismus Sudden, rapid extension of a limb.

ballistophobia Abnormal fear of missiles.

balmy Lay term for crazy in the United States. Based on the mispronounciation of *barmy,* derived from Barming (Kent County, England), the site of a large psychiatric hospital.

balneology *Obs.* Study of waters used in baths.

balneum calidum *Obs.* Hot bath.

balneum frigidum *Obs.* Cold bath.

Baló's disease Concentric demyelination. See *sclerosis, diffuse.*

bangungut A culture-specific syndrome reported among male Filipino and Laotian youths; death from cardiac arrhythmia initiated by frightening dreams; also called *Oriental nightmare-death syndrome.*

baquet See *Mesmer.*

baragnosis (bar-ag-nō'sis) Absence of ability to recognize weight of objects, generally tested by placing objects in the hand; indicative of parietal lobe lesion.

barbiturates A group of central nervous system depressants that are chemical derivatives of barbituric acid (malonyl-urea); among them are phenobarbital, Amytal, pentobarbital, Seconal, Evipal, and Pentothal. There are many similarly acting sedative and hypnotic drugs that produce the same kinds of complications, abuse, and dependency as seen with the barbiturates; among them are minor tranquilizers (e.g. chlordiazepoxide, diazepam, meprobamate, oxazepam) and hypnotics (e.g. chloral hydrate, ethchlorvynol, flurazepam, glutethimide, methaqualone, methyprylon, paraldehyde).

Of particular interest in psychiatry is the increasingly important role the sedatives and hypnotics have been playing as addicting drugs. They are classified within psychoactive *substance abuse and dependence disorders* (q.v.) because they are associated with both abuse and dependence. Abuse is characterized by continuous or episodic use of the drug(s) for at least one month, impairment in social or occupational functioning, psychological dependence (dyscontrol) manifested in a compulsive craving for them or an inability to reduce, stop or otherwise regulate their use; and in many abusers a grossly pathologic pattern of use, such as remaining intoxicated throughout the day, using very high dosages, or having two or more blackouts (amnesic periods without loss of consciousness while using the substance). Dependence on the drug(s) further involves tolerance (increasing amounts of the substance are required to achieve the desired effect; a daily intake of 100 capsules of 1½ grains strength of barbiturate is not unheard of) and/or development of withdrawal symptoms after cessation or reduction of intake.

In DSM-III-R the distinction between drug abuse and drug dependence is no longer drawn. Instead, dependence includes all clinically significant behaviors that indicate a serious degree of involvement with the drug. Barbiturate dependence is within the category of "sedative or hypnotic dependence." See *dependence, drug.*

Symptoms of intoxication (i.e. indicators of abuse or dependence) include lability of mood, disinhibition of sexual and aggressive impulses, irritability, garrulity, slurred speech, poor coordination, unsteady gait, impaired attention or memory, impaired judgment, failure to meet responsibilities, and other signs of impaired social, occupational, or academic functioning.

Withdrawal symptoms follow cessation or reduction of use in persons dependent on the substance(s): nausea, vomiting, malaise, weakness, autonomic hyperactivity (sweating, rapid pulse, elevated blood pressure), insomnia, orthostatic hypotension, coarse tremor of hands, tongue, or eyelids, and grand mal seizures (in 75% of those with barbiturate dependence who withdraw abruptly).

A withdrawal delirium occurs in some (in as many as 60% of abrupt barbiturate withdrawals), manifested by autonomic hyperactivity, disturbance of attention, and inability to sustain goal-directed thinking or behavior, impaired memory and orientation, altered sleeping/waking pattern and level of psychomotor activity, and perceptual disturbances manifested as simple misinterpretation, illusions, or hallucinations.

Prolonged heavy use of this group of substances may be associated with an amnestic syndrome, characterized by impairment of short-term memory (leading to failure to store memory, inability to retrieve memories and, sometimes, confabulation), but retention of immediate memory. More extensive impairment is seen with barbiturate *dementia* (q.v.).

baresthesia (bàr-es-thē′zē-à) Pressure sense.

barognosis (bar-og-nō′sis) The sense of weight-differences, usually by lifting objects in the hand.

barophobia Fear of gravity.

Barr bodies Sex chromatin; a densely staining chromatin patch on the inner surface of the nuclear membrane, first described by Barr and Bertram in 1949. It was originally believed that the sex chromatin consisted of parts of both of the X chromosomes that the female possesses, but currently most workers subscribe to the "Lyon hypothesis"—early in the embryonic development of the female one X chromosome in each cell is inactivated and becomes the sex chromatin. The number of Barr bodies is always less than the number of X chromosomes possessed.

barrier Boundary; limit; obstruction; separation. In psychiatry, the word is generally used in three contexts: (1) the neurophysiologic, to refer to the functional obstruction of the free flow of constituents of the blood into the brain (see *barrier, blood-brain*); (2) the interpersonal, to refer to an absent or defective ability to form adequate relationships with people—the *schizophrenic barrier* is thus considered a type of autistic behavior based on an ego

defect, although the phrase is on occasion used to refer to lack of relatedness between different parts of the schizophrenic's personality; and (3) in projective testing where *barrier response* is used to indicate a response that emphasizes the periphery of a percept and highlights the boundary (e.g. "turtle with shell," "man in armor"). Responses that emphasize weakness and permeability (e.g. "a gaping wound," "a torn rug") are called *penetration responses*. Schizophrenic patients tend to have fewer barrier responses and more penetration responses than neurotic or "normal" subjects.

barrier, blood-brain A hypothesized resistance or obstruction to the free flow of various constituents of the blood into the brain; also known as *hematoencephalic barrier*, it is the interface between capillaries and the glial protoplasm (of astrocytes and/or dendroglia). It is probable that many other factors influence entry of metabolites into the brain, such as carbon dioxide content of blood (which affects permeability of brain capillaries) and circulating antibodies. "The term barrier-antibody system is thus proposed to denote both fixed and circulating barrier components, whose functions are defense, and the maintenance of a selective internal environment for the brain." (Bogoch, S. *Archives of Neurology and Psychiatry 80,* 1958)

barrier, incest The ego's defenses against incestuous impulses, which are formed mainly in the latency period by deflection of infantile impulses from their sexual aims, with resultant desexualization of impulses.

Bartley v. Kremens See *consumerism.*

baryglossia *Obs.* Thick, heavy speech, usually implying a disorder of the tongue.

barylalia An indistinct and thick speech, observed principally in patients with an organic lesion, often in the central nervous system (Broca's area). It is common in advanced states of general paresis.

baryphonia A heavy quality of voice; generally deep and hoarse.

barythymia *Rare.* Depression of emotions. It is generally accompanied by difficulty in thinking and acting.

basal ganglia Masses of gray matter lying deep within each cerebral hemisphere.

The basal ganglia are composed of (1) corpus striatum, including (a) pallidum (globus pallidus), (b) neostriatum (putamen and caudate nucleus), and (c) amygdala and claustrum; and (2) the internal capsule. The lenticular nucleus is used to refer to the outer putamen and the globus pallidus. The corpus striatum is an important unit of the *extrapyramidal system* (q.v.). The neostriatum receives fibers from the thalamus and the cortex (frontal cortex and pyramidal tract) and sends efferents mainly to the pallidum. The pallidum sends efferents to the thalamus, hypothalamus, subthalamus, substantia nigra, midbrain, pons, and medulla. (Authors vary as to what is included in the basal ganglia, and some include any or all of the following: substantia nigra, subthalamic nucleus of Luys, amygdala, cerebellum, locus coeruleus, red nucleus, and thalamus.)

Lesions in the corpus striatum may cause various symptoms, including muscular rigidity, involuntary movements (e.g. tremor, chorea, athetosis), and hypotonia. Lesions of the globus pallidus or substantia nigra are most commonly associated with muscular rigidity and tremor, as in Parkinsonism.

The internal capsule is a band of white fiber tracts separating the lenticular nucleus from the caudate and thalamus. It contains all the fibers that ascend to and descend from the cortex: pyramidal tract, thalamocortical fibers, optic radiation from the lateral geniculate body, auditory radiation from the medial geniculate body, fronto- and temporopontine tracts, fibers of the corpus striatum, and the corticothalamic tracts. Lesions in the internal capsule, common in cerebrovascular accidents, result in contralateral spastic hemiplegia.

Basedow's disease Hyperthyroidism or overactivity of the thyroid gland. Karl A. von Basedow, German physician (1799–1854), described the disease exophthalmic goiter in 1840. It is characterized by enlargement of the thyroid gland, protrusion of the eyeballs, rapid heart action, fine muscular tremors, and so-called general nervousness. It is as commonly called Grave's disease and less frequently Begbie's, Marsh's, Parry's, Parsons', or Flajani's disease.

basic anxiety See *anxiety, basic*.

basic assumptions group See *group, basic assumptions*.

basic fault See *fault, basic*.

BASIC-ID An acronym devised to refer to what A. Lazarus, the originator of *multimodal therapy*, considers the core elements in human life and conduct: **b**ehaviors, **a**ffective processes, **s**ensations, **i**mages, **c**ognitions, and **i**nterpersonal relationships springing from a biologic matrix. For mnemonic reasons, the biologic is represented by **d**rugs, and the second part of the acronym becomes **ID** as in identity.

Multimodal therapy, also known as *multimodal behavior therapy*, is a form of brief psychotherapy that utilizes many techniques drawn from different sources without necessarily accepting the theory or system underlying each technique. In multimodal therapy, a *modality profile* is constructed for the patient that consists of a chart listing both problems and proposed treatments for each of the elements in the BASIC-ID. This enables the therapist to devise the best method or combination of treatment approaches for each patient and avoids the difficulties inherent in trying to fit every patient into the same form of therapy.

basic mistakes In Adlerian psychology, incidents, concepts, and attitudes of early childhood that have determined or contributed to a person's lifestyle, which must be corrected if the patient is to be helped. They are revealed through exploration in psychotherapy of the patient's early recollections. See *constancy*.

basic trust See *relatedness*.

basiphobia Morbid fear of walking. It is common in the psychoneuroses, less so in the psychoses. Generally it is related to fear of collapse and death, rather than to fear of objects while walking.

basistasiphobia *Stasibasiphobia* (q.v.).

basophobia *Basiphobia* (q.v.).

basostasophobia *Stasibasiphobia* (q.v.).

Bastian's law (Henry C. Bastian, English neurologist, 1837–1915) In severe crush or complete interruption of the spinal cord, there results a total and permanent loss of reflexes with flaccid paralysis; death ensues within a few days or weeks.

bath, continuous "The *continuous bath* is a valuable therapeutic agent in the management of the very excited, delirious, and exhausted patients. The tub is arranged for a continuous inflow and outflow of water at a constant temperature of approximately 98°F. The patient is permitted to lie comfortably in a canvas suspended in the the tub, and the body immersed in water." (Sands, I.J. *Nervous and Mental Diseases for Nurses*, 1937)

bathophobia Morbid dread of depths. The term commonly refers to fear of height, that is, fear of losing control of oneself while in a high place; it is a fear of falling from the height and of thus being killed. The fear is common among normal people, but they can control the impulse without much anxiety. It is morbid when the anxiety is intense and lasting and leads to measures to avoid high places. Common to many psychiatric conditions, it gains particular prominence among psychoneurotic subjects. It is symbolic of an unconscious impulse, the nature of which is unknown to the person ruled by the fear.

bathyesthesia (ba-thē-es-thē′z[h]ē-à) Deep sensibility; sensibility of the parts of the body beneath the surface. "Here deep pressure pain, muscle and joint sense and bony sensibility are to be tested. Deep pressure with the thumb and fingers, or a special instrument (baresthesiometer) is used. The pressure should be sufficient to cause pain." (Jelliffe & White, *DNS*)

batophobia Fear of (being on or passing) high objects or buildings.

batrachophobia Fear of frogs.

battarismus (bat-ar-iz′mus) *Stammering; stuttering* (qq.v.); hesitating speech.

battered child See *syndrome, battered child.*

Battery, Quantitative Electrophysiological Often referred to as *QEB;* a computer analysis of the evoked potentials of the brain as the subject is confronted during a 15- to 50-minute session by a series of changes in his environment (*challenges*); devised by E. Roy John and his co-workers as part of a methodology they term *neurometrics* (q.v.).

battle fatigue See *shell shock.*

Battle sign (William Henry Battle, London surgeon, 1855–1936) Postauricular and subconjunctival ecchymosis in cases of fracture of the base of the skull.

Bayle's disease Antoine Bayle, French physician (1799–1858), first described it in 1822. *Obs.* Commonly known as general paralysis or *paresis;* dementia paralytica.

β-CCE β-carboline-3-carboxylic acid ethyl ester, a high-affinity benzodiazepine-receptor ligand that blocks the anticonvulsant, anxiolytic, and sedative-hypnotic actions of benzodiazepines.

bdelygmia (dē-lig′mē-à) A Hippocratic term referring to a morbid loathing of food.

BDI *Beck Depression Inventory* (q.v.).

BEAM Brain electrical activity mapping, an imaging technique that provides a topographic display of scalp-recorded signals from the EEG electrodes. It is sometimes called *spectral photography.* See *neurometrics.*

Beard, George Miller (1840–83) American psychiatrist; introduced the term *neurasthenia* in a paper, "Neurasthenia or Nervous Exhaustion," *Boston Medical and Surgical Journal LXXX,* 1869.

beating Flagellation. Beating phantasies accompanying masturbation were discussed as a form of perversion by Freud. In the girl, beating phantasies typically go through three stages of development; first the father is beating a sibling, next he beats the girl herself, and finally he beats the other children again, but these are boys and need not be siblings. In the boy, beating phantasies develop in two stages: in the first, the father is beating the boy, and in the second it is the mother who is beating him. In both sexes, the phantasies originate from an incestuous attachment to the father; the boy evades the threat of homosexuality by transforming the beating father into the beating mother, while the girl transforms herself in phantasy into a man and derives masochistic pleasure from what appears on the surface to be a sadistic phantasy.

Bechtereff-Mendel reflex (V.M. Bechtereff, Russian neurologist, 1857–1927 and Kurt Mendel, German physician, 1874–1946) Also known as the cuboidodigital or dorsocuboidal reflex; by striking the outer part of the dorsum of the foot, there results normally a dorsal flexion of the toes; in abnormal conditions such as pyramidal tract disease, there is plantar flexion.

Beck Depression Inventory (BDI) A scale of 21 items designed to provide a quantitative assessment of depressive disorders. The subject is asked to rate each statement on a scale from zero to three to indicate the severity of depression.

Bedlam The name of the Priory of St. Mary of Bethlehem, founded in London in 1247, turned into a mental hospital in 1402 and incorporated in 1547 as the Hospital of St. Mary of Bethlehem. The proper name of this first English "lunatic asylum" became a common appellation for "lunatic asylum" in general and, still later, synonymous with states of frenzy, excitement, wild tumult, pandemonium.

bedlamism *Rare.* A word or act that is characteristic of psychosis or of psychotic individuals; a trait of psychosis.

bedlamite *Obs.* Psychotic person.

Beers, Clifford W. (American layman, 1876–1943) In 1909 founded National Committee for Mental Hygiene (now called National Association for Mental Health); wrote *A Mind That Found Itself.*

Beevor's sign (Charles Edward Beevor, British neurologist, 1854–1908) Upward excursion of the umbilicus, observed when the lower half of the abdominal muscles are paralyzed.

beggar, emotional A term describing that type of person who is always "holding his mental palm out to people, yet always expecting it to be slapped down." The emotional beggar has been unable to detach himself from his parents (usually the parent of the opposite sex). "He cannot get away from the desire to possess and be possessed" by the parent and "is always seeking more, no matter how close to the parent he has managed to attach himself emotionally. This impulse usually begins in infancy, the person never having been weaned physically or emotionally. "His general reaction to people is a suckling one." (Hinsie, *UP*)

behavior The manner in which anything acts or operates. With regard to the human being the term usually refers to the action of the individual as a unit. He may be, and ordinarily is, acting in response to some given organ or impulse, but it is his general reaction that gives rise to the concept *behavior*. Each component of the body has its own special way of reacting; when the action of individual parts is meant, terms such as physiology and pathology are used. A hungry man seeks food; the seeking constitutes behavior. Food gets into his stomach; the stomach acts and reacts, that is, it exhibits physiology or pathology.

behavior, catastrophic A term introduced by Kurt Goldstein in 1939 to describe a type of behavior disorder that seemed more or less characteristic, or specific, for patients suffering from those disturbances of language and thought that had been grouped under the general diagnostic term *aphasia*. This symptomatic behavior takes the form of an inability to carry on a simple course of action once it is interrupted. The patients "become agitated and fearful and more than usually inept when presented with once simple tasks that they can no longer do." Goldstein interprets such traits of behavior as characteristic of a trend toward fanatical orderliness and the reaction of disinterest and aversion as defensive methods of avoiding "catastrophic" embarrassment. It would seem that the catastrophic reaction stems from the personality (or psychological) responses to the organic brain injury that underlies so many aphasia cases. (Hunt, *PBD*)

behavior, chaotic An extreme disorderliness in organizing one's humdrum affairs, with respect to the time to be made available for different needs, the necessary money for various expenditures, or the disposition of personal effects—all suggesting or betokening a straying from mental health. Fenichel states that chaotic behavior appears usually as a character trait of hysterical individuals. He explains that chaotic behavior "represents a striving to get rid of traumatic impressions by actively repeating them." (*PTN*)

behavior, collective The behavior that results when every individual in a group, an assemblage, or a public is moved to think and act under the influence of a mood or state of mind, in which each shares and to which each contributes.

In the broadest sense all group behavior is collective behavior. In the narrow sense collective behavior is applied not so much to customary and conventional behavior as to the emergence of new forms of behavior under conditions of interstimulation wherein "individuals reflect one another's states of feeling and in so doing intensify this feeling." (Blumer, H.E. in *Principles of Sociology*, ed. R. E. Park, 1939)

Elementary forms of collective behavior are to be observed in the street crowd, the acting crowd, the expressive crowd, the mob, the gang, the panic, the riot, the stampede, and the mutiny; intermediate forms in mass behavior, the public, public opinion, the party, and crusades; and more highly organized forms in propaganda, advertising, religious movements, nationalistic movements, fashion, reform, and revolution.

behavior contract A negotiated agreement that details in writing the conditions under which a person will do something for another person; often useful in promoting an exchange of positive reinforcement among family members. See *therapy, contract.*

behavior control See *forced treatment.*

behavior, criminotic Terms such as criminotic, criminotic behavior, criminosis have been introduced into psychiatric literature by A. Foxe. The word criminosis is coined on the pattern of neurosis and psychosis in regard to form, but differs in meaning in that it does not specifically connote mental illness. The criminotic is not necessarily mentally or emotionally ill, but the term criminosis would imply or describe his condition. And the term criminotic behavior would refer to the crime-committing activities of that person, as constituting the evidences of criminality or *criminosis* (q.v.).

behavior disorders A group of psychiatric disorders in children and adolescents which are not secondary to somatic diseases or defects or to convulsive disorders and which are not part of a well-defined psychosis or psychoneurosis (see *conduct disorders*). The primary behavior disorders are considered to be reactions to an unfavorable environment; they appear as problems of personality development, as persisting undesirable traits or unfavorable habits (the so-called habit disorders, including nail-biting, thumb-sucking, enuresis, masturbation, and temper tantrums), as delinquency or conduct disorders (truancy, fighting and quarreling, disobedience, untruthfulness, stealing, forgery, setting fires, destruction of property, use of alcohol, use of drugs, cruelty, sex offenses, vagrancy, etc.), as certain neurotic traits (such as tics and habit spasms, sleepwalking, overactivity, and fears), and as problems of school and general educa-

tional or vocational difficulties. In the past, children with such disorders were referred to as "problem children." See *oppositional disorder.*

behavior, expiatory See *expiation.*

behavior genetics Behavioral genetics. See *genetics.*

behavior, intentional unvoluntary See *intentional unvoluntary behavior.*

behavior language This term means that the actions of the child, before he learns to speak, constitute a real language or means of expression. The crying, fretting, anxiety, quiescence, satiety, smiling, and self-activity are the words of a language the infant uses before acquiring the capacity of producing articulate sounds. See *jargon, organ.*

behavior modeling See *modeling, behavior.*

behavior modification See *therapy, behavior.*

behavior, multidetermined Human behavior, healthy or disordered, can be conceived of as being carried out at four fundamental levels: (1) the eugenical, (2) the physiological, (3) the psychological, and (4) the environmental. Multitudinous factors stemming from past experience on the one hand, and the current, present environmental situation on the other, constantly interact and interreact to determine the current behavior at the present cross-sectional level.

In the field of prevention, this important concept of the multidetermined origin of human behavior is the basis for the "all out," "gun shot," "total push," eclectic methods of approach toward psychiatric treatment and prevention.

behavior, nodal In group therapy, the peak of hyperaggressivity and hilarity on the part of children. This high peak is always followed by a period of quietude, which is the *antinodal phase.* This alternation of quiet and action occurs in cycles. The frequency of this manifestation decreases as therapy progresses.

behavior reversal A behavior technique in which more desirable responses to interpersonal conflict situations are practiced under the therapist's supervision.

behavior theory A theory of the genesis of neurotic behavior, based on learning theory; among its leading exponents are Eysenck, Jones, and Wolpe. The theory postulates that neurotic symptoms are learned patterns of behavior which are unadaptive. If neurotic symptoms are learned, then they should be amenable to "unlearning," and behavior therapy is directed to the inhibition and/or extinction of the learned neurotic responses. One form of behavior therapy is J. Wolpe's *reciprocal inhibition psychotherapy:* "If a response antagonistic to anxiety can be made to occur in the presence of anxiety-evoking stimuli so that it is accompanied by a complete or partial suppression of the anxiety responses, the bond between these stimuli and the anxiety responses will be weakened." (*Psychotherapy by Reciprocal Inhibition,* 1958)

Particular forms of behavior therapy include assertiveness training, aversive therapy, biofeedback, conditioning, contract therapy, delay therapy, flooding, implosion, modeling, reciprocal inhibition and desensitization, shaping, system substitution, and systematic desensitization. See *BASIC-ID; behaviorism.*

behavior therapy See *behavior theory; therapy, behavior.*

behavior, type A See *type A.*

behavior utilization See *utilization behavior.*

behavioral ecology See *ecology.*

behavioral genetics See *genetics.*

behavioral medicine See *medicine, behavioral; psychosomatic medicine.*

behavioral neurochemistry Study of the relations between chemical substances in the brain and behavior—including neuroregulatory substances, genetic control of transmitter agents, different roles of compounds in different areas of brain, pharmacogenetics, biochemical effects of receptor excitation, interactions between different agents within the brain, actions of drugs on enzymatic and metabolic processes within the brain, and the relation of all such biochemical events to psychological events and behavior.

behavioral neurology See *neurology, behavioral.*

behavioral reaction See *personality disorders.*

behavioral rehearsal See *therapy, behavior.*

behavioral sciences "A multidisciplinary pursuit of knowledge about behavior in its roots and manifestations, in man and animals, in individuals, groups, and cultures, and in all conditions, normal, exceptional, and pathological. Behavioral scientists re-

main specialists in their respective fields, while striving to unify their diverse theories and concepts." (Bry, I., et al. *Mental Health Book Review Index,* January 1960) Among the many disciplines contributing to the behavioral sciences are all those ordinarily subsumed under the following groupings: "The Natural Sciences, which explore the inanimate and animate universe in which man finds himself; the Social Sciences, concerned with the political, social, legal, and economic structure he has given to the world around him; and the Humanities, the study of man's lasting intellectual and artistic creations." (Ibid.)

behaviorism A term coined by J.B. Watson in 1913 to indicate that all habits may be explained in terms of conditioned glandular and motor reaction.

"Behaviorism, on the contrary, holds that the subject matter of human psychology is the *behavior or activities of the human being.* Behaviorism claims that 'consciousness' is neither a definable nor a usable concept; that it is merely another word for the 'soul' of more ancient times." (*Behaviorism,* 1924)

Classical behaviorism asserted that all behavior is to be understood in terms of the stimulus-response formula; the organism thus is essentially passive and can only react to stimulation. Modern behaviorism, as exemplified by Skinner's *operant behaviorism,* eschews a mechanistic view of human nature. It claims that organisms can initiate action as well as react to stimulation. Because it does not insist that the specific cause of any original action can be demonstrated, it need not invent questionable mechanisms to explain how activity can originate.

The core theme of Skinner's operant behaviorism is that activities of the organism bring consequences that shape and influence further action. It is the environment that produces the consequences, so it is the environment that shapes, influences, and determines a person's behavior. Behavior that elicits positive consequences (rewards) will tend to be repeated—*positive reinforcement* in Skinner's terminology. Negative consequences (punishment, in the form of either aversive stimulation or withdrawal of a positive stimulus) will tend to be avoided, and behavior that removes aversive stimulation will tend to be repeated (*negative reinforcement*). Operant behavior, which produces changes in (operates on) the environment, is roughly equivalent to voluntary behavior, which itself is modified by environmental feedback. *Behavioral engineering* refers to systematic control of the environmental conditions that shape the behavior of people. Skinner contends that such control proffers the greatest hope for improving the human condition. (Skinner, B.F. *Walden Two,* 1948; *Science and Human Behavior,* 1953; *Beyond Freedom and Dignity,* 1971) See *conditionalism.*

Bell, Luther V. (1806–62) American psychiatrist; one of the "original thirteen" founders of the Association of Medical Superintendents of America (the forerunner of The American Psychiatric Association); *Bell's mania* (q.v.).

belle indifference See *hysteria.*

Bell's mania Luther V. Bell (*American Journal of Insanity 6,* 1849) described 10 patients who died suddenly and whose autopsies failed to reveal an adequate explanation; the term Bell's mania was used to describe this entity, although later it was more commonly called *lethal catatonia, exhaustion death,* or *deadly catatonia.* The clinical picture consists of severe agitation, mutism, high fever, dehydration, delusions, hallucinations, and rapid death.

In recent years, phenothiazine deaths have also been described: sudden deaths or sudden cardiovascular collapse without physical or autopsy findings that explain the death. R. Peele and I.S. Von Loetzen (*American Journal of Psychiatry 130,* 1973) present evidence suggesting that " 'phenothiazine death' includes two previously known types of sudden, unexplained, autopsy-negative deaths: cardiac deaths among the general population and lethal catatonia among the mentally ill."

Bell's palsy See *nerve, facial.*

belonephobia Fear of needles.

belongingness A feeling of being a part of and/or being accepted by another person or group. A lack of this feeling is often a complaint of schizophrenic patients. See *autism.*

Benda, Clemens E. (1899–1975) German-born neuropathologist and psychiatrist who came to the United States in 1936;

mental retardation, especially mongolism. See *syndrome, Down.*

Bender, Lauretta (1897–1987) American neuropsychiatrist; Visual Motor Gestalt test; child psychiatry, especially schizophrenia and brain damage.

bends, the See *disease, caisson.*

Benedikt's syndrome (Moritz Benedikt, Austrian physician, 1835–1920) The symptoms following a lesion of the red nucleus in the midbrain involve the oculomotor fibers passing through the midbrain: homolateral oculomotor paralysis, contralateral hyperkinesis.

beneficence Goodness, kindness, or the performance of such acts toward others. In medical ethics beneficence generally refers to preventing harm from befalling others (*nonmalfeasance*) and, in addition, acting to promote the well-being of others.

benign In psychiatry, referring to a disorder with good prognosis. It does not refer to the intensity of the clinical syndrome. A benign psychosis may be extremely intense, as the benign stupor state, from which the patient generally recovers or experiences appreciable amelioration.

Benommenheit (be-nom'en-hīt) Literally, a benumbing; Bleuler's term for one of the acute syndromes of the schizophrenias in which there is a slowing of all psychic processes but no dejection of mood or self-depreciatory ideas. Patients with Benommenheit are unable to deal with any relatively complicated or unusual situation; they make mistakes and show marked apraxia and impaired comprehension. This syndrome may persist but it is not otherwise indicative of poor prognosis.

Benzedrine dependency Symptoms include an inability to abstain from the drug, need for increasing dosage (high tolerance is developed, e.g. 1500 mg may be the usual daily dose), insomnia, restlessness, irritability, gross errors in judgment, loss of impulse control (especially aggressive impulses), ideas of reference and delusions of persecution, and hallucinosis with auditory and visual hallucinations. The hallucinosis usually clears within four or five weeks; males are much more prone to develop such symptoms than females.

benzodiazepine See *psychotropics.*

BEP Brief and emergency psychotherapy. See *psychotherapy, brief and emergency.*

berdache Transvestite; a respected gay man with clearly defined role(s). The respect accorded the berdache of some American Indian tribes—and apparently this was also the case among the Germanic peoples of the early Middle Ages—depended at least in part on acceptance and successful adoption of the defined role, such as the "passive" partner or "wife" in a homosexual union.

bereavement Loss, most often used to refer to the loss of a loved one through death. The feelings of anguish and desolation and accompanying symptoms and signs constitute a psychiatric syndrome of depression (at least by DSM-III standards) even though the affective state is a normal reaction to loss. In the older literature, the distinction was often drawn between normal *mourning* and the pathological states of *melancholia* and *depression* (qq.v.).

Three stages of bereavement have been described: (1) a feeling of numbness and unreality, which lasts from a few hours to several days; (2) dejection and sadness, typically with insomnia and loss of appetite; about a third of bereaved people feel they did not do enough for the dead person, and about a fifth blame some other person(s) for their loss; (3) a stage of acceptance, with gradual abatement of stage 2 symptoms.

Even though bereavement is normal, studies have shown that bereaved subjects are immunosuppressed and may be vulnerable to physical illness. Older widowers have increased mortality during the first six months of bereavement, due mainly to cancer, cardiovascular disease, accidents, suicide, and cirrhosis of the liver. The particular illnesses associated with the increased mortality suggest that lifestyle factors, such as increased use of tobacco and alcohol, may be the responsible agents.

bereavement, feigned A false tale of death of a relative or loved one presented by the subject as a major factor in development of the grief of which he complains. It is probably a variant of the Munchhausen syndrome. See *syndrome, Munchhausen.*

Bergen's fraction A plasma factor claimed by some to be characteristic of schizophrenia; its effect, when injected into trained rats, is to impede their rope-climbing performance. The name comes from J.R. Bergen and his colleagues at the Worcester Foundation. Bergen suggested (1968) that the *Frohman factor* (q.v.) is identical to Bergen's fraction, and that both are an alpha-2-globulin.

Berger rhythm, Berger wave See *electroencephalogram.*

Berne, Eric (1910–70) Canadian-born psychoanalyst, in United States after 1936; transactional analysis, group treatment.

Bernheim, Hippolyte-Marie (1840–1919) French psychotherapist; hypnotism and suggestibility.

Bessman-Baldwin syndrome See *syndrome, imidazole.*

best interests doctrine See *custody.*

bestiality Any type of human behavior that resembles that of beasts; more specifically, sexual congress between humans and animals.

beta alcoholism See *alcoholism.*

beta arc See *alpha arc.*

beta error See *error, beta.*

beta rhythm or **wave** See *electroencephalogram.*

Betz cell (Vladimir Aleksandrovich Betz, Russian anatomist, 1834–95) See *lobe, frontal.*

bewildered A term often used to describe the lost, dazed, perplexed, puzzled patient who appears to be confused but shows a sort of numb apathy about his confusion. Bewilderment is often associated with conscious ambivalence, with dereistic or autistic thinking, with preoccupation, and with vacuity or sterility of thinking. See *Benommenheit.*

β-glucuronidase deficiency See *mucopolysaccharidosis.*

bhang The Hindu name for cannabis. See *marihuana.*

Bianchi, Leonardo (bē-äng′kē) (1848–1927) Italian psychiatrist and neurologist. See *syndrome, Bianchi's.*

bias A tendency to err, usually because the sample from which conclusions are drawn is not representative of the group to which the conclusions are applied.

bias, antitechnology See *Frankenstein factor.*

biased apperception Seeing things only as one wants to see them, considered by Adler a prerequisite for social participation since, without it, social movements would be stifled by indecisiveness. The person who cannot make a move unless he is certain to be right, for example, cannot usually move very much. The normal person, by contrast, takes a chance and chooses in accordance with his preferences and his subjective evaluation of the situation.

biblioclast One who destroys or mutilates books.

"Among biblioclasts some act in groups *cornering* copies of a rare book and making a *'pool' of any volumes which are not immaculate;* from among these they *complete or perfect* as many copies as possible, and destroy the remainder." (Jackson, H. *The Anatomy of Bibliomania,* 1932)

biblioklept One who steals books.

bibliokleptomania Morbid tendency to steal books.

bibliomania Book-madness; an intense desire to collect and possess books, especially rare and curious ones.

bibliophobia A morbid dread or hatred of books.

bibliotherapy Utilization of reading as an adjunct to psychotherapy. Books may be recommended to patients for the following reasons: (1) to help the patient understand better his own psychological and physiological reactions to frustration; (2) to remedy insufficient or erroneous knowledge; (3) to facilitate communication between patient and therapist by helping the patient understand the terminology of therapy; (4) to stimulate the patient to discuss and verbalize certain problems by helping to remove the fear, shame, or guilt related to those problems; (5) to stimulate the patient to think constructively between interviews; (6) to reinforce accepted social and cultural patterns and thereby inhibit certain infantile patterns of behavior; (7) to stimulate the patient's imagination and give him vicarious satisfactions which reality cannot afford without danger; (8) to enlarge the patient's sphere of interest; (9) as an adjunct to a program of vocational rehabilitation. The reading matter recommended must, of course, be selected individually for the specific patient, depending on the goals of therapy, the intellectual capacities of the patient, and his stage of achievement in therapy.

Bichat, Law of (Marie Francois Xavier Bichat, French anatomist, 1771–1802) According to Bichat there are two great body

systems, called by him the vegetative and the animal. The former provides for assimilation and augmentation of mass, while the latter provides for the transformation of energy, "that is, for the relations with the environment." The two systems "are in inverse ratio of the development in ontogenetic evolution—the greater the development of the vegetative system, the less developed is the system of relation." (Pende, N. *Constitutional Inadequacies,* 1928)

Biedl-Moon-Laurence syndrome See *syndrome, Laurence-Moon-Biedl.*

Bielschowsky's disease (Max Bielschowsky, German neuropathologist, 1869–1940) See *Tay-Sachs disease.*

bill of rights For psychiatric patients (and inpatients in particular), a listing of the civil rights that merit particular attention and protection, including the right to treatment (including the right not to be confined in a mental institution if only custodial care and not active treatment is provided), the right to refuse treament, the right to have the least amount of and the least invasive treatment (this includes the least restrictive environment and related concepts), the right not to be subjected to unusual or cruel or hazardous treatments without express and informed consent, the right of due-process protection (for children as well as adults), the right to legal counsel, the right to a humane environment with adequate staffing, etc. See *consumerism.*

bimodality The potentiality of functioning in two ways, most often used to refer to cerebral dominance or lateralization. See *dominance, cerebral.*

bind, double This term is approximately equivalent to dilemma and is used particularly to refer to a type of interaction said to be characteristic of families containing schizophrenic members. The parent of a schizophrenic, for example, is perceived by the patient as emitting "signals of an incongruent nature. This incongruence is perhaps most clear when one half of the parent's behavior precedes an act of the patient and the other half follows. The parent will, for example, invite the patient to express a courageous opinion, and when that opinion is expressed, will disparage it as unloving, disloyal, disobedient, etc." (Bateson, G. in *Schizophrenia—An Integrated Approach,* ed. A. Auerback, 1959) As a result of repeated entrapment in the double-bind, which he can neither ignore nor attack directly by commenting on the incongruity, the schizophrenic learns to strip all his communications of material that might be maltreated in this way. This is believed by some to be the mode of development of certain of the schizophrenic's fundamental symptoms.

J.H. Weakland and D.D. Jackson (*Archives of Neurology and Psychiatry 79,* 1958) define the double bind as "a hostile dependent involvement where one of the parties insists on a response to multiple orders of messages which are mutually contradictory, and the other (the schizophrenic patient to be) cannot comment on these contradictions or escape from the situation."

A. Ferreira (*Archives of General Psychiatry* 1960) terms the double bind described above a "unipolar message." He notes that the double bind is not confined to the schizophrenogenic relationship. But what is seemingly characteristic of schizophrenics is that the contradictory messages emanate from a single (unipolar) source, usually the mother. In delinquent behavior, on the other hand, the source of the messages is split (bipolar), with message A emanating from the father and message B (a comment about message A with the effect of opposing or destroying it) emanating from the mother, or vice versa. Ferreira calls this the "split double bind."

Binet-Simon tests See *tests, Binet-Simon.*

binge-buying, binge spending *Oniomania* (q.v.).

binge eating See *bulimia; syndrome, night-eating.*

Binger, Carl A.L. (1890–1976) American psychoanalyst; psychosomatic medicine.

Bini, Lucio (1908–64) Italian psychiatrist. Co-discoverer (with Ugo Cerletti) of electric convulsive therapy, first demonstrated in Rome on March 28, 1938. The idea of inducing convulsions electrically rather than pharmacologically was Cerletti's, but the elaboration of the technique and bitemporal placement of the electrodes was Bini's.

Binswanger, Otto (bēn'sväng-gēr) (1852–1929) German neurologist and psychiatrist; originated concept of presenile dementia.

Binswanger's disease See *encephalopathy, subcortical arteriosclerotic; lacuna.*

bioanalysis "The question presents itself to me whether the term psychoanalysis is really broad enough and whether another more comprehensive and more all-inclusive term, such as *bioanalysis* or *psychobioanalysis* should not be substituted for it, especially if we would include the analysis of the somatic symptoms of the psychoneuroses, psychoses, and other psychic states as well as the multiform conduct of man at every stage of evolution and development." (Solomon, M. *Psychoanalytic Review 2,* 1915)

bioavailability The degree to which a drug administered is distributed throughout the body and thus available for action at the desired receptor sites.

biobehavioral shift See *shift, biobehavioral.*

biodynamics J.H. Masserman's system of psychoanalytic psychiatry: "biodynamics derives some of its essential dynamic orientations from analysis, and serves no greater practical function than to generalize fundamental analytic concepts and to demonstrate their theoretical, experimental and clinical applicability to a wide range of phenomena in animal and human behavior." *The Practice of Dynamic Psychiatry,* 1955) The four principles of biodynamics—motivation, milieu, adaptation, and conflict—are stated as follows: (1) all organisms are actuated by their physiologic needs; (2) every organism reacts to its own interpretations of its milieu in terms of its individual needs, special capacities, and unique experiences; (3) whenever an organism's goal-directed activities are frustrated by external obstacles, the organism either changes its techniques to reach that same goal or changes its goal; (4) when two or more urgent motivations conflict so that the adaptive patterns attendant to each are mutually exclusive, the organism experiences anxiety and its somatic and muscular behavior becomes either ambivalent, poorly adaptive, and ineffectively substitutive (neurotic), or progressively more disorganized, regressive, and bizarrely symbolic (psychotic).

bioethics See *ethics, biomedical.*

biofeedback "An instrumental procedure that senses, records, and provides the subject with information about those physiological functions in relation to which there is usually no awareness or voluntary control." (Moldofsky, H. in *Psychiatry Update III*, ed. L. Grinspoon, 1984.) Even though they are not conscious, such autonomic nervous system functions are subject to learning (visceral learning, physiologic self-regulation, learned automatic control). In theory, a subject can learn to control his internal organs and vital functions; it might therefore be possible for a patient with essential hypertension to learn how to reduce his blood pressure. Vital functions, such as blood pressure, are not maintained at a constant level, hence their fluctuations can be treated as responses and reinforced appropriately. The use of biofeedback and operant reinforcement (see *conditioning, operant*) has been successful in regulating a number of bodily processes in laboratory experiments; attempts to transfer the learned visceral responses to real-life situations, however, have often failed. See *therapy, behavior.*

biofidelity The quality of being lifelike in appearance or responses; often refers to dummies used in safety investigations of motor vehicles or in demonstrations of cardiopulmonary resuscitation.

biogenetic law of Haeckel See *law, biogenetic mental.*

biogenetics See *genetics.*

biogenic amines See *amine.*

biography in depth The use of established psychoanalytic knowledge to contribute to the understanding of the personality of the subject being studied. See *pathography, psychoanalytic.*

biohazard Potential danger from biological sources, as opposed to chemical or mechanical dangers. The alleged dangers of recombinant DNA research, for example, are biohazards of molecular biological research.

biological clock See *clock, biological.*

biology, mathematical That branch of biology concerned with the development of conceptual or mathematical models of various biological phenomena. From those models, various mathematical consequences are deduced that are then compared to actual experiments or other observed phenomena. Successful mathematical theories have been developed for a large number of biological phenomena, including nerve excitation, endocrine secretions, conditioning, and learning.

biomedical ethics See *ethics, biomedical.*

biometry The measurement of life; specifically, calculation of the probable duration of life and study of all the factors, endogenous and exogenous, that enter into the determination of the duration of life.

bion The energy vesicles through which the orgone (life energy) manifests itself, according to Wilhelm Reich's theory. See *orgone.*

bionegativity A personality constellation in which one or more part processes disturb the total function of the organism. In an entirely healthy organism the various part processes are integrated in such a way that they subserve and promote the total function of the organism, while in an abnormal condition the integration is impaired and one or more part functions impede or disturb instead of promoting the total function. Instead of being viewed as an abnormality such an impairment is therefore conceived as an integrational state, a specific relation between part and whole, and is called bionegativity.

bionics The study of biological functions and mechanisms from the point of view of applying them to electronic devices, such as computers.

bionomics *Ecology* (q.v.); bionomic factors are those external, environmental factors that limit the development of an organism.

biophilia Instinct of self-preservation.

biopsy, chorion *Chorionic villus biopsy; CVS* (chorionic villus sampling); excision of chorionic (placental) tissue to obtain a sampling of fetal cells that are then examined for chromosome abnormalities. The technique is painless, and tissue is taken directly through the cervix rather than by means of a needle biopsy through the abdominal wall, as in amniocentesis. Chorion biopsy can provide a larger sample of fetal tissue than can be obtained by amniocentesis, and the test can be performed earlier. Further, it provides material for immediate examination in contrast to amniocentesis, where the sample of amniotic fluid must first be cultured before it can be analyzed for chromosomal irregularities. Some studies have suggested, however, that the technique may be associated with a higher incidence of spontaneous abortion.

Coupled with DNA *probes* (q.v.), new techniques for analyzing human genetic material through recombinant DNA methods, chorion biopsy may make it possible to detect almost any of the 3,800 different genetic disorders for which a faulty gene is known to exist (among them cystic fibrosis, phenylketonuria, and galactosemia, three of the most important genetic disorders among white Americans; sickle cell anemia, various forms of thalassemia or Cooley's anemia, hemophilia, and Duchenne's muscular dystrophy.)

biosphere The realm or sphere of life in which the total biological process takes place. The biosphere includes both the individual and his environment not as interacting parts of constituents that have an independent existence, but as aspects of a single reality that can be mentally separated only by abstraction. The limits of life extend as far as the organism is able to exert an influence on the events outside of him. (Biosphere corresponds to the German term *Lebenskreis*.)

biostatistics Vital statistics; the numerical representation of conditions associated with life.

biotaxis See *network; taxis.*

biothanatos *Obs.* Suicide.

biotype All individuals who equal each other *genotypically*, whether or not their *phenotypical* appearance may show any obvious resemblance. The phenotypical features of two individuals belonging to the same biotype may be dissimilar to a considerable extent, since every hereditary predisposition has a certain amount of variability of manifestation.

biotypogram In Pende's system of constitutional medicine, a variety of constitutional formulas as they are to be recorded in the individual's "book of health" for the purpose of a "diagrammatic representation" describing the various types in all their somatic and psychological aspects.

biotypology The systematic study or doctrine of biotypes. Although the genetic concept of biotype applies to individuals equaling each other *genotypically*, it has been taken in the field of constitutional studies, especially by the Italian school, to

indicate the phenotypical constellation of all characteristics making up the "somatic-psychic individuality" of a human being, including the morphological, physiological, and psychological aspects of the given type.

bipolar illness *Bipolar disorders;* affective disorder characterized by episodes of both mania and depression; manic-depressive disorder, mixed type.

Dunner and others differentiate between *bipolar I*—affective illness that has included mania of severe enough degree to require hospitalization, and *bipolar II*—affective illness with a history of hospitalization for depression and a history of hypomania, but the manic element has not been severe enough to require hospitalization. In some classifications, *cyclothymic disorder* is included within the bipolar II category, which is viewed as an intermediate phenomenological type that lies between unipolar II depression and bipolar I. In DSM-III-R, bipolar disorders include manic, depressed, and mixed forms as well as cyclothymia. See *affective disorders; cyclothymia; depression, unipolar; mania; psychosis, manic-depressive.*

bipolar double bind See *bind, double.*

bipolarity *Ambivalence* (q.v.).

Birnbaum, Karl (1878–1950) German psychiatrist; forensic psychiatry.

birth, anal In psychoanalytic theory this term refers to the sexual fantasies or dreams directly connected with anal erotism when these phantasies or dreams are expressed in the symbolic form of a wish to be reborn through the anus. In this respect, Freud gave the following dream as example: "Spending the summer beside Lake ——— she flings herself into the dark waters at the place where the pale moon is mirrored." Freud defined this dream as an expression of anal birth. The interpretation of the dream reveals that "she flings herself into the water" means "she comes out of the water," that is to say, "that she is born." The moon represents an anal symbol derived from the French language in which the "derriere" (the "behind") is vulgarly spoken of as "la lune" (the moon).

birth control Regulation of the number or spacing of offspring, either by measures designed to prevent conception or by termination of pregnancy once conception has taken place. Two factors have significantly altered the complexion of birth control in recent years. One is the development in the 1960s of intrauterine contraceptive devices and of the contraceptive pill. The other is the 1972 decision of the United States Supreme Court that invalidated restrictive abortion laws. Those two developments made both contraception and termination of pregnancy easier and safer to achieve, with relative certainty, and removed from the realm of criminal behavior. The last aspect is of particular relevance to psychiatry since before the 1972 decision the major legal rationale for abortion was danger to the prospective mother's mental health, a danger that society expected the psychiatrist to foretell.

For the sexually active and fertile female, the changes were even more profound. Effective contraceptive measures that need neither the cooperation and skill of the sex partner nor the interference of a mechanical contrivance with the natural progression of the sex act have given the woman a new freedom in sexuality. No longer is her sexual activity limited by fears of pregnancy or doubts about the suitability of a sex partner as a lifetime spouse. She is as free to choose when to have sex, and with whom, as men have always been. The decision to terminate pregnancy is now hers alone to make, and not a permission granted reluctantly by an ambivalent society.

birth injury Any damage to the fetus-neonate as a result of the birth process; often used in a more limited way to refer to brain damage due to the birth process (including that due to instrument delivery). See *brain damage*.

birth, multiple In biology and vital statistics the term applies to all instances in which women produce more than one child at the same birth. The tendency to multiple births seems to run in certain families, although it has not yet been proved that it is based on a specific hereditary factor.

Twins come about once in every 90 births in most of the American and European countries. The proportion of fraternal to identical twins is approximately 3:1 (see *twins*).

Triplets occur once in about 8,000 births. They also may be identical or "un-matched" multiples, that is, developed either from one egg or from three separate eggs. The third possibility is that only two members of a set of triplets are identical, developed from one egg, and the third is a fraternal, developed from a different egg.

Quadruplets are reported by Scheinfeld to occur once in about 700,000 births, with only a few sets surviving. Here the following combinations are possible: (1) all four identicals; (2) three identicals and one fraternal; (3) two identicals and two fraternal; and (4) most rarely, all four fraternals.

The birth of five humans at one time is believed to have occurred spontaneously not more than 60 times in the last 500 years. In most cases, however, these *quintuplets* perished soon after birth.

With the increasing use of *fertility-inducing drugs* since the 1960s, there has been an increase in multiple births. The drugs used are those that stimulate the pituitary to produce gonadotropins or, if the pituitary produces none, gonadotropins themselves are used in an attempt to stimulate the ovary directly. It has been estimated that multiple births occur in about 20% of women treated with such drugs.

bisexuality The presence of the qualities of both sexes in the same person. The term is synonymous with hermaphroditism, though the latter term appears to have gained almost exclusive reference to the organic manifestations of the condition. The term intersex, introduced by Goldschmidt, is used "to designate hermaphrodites as individuals who started out either male or female from a genetic standpoint but who after a certain period completed their sexual development in the opposite direction. In the intersex there is first a female phase and later a male phase, or vice versa, and in the second phase a typical mixture of both sexes exists." (Young, H.H. *Genital Abnormalities, Hermaphroditism and Related Adrenal Diseases,* 1937)

In the classical sense a bisexual or hermaphroditic individual is one "who has the gonads and external genitalia of both sexes and is capable of living as either a man or a woman." (ibid.)

Bisexuality manifests itself also in the psyche. "It would seem palpably obvious that the repression and the formation of the neurosis must have originated out of the conflict between masculine and feminine tendencies, that is, out of bisexuality." (Freud, *BW*)

At the present time there is a tendency to use the term in a more limited fashion, to describe persons who, for a significant time after the period of adolescence, consciously feel, think and alternately react psychically, erotically, and/or orgastically to members both of the same and of the opposite sex. See *androgyneity; gender identity; gender role.*

bivalence (bī-vā′lens, biv′à-lens) See *ambivalence.*

bizarreness Striking incongruity or eccentricity; discordant, disharmonious, contradictory behavior such as is seen most commonly in schizophrenic patients.

blackout 1. Loss of consciousness, usually secondary to brain anemia or oxygen deprivation. When the loss of consciousness is only partial, *gray-out* is the term applied; this is seen frequently in pilots when they rapidly change altitude, as in a dive.

2. The alcoholic's amnesia for his behavior during drinking episodes (sometimes termed *dim-out* to differentiate it from the acute syncopal episode described above). Such blackouts are indicative of beginning, but still reversible, brain damage *(intermediate brain syndrome due to alcohol).* Typically, the blackout follows moderate drinking, and the drinker converses reasonably and carries out elaborate activities without signs of intoxication, but the next day he has no memory of what he said or did.

Such blackouts appear to be due mainly to a failure of memory consolidation and, to a lesser extent, retrieval. They precede by months or years the other two major hallmarks of alcohol addiction: loss of control and prolonged drinking bouts. See *alcoholism.*

bladder, automatic The filling and spontaneous evacuation of the urinary bladder occurring in cases of transsection of the spinal cord.

blaesus (blē′sus) *Obs.* General paralysis.

-blast, blasto- Combining form meaning sprout, shoot, germ, embryonic; from Gr. *blastós,* sprout, shoot, twig.

blast concussion See *neurosis, postconcussion.*

blastomere Cell(s) formed by the first cell divisions of a fertilized egg undergoing the process of *cleavage* (q.v.).

blastophthoria (blas-tof-thōr′ē-à) Degenerative effect on germ cells of poisons such as alcohol and lead; many temperance adherents claim that alcohol has a blastophthoric effect that is manifested in mental retardation in the alcoholic's children. See *syndrome, fetal alcohol.*

blastopore See *gastrulation.*

blastula (blas′chū-là) In this embryological stage of a human organism, there is continued cell division beyond the 32-cell stage and the appearance of an enlarging central cavity, the blastocele, in the fertilized egg undergoing the segmenting process of *cleavage* (q.v.).

At first the blastula is a hollow sphere whose wall is a single layer of morphologically and functionally identical cells, the primitive *ectoderm* (q.v.). Only in the later stages of this *monodermic* blastula condition one finds those larger cells at the pole opposite that of the location of the polar bodies, which foreshadow the future *entoderm* (q.v.).

blepharospasm (blef′à-rō-spaz′m) Spasmoid closing of the orbicular muscle; a winking tic; *blinking* (q.v.).

Bleuler, Eugen (1857–1939) Swiss psychiatrist; schizophrenia. In 1911, Bleuler suggested the term *schizophrenia* to replace dementia praecox. His monumental treatise, *Dementia Praecox or the Group of Schizophrenias,* differentiated between the fundamental and the accessory symptoms of schizophrenia, and it remains today the authoritative source book on the development and manifestations of schizophrenic symptoms.

blind, double See *double blind.*

blindism Mannerisms and habitual movements seen in blind patients, and particularly in children, such as repeated rubbing of the eyes, shaking and rolling the body, poking at the eyes or ears, shaking the hands when excited and, if there is some vision, fanning the fingers in front of the eyes. Usually the blindism is given up as the child grows older.

blindness, circumferential See *field defect.*

blindness, cortical psychic A condition usually due to bilateral occipital lobe lesions producing a loss of topographical orientation, optic memory image, and spatial orientation.

blindness, hysterical Blindness as a symptom of conversion hysteria. In principle it bears out the popular belief that we see what we want to see and are blind to the things we do not want to see. Hysterical blindness is of the same order. A young woman, inordinately fond of her father, tried frantically to drive him out of her mind. Realizing the unnaturalness of her love for him, she became blind, owing to her strong sense of guilt and because she could no longer look upon her father.

blindness, mind Psychic blindness; objects and space dimensions are seen by the eye, but the patient has an erroneous idea of the size of objects and the three dimensions of space. Sometimes he sees objects as flat, or as small (see *micropsia*). Uncertainty over object relationships may be a basic element in the development of such symptoms. P. Schilder described the case of a patient who, during analytical treatment, had the impression of seeing the analyst seated in a chair very far away. In anxiety cases the distance between the subject and the beloved person is the only space that seems real to the patient. Accordingly, when the beloved person is away, or out of sight, the space seems to become immense. "In some phobias connected with walking the patients occasionally dream that their feet do not touch the ground." This, according to the psychoanalytical interpretation of Schilder, symbolizes the distance of their genitals from their mother. (*Mind, Perception and Thought*, 1942)

blinking Quick, involuntary, apparently purposeless and repetitious movement of the eyelids (alone or associated with similar movements involving other groups of muscles and belonging to the category of tics or habit spasms) observed in nervous children. See *blepharospasm*.

BLM Bucco-lingual-masticatory syndrome, the most common form of tardive dyskinesia. See *dyskinesia, tardive*.

block See *chromosome*.

block, affect Inability to discharge emotions adequately or appropriately, seen typically in obsessive-compulsives, who often appear cold, unfeeling, and emotionally stiff and overcontrolled, and also in some schizophrenics. Freud termed this "isolation of affect." "In such cases a fantasy connected with a wish or a crucial memory from the past may have ready access to consciousness, but the emotion, usually a painful one, which should be connected with it does not become conscious. Moreover, such patients usually manage to keep from feeling too much emotion of any sort. . . . However, in some unfortunate individuals it goes so far that in the end the individual has hardly any awareness of emotions of any kind and seems like a caricature of that equanimity which ancient philosophers put forward as an ideal." (Brenner, C. *An Elementary Textbook of Psychoanalysis*, 1955)

block, partial genetic See *disease, genetotrophic*.

blockade, narcotic Inhibition, removal, or diminution of the euphoria produced by narcotic drugs such as heroin. Some have advocated the use of methadone in narcotic addicts to produce blockade, but others have pointed out that a search for euphoria or avoidance of withdrawal symptoms may not be the only determinant in addiction to narcotics.

blocking Sudden cessation in the train of thought or in the midst of a sentence. The patient is unable to explain the reason for the sudden stoppage, which may occur in the absence of intellectual defect or sensorial disorder. "Often thinking stops in the middle of a thought; or in the attempt to pass to another idea, it may suddenly cease altogether, at least as far as it is a conscious process (blocking). Instead of continuing the thought, new ideas crop up which neither the patient nor the observer can bring into any connection with the previous stream of thought." (Bleuler, E. *Dementia Praecox or the Group of Schizophrenias*, 1950) Blocking is also known as "thought-deprivation." It is usually experienced by the patient as unpleasant. Bleuler considered a positive response by a patient to the question of whether or not he had ever experienced thought-deprivation pathognomonic of schizophrenic association disorder. See *obstruction*.

In experimental psychology, blocking consists of temporary complete cessation of work during a period of continuous practice. Blockings of this sort are more frequent in schizophrenics than in others.

blocking, counterimpulse in The opposite of the impulse that is blocked. Kraepelin particularly stressed that counterdrives may cause blocking. Bleuler points out that "the denial of any impulse is so very often associated with a counter-impulse that, in stressing the counter-impulse, we only emphasize a different aspect of the same process, but we do not gain a new perspective." (*Dementia Praecox or the Group of Schizophrenias*, 1950) One schizophrenic demonstrated blocking whenever he was asked about his father. Further investigation indicated that the patient had marked ambivalence toward his father, and questioning him touched upon his hatred for the father and at the same time upon his love for the father. Here the impulse appeared to be canceled out, as it were, by the counterimpulse, and blocking resulted.

boarding-out system See *system, boarding out*.

bodies, geniculate See *geniculate bodies*.

body buffer zone The degree of physical proximity to a second person that is experienced as uncomfortable by the subject. For most persons, the body buffer zone to the rear is significantly larger than frontal distances. Several studies have also indicated that a positive correlation exists between size of body buffer zone and degree of aggressivity.

body build, index of A standard devised by Eysenck in his studies on the relationship between somatotype and psychosis. The IB consists of a measurement of stature and transverse chest diameter:

$$IB = \frac{\text{stature} \times 100}{\text{transverse chest diameter} \times 6}$$

body cell See *cell, body*.

body-centered therapy A host of therapies whose common goal is the altering of self-image or personality through work with the physical body, either exclusively or as a major component of the therapy. Among the major ones are *bioenergetics*, *Rolfing (structural integration)*, *Feldenkrais method (functional integration)*, *body-centered psychotherapy* (a major form of which is called *Hakomi method*), *psychomotor therapy* (developed by Albert Pesso), *Lomi work* (developed by Robert Hall, Ellisa Hall, Cather-

ine Flaxman, and Richard Heckler), *Alexander technique* (developed by F. Mathius Alexander).

The various body-centered therapies work with the body in different ways: (1) slow, precise movements, as in the Feldenkrais method, t'ai chi, and Alexander technique; (2) expressive movements and stressful postures, used to access emotionally charged material, as in bioenergetics and dance therapy; (3) the manipulation of body tissue, as in Rolfing; (4) the body as an expression of character, as in bioenergetics, body-centered psychotherapy, and psychomotor therapy; (5) general conditioning and toning of the body to enhance health, feelings of well-being, and the development of the skills of self-defense and personal control, as in yoga and the oriental martial arts.

Bioenergetics is an offshoot of Reichian therapy developed by Alexander Lowen and John Perrakos.

In Rolfing, the intention is to create changes in the subject's self-image and personal feelings through integration of the myofacial system (the system that binds and gives shape to the muscles of the body) and the integration of the whole body to the field of gravity.

The Feldenkrais method uses heightened attention to the fine details of slow, gentle movement, whether the practitioner manipulates the subject's limbs or the subject makes the movements guided by a leader. The object is to enhance the subject's body image and thereby improve movement functions. (Feldenkrais, M. *Awareness Through Movement*, 1972)

Body-centered psychotherapy is the most directly psychological method. In both the Hakomi method, developed by Ron Kurtz, and the psychomotor therapy of Pesso, the therapist combines discussion, action, and awareness as a way of gaining access to important emotional material.

body image See *ego, body; image, body*.

body language The expression of feelings or thoughts by means of bodily movements. See *language, primitive psychosomatic*.

body/mind perception, altered See *perception, altered mind/body*.

body-mindedness Psychosomatic (q.v.).

body of Luys (Jules Bernard Luys, French physician, 1828–98) See *subthalamus*.

body packer See *syndrome, body-packer.*

body, polar In sexual reproduction, the female germ cells or oogonia divide into two unequal daughter cells, the smaller of which is called the first or second polar body, according to whether it is produced by the first or second meiotic division. Only the larger cells or oocytes have a reproductive function, whereas the polar bodies gradually disintegrate and disappear.

body protest See *protest, body.*

body scheme See *ego, body.*

bogeyman A spirit or goblin who will punish the child for misbehavior; often interpreted psychoanalytically as externalized pre-superego, i.e. a projection onto persons in the external world of the internalized parental prohibitions that are the forerunners of the *superego* (q.v.).

bombesin A gastric peptide that may be the hormonal signal of gastric satiety; in humans, it produces a potent inhibition of normal feeding.

bond, peptide See *peptide, brain.*

bondage A form of overt sexual masochism in which erotic pleasure depends on the subject's being humiliated, endangered and enslaved; bondage appears to be more frequent in men and more often than not with a homosexual orientation. Bondage may account for as many as 50 deaths annually in the United States, typically through a combination of suicidal wishes and accident.

bonding Interaction; mutual dependency; often used to refer to the mother-infant relationship before *separation-individuation* (q.v.) has been completed. See *attachment; fault, basic; spacing.*

bone-pointing Death produced by a magic spell cast by a witch doctor into the victim's spirit. Pointing the bone is to some extent analogous to those patients with malignant disease whose realization of impending death is so terrible a blow that they die before the disease appears to have advanced enough to cause death.

Bonhoeffer, Karl (1868–1949) Berlin psychiatrist; symptomatic (organic) psychoses, acute exogenous reactions. *Bonhoeffer's sign* is the loss of normal muscle tone in chorea.

Bonnier's syndrome (Pierre Bonnier, French physician, 1861–1918) Symptoms resulting from a lesion involving the acoustic, glossopharyngeal, and vagus nerves: paroxysmal vertigo (Ménière's disease), contralateral hemiplegia, aphonia, dysphagia, and loss of gag reflex.

borderline personality Although the term has been used to refer to preschizophrenic or latent schizophrenic patients (see *borderline psychosis*), it has also been used as a description of one group of *personality disorders* (q.v.). It can thus best be regarded as a group of disorders whose lines of demarcation from other disorders is uncertain and varying. Among the characteristics that have been considered "typical" of borderline personality are lack of synthetic capacity, defective regulatory control of inner states; alternation and dissociation of ego states; sense of self-fragmentation; loss of sense of self and conflict of the self with objects; identity diffusion; instability of cohesive self; defects in autonomy; predominance of oral motifs; predominance of aggression; failure of phase dominance, and especially of libidinal-phase dominance; peculiar mixture of pregenital and genital defensive organization; polymorphous perverse sexual manifestations; narcissism, with tendencies to idealization and devaluation; significant role of projection; defects in object relations; impaired reality testing; sense of entitlement and specialness; sense of worthlessness, emptiness, vulnerability; controlling behavior; tendency to volatility; hypomanic behavior; destructive, annihilatory anger. Persons with borderline personality have also been described as having failed to achieve a stable evocative memory capacity, as a result of which the stress of rage abolishes their memories and phantasies of significant persons and they feel a sense of aloneness and abandonment; they are unable to maintain a therapeutic alliance, which is disrupted by overwhelming feelings.

borderline psychosis An inexact term, often used to describe a patient who is potentially psychotic (usually schizophrenic) but has not, as yet, broken with reality. See *schizophrenia, ambulatory; schizophrenia, pseudoneurotic.* "There are neurotic persons who, without developing a complete psychosis, have certain psychotic trends, or have a readiness to employ schizophrenic mechanisms whenever frustrations occur.... To this group belong queer psychopaths, abortive paranoids, the many 'apathic' individuals whom one may call hebephrenoid personalities, all the types who, as adults, retain or regain a large part of their primitive narcissism because they are able to answer narcissistic hurts with simple denials and with protective increase in their narcissism; they tend to react to frustrations with the loss of object relationships, although this loss frequently is only partial and temporary." (Fenichel, *PTN*)

The term "borderline" was originally used to describe patients who were not overtly psychotic (and thus by definition too ill to be placed on the couch) and yet did not respond well to classical psychoanalytic treatment. The term was extended to include several groups of patients who had been described and labeled by various clinicians: as if personality (Deutsch), ambulatory schizophrenia (Zilboorg), preschizophrenic disorder (Rapaport, Gill, Schafer), pseudoneurotic schizophrenia (Hoch, Polatin), latent schizophrenia (Federn), latent psychosis (Bychowski), and borderline schizophrenia (Kety, Rosenthal). R. Grinker, B. Werble, and R. Drye (*The Borderline Syndrome*, 1968) applied the term to patients they did not consider schizophrenic or preschizophrenic; since then the concept of borderline personality disorder that is distinct from the psychoses and also from other *personality disorders* (q.v.) has gained wide acceptance. Some authors hypothesize that borderline personality disorder may be more closely related to affective disorders than to schizophrenic disorders. See *borderline personality*.

Characteristic lifelong features include some or all of the following: (1) prominent anger, with behavior that is inexplicably rude, argumentative, sarcastic, demanding, or difficult; (2) unstable and stormy interpersonal relationships, lack of regard or concern for others and narcissistic preoccupation with self, feelings of entitlement or of being special, exploitative, and manipulative toward others; (3) impulsivity and unpredictable behavior, such as periodic binge eating or drug/alcohol abuse, promiscuity, shoplifting,

episodes of destroying property; (4) unstable, labile affect; (5) feelings of emptiness, loneliness, anhedonia; (6) fears of being alone, low frustration tolerance, tendency to act out; (7) lack of a consistent sense of personal identity, contradictory views of self and others; and (8) self-destructive actions, suicidal gestures, and recurrent accidents.

boredom A feeling of unpleasantness due to a need for more activity, or a lack of meaningful stimuli, or an inability to become stimulated. The last form is generally considered pathological and may be expressed as a need to maintain the status quo and as a stubborn clinging to stimuli that are without interest or meaning to the subject. Pathological boredom usually represents a defense against libidinal or aggressive strivings.

bouffées délirantes In the French nomenclature, acute delusional psychoses with a favorable outcome and no evidence of a strong genetic link to schizophrenia. See *psychosis, reactive*.

boundary, ego A concept introduced by Federn to refer to "the peripheral sense organ of the ego." The ego boundary discriminates what is real from what is unreal. Because the boundary is flexible and dynamic, it will vary in accordance with different ego states. There are two main ego boundaries, the inner and the outer. The inner ego bowndary is the boundary toward the repressed unconscious. This is strengthened by countercathexes (anticathexes) and thus is able to prevent the entrance of repressed material. Its flexibility is demonstrable in hypnagogic states and in normal falling asleep, where the ego and its boundaries lose cathexis and unegotized material enters. The external or outer ego boundary is the boundary toward stimuli of the external world. The external ego boundary includes the sense organs but it is more than mere summation of these, for the sense of reality of an object comes not alone by stimulation of a sense organ but further requires that the non-ego material impinges upon a well-cathected external ego boundary. If the boundary loses cathexis, these perceptions, no matter how vivid, will have a strange, unfamiliar, or even unreal quality. See *derealization*.

bouquet de malades (boo-kā' dĕ málåd')The distinctive odor said to be characteristic of psychiatric patients.

Bourneville's disease (Désiré-Magloire Bourneville, Paris neurologist, 1840–1909) Tuberous sclerosis. See *sclerosis, tuberous.*

bouton Terminal outpuching of the axon. See *neurotransmitter; synapse.*

bouts of ritual making See *ritual-making.*

Bovarism (From the title character in the novel *Madame Bovary*, by Gustave Flaubert) Confusion of daydreaming with the facts of the perceptual world; failure to differentiate between phantasy and reality.

bovina fames *Obs.* (L. "oxlike hunger") Bulimia.

boxer's traumatic encephalopathy See *dementia, boxer's.*

brachuna (brà-kū'nà) Acrai; nymphomania and/or satyriasis.

brachy- (brăk'i-) Combining form meaning (abnormally) short.

brachycephaly, brachycephalism A skull with shortened anteroposterior diameter. See *index, cephalic.*

brachylineal Brachymorphic.

brachymorphic Relating to or characterized by brachymorphy; a constitutional type that is shorter and broader than the normal, corresponding roughly to the *pyknic* type of Kretschmer or the *megalosplanchnic* type of Viola.

brachymorphy Shortness of stature. See *brachymorphic.*

brachyskelic Characterized by an excessive shortness of the legs. See *type, pyknic.*

brachytypical Synonymous with *brevilineal* and *brachymorphic* (qq.v.).

brady- (brăd'i-) Combining form meaning slow, from Gr. *bradys.*

bradyarthria Slowness of speech, due to some disorder in the central or peripheral apparatus connected with speech. See *bradylogia*, the implication of which is psychological (emotional) origin.

bradyglossia Slowness of speech because of impaired mobility of the tongue, which may be due to local tongue or mouth pathology or to more distant neural lesions (e.g. hypoglossal nerve, cerebellum, cerebrum).

bradykinesis, bradykinesia Slow or retarded movement; it may be organically or psychically determined. It is common in depressive states and is often observed in schizophrenia.

bradylalia Abnormal slowness of speech; *bradyarthria.* It may, like bradylexia, be occasioned by organic or psychological pathology or both. It is common in depressed states.

bradylexia Abnormal slowness in reading; it may be associated with mental retardation or other brain dysfunction, or it may be one manifestation of psychomotor retardation in depressive states.

bradylogia Slowness of speech; *bradyarthria.* Some use the terms interchangeably; others use bradyarthria to refer to organically determined slowness of speech and bradylogia for slowness determined by psychologic (emotional) factors.

bradyphasia Slowness of speech.

bradyphrasia Slowness of thought.

bradyphrenia Sluggish mentality. It is used by some as the equivalent of mental retardation, by others as the equivalent of psychomotor retardation.

Bradyphrenia may be symptomatic of any acquired disorder that interrupts the functioning of intelligence.

Bradyphrenia is focal when there is retardation in the presence only of disagreeable or painful ideas; it is diffuse when it is vague and unvarying irrespective of the topic in mind.

Slowness in thinking is often associated with states of intense emotion, as in severe anxieties and depressions; in the latter there may be a marked paucity or such a profusion of ideas as to lead to great difficulty in concentrated thinking. Bradyphrenia, like intellectual retardation, may be initial, that is, slowness in starting, or consistent, that is, slowness in continuing.

bradypragia Slowness of action, with the implication that the cause is organic (as generalized slowing in myxedema or other deficiency states). Some use the term also for psychomotor retardation of psychologic origin, which most would term *bradyphrenia* (q.v.).

bradytrophism Bouchard's term in constitutional medicine to designate a syndrome that is caused by a slowing down of the nutritive movement. The condition may be generalized or localized and is characteristic of such diseases as gout, diabetes, asthma, various chronic or recurrent rheumatisms, and various forms of lithiasis and of pruritic and chronic or recurrent desquamative dermatosis.

General bradytrophism results in products of imperfect metabolism and chronic autotoxemia. *Local* bradytrophism is best understood as a nutritive torpor of the organs that leads to the accumulation of lymph and waste material in their interstitium and gradually produces fatty infiltration, sclerosis, and early aging of the organs.

braid-cutting A perversion (paraphilia), relatively rare nowadays, consisting of the cutting of the hair from the victim. This perversion is a form of sadism combined with a fetishistic preference for hair. Psychoanalytically, it is interpreted as expressing the idea, "I am the castrator, not the castrated one," and often also the complementary idea, "I am only a pseudocastrator, not a real castrator." The knowledge that the hair will grow back is an important part of the reassurance that the subject gains from the act in that it proves to him that castration need not be final.

braidism (brād′iz'm) The theory of hypnosis named after James Braid, English surgeon (1795–1861), who in 1843 published *Neurypnology, or, the Rationale of Nervous Sleep, considered in relation with animal magnetism.*

brain The part of the nervous system within the skull; it includes the cerebrum, midbrain, cerebellum, pons, and medulla. See *neurochemistry.*

brain control Affecting behavior by physical manipulation of the brain; includes electrical or chemical stimulation of discrete areas of the brain, electroconvulsive treatment and psychosurgery (which is also known as functional neurosurgery, sedative neurosurgery, psychiatric surgery, etc.). As distinguished from neurosurgery, *psychosurgery* (q.v.) refers to the selective destruction of areas of the brain for the primary purpose of altering thoughts, emotional reactions, personality characteristics, or social response patterns. (Valenstein, E.S. *Brain Control,* 1973)

brain damage Intracranial birth injury and/or its results; among the most important causes are excessive or otherwise abnormal compression due to abnormal presentations, contracted pelvis, or instrumentation; excessive longitudinal stress produc-

ing tears of the dura and rupture of venous sinuses; certain methods of resuscitation, which predispose to sinus rupture; prematurity, which predisposes to intracranial hemorrhage. See *syndrome, organic.*

brain-damage behavior syndrome See *impulse disorder, hyperkinetic; syndrome, organic.*

brain disorder In DSM-I, any psychiatric syndrome caused by or related to impairment of brain tissue function, corresponding to what are termed *organic psychoses, organic reaction types, organic brain syndromes (OBS)* in DSM-II, or *organic mental disorders* in DSM-III. See *syndrome, organic.*

brain scan See *encephalography, radioisotopic; tomography.*

brain stem This term includes both the *pons* (q.v.) and the *medulla oblongata* (q.v.).

brain syndrome associated with systemic infection Organic reaction occurring as a complication of the acute or convalescent stages of such disorders as pneumonia, typhoid fever, rheumatic fever, scarlet fever, malaria, influenza, smallpox, and typhus; also known as infective-exhaustive psychosis, acute toxic encephalopathy, acute toxic encephalitis, and acute serous encephalitis. The chief types of reaction, which occur mainly in children, are delirious, epileptiform, stuporous or comatose, hallucinatory, and confusional. The most common form is the toxic delirium.

brain trauma See *brain damage; compression, cerebral; concussion; contusion, brain; syndrome, organic.*

brain tumor See *tumor, intracranial.*

brain, visceral See *rhinencephalon.*

brain wave See *electroencephalogram; neurometrics.*

brainstorm An inspirational thought or new perception of the world, often accompanying bursts of electrical activity within the limbic system. Such limbic seizural activity may be precipitated by psychologic stress and also by toxins and any metabolic imbalance.

Brainstorm has also been used to refer to any sudden disturbance in brain functioning and, more recently, to any sudden insight or new idea. The latter meaning is retained in the popular use of brainstorm as a verb, meaning to meet with others to exchange ideas in an atmosphere free of the ordinary constraints of logic and orthodoxy, in the hope that such freedom of associations will encourage new insights or creative solutions to problems.

brain washing See *deprivation, sensory; menticide.*

break-off A phenomenon that occurs in aviators when flying alone, at high altitudes, and when relatively unconcerned about flying details; the phenomenon consists of a feeling of physical separation from the earth. It is more frequent in emotionally unstable flyers and can itself precipitate an acute phobic reaction that may develop into a general fear of flying.

breakdown, nervous A popular, inexact term for the appearance of neurotic or psychotic symptoms of enough severity to impair significantly the person's ability to cope with the demands of his current life. The term implies a relatively sudden onset of disability and/or a readily discernible fall from a previously maintained level of performance or adaptation.

breakdown, social See *syndrome, social breakdown.*

breakthrough Sudden resumption of progress within psychoanalytic therapy after a period of doldrums, resistance, or inactivity. See *working-through.*

breeder hypothesis The theory that schizophrenia is caused by the social conditions under which many schizophrenics live: poverty, isolation, being single and/or an unskilled worker, living in the center of cities, etc. In opposition to the breeder hypothesis is the drift hypothesis: it is the schizophrenic illness that propels the patient into such conditions as social isolation and poverty.

Breuer, Joseph (1841–1925) Viennese neurologist; published (1895), with Freud, *Studien über Hysterie.*

brevilineal One of the two constitutional types distinguished by Manouvrier on the basis of the configuration of the body as a whole. In contradistinction to the longilineal type, it designates the type built along lines that are shorter and broader than the average figure.

Persons of this type correspond roughly to the *pyknic* type of Kretschmer, the *brachymorphic* type of Pende, and to their equivalents in other systems.

bribe In psychoanalysis, a compromise. The symptoms of a neurosis are regarded as symbolic representations of repressed impulses. At first the ego rejects the symptoms; later it becomes reconciled with them, since they afford a certain protection to the security of the ego. The symptoms are accepted by the ego in the nature of a bribe, but the acceptance carries certain favorable elements. For instance, there is the so-called secondary gain from suffering. The repressed impulse is released in the guise of symptoms; the patient does not recognize the released impulse in its new manner of expression. Moreover, in order to placate the *superego,* or inner conscience, the ego bribes it by suffering. "Thus, forbidden pleasure gratification, by being presented to the Ego as a punishment, is made acceptable. At the same time, the Super-Ego itself, which recognizes the latent meaning of the symptom in spite of disguise, is 'bribed with suffering.' " (Healy et al., *SMP*)

Brickner, Richard (1896–1959) American neurologist; multiple sclerosis, physiology of the frontal lobes.

bridging In multimodal behavior therapy, accepting the patient's interpretation or viewpoint and discussing it before branching off into a modality that the therapist believes is more likely to be significant. This is in contrast to confrontation techniques that try, for example, to challenge the patient's rationalizations or denial and arouse intense emotions. The bridging technique ultimately gets to the same significant modality—whether behavior, affect, imagery, or any other—but in doing so it takes care not to dismiss the patient's initial productions as irrelevant, trivial, or resistant. See *BASIC-ID.*

brief psychotherapy See *psychotherapy, brief.*

brief reactive psychosis Any reaction to major stress that is of psychotic proportions, with impaired reality testing and emotional turmoil, and a return to the premorbid level of functioning within one month. See *schizophreniform disorder.*

Briggs's law See *law, Briggs's.*

Brigham, Amariah (1798–1849) American physician and alienist; founded *American Journal of Insanity* (1844), now the *American Journal of Psychiatry;* "moral treatment."

Brill, A.A. (1874–1948) First American psychoanalyst; translated Freud's works into English.

Briquet, Paul (brē-kā′) (1796–1881) French psychiatrist; author of a monumental treatise on hysteria (1859), which is consequently termed Briquet's syndrome.

Brissaud's syndrome (brē-sō′) (Edouard Brissaud, French physician, 1852–1909) Infantilism due to thyroid dysfunction; cretinism.

broadcasting, thought See *symptoms, first-rank.*

Broca's speech area (Paul Broca, Parisian anthropologist and surgeon, 1824–80) The motor speech area; areas 44 and 45 of Brodmann; the inferior end of the motor area in the third left frontal convolution. Lesions here in a right-handed subject result in motor aphasia; in pure motor aphasia, the patient is able to write or otherwise indicate his desires, but articulate speech either is impossible or is restricted to a few ill-pronounced expletives.

bromidism Bromide intoxication that may be manifested in several ways: (1) simple intoxication, with mental dulling, memory disturbances, enfeeblement, tremor (especially of the hands, face, and tongue), ataxia, incoordination, acneform dermatitis, fetid breath, and coated tongue; (2) delirium, with disorientation in all spheres; (3) hallucinosis, with marked fear reactions; in contrast to delirium tremens, bromide hallucinosis lasts weeks rather than days; (4) schizophreniform psychosis; or (5) pseudoepilepsy.

bromidrosiphobia Morbid dread of the alleged offensive odors of the body.

bromidrosis Perspiration with foul odor.

brontophobia Fear of thunder; astraphobia. It is related in part to the dread of allegedly demonical phenomena of nature, akin to personalization of such phenomena by primitive man; it may also be related to fear of real persons, and especially of the father or father figure.

brooding Anxious or moody pondering, usually about very abstract matters. Brooding is seen frequently in obsessive-compulsive neurotics as a *thinking compulsion,* a need to worry very much about apparently insignificant things. This is a form of displacement onto a small detail and represents an attempt to avoid objectionable impulses or affects by escaping from the world of emotions into a world of intellectual concepts and words; also

termed intellectualization or *Grübelsucht* (q.v.).

brooding spells One of Rado's subdivisions of obsessive attacks is called *spells of doubting and brooding:* a swinging back and forth between the same pros and the same cons without reaching a decision. Since this may invade any mental activity, the patient soon finds he can trust no belief, no memory, not even his own observations, and as a result he must check and recheck his every move, to make sure that it has been right. See *obsessive-compulsive psychoneurosis.*

Brown-Séquard's syndrome (brown-sakȧr′) (Charles Brown-Séquard, French neurologist, 1817–94) Hemisection of the spinal cord (as in cord tumor, syringomyelia, stab wound, etc.) producing homolateral lower motor neuron paralysis in the segment of the lesion, homolateral upper motor neuron paralysis below the lesion, homolateral anesthesia in the segment of the lesion, homolateral hyperesthesia below the lesion, homolateral loss of proprioception, vibratory and two-point discrimination below the lesion, contralateral hyperesthesia in the segment of the lesion, and contralateral loss of pain and temperature below the lesion.

Brudzinski sign See *sign, Brudzinski.*

Brueghel's syndrome See *syndrome, Meige.*

Bruns's sign (Ludwig Bruns, German neurologist, 1858–1916) Headache, vertigo, and vomiting associated with sudden movements of the head, occurring in cases of tumor of the fourth ventricle.

bruxer A term suggested for a person with bruxism.

bruxing Grinding the teeth.

bruxism (bruk′siz′m) Gnashing or grinding of the teeth that occurs typically at night, during sleep. It is said to be especially common in alcoholics and to indicate repressed aggressivity or hostility.

bruxomania Grinding, pounding, or setting of the teeth apart from the normal activity of mastication. There results a loosening of the teeth and a bleeding of the gums.

BSEP Brain stem-evoked potential. See *neurometrics.*

BST Brief stimulus therapy. See *therapy, brief stimulus.*

budgeting, functional See *functional budgeting.*

buffoonery psychosis See *psychosis, buffoonery.*

bufotenin (bu-fō′te-nin) Dimethylserotonin. An analogue of serotonin that, unlike serotonin itself, is psychotomimetic in the cat, monkey, and man and produces effects similar to those seen following lysergic acid or mescaline administration. It has been suggested that conversion of serotonin into bufotenin rather than breakdown by monoamine oxidase into 5-hydroxyindole acetic acid may be of significance in the etiology of endogenous psychoses.

bug, cocaine One of the more common unpleasant tactual paresthesiae that may appear during withdrawal of cocaine in a cocaine addict. Also known as *formication.* The patient typically interprets the sensation as an itching, biting, crawling, or sticking due to an insect. See *sign, Magnan.*

bugger Colloquial for a homosexual who practices anal intercourse, from *bougre,* a French word for heretics, and particularly for certain types of Bulgarian origin; later it came to refer to a person who practiced sodomy, or to a homosexual male. In modern French, the word has no sexual implication.

bulbar Referring to the bulb (see *medulla oblongata*).

bulbocapnine One of the drugs used relatively early in the many experiments of H.H. DeJong in experimental production of catatonia.

bulbotegmental reticular formation See *formation, reticular.*

bulesis The motivational or volitional apparatus; the will. See *abulia.*

bulimarexia See *restricters.*

bulimia (bū-lēm′ē-à) Insatiable hunger; also known as bulimia nervosa, fames canina, phagedena, phagomania, polyphagia. Bulimia is the type of *eating disorder* (q.v.) characterized by a pattern of eating binges during which a large amount of food is ingested in a short period of time (usually less than two hours). Each binge is typically followed with depression in mood and disparaging self-criticism and, in some, imposition of a rigid diet. Bulimia occurs most frequently in females, beginning in adolescence or early adulthood, and extending over a period of many years.

bulimia nervosa A chronic phase of anorexia nervosa characterized by self-induced vomiting and purging following eating (which is usually of the binge eating variety). The resulting loss of body fluids and electrolytes may lead to EKG abnormalities, muscle weakness, tetany, and other disturbances. Bulimia nervosa is often used interchangeably with *bulimia* (q.v.), but in practice the term emphasizes the physiologic results of binge eating while bulimia alone emphasizes the eating behavior. See *restricters.*

Bumke, Oswald (1877–1950) German psychiatrist and neurologist.

burnout A syndrome of physical, emotional, or attitudinal exhaustion characterized by impaired work performance, fatigue, insomnia, depression, increased susceptibility to physical illness, reliance on alcohol or other drugs of abuse for temporary relief with a tendency to escalation into physiologic dependency, and in many cases suicide. The syndrome is generally considered to be a stress reaction to unrelenting performance and emotional demands stemming from one's occupation. See *life, noon of.*

Burrow, Trigant (1875–1951) American psychoanalyst; developed *phyloanalysis* (q.v.).

Butler, John S. (1803–90) American psychiatrist; one of the "original thirteen" founders of Association of Medical Superintendents of America (forerunner of American Psychiatric Association).

buying spree Oniomania.

BWAM Brain wave activity measurement. See *neurometrics.*

BWS Battered wife syndrome. See *wife battering.*

by-idea The secondary or manifest thought, concept, symbol, or idea onto which the primary or latent idea is displaced. While discussing speech disorders in dreams, Kraepelin (*DP*) said: "The common feature in all these observations (dream paraphasias) is the displacement of the basic thought by the entrance of a by-association, for an essential link of the chain of ideas. The derailment of speech or of thought to a by-association is due, in my opinion, to lack of distinctness in the ideas." He also said: "The by-idea causing the displacement of thought was distinctly a narrower and more comprehensive idea which suppressed the more general and more shadowy one." He referred to this condition as *metaphoric paralogia.*

C

C In Rorschach scoring, a color response, i.e. response of an object imagined to have the same chromatic colors as those which stimulated the response. The color responses measure the degree of emotional responsiveness to the environment, whether positive or negative. The greater the role of the form element in color responses (scored as *FC*), the more the subject considers others in his emotional attitudes. The greater the role of color in relation to form (the *CF* responses), the more blind, self-centered and inconsiderate is the subject in his emotional reactions. A lack of *C* responses indicates apathy and flatness of emotions.

c In Rorschach scoring, that type of shading response determined by the light shades of gray on the blots and uninfluenced by the form of the area. See *ShR.*

c' In Rorschach scoring, that type of shading response determined by the dark or black areas and uninfluenced by the form of the area. See *ShR.*

C-L Consultation-liaison. See *consultant.*

CA 1. Abbreviation for chronological age. 2. Catecholamine.

cacergasia *Obs.* Inadequate functioning of body or mind.

cachectin See *cachexia.*

cachexia A chronic catabolic state, associated with certain infections and malignancies, characterized by weight loss that continues despite consumption of an adequate diet. A factor or factors—termed *cachectin*—produced by endotoxin-stimulated macrophages inhibits the activity of lipogenic (fat-producing) enzymes, and triglycerides are mobilized from adipose tissue with resultant weight loss. See *anorexia nervosa; cachexia, hypophysial.*

cachexia, hypophysial A condition due to necrosis or other destruction of the anterior lobe of the pituitary gland, occurring most commonly in women. Characteristic symptoms are marked asthenia, great loss of weight with extreme emaciation, chilliness, slow pulse, anemia, low basal metabolic rate, loss of hair, amenorrhea or impotence, somnolence, apathy, poor memory, and occasionally hallucinations and delirium. Also known as *Simmonds' disease* (q.v.). See *anorexia nervosa.*

cachinnation (kak-i-nā'shun) Inordinate laughter without apparent cause; it is common in the hebephrenic form of schizophrenia.

caco- (kak'ō-) Combining form meaning bad, vitiated, distorted; from Gr. *kakós*, bad, evil.

cacodaemonomania A condition in which the patient believes himself to be, or to be inhabited by, or possessed of, a devil or some evil spirit; it may be a symptom of the hebephrenic form of schizophrenia.

cacogenic The term (the opposite of *aristogenic* or *eugenic*, qq.v.) means "giving rise to a deteriorated race" and refers to deteriorating agencies in heredity.

cacogeusia (-gū'sē-à) A bad taste; a frequent complaint in idiopathic epilepsy, in patients receiving tranquilizer therapy, and in somatic delusional states.

cacolalia *Coprolalia; coprophrasia* (qq.v.).

cacopathia *Obs.* A Hippocratic designation for a severe mental disorder.

cacophoria See *euphoria.*

cacosomnia *Obs.* Sleeplessness.

cacothymia *Obs.* Any mental affection with depravation of the morals. (Tuke, *DPM*)

cadiva insania (L. "falling or epileptic insanity") *Obs.* Epilepsy.

caduca passio (L. "falling disease") *Obs.* Epilepsy.

caducus morbus (L. "falling sickness.") *Obs.* Epilepsy.

caelotherapy Pastoral counseling. See *counseling, pastoral*.

cafard (ka-far') *Depression* (q.v.) of severe degree, such as acute depression in Kraepelin's terminology or melancholia in DSM-III.

caffeine intoxication Caffeinism, caused by the ingestion of substances containing caffeine (coffee, tea, cola drinks, hot chocolate, cocoa, cold remedies, some analgesics, etc.). Symptoms of intoxication may appear with intake of 250 mg of caffeine per day (coffee contains 100–150 mg of caffeine per cup, tea about half as much, cola about one third as much); they include restlessness, excitement, insomnia, flushing, diuresis, and a feeling of nervousness. Above levels of 1 g per day there may be muscle twitchings, increased psychomotor activity, rambling thought and speech, cardiac arrhythmias, ringing in the ears and other sensory disturbances. Convulsions, respiratory failure and death have been reported with doses above 10 g.

CAGE A four-question screening instrument for the detection of alcoholism devised by Ewing and Rouse; the letters of the acronym refer to the key word in each question—(1) Have you ever felt you should *Cut* down on your drinking? (2) Have people *Annoyed* you by criticizing your drinking? (3) Have you ever felt bad or *Guilty* about your drinking? (4) Have you ever used a drink as an *Eye*-opener (a drink first thing in the morning to steady your nerves or get rid of a hangover)?

cainophobia, cainotophobia See *kainotophobia; neophobia*.

Cairns' stupor Akinetic or diencephalic stupor: stupor, rigidity, postural catatonia, absence of spontaneous movement and emotion. See *mutism, akinetic*.

caisson disease See *disease, caisson*.

calamitous relationship See *group tension, common*.

calcarine area See *lobe, occipital*.

calcium channel blockade See *verapamil*.

callipedia *Obs.* The desire to give birth to a beautiful child.

callomania *Obs.* Love of beauty and grace; the delusion that one is beautiful.

callosal gyrus *Cingulate gyrus* (q.v.).

camisole A canvas shirt with very long sleeves, used to restrain a violently psychotic person; popularly known as a strait-jacket. The shirt is put on and securely laced, and then the patient's arms are folded and the ends of the sleeves are fastened behind the back; sometimes simply a square of canvas fastened behind with a buckle, binding the arms to the sides of body.

camouflage, neurotic A term for neurotic endeavor to disguise. "It represents an attempt to reconcile two psychic processes which tend to go in opposite directions. The patient wishes to be obedient to the compulsion imposed by the neurosis, but at the same time he feels impelled to heed the psychic necessity of making his behavior conform to the requirements of his social milieu.... I venture to assert that social camouflage constitutes a typical feature in the behavior of all psychoneurotics at a certain stage of development of their neurosis." (Reik, T. *American Imago 2*, 1941) The neurotic camouflage is particularly evident in the obsessive-compulsive patient, whose need to conform often drives him to obsessional rehearsal. See *rehearsal, obsessional*.

cAMP See *adenyl cyclase*.

campimeter A chart upon which the visual field is plotted or projected. See *field defect*.

camptocormia (kamp-tō-kōr'mē-à) Functional bent back; first described by Brodie in 1837, named camptocormia by Souques in 1915. It consists of persistent lumbar pain, anterior bending of the trunk of the body, and an anthropoid posture with head and trunk parallel with the ground and the arms swinging. Often there is a history of trauma, and almost always there is an accompanying psychic impotence. Most cases reported have been in soldiers; Kosbab reported the only known case in a woman, in 1961. In many of the cases the symptom has served as a conversion defense against an underlying schizophrenic process.

canalization Restriction of behavior patterns, and particularly the choice of one way of satisfying a drive in preference to all other possible ways. Janet used the term to refer to substitutive discharge of tension.

cancer, fear of The fear of cancer occurs quite frequently, especially in older persons, but sometimes it is seen as a phobia in younger persons too. It may represent a fear of castration and/or a fear of being devoured by an introjected object.

canchasmus (kang-kaz′mus) *Obs.* Inordinate laughter sometimes observed in hysterical and schizophrenic patients.

canina appetentia (L. "dog-appetite") *Obs.* Bulimia.

cannabis organic mental disorders Those mental disorders associated with cannabis abuse and cannabis dependence (see *mari-huana*). Included are (1) cannabis intoxication—euphoria, intensified perceptions, a feeling of time slowing down, tachycardia, conjunctival injection, increased appetite, and maladaptive behavioral effects such as paranoid ideas, panic attacks, a fear of "going crazy"; (2) delusional syndrome—persists only a few hours and may be only an extension of the paranoid ideas of cannabis intoxication; (3) delirium.

cannibalistic In psychoanalysis, referring to the hostile, sadistic aspects of (usually oral) introjection or incorporation.

Cannon hypothalamic theory of emotion Cannon and Bard offered a more modern version of Head's thalamic theory: afferent impulses from peripheral receptors may evoke patterned efferent "emotional" responses directly through reflex pathways at the thalamic level and/or indirectly through arousal of "conditioned responses" at the cortical level, which in turn release diencephalically integrated patterns of emotional response from cortical inhibition. At the same time, upward discharges from the activated diencephalon reach the cortex, thus adding a patterned "quale" to the sensory experience and transforming the "object-simply-apprehended" to the "object-emotionally-felt."

Cannon, Walter B. (1871–1945) American physiologist, whose broad-ranging studies led ultimately to enunciation of the principles of homeostasis ("wisdom of the body"). His experiments in diagnostic roentgenography stimulated his interest in esophageal and gastrointestinal motility and subsequently to recognition of the role of the autonomic nervous system, humoral transmission, and "sympathin." From that point he turned to a study of shock and the role of the adrenal medulla and then to investigation of the central nervous system basis for emotion.

Capgras, Jean Marie Joseph (1873–1950) French psychiatrist. See *syndrome, Capgras's.*

capsule, internal See *basal ganglia.*

captation *Obs.* Used by Descourtis to denote the first stage in hypnosis.

captivation Max Hirsch's term for the state of light hypnosis; Hirschlaff called the state one of pseudohypnosis.

caput obstipum *Obs.* See *torticollis.*

carbon dioxide inhalation See *therapy, carbon dioxide inhalation.*

card sorting See *tests, sorting.*

cardiazol (kär′dē-à-zōl) Metrazol.

cardiopathia adolescentium *Obs.* Immaturity or inadequate development of the heart, seen frequently in asthenic body types.

care, alternate level of See *ALC.*

care, custodial Any of a continuum of services in which protection and monitoring of the patient, or protection of others from the patient's aggressive potential, is of paramount importance. Custodial care may include active medical intervention, but most often it is needed for chronically ill patients whose level of functioning is unlikely to change appreciably for the better, even though they may require continuing drug treatment and milieu therapy to prevent or retard further deterioration.

care, intermediate Residential program providing rehabilitation rather than acute inpatient or skilled nursing care. Included are halfway houses, quarterway houses, and recovery homes that are usually community based, and especially for alcoholism and drug abuse programs peer-group oriented services that provide food, shelter, and supportive services in an alcohol- or drug-free environment.

care, long-term All those habilitation and rehabilitation services and social restructuring that are required to maintain a patient at the highest level of functioning possible within the limitations imposed by chronic mental illness. Such services may include custodial care within a mental hospital, partial hospitalization, or a spectrum of domiciliary settings ranging from highly structured skilled nursing facilities through halfway houses to *satellite housing* (q.v.) with minimal supervision. Almost always, they also include psychopharmacologic treatment, which, in combination with the foregoing organization technology, aims to prevent symptomatic relapse and enable the patient to perform appropriately within the social unit of which he is a part. See *rehabilitation.*

carebaria Unpleasant head sensations, such as pressure or heaviness in the head.

caregiver Any person involved in the identification or treatment or prevention of illness, and in the rehabilitation of patients. The *primary physician* (typically, the general practitioner in the community to whom the patient comes for help, no matter what the nature of the problem or illness) is often termed the front-line caregiver. Another type of caregiver is the *indigenous worker*—the person from the population being serviced who has had special training in diagnostic or treatment techniques and whose function is "to find out from the residents of the neighborhood how they saw their needs, and to explore with them the ways in which we [i.e. the professionals of the Community Mental Health Center] could or could not be helpful." (Peck, H.B., Roman, M., & Kaplan, S.R. *Psychiatric Research Report 21,* APA, April 1967) A third type of caregiver, the *indigenous therapist,* is a member of a community who uses sociologic circumstances peculiar to the predominant ethnic and culture groups of that community in an attempt to correct, ameliorate, or modify physical and/or mental disorders. See *enabler.*

carezza Also karezza; coitus prolongatus, *coitus reservatus* (q.v.).

carotodynia Pain in the malar (cheek) region, in the back of the neck, and about the eyes due to pressure on the common carotid artery.

carpal tunnel syndrome See *syndrome, carpal tunnel.*

carphology *Trichologia;* aimless picking or plucking at the clothes or bed coverings, seen often in patients with primary dementia and in deliria.

carrier See *taint carrier; trait carrier.*

carrier screening See *screening, genetic.*

carus catalepsia *Obs.* Catalepsy.

carus lethargus *Obs.* Lethargy.

case-control study See *methodology.*

case ethics See *casuistry.*

case index In genetics and epidemiology, the person in a family or group who is the subject of investigation.

case mix The relative frequency of different types of patients treated at a particular site. In prospective payment approaches, a hospital's case mix is determined by principal and secondary diagnoses, age, discharge status, operating room procedures, and significant or substantial comorbidities and complications.

casework, social One of the major divisions of social work along with social group work and community organization or social welfare planning. Its concern is with social relationships and its disciplines directed toward the release of individual capacities and the relieving of environmental pressures.

castration Surgical removal of the ovaries (*ovariectomy, oophorectomy*) or of the testes (*orchidectomy*). The result in females is loss of the ablility to produce ova and elimination of estrus, and in males loss of the ability to produce sperm. Castration is now used only for medical reasons (e.g. control of prostatic and breast carcinomas). For eugenic purposes, sterilization by *vasectomy* or *salpingectomy* is preferred to castration, since they affect only reproductive capacity whereas castration affects both reproductive capacity and secondary sex characteristics.

When performed or occurring *after* puberty, castration has in neither sex such drastic effects as are observed following surgical removal of the sex organs in early life, when the secondary sex characters of the organism have not yet developed. Castration *before* puberty results in *eunuchoidism* or *eunuchism*—the development of the secondary sexual characteristics of the opposite sex. *Eunuchoid women* are recognizable by male body proportions, deep voice, and hairiness of body and face, and *eunuchoid men* by large hips, narrow sloping shoulders, absence of beard and body hair, high-pitched voice, etc.

In psychoanalytic theory castration means loss of the penis, and the *castration complex* refers to the boy's fear of loss or injury to his penis, and the girl's concern that she lacks a penis. The castration complex is typically associated with the phallic stage of psychosexual development, and the manner in which the castration complex is handled determines in large part the fate of the Oedipus complex. See *complex, Oedipus; envy, penis; ontogeny, psychic.*

castrophilia *Obs.* See *transvestitism.*

castrophenia *Nooklopia* (q.v.).

casuistry The science of dealing with matters of conscience and deciding on questions of right and wrong in conduct. The term is often used in a derogatory sense to refer to the highly specific quality of rules used by casuists and the certainty they express about the acceptablility or unacceptability of specific types of conduct. The casuist's approach to case ethics is to apply practical traditions (e.g., the Jewish *halachah,* the Catholic *casus conscientiae,* Protestant case morality, Anglo-American common law), based on experience with concrete modes of behavior, rather than to try to develop abstract and general principles.

cat cry syndrome See *syndrome, cat cry.*

CAT scan Computerized axial tomography scan; see *encephalography, radioisotopic; tomography.*

catabolic Pertaining to, or characterized by, *catabolism* (q.v.). In constitutional medicine the term applies to the *anabolic-catabolic balance,* which, according to the theories of Pende, is the most fundamental criterion in describing or typing human beings (see *anabolic*).

On the basis of this concept, the *catabolic biotype* constitutes the fundamental underlying type to which the more superficial characterizations of the types called *microsplanchnic, dolichomorphic,* and *sympathicotonic* (qq.v.), among others, apply.

catabolism In physiology and general medicine, this means *destructive metabolism* or a downward series of changes by which complex bodies are broken down into simpler forms. In certain cases, of course, catabolism can be constructive, especially in botany. See *metabolism, destructive.*

catabythismus *Obs.* Suicide by drowning.

cataclonia, cataclonus Rhythmic convulsive movements, especially when psychically determined.

catagelophobia Fear of ridicule. See *agoraphobia.*

catalentia *Obs.* A Paracelsian term for epilepsy.

catalepsia cerea *Obs.* Catalepsy.

catalepsy Inordinate maintenance of postures or physical attitudes. The term is usually synonymous with *flexibilitas cerea.*

"The muscular system may be in a condition of *waxy flexibility,* permitting of the molding of the limbs into any position where they remain indefinitely—*catalepsy.*" (Jelliffe & White, *DNS*) Catalepsy is regarded as a high degree of suggestibility and is often associated with other forms of suggestibility, such as echopraxia, echolalia, command automatism, etc.

Waxlike postures may also appear with rigid rather than flexible musculature, so-called *rigid catalepsy.*

Cataleptic states may appear in a wide variety of clinical syndromes, but are most common in schizophrenia, epilepsy, and hysteria. It may be psychically induced through hypnotism. "Cerebellar patients, also, and certain types of cases with fronto-cerebellar pathway disturbances show what is known as *cataleptic rigidity* in this (erect) position." (Ibid.)

catalepsy, artificial Catalepsy occurring during induced hypnosis.

catalepsy, epidemic Cataleptic states appearing simultaneously in many persons, as a consequence of imitation or identification.

catalepsy, rigid See *catalepsy.*

catalexia A type of reading disability characterized by a tendency to reread words and phrases.

catalogia *Catalexia; cataphasia; logoclonia; verbigeration* (qq.v.).

catalysator, catalyzator (kat′à-li-zā-tēr) An external stimulus that serves to loosen inhibitions; a catalyzer.

catamite *Rare.* A male (the term implies a young boy) who adopts a passive or receptive role in homosexual activity. See *active.*

catamnesis (kat-am-nē′sis) The medical history of a patient following a given illness, the so-called follow-up history; sometimes used to refer to the history of the patient and his illness following the initial examination.

cataphasia The repetition of words or phrases, seen in pronounced form in the catatonic form of schizophrenia. See *stereotypy; verbigeration.*

cataphora (kà-taf′ō-rà) A form of coma that may be interrupted by transitory states of partial consciousness; coma somnolentium.

cataphrenia *Pseudodementia* (q.v.).

cataplectic attack See *cataplexy.*

cataplexy (kat′a-plek-sē) Temporary paralysis or immobilization. "Cataplexy denotes paroxysmal attacks of loss of muscle tone (often without loss of consciousness), so that the patient sinks to the ground. It is usually associated with narcoleptic attacks (paroxysms of sleep)." (Henderson, D.K., & Gillespie, R.D. *A Text-Book of Psychiatry*, 1936)

cataplexy of awakening See *paralysis, sleep.*

cataptosis Galen's term for an epileptic or apoplectic seizure.

catastrophe See *behavior, catastrophic; theory, catastrophe.*

catathymia In psychoanalysis, the existence in the unconscious of a complex that is sufficiently charged with affects to produce effects in consciousness.

catatonia, deadly See *Bell's mania.*

catatonia, depressive Synonymous with, but rarely used today for catatonic stupor. See *schizophrenia, catatonic.*

catatonia, katatonia A lowering of tension. From the clinical point of view many different syndromes have been called catatonia. Modern descriptions of the clinical condition were first given by Kahlbaum in 1874 and the general concepts laid down by him have prevailed, save for minor changes. Kahlbaum regarded catatonia as a nosologic entity, but since the later works of Kraepelin it has been looked upon as a subdivision of schizophrenia (see *schizophrenia, catatonic*). It is true that catatonic or rather cataleptoid syndromes are not infrequently a part of other diagnostic groups (e.g. hysteria and manic-depressive psychosis), but the tendency is to restrict the term catatonia to the schizophrenic group. Cataleptoid states may also be observed in association with organic pathology, as is found, for example, in lethargic encephalitis.

The clinical syndrome called *catatonia* is characterized as a rule by (1) stupor, associated with either marked rigidity or flexibility of the musculature or (2) overactivity in conjunction with various manifestations of stereotypy.

catatonia, lethal See *Bell's mania.*

catatonia, manic *Rare.* Catatonic excitement. See *schizophrenia, catatonic.*

catatonia mitis (mē′tēs) A mild and relatively short course of catatonia, with stupor and immobility as the principal symptoms.

When the catatonic syndrome is more extensive, resembling that described un-

der the heading *schizophrenia, catatonic,* the expression catatonia protracta is sometimes used.

catatonia, periodic In Leonhard's classification, a subtype of nonsystematic schizophrenia characterized by acute episodes of akinetic symptoms, sometimes interrupted by hyperkinetic symptoms, and regular remissions between episodes. See *schizophrenia, systematic.*

catatonia protracta See *catatonia mitis.*

catatonia, Stauder's lethal See *paralysis, catatonic cerebral.*

catatonic cerebral paralysis See *paralysis, catatonic cerebral.*

catatonic schizophrenia See *schizophrenia, catatonic.*

catatony (kà-tat′ō-nē) A rarely used Anglicized form of catatonia.

catchment area See *psychiatry, community.*

catecholamine See *epinephrine.*

catecholamine hypothesis In relation to affective disorders, the hypothesis states that some or all depressions are associated with a relative deficiency of norepinephrine at functionally important adrenergic receptor sites in the brain and that elations (manias) are associated with an excess of such amines. Confirmation of the hypothesis will require direct demonstration of such a biochemical abnormality in the naturally occurring illness and that has not yet been achieved. However, even were such a biochemical abnormality demonstrated, it would not necessarily imply a genetic or constitutional etiology of affective disorders, for early experiences of the infant or child may also cause enduring biochemical changes that predispose to affective disorders in adulthood. (Schildkraut, J.J., & Kety, S.S. *Science 156,* 1967)

categorical attitude *Abstract attitude* (q.v.).

categorization, symbolic A type of abstract thinking that requires the subject to make a mental diagram of relationships in order to answer the question posed; it is used as a measure of dominant parietal lobe functioning. An example is: What is the relationship to you of your brother's mother? Of your brother's mother-in-law?

category mistake See *mistake, category.*

catharsis In psychiatry the term was first used by Freud to designate a type of psychotherapy. He tried through the methods of free association and hypnosis to bring so-called traumatic experiences and their affective associations into consciousness. Psychiatric symptoms or symbols are looked upon as disguised representations of forgotten and repressed ideas or experiences. When the latter are brought back into the sphere of consciousness and lived out fully (in a therapeutic sense), the method is called catharsis.

Abreaction and *catharsis* are often used synonymously.

catharsis, activity In psychotherapy, especially in activity group psychotherapy, a catharsis in which the patients convey their unconscious preoccupations and conscious intent through *action* rather than through language.

catharsis, community Abreaction in a group, as in *psychodrama* (q.v.).

catharsis, emotional *Catharsis; abreaction* (qq.v.).

catharsis, psychodramatic See *psychodrama.*

cathect, cathecticize To charge with, to infuse with psychic energy. See *cathexis.*

cathexis Concentration of psychic energy on a given object. Investment of the psychic energy of a drive in a conscious or unconscious mental representation such as a concept, idea, image, phantasy, or symbol.

From the standpoint of general location of cathexis psychoanalysts refer to three terms:

1. *Ego-cathexis*—when the psychic energy is attached to the conscious division of the ego. Hence, the expressions ego-libido and narcissism arise. Some use the term *self-libido* or *autolibido* in contradistinction to *object-libido.*

2. *Phantasy-cathexis*—when psychic energy is attached to wish-formations or phantasies or to their original sources in the unconscious. Both ego-cathexis and phantasy-cathexis are associated with primary narcissism.

3. *Object-cathexis*—the expression employed to refer to psychic energy that is attached to some object outside of the subject himself or to its representation in the mind of the person. Object-cathexis is less stable or fixed than the other forms, because it is associated with manifestations of secondary narcissism, which, in turn, are less durable than those of the primary kind.

When there is an overcharge of psychic energy in an object, the term *hypercathexis* is used; when an undercharge, *hypocathexis.*

Other words are often prefixed to the term cathexis: (1) to signify the quality of the charge—adjectives, as in affective-cathexis, libidinal-cathexis, erotic-cathexis, instinctual cathexis; nouns, as in word-cathexis, thought-cathexis, thing-cathexis, or (2) to express the degree of cathexis, as in hypercathexis, hypocathexis, acathexis.

catochus (kat'ō-kus) *Obs.* Catalepsy, especially that phase of ecstasy or trance in which the patient is conscious but cannot move or speak.

caudate nucleus (kaw'dāt) See *basal ganglia.*

causalgia (kaw-sal'jē-à) Sensation of burning pain in the distribution of a peripheral nerve, associated with glossy skin devoid of hair or wrinkles. Other associated changes include swelling, redness, sweating, and curling of the nails. Causalgia is usually due to irritation of a nerve by injury; the median or sciatic nerves are most commonly involved.

cause, distinct sustaining See *sustaining cause, distinct.*

CAVD A measure of intelligence, devised by Thorndike, consisting of a battery of four tests: completion, arithmetic, vocabulary, and direction-following.

CBA See *analysis, cost/benefit.*

CCC Citrated calcium carbamide; sometimes used as a substitute for Antabuse (disulfiram) in the treatment of alcoholism.

Cd In Rorschach scoring, color denial, i.e. protestation that the color had nothing to do with the percept or that the color on the blot is wrong. Color denial indicates a neurotic avoidance of realistic attitudes and a wish for more intense emotional experiences.

CEA See *analysis, cost-effectiveness.*

cell In biology, the term denotes those minute structural units of protoplasmic nature that determine the different organic qualities of plant and animal bodies. Cells are ubiquitous and represent the fundamental elements of all organisms. They are so small—ranging ordinarily from 0.01 to 0.1 mm in diameter—that there may be billions of them in a cubic inch of tissue.

Each cell consists of a denser protoplasmic body, the *nucleus,* which exerts a governing influence over all cellular activities, and the surrounding *cytoplasm*. All development from seed or egg involves cells, and each phase of hereditary transmission is guided and affected by cellular elements.

In the many-celled animals there are two genetically different classes of cells, the *somatic* or *body* cells, which are directly responsible for the actual manifestation of inherited characters but have nothing to do with their transmission, except in primitive types of reproduction; and the *germ* cells, which perform the transmission from generation to generation in the higher forms of reproduction. In animals, the somatic cells produce germ cells only very rarely, while the germ cells give rise in every generation to both somatic and germ cells, thus constituting a reserve out of which the genetic continuity of the germ cells and the repetition of the production of bodies in each generation are maintained.

The process of cell division is initiated and controlled largely by the nucleus and is commonly called *mitosis*.

cell, body That type of somatic cell that forms the somatoplasm of higher animals and does not produce germ cells. According to Weismann's germ plasm theory, the body cells have nothing to do with the hereditary transmission of inherited characters but are responsible only for their phenotypical manifestations, at least in the higher forms of reproduction. See *plasm, germ; somatoplasm*.

cell, germ That type of cell that transmits inherited characteristics from generation to generation. See *cell*.

cell, padded An older term for what is nowadays more commonly called a *seclusion room* or *quiet room*, used as a form of physical restraint in the management of disturbed or violent patients who are a danger to themselves or others, and for patients who ask for help in gaining control over destructive impulses. The older term emphasized the physical features of the room that ensured the patient's safety: a large mattress on the floor and padding on the walls.

cell, Purkinje (Johannes Evangelista Purkinje, Bohemian physiologist, 1787–1869) See *cerebellum*.

celom, coelom (sē'lom) In the tridermic stage of embryological development, the splitlike cavity formed by the lateral plates of the middle germ layer or *mesoderm* (q.v.).

cene-, coene- Combining form meaning common or general, from Gr. *koinós*.

cenesthesia (sē-nes thē'zē-à) The general sense of bodily existence (and especially the general feeling of well-being or malaise), presumably dependent on multiple stimuli coming from various parts of the body, including sensations of internal organ activity even though these are not necessarily on a conscious level.

cenesthesic Relating to mental constituents caused by stimuli from organs other than the one in which the constituent appears.

cenesthopathy Any localized distortion of body awareness, such as the feeling that a hand has become like jelly; less commonly the term is used to refer to a feeling of general physical ill-being.

cenophobia See *kenophobia*.

cenotrope, coenotrope Instinct; behavior characteristic of all members of a group having the same biological and experiential background.

censor, endopsychic See *censorship*.

censorship A nonspecific term referring to the critical and evaluative scrutiny to which any instinctual quality or drive impulse is subjected before it is allowed to pass into a higher level of mental organization. Both ego and superego have censorship functions and most typically, at least in the adult, these require some modification of the original drive.

censorship, dream Dreams are highly disguised representations of unconscious impulses. They are under the constant rule of censoring influences. "The stricter the domination of the censorship, the more thorough becomes the disguise, and, often enough, the more ingenious the means employed to put the reader on the track of the actual meaning." (Freud, *ID*)

Center, Community Mental Health See *psychiatry, community*.

center, psychical *Obs.* The hypothesized localization of mental and intellectual functions in one or more specific sites in the brain.

center, psychomotor The part of the cerebral cortex around the central fissure, embracing the centers of voluntary muscular movement; psychocortical center.

centering Goldstein's term for perfect integration of the organism with its environment.

central constant See *constant, central.*

central excitatory state See *summation.*

central integrative field factor The sum total of previous experience that forms the basis for *apperception* (q.v.) and incorporation of new experiences.

central issue See *issue, central.*

central nervous system deviation See *impulse disorder, hyperkinetic.*

centration Piaget's term for prolonged involuntary attachment of a sensory modality to one part of a field, producing perceptual errors of exaggerations and distortions. Motor behavior based on perception (such as drawing tasks) is often secondarily affected and may thus be used to differentiate between the neurologically impaired, with perceptual distortions, and the emotionally disturbed, with thought disturbances.

centrencephalic system See *system, centrencephalic.*

centrifugal Radiating or flying off from a center. See *centripetal.*

centripetal Directed toward the center. In psychiatry the term implies a moving toward the psyche. It is said, for example, that the psychoanalysis of Freud is essentially a centripetal psychology. "For Freud the aims of empirical science, with its centripetal bias towards a minute and detailed analysis of observable facts, were absolute; whereas for Jung a purely objective psychology was not enough, in that it entirely omitted the undeniable reality and power of the idea." (Baynes, H.G. Translator's Preface to Jung's *Psychological Types,* 1923)

The opposite of centripetal forces (of the mind) are *centrifugal* ones. Jung is today the outstanding upholder of the centrifugal point of view, the principal representation of which is his *collective unconscious.* "To Jung the psyche is a world which contains all the elements of the greater world, with the same destructive and constructive forces—a pluralistic universe in which the individual either fulfils or neglects his essential role of creator." (Ibid.)

centrolobar sclerosis See *sclerosis, diffuse.*

centrosome Central body; a central cytoplasmic particle that is thought to be important in the mechanism of cell division. See *cytoplasm.*

cephalalgia (sef-al-al′jē-à) Headache, sometimes a *somatoform disorder* (q.v.).

cephalalgia, histaminic See *histamine.*

cephalea, epileptic (sef-à-lē′à) A type of visceral epilepsy, more common in children than adults, in which paroxysmal headache is the most prominent symptom.

cephalogenesis In embryological development, the stage that follows *notogenesis* (q.v.) and is associated with the origin of the primordia of the head.

This stage is initiated by the appearance of the *neural plate,* the primordium of the nervous system, and the formation of the head fold that delimits the head end of the embryo from the extraembryonic blastoderm. The neural plate forms the floor of the *neural groove,* which is bounded along both borders by a *neural fold* developing subsequently into the *neural tube,* lined with neural ectoderm, from an overlying epidermal ectoderm. The cephalic portion of a neural tube produces three dilatations that later become forebrain, midbrain, and hindbrain, the primordia of the future cerebrum, cerebellum, and pons and medulla oblongata. The later steps in cephalogenesis lead to the formation of the face and the head as well as of the eyes and the ears.

ceraunophobia See *keraunophobia.*

cerchnus (sērk′nus) *Obs.* Hoarseness.

cerea flexibilitas See *catalepsy.*

cerebellum A large, oval structure with a laminated appearance that lies in the posterior fossa of the skull behind the pons and medulla oblongata. It is joined to the brainstem by three peduncles, the superior, middle, and inferior, and appears grossly to be divided into two lateral lobes (the cerebellar hemispheres) and an unpaired median lobe (the vermis). Morphologically, however, "the cerebellum has two primary divisions: (1) the flocculonodular lobe, the most primitive part, with connections which are entirely vestibular, and (2) the corpus cerebelli, itself divided into (i) a palaeocerebellar division, receiving vestibular and spinocerebellar fibres, and composed anteriorly of lingula, centralis, and culmen, and posteriorly of pyramis, uvula, and paraflocculi, and (ii) a neocerebellar division, constituting the greater part of the corpus cerebelli, with connections mainly corticopontine.

"The cerebellum consists mainly of white matter which is covered with a thin layer of grey matter, the cerebellar cortex, and contains several grey masses, the nuclei. These are divided into lateral nuclei, the nuclei dentatus and emboliformis, and middle and roof nuclei, the nuclei globosus and fastigii.

"Microscopically the cortex consists of three principal layers of cells, the molecular layer, which lies most superficially, the granular layer, which is the deepest, and the layer of Purkinje cells, which lies between the two." (Brain, *DNS*) "The neocerebellum is essentially a reinforcing and coordinating organ which plays an important part in graduating and harmonizing muscular contraction, both in voluntary movement and in the maintenance of posture.

"The anterior lobe and the roof nuclei are concerned with the regulation of stretch reflexes and the anti-gravity posture. The flocculonodular lobe is an important equilibratory centre and lesions of this region cause swaying, staggering, and titubation. The neocerebellum regulates voluntary movement." (ibid.) Thus the cerebellum maintains orientation in space and it brakes volitional movements, especially those requiring checking or halting, and the fine movement of the hands.

Lesions of the cerebellum may produce the following symptoms: dysmetria, intention tremor, inability to perform alternating movements (dysdiadochokinesia), ataxia, decomposition of movement, rebound, nystagmus, vertigo, dysarthria, plurosthotonus, hypotonia, skew deviation of the eyes, and cerebellar "fits." To a considerable extent, however, other parts of the nervous system are able to compensate for loss of cerebellar function.

cerebral embolism (ser'e-bral em'bō-liz'm) See *accident, cerebrovascular.*

cerebral hemorrhage See *accident, cerebrovascular.*

cerebral palsy *Little's disease* (q.v.).

cerebral peduncle See *midbrain.*

cerebral syphilis See *syphilis, cerebral.*

cerebral thrombosis See *accident, cerebrovascular.*

cerebrasthenia *Obs.* Neurasthenia relating to the head.

cerebration Lewes used this term for "cerebral actions consecutive on a perception"; today it generally means any kind of conscious thinking.

cerebration, unconscious *Obs.* Mental activity occurring without conscious direction; latent thought.

cerebria Pinel's term for mental derangement in general.

cerebria acuta (L. "acute mental derangement") Pinel's term for mania.

cerebria chronica (L. "chronic mental derangement") *Obs.* Imbecility.

cerebria partialis (L. "partial mental derangement") *Obs.* Monomania.

cerebria sympathetica (L. "sympathetic mental derangement") *Obs.* Hypochondriasis or hysteria.

cerebropsychosis *Obs.* Those forms of mental disturbance that result from disease of the psychic centers, such as mania and general paralysis. Also used in a generic sense for all mental affections. (Tuke, *DPM*)

cerebrotonia A personality type, described by Sheldon, associated with the ectomorphic body build and characterized by restraint, inhibition, alertness, and a predominantly intellectual approach to reality.

cerebrovascular accident See *accident, cerebrovascular.*

cerebrum The major portion of the brain; the *forebrain* (q.v.) or prosencephalon.

ceremonial, compulsive A term used to describe the ritualistic behavior that is characteristic of the obsessive-compulsive. As in all neurotic symptoms, the compulsive ceremonials defend against certain unconscious instinctual demands that are threatening to the ego. According to Freud, this ritualistic behavior demonstrates the use of two types of defense mechanisms in particular: "undoing" and "isolation." Through motor means, that is, by a gesture or act that is symbolic and is repeated countless times, the patient tries to undo an undesirable or traumatic experience. For example, a patient with a washing compulsion is undoing a previous dirtying action (either real or imaginary). The dirtying action is usually masturbation, which by anal regression (characteristic of the obsessive-compulsive) is conceived of as dirty. Through order, routine, and system the obsessive-compulsive tries to isolate his experiences and rid them of their emotional concomitants. In analysis he finds it extremely difficult to associate or to experience any emotional reactions no matter how exciting his ideas may be.

The mechanism of isolation is seen most vividly in compulsive ceremonials that center around the taboo of touching. Many obsessive-compulsives have routines concerning which objects should not be touched and which should, and, in the latter case, in which order the objects should be touched. These rituals frequently concern routines to be followed in washing or bathing, but they may involve any ordinary daily activity such as crossing thresholds or handling doorknobs.

ceremonial defensive A more or less elaborate pattern of actions unconsciously devised by a person as a defense against anxiety and compulsively executed by him whenever this anxiety threatens.

In traumatic neuroses, for example, "a large group of patients have symptoms that are chiefly unconscious defense reactions against the original trauma." For example, "the symptom may be a more complete elaboration of a defensive reaction that was not carried out on the original traumatic occasion." (Kardiner, A., & Spiegel, H. *War and Stress and Neurotic Illness,* 1947) Whatever actions might be gone through in this elaboration of the incompleted defensive reaction would constitute a defensive ceremonial.

A "defense ceremonial has the nature of a compulsory act which the patient carries out without knowing exactly why, but which relieves him of anxiety." It is "usually carried out with no more control of the will than is shown in the ordinary compulsive ritual. . . . The ceremonial which the patient unconsciously devises takes form some years after the original traumatic event." (Ibid.)

Cerletti, Ugo (1877–1963) Italian neuropsychiatrist; in 1938, with L. Bini, introduced electrical form of convulsive therapy.

certification Designation of competence by a professional review body; those so certified by the American Board of Psychiatry and Neurology, Inc. (ABPN) are issued diplomas indicating that they have passed

the required examinations and hence are termed *diplomates.*

In Utilization Review procedures, the *certification process* refers to review of the case record to determine whether health care is necessary, and if the type or level of care and the site in which it is rendered are appropriate.

Certification is also used to refer to the process of completing the necessary documents in *commitment* proceedings (q.v.).

certification, admission See *review.*

certify To formally declare a person insane.

ceruloplasmin An alpha-globulin that contains almost all the copper in blood serum. Among other substrates, ceruloplasmin acts on serotonin and norepinephrine. One theory, no longer considered tenable, was that schizophrenia is due to a genetic defect or metabolic error that produces an abnormal ceruloplasmin, *taraxein,* which fails to neutralize noxious metabolites such as adrenoxine and adrenolutin.

cervical migraine See *migraine, cervical.*

c.e.s. Central excitatory state. See *summation.*

CET 1. Cerebral electrotherapy; *electrosleep* (q.v.). Low-intensity pulses of direct current that some have claimed to be of value in the treatment of depression, anxiety, and insomnia. 2. Computer electroencephalographic tomography.

ceteris paribus Other things being equal.

CF Rorschach scoring symbol for a response determined by color and form, with color dominant.

Chakrabarty The defendant in *Diamond Commissioner of Patents and Trademarks v. Chakrabarty.* Ananda Chakrabarty was a molecular biologist who invented a genetically engineered bacterium capable of breaking down crude oil, and in 1960 the U.S. Supreme Court held that such a live, human-made microorganism is patentable subjected matter.

chalasis (kal'à-sis) Inhibition of resting posture. Hines, in her studies on the maturation of excitability in the precentral gyrus, describes chalastic foci that cause inhibition of resting posture.

chalastic fits, postdormital See *paralysis, sleep.*

challenge, lactate See *lactate challenge.*

chance action An action that is executed by mere chance and has no conscious aim or purpose, but nevertheless subserves the execution of an unconscious intention. Under this heading Freud distinguishes three separate categories: (1) habitual actions such as fingering one's hair; (2) actions that are usual under certain circumstances, such as doodling and coin-jingling; and (3) isolated chance actions. One example of the last variety might be the loss of a wedding ring on the honeymoon, indicating an unconscious wish to dissolve the marriage. Another might be the leaving of personal articles such as gloves or a cigarette lighter in the psychotherapist's office, indicating a patient's difficulty in tearing himself away.

Freud separates these "symptomatic" or "chance" actions from those carried out erroneously. In the latter we have to do with an action that has a conscious intention but is carried out erroneously in a way that reflects the person's unconscious intention. Manifestly, the line of demarcation between these two categories is not definite.

change agent See *psychiatry, community.*

changing, compulsive A symptom found in some obsessive-compulsives expressing itself in a tendency to change continuously. This changing apparently has no limitations and may involve anything anywhere: personal habits, dress, work, social relations, opinions, etc. The changing is an effort to bring the world into accord with the patient's system. Apparently through compulsive changing the patient can avoid the reality that the world does not obey his compulsive system.

channels of communication See *communication.*

chaotic families See *family types.*

character In current usage, approximately equivalent to *personality;* it consists of the totality of objectively observable behavior and subjectively reportable inner experience. It includes the characteristic (and to some extent predictable) behavior-response patterns that each person evolves, both consciously and unconsciously, as his style of life or way of being in adapting to his environment and in maintaining a stable, reciprocal relationship with the human and nonhuman environment. The character or personality reflects the nature of the person's psychologic defense system, his autoplastic and alloplastic maneuvers,

and the ego defenses that he automatically and customarily employs to maintain intrapsychic stability. The character is the agency through which inner personal and outer environmental forces are brought together, critically evaluated, and acted upon; it is, in other words, a compromise between inner drives, the claims of the superego, and reality demands. Because the character or the personality is egosyntonic, it must be recognized that any diagnosis of *character disorder* or *personality disturbance* is fundamentally a social diagnosis, and made by people other than the subject himself, whose behavior is perceived by others as destructive, frightening, nonconforming, or otherwise deviant.

Some authorities define character as learned attributes originating primarily in early life experience and personality as the combination of temperament and character. See *defense, character; structure, character;* and the multiple listings under *constitution; disposition; personality; temperament.*

character, anal Obsessive-compulsive personality disorder. The anal character is made up of three cardinal traits. The first is orderliness (reliability, conscientiousness, punctuality, etc.); the second is parsimony, which may be expressed as avarice; the third is obstinacy and its closely allied traits (defiance, vindictiveness, irascibility, etc.). See *anal erotism; defense, character; phase, anal.*

character, ascetic A mode of life characterized by rigor, self-denial, and mortification of the flesh. Asceticism is seen typically as a phase in puberty, where it indicates a fear of sexuality and a simultaneous defense against sexuality. Asceticism is also seen as an extreme type of masochistic character disorder, where almost all activity is forbidden because it represents intolerable instinctual demands. In such cases, the very act of mortifying may become a distorted expression of the blocked sexuality and produce masochistic pleasure. An example of this is the eccentric who devotes his life to the combating of some particular evil that unconsciously represents his own instinctual demands.

character, daemonic The person who is his own worst enemy and throughout his life (unconsciously) brings ill-fortune upon himself. See *masochism; proneness, accident.*

character, epileptic See *personality, epileptic.*

character, exploitative Fromm's term for a new presentation of the character pattern described by Abraham as *oral aggressive* (see *defense, character*), in agreement with the so-called cultural school of psychoanalysis, which has made its own classification of character types. Instead of viewing character structure as the result of libido sublimation or reaction formation, this school sees the character types as basic attitudes in the process of socialization and coping with each particular life situation. Accordingly, Fromm believes that such a person develops in a frustrating atmosphere and hence comes to feel that one can have only what one takes and that the only source of security lies in exploiting others. When threatened with danger, the exploitative character tries to manipulate the situation by flattery, cajoling, aggression, or any other means.

character, genital The genital character is the resultant of those character traits (handed down from the pregenital levels) that serve the interest of genitality and of the traits that issue from the Oedipus complex. During the pregenital stages the management of instinctual energies was largely of an autoerotic and narcissistic character; now, since the object of the genital impulses is outside of the person himself, the instincts strive toward alloerotic (homosexual and heterosexual) expression.

In the normal person the final formation of the genital character is relatively unnarcissistic and unambivalent. "Generally speaking, we may say that when the child has been able to subdue his Oedipus complex with all its constituents, he has made the most important step toward overcoming his original narcism, and his hostile tendencies; and at the same time he has broken the power of the pleasure principle to dominate the conduct of his life." (Abraham, *SP*)

character, hysterical See *defense, character.*

character, neurotic See *neurosis, character.*

character, oral The personality traits based on the two stages of oral erotism. According to Abraham there are two principal ways of expressing oral activity: (1) sucking, in the first stage, and (2) biting, in the second, and from each of these arise definite types of personality.

If the infant suffered no difficulties or privations during the sucking period, if the sucking phase was largely pleasurable, it is believed that the pleasure is carried over as a character trait, leading to the optimistic type of person who believes that he will succeed in any undertaking. Moreover, such people may exhibit carefree indifference and perhaps inactivity. The mother's breast will "flow for them eternally." Because the infant was treated so generously, identification with the mother gives rise to generosity as an important trait in the child.

If, on the other hand, the infant failed to achieve gratification during the sucking period, it develops a pessimistic attitude. In later life the child is apprehensive and demanding; he is never satisfied and comes to believe he never will be.

The second or biting stage is said also to lead to development of character traits: to a tendency to hate and to destroy. "This fundamental difference extends to the smallest details of a person's behavior." (Abraham, *SP*)

character, paranoiac In this personality type, projection mechanisms are foremost, in that the subject constantly blames the environment for his difficulties. Moreover, he generally has greatest trouble in getting along with members of his own sex. The paranoiac usually superimposes his false claims on some real circumstances in the environment, thus giving some degree of plausibility to his delusional formations.

The *paranoid personality* possesses the same fundamental traits, but to a more marked degree. Furthermore, it is usually easy to detect the delusional basis for his trouble. See *personality disorders.*

character, receptive A type described by Fromm; such a person is passive, dependent, clinging, and compliant. This type is similar to the passive-oral or passive-dependent type of other writers.

character, reformation of A psychoanalytic term referring to a form of defense that occurs in everday life and also frequently as a way station in the course of the psychoanalytic procedure. In this form of defense the patient leans over backward in the proverbial "reformed rake" fashion. By his meticulosity and carefully guarded behavior, he denies the presence of the "old" recently uncovered "bad " traits and "bad" instinctual desires. He is constantly preoccupied with "selling" the picture of himself, as a reformed character, to himself, the analyst, and the world. The change is no more than temporary reaction formation, however, and further analytic work is required to uncover the sources of the anxiety against which that defense has been erected.

character structure See *defense, character; structure, character.*

character, unit See *unit-character.*

character, urethral A character type, mentioned briefly by Freud and Ferenczi and belonging to the classificatory group that stresses the libido origin of character structure (see *defense, character*). The urethral character commonly gives a history of bedwetting beyond the usual age. The behavioral characteristics of this type depend on reaction formation in relation to the specific fear of urethral eroticism, which is shame. Burning ambition, a need to boast of achievement, and great impatience are typical traits.

Charcot, Jean-Martin (shàr-kō') (1825–93) French neurologist and psychiatrist; localization of function in cerebral disease; hysteria; hypnosis; the first modern physician to make a serious attempt to treat emotional disorders on an individual psychotherapeutic basis.

Charcot-Marie-Tooth's disease (Jean-Martin Charcot, q.v.; Pierre Marie, French physician, 1853–1940; and Howard Henry Tooth, English physician, 1856–1926) See *atrophy, peroneal muscular.*

Charcot triad See *sclerosis, multiple.*

Charcot's syndrome Multiple sclerosis.

charge, mental *Cathexis* (q.v.).

charm Light hypnosis; *hypotaxia* (q.v.).

chart, life See *sketch, biographic.*

chastity, conjugal The state of husband and wife living in celibacy.

cheese effect Hypertensive crisis due to the interaction of monoamine oxidase inhibitors with tyramine, a potent vasopressor. Tyramine is formed when bacteria in food provide the enzyme that decarboxylates the amino acid tyrosine. Many foods contain tyrosine, but over 75% of the hypertensive reactions reported with MAOI use, and almost all the resultant deaths, have been associated with the ingestion of cheese.

cheimaphobia Fear of cold.

cheiro- See *chiro-.*

chelation The act of binding, fixing, or attaching chemically; specifically, formation of a bond between a metal ion and another molecule, as in the chelation of the iron ion by the porphyrin ring in heme. Chelating agents, such as British anti-Lewisite (see *BAL*) and/or versenate, are used in the treatment of heavy metal poisoning to form stable compounds with the toxic metal, which can then be eliminated safely from the body without exerting their toxic effects on tissues.

chemical aversion therapy See *aversion therapy.*

chemical neuroanatomy See *neuroanatomy, chemical.*

chemopallidectomy Injection of small amounts of alcohol into the globus pallidus, used in the therapy of basal ganglia hyperkinetic disorders.

chemopsychiatry A psychiatric term intended to designate the application and effect of chemical substances in psychiatry. See *psychotropics.*

cheromania The manic form of bipolar (manic-depressive) illness.

child abuse See *syndrome, battered child.*

child, battered See *syndrome, battered child.*

child, bright A child of superior ability; some writers make the following distinction: (1) *bright child*—a child of average intellectual endowment with an ability to perceive, grasp, and absorb communicated knowledge more quickly than his peers; (2) *superior child*—one with an extraordinary capability in some special field; (3) *gifted child*—one with a specific talent, usually overdeveloped in relation to other abilities which may be at a bright, average, or dull level; (4) *prodigy*—a rare type of superior child who from the earliest stage of life shows an unusual and practically untrained capability in one or more fields.

child-centered In educational psychology, a school whose primary concern is fulfilling the child's present needs rather than preparing him for adult life.

Child ego state See *transactional analysis.*

child, emotionally handicapped See *handicap, emotional.*

child, gifted See *child, bright.*

child guidance Preventive or prophylactic measures directed toward the goal of minimizing the chances of mental and emotional disorders developing in adult life. Child guidance strives to influence the child's developmental familial and social milieu mainly through education, support, insight, and understanding, directed toward both the child's immediate family and such influential parent surrogates as the family physician or pediatrician, the school nurse, the teacher, and the minister.

"child is being beaten" See *beating.*

child, problem See *behavior disorders; developmental disorders.*

child prodigy See *child, bright.*

child psychiatry The branch of psychiatry dealing with disorders of children and adolescents, including the study of normal psychological, physical, and social development, parenting, education, and learning. Basic research in child development has focused on studies of object attachment, cognition, psycholinguistics, affective states, and bonding. Clinical research has extended the understanding of the pervasive developmental disorders, learning disorders, Tourette syndrome, eating disorders, classification and epidemiology of psychiatric disorders in childhood, affective disorders and suicide, and the rights of the child in the juvenile justice systems.

childbirth, envy of According to some authorities the boy has an envy of the girl's ability to bear children, which in its intensity matches the girl's envy of the boy's penis. Fenichel does not believe this to be the case. He points out that both boys and girls may have a "passionate wish to give birth to babies, a wish that is doomed to frustration," since little girls can in no possible way bear children any better than can little boys. (Fenichel, *PTN*)

childhood The period of life from birth to puberty. See *developmental levels.*

childhood, land of Jung's expression to describe "that time in which the rational consciousness of the present was not yet separated from the 'historical soul,' the collective unconscious, and thus not only into that land where the complexes of childhood have their origin but into a prehistorical one that was the cradle of us all. The individual's separation from the 'land of childhood' is unavoidable, although it leads to such a removal from the twilit psyche of primordial time that a loss

of the natural instincts thereby occurs." (Jacobi, J. *The Psychology of C.G. Jung,* 1942)

childhood psychosis See *atypical childhood psychosis; developmental disorders, pervasive.*

children at risk See *risk.*

children, ego deviant Beres's diagnostic label for those children whom others would classify as having childhood schizophrenia or early infantile autism.

China white *MPTP* (q.v.).

Chinese menu approach Use of checklist(s) as a means of describing clinical phenomena or generating diagnoses on the basis of objective phenomena that can easily be identified or recognized. The technique is often viewed as sacrificing the intuitive aspect of clinical practice for the reproducible certainty of counting bits of information that may be irrelevant to the patient's condition.

chionophobia Fear of snow.

chipping Controlled use of opiates; it is believed that long-term chippers account for a large number of opiate users.

chiro- Combining form meaning hand, from Gr. *cheir.*

chiromania *Obs.* Masturbatic psychosis; morbid impulse to masturbate.

choc fortuit *Obs.* (F. "accidental shock") Binet's term (1887) to denote an accidental shock to the psyche. The shock or psychic trauma is usually of a sexual character and is influential in modifying to a greater or lesser degree the subsequent adjustment of the person.

choice of neurosis See *compliance, somatic.*

cholecystokinin A neuropeptide that is found in the gut as well as in the central and peripheral nervous systems. It is believed to play an important role in regulation of satiety.

choleric See *type, choleric.*

cholinergic A term used for all nerves that release acetylcholine at their terminals: all postganglionic parasympathetic nerves, all autonomic preganglionic fibers whether parasympathetic or sympathetic, and postganglionic sympathetic nerves to sweat glands and certain blood vessels, and the somatic nerves to skeletal muscles.

cholinesterase See *acetylcholine; process, elementary.*

chorea (kō-rē′à) A movement disorder characterized by irregular, spasmodic, involuntary movements of the limbs or facial muscles. Choreic movements are jerky, irregular, and quasi-purposive. Unless otherwise modified, chorea usually means Sydenham's chorea, or St. Vitus' dance. See *chorea, Sydenham's*.

chorea, epidemic The convulsive dances of the Middle Ages that spread among the population like an epidemic. See *choreomania*.

chorea, Huntington's (G. Huntington, U.S. neurologist, 1850–1916) Chronic progressive chorea; adult chorea; currently known as Huntington disease. A rare hereditary disorder of the basal ganglia and cortex, often grouped with the presenile dementias. Many cases in the United States have been traced to two brothers from England who settled in Long Island about the year 1630. Huntington disease is transmitted by a single autosomal dominant gene; although 50% of offspring can thus be expected to develop the disease, some gaps occur because of the relatively late onset of the disorder.

Mean age of onset is 35 years, with choreic movements; when the disorder begins in the twenties striate rigidity is generally the first symptom, and when it begins after the twenties the leading disability is usually an intention tremor.

Involuntary movements usually begin in the face, hands, and shoulders. The patient becomes clumsy and fidgety, and soon his restlessness acquires the characteristic jerking quality. The choreic movements are typically exploited to serve voluntary actions of a quite unnecessary kind (e.g. a person with a forward arm jerk tries to make it look like part of an intended movement to smooth down his hair). The face takes on a grotesque expression because it is in constant, writhing contortion. With progression, movement becomes increasingly disorganized, and jerking of the diaphragm produces abrupt, staccato speech with rapid modulations in tone and tempo.

Mental changes progress side by side with the movement disorder. The patient becomes increasingly apathetic, muddled in his thinking, disoriented, and markedly distractible. Memory may be fairly well retained even when the dementia is well established, although finally the patient presents a picture of complete fatuity unin-

fluenced by any change in his environment. The most common psychosis is a shallow, ill-sustained depression.

Average duration of the disorder is 10 to 15 years, with death before the age of 60; some families, however, are notable for the much slower progression of the disorder in their affected members.

The affected offspring are said to have significantly more personality abnormalities than the nonaffected: alcoholism, criminality, impulsive and unpredictable behavior, outbursts of explosive rage and violence, and/or sexual promiscuity. There is a marked familial trend toward suicide, and mental symptoms such as a morose and truculent discontent or delusions of reference frequently precede the development of neurological symptoms.

Pathology consists of extensive meningitis, brain atrophy most marked in the fronto-Rolandic areas, and secondary hydrocephalus with gross dilation of the ventricular system. Cellular degeneration is greatest in the third and fourth cortical laminae, the caudate nucleus, and the putamen. Some studies suggest that the basis of the disorder may be abnormalities in the metabolism of γ-aminobutyric acid and perhaps of acetylcholine.

chorea, maniacal *Obs.* See *chorea, Sydenham's*.

chorea nutans A hysterical symptom characterized by rhythmical nodding; also called *chorea oscillatoria*, though the latter term refers to rhythmical hysterical movements seen in any part of the body.

chorea oscillatoria See *chorea nutans*.

chorea saltatoria (sȧl-tȧ-tō′rē-ȧ) A form of chorea in which the patient involuntarily jumps rhythmically or irregularly.

chorea, senile A severe, progressive dyskinesia that occurs in elderly persons; it resembles *Huntington's chorea* but is sometimes mistaken for *tardive dyskinesia* in patients who have been on antipsychotic drugs for long periods.

chorea, Sydenham's (sī′den-hams) (Thomas Sydenham, English physician, 1624–1689) St. Vitus' dance; an acute toxic disorder of the central nervous system secondary to rheumatic infection (although it has also been reported in association with other infections, e.g. scarlet fever, diphtheria, and chickenpox). It occurs chiefly in children and young adolescents, in females more than in males. Chief symptoms are involuntary movements that resemble fragments of purposive movements haphazardly performed, hypotonia and hyperextensibility, and often emotional instability of an agitated, overactive kind. On occasion, persistent excitement and insomnia are seen—*maniacal chorea*. Recovery is the rule, although the patient may have several recurrences. Sedatives and cortisone are of value in treatment.

chorea, tetanoid See *degeneration, hepatolenticular.*

choreatiform syndrome See *impulse disorder, hyperkinetic.*

choreiform Resembling chorea, choreoid.

choreo-athetosis A combination of the clinical features of *chorea* (q.v.) and *athetosis* (q.v.) . Both chorea and athetosis physiologically present features that are the opposite of the symptoms of Parkinsonism, and it has therefore been suggested that while Parkinsonism represents a loss of function of the corpus striatum, chorea and athetosis are due to lesions involving especially the caudate nucleus and the putamen.

choreomania Dancing mania; epidemic chorea. At different times in different countries epidemics of frenzied dancing have taken place. During the fourteenth and fifteenth centuries such epidemics were prominent in western Germany, where they were known as *Tanzwut;* later they were called *chorea Germanorum* to distinguish the condition from *chorea Anglorum* or the form of chorea first described by Sydenham.

choriomeningitis, acute lymphocytic A virus infection, spread by mice, involving the leptomeninges, the ependyma of the ventricles and the choroid plexuses, and ganglion cells of the brain. Children are most commonly affected, and complete recovery is the rule.

chorion biopsy See *biopsy, chorion.*

chorionic villus biopsy See *biopsy, chorion.*

chrematophobia Fear of money; rare in the United States, where chrematomania is the more common condition.

chrematorrhea Spending spree.

chromatic In genetics the term relates to the protoplasmic cell substance called *chromatin* that stains the nuclear network and constitutes the morphological basis of heredity.

chromatid Each of the two daughter chromosomes formed during the prophase of mitosis or meiosis from the original chromosome; each chromatid will become a chromosome in the next generation of cells.

chromatin *Biol.* Stainable tissue. This collective biological term refers to a reticulum of protein substances in the nucleus of a cell, which are readily stainable and render the nucleus conspicuous in dyed tissues. See *chromosome.*

chromatophobia Morbid dread of certain color or colors.

chromesthesia A form of synesthesia in which colors are seen in association with the other forms of sensation, and especially in association with sounds (colored hearing).

chromidial neuroplasm See *neuron.*

chromidrosis Colored perspiration.

chromomere Minute nodules in the chromosomes of a cell nucleus that form a chain of chromatic bodies, particularly in the early stages of mitosis, and are strung like beads on a fine thread. They show persistent differences in size and distribution and presumably have also different chemical compositions. There are sound reasons for believing that many chromomeric nodules are too small to be visible. See *chromosome.*

chromophobia Fear of color(s).

chromosomal, chromosomic, chromosomatic The adjectives not only refer to the minute chromosome particles themselves into which the scattered chromatin of a cell nucleus separates at the beginning of cell division, but are also used to characterize that part of the mechanism of heredity that is based on the activities of the chromosomes.

chromosome A dark staining structure in the nucleus of the cell that contains deoxyribonucleic acid (DNA) and ribonucleic acid (RNA) attached to a protein core. The components in the linear thread of DNA molecules—the chromosomes and the genes—determine the genetic information that will be passed on to the next generation of cells.

In the human, there are 46 chromosomes, arranged as 22 pairs of *autosomes* and a pair of sex chromosomes, or *heterosomes* (XX in the female and XY in the male). The identical members of a pair of chromosomes are known as homologues. The full complement of 46 chromosomes is the *diploid* number.

In sexual reproduction, two germ cells, or *gametes,* one from the paternal side and the other from the maternal side, join to form a single new cell. To maintain the correct number of chromosomes in the new cell, each gamete must contain only half the full number of chromosomes. The reduction to the *haploid* number of chromosomes occurs during the stage of cell division called *meiosis.* The resultant gamete with the haploid number is then ready to unite with the gamete from the other parent (which also has the haploid number) to form the *zygote.* The union of the two gametes restores the diploid number of chromosomes to the zygote, half of them having come from the mother and the other half from the father.

The genetic information or hereditary coding is carried by DNA, whose structure resembles a twisted ladder, or double helix. The sides of the ladder do little more than hold the structure together; they carry almost no genetic information and are composed of monotonously repeating sugar molecules joined by phosphate bonds. It is the DNA that contains the chemical language of heredity, telling every cell what it can do and what its progeny can become. The alphabet of the hereditary language is in the rungs of the ladder. Each rung consists of a pair of nucleotide bases (one base from each side of the ladder, loosely held together by a hydrogen bond). The nucleotides are only four in number, and they always pair with the same partner to form a rung—an adenine and thymine pair (A-T or T-A), or a guanine and cytosine pair (G-C or C-G).

The order in which the base pairs appear controls the manufacture of proteins in each cell in the body. Even though there are only four "letters" in the alphabet, the haploid chain in the human contains about 3 billion base pairs. These base pairs form the chromosomes. The largest human chromosome consists of 250 million base pairs, and the smallest is roughly 48 million base pairs. Genes, the basic units of inheritance, are submicroscopic entities located at various points along the chromo-

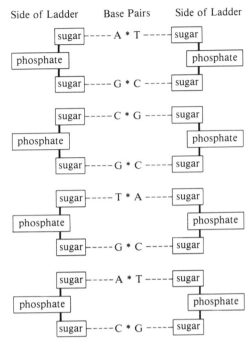

Schematic representation of DNA. Instead of the 8 base pairs shown, however, DNA contains approximately 3 billion base pairs. *Key:* * = weak hydrogen bond; A = adenine (a purine); T = thymine (a pyrimidine); G = guanine (a purine); C = cytosine (a pyrimidine).

somes. The zygote receives either one of the pair of homologous chromosomes, along with the genes it carries, but not both chromosomes. Genes are DNA, and the DNA molecule constitutes a tape of coded instructions with almost infinite variations. The average human gene covers about 30,000 base pairs; there are approximately 100,000 genes carried by each human. See *gene.*

Translating the genetic coding into action requires that the sequence of base pairs in DNA be converted into the sequence of amino acids in a protein. The necessary conversion is achieved through the medium of concerted action of different species of RNA, including messenger RNA and transfer RNA, which translate the code into a message that can be recoded into a message comprehensible to the next "translator" along the way. The sequence of genetic messages in DNA orders the corresponding sequence in RNA as well as the sequence of the amino acids attached to RNA. Peptide bonds are formed between the aligned amino acids and a new protein is constructed.

The gene exerts its action through its chemical properties—it instructs the cells or metabolic processes under its influence by means of a chemical code. In the many chains of chemical events that constitute metabolism, each gene directs one specific action—a particular polypeptide chain. Genetic disorders arise when the gene's chemical code is misinterpreted at any step in its conversion into the specific order of amino acids that will form protein.

Mutations, whether naturally occurring or induced by mutagens, arise if the alphabet code is misread at any step along the way. Wrong nucleotides may be added, others may be deleted, or substitution or rearrangements of nucleotides may occur. Any of these possibilities will alter or erase a polypeptide or enzyme that is essential for one step in a metabolic pathway; consequently, a biochemical *block* develops at the expected site of action. The absence of the usual end product of the metabolic pathway may produce disease, and/or the accumulation of intermediate products (that would ordinarily have been broken down and removed) may produce disease. An example of the former kind of heritable deficiency is succinylcholine sensitivity, due to absence of the enzyme pseudocholinesterase. Phenylketonuria and galactosemia, on the other hand, are examples of the second kind of mutation, where accumulation of an intermediate metabolic substance (or a derivative) is responsible for development of the symptoms characteristic of the disorder.

Since the entire process of transmitting the instructions carried within DNA to amino acids is a mechanical one, once a mutation has occurred it will be copied faithfully forever after. See *heredity; law, Mendelian; Mendelism; mutation.*

It is estimated that over 15 million Americans suffer from one or more birth defects, 80% of which are thought to be caused by genetic changes. Genetic factors are responsible for 50% of all miscar-

riages, for at least 40% of all infant deaths, and for 80% of mental retardation in the United States. As many as 30% of all pediatric and 10% of all adult hospital admissions in the United States and Canada stem directly from genetic disorders.

The most common of the lethal genetic diseases is cystic fibrosis, which affects 1 in every 1,800 births in the United States. Duchenne's muscular dystrophy, one of the most common sex-linked disorders, affects 1 of every 3,000 males born in the United States. Huntington disease affects 1 in every 10,000 births. Phenylketonuria (PKU) affects 1 in every 12,000 births. Type A hemophilia affects 1 of every 10,000 males.

Among the 3,500 or more diseases recognized as genetic disorders are albinism, alkaptonuria, cystinuria, pentosuria, galactosemia, anidiria, microphthalmus, arachnodactyly, adenosine deaminase deficiency, Lesch-Nyhan syndrome, chondrodystrophy, sickle cell disorder, color blindness, epiloia, Tay-Sachs disease, Wilson's disease, retinoblastoma, and neurofibromatosis. Some believe that certain forms of epilepsy, manic-depressive (bipolar) disorder, schizophrenia, Pick's disease, Alzheimer's disease, and some forms of alcoholism are largely of genetic origin. Hormonal abnormalities that are recognized as genetically determined are diabetes insipidus, diabetes mellitus, and one form of goitrous cretinism. Diseases known to be due to gross chromosome abnormalities are Down syndrome, Turner's syndrome (with XO sex chromosomes instead of XX or XY), Klinefelter's syndrome (XXY), superfemale (XXX), and chronic granulocytic leukemia.

chromosome, fragile X See *syndrome, fragile X.*

chromosome, sex See *sex chromosome.*

chromotopsia A condition, most often due to ingestion of certain drugs, in which all objects appear to be of the same color or hue.

chronaxia, chronaxy The shortest duration a current of a certain defined strength takes to flow through a nerve in order produce a muscular contraction.

chronic brain syndrome See *brain disorder; syndrome, organic.*

chronic mentally ill A generic term for patients with severe mental illness (most often schizophrenic and organic disorders), who need continuing care for long periods and at varying levels of intensity in accordance with their changing needs and their responsiveness (or lack of it) to treatment measures. Their plight was highlighted by *deinstitutionalization* (q.v.), since it was recognized that for many patients what had happened was appropriately termed *transinstitutionalization*—a shift out of the hospital and into other institutions such as jails, nursing homes, and other *domiciles* (q.v.). *The young adult chronic patient* is a subgroup of patients between 18 and 35 years of age with severe and persistent dysfunctions combined with alternating abuse and underutilization of mental health services. As generally reported, over half of the patients in this group are diagnosed schizophrenic; others are diagnosed severe personality disorder or neurosis, organic mental disorder, mental retardation, or specific learning disability.

chronograph, interaction A mechanical device, developed by E.D. Chapple, that enables the observer of a standardized psychiatric interview to record certain temporal aspects of verbal and gestural interactions between interviewer and subject. Chapple's interaction theory of personality assumes that personality can be assessed without recourse to intrapsychic or other psychodynamic formulations, and that its assessment involves merely the process of observing the time relations in the interaction patterns of the subject.

chronophobia A neurotic fear of time. This is the most common psychiatric disorder in prison inmates, and sooner or later almost all prisoners suffer chronophobia to some degree; it occurs in every potential neurotic who goes to prison. The duration and immensity of time are terrifying to the patient, and the passage of time throws him into a panic. The frequency of chronophobia in prisoners has led to the condition's being called *prison neurosis*.

Chronophobia appears suddenly, without warning, at the time the inmate comes to grips with his sentence. The introductory phase of imprisonment is ordinarily marked by hopes and plans for a new trial or the like, by uncertainty, and by a studied indifference or carefree attitude. After the novelty of prison has worn off and the real length of the sentence is felt, chronophobia sets in. The prisoner goes into a panic, usually while in his cell, and fears his enclosure and restraint, but this apparent claustrophobia arises from fear of time, as represented by the prison. After the first attack, more or less constant anxiety, restlessness, insomnia, dissatisfaction with life, numerous hypochondriacal complaints, and progressive inability to adjust himself to his surroundings appear. The intensity of the crisis usually passes within a few weeks or months, though mild relapses may occur. But the prisoner becomes essentially a phlegmatic, indifferent automaton who serves the rest of his sentence by the clock and lives wholly in the present, one day at a time.

chronotaraxis (kron-ō-târ-ak′sis) Confusion for time, as for date, seasop of year, time of day, and overestimation or underestimation of duration of time; this symptom has been reported as occurring as a result of bilateral lesions of the dorsomedial and anterior thalamic nuclei.

chronotherapy Treatment of delayed sleep phase syndrome (DSPS) based on a sleep-wake phase angle physiology. The complaint is that the subject cannot fall asleep at the desired time and has difficulty awakening in the morning. It is believed that such subjects are unable to phase advance; i.e. they cannot move their sleep times ahead to earlier, more conventional hours. Treatment consists of a phase delay of approximately three hours on each consecutive day. The schedule must be rigidly maintained, for if the subject is allowed a late night, the original complaints recur. See *sleep-wake schedule disorders*.

chthonic (thon′ik) Relating to the depths of the earth. Jung likens the psyche to the earth. Speaking of psychic archetypes, he says that "they are essentially the chthonic portion of the mind—if we may use this expression—that portion through which the mind is linked to nature, or in which, at least, its relatedness to the earth and the universe seems most comprehensible." (Jung, *CAP*)

Chubby Puffer See *syndrome, Chubby Puffer*.

chunking A type of cognitive therapy that has been found useful for the insomnia of ruminative, intrusive thinkers; the patient is trained to connect the randomly occurring thoughts into logical groups, which then become easier to control.

cibophobia Fear of food; sitophobia.

ciliospinal reflex A superficial reflex; scratching or pinching of the skin on the side of the neck produces dilation of the pupil; strong light and accommodation must be avoided in this test.

cinaedi Males who adopt the passive or receptive role in homosexual activity. See *active*.

cineseismography. A photographic system for recording and measuring abnormal involuntary movements; its great advantage is that it obviates the need to attach any devices to the subject.

cingulate gyrus (sin'gū-lāt jī'rus) The arched, crescent-shaped convolution on the medial surface of the cerebral hemisphere that lies immediately above the corpus callosum. Also known as gyrus cinguli; callosal gyrus. Part of "Papez's circle." See *emotion, Papez's theory of*.

cingulumotomy A type of *psychosurgery* (q.v.) in which small portions of the cingulum bundle are coagulated bilaterally; the procedure is said to be beneficial in chronic psychosis that has not responded to other forms of treatment, and also in chronic alcoholism and drug addiction.

cipher method A method in secret writing. While writing on the question of dream interpretation Freud refers to the "cipher method," which "treats the dream as a kind of secret code in which every sign is translated into another sign of known meaning, according to an established key." (Freud, *ID*) The method is said by psychiatrists to possess no scientific value.

circadian See *rhythms, biologic*.

circadian desynchronosis Jet lag, typically including fatigue, irritability, short-term memory loss, and shortened attention span.

circle, closed See *theory, immanence*.

circle, Papez's See *emotion, Papez's theory of*.

circuit, reverberating Lorente de No's hypothesis to explain enduring reflex responses to a single stimulus; the hypothesis assumes that several internuncial neurons are intercalated between the sensory fibers and the anterior horn cells and that these several neurons discharge in sequence rather than simultaneously and thus produce an enduring *cerebral excitatory state* and enduring reflex discharge.

circular In psychiatry the term is used in characterizing manic-depressive psychosis, because the psychosis is often characterized by cycles of mania and depression.

circulatory state, hyperdynamic β-adrenergic Panic disorder or generalized anxiety disorder in which cardiac symptoms occupy the forefront of complaints: chest pain, palpitations, breathlessness, a feeling of oppression, dizziness, sweating, fatigue, headache, tremor, and nervousness. As described, it is approximately equivalent to cardiac anxiety state, cardiac neurosis, da Costa's syndrome, or effort syndrome.

circumscription, monosymptomatic When a patient has but a single symptom psychiatrists speak of monosymptomatic circumscription. See *monoideism; monomania*.

circumstantiality A disorder of associations seen in schizophrenics in which too many associated ideas come to consciousness because of too little selective suppression. Many things that are implicit in ordinary conversation are explicitly communicated and, typically, to an absurd and bizarre degree. One of Bleuler's patients, for example, wrote the following letter to his mother: "I am writing on paper. The pen I use for it is from a factory called Perry & Co., the factory is in England. I am assuming that. After the name Perry Co. the city of London is scratched in; but not the country. The city of London is in England. That I know from school." Some patients who are aware of their circumstantiality will describe an accompanying subjective experience of feeling that the central idea has not been communicated until all of its facets have been considered in detail. This same sort of uncertainty and doubt about adequacy of communication may be seen in obsessional disorders where it usually appears as overmeticulousness, precision, or ostentatious honesty. See *Klebenbleiben*.

Circumstantiality also occurs in epileptic dementia.

cistern puncture See *puncture, cistern*.

cisvestitism Dressing in the clothes of one's own sex, but in clothes inappropriate to one's station of life, as when an adult dresses as a child, or a child as an adult, or a civilian as an army officer. See *transvestitism*.

cittosis *Pica* (q.v.).

CJD *Creutzfeldt-Jakob's disease* (q.v.).

claim, neurotic Horney's term for the belief held by certain patients (whom Freud called "the exceptions") that they are in some way superior and that others should fulfill their wishes and needs.

claims review See *audit; review.*

CLAMS Clinical Linguistic and Auditory Milestone Scale, a screening test for defects in language development, developed by Arnold Capute, Bruce Shapiro, and Frederick Palmer. The test compares the child's language development with standardized receptive and expressive milestones for the age period between 1 week and 36 months.

clang See *association, clang.*

clarification See *interpretation.*

clasp-knife phenomenon See *rigidity, decerebrate.*

class, social Rank, estate, station, or status within a society or group; a grouping of people on the basis of similarity in income, education, vocation, etc.

In the United States, Howard Waitzkin (*Annals of Internal Medicine 89,* 1978) offered the following description of class by income:

Corporate class—the major owners and controllers of wealth, who constitute 1% of the population and own 80% of all corporate stock; their median annual income (in 1975) was between $114,000 and $142,000.

Upper middle class—(a) professionals, who constitute 14% of the population, with a median income of about $25,600; and (b) middle level executives, who constitute 6% of the population, with a median income of about $22,700.

Lower middle class—(a) shopkeepers, artisans, and craftsmen, who constitute 7% of the population, with a median income of $12,100; and (b) clerical and sales workers, who constitute 23% of the population, with a median income of $9,200.

Working class—manual laborers, service and farm workers, who constitute 49% of the population, with a median income of $8,500 or less

While some sociologists define social class (or stratum) largely in economic terms, others stress similarity of lifestyle, attitudes, or prestige. A.B. Hollingshead and Fritz C. Redlich (*American Social Review 18,* 1953) studied the urbanized community of New Haven, Connecticut, in 1950 and 1951, in an attempt to define the relationship between social class and mental illness. They used the following categories:

Class I—business and professional leaders, including a long-established core group of interrelated families and a smaller upwardly mobile group of new people.

Class II—managers or less ranking professions; four of five in this category are upwardly mobile.

Class III—salaried administrative and clerical workers; small business owners.

Class IV—working class; semiskilled or skilled manual workers; education within this class usually ends with graduation from grammar school.

Class V—semiskilled factory workers or unskilled laborers, who usually have not completed elementary school.

Hollingshead and Redlich found an inverse relationship between social class and mental illness; the significant division was between Class V and all the other classes. See *neuroses, class differences in.*

classical technique See *parameter.*

classification See *DSM-III; nomenclature; nosology.*

classification, multiaxial See *DSM-III.*

classification of disordered behavior (Rado) See *disordered behavior, classification of.*

claudication, cerebral intermittent A vasomotor phenomenon in which transient spasm and closure of the lumen of an artery occurs, temporarily depriving a part of the brain of its blood supply, producing transitory hemiplegia. This condition is usually observed in the course of cerebral arteriosclerosis.

claudication, mental Transitory spasm of the blood vessels of the brain. Some authors hold that mental claudication may be responsible for sudden fleeting episodes of mental confusion.

claustrophilia A pathological desire to be confined and enclosed with a small space— the exact opposite of *claustrophobia.* Claustrophilia is a manifestation of a strong tendency to withdraw in a somatic way and is seen in many catatonic episodes. It has been suggested that certain criminals have adopted a psychopathic reaction pattern, thus inviting incarceration, which represents a protected withdrawal from unbearable environmental tension. In these cases claustrophilia is interpreted psychoanalytically as an escape from the world and a tendency to return to the womb. A disposition to claustrophilia is often seen in asthmatics, who symptomatically withdraw into their own respiratory cavities. Such patients show a predilection for introversion and isolation, often with a strong need for solitude and silence.

claustrophobia Fear of being locked or shut in; fear of enclosed places, such as tunnels, elevators, theaters, classrooms, boats, or narrow streets. Like all phobias, this fear may represent a feared temptation (e.g. a fear of sexual excitement which in some patients is manifested in feelings of constriction and painful vegetative sensations, or a fear of phantasies of being in the mother's womb, or a fear that one might not escape his own excitement once it has reached a certain intensity), or it may represent punishment for yielding to temptation, or (as is most common) it may represent a combination of both the foregoing. See *agoraphobia; anxiety-hysteria.*

claustrophoboid Lewin's term for a person afflicted with claustrophobia; *claustrophobiac* is the more correct form.

claustrum See *basal ganglia.*

clavus Severe head pain, sharply defined, and typically described as feeling like a nail is being driven into the head; usually regarded as a conversion symptom.

cleft, synaptic See *neurotransmitter; synapse.*

Clérambault-Kandinsky complex See *complex, Clérambault-Kandinsky.*

client A purchaser of services or goods; in nonmedical settings used instead of *patient* to refer to the recipient of mental health care.

client-centered therapy See *therapy, client-centered.*

climacophobia Fear of stairs.

climacteric Of or pertaining to the so-called involutional period of life, characterized in the woman by the cessation of the menses and less definitely characterized in men.

climacterium A critical period of life; most commonly, in present-day usage, that period generally designated as the involutional period when the endocrine and reproductive glands undergo a decrease in functional activity. In the male, the cli-

macterium is generally considered to fall between the ages of 50 and 65 years; in the female, between 40 and 55 years. See *developmental levels; psychosis, involutional.*

climacterium, male An ill-defined syndrome in males, in middle life, and thought of as analogous to the menopause in females. The major symptoms are usually nocturnal frequency, fatigue, indecision, flushes, decreased sexual desire, and decreased erective and intromissive potency. Various other symptoms may be present also. It is a moot question whether this syndrome constitutes a separate and distinct clinical entity, or whether it is a symptomatic manifestation of a psychoneurotic breakdown in middle life, revolving, in the main, around psychogenic impotence and anxiety. In a very small percentage of cases, a true organic, or gonadal, endocrine etiology, secondary to testicular atrophy and degeneration, has been diagnostically validated by means of the therapeutic test with androgens and gonadotrophic assays of the urine.

climax Peak; acme; often used synonymously with *orgasm* (q.v.).

clinical algorithm See *algorithm, clinical.*

clinical poverty syndrome See *syndrome, clinical poverty.*

clinical psychologist See *psychologist.*

clinical trial See *trial, clinical.*

clitoris A female sex organ. It is about an inch and a half in length and is composed of two corpora cavernosa capped by a glans. It is part of the external genitalia.

According to psychoanalysis, the first genital belief of the child is that everyone possesses a penis. The little girl regards her clitoris as an undeveloped penis. Deutsch stresses that in the beginning of the phallic stage the clitoris possesses for the girl the same pleasure-giving capacities as the penis has for the boy. There is clitoral primacy just as there is phallic primacy.

clitoromania *Obs.* Nymphomania.

cloaca (klō-ā'kà) The cloaca is an embryological organization of the rectum and urogenital sinus. In the embryo the rectum and the urethra have a common opening. Later when the anal membrane ruptures, the rectum acquires its own orifice.

In psychoanalysis emphasis is placed on the child's cloaca phantasy, the so-called cloaca theory, that babies are expelled by way of the anal aperture. At the time that children develop this concept their interests are largely coprophilic; hence there is nothing illogical to them in the belief that babies follow the same anatomical course as feces. Nor do children at this early age know that only females bear children; they believe both sexes can perform that function.

clock, aging See *aging, theories of.*

clock, biologic(al) A neural mechanism, perhaps located in the suprachiasmatic nucleus (SCN) of the inferior hypothalamus, that regulates the internal temporal order and timing of hormonal, physiologic, and behavioral rhythms. Jet lag and the effect of changes in work shift reflect physiological derangements of circadian organization, and it is hypothesized that the same neural mechanism is responsible for the periodicity of various neuropsychiatric disorders. See *aging, theories of; rhythms, biologic.*

clock-driven behavior Endogenous rhythmic behavior. See *clock, biologic; rhythms, biologic.*

clone (klōn) A group of organisms that have originated from a single individual by asexual reproduction. Since all these organisms must be endowed with the same hereditary equipment, it may generally be assumed that differences in their phenotypical appearance are due to modifying conditions of their environment. See *modification.*

cloning, molecular The series of procedures involved in inserting DNA from one organism to another; the process of producing *recombinant DNA* (q.v.).

clonus A rhythmical series of contractions in response to the maintenance of tension in a muscle, often appearing in pyramidal lesions as a manifestation of exaggerated tendon reflexes.

clonus, ankle A clonic rhythmical tremor of the foot elicited by placing the leg in semiflexion, holding the leg with one hand, grasping the foot with the other, and briskly dorsiflexing the foot one or more times. See *clonus.*

clonus, patellar Patellar clonus is elicited by extending the leg, grasping the patella (knee cap) between index finger and thumb, and briskly pushing the cap down one or several times. See *clonus.*

closing-in A symptom of constructive apraxia in which the patient tends to close in on the model when performing constructive tasks. For example, when attempting to copy from a model, the patient moves toward the model; or, in setting-up exercises, he will bring his hands ever closer to those of the demonstrator. The symptom, which becomes worse with an increase in the difficulty of the task, may be the result of a fear of empty space, but more likely it represents an attempt to perform better when there is a disturbance in the ability to make an abstract copy from a concrete model.

closure Conclusion, resolution, ending; the process of reaching a decision or ending a debate.

closure, law of and life-course A person's course of life is described by a general law of Gestalt dynamics, the law of closure. This means that every uncompleted whole tends to a kind of continuation that is in accordance with the inherent system of that given whole. In the early phase of life only a few initial lines of the life patterns are apparent, and the continuation patterns may take many different directions. The more the pattern nears completion, the less variation in the pattern continuation is possible.

clouded states, epileptic See *epileptic clouded states.*

cloudiness See *sensorium.*

clouding (of consciousness) A condition, seen most commonly in the acute and chronic brain disorders (the organic reaction types), in which there is impairment of orientation, perception, and attention. The subject appears drowsy, slow to react, muddled in thinking, and sometimes misinterprets external events.

Clouston, Sir Thomas Smith (1840–1915) British psychiatrist and neurologist.

clownism A popular term denoting clownish, grotesque attitudes assumed by certain psychiatric patients; seen especially in the so-called *Faxenpsychosis* (q.v.) and buffoonery psychosis and, to a lesser extent, in Ganser state. See *psychosis, buffoonery; syndrome, Ganser.*

clumsiness Difficulty in performing skilled movements that a normal subject of the same age could perform with ease; the difficulty is not due to cognitive, intellectual, or gross sensory deficits. Clumsiness in children is sometimes called *developmental apraxia* and is often associated with speech or reading problems, as in attention deficit disorder or minimal brain dysfunction. See *impulse disorder, hyperkinetic*.

clumsiness, arranged An unconsciously prepared inaptitude through which the neurotic prevents himself from properly performing certain acts that he secretly fears. In a general sense, arranged clumsiness is an escape mechanism by means of which the performance of certain acts is avoided through the pretence of lack of skill. In a more specific way, this expression is used in relation to the unconsciously prearranged inability to find the vaginal entrance in an attempt to perform coitus, and to other inadequacies in the performance of sexual acts.

cluster headache See *headache, cluster*.

cluttering Rapid, jerky speech with faulty phrasing patterns, as a result of which the child's language is at times unintelligible. Cluttering is a language and speech disorder within the group "specific developmental disorders" in DSM-III-R. It is commonly associated with motor awkwardness and personality and behavior changes (e.g. behavior is erratic, disorganized, impulsive, untidy). Other language disorders such as delay in beginning to speak, reading disability, and spelling disability are common. Family history frequently reveals clutterers in the same family and the condition is often mistaken for stammering. Like stammering, it is more common in boys, but cluttering tends to persist throughout life and the cluttered speech is characteristic. It is hurried, even precipitate (tachylalia), and confused.

Probably the most famous clutterer was the Reverend W.A. Spooner, Warden of New College, Oxford, whose word confusions have come to be known as *spoonerisms*. Typical examples include "The two great English poets, Kelly and Sheets" (for "Shelley and Keats") and "The Lord is a shoving leopard" (for "loving shepherd").

Cluttering is also sometimes called *agitolalia*.

CMCHS Civilian-Military Contingency Hospital System, a plan to supplement the capabilities of the military health care system with the use of civilian hospitals in the event of the sudden production of war casualties at a higher rate than can be absorbed by the military system.

CME Continuing medical education.

CMHC Community Mental Health Center. See *psychiatry, community*.

CMI Case-mix index, a pooling of different kinds of cases so that the assigned average reimbursement rate per case over a year or some other period would not penalize the treating facility.

CMMS Columbia Mental Maturity Scale, designed primarily for use with patients with cerebral palsy.

CMP Competitive medical plan; chronic mental patient; see *chronic mentally ill*.

Cn In Rorschach scoring, color naming, i.e. the naming of a chromatic color that is proffered by the patient as a complete response requiring no further elaboration. The *Cn* indicate superficial, labile affectivity and are produced most commonly by organic brain cases.

CNV Contingent negative variation; in testing event-related potentials (see *ERP*), the negative voltage that builds slowly in the subject who is warned of the imminence of a target. The CNV is generally interpreted as an indicator of arousal or anticipation. It is reduced in amplitude in many schizophrenics and in other disorders as well, but in the latter it returns to normal when patients are in clinical remission while it remains abnormal in schizophrenics in remission.

CO Community organization, community organizer. See *social policy planning*.

co-conscious, co-consciousness "Conscious states that we are not aware of, simply because [they are] not in the focus of attention but in the fringe of the content of consciousness. The term would also include pathologically split-off and independently acting co-conscious ideas or systems of ideas such as occur in hysteria, reaching their apogee in conscious personalities and in automatic writings." (Prince, M. *The Unconscious*, 1916)

In psychoanalysis the term preconscious is in general equivalent to co-conscious.

co-twin control See *control, co-twin*.

cocaine An alkaloid obtained from coca leaves (Bolivia, Peru), sometimes used as a topical anesthetic. Nowadays it is mainly a drug of abuse and dependence. Cocaine intoxication is manifested in the following symptoms: psychomotor excitement, garrulousness, feelings of elation and grandiosity, a sense of heightened awareness, dilated pupils, tachycardia, sweats or chills, anorexia, nausea, insomnia; there may be ideas of reference, impaired judgment, hallucinations (usually auditory). When taken intravenously, cocaine produces a "rush"—a feeling of intense well-being and confidence. After an hour or so the effects begin to wear off and during this period of "crashing" feelings of irritability, anxiety, or depression may emerge, along with a strong desire for more cocaine. See *crack*.

cocaine bug See *sign, Magnan*.

cocainism Cocaine poisoning or cocaine dependency; symptoms are referable to sympathomimetic discharge (e.g. rise in blood pressure, sweating) and to central nervous system excitation (subject is more active mentally, overestimates his physical and mental capacities, may have pleasurable illusions and hallucinations that may be of the Lilliputian variety). After these effects wear off, there may be motor incoordination, moroseness and suspiciousness, and sometimes convulsions. See *dependency, drug*.

cocainomania Morbid craving for cocaine.

coccygodynia (kok-sig-ō-din′ē-à) Pain at the tip of the coccyx.

cochlear nerve See *nerve, acoustic*.

cocktail, lytic A mixture of neuroleptic drugs (usually chlorpromazine, promethazine, Hydergine, atropine, etc.) used in the treatment of acute or impending delirium.

code of ethics See *ethics*.

code, professional An articulated statement of role morality as perceived and agreed on by the members of the profession itself. Such codes are often criticized as lacking adequacy and comprehensiveness because they emphasize a limited number of moral principles but ignore others. Specifically in medicine, at least in the past, they have tended to focus on the obligations of the professional but have managed at the same time to ignore patient autonomy.

codification The act of systematizing or classifying; in communications theory, the phrasing of signals in such terms as to be understandable to others.

coefficient, correlation See *correlation*.

coefficient, regression See *correlation*.

coelom See *celom*.

coene- See *cene-*.

coercion Any threat of sufficient force that no rational person would reasonably be expected to resist it. Strong or forceful recommendations, particularly when given so as to overcome a patient's irrational fear about a procedure or plan for treatment, do not ordinarily consititute coercion. Threatening to commit a patient or hospitalize him involuntarily if he does not accept the proffered treatment, however, often falls within the definition of coercion in that it has removed the patient's freedom of choice. Because even under identical conditions, and given identical choices, not all would choose the same course of action, valid consent must include freedom of choice and lack of coercion to make one choice, provided that more than one course of action is available. Physicians tend to rank survival as the most important choice, no matter what the alternatives, whereas many patients consider pain or disability more significant in determining choice than the prospect of mere survival. See *consent, informed*.

coercive philosophy See *philosophy, coercive*.

coercive treatment See *forced treatment*.

cognition, paranormal Obtaining knowledge by means outside of the normal process of perceiving or thinking, as in extrasensory perception. See *perception, extrasensory*.

cognition, primary The earliest way of viewing the world, when there is no clear distinction between self and non-self, inside and outside. Arieti relates the primary process to this level of cognitive organization and suggests that schizophrenia consists of regression to the level of primary cognition as a way of interpreting the world and the self-image in less frightening ways. See *process, primary psychic*.

cognitions In cognitive therapy, the thoughts or images in consciousness that appear almost automatically when one is confronted with a situation; what a person thinks in a situation and not what he thinks about a situation. Cognitions are differentiated from *schemata*, the silent assumptions or beliefs based on past experience that direct a person to attend to certain stimuli, to ignore others, and to value and perceive events in a certain way. Schemata thus account for cognitions, and analysis of a series of cognitions enables the therapist to infer the schema. See *therapy, cognitive.*

cognitions, depressive The characteristic thought content of patients with clinical *depression* (q.v.): ideas of present failure and inadequacy, hopelessness about the future, and ruminations about past misdeeds.

cognitive See *conation.*

cognitive anthropology Ethnoscience (q.v.).

cognitive control See *style, cognitive.*

cognitive defects See *defects, cognitive.*

cognitive dissonance In information theory, *incongruity* (q.v.).

cognitive functioning The way a person thinks and particularly how one's intrapsychic constructs prepare that person to assess and deal with external reality. See *style, cognitive.*

cognitive psychology See *style, cognitive; therapy, cognitive.*

cognitive restructuring Cognitive behavior therapy. See *therapy, behavior; therapy, cognitive.*

cognitive science The attempt to comprehend the structure of higher mental processes and the nature of knowledge, typically using the electronic computer as model and blending contributions from various disciplines such as artificial intelligence, linguistics, psychology, anthropology, philosophy, and the neurosciences. To some extent cognitive science developed as a reaction against behaviorism and neurophysiology, both of which tried to explain complexly organized behaviors such as speaking as a consequence of environmental promptings. The currently dominant theory of human cognition is based on symbolic computation and emphasizes that organization stems from the organism itself, that central brain processes precede and determine the ways in which an organism carries out complex behavior. Patterns of generic relations, or schemata, are used to organize information, and cognitive skills are composed of rules that can be represented symbolically in the form, "If this, then that." See *connectionism; style, cognitive.*

cognitive slippage P.E. Meehl's term for loosening of associations that he considers a core element in schizophrenia. (*American Psychologist 17*, 1962)

cognitive style See *style, cognitive.*

cognitive therapy See *therapy, cognitive.*

cohabitation See *coitus.*

cohesion, social See *hedonism.*

cohesive self See *autonomy, sense of.*

cohort A group of subjects who share one or more characteristics, such as having experienced the same event during the same period of time. *Cohort analysis* is the use of such a group as a way to study how differences develop over time in the persons who make up the cohort. A birth cohort, for example, comprises individuals born at the same time (day, month, or year), and analysis of that cohort is concerned with how the persons who were alike at the start turn out to be significantly different from each other at the end of the study. Cohort analysis thus emphasizes the socioenvironmental context within which individual differences develop. See *methodology.*

coitophobia Fear of the sexual act.

coitus a tergo See *coitus more ferarum; pederasty.*

coitus, coition Sexual intercourse per vaginam between male and female.

In medicine *coitus, copulation, cohabitation,* and *sexual intercourse* are used synonymously, though the words have a widely different meaning in their original context.

coitus, external Perineal coitus.

coitus, incomplete *Coitus interruptus* (q.v.).

coitus inter femora *Obs.* Sexual relations by the insertion of the penis between the thighs of the partner.

coitus interruptus Cessation of sexual intercourse before emission; synonymous with *onanism.* (Popular usage, however, has equated onanism with masturbation.)

coitus more ferarum *Obs.* (L. "sexual intercourse in the manner of wild beasts") The carrying out of the act of heterosexual intercourse in the "natural" position of lower animals, that is, from the rear, and usually with the female on hands and knees. The penis is inserted into the vagina; when it is inserted into the rectum, the act is called anal intercourse. This latter practice is called *pederasty* (q.v.) when the partner is a boy, and *sodomy* (q.v.) when the sexual relation is with an animal through the vagina.

Coitus more ferarum is not sodomy, but is thought of as primitive. The axis of the vagina, in this position, is in direct correspondence with the axis of the penis in erection. This might indicate the primitive biological congruity of this position. Certain elements of tenderness, which are dominant in the so-called normal, or face-to-face, position, are, however, excluded in this approach.

coitus oralis *Obs. Fellatio* (q.v.).

coitus per anum *Pederasty* (q.v.).

coitus, perineal External coitus; Lacassagne coined the expression for the act of rubbing the penis against the perineal region.

coitus reservatus Sexual intercourse in which the male partner delays or withholds his orgasm until the female partner has hers, or indefinitely as a means of birth control.

COLA Cost of living adjustment, tied in with supplemental security income (SSI), social security benefits.

collaboration As used by Sullivan, a type of interpersonal relationship in which there is not only cooperation but also sensitivity to the needs of the other person.

collateral Any person related by blood to a series of siblings, but not descended from the same line of immediate ancestors. A first cousin is the most closely related instance of a collateral.

The term also means "indirect" when applied to this line of descent of an individual or to the form of inheritance of a Mendelian factor as characteristic of *recessiveness* (q.v.), that is, the transmission of a trait to the descendants of the siblings of a trait carrier.

colleague-centered consultation See *consultant*.

collecting, collection See *soteria; mania, collecting*.

collection The impulse to collect is given much prominence in psychoanalysis. "A passion for collection is frequently a direct surrogate for a sexual desire; and in that case a delicate symbolism is often concealed behind the choice of objects collected." (Abraham, *SP*)

It is the belief of psychoanalysts that the desire to possess and control is a reflection also of early oral and anal conditions. In the oral stage the motive is to gain, in the anal it is to hold. "The possessiveness of anal love shows itself clearly in the collector; the objects collected are associated symbolically with excrement." (Healy et al., *SMP*)

collective life handicap See *handicap, collective life*.

collective unconscious "All those psychic contents I term collective which are peculiar not to one individual, but to many, at the same time, i.e., either to a society, a people, or to mankind in general. Such contents are the 'mystical collective ideas' ('representation collectives') of the primitive described by Levy-Bruhl; they include also the *general concepts* of right, the State, religion, science, etc., current among civilized men. . . . The antithesis of *collective* is *individual*."

Jung refers to two divisions of the unconscious, the *personal* and the *collective*. The former "embraces all the acquisitions of the personal existence—hence the forgotten, the repressed, the subliminally perceived, thought and felt. But, in addition to these personal unconscious contents, there exist other contents which do not originate in personal acquisitions but in the inherited possibility of psychic functioning in general, viz. in the inherited brain-structure. These are the mythological associations—those motives and images which can spring anew in every age and clime, without historical tradition or migration. I term these contents the *collective unconscious*." (Jung, *CAP*) See *analytic psychology*.

college, invisible A collection of individuals or of scientists with a feeling of allegiance to another and with frequent professional and social interactions. Although the term originated in the 17th century, it is now used to refer to a group of scientists who live in "disparate geographical locations, but who often attend the same conferences, who publish in the same journals, who invite each to give presentations in their home institutions, and who share preprint of their research endeavors. It is through the political power of such "colleges" that many of the changes in science are made." (Blashfield, R.K. *Schizophrenia Bulletin 8*, 1982)

colloidal gold reaction See *Lange's colloidal gold reaction*.

colloidoclastic diathesis See *diathesis, colloidoclastic*.

coloboma A cleft or defect, especially of the eye; of significance in neuropsychiatry in that choroidoretinal coloboma is one of the elements of a familial syndrome that also includes dysplastic body build and mental retardation. The coloboma appears as a white patch of exposed sclera below the optic disc and causes a scotoma in that region.

colony, Gheel See *Gheel colony.*

Columbia Mental Maturity Scale See *CMMS.*

coma The profoundest degree of stupor in which all consciousness is lost and there is no voluntary activity of any kind. Among the various conditions that may produce coma the most common are encephalitis, cerebral hemorrhage, cerebral thrombosis, cerebral embolism, subarachnoid hemorrhage, intracranial tumor, head injury, postepileptic coma, diabetic coma, hypoglycemic coma, hypertensive encephalopathy, uremic coma, acute alcoholism, intoxication with opiates or other sedatives, hypothalamic lesions, congestive attacks of general paralysis, hysterical trance, and catatonic stupor.

coma somnolentium (L. "coma of the somnolent") *Cataphora* (q.v.).

coma vigil Coma in which the eyes remain open. Coma vigil occurs in certain acute brain syndromes associated with systemic infection (the infective-exhaustive psychoses, also known as acute toxic encephalopathy, acute toxic encephalitis, or acute serous encephalitis). See *mutism, akinetic.*

combat exhaustion Same as *combat fatigue.* See *shell shock.*

combination In genetics, this term refers to the hereditary variations that represent the effect of *hybridization* and that occur in crossbred products originating from the union between two individuals with unlike hereditary equipment. The formation of new hereditary combinations that account for the majority of genetic differences among animals and plants, and also explain why hybrids do not breed true, takes place in accordance with the *Mendelian law,* which governs the reassortment of the different genetic factors involved in a given cross (see *variation*).

Pearson used this term to refer to what he considers the earliest mechanism of learning: the unification of sensory impressions from the outside with perceptions arising from instinctual (internal) stimuli.

combined degeneration of the spinal cord See *sclerosis, posterolateral.*

combining forms See listing of frequently used combining forms (e.g., brady-, dys-, hyper-, tachy-) under *speech disorders.*

cometophobia Pathologic fear of comets.

coming out Open acknowledgment of one's homosexuality; less commonly used to refer to admission of any kind of pathology or variance from the norm (e.g. binge eating, agoraphobia).

command negativism See *negativism.*

commensalism See *symbiosis.*

commissure Transverse or commissural fibers; those portions of the white substance of the cerebral hemispheres made up of medullated nerve fibers connecting the two hemispheres. The commissural fibers are to be distinguished from the two other types of myelinated nerve fibers found in the white matter: *projection fibers,* which connect the cerebral cortex with lower portions of the brain and spinal cord, and *association fibers,* which connect different portions of the same hemisphere.

commitment Depriving a person of his liberty by putting him under the guardianship of another (whether mental hospital, prison, or other institution, or in the custody of a probation officer). In psychiatry, commitment is a process whereby one or more doctors explain to a court why a patient's mental problems necessitate forfeiture of his freedom. Such explanation is usually in the form of a certificate signed by the examining physician(s), and it is the process of completing this certificate that is properly labeled *certification.* In practice, however, the terms commitment and certification are interchangeable.

communication The process of transmitting information from sender (*encoder*) to receiver (*decoder*). "The encoder is the originator of the message; the decoder is the recipient of the message; and the message is a response of an encoder which may be the stimulus for a decoder. Communication results when a response of an encoder is received as a stimulus for a decoder."

Channels of communication are differentiated according to the source and destination of the message. "The six major channels of human 'face to face' communication, defined in terms of their source and destination, are: speech (*source:* vocal tract; *destination:* ear), kinesics (body movement; eye), odor (chemical processes;

nose), touch (body surface; skin), observation (body surface; eye), and proxemics (body placement; eye)." (Kiesler, D.J. *The Process of Psychotherapy*, 1973) See *empathy*.

The foregoing describes an informational approach to communication, emphasizing the content or meaning. Another approach is the interactional, which defines communication not as a transaction but as a way of structuring and managing social occasions by behavioral means. Such an approach is concerned with how behavior is organized rather than what it means.

The relational approach considers communication to be the overall system of relationships that are developed between people and by those people with their community and their habitat. An outgrowth of the relational approach is the double-bind model of psychopathology, which views schizophrenia as a distortion in the pattern of relationships between the subject and other persons rather than as a distortion in the behavior of the subject. See *bind, double*.

communication deviance Tendency toward a fragmented or amorphous conversational style, noted to be frequent in parents of schizophrenic offspring. Although first interpreted as a parental disturbance that predisposed to the development of schizophrenia, it is now recognized as a reaction of families to a schizophrenic member, a reaction that may secondarily aggravate the offspring's illness.

communication, disordered Altered ability to transmit a message, believed by some workers to be a characteristic of the families of schizophrenics. Among the patterns described are *amorphous communications,* which are vague, loose, and indefinite, and *fragmented communications,* which lack closure and are easily disrupted and poorly integrated.

communication, nonverbal Transmittal of information by means other than formal language. As with verbal communication, nonverbal messages may be factual, *indexical* (conveying information about the nature of the sender), or interactional. Erving Goffman, (*The Presentation of Self in Everyday Life,* 1969) described four basic types of communicational relations: direct (the sender conveys a message through signals known to be understood by the receiver) and indirect (the message must

be decoded by the receiver); symmetrical (sender and receiver send messages back and forth to each other) and assymetrical (the sender and receiver roles are not reversible).

communication, physiognomonic Nonverbal communication, such as by gesture, mime, facial expression, and/or any number of minimal cues by which meaning is transmitted from one organism to another.

communication, privileged Information that a patient discloses to his physician while the latter is attending him in a professional capacity; such information is termed privileged because in some states and according to ethical precepts of the medical profession the physician is not allowed to divulge such information without the patient's consent. This is, in other words, the patient's privilege of silence in regard to confidential matters on the part of his physician. See *confidentiality*.

communication unit The essential components of transmission of information from one person to another; these components are the *source* (the person sending the message), the *transmitter* (the motor apparatus through which the message will be expressed), and the *destination* (the person to whom the message is sent, who picks up the message through his receiver, or sensory apparatus). See *information theory*.

communion, magical According to psychoanalytic theory, in unconscious thinking, "by incorporating objects one becomes united with them." That is, to eat something or be eaten by someone is an unconscious way of achieving union with that object. In countless experiences of everyday living one shares ideas, emotions, activities with others. Some of these experiences of sharing with others present as their unconscious significance, psychoanalytically, the type of mystical or magical union described above. This magical communion of "becoming the same substance" takes place when the same food is jointly eaten or the respective bloods of the individuals involved are mixed. The latter type of communion is seen in many tribal rites of friendship, and, symbolically, in our custom of handshaking. The magical union mediated through food is seen not only in the old idea that friendship and hospitality are associated with breaking bread together, but also and particularly in the well-known religious rites of the Eucharist, the bread and wine (distributed to the parishioners) symbolizing, as in the Last Supper, Christ's body and blood. (Fenichel, *PTN*)

community care See *domicile; rehabilitation.*

community divorce See *divorce, stations of.*

community feeling The sense of relationship between the individual and the community. Adler states that out of community feelings "are developed tenderness, love of neighbour, friendship and love, the desire for power unfolding itself in a veiled manner and seeking secretly to push its way along the path of group consciousness." (Adler, A. *The Practice and Theory of Individual Psychology,* 1924)

Community Mental Health Center See *psychiatry, community.*

community organization See *social policy planning.*

community, therapeutic 1. A psychiatric or mental hospital that emphasizes the importance of socioenvironmental and interpersonal influences in the therapy, management, resocialization, and rehabilitation of the long-term patient. Self-control, dignity, and trust are employed rather than excessive imposed controls, restrictions, regimentation, and meaningless rituals.

The therapeutic community requires an organized social structure that becomes a therapeutic culture in which the living-learning-confrontation aspect engenders increasingly open communication between patients and staff and the opportunity for immediate feedback about patients' behavior and interactions. See *culture, therapeutic.*

2. A residential setting for the rehabilitation of drug abusers, consisting of a drugfree program combined with provocative encounter-group sessions with peers and drug counselors.

comorbidity Occurrence or existence of more than one disease at the same time in the same subject. The comorbidity hypothesis of schizoaffective disorder postulates that it represents the chance association in one subject of all the factors responsible for two different disorders, schizophrenia and affective disorder.

Particularly in utilization review and in reimbursement guidelines, comorbidity is also termed *substantial comorbidity* and de-

fined as a preexisting condition that, because of its presence with a specific principal diagnosis, causes an increase in length of hospital stay by at least one day in approximately 75% of cases.

companion, imaginary It has often been observed that a child will create an imaginary companion and will endow this product of phantasy with the qualities of reality. The imaginary companion will have a name, a definite appearance and personality—even an imaginary family created for it, and so on.

Imaginary companions are created mostly by only children, or by children whose siblings are much older, or who for any reason are without real playmates. The imaginary companion thus fulfills the child's need for intimate companionship and friendship and serves an important function in his emotional life. For the imaginary companion is freely taken into confidences from which parents are distinctly barred and becomes "someone to tell troubles to" and "to share secret pleasures with." In general, the imaginary companion is so created by the child that it has everything the child desires but lacks. The play *Harvey* presents an amusing and not dissimilar instance of this imagery, a huge white rabbit created as an imaginary companion. Though it is an animal and the imaginary creation of an adult, its origin and function are much the same as those of the imaginary companions of children. See *Doppelganger; game, hallucinatory.*

companion, phobic See *agoraphobia.*

compartmentalization Isolation; keeping separate parts of one's personality that should be kept together; psychic fragmentation.

compensation Counterbalancing an inequity, making restitution for a loss, correcting an inferiority or loss (in somatopathology, typically by hypertrophy of tissue or by increased functioning of the organ or system in question), providing a substitute for something that is unacceptable or unattainable. See *overcompensation.*

compensation-ideal Adler's term for substitution of some superior image in dreams or phantasy for an inferior one, a reflection of the desire for power and mastery.

compensation neurosis See *neurosis, compensation.*

competence In forensic psychiatry, ability to perform or accomplish an action or task that another person of similar background and training, or any human being, could reasonably be expected to perform. Almost always the term refers to mental capacity. Ordinarily a person is not deemed incompetent on the basis of a physical defect that impairs performance. See *incompetent.*

competition The struggle for existence and for a livelihood. Competition may be either unconscious or conscious; as it becomes self-conscious it tends to pass over into social conflict.

competitive inhibition See *antagonistic, narcotic.*

complacency, principle of W.B. Cannon formulated the thesis that "instincts" and "drives" are in a sense attempts on the part of the organism to maintain its optimal body economy (homeostasis). R.B. Raup called it the principle of complacency, thereby indicating that every organism is a physiological system that tends to preserve its stationary condition or to restore the stationary condition as soon as it is disturbed by any variation occurring within or outside the organism. In a sense all needs and desires are behavior patterns, such as withdrawal, or attack, or flight, in direct or indirect consequence of this general tendency to keep a physiological condition constant.

complaint habit *Hypochondriasis* (q.v.).

complementarity A state of harmony or balance between the emotional needs of the interacting members of a group, or the degree to which such a balance has been achieved. N.W. Ackerman (*The Psychodynamics of Family Life,* 1958) describes a *minus form* of complementarity in family role relations that is limited to neutralization of the disintegrating effects of conflict and anxiety. The *plus form,* in addition to such neutralization, promotes further growth and creative development in the family unit and in the individual members of the unit.

complementarity, reciprocal In sociology, the postulate that moral and social codes, rather than being arbitrary conventionalities that are antagonistic to emotional drives, are an intrinsic factor in human functioning and that homeostasis exists in relation to the social environment fully as much as it exists in relation to the internal milieu.

complementary Mutually supplying each other's lack; used most often to refer to a type of relationship within a family, or between husband and wife. "In a *complementary* relationship, behavior of one sort by one partner—such as dominance—is met by behavior of another sort, in this case submission, by the spouse. In a *symmetrical* relationship, both partners exchange the same kind of behavior—both are giving, or both are domineering, for example. In contemporary America, a husband often has to deal with a wife who demands a symmetrical relationship on the one hand, and insists that she be treated as an equal, but at the same time demands that her husband dominate her in a complementary relationship. Such an incompatibility of messages constitutes paradoxical communication, or what has been termed by Bateson, Jackson, and their co-workers, a 'double bind.' " (Campbell, R.J. in *Marriage: A Psychological and Moral Approach,* ed. W. Bier, 1964)

complex A group of repressed ideas interlinked into a complex whole, which besets the individual, impelling him to think, feel, and perhaps act after a habitual pattern. Jung, who introduced the term *complex* to psychiatry, describes it as the grouping "of psychic elements about emotionally-toned contents." He adds that it "consists of a nuclear element and a great number of secondarily constellated associations." Jones defines a complex as "a group of emotionally invested ideas partially or entirely repressed." (Jones, E. *Papers on Psycho-Analysis,* 1938)

In general it may be said that fundamental psychic conflicts, usually those derived during the stages of infantile sexuality, may give rise to a complex. Thus one speaks of the Oedipus, Electra, and castration complexes.

complex, active castration The ideas centered around the fear of losing the penis and the emotions linked with these ideas. The passive castration complex is the idea that the penis has already been lost and/or the wish to lose the penis.

complex, apprentice The time in a boy's life when he aims to be like his father and will act as a pupil or apprentice: in psychoanalytic terms, will have a penis like his father. To achieve this, he is submissive, passive, with the idea or phantasy that by this method, in the future, he will be prepared to be masculine and active, like his father.

complex, Atreus See *complex, Medea.*

complex, authority A group of emotionally invested ideas centering around the concept of authority. These emotions are entirely or partly repressed together with the original ideas concerning authority to which they are attached. If a person's earliest experiences with authority have been sufficiently painful, it is likely that both the experiences and the associated affects have undergone repression. The material thus repressed constitutes a complex and is termed an authority complex. The person will always react to authority just as he did originally, although he will not be aware of this fact. Unconsciously overdetermined reactions to authority either in the direction of rebellion against it or in submission to it are common in neurotic patients.

complex, autonomous "All those psychic formations which at first are developed quite unconsciously, and only from the moment when they attain threshold-value are able to break through into consciousness. The association which they then make with consciousness has not the importance of an assimilation, but rather of a perception; which means to say, that the autonomous complex, although certainly perceived, cannot be subjected to conscious control, whether in the form of inhibition or of voluntary reproduction. The autonomy of the complex reveals itself in the fact that it appears or vanishes when and in such guise as accords with its own intrinsic tendency; it is independent of the option of consciousness." (Jung, *CAP*)

complex, breast Psychoanalytic term for substitution of the possessed penis for the mother's breast that has been denied or withheld from the boy. The breast complex may be expressed in the phantasy of vagina dentata (a vagina with teeth), where the vagina represents the mouth that originally wanted to tear off the mother's breast. The complex may also be expressed in breast envy, which in turn may be expressed in that type of overt homosexuality in which the penis of the subject and/or his partner unconsciously represents the breast.

complex, brother See *complex, Cain.*

complex, Cain An expression synonymous with *brother complex;* rivalry, competition, aggression, or destructive impulses directed against a brother.

complex, castration See *castration.*

complex, chronological See *complex, subject.*

complex, Clérambault-Kandinsky (klā′-räN-bô kän-dēn′ski) (Gatian G. de Clérambault, 1872–1934, French psychiatrist) *Erotomania* (q.v.).

complex, Clytemnestra This refers to the wife who kills her husband so that she may possess one of his male relatives.

complex, dart and dome The spike and wave type of electroencephalographic tracing seen in petit mal epilepsy. See *epilepsy.*

complex, Demosthenes The neurotic need to achieve mastery over inferiority feelings through words and language in the process of speaking. See *overcompensation.*

complex, Diana The wish of a female to be a male. See *transsexualism.*

complex, Electra *Obs.* The female Oedipus complex. Electra, the daughter of Agamemnon, induced her brother Orestes to wreak vengeance on their mother, Clytemnestra, and her new husband, Agamemnon's brother, for having together murdered Agamemnon. The dark broodings over the fate of her beloved hero-father possessed the wedlock-scorning Electra till death.

complex, femininity Psychoanalysts believe that, in the infantile life of the boy, there is a phase equivalent to the "penis" phase in the little girl. Girls believe that they once possessed a phallus just like the one that boys have, but through some misdeed on their part it was taken from them. The male child develops the same fear or frustration (castration phantasy), which Klein calls a *femininity complex.* In essence it is the inferiority complex of Adler. The boy thinks that the mother is the castrator. In order to save his phallus from the fate suffered by girls he identifies himself with his mother and wishes for a vagina and breasts. There is thus "vaginal envy" in boys as there is "penis envy" in girls. At the same time there is a dread on his part of the feminine role that castration would bring about. The dread may appear as its opposite, aggression. "A tendency to excess in the direction of aggression which very frequently occurs has its source in the femininity-complex." (Klein, M. *The Psycho-Analysis of Children*, 1932)

complex, function In Jung's analytic psychology, a mechanism through which a function operates. Jung identified four function types: thinking, feeling, intuition, and sensation. No matter what function predominates in a person, daily living requires many ad hoc adjustments. One such is the function complex called the *persona* (q.v.), a mask or outer appearance that is adopted as a temporary expedient to fit in with the environment. The persona and other function complexes may be used by any of the function types.

complex, Griselda (Griselda, or Griselidis, was a paragon of womanly purity, virtue, and endless patience, widely celebrated in medieval romances) The name given by Putnam to the father's complex in regard to his daughter. In the father-daughter complex the father unconsciously grudges giving up his daughter to another man, not wishing to part with her himself. Contemplation of the marriage of his daughter—the future mother—reactivates the older oedipal yearning for his own mother. The father's reluctance to give up his daughter to another man is often thinly disguised under the pretext of altruistic solicitude for the daughter's welfare.

complex, heir of the Oedipus See *superego.*

complex, Heracles The hatred of a father for his children. See *complex, Medea.*

complex, incest See *incest.*

complex, inferiority See *inferiority; inferiority, feeling of.*

complex, Jocasta The term proposed by Raymond de Saussure (1920) for the morbid attachment of a mother for her own son—from the marriage of Jocasta to her son Oedipus (see *complex, Oedipus*). The Jocasta complex represents a type of perverted mother love and has various degrees of intensity—from the maternal instinct slightly deformed to a frank sexual attachment in which both physical and psychic satisfaction is found. See *complex, Phaedra.*

complex, masculinity Rebellion against castration in the girl, leading to masculine attitudes and behavior. This term is used by Freudian psychoanalysts in much the same way that Adler uses *masculine attitude in female neurotics* (q.v.).

complex, Medea The hatred and/or homicidal wishes of the mother toward her child. The death wishes against the offspring are usually motivated unconsciously by a desire for revenge against her husband. Fritz Wittels used the term in a more limited way to indicate a mother's death wish against her daughter. Strictly speaking, this is not correct, for the Medea of Euripides had only sons. The term Atreus complex has been suggested for a father's death wishes against his offspring.

complex, nuclear In psychoanalysis, synonymous with Oedipus complex.

complex, Oedipus Oedipus was a son of Laius, King of Thebes, and Jocasta, his wife. The King learned from an oracle that he was fated to be killed by his son. When a boy was born, the King gave him to a shepherd to leave him on Mt. Kithaeron to die. However, the compassionate shepherd gave the infant to the childless King of Corinth, Polybus. When Oedipus reached the age of puberty and an oracle told him that he would kill his father and form an incestuous union with his mother, he decided not to return to Corinth to his alleged father. In his journey he met Laius, whom he slew in a quarrel. When Oedipus arrived at Thebes the Sphinx presented a riddle for solution. Oedipus solved the riddle and the Thebans in gratitude gave him Jocasta as wife. When finally he discovered the relationship between him and his wife he blinded himself, while Jocasta hanged herself. Oedipus wandered away, accompanied by his daughter, Antigone. Finally he was destroyed by the avenging deities, the Eumenides.

The principles of the Oedipus situation are regarded by psychoanalysts as characteristic of all persons. During the phase of late infancy, the child shifts a quantum of energy into sexual interests in the parents. Normally the boy becomes chiefly attached to his mother, the girl to her father. The solution of the struggle determines the character of the child's later reactions. During the latency period the Oedipus complex is normally relinquished in favor of extraparental activities and interests. With the advent of puberty the original, infantile

Oedipus situation is again aroused, and is normally dissolved by the centering of interests in others.

However, the average psychiatric patient never successfully manages his Oedipus complex. Schizophrenia serves as an excellent example. A schizophrenic patient believed implicitly that he was not the child of his parents, that his mother was his wife and that his brothers and sisters were his children; he maintained that his father did not exist. The same patient also insisted that he was blind; on other occasions he spoke of having been castrated. The schizophrenic patient relives the Sophoclean tragedy often with minute precision, even to the point of claiming royal birth.

The same theme is common to psychoneurotic patients, but it is often highly symbolized as a fear, a compulsion, or a conversion phenomenon.

Freud is responsible for the introduction of the Oedipus concept into psychiatry. "One says rightly that the Oedipus complex is the nuclear concept of the neuroses, that it represents the essential part in the content of the neuroses. It is the culminating point of infantile sexuality, which through its after-effects decisively influences the sexuality of the adult." (Freud, S. *Three Contributions to the Theory of Sex*, 1930)

complex, Orestes (Orestes, the son of the Mycenaean King Agamemnon, who killed his own mother, Clytemnestra, and her paramour, Aegisthus, for murdering her husband, Agamemnon) The psychiatric term proposed for a son's killing, or desire to kill, his own mother. F. Wertham believes this is a universal complex, like the Oedipus complex. The majority of psychoanalysts disagree with this view and feel, instead, that when it occurs the Orestes complex is an outgrowth of the Oedipus complex and is a reaction by the male child to rejection or frustration by the oedipal love object, the mother.

complex partial seizures Temporal lobe epilepsy; psychomotor seizures. See *epilepsy*.

complex, perceptual Predominance of images and concrete objects in thinking, with resultant distortions and condensations that run counter to logical, rational thinking; concretistic thinking; *paleologic* (q.v.).

complex, Phaedra This refers to the mother who is in love with her son. The term is also used to refer to a nonpathologic attraction between step-parent and step-child, a counterpart of the Oedipus relationship that is seen more frequently as a result of increasing rates of divorce and remarriage. See *complex, Jocasta*.

complex, Polycrates *Polycratism* (q.v.).

complex, power "The total complex of all those ideas and strivings whose tendency it is to range the ego above other influences, thus subordinating all such influences to the ego, quite irrespective of whether they have their source in men and objective conditions, or spring from one's own subjective impulses, feelings, and thoughts." (Jung, *PT*)

complex, Pygmalion *Pygmalionism* (q.v.).

complex, Quasimodo Emotional conflict, personality disorder, or social maladaptation developing as a result of disfigurement or deformity.

complex, receptor See *receptor complex, supramolecular*.

complex, small penis Concern that one's penis is inadequate because of its size. "What such a man is really ashamed of is not that his penis is 'small,' but the reasons *why* it is 'small.' " (Jones, E. *Papers on Psycho-Analysis*, 1938)

complex, spike and wave The dart and dome type of electroencephalographic tracing seen in petit mal epilepsy. See *epilepsy*.

complex, subject See *complex, systematized*.

complex, symptom See *syndrome*. Syndromes are complexes of symptoms that belong together genetically. (Bleuler, *TP*)

complex, systematized *Obs.* A grouping of associated experiences or mental events that becomes relatively fixed over time and predisposes the person to behave or respond in a particular way. Character and personality traits are examples of systematized complexes.

M. Prince differentiated among *subject complexes* or systems, related to certain types of experience, *chronological complexes* or systems, related to experiences during a particular time of life, and *disposition* or *mood complexes*, related to particular emotions or feeling tones. (*The Unconscious*, 1916)

compliance Self-effacing submission or obedience to the overt or implied demands of others; when used in clinical psychiatry the term implies a neurotic degree of over-submissiveness. It is seen most commonly as a part of the obsessive-compulsive character's defensive system.

compliance, motor A type of response noted in many schizophrenic children, in whom light palm contact is enough to make them turn or change position. Such children show marked dependence on contact with others—they melt into the lap of the examiner and show many disturbances in motility. See *schizophrenia, childhood.*

compliance, patient Adherence to the prescribed treatment regimen, used most commonly in reference to taking medications in the amount and frequency recommended. Lack of compliance is a major factor in apparent treatment failures and in relapse of chronic patients.

compliance, somatic The degree to which the individual's organic structure coincides with his psychological mechanism in the symptomatic expression of his pathological defenses. In conversion symptoms, for instance, the entire cathexis of the objectionable impulses is condensed onto a definite physical function. The ability of the affected function to adsorb this cathexis is its somatic compliance. The function may be chosen because the organ in question presents a locus minoris resistentiae (see *inferiority, organ*), or because the erogeneity of the afflicted part corresponds to the unconscious phantasies seeking expression (as in the case of a person with oral fixations who, when symptoms are developed, will show primarily oral symptoms), or because of the situation in which the decisive repression occurred (the organ or function under highest tension at the decisive moment is likely to become the seat of disturbance), or because of the organ's ability to symbolize the unconscious drive in question (thus convex organs such as the hand, nose, and breasts may symbolize the penis and represent masculine wishes).

compliance, strategic In paradoxical therapy, change based on the patient's acceptance of or obedience to the therapist's directive. A well-known compliance-induction procedure is the *Devil's Pact*, in which the patient is induced to promise that he will carry out a plan before he is told what the plan is. See *therapy, paradoxical.*

componential analysis *Ethnoscience* (q.v.).

component-instinct *Part-instinct* (q.v.); component impulse. See *impulse, component.*

compos mentis L. "sound of mind."

comprehension Understanding, especially as opposed to mere apprehending or cognition. In examining the sensorium, mental grasp, and capacity of a patient, the examiner often presents him with a *comprehension test*, which commonly consists of having the patient read or listen to a narrative paragraph and then asking him questions to determine how much he grasped of the significance of the story.

compression *Condensation* (q.v.).

compression, cerebral This term is used to refer to any degree of head injury (concussion, brain contusion, or cerebral laceration) that is followed by intracranial hemorrhage. The latter may be subdural (which is twice as common) or extradural. Acute subdural hemorrhage is usually the result of severe cerebral laceration; extradural hemorrhage is usually due to laceration of the middle meningeal artery by fractured bone, and in this case the posterior branches of the artery are more frequently involved than the anterior.

compromise-distortion In contradistinction to *compromise-formation* that occurs in normal and neurotic development, Freud used the term *compromise-distortion* to describe an analogous process in a psychosis. Owing to a compromise between the resistance of the ego and the strength of the idea under repression, the return of the repressed idea becomes distorted into a delusion or a hallucination. "A circumstance quite peculiar to paranoia . . . is that the repressed reproaches return as thoughts spoken aloud. They must thereby suffer a two-fold distortion, first, through a censorship, which leads to their substitution by other associated ideas or to a disguise by indefinite kinds of expressions, and secondly, through their relation to current experiences which are merely analogous to the original." (Freud, *CP*)

compromise-formation In psychoanalysis, a substitutive idea or act representing a repressed conflict. Freud held that as a consequence of the ego's contacts with reality, four typical danger situations arise, each derived from some stage of infantile sexuality. They are (1) danger of separation, i.e. loss of the love object; (2) danger of the loss of love; (3) danger of castration; and (4) danger of the loss of superego approval, i.e. guilt. See *anxiety.*

All psychogenic symptoms are compromises, for they arise on the basis of repressed material and thus serve to give release to the pressure or tension resident in the repressed complex.

compulsion A repetitive, stereotyped, and often trivial motor action, the need for whose performance insistently forces itself into consciousness even though the subject does not wish to perform the act. Failure to perform the act generates increasing anxiety; completion of the act gives at least temporary surcease of tension. Compulsions are obsessions in action and, like the latter, are ego-alien and therefore always resisted. See *obsession.*

The compulsion involves a volitional disability in that the subject acts intentionally but not voluntarily, and although he can perform the action he cannot refrain from performing it even though he has good reason to do so. The compulsion is an intentional but involuntary action. See *volition.*

compulsion, masked A mental mechanism by which the neurotic person hides his real obsessive idea behind a compulsion. This compulsion acts only as a disguise (= mask) for the obsessive idea. Such is the case of the patient who has the compulsion of constantly complaining of pain when, in reality, what he is trying to do is to avoid the knowledge of the real cause of his trouble, which is produced by the existence of obsessive ideas. The patient complains of pain instead of obsessions because in this way he can continue with these same obsessions.

compulsion, thinking See *brooding.*

compulsive-obsessive psychoneurosis See *obsessive-compulsive psychoneurosis.*

compulsive personality See *defense, character; personality trait disturbance.*

computation, symbolic See *cognitive science.*

conarium (kō-nā′ri-um) The point of contact of mind and body in Cartesian philosophy. The basic tenet of this philosophy is that the human mind is a thinking substance in intimate association with the body. The Cartesian conarium was renamed the *id* by Freud, who regarded it as

the place in which the instincts in both their organic and their psychic manifestations are localized and from which they spread to diverse sections of the body and the mind.

conation Striving, inclination, tendency to do actively or purposively. Many psychologists distinguish among three categories of mental functioning: the cognitive (perceptual or intellectual), the emotional, and the conative. Conation includes instincts, drives, wishes, and cravings.

concentration See *attention.*

concentric demyelination Balo's disease. See *sclerosis, diffuse.*

concept, body See *image, body.*

concept, feces-child-penis According to psychoanalysis, many factors connected with the anal stage have significant bearing upon the Oedipus and castration complexes. As Freud says: "The handing over of feces for the sake of (out of love for) someone else becomes a prototype of castration; it is the first occasion upon which an individual gives up a piece of his own body (it is such that feces are invariably treated by children) in order to gain the favor of some person whom he loves. So that a person's love for his own penis, which is in other respects narcissistic, is not without an element of anal-erotism." The same reasoning applies to the concept of child and the breast, and the symbolic equation breast-feces-penis-child is at the root of many pregnancy phantasies. (Freud, *CP*)

conception-hallucination. See *hallucination of perception.*

concordance Agreement; in statistics, used primarily in twin studies to refer to the proportion of a representative sample of affected twins whose co-twins are or will be similarly affected. To be contrasted with *frequency*, which refers only to incidence of illness among twins, without regard to incidence in their co-twins.

concordance, probandwise The risk of illness in co-twins of proband twins.

concrete attitude See *abstract attitude.*

concrete operations See *adolescence.*

concrete thinking See *thinking, concrete.*

concretism In analytic psychology concretism is defined as "a definite peculiarity of *thought* and *feeling* which represents the antithesis of abstraction. The actual meaning of concrete is 'grown together.' A concretely-thought concept is one that has grown together or coalesced with other concepts. Such a concept is not abstract, not isolated, and independently thought, but always impure and related. It is not a differentiated concept, but is still embedded in the sense-conveyed material of perception. Concretistic thinking moves among exclusively concrete concepts and views; it is constantly related to sensation." (Jung, *PT*)

concretization The act of making or being concrete and specific, as opposed to general and abstract. In psychiatry, the term generally connotes an overemphasis on specific detail and on the events of immediate experience especially in the subject's verbal productions, in which case the concretization is considered to be an association defect. See *associations, disturbances of; reification*.

For example, a university student with an IQ of 134 gave the following concretistic responses to a word association test: "My father always 'has a head and shoulders' " and "If I were queen I would 'be seated and have a scepter.' "

concurrent review See *review*.

concussion Widespread paralysis of brain function, due to a blow on the head, with a strong tendency to spontaneous recovery, and not necessarily associated with gross organic brain damage. Experimental evidence suggests that this functional disturbance is due to a direct physical injury to the neuron that is reversible, the rate of recovery being proportional to the severity of the injury. See *compression, cerebral*.

concussion, blast See *neurosis, postconcussion*.

condemnation Freudian term meaning "rejection based on judgment." In his discussion of the fate of libido, Freud says that one cannot flee from internal stimuli: "With an instinct, flight is of no avail, for the ego cannot escape from itself. Later on, rejection based on judgment (*condemnation*) will be found to be a good weapon against the impulse." (*CP*)

condensation The process whereby an idea is made to contain all the emotion associated with a group of ideas. A single word or phrase may be overcathected or overcharged with emotion when it stands for something else of a much larger order.

One person in a dream, for instance, may be a fusion of the memories of many people. Similarly, a phobia symbolizes a chain of circumstances rather than a single event.

conditionalism Approximately equivalent to the Jungian concept of determinism and to the Skinnerian concept of *contingency*. Causality is relative rather than absolute, and effects are dependent upon (contingent upon, conditional upon) certain other things occurring. Those other things increase the probability that such effects will be produced; they are necessary but not always sufficient to elicit the results. Turning a key in the ignition may be a necessary condition to start a motor, but it will not always start even when the key is turned. See *behaviorism; therapy, behavior*.

conditioning A procedure in which an adequate stimulus (e.g. presentation of food, causing salivation in the experimental animal) is paired with an inadequate stimulus (e.g. ringing of a bell, which of itself has no effect on salivation) until the previously inadequate stimulus is by itself able to evoke the response. The original, adequate stimulus (food, in the above example) is termed the unconditional stimulus (US), and the response to the unconditional stimulus is termed the unconditional response (UR). The other stimulus (ringing of a bell in the above example) is termed the conditioned or conditional stimulus (CS), and the response to it once conditioning is established is termed the conditioned or conditional response (CR). Because conditioning as thus defined was first described by I.P. Pavlov, it is often known as *Pavlovian conditioning*. It is also known as *classical conditioning or respondent conditioning*.

conditioning, aversive See *therapy, aversion*.

conditioning, cognitive A form of *conditioning* (q.v.) in which an aversive stimulus is paired with a thought, phantasy, or memory of the behavior to be modified or eliminated. In one method of treating smoking, alcoholism, and other addictive behaviors, the subject imagines vividly that he is smoking, drinking, etc., and while doing so administers an electric shock to himself. In time, the thought alone serves as a cognitive shock that discourages the behavior.

conditioning, operant Consequence-governed behavior; B.F. Skinner's term for the process of reinforcing a subject's spontaneous activities. The behaviorist waits for the subject to perform an action, and once the deed is done the subject is rewarded. It has been suggested that many forms of psychotherapy are applications of operant conditioning, in that the patient's speech is rewarded by (reinforced by) remarks or other behavior on the part of the therapist. The patient learns what the therapist expects or wants to hear, and he modifies his own speech and behavior accordingly. See *behaviorism; biofeedback; therapy, behavior.*

conduct 1. As a rule the word conduct refers to the action or behavior of the total individual rather than to parts of him (such as movement of an extremity as an isolated act). Conduct implies psychic as well as somatic activity.

2. Self-conscious behavior as determined by the standards set for the person by his social environment.

conduct disorders *Behavior disorders* (q.v.); a group of childhood disturbances consisting of repetitive and persistent antisocial activities that violate the rights of others and are clearly beyond the usual pranks of childhood. Included are (1) aggressive type, with verbal or physical aggression directed against adults and peers, initiated by the subject; and (2) group delinquent type, where the behavior occurs mainly as group activity among peers with similar conduct problems. The most typical symptoms are stealing, running away from home, lying, fire setting, truancy, breaking into someone else's house, destruction of others' property, physical cruelty to animals or people, forcing another into sexual activity, using a weapon in a fight, and initiating fights. See *oppositional disorder.*

conduction, avalanche Spread of nerve impulse to many more neurons so that an effect disproportionate to the initial stimulus is produced. See *law of avalanche.*

conduction, nerve Electrochemical transmittal of information from one end of the neuron to the other. Transmittal of information from one neuron to another is a chemical process that begins with the release of *neurotransmitter* (q.v.) from the neuronal terminals when they are depolarized. See *synapse.*

Nerve conduction is dependent on a *sodium pump* within the neuronal membrane that secretes two ions of sodium for every potassium ion pumped into the neuron. During conduction, sodium ions enter and potassium ions leave the nerve cell. The resulting shift in membrane potential eventually causes conduction to cease and excitability is restored by the sodium pump, which transports sodium and potassium ions across the nerve membrane in the opposite direction. The sodium pump consists of a membrane-bound enzyme, the sodium ion-dependent adenosine triphosphate.

confabulation Falsification of memory occurring in clear consciousness in association with an organically determined amnesia. In psychiatry, the act of replacing memory loss by phantasy or by reality that is not true for the occasion. The gaps in memory are filled by all sorts of *confabulations* or *fabrications* that are narrated in great detail and with perfect appearance of lucidity (thus sometimes termed *opportune confabulation*). See *amnesia; amnestic syndrome.*

The term implies also lack of insight, in the sense that the subject fully believes his answers to be correct. Confabulation is found in organic brain diseases in which intellectual impairment is a prominent feature. For example, the patient with a Korsakoff syndrome often fills in the memory gaps with incorrect details. A patient, bed-ridden in the hospital for months, said that he had just returned from a European journey and gave many details of the trip, believing thoroughly in his account. See *syndrome, Wernicke-Korsakoff.*

Confabulation is to be differentiated from *pseudologia fantastica* (q.v.), which occurs mainly in the "psychopathic" group and in other conditions in which acting-out is prominent. In pseudologia fantastica, the phantasy is believed only momentarily and will quickly be dropped if the patient is confronted with contradictory evidence. The confabulator, in contrast, will stick steadfastly to his story.

In describing the perceptual, thought, and language disturbances of schizophrenic children, W. Goldfarb terms *confabulations* those misconceptions that the child is seeing different people when he is really seeing the same person in different settings.

confabulation, suggestion *Confabulation* (q.v.) that incorporates data from questions posed or statements made to the subject, even though such data may contradict other portions of the fabrication.

confabulosis A type of symptomatic psychosis characterized by systematized confabulations in a setting of relatively clear consciousness; other than confabulations, memory disturbances are mild, and orientation is relatively intact. Confabulosis typically occurs at the stage of recovery from an acute brain syndrome.

Conferences, A.K. Rice Group Relations Offshoots in the United States of the group relations conferences sponsored by the Tavistock Clinic in Leicester, England. Based on Rice's systems theory of organizations, the conferences provide a means of learning group, organizational, administrative, and leadership functions. They last a few days to two weeks and include *study groups* (small group meetings, organized around specific events), large group meetings, *intergroup exercises* (in which the entire group is brought together and is organized into ad hoc task forces to react with other groups, management, staff, etc.), lectures on group theory, and *application groups*, which provide participants the opportunity to discuss their home organizations and how to apply what they have learned to their own situations.

confidence, diagnostic See *sensitivity.*

confidence, level of A quantitative expression of the degree of reliability of an inference; a 5% level of confidence, for example, is a statement that the particular inference would be wrong 5% of the time. Thus the percentage specified is seen to be negatively related to the degree of confidence involved, and a small percentage denotes a high degree of confidence or a low degree of uncertainty.

confidentiality The expectation of both patient and physician that what happens between them is private and that the information revealed during their interactions will not be divulged to others under ordinary circumstances. The limits of privacy are defined by medical ethics, which recognize privacy as essential to diagnosis and treatment, and by the law, whose concern is the patient's right (the physician-patient privilege) to withhold evidence that emerged within the context of medical treatment.

Some states have enacted medical confidentiality laws that define specifically the limits of the patient's right to privacy. To some extent, legal and traditional safeguards of that right are rendered less effective when the physician-patient relationship is altered by a third-party—an employer or a relative who is paying the bill, an insurance company that wants to know if the treatments rendered were necessary and appropriate, or a government that is funding the program under which the patient is being treated. See *consent, informed; privacy.*

configuration 1. Gestalt. See *psychology, gestalt.*

2. In the card-sorting tests devised by David Reiss and his colleagues to measure the *indigenous family culture*, the amount of information on the cards that is used by the family members as they work at the task together. High-configuration families recognize subtle patterns and sort the cards accordingly. High configuration does not depend on intelligence or education but is rather a reflection of the family's optimism about it's ability to solve a problem through diligent work. (Reiss, D. *The Family's Construction of Reality*, 1981) See *family culture, indigenous.*

conflict Inability to complete a response, either because it is blocked by some environmental condition (frustration) or because the response is incompatible with other response tendencies of the subject (intrapsychic conflict). See *frustration.*

conflict, actual A conflict precipitating the crisis. It occurs when the struggle begins between the conscious and unconscious forces. This must be differentiated from *root conflict*, the early source of the struggle, which has been dormant in the unconscious since childhood and repressed. (London, L.S. *Libido and Delusion*, 1946)

conflict, basic Horney's term for the intrapsychic struggle between opposing neurotic trends, such as self-effacing vs. expansive solutions, or proud self vs. despised self. See *conflict, central.*

conflict, central Horney's term for the intrapsychic struggle between the healthy, constructive forces of the real self and the neurotic, obstructive forces of the idealized self. In general, the central conflict involves the whole self (and not just part of the self, as is the case with basic conflict), is more severe than basic conflict, and is encountered during the course of psychoanalytic treatment.

conflict detouring See *scapegoating*.

conflict, experimental An artificial situation created through hypnotic suggestion in order to demonstrate to the patient his inner attitude toward the real conflict. Accordingly one may refer to it as "an experimental neurosis" deliberately induced by the hypnotist so as to direct his patient toward awareness of the true motivations of his real neuroses. See *neurosis, experimental*.

conflict of interest See *consent, informed*.

conflict, root In psychoanalysis, a term that refers to the earliest source of the patient's struggle, lying at the root of the conflict. See *conflict, actual*.

confluence Used in individual psychology (Adler) to refer to the flowing together of several instincts into a single object. In genetics, the combined influence of heredity and environment.

conformity, automaton The course of blindly adopting the pattern of culture of one's environment and bowing submissively to its dictates: the person accepts the way to live, to feel, and to think as implicitly or explicitly recommended by the group. The effects of culture on personality were greatly emphasized by Fromm. Man has tmday become aware of himself as a separate entity. The growing realization of his separateness gives him a sense of isolation and a longing to return to the earlier feeling of solidarity with others. So he uses certain irrational methods of relating back to the group. These are termed mechanisms of escape and include sadomasochism, destructiveness, and automaton conformity.

confrontation See *interpretation*.

confrontation, reality See *therapy, social*.

confusion A state of disordered orientation; a disturbance of consciousness in the sense that awareness of time, place, or person is unclear. Confusion may be occasioned by organic or psychic causes. See *syndrome, organic*.

Some clinicians differentiate between anamnestic and deliriant confusion. *Anamnestic confusion* consists of a disturbance of orientation and perception secondary to domestic dislocation, such as transfer of an older person to a nursing home. Such confusion can sometimes be prevented by informing, describing, or demonstrating in advance the changes the person is likely to encounter.

Deliriant confusion occurs mainly at night and may be accompanied by severe agitation. Usually it is due to inadequate cerebral oxygenation, as when an already embarrassed cardiovascular or cerebrovascular system is compromised by nocturnal vagotonia combined with hypnotic medication. Because those with deliriant confusion appear to have relatively normal mental functioning during the day and develop confusional episodes only at night, they are sometimes referred to as *sundowners*.

confusion psychosis See *cycloid psychosis*.

confusion, role See *identity crisis; ontogeny, psychic*.

confusional state, acute An acute stress reaction, occurring typically in adolescents when they are placed in an unfamiliar environment, such as college, and are expected to manifest a degree of psychological maturity that they have not as yet achieved. The reaction is precipitated by some minor frustration and is characterized by rage, followed by the confusional state itself (inability to concentrate, estrangement, depersonalization, feelings of loneliness, sometimes impulsive suicidal attempts). Unless the subject is otherwise predisposed to the development of psychosis, the acute confusional state is self-limiting and the subject slowly reintegrates his ego defenses.

congelatio *Obs*. Rigid state of the body in catalepsy; same as *gelatio*. See *catalepsy*.

congenital Existing or possessed since birth. In biology applied to an attribute, or anomaly, possessed and manifested by an individual since birth. See *hereditary; teratology*.

congophilic Having an affinity to Congo red dye, such as the amyloid deposits within the senile plaques of *Alzheimer's disease* (q.v.).

congruent Consistent, dependable; in harmony with or concordant with what would generally be considered proper, reasonable, or appropriate. Rogers emphasizes the need for the therapist to be congruent; that is, to be dependably real and to act in accordance with the feelings or attitudes he is in fact experiencing, rather than to adopt a stereotyped demeanor (e.g. of loving acceptance) that is rigidly maintained no matter what happens between him and his client. See *mood, congruent.*

conjoint marital therapy See *matrix, therapeutic.*

conjugal paranoia See *jealousy, morbid.*

conjugal unit, isolated The expected and usual pattern of marriage in the United States, in which young men and women mingle freely, choose their own partners, and set up their own household separate from relatives. Such a unit is in marked contrast to the *extended family,* characteristic of most of the rest of the world, where a new family is received into a group that is economically, psychologically, and socially experienced in family living. The extended family includes parents, children, and persons united by kinship or marital ties; the *nuclear family* is limited to parents and their children.

conjunctive Sullivan's term for that which promotes harmony among different and even contradictory factors and situations.

connectionism An associationist theory of human cognition which assumes that the mind is a large set of simple units connected with one another in a network. The interconnected units excite and inhibit each other throughout the network simultaneously, in parallel operations rather than in a sequence. Knowledge consists of the connections between pairs of units that are distributed throughout the network rather than being stored in localized structures. Because of those assumed characteristics, the theory is sometimes referred to as *parallel distributed processing.* See *cognitive science.*

connotation The significance of a word as it applies to a whole class rather than to a specific or concrete embodiment of the word. Thus the connotative meaning of the word *chair* would include all the qualities essential to any chair and would be most closely indicated by the phrase *chair in general as a physical entity.* This is to be distinguished from *denotation,* or denotative meaning, which (in this case) would refer to certain chairs or to a specific chair.

It has been noted that schizophrenics typically demonstrate a reduction in their connotation ability and are able to define words only as they apply to specific objects and not in their general sense as representative of a group or class. As a result, there is relative overemphasis on denotation and thinking comes to be pathologically concretized (see *concretization; holophrastic*). This would also appear to be an important factor in the schizophrenic's overliteralness and inability to use metaphor.

Conn's syndrome *Aldosteronism* (q.v.).

Conolly, John (c.1794–1866) British psychiatrist; psychotherapy.

conquassationes animi (L. "severe shakings of the soul") *Obs.* Mental derangement.

consanguinity In contradistinction to affinity or the relation by marriage, consanguinity means relation by blood or descent from a common ancestor within the same family stock. See *kinship.*

conscience Those psychical organizations that stand in opposition to the expression of instinctual actions. Conscience relates to the moral and esthetic and ethical attitudes of the individual. According to psychoanalysis, when the parental attitudes, prohibitions, and commands take up their position in the unconscious to form the superego, it is the superego that is conscience. Later in development, when the child begins to emulate others outside the family circle and develops an ego-ideal, he acquires another conscience. There is, however, a continuity between the two. See *superego.*

The function of conscience is to warn the ego to avoid the pains of intense guilt feelings. "Conscience becomes pathological when it (a) functions in too rigid or too automatic a manner, so that realistic judgment about the actual outcome of intended actions is disturbed ('archaic superego') or (b) when the breakdown toward 'panic' occurs and a greater or lesser sense of complete annihilation is experienced instead of a warning signal, which is the case in severe depressions." (Fenichel, *PTN*)

conscience, outer A term used by L.E. Hinsie to designate the ego-ideal. The ego-ideal is a mental organization formed by the child's teachers, playmates, and other associates. This organization constitutes a conscious standard guiding the individual. Through the formation of the ego-ideal or outer conscience some of the individual's mental energy is diverted from the parents to others. (*UP*)

conscious 1. As a noun, the conscious denotes a particular division of the psyche. In such use it is practically synonymous with *consciousness*. 2. It is used less frequently as an adjective descriptive of a function of consciousness or of the conscious realm as a perceptive faculty. As such, it is synonymous with aware, having knowledge of, present in the field (or realm) of consciousness.

consciousness The term includes (1) vigilance—a biologic concept, referring to the degree of reactivity ranging from coma to optimal consciousness, related to reticular formation functioning; (2) reactions to the environment, including those of lower animals, that may be related to hippocampus functioning; simple awareness of objects in the environment is termed *sentience;* (3) awareness of facts and the content of mental phenomena. See *conscious.* Different levels of consciousness are often differentiated clinically: alert wakefulness, lethargy, obtundation, stupor, and coma.

consciousness, clouding of See *sensorium.*

consciousness, disintegration of "The vast majority of mental diseases, in so far as they are not of a definitely organic nature, are due to a disintegration of consciousness caused by an irresistible inundation of unconscious contents." (Jung, *CAP*) This means that material from the unconscious more or less gradually causes the disruption and disintegration of the contents of consciousness.

consciousness, double, dual See *personality, alternating.*

consciousness, dream See *ego, dream.*

consciousness raising The process of increasing a subject's awareness of himself—including recognition not only of the subject's needs but also of how the subject relates to his environment and how the culture of which he is a part fosters attitudes and stereotypes about people and subgroups within the culture. Most commonly, consciousness raising is a group process that may use discussion groups (*rap sessions*) as its primary vehicle.

consciousness, splitting of When a set of experiences, a mental constellation, exists, as in hysteria, essentially alone in consciousness, without associations with other components of consciousness, it is said that there is a splitting of consciousness.

consciousness, subliminal See *cue, minimal.*

consensual light reflex When light enters the pupil of one eye only, causing the iris of the other eye to contract.

consensual validation See *distortion, parataxic.*

consent, informed Competent, knowing, and voluntary agreement to a therapeutic or experimental intervention. Despite the increasing tendency of the courts and the legislatures to mandate "fully informed consent" in all types and stages of medical and research intervention, it remains highly questionable if that ever is possible, particularly since researchers themselves often do not understand fully the potential harm (or benefit) of their work. The situation is even more difficult in psychiatry where there is continuing debate about whether mental patients (or children) have the capacity to understand the information given them, about who may consent for them (family, guardian, or court?), and about what degree of description of possible dangers or rare side-effects is advisable or necessary. In reaction to clearcut demonstrations of abuses in the past, regulations have been proposed that would impose such stringent limitations that no meaningful research could be done. See *ethics.*

Bioethicists, in particular, prefer the term *valid consent*, which in addition to the concept that adequate information is meaningfully imparted also includes the notions of coercion and competence. Valid consent in medicine is no different from valid consent in law or any other area, although the amount of information required to make the consent valid, and the condition of the patient that may interfere with his understanding of the information that should be imparted, may render the process of obtaining it more difficult. Under ideal conditions, the patient should know or be informed of everything that would affect his personal decision concerning which of the courses of treatment available to him he should choose. Because valid consent must always refer to an individual decision, it must allow for the ways in which the patient's religious beliefs, cultural beliefs, or even superstitions might affect his decision.

Informed consent is a slippery concept whose shape changes with the context. Legal informed consent entails two separate questions: Has the physician discharged his duty to disclose and has the patient comprehended enough. U.S. Supreme Court Justice Blackmun's rudimentary definition—the giving of information to the patient as to just what would be done and as to its consequences—is clearly not adequate to many conditions, particularly in psychiatry. Yet no definition has been fully satisfactory, and all are compromises between ideals and economic realities.

Double-agentry is a specific ethical problem within the area of informed consent; the term refers to the conflict of interest inherent in the situation where a psychiatrist in the employ of a hospital, governmental agency, or some other authority examines a patient. Is the psychiatrist's obligation to the patient first or only to the agency that employs him? It is generally agreed that the "patient" must be informed that he is not really a patient when the physician's responsibility is in fact to the Army, hospital, court, etc. In similar fashion, most psychiatrists agree that the patient should know under what conditions the psychiatrist will feel it justifiable, warranted, or necessary to inform any other person or agency of information divulged by the patient within the therapeutic setting. See *confidentiality; consumerism.*

conservator Protector; guardian; a person or institution designated to protect the interests of another. The conservatorship procedure is a way of protecting and preserving the property of persons with a serious debility (mental and/or physical), whose condition falls short of incompetency or, if actual incompetency exists, where there is a disinclination to declare the person incompetent because of the stigma attached thereto.

consolidation See *memory.*

constancy Steadfastness or stability; Adler assumed a constancy of personality, i.e. that a person remains fundamentally the same once his personality has been well established in early childhood. Such constancy of personality constitutes the *lifestyle* of the person, the characteristic way in which he pursues his long-range goals. See *psychology, individual.*

In object relations theory, constancy refers to an inner coherence underlying the changes and unpredictablility of perceptions and sensations; the cognitive processes underlying rule extraction, cognitive integration, and elaboration organization of the world perceived and the objects within it as enduring and stable, despite their moment-to-moment variations; stable and internal representations of self and others; ordering and analyzing symbolic representations; keeping the "word" and the "thing" clearly defined and appropriately separated. See *identity diffusion; object relations theory; separation-individuation.*

constancy, object See *autonomy, sense of; object constancy.*

constant, central T. Burrow's term for the primary principle governing the organism's total action pattern. Essentially homeostatic, this principle, on the basis of phyloorganismic behavior, relates the organism of man-as-a-species to its environment. A synonym is *intrinsic constant.* (*The Biology of Human Conflict,* 1937)

constant, extrinsic Burrow's term for the secondary, symbolic principle in organism-environment relationship. It refers to the partial reaction patterns mediated through the cortex and conforms symbolically to the consistency of phenomena throughout the external world. The organism's extrinsic constant regulates the secondary, partial system of word-conditioned reflexes, and is subordinate to the organism's primary principle or central constant. (*The Biology of Human Conflict,* 1937)

constant, intrinsic See *constant, central.*

constellation A group of allied thoughts, centering around a nuclear idea. "The nuclear element has a constellating power corresponding to its energic value. From this power there follows a specific constellation of the psychic contents; and thus is developed the complex, which is a constellation of psychic contents dynamically conditioned by the energic value." (Jung, *CAP*)

constitution The relatively constant physiological composition and biological makeup of the human organism that determines the individual's reaction, successful or unsuccessful, to the stress of environment.

Few expressions in contemporary medical literature are applied with so little unanimity and exactness as is the term *constitution*. Its identification with the phenotype, body build, or genotype of an individual is almost as common as its usage—with or without the epithet "hereditary"—for denoting the general biological make-up or the particular genetic structure of an organism. Many authors still use the term "constitutional" in connection with diseases that are caused "internally" or affect, as do gout and diabetes, the whole organism. Another school describes the constitution in terms of the different types of physique and seeks in them the primary etiologic basis of variations in clinical pathology.

From Hippocrates to the present there have been systems of constitutional types and diseases, which changed in content and could be more finely subdivided when further knowledge was added. Up to the 19th century, all diseases not localized in the pathology of a single organ were constitutional. When the knowledge of pathogenesis advanced, the number of these so-called constitutional diseases was correspondingly reduced. (See listings below and also under *type*.)

Following the discovery of the physiological and chemical cell processes in the bacteriological era, constitutional research was almost forgotten and had to retreat to the classification of different physical types. Although these studies were to some extent successful, especially in psychiatry and under the influence of Kretschmer's systematic work, there were many disappointments in other fields of medicine so long as the study of constitution was confined to purely anthropological investigation of the individual and the concept of constitution was not founded on accurate genetic principles. The classification of constitutional disease groups as clinical entities was bound to remain useless, because there is no disease that is purely constitutional, and there is no constitutional system that is alone the basis for a specific pathology.

According to the principles of modern physiological genetics the furthest one can go is to distinguish between predominantly hereditary and predominantly peristatic diseases (see *peristasis*). Consequently, the concepts of heredity and constitution have become practically inseparable, although it is clear that the constitution is not to be identified with either the genotypical structure or the phenotypical makeup of a person. While the phenotype is the *changeable* picture of the manifest appearance of an organism and is always modified by its external life-situation, constitution represents a *relatively constant* state of the person and classifies this person according to his biological values. It is therefore best understood as an auxiliary concept of medical classification and general pathology. See *medicine, constitutional.*

constitution, carcinomatous *Obs.* A constitutional type believed to be predisposed to carcinoma by a particular physique, practically identical with the *neoplastic diathesis.*

constitution, epileptic psychopathic See *epilepsy; personality, epileptic.*

constitution, hydropic A form of *exudative diathesis* in children characterized by thermic lability, instability of body weight, a tendency to edema and the accumulation of water and salt in the tissues, and a marked instability of the combining property of water in the tissues themselves. These features are often supplemented by the development of vegetative nervous system disorders.

constitution, hyperadrenal A type associated with oversecretion of the adrenal gland (medullary portion?). The type's physical characteristics are an apoplectic habitus with muscular overdevelopment and hypertonia, marked muscular strength, hypertonic peripheral arteries with a blood pressure above the average, hypertrichosis, hyperglycemia, and hypercholesteremia. The psychological features are said to be characterized by euphoria and great moral and intellectual energy.

constitution, hyperpituitary A type characterized by oversecretion of the pituitary gland occurring after or toward the end of the period of normal growth, as compared with such oversecretion occurring earlier in life and producing *gigantism.*

The general constitutional aspects of this *hyperpituitary* type correspond to Kretschmer's *athletic* type with *dysplastic* features and mainly consist of strong long bones, massive face, hands, and feet, thick oily skin, scanty scalp with seborrhea, large external genitalia, a tendency to tachycardia, hypertension, and arteriosclerosis, increased basal metabolism, a hypervigilant mental attitude, and a tendency to control emotions through intellectualization.

constitution, hyperthymic In the system of constitutional types described by Pende and Berman, this term denotes a type associated with overdevelopment of the thymus gland and its persistence into adulthood.

In infancy, this constitutional type is represented by the angelic child, with pretty and well-proportioned features, delicate body proportions, exceptional grace of motion, and an alert mind. These children are models of beauty, but they fall easy victims to tuberculosis, meningitis, and other infections.

After puberty, all hyperthymic constitutions are distinguished by hypoplastic hearts and arteries, insufficient muscular strength, and a tendency to sudden circulatory imbalance that often leads to sudden death or a rupture of the hypoplastic arteries. While the *male* hyperthymic is characterized by elegant feminine body outlines, long thorax, rounded pelvis, soft skin, and milky color, the *female* type shows delicate skin and nails, little hair, deficient mammary development, delayed menstruation, and, in some cases, a certain persistent adiposity and juvenility.

On the psychic side, there are impulsiveness, incapability for adaptation to the difficulties of social life, and a tendency to suicide.

constitution, hyperthyroid This constitutional type is associated with excessive secretion of the thyroid gland and is said to be characterized by youthfulness, well-developed sexual characteristics, well-formed nails and teeth, large brilliant and sometimes rather prominent eyes, hyperpigmentation of the skin, slightly enlarged thyroid, swiftness of all functional reactions, marked irritability of the sympathetic nervous system, and general hyperemotivity and instability. The physical and psychological aspects of this type correspond to those of the *asthenic.*

constitution, hypoadrenal The constitutional type associated with a deficient secretion of the adrenal gland (medullary portion?) and described by N. Pende as characterized by a hypoplastic trunk, slender bones, habitual leanness, marked developmental deficiency of both skeletal and smooth muscles, an accentuated universal lymphatism with or without hyperplasia of the thymus, marked arterial hypotension, lymphocytosis, and a hypotrophic skin with increased pigmentation, especially on the exposed parts of the body, and often an abundance of pigmented moles. "Psychologically there is a tendency to melancholia, while the intelligence is normal or supernormal." (*Constitutional Inadequacies,* 1928)

constitution, hypopancreatic See *constitution, hypoparathyroid.*

constitution, hypoparathyroid This constitutional type is distinguished by deficient secretion of the parathyroid glands and is said by Pende to be characterized by hyperkinesis and hyperreflexia of the striated as well as the smooth muscles, sensory hyperexcitability, fragility of the incisors, a tendency to rickets in infancy, and anomalies of the calcium metabolism. There is also a frequent association of this type with the *hypopancreatic* constitution, which results from a diminished tolerance for carbohydrates and constitutes a transition to true diabetes.

constitution, hypopituitary A type described by Pende associated with deficient secretion of the pituitary gland. The general constitutional aspects of this type correspond to the *hypoplastic* group in Kretschmer's system, although age and sex considerably modify them.

The *infant* type is characterized (1) in *both sexes,* by defective stature and growth, increased adiposity, small head, short bones, irregular dentition, thin lips, poorly spaced eyes with scanty eyebrows, small hands, and circular mouth; (2) in the *male,* by small external genitals and, sometimes, by cryptorchidism; and (3) in the *female,* by a feminine appearance even in early childhood.

The *adult* (adolescent) type is characterized (1) in the *male,* by delicate facial features, smooth bony contours, silky hair, large pelvis, feminine distribution of fat and pubic hair, hairless trunk and extremities, small hands, and defective sex activity; (2) in the *female*, by small breasts, frigidity, and the tendency to sterility and masculinism; and (3) in *both sexes*, by low blood pressure, slow pulse, increased carbohydrate tolerance, polyuria, and general mental torpor.

constitution, hypothyroid In constitutional medicine, this term refers to a type with a deficient secretion of the thyroid gland. While the body build of this type generally corresponds to that of a *pyknic* or *megalosplanchnic* individual, its further characteristics mainly consist of generalized adiposity with special fatty deposits on face and neck, large head, thick neck, short and stubby hands, small and expressionless eyes, short and thick nose, round face with poorly marked features, poor pigmentation of the skin, premature baldness, dystrophic teeth and nails, torpid vasomotor reactions, normal sex development, acrocyanosis, habitual hypoglycemia with great carbohydrate tolerance, diminished basal metabolism, and a torpid and apathetic mental attitude.

constitution, paranoid See *character, paranoiac*.

constitution, post-traumatic The clinical syndromes subsumed under this heading vary from person to person; the symptoms are often a mixture of both neurotic and psychotic phenomena. *Friedmann's complex* is one of the most common syndromes; it is said to be due to cerebral vasomotor disturbance and is characterized by headache, dizziness, insomnia, easy fatigue, irritability, and other character changes.

See *post-traumatic and postencephalitic syndromes, classification of*.

constitution, psychic The original structure and function laid down in the individual as distinguished from acquired modifications, i.e. the phylogenetic inheritance of the psyche such as, in Jung's terms, the *collective unconscious* (q.v.).

constitution, psychopathic See *psychopathic personality*.

constitutional Pertaining to those elements in the biologic and physiologic makeup of an organism that are inherent and relatively constant. See *hereditary*. The concept of constitution is based on the differentiation of three factors determining the final nature of the organism: the inherited elements that make up the *genotype* and are again transmissible, the *peristatic* conditions of the environment, and the *dispositional response* of the individual organism. A change in any of these factors is bound to modify the phenotypical appearance of the organism, although the genotypical structure is of primary importance to the prospective biological development in that it expresses the actual equipment of the individual as a classified member of a particular species or group, and demarcates the limits and qualities of all future reactions of the given organism to its individual life situation. See listings under *constitution* and *type*.

constitutional mania See *disposition, constitutional manic*.

constitutional psychology The theory that personality and other specific psychologic characteristics are associated with particular types of physical constitution.

constitutional type See *type, constitutional*.

constraint of thought The idea, expressed especially by patients with schizophrenia, that one's thoughts are under the influence of others.

When the same idea of constraint prevails as regards movements, one speaks of *constraint of movement*.

It is to be noted that psychiatric usage differentiates between constraint and *constriction* (q.v.).

constriction When applied to thinking or movement, this term implies a reduction in range or variability. Constriction is associated with diminished spontaneity. Psychiatric usage differentiates between constriction and *constraint* (q.v.).

constructive Synthetic, as opposed to reductive. "The constructive method is concerned with the elaboration of unconscious products (dreams, phantasies, etc.). It takes the unconscious product as a basis or starting point, as a *symbolical* expression, which, stretching on ahead, as it were, represents a coming phase of psychological development," (Jung, *PT*)

consultant In traditional medicine and psychiatry, an advisor to the treating physician on matters of diagnosis, treatment, rehabilitation, etc. Ordinarily, the consultant is a specialist whose expert advice is sought by the attending physician or, sometimes, by the patient. The consultant may or may not meet directly with the patient, but ordinarily he does not take actual charge of a case; instead, he advises or counsels the attending physician, although his advice is *patient-oriented.*

Another type of consultation is *colleague-centered;* here the consultant-specialist meets with one or more colleagues to advise, counsel, or educate them in the area of his specialized knowledge. Questions about the management of specific patients may legitimately be raised during the course of colleague-centered consultation, but the primary focus of the consultant is not a single patient, but the other physician(s). In psychiatric colleague-centered consultation, for example, the implicit goal is that the nonpsychiatrist physician will understand and be sensitive to the emotional needs of the patient, to his family and the other biosocial systems with which he relates; that the physician will develop skills to meet those needs and thereby foster emotional growth and mental health in his patient; and that the physician will utilize collateral resources appropriate to those ends.

Still another type of consultation is *agency-centered;* here it is the entire organization or agency with whom the consultant meets and tries to help.

Consultation psychiatry may refer to any of the above types of consultation performed by a psychiatrist. Often, however, it is limited to the activity of the psychiatrist (diagnostic, therapeutic, teaching, research, etc.) in the nonpsychiatric parts of a general hospital; when used in this sense, it is synonymous with *liaison psychiatry.* *Consultation-liaison psychiatry* (C-L psychiatry) is concerned primarily with psychiatric and psychosocial problems associated with physical illness.

G. Caplan (*The Theory and Practice of Mental Health Consultation,* 1970) views consultation as a process of interaction between two professionals, the mental health consultant and the *consultee,* who seeks the consultant's help in regard to a current work problem. Caplan limits the term consultation to a coordinate relationship between the two professionals and to that type of interaction in which the consultant accepts no direct responsibility for implementing remedial actions for the client.

To preserve the coordinate relationship, the consultant ought not to be of the same discipline as the consultee. Caplan subdivides consultation into the following types:

A. Case Consultation—the focus is a specific client/patient
 1. Client-centered: the consultant sees the client to gain an understanding of his makeup, and then offers recommendations to the consultee about how the latter might manage the client.
 2. Consultee-centered: the consultant ordinarily does not see the client but instead tries to understand what biases, misperceptions, distortions, etc., of the consultee are interfering with the latter's management of the client.

B. Administrative Consultation—the focus is on the policy setting, planning, program, etc., of the organization or agency
 1. Program- or policy-centered: the consultant deals with a group of professionals, typically about what might be done to develop a new program or improve an existing one.
 2. Consultee-centered: the focus is on the problems of programming and organization created by problems within the consultees themselves.

consultation-liaison In the 1980s the favored term for what had previously been called consultation psychiatry and liaison psychiatry; it is the subspecialty of psychiatry that focuses on psychiatric morbidity among physically ill and somatizing patients, and on the provision of consultation and education for nonpsychiatric health workers in general hospitals or any other clinical setting. See *consultant.*

consultee See *consultant.*

consumerism In medicine, the movement to guarantee high quality of care and protection of the rights of patients (see *advocacy*). In psychiatry, consumerism has focused on the civil rights of patients, and particularly on the *right to treatment,* enunciated by Dr. M. Birnbaum, who noted in 1960 that the due process of law does not allow the mentally ill person who has committed no crime to be deprived of his liberty by indefinitely institutionalizing him without medical treatment.

Judge D. Bazelon's decisions (1966) in *Rouse v. Cameron* and *Lake v. Cameron* emphasized that the *least restrictive alterna-*

tive is the desideratum, that less treatment, rather than more, is the acceptable objective.

In *Wyatt v. Stickney* (1972), the court concluded that treatment requires a humane environment and "adequate" staffing (as defined by standards of staff/patient ratios, floor space, individualized treatment plans, etc.). One of the standards stated that patients have the right not to be subjected to unusual or hazardous treatment procedures without their expressed and *informed consent*. This led ultimately to the establishment of a *bill of rights* for patients, limiting the incursions that can be made into patients' freedoms in the name of treatment (see *consent, informed*). The *Willowbrook Consent* (1972) ruled that the mentally retarded also have a right to protection from harm, and their rights were spelled out in 23 steps, standards and procedures dealing with programming, staffing, and the environment.

In *O'Connor v. Donaldson* (1975), the court ruled that no nondangerous person can be custodially confined if he can survive safely in freedom. In *Bartley v. Kremens* (1976), the Pennsylvania court extended due process protections and provision of legal counsel to children committed to mental facilities by their parents.

In a number of decisions subsequent to the foregoing, the right of patients not to be subjected to unusual or hazardous treatment has been extended to include the *right to refuse treatment,* concern for which has been heightened by a growing awareness of the potential misuse of psychotechnology as a means of social control. At issue also is what the courts consider to be unusual, invasive, intrusive, or high risk treatments—judgments that seem to the physician to ignore very often the clinical and human realities with which he must deal.

contamination *Agglutination;* an error of speech characterized by amalgamating a part of one word with that of another (Freud). Bleuler gives as an example the neologism "gruesor," derived from gruesome and sorrowful. Apparently the result of contamination is a neologism. Freud states that contamination is the first step in the process of condensation.

In Rorschach interpretation, contamina-

tion is a pathological response, pathognomonic of schizophrenia, characterized by the following: "First the patient is unaware of what he is doing; second, the resulting response is perceptually unintelligible; third, at least two different percepts overlap so that the same area is covered by different percepts simultaneously; and fourth, the patient is unable to disjoin the condensed percepts at will and with clarity." (Piotrowski, Z.A. *Perceptanalysis,* 1957)

content, dream See *content, latent; dream-content.*

content, latent This concept, particularly emphasized and developed by Freud, refers to the consideration that the bulk of psychiatric phenomena is made up of symbolic expressions—phobias, compulsive-obsessive symptoms, delusions, hallucinations, conversion symptoms, dreams, etc.—which, in themselves, do not reveal the nature of the disorder. They constitute what is called the *manifest content.* The real meaning of the symptoms or symbols is concealed and unconscious, that is, latent.

content, manifest See *content, latent.*

contentious Quarrelsome. Some patients, particularly those with a manic syndrome and those in the early stages of a paranoid reaction, feel that they and others are being treated unfairly; they see slights when none is present or intended, as a result of which they incessantly quarrel about discrimination.

contextualism The theory that the quality of experience is as significant as the events themselves in determining the memory of the experience. The older *associationism* theory held that memory and other mental structures were assemblies or clusters of linkages, and that simple addition of one subassembly to another produced behavior that was more complicated but not different in kind.

contingency See *conditionalism.*

contingency contracting See *therapy, contract.*

contingency management See *therapy, behavior.*

continuation maintenance therapy See *preventive therapy, long-term.*

continued stay review See *review.*

continuity of care See *psychiatry, community.*

continuity, social The maintenance of cultural forms in succeeding generations. The family, school, play group, and church are some of the major agencies involved.

continuity theory of aging A person's predispositions, an outgrowth of his experiences in life which reflect the interaction between biologic and psychologic factors as well as socioeconomic opportunities, determine whether he disengages or remains active in old age. This is in contrast to the *life-event stress theory*, which holds that major life events are inevitable and that they determine the subject's attitudes toward and activities during old age. See *disengagement*.

contract, interactional See *contracting*.

contracting Agreeing that if no one person engages in certain behaviors, the other person will engage in certain other behaviors. In Sager's model, a contract is a set of assumptions and expectations of the self and partner with which each person approaches the relationship. They come from various aspects of childhood development, cultural norms, need and wishes of the family of origin, and internal dynamically based needs. From these individual contracts, couples join to form a system with its own dyadic rules, the *interactional contract*. See *therapy, contract*.

contraction, habit See *tic*.

contraindication A reason for not doing something; more specifically, a feature or complication of a condition that countermands the use of a therapeutic agent that might otherwise be applied. Active pulmonary tuberculosis and aortic valvular insufficiency, for example, are ordinarily considered to be contraindications to the use of electroconvulsive therapy in depression.

contrary sexual A homosexual; *homosexuality* (q.v.).

contrasexual Jacobi's term for the "repressed side" in Jung's theory of analytical psychology. Jung maintains that there is a male and a female side to everyone, the side that is not dominant being repressed; i.e. in the male the female side is repressed and vice versa. "The second stage of the individuation process [self-realization through Jungian analysis] is characterized by the meeting with the figure of the 'soul-image,' named by Jung the *anima* in the man, the *animus* in the woman. The archetypal figure of the soul-image stands for the respective contrasexual portion of the psyche, showing partly how our personal relation thereto is constituted, partly the precipitate of all human experience pertaining to the opposite sex. In other words, it is the image of the other sex that we carry in us, both as individuals and as representatives of a species. One experiences the elements of the opposite sex that are present in one's own psyche *in the other person*. One chooses another, one binds one's self to another, who represents the qualities of one's own soul." (J. Jacobi, *The Psychology of C.G. Jung*, 1942)

contrasuggestibility *Negativism* (q.v.).

contrectation Tumescence or the swelling of the penis; erection.

control In clinical psychiatry, control usually refers to conscious limitation of impulses, wishes, tendencies, etc., that is, to suppression of instincts and affects.

In experimental psychiatry, control refers to regulation of all known variables in the experimental situation except the variable that is under investigation. This is an attempt to insure that whatever effects are produced will be a function of the experimental variable and not due to extraneous factors. In assessing the value of a particular drug in the treatment of depression, for instance, a "control group" may be formed by patients matched in age, clinical condition, and treatment conditions to the "experimental group," the only difference being that the control group does not receive the drug while the experimental group does. In such an experiment, a *placebo* (q.v.) may be used in place of the drug under investigation to mimic more closely all the extraneous factors that may influence the response of the experimental group to the experimental drug.

control analysis See *analysis, control*.

control, co-twin A method used in biogenetics in which one member of an identical twinship is trained, treated, etc., while the other is not.

control, loss of See *alcoholism*.

control, social The influence upon the behavior of a person exerted by other persons, particularly as members of a social group or of a society.

The formal control of society over its members exemplified by law and by institutions derives its effectiveness in large part from their conformity to the folkways, the mores, and public opinion. See *dilemma, Scull's*.

control training Any treatment and rehabilitation program that aims to teach the alcohol abuser techniques of handling drinking problems. Such an approach is open to goals other than total abstinence and recognizes that some alcohol abusers can both reduce alcohol intake and reduce problems connected with drinking without maintaining total abstinence for the rest of their lives.

controlled clinical trial See *randomized clinical trial.*

contusion, brain A diffuse disturbance of the brain, secondary to head trauma, with edema and multiple intracerebral hemorrhages, most commonly at the poles of the hemispheres. Typically, cerebrospinal fluid pressure is raised and this plays an important part in the production of symptoms (coma, stupor, drowsiness, or confusion). A late result of the edema of the brain may be localized, severe demyelination. Although a patient may recover rapidly and completely from cerebral contusion, persistent disabling symptoms are extremely common. The three cardinal late symptoms are headache, dizziness, and mental disturbances (typically, a mild dementia, with inability to concentrate, memory impairment, and anxiety). See *constitution, post-traumatic; post-traumatic and postencephalitic syndromes, classification of.*

conventional virus See *virus infections.*

convergence See *accommodation.*

conversion Symbolic representation of psychical conflict in terms of motor or sensory manifestations. The symbolization is the means by which repressed instinctual tendencies gain external expression; usually, as for instance in hysteria, the symbolization also contains the defense set up against the instinctual impulses.

There is probably no psychiatric disorder in which conversion symptoms may not appear. See *hysteria.*

conversion hysteria See *conversion; hysteria.*

conversion reaction See *conversion; hysteria.*

convexity syndrome See *syndrome, convexity.*

convulsion An involuntary, violent muscular contraction; a fit. See *epilepsy.*

convulsion, clonic Convulsion characterized by alternate contraction and relaxation of muscular tissue.

convulsion, static Special forms of motor aurae of epilepsy, such as procursive epilepsy. See *epilepsy, procursive.*

convulsion, tonic Sustained contraction of a muscle.

cooperation, antagonistic Alexander uses this term to describe the organizational nature of our present-day society. He says that in our "laissez-faire," competitive society we are at one and the same time both friends and rivals; we live in an antagonistic cooperation with our fellowmen. This life pattern can lead to fears and hostility, frustrations and thwarted hopes, exaggerated ambitions and discouragement, all of which can cause disturbed human relations and can lead to mental and nervous symptoms. (Alexander, F., & French, T.M. *Studies in Psychosomatic Medicine,* 1948)

coordination In group and family therapy, the amount of agreement and cooperation between subjects who are asked to solve a problem or work at a task together. In family therapy, coordination has been observed to reflect the family's conception of how it is treated by the outside world, high coordination indicating its feeling that the world treats is as a unitary group and that whatever one member does reflects on the entire family. See *family culture, indigenous.*

coordination disorder A motor skills disorder (within the group, specific developmental disorders, and not secondary to known physical disorder such as cerebral palsy) consisting of clumsiness, delays in achieving motor milestones (crawling, sitting), poor performance in sports, poor handwriting, etc.

coparental divorce See *divorce, stations of.*

coping Adjusting; adapting; successfully meeting a challenge. Coping mechanisms are all the ways, both conscious and unconscious, that a person uses in adjusting to environmental demands without altering his goals or purposes.

copro- (kop′rō) Combining form meaning feces, filth, from Gr. *kopros.*

coprolagnia Sexual pleasure from handling feces. See *anal erotism; sadism, anal.*

coprolalia Literally, fecal speech; the involuntary utterance of vulgar or obscene words, seen in some schizophrenics who play with words as though they were feces. See *syndrome, Gilles de la Tourette.*

coprophagy (kop-rof′à-jē) The ingestion of feces.

coprophemia Obscene speech; scatalogia; most commonly presenting as a type of *paraphilia* (q.v.) in which uttering obscene words or phrases is a necessary condition for sexual excitement in the subject.

coprophilia Love of feces or filth; see *sexual disorders*. According to psychoanalysis, *anal erotism* (q.v.) possesses two chief aspects, the first concerned with the retention and expulsion of fecal material, and the second with pleasure in the product itself. During the stage of sphincter training the aim is twofold—to perform regularly and not to soil. The discipline associated with so-called anal training is later carried over in the form of character traits, while a certain quantum of libido remains fixed in its original form. A third possibility exists, namely, that the interest in the product is later transferred to other objects that resemble or symbolize feces, even though there may be no conscious awareness of the resemblance. Thus Ferenczi traces the development from feces through its various forms of symbolizations: mud pies, sand, pebbles, marbles, buttons, jewels, coins, currency, securities, etc. Hence ownership of valuables is traced chiefly, but not exclusively, to early anal interests; that is, it is a coprophilic interest. See *mania, collecting; soteria.*

Coprophilic interest may also be sublimated in such forms as painting, sculpting, or cooking. Some patients exhibit coprophilia more literally. Thus one patient hoarded his feces as earlier he had hoarded his money. Another "decorated" himself, as he put it, with feces. A third said she loved her feces "as if it were her child." A fourth could experience sexual potency only when thinking of feces.

coprophobia Fear of rectal excreta, sometimes seen in obsessive-compulsive psychoneurosis. More typically, the fear is expressed symbolically, as fear of dirt or of contamination (e.g. fear of an infectious disease, or fearing to touch anything lest the patient acquire some ailment). Coprophobia is generally a reaction-formation against unconscious coprophilic impulses, which are derivatives of the anal stage. See *anal erotism.*

coprophrasia *Coprolalia* (q.v.).

copying mania *Amurakh; echopraxia* (qq.v.).

coronary-prone See *type A.*

corpora quadrigemina Four raised eminences, arranged in pairs, on the dorsal surface (tectum) of the midbrain. The two superior colliculi and the two inferior colliculi make up the four corpora. The superior colliculi are optic reflex centers and receive fibers from the lateral geniculate body via the superior quadrigeminal brachium. The more prominent inferior colliculi are associated with the auditory system and are the termination of the lateral lemniscus. The inferior colliculi project to the medial geniculate body via the inferior quadrigeminal brachium.

corporate class See *class, social.*

corpus callosum (kor′poos ka-lō′soom) A broad, white fiber tract that connects the cerebral hemispheres and forms the roof of the lateral and 3rd ventricles. Most of its fibers arise in various parts of one hemisphere and terminate in the symmetrical area of the opposite hemisphere.

The following syndromes have been described in association with lesions of the corpus callosum: (1) anterior lesion—dyspraxia in the left hand of a right-handed person and in the right hand of a left-handed person; and (2) posterior (splenium) lesion—alexia of the field of vision opposite to that of the side of the lesion. Mental changes are more frequently observed in cases of tumor of the corpus callosum than in any other part of the brain, including the frontal lobe. Apathy, drowsiness, and memory defect are the most common disturbances, but there may be depression, anxiety, and epileptiform convulsions.

corpus striatum See *basal ganglia.*

corrective emotional experience See *experience, corrective emotional.*

correlation Mutual relation. Tendency to concomitant change in two variables. If the change, whether positive or negative, in one is accompanied by a like (i.e. in the same direction) change in the other variable, the correlation is positive with a maximal coefficient of $+1$. If an increase in one corresponds to a decrease in the other (or, vice versa, a decrease in one corresponds to an increase in the other) the correlation is negative, with a maximal coefficient of −1. If there is no change in the second variable, the correlation is 0.

The principle of correlation is frequently useful as evidence of heredity when other signs fail. It indicates a connection between two properties of the individuals of a population such that, as one of the properties varies, the other tends to vary. If as one property increases the other tends to increase, the correlation is *positive*. If as the one property increases the other tends to decrease, the correlation is *negative*. Positive correlation means that the two qualities have part of their physiological bases in common, and their physiological bases are frequently genetic.

The most commonly used measure of correlation is Pearson's coefficient of correlation, while the best method describing an individual in terms of the degree to which he possesses the factors that vary *independently* of one another is constituted by the analysis of a person according to "independent variables" as devised by Spearman, Cohen, and others (see *type, constitutional*).

With factors that are related, the change that takes place in one factor for a unit change in the other can be computed; this statistic is known as the *regression coefficient*. Computation of this allows the value of one factor to be estimated when the value of the other factor is known. Even when the correlation is very high, however, the error of this estimate may be large.

To be noted in any consideration of correlation is the fact that evidence of association is not necessarily evidence of causation, and the possible influence of other factors common to the ones for which correlation is discovered must always be remembered in interpreting correlation coefficients. "*Correlation does not imply direct causation* and must not under any circumstances be so interpreted without *additional experimental proof*." (Eysenck, H.J. *Handbook of Abnormal Psychology*, 1960)

Eysenck cites a study of the relationship between early weaning and the later appearance of oral aggressive character traits (see *defense, character*). The finding that mothers who practiced early weaning had children who developed oral aggressive traits was interpreted as evidence that early weaning causes aggression. But "this argument clearly has no logical validity at all; there are many other alternative hypotheses which account equally well for the observed facts. One alternative . . . may be called the hereditary theory. Using the same facts as before we may argue that aggressive parents wean their children early, and that the children inherit the parents' aggressiveness. . . . The second alternative theory can be called the reaction theory. According to this hypothesis, aggressive children behave aggressively to their mothers, reject the breast, etc. They therefore cause their mothers to wean them early. . . . Many other possibilities could be envisaged, but these two will suffice to show that the known facts cannot be used to support the environmental theory in any unequivocal manner. Essentially, the facts offered are *correlational*." (ibid.)

correlative Pertaining to the values of a reciprocal relation between biological phenomena as indicated by the method of *correlation* (q.v.).

cortex, cerebral The most anterior portion of the telencephalon; the cerebral cortex is made up of the two cerebral hemispheres, each of which is subdivided into the frontal lobe, parietal lobe, occipital lobe, temporal lobe, and insula. Strictly speaking, the rhinencephalon is not considered part of the cerebral cortex, although by implication the rhinencephalon is included where the term cerebral cortex (or cerebrum) is used.

For a more detailed description of function, see under the various divisions of the cortex—e.g. *lobe, frontal*. See also *isocortex*.

cortex, motor See *motor cortex*.

cortex, olfactory See *rhinencephalon*.

cortex, visual See *lobe, occipital*.

corticalization *Encephalization* (q.v.).

cosmic identification See *identification, cosmic*.

cost/benefit analysis See *analysis, cost/benefit*.

cost-effectiveness analysis See *analysis, cost-effectiveness*.

cost shifting In health care delivery systems, charging one patient group (e.g. private patients) more in order to balance losses incurred from caring for other patients (e.g. patients in federal programs such as Medicare)

costal stigma See *sign, Stiller's*.

Cotard's syndrome See *syndrome, Cotard's.*

cotherapy See *psychotherapy, multiple.*

cough, convulsive, of puberty A condition characterized by paroxysms of coughing, lasting about a minute, and based, presumably, on hysterical mechanisms. Sometimes called *cynobex hebetis.*

counseling *Guidance* (q.v.); a type of psychotherapy of the supportive or reeducative variety; often the term is applied to behavioral problems not strictly classifiable as mental illness, such as vocational or school or marriage problems. See *psychotherapy.*

counseling, genetic Application of the knowledge of genetics to those who may be at risk for the occurrence or recurrence of birth defects, chromosomal aberrations, or other genetic disorders. Because it is now possible to predict with relative accuracy the likelihood of occurrence or recurrence of such disorders, health professionals with special training in genetic principles can bring that specialized knowledge to assist in family planning for future offspring and to promote the best adjustment possible within a family already affected by a birth defect or other genetic disorder. It has been estimated that over 17 million Americans have some form of genetic disorder; that 0.5% of newborns have some kind of chromosome aberration; that 5% of newborns have major congenital malformations; that from 10 to 25% of admissions to pediatric hospitals are cases of clearly genetic etiology.

The essentials of genetic counseling are a thorough knowledge of genetics, accurate diagnosis, communication of the scientific and medical facts in such a way that they will be understood and assimilated, and dealing with the many human problems associated with the possibility or reality of occurrence of a genetic disorder within a family.

Genetic counseling is also known as *family counseling* or *genetic guidance.*

counseling, marriage "The process through which a trained counselor assists two persons to develop abilities in resolving, to some workable degree, the problems that trouble them in their interpersonal relationships. A basic assumption is that all individuals grow to greater adequacy and maturity in their relationships if not blocked by such obstacles as loneliness, fear, hostility, guilt and their displacements, or transferences which prevent a person from experiencing the present as it really is and hence behaving effectively. New experience in communication is offered, and a search for more realistic solutions of present difficulties is made in an atmosphere of acceptance and understanding. The process is not encumbered with detailed consideration of conflicts in the past, their devious and disguised transferences, or with intense and difficult ventilations of feeling." (Appel, K.E., et al. *American Journal of Psychiatry 117,* 1961)

counseling, pastoral The application of the principles of mental health by the cleric to the management of the problems presented by those who seek help. Pastoral counseling is a type of supportive or guidance therapy in which the cleric, in the role of interpreter of personal and societal values, attempts to relate the contributions of the behavioral sciences and the resources of religion to the needs of parishioners.

counteraffect See *affect, inversion of.*

countercathexis *Anticathexis* (q.v.).

countercompulsion A compulsion secondarily developed to fight the original compulsion, when the patient finds himself deprived of the means to continue the performance of such original compulsion. The patient supplants the original compulsion with the new one in order to continue his compulsive behavior. In the opinion of Stekel (*CD*), "Every compulsion causes a counter-compulsion in the same way that every pressure causes a counterpressure." The compulsion to keep silent is in opposition to the compulsion to talk.

counterego Stekel's term for the unconscious part of the self which acts antagonistically toward the ego proper or consciousness.

counterformula A new formula often resorted to by a compulsive patient under certain (insurmountable) circumstances and consisting of the *exact opposite* of his hitherto established *tenet.* A tenet characteristic might be: "If I do not perform this action my father will die." Very often, however, it is impossible to carry out the particular action. When such an impossibility is encountered, the patient goes through a series of compulsions and obsessions until he eventually finds a solution, by amending his formula in the following manner: "My father will die if I *do* perform this action." The final version is called the counterformula. (Stekel, *CD*)

counteridentification A form of *countertransference* (q.v.) in which the analyst identifies with the analysand.

counterimpulse See *blocking, counterimpulse in.*

counterinvestment *Anticathexis* (q.v.).

counterphobia Preference for or seeking of the very situation which the phobic person is, or was, afraid of. Probably the basic component of the pleasure derived from the counterphobia is the gratification that the person takes in the fact that indulging in the particular pleasure is now possible without anxiety. The counterphobic attitude is similar to the mechanism (seen normally in childhood and frequently in cases of traumatic neurosis) of striving to master excess anxiety through repeated coping with danger. Such repetition makes possible the transformation of passivity into activity; and it may also indicate libidinization of the anxiety or a flight into health.

countershock Nonconvulsive electrical stimulation usually applied for a one-minute period immediately after an electroconvulsive shock. Some claim that countershock relieves postconvulsive amnesia or confusion; others find that countershock may even increase amnesia.

countertransference Annie Reich (*International Journal of Psychoanalysis 32,* 1951) defines countertransference as the effects on his understanding or technique of the analyst's unconscious needs and conflict. The patient's personality, or the material he produces, or the analytic situation as such represents an object from the analyst's past, onto which the analyst's past feelings and wishes are projected. A broader definition would include not only situations in which the patient serves as a real object onto whom something is transferred, but also those where the patient serves merely as a tool to gratify some need of the analyst, such as alleviation of anxiety or mastery of guilt feelings. Countertransference is a necessary part of psychoanalytic therapy, for it is within the framework of countertransference that the analyst's unconscious perception and understanding of his patient's production

come about, typically by means of partial and short-lived identifications with the patient at which points the analyst gains insight and comprehension of the patient's previously incomprehensible and confusing productions. But the analyst must be able to give up this identification and swing back into his objective role, thereby preserving the neutrality of his reactions to the patient's emotions, which makes the patient's transference possible.

Ideally, the analyst's unconscious mechanisms will be sublimated successfully into the qualities necessary for the practice of psychoanalytic technique. If this has not occurred, however, there may appear various undesirable countertransference manifestations. These may be acute, temporary, and short-lived, and such manifestations are often based on identification with the patient or on reactions to the specific content of the patient's productions. As an example of the former, Reich cites the case of the analyst who was in pain and taking analgesics. His patient began to make aggressive demands for attention, which irked the analyst because he was himself in a situation that would justify similar demands, but he was forced to control himself. As an instance of reaction to specific content, Reich describes the analyst who became sleepy and found it hard to concentrate or remember when his patient produced material which he perceived as relating to the primal scene; in the therapeutic situation, he reacted with the same defenses that he had himself used as a child when exposed to the primal scene.

More serious, however, are long lasting, frequently recurring, or even permanent manifestations of countertransference; these are usually based on deeply ingrained personality disturbances. Thus passive masochistic wishes in the analyst may make it impossible for him to analyze resistances in the patient; instead, he accepts them at face value and lets the patient accuse and mistreat him. Or unconscious aggression may make the analyst overconciliatory, hesitant, and unable to be firm. Unconscious guilt feelings may lead to boredom or therapeutic overeagerness.

A not uncommon type of countertransference is based on a paranoid attitude in the analyst so that he unearths in the patient what he wants not to see in himself, even if such content exists in only a small degree in the patient. A need to show that he is unafraid of the unconscious and its manifestations may produce a compulsion in the analyst to understand the unconscious intellectually, but such isolation renders him unable to understand defense mechanisms. If the analyst doubts the veracity of unconscious expressions, he may be afraid to make any interpretations, or he may overcompensate by making too early and too deep interpretations whenever any small bit of unconscious material is recognized. When analysis represents mainly a source of narcissistic gratification for the analyst, he will see himself as a magic healer who restores potency and heals castrations; this will lead to therapeutic overambitiousness, overestimation of patients, and hostility toward patients who do not improve. A pedagogic attitude in the analyst results in reassurance therapy rather than analytic therapy, for in essence he is saying to the patient: "You see the world is not as bad as you think, and I do not mistreat you as you were mistreated in childhood."

countervolition Counterwill, as is evidenced frequently in dreams in the form of being physically unable to perform some action (such as running away) or being unable to attain some goal by reason of the particular dream situation (e.g. the dreamer wishes to visit his sweetheart but is unable to find her house, even though he has been there many times before).

counterwill, hysterical An impulse or a wish, unconsciously determined, that expresses the opposite of a conscious wish.

"A child who is very ill at last falls asleep, and its mother tries her utmost to keep quiet and not to wake it; but just in consequence of this resolution (hysterical counterwill) she makes a clucking noise with her tongue." (Freud, *CP*)

counting, compulsive See *arithmomania*.

coupling The capacity of hereditary characters to remain associated in several generations, without regard to the Mendelian principle of independent assortment. See *linkage*.

cousin marriage See *intermarriage*.

couvade (koo-vàd′) A custom, found in some primitive tribes, consisting of the father taking to his bed during or shortly after the birth of his child, as though he himself had given birth to the child.

cover-memory See *memory, screen; screen*.

Cp In Rorschach scoring, color projection, i.e. a response of color to an area of the blot that contains only gray. Color projection seems to reflect a conscious determination to appear happy despite inner sadness; it occurs most frequently in organic brain disorders and in mild or early schizophrenias.

CPR Cardiopulmonary resuscitation.

CR 1. Conditional response. See *conditioning*. 2. Critical ratio; a measure of the significance or stability of a statistic, obtained by comparing the statistic to its standard error.

crack Alkaloidal cocaine (free base) in a form suitable for smoking. This almost pure form of cocaine is made by preparing an aqueous solution of cocaine HCl and adding ammonia (with or without baking soda) to alkalinize the solution and precipitate alkaloidal cocaine. It is usually sold as pure beige crystals (*rocks*). Crack melts at 98°C and vaporizes at higher temperatures, making it suitable for smoking (see *freebasing*) in a "base pipe." Its name derives from the crackling noise it makes when heated. The rock can also be crushed, mixed with tobacco, and smoked in a cigarette.

Unlike *freebasing* (q.v.), crack smoking does not require preliminary mixing of the substance with a solvent to clear it of contaminants. The "high" it gives is more intense and more rapidly reached than that attained by snorting (inhaling) or injecting other forms of cocaine. Effects appear 4 to 6 seconds after inhalation and last 5 to 7 minutes; snorting, in contrast, produces effects in 1 to 3 minutes and they last 20 to 30 minutes. The intense, short high produced by crack is followed by a period of deep depression, so the user is compelled to continue use of the drug in order to regain the exhilaration, euphoria, and feelings of power and superiority it bestows.

Overdosage is frequent with crack. Cocaine is a central nervous system stimulant that increases heart rate and blood pressure. It may cause hyperpyrexia, seizures, angina pectoris, myocardial infarction, and ventricular arrhythmia. Many of the deaths caused by cocaine are believed to be due to seizures leading to anoxia. Other possible side-effects include extreme anxiety, tactile hallucinations, loss of consciousness, and paranoid psychosis.

crack house Base house; the place where sales of *crack* (q.v.) are made and where users gather to indulge in smoking binges that may last for hours or days.

cramp, memory Constant and annoying recurrence of certain tunes, melodies, phrases, verses of poetry, etc.

cramp, occupational See *neurosis, occupational.*

craniosynostosis A congenital anomaly in which there is premature closure of the cranial sutures, resulting in oxycephaly (the most frequent form, due to closure of the coronal and lambdoid sutures), scaphocephaly (due to closure of the sagittal suture), or acrocephaly (due to closure of the coronal suture).

crash, depressive See *depressive crash.*

crashing See *cocaine.*

cratomania *Obs.* The monomania of power, preeminence, and superiority. (Tuke, *DPM*)

craving, autonomic-affective *Obs.* An expression peculiar to the psychopathology of E. Kempf (*PP*) "The postural tensions of the hollow viscera give rise to a continuous, complex, converging affective stream from all parts of the autonomic musculature. Most of the time this afferent affective stream is subliminally active and does not cause the organism to become conscious of the segment's activities. When, however, the tension of some viscus is increased, the sensory stream is felt in the form of *craving.*"

creation, replacement Any symptom formed by means of displacement of drive energy. Replacement creations take the place in consciousness of the painful and repressed complexes.

creative self See *psychology, individual.*

creativity The ability to create something new, presumed to be a derivative of sublimation.

cremnophobia Fear of precipices.

cretinism Hypothyroidism in infancy. Mental and physical signs usually appear at about the sixth month of life: apathy, lethargy, protrusion of the tongue, skin changes, thickening of features, prominence of abdomen, breathing difficulties (the 'leathery" cry), defective speech, difficulty in posture and gait, generalized underdevelopment, and intellectual impairment (a form of deprivative amentia).

Creutzfeldt, Hans Gerhard (1885–1964) German psychiatrist; *Creutzfeld-Jakob's disease* (q.v.).

Creutzfeldt-Jakob's disease (CJD) *Spastic pseudosclerosis; cortico-striato-spinal degeneration;* a rare (approximately one case per million population), transmissible virus dementia, beginning typically in the midfifties, with associated pyramidal, extrapyramidal, and occasionally cerebellar motor disturbances. It is two or three times more frequent in males than in females. It usually appears sporadically, although in about 10% of cases there is a familial pattern. The incubation period is variable; in most cases it is approximately 2 years, but in a few it appears to have been as long as 50 years.

CJD may begin with specific agnosias (e.g. symptoms began in a choreographer with inablility to pirouette to the right while standing on his left leg although he could perform the action while standing on his right leg). Later there are widespread neurologic disturbances such as gross ataxia, dysarthria, growing spasticity of the limbs, grotesque extrapyramidal movements, and myoclonus.

Once it becomes clinically manifest, the dementia develops rapidly, with inertia, failure of attention, markedly defective registration and retention of recent experiences, and a tendency to confabulation. Speech becomes an incoherent jumble, sphincter control is lost, and death ensues (on the average, in 11 months, with a range of 4 to 24 months) in a state of extreme emaciation.

cri-du-chat See *syndrome, cat cry.*

crime à deux (krēm à dü) *Folie à deux* (q.v.) in which one or more crimes are committed as part of the psychotic behavioral pattern. The term was introduced by Moreau de Tours in 1893.

crime and mental disorder There is no invariable relationship between crime and mental disorder, although criminals as a group have a greater incidence of psychiatric abnormalities than noncriminals.

Many studies have shown that some degree of mental retardation is found in unexpectedly high frequency in prison inmates (20 to 25%, as opposed to the expected 1 to 3%); although such findings may indicate that the retardate is defective in his ability to control aggressive or other antisocial impulses, it may equally indicate that the retardate is less adept in escaping detection, more likely because of his suggestibility to be influenced by others to act against society, and/or is poorly equipped to defend himself once he is brought to trial.

Other disorders with a higher than expected incidence of crime are schizophrenia, epilepsy and other organic brain disorders, alcoholism (especially states of acute and pathological intoxication), drug use and abuse, amnesic episodes, and fugue states. The greatest proportion of habitual offenders, however, rather than belonging to any of these categories, fall instead into the group labeled antisocial or psychopathic personality. Many of these have had an arrested emotional development, have learned a style of delinquent life in unfavorable psychosocial settings, have had no proper models for constructive identification and have had to resort to models from disapproved subcultures (in Erikson's terminology, *malignant identity diffusion*), and/or have been reared in a society that aroused expectations in them but then denied them opportunity to fulfill those expectations

One of the major interests of the psychiatrist in crime and mental disorder, and in the *criminally insane*, revolves about the question of responsibility of the accused for the criminal action he is alleged to have committed. See *responsibility, criminal*.

criminal from sense of guilt A person with an unconscious need for punishment stemming from repressed oedipal wishes; this unconscious need propels him into commission of a crime for which punishment is certain.

criminal intent See *intent, criminal*.

criminalism, compulsive Frequent repetition of criminal acts in a compulsive manner. Like most symptoms of the obsessive-compulsive, such antisocial acts are closely related to feelings of hostility and aggression, often against the father. Because

these acts are symptomatic, they afford only temporary relief and are therefore repeated. One patient with compulsive criminalism was apprehended after breaking into a hardware store and stealing money. He later confessed to many similar incidents over the preceding two years. He did not need the money and stole only for the sake of stealing.

criminally insane See *crime and mental disorder*.

criminosis Antisocial behavior; criminality. The word is patterned after neurosis and psychosis in form, but differs in that it does not specifically connote mental illness. It suggests instead that criminals be classified on the basis of the behavior they demonstrate unless they show clearcut evidence of mental disorder.

crises, urban See *social policy planning*.

crisis, adolescent The emotional changes that take place during adolescence; the psychological events during this period constitute a kind of crisis, the last battle fought by the individual before reaching maturity. The ego must achieve independence, the old emotional ties must be cast off and new attachments made. Biological development brings in its train great qualitative and quantitative changes, in both the physiologic and the psychologic fields, and as a result the adolescent ego is confronted with new difficulties. Because they are closely connected with instinctual life, the emotions are affected more than is any other part of the personality by the problems of growth and therefore represent a challenging problem for the adolescent.

crisis, catathymic Usually, an isolated, nonrepetitive act of violence that, though occurring suddenly, develops from a background of intolerable tension. See *disorders of impulse control*.

crisis, hemoclastic Reversal of the normal white blood cell and blood pressure response to the ingestion of protein. In the normal, ingestion of protein results in leukocytosis and rise of blood pressure. In contrast, hemoclastic patients show a fall in blood pressure, leukopenia, altered differential white blood count, and a reduction in the refractive index of the blood. Hemoclastic crisis is said to be particularly frequent in schizophrenia, depression, and anxiety states, and to be correlated with a poorer prognosis than in patients with a normal response.

crisis intervention Brief psychotherapy used to aid a person or group in coping with unusual or unforeseen demands on functioning capacity, such as during developmental crises (adolescence, parenthood, retirement, etc.) or accidental crises (bereavement, disaster, etc.). See *psychiatry, community*.

crisis, oculogyric See *spasm, oculogyric*.

crisis, physiologic Bender's term for any sudden change, endogenously produced, that occurs in the course of apparently normal maturation and development. Physiologic crisis is always seen in the history of childhood schizophrenics and is often a precipitating factor in onset of psychosis. The physiologic crisis appears to depend upon embryonal plasticity and a maturational lag.

crisis, psycholeptic Eruption of irrational unconscious elements into consciousness. H. Baynes analogizes breaking in of unconscious material with the psycholeptic outbreak, which is essentially the feeling of a catastrophe, namely, the end of the world. Epileptics often have ideas of impending destruction. There, too, the breaking of unconscious material into the consciousness is assumed to be responsible for this ideation. (*Mythology of the Soul*, 1940) See *psycholepsy*.

crispation Slight spasmodic or convulsive muscle contraction. A synonym for *dysphoria nervosa* (q.v.).

criterion-referenced See *test*.

critical flicker (fusion) frequency See *flicker*.

critical judgment See *judgment*.

criticizing faculty See *superego*.

crocidismus *Carphology* (q.v.).

Crocodile Man A person whose murderous assaults were likened by his defense lawyers to attacks by a crocodile and attributed to a limbic system disorder that released impulses over which the subject had no control. See *dyscontrol, episodic; explosive disorder*.

crocodile tears See *syndrome, Bogorad's*.

cross-association, telepathic The phenomenon that occurs when a thought or phantasy in one mind suddenly intersects a thought or phantasy articulated by another. It is assumed that such factors as coincidence, intuition, suggestion, or sym-

pathetic identification of the one individual with the other are not at play.

cross-cultural Referring to the comparative study of phenomena as they appear in different societies, nations, and cultures. Cultural or cross-cultural psychiatry is concerned with mental illness in relation to the cultural setting in which it occurs. What is regarded in one culture as clearly pathologic may be regarded as normal or even desirable in another. See *syndromes, culture-specific*.

cross-dressing *Transvestitism* (q.v.).

cross-fostering A strategy for investigating genetic factors in the development of any disorder in which offspring of normal biologic parents are reared by adopting parents who manifest the trait or disorder under investigation. Most commonly, the cross-fostered subjects are compared with two other groups—one group consisting of offspring of parents with the disorder reared by normal adopting parents (*index adoptees*), the other consisting of offspring of normal parents reared by normal adopting parents (*control adoptees*).

cross-gender disorder, nontranssexual See *transsexualism*.

cross-linkage theory See *aging, theories of*.

crossing over The genetic mechanism by which a chromosomal linkage group is broken up, so that some of the linked genes are able to separate and to enter different gametes and new *recombinations*. Since this interchange of genes between members of a pair of homologous chromosomes tends to involve large parts of chromosomes, that is, blocks of genes rather than single genes, mixed chromosomes, composed of both paternal and maternal gene units, originate either by *single* or *double* crossing over.

That crossing over occurs only between chromatids is due to the fact that it does not take place until after the chromosomes have each split into a pair of chromatids, early in prophase.

The new linkage groups are again as permanent as those that preceded them. It is clear, however, that a second crossing over not only undoes the genetic effect of a single crossing over, but also prevents single crossings over from occurring in more than 50%. If exactly 50% of crossing over took place, the numerical result would be the same as if free assortment were operating.

If there is only little crossing over between two genes, the linkage is said to be *strong* or *close*. If there is much crossing over taking place, it is said that the linkage is *weak* or *loose*. See *linkage*.

crossover See *recombination*.

Crow type I schizophrenia T.J. Crow (*British Medical Journal 280*, 1980) hypothesized that schizophrenia is a composite of two syndromes: type I, characterized by reversible delusions, hallucinations, and thought disorder with good response to neuroleptic treatment and possibly due to increased numbers of striatal and limbic dopamine receptors; and type II, characterized by frequently unremitting negative symptoms (flat affect, social withdrawal, poverty of thought content), poor response to neuroleptics, and a presumptive etiology of cell loss and structural brain damage, possibly due to a virus. See *symptoms, negative*.

crowding See *spacing*.

crowding, thought By this expression Bleuler (*TP*) denotes what may be called enforced thinking. "In superficial contradistinction to obstruction, schizophrenics often feel a 'crowding of thoughts'; they are forced to think." Bleuler adds that it is to be distinguished from obsessive thinking in that "in the former the obsession lies in the subject-matter, while in the latter it is in the process."

cruciata, hemiplegia See *hemiplegia cruciata*.

cry, epileptic A peculiar discordant cry or yell occasionally uttered at the beginning of an epileptic fit, just before respiration is arrested. It is believed to be due to the expulsion of air through the glottis, which is narrowed at the time of the tonic spasm. The epileptic cry is sometimes referred to as the *initial cry*.

cry, initial See *cry, epileptic*.

crying cat syndrome See *syndrome, cat cry*.

cryogenic Relating to refrigeration, and especially to methods of producing very low temperatures. In neuropsychiatry, used particularly to describe methods of producing brain lesions; the technique is generally reported to produce less severe blood loss and lower mortality than other types of surgery.

cryptesthesia A general term for clairvoyance, clairaudience, and other types of

paranormal cognition in which the sensory stimulus is unknown. See *paranormal; perception, extrasensory*.

cryptomnesia When a forgotten experience is recalled, but it appears to the subject that the experience is completely new, the condition is known as cryptomnesia.

crystallized Referring to the state that develops in some chronic users of phencyclidine (PCP): poor attention, dulling of thinking and reactions, loss of recent memory, decreased impulse control, lethargy, and depression.

crystallophobia Fear of glass.

CS Conditional stimulus. See *conditioning*.

Cs *Conscious* (q.v.).

CSR Continued stay review. See *review*.

CT 1. Computerized tomography scan. See *NMR; tomography*. 2. Conduction time.

CTS See *syndrome, carpal tunnel*.

cue, minimal The smallest quantum or most elemental aspect of a stimulus presentation that will elicit a response or a major portion of the total response. The responder is typically unaware of the significance or even the presence of the stimulus, and his response in many respects is similar to the conditional response in clinical or operant *conditioning* (q.v.). The mechanisms involved, at least at times, are also analogous to those operative in the production of temporal *summation* (q.v.) through subliminal excitation.

cued memory See *memory*.

Cullen, William (1710–90) A Scottish physician who emphasized the endogenous nature of mental disorders and their relationship to irritability of the nervous system; Dr. Benjamin Rush was among his students.

culmen See *cerebellum*.

cult A group of people or a movement with a distinctive doctrine or set of strongly held beliefs whose dogma and ritual are typically contrary to the established one(s) within the community. In what has been termed a *totalist cult*, the characteristic dedication to the dogma and the leadership of the movement may lead to the use of unethically manipulative techniques of persuasion and control in order to fulfill the goals of the leaders and recruit new members.

cultural psychiatry See *psychiatry, comparative*.

culture The totality of all the individual artifacts, behaviors, and mental concepts transmitted among the members of society by learning; what remains of man's past working on his present to shape his future.

The distinction is made between *material* culture, including tools, shelter, goods, technology; and *nonmaterial* culture, as values, customs, institutions, and social organization. According to H.W. Dunham (*Archives of General Psychiatry 24*, 1971), culture is a total way of life in a group of human beings, including shared patterns of belief, feeling, and adaptation, which serves as a guide of conduct in the definition of reality.

culture-bound *Culture-specific;* characteristic of or confined to a particular ethnic or cultural population. See *syndromes, culture-specific.*

culture shock A type of interface shock. See *network.*

culture, therapeutic A concept basic to the therapeutic community, referring to the requirement that all activities and actions within the community relate to the goal of reeducation and social rehabilitation of the patients. See *community, therapeutic.*

cunnilinction Apposition of the mouth to the female genitals.

cunnilingus Apposition of the mouth to the vulva or to any part of the external female genitals, usually clitoris.

cunnus (kun'us) Pudenda; vulva; female external genitalia.

curanderismo *Folk healing* (q.v.) among Spanish-speaking people and, in particular, among Mexican-Americans. The folk healers themselves are curanderos (males) and curanderas (females). The curanderos are believed to have derived their calling as well as their rituals from divine inspiration. Their techniques typically involve herbal infusions, dramatic healing rituals, and prayer directed against a variety of physical and psychological symptoms such as *embrujo* (witchcraft), *empacho* (intestinal distress), *mal ojo* (evil eye), *mal puesto* (hexing), and *susto* (soul loss). Curanderismo is not viewed as competitive with or antithetical to medical treatment, which may be sought and followed concurrently. See *folk medicine.*

curdling *Rare.* A term, coined by Masselon, for emotional dementia; it refers to the fixation of affects upon infantile or early childhood experiences.

cure, transference See *flight into health.*

curiosity, infantile Curiosity concerning matters of a directly sexual nature, indulged in by most children at one time or another. Some children exhibit a kind of foolish, witless behavior, in order to delude their elders into regarding them as being "too young to understand" or even into altogether disregarding their presence. The purpose of the artifice is that by these means children can view and overhear various private things which they are not supposed to. See *pseudoimbecility.*

current, action See *action current.*

curse, psychotic Profane speech in a mentally ill person, as in Gilles de la Tourette syndrome or as a complication of neuroleptic treatment of the syndrome.

curve, Lange's colloidal gold See *Lange's colloidal gold reaction.*

Cushing's syndrome (Harvey William Cushing, American surgeon and neurologist, 1869–1939) Hyperadrenocorticism. See *adenoma, basophile.*

custody Safekeeping, guardianship, protectorship, or the state of being guarded or protected. See *care, custodial.*

Most typically, the term is applied to children in the sense of which parent retains the control of and responsibility for the child in cases of divorce. Historically, custody has meant both ownership and protectorship. Until the middle of the 19th century, the father was usually awarded custody of the child in the same way that he had absolute control over all family property. With the Victorian era came the *tender years presumption,* that the young child needed the ministrations of a gentle mother more than the firmness and discipline that a father could provide. Children of prelatency years were generally awarded to their mothers, but it was not unheard of that as they grew older they would be shifted to the father's care. The approach in favor during most of the 20th century emphasizes the rights of children and would assign custody on the basis of what is in the best interest of the child—the *best interests doctrine.*

Joint custody refers to the sharing of custody by both parents, such as joint *legal* custody (the parents share decision making in all or specified areas, while the child resides with one parent), joint *physical* custody (the child spends a specified amount of time with each parent), or various other arrangements.

Cutter, Nehemiah (1787–1859) American psychiatrist; one of the "original thirteen" founders of Association of Medical Superintendents of America (forerunner of American Psychiatric Association).

cutting See *self-mutilation.*

CVA Cerebrovascular accident. See *accident, cerebrovascular.*

CVS Chorionic villus sampling; see *biopsy, chorion.*

CWF Cornell Word Form. See *test, Cornell Word Form.*

cybernetics The study of messages and communication in humans, social groups, machines, etc., especially in reference to regulation and control mechanisms such as *feedback* (q.v.). The field of cybernetics is particularly associated with the name of Norbert Wiener, who hypothesizes a similarity between the human nervous system and electronic machines. See *information theory.*

cyberphobia Pathologic fear of direction or authority; fear of control, especially mind control (see *brain control; menticide*); fear of computers, computer technology, or the possibility that computer intelligence will supplant human intelligence.

Cyclazocine See *methadone.*

cycle length In recurrent disorders such as major depressive disorder or bipolar disorder (manic-depressive psychosis), the period between the onset of one episode and the onset of the next, including the period of the first episode.

cycle, life See *developmental levels.*

cycle, manic-depressive See *psychosis, manic-depressive.*

cycloid The type of personality characterized by alternating states of increased psychic and motor activity, usually with feelings of well-being, and of diminution of the same factors. The personality is said to alternate from the one to the other. *Cycloid* commonly describes the normal or usual personality of many who subsequently develop manic-depressive psychosis, although the development of the psychosis is not a necessary result of such a personality.

Cycloid and cyclothymia are regarded by many as synonymous, although the latter term generally refers to personality problems that are more than cycloid and less than manic-depressive reactions. See *affective disorders.*

cycloid psychosis As used by Karl Kleist, *cycloid marginal psychosis* referred to an episode of atypical psychosis that did not fit clearly into either the schizophrenic or the manic-depressive category.

Leonhard and Perris used *cycloid psychosis* to denote atypical psychosis with delusions or hallucinations or both, with bipolar manifestations, and with good outcome (i.e. no chronic or residual defect state). Other symptoms, in order of frequency, are perplexity (the most frequent), motility disturbances, pananxiety, and ecstasy. Leonhard distinguished three forms, depending on which symptoms were predominant: *anxiety elation psychosis,* with anxiety at one pole and elation, often of ecstatic nature, at the other; *confusion psychosis,* with thought disorder prominent, ranging from excitement at one pole to underactivity and poverty of speech at the other; and *motility psychosis,* with psychomotor symptoms predominant.

As described, cycloid psychoses are more frequent in females than in males, and affected patients are younger at the time of first admission than unipolars. Rates of both schizophrenia and affective illness in subjects' relatives are intermediate between the rates found in schizophrenics' and affectives' families. Although recurrences are frequent, they tend to be short-lived. See *reactive psychosis.*

cyclophrenia *Rare.* Manic-depressive psychosis; thymergasia. See *psychosis, manic-depressive.*

cycloplegic See *mydriasis.*

cyclothymia, -themia Mild fluctuations of the manic-depressive type that almost have the stamp of normal mood shifts come under the heading of cyclothymia. There need not be fluctuations from psychomotor overactivity to underactivity. Some cases give a history only of periodic excitements, while others have one of periodic depressions. See *affective disorders*

The depressive phase may be clouded by the predominance of physical complaints, to which the term *neurasthenia* has been applied.

In DSM-III-R cyclothymia is classified as one of the *bipolar disorders* and is described as recurrent periods of abnormally elevated or expansive mood and of abnormally dejected mood or loss of interest or pleasure; the abnormal mood shifts must have continued for a minimum of two years, but they are not of such quality or severity as to meet the criteria for manic episode or major depressive episode.

cyclothymic personality See *personality disorders.*

cyclothymosis A term suggested by Southard for manic-depressive reactions.

cynanthropy *Obs.* A symptom in which the patient believes himself to be a dog; it is sometimes seen in the hebephrenic form of schizophrenia.

cynobex hebetis See *cough, convulsive, of puberty.*

cynophobia Fear of a dog, or of rabies, sometimes called pseudohydrophobia; a morbid mental state, usually hysterical in character, sometimes precipitated by the bite of a dog.

cynorexia Dog's appetite. *Bulimia* (q.v.).

cypri(do)phobia Pathologic fear of sexual intercourse and, in particular, of venereal disease as a consequence of sexual activity.

cystathianineuria (sist-à-thī-à-nēn-ūr′ē-à) A metabolic defect associated with mental retardation.

cytheromania *Nymphomania* (q.v.).

cytoarchitecture Cell structure; used primarily in neurohistology. See *isocortex.*

cytogenetics That branch of biology dealing with heredity and variation at the cellular level; specifically, the study of the chemical structure of genes, the specific arrangement of gene units on chromosomes, and effects of quantitative chromosomal irregularities. See *gene; chromosome.*

cytomegalic disease Congenital cytomegalic inclusion body disease is a viral disorder that may infect the fetus and produce mental retardation; inclusion bodies are demonstrable in the cells of cerebrospinal fluid, tissues, and urine. About one of every 200 live births is infected with the virus, and it has been estimated that at least 10% of those infected at birth will become mentally retarded.

cytoplasm The outer protoplasmic substance of a cell, exclusive of the nucleus and the cell wall. The matrix or ground substance contains numerous enzymes, most of the soluble precursors of the cellular pool, and various differentiated structures (organelles), including centriole, around which spindle microtubules are organized; centromere, with which spindle fibers become associated during mitosis and meiosis; Golgi apparatus, concerned with the elaboration or storage of various substances within the cell; lysosomes, containing hydrolytic enzymes that act on substances taken up by the cell; mitochondria, whose major function is phosphorylation; and ribosomes, containing proteins and several kinds of ribosomal RNA that are of central importance in genetic translation.

The cytoplasm provides the substrate for gene action and regulates the expression of genetic information through chromosomal inheritance. In addition it contains the elements (e.g. mitochondria and other inclusion particles) responsible for extrachromosomal inheritance, which consequently is termed cytoplasmic inheritance.

D

D In Rorschach scoring, a response to details of the ink blot that are selected frequently by healthy subjects. Piotrowski considers the *D* to be a measure of practical intelligence.

d In Rorschach scoring, a rare-detail response, i.e. a response to a part of the ink blot that is neither a *W*, a *D*, nor a *Dr* (qq.v.). Numerous *d* in a record indicate the subject's tendency to alleviate anxiety by occupying himself with small, precise, exacting tasks; such records are most commonly seen in schizophrenics, organic brain disorders, and obsessive neurotics.

D-O psychiatrist Directive-organic psychiatrist; Hollingshead and Redlich so designated that group of psychiatrists whose orientation is biological and whose psychotherapeutic approach is directive and authoritarian. In contrast to the *A-P psychiatrist* (q.v.), the D-O psychiatrist is often outspokenly antagonistic to psychoanalytic theory.

DA Dopamine.

Da Costa's syndrome Effort syndrome; neurocirculatory asthenia; soldier's heart. See *asthenia, neurocirculatory*.

dacrygelosis (dak-rē-je-lō′sis) *Obs.* Condition characterized by spells of alternate weeping and laughing; seen most frequently in hebephrenic schizophrenia.

daemonophobia A morbid fear of ghosts, spirits, devils, etc.

DAF Delayed auditory feedback. See *feedback*.

DAH Disordered action of the heart; the syndrome is known as neurocirculatory asthenia or effort syndrome.

Dale's law The principle that each neuron utilizes only one transmitter. It is now known that more than one *neurotransmitter* (q.v.) may be contained in and released by a single neuron; most often, the combination involves a biogenic amine or amino acid neurotransmitter with a neuropeptide as cotransmitter. The cotransmitter exerts a long-term modulatory effect on adjacent cells. Although approximately 30 neurotransmitters were known by 1987, the fact that they work in combination indicates that any satisfactory description of neurotransmission must make allowance for the 435 combinations of these transmitters that might occur.

Daltonism Red-green color blindness.

dance, St. Vitus' See *chorea, Sydenham's*.

dancing mania *Choreomania* (q.v.).

danger situation See *anxiety*.

DAP Draw-a-person. See *test, draw-a-person*.

dart and dome The spike and wave type of electroencephalographic tracing seen in petit mal epilepsy. See *epilepsy*.

Darwin, Charles Robert (1809–82) British naturalist; his demonstration of breeding experiments as a means of settling problems of ancestry anticipated modern *genetics;* in *On the Origin of Species by means of Natural Selection or the Preservation of Favored Races in the Struggle for Life* (1859) he enunciated his theory of *evolution* (q.v.).

Darwinism, Darwinianism Both terms relate to the branch of biology that deals with, or is in favor of, the doctrine of Charles Darwin postulating the evolution of all forms of living organisms from a few forms of primitive life (see *evolution*).

Dasein (dä-sīn′) "A being who is here"; a term used in *existentialism* (q.v.) to refer to the distinctive character of human existence, the capacity to become aware of one's own being at any particular point in time and in space and thereby to accept responsibility for what one is to become in the immediate future.

DAT Dementia of the Alzheimer type. See *Alzheimer's disease.*

data base See *problem-oriented record.*

Dauerschlaf (dow'er-shlaf) Prolonged sleep treatment with drugs (usually barbiturates), used mainly in status epilepticus, acute psychotic episodes, and drug addiction.

day center An outpatient or aftercare unit, ordinarily with a nonmedical staff, designed to provide company for the lonely, occupation for the handicapped, and meals for people unable to shop or cook for themselves.

day hospital A type of treatment for mentally ill patients consisting of a psychiatric hospital program (including individual and group psychotherapy, somatic treatment, nursing care, social case work, psychological evaluation, occupational and recreational therapy) in which the patient participates during the day but, at night, returns to home, family, and community. The first day hospital was set up by Dr. Ewen Cameron at the Allan Memorial Institute, Montreal, in 1946. In 1954, the first *night hospital* (with patients partaking of hospital care at night but returning to their homes and occupations during the day) was established at the Montreal General Hospital.

Both the day hospital and the night hospital are types of *partial hospitalization,* another form of which is the weekend hospital. See *psychiatry, community.*

daydream Phantasy; idle indulgence of the fancy during the waking hours; wishful thinking. Often, as in schizophrenia, daydreams assume preeminence in the mind of the subject, in whom they take the place of action in the real environment. In schizophrenia daydreams acquire the value of reality for the patient; that is, they become symptoms of the psychosis. When the latter takes place one no longer speaks of the phantasies as daydreams, because reality has been abandoned for the unconscious strivings and their presentation in the form of symptoms.

Freud says that daydreams hover in a curious medley of the past, present, and future. Some thought of the present creates a desire; the desire courses back to some earlier pleasant experience, which is lived out again in the mind with the idea of future fulfillment.

The driving force behind daydreaming is a conscious or unconscious wish or striving. Daydreams serve an appeasing function, in that they give partial release to strong, unconscious affects. The process involved is in the nature of abreaction. Federn says that abnormal daydreaming is analogous to sexual forepleasure in that neither represents the fulfillment of the final aim. See *phantasy life.*

daymare Anxiety-attack; panic attack.

Dd Rorschach scoring symbol for an unusual detail response.

dD In Rorschach scoring, a confabulated detail response; it is the use of a single, small detail as the basis for interpretation of a larger area of the inkblot. Such responses are always poorly conceived and thus of poor form quality.

dd Rorschach scoring symbol for a very small detail response.

Dds Rorschach scoring symbol for a detail response to a small white space on the card.

DdW Rorschach scoring symbol for an unusual detail response that is elaborated in such a way that the whole is perceived in the form of the detail.

de Rorschach scoring symbol for edge detail.

de-analize Instincts are said to be *de-analized* when they are shifted from the anal region to another object or form of expression. For example, interests in feces may later be expressed as interests in mud, still later in money, securities, etc. Part of the interests may be expressed as a character trait (e.g. cleanliness).

deadly nightshade poisoning See *poisoning, deadly nightshade.*

deafferented state See *mutism, akinetic.*

deafferentiation Elimination or loss of afferent stimuli. Sleep was once believed to be a temporary shutting down of mental and biological activity due to deafferentiation.

deafness, prelingual Hearing impairment that develops before speech is learned. Prelingual deafness interferes markedly with speech and language development.

deafness, word Auditory aphasia. See *aphasia, auditory.*

death Cessation of life, physical and mental; total and permanent cessation of the functions or vital actions of an organism. Among certain psychiatric patients the term "death" does not imply cessation of life, save in the sense that the patient ceases to continue in the environment in which he lives. Death is regarded simply as a preliminary step to rebirth, without any essential alteration of the body or psyche. This concept is common in schizophrenia.

In others (e.g. hysterical persons), death may represent punishment for carrying out a forbidden impulse, such as incest. Or it may represent reunion with the Oedipal love object.

Another symbolic meaning of death occurs in depressive states, in which suicide unconsciously represents the means by which the death of another is accomplished.

With the development of technology that permits life-support of patients for long periods of time after they might otherwise have died, many new questions about death have arisen. There is continuing controversy in both medicine and law concerning the definition of death, whether death is to be defined in terms of cessation of brain activity or cessation of measurable cardiac function, whether artificial or technologic mimicry of certain "essential" functions can be equated with life, etc. In some states in the United States, death has been defined in statutes in an attempt to provide a societal determination of the answer to the ethical questions surrounding the controversy.

death, autopsy negative See *Bell's mania.*

death instinct See *instinct, death.*

death, phenothiazine See *Bell's mania.*

death rate See *rate, death.*

death trance A state of apparent death; so-called suspended animation as may be seen in hysteria and catatonic schizophrenia.

death trend See *suicide.*

debilitas animi *Obs.* (L. "infirmity of the spirit") Imbecility.

debility Asthenia.

decadence The retrogression of a person or society that results from social rather than from physical or biological change. See *degeneration.*

decades, involutional Roughly, the period from 40 to 60 years of age; in women, the involutional period is usually considered to include the years between 40 and 55, in men the years between 50 and 65.

decapitation, fear of Castration anxiety may take many forms depending on the history of the particular person, and one of these forms is a fear of decapitation.

decarceration See *dilemma, Scull's.*

deception Simulation; *malingering* (q.v.).

deception, reduplicative memory Pick's term for a form of false memory sometimes observed in patients with organic brain disease. The patient claims, for instance, that he has already been examined by the same doctor, in the same examining room, with the same nurse in attendance, although the entire situation is in fact new to him. See *confabulation; déjà fait.*

decerebrate rigidity See *rigidity, decerebrate.*

decidentia (dā-kē-den'tē-à) *Obs.* Epilepsy.

decision support system See *information system, executive.*

decision tree See *algorithm, clinical.*

decompensation Recurrence or exacerbation of an illness, and in particular schizophrenia, because the mechanisms that had served to correct it are no longer adequate to maintain an acceptable or desirable level of functioning. See *personality, multiplication of.*

decompose To divide oneself or another into separate and distinct personalities.

decomposition Division of a person into separate components, or, more correctly, personalities. It is often observed among patients with the paranoid form of schizophrenia that they decompose or split the persecutor into separate entities.

decomposition, in dreams The gradual dissolution of the whole structure (i.e. its manifest content) of the dream into its component parts (i.e. its latent content) by the process of free association.

decomposition of ego See *ego, decomposition of.*

decomposition of movement This condition, described by Babinski, is characterized by irregularity in the successive flexion or extension at the various joints, instead of steady, well-timed movements. See *cerebellum; disorganization.*

decriminalization The act or process of removing acts or deeds from the category of criminal behavior. Decriminalization programs are those which remove certain types of juvenile offenders from the juvenile justice system and handle them instead under a child welfare or other noncourt system. The term has also been applied to the 20th-century tendency to label as sickness many behaviors that in earlier times were considered criminal or immoral.

dedifferentiation Loss of higher levels of organization and function; regression; usually applied to the simultaneous acceleration and retardation of development found in schizophrenic children and approximately equivalent to what Bergmann and Escalona termed *fragmentation of the ego*, to Erikson's *interference with psychoembryological schedule of ego functions*, to what Eckstein and Wallerstein termed *fluctuating ego states*, and to Rank's *atypical development*. See *personality, multiplication of.*

deemed status Certification that a facility or unit has satisfied appropriate standards in consequence of which it can be delegated to perform self-regulation and monitoring that would ordinarily be the responsibility of an external regulatory agency.

deep interpretation See *interpretation, deep.*

deerotize To remove libidinal cathexis from the psychic representation of an object.

defaulter Also *drug defaulter;* the patient who does not follow the recommended dosages of prescribed drugs.

defect See *disease.*

defect, field See *field defect.*

defectio animi (L. "deficiency of mind") *Obs.* Mental deficiency.

defective, mental One who is subnormal intellectually; feebleminded. See *retardation, mental.*

defects, cognitive Any of those signs and symptoms indicating impairment in the ability to recognize and understand reality; difficulties in perceiving, recognizing, judging, and reasoning are characteristic of organic mental disorders. When the degree of intellectual deterioration is such as to interfere with social or occupational functioning, the term *dementia* (q.v.) is often applied. The most common cognitive defects are impaired abstract thinking (as manifested in abnormally concrete interpretation of proverbs or inability to recognize the similarity between related objects), constructional difficulty (as in inability to reproduce geometrical designs), apraxia (inability to perform motor acts in the absence of paralysis or sensory disturbance), impaired ability to name objects and similar aphasic disturbances. See *syndrome, organic.*

defemination See *eviration.*

defense (defence) A mental attribute or mechanism or dynamism, which serves to protect the person against danger arising from his impulses or affects. See *anxiety.*

The ego arises in response to the frustrations and demands of reality on the organism; it learns to follow the reality principle. But the id follows the pleasure principle only, so that often there are conflicts between the two. This is the essential neurotic conflict. The superego may take either side, and if the world and external reality appear to the ego to be sources of temptation, the conflict may appear to be between the world and the ego.

The mechanisms of defense are developed as a means of controlling or holding in check the impulses or affects which might occasion such conflicts. The various motives for the development of defense mechanisms are (1) anxiety, arising when the ego believes the instinct is dangerous; (2) guilt, with anxiety of the ego toward the superego and fear of annihilation or decrease of narcissistic supplies; (3) disgust, when the ego must reject the impulse or it will have to be vomited out; and (4) shame, a fear of being looked at and despised if the impulse is not rejected.

Various defense mechanisms have been described. Anna Freud (*The Ego and the Mechanisms of Defence,* 1948) lists the following: regression, repression, reaction-formation, isolation, undoing, projection, introjection, turning against the self, reversal, and sublimation or displacement of instinctual aims. O. Fenichel (*PTN*) includes regression, repression, reaction-formation, isolation, undoing, projection, introjection, sublimation, displacement, denial, postponement of affects, affect equivalents, and change in the quality of affects.

Evidently both Anna Freud and Fenichel use introjection and identification interchangeably, although technically introjection is the mechanism by which *identification* (q.v.) is accomplished.

defense, character Personality, viewed as a grouping of defenses that have been developed by the subject as a routine way of coping with reality. In the early 1920s, many psychoanalysts had become pessimistic about the value of therapy. Reich (*Char-*

acter Analysis, 1949) pointed out that many chaotic analyses are the result of failure to recognize a latent negative *transference* (q.v.).

This negative transference is commonly hidden behind the character traits of the person, which serve as a protective armor against stimuli from the outer world and against his own libidinous strivings. In the course of the conflict between instinctual demands and the frustrating outer world, the character armor develops in the ego and becomes a habitual pattern of reaction to threatened or actual frustration from the outer world. Also, in psychoanalytic treatment the character armor serves as a compact defense mechanism, and this character resistance or character defense must be overcome if the analysis is to proceed properly. The ego employs other mechanisms of defense, such as repression, regression, reaction-formation, isolation, undoing, introjection, turning against the self, reversal, and sublimation. Although any or all of these mechanisms may be involved in the development of the character defense, they correspond essentially to a single experience, whereas the character represents a specific way of being and is an expression of the total past.

Reich described four main types of character defense: (1) hysterical; (2) compulsive; (3) phallic-narcissistic; and (4) masochistic.

1. In the *hysterical* (which includes the passive-feminine) character obvious sexual behavior is combined with a specific kind of bodily agility that has a definitely sexual nuance. Such behavior traits are combined with outspoken apprehensiveness, which is increased when the sexual behavior comes close to attaining its goal. The hysterical character represents an apprehensive defense against incest wishes inhibited by the anxiety related to any genital expression.

2. The *compulsive* character (or *anankastic personality*) has a pedantic concern for orderliness, a tendency to collect things, and thriftiness or avarice. Thinking is circumstantial and ruminative in type. This character armor is a defense against sadistic and aggressive impulses. See *phase, anal.*

3. The *phallic-narcissistic* character appears self-confident and arrogant; behavior is either cold and reserved or derisively aggressive. Most forms of active homosexuality and of schizophrenia fall into this group. Phallic-narcissistic attitudes in men are a defense against passive-feminine tendencies and represent an unconscious tendency of revenge against the opposite sex. The character resistance is seen in aggressive deprecation of the analysis and a tendency to take over the interpretation work.

4. The *masochistic* character shows chronic tendencies to self-damage and self-deprecation and subjectively has a chronic sensation of suffering. The masochistic self-punishment is a defense against punishment and anxiety in that it represents a milder substitute punishment. The masochistic character avoids anxiety by wanting to be loved, but the excessive demand for love is disguised in grandiose provocation of the love object. The purpose of this is to make the provoked person react with behavior that will justify the reproach: "See how badly you treat me."

The classification above is in terms of the clinical picture. There is another classification that stresses the libido origin of character. In this system, the character attitudes are assumed to be reaction-formations or sublimations of the libido of the stage in question. Thus:

1. The *oral receptive* character is considered a sublimation of the earliest sucking stage of life. Such people are characterized by friendliness, optimism, and generosity and expect the whole world to mother them. When frustrated they become pessimistic and act as if the bottom had fallen out of the world.

2. The *oral aggressive* character represents a sublimation of the oral biting stage. Aggressiveness, envy, ambition, and a tendency to exploit others are typical features.

3. The *anal* character corresponds to the compulsive character described as (2) in the other classification above.

4. The *phallic* character has also been described.

5. The *urethral* character has burning ambition and a need to boast of achievement, and is impatient; there is often a history of bedwetting beyond the usual age.

6. The mature or *genital* character is no

longer dominated by the pleasure principle, shows features characteristic of the preceding stages, but in a combination conducive to the greatest effectiveness. The mature character is able to care for and contribute to the welfare of another.

defense mechanism The means by which the organism protects itself against impulses and affects. See *defense.*

defense neuropsychosis See *psychosis, defense.*

defense, pathogenic A defense against instinctual demands, pathogenic in its nature, because the opposed unconscious impulse cannot find discharge.

For many reasons, as the person develops, he learns to "ward off" his own impulses, his instinctual drives. First, as an infant he required external help to satisfy these demands and since this help was not always immediately at hand, the infant found himself in traumatic situations as a result of his instinctual excitations. Second, both education and nature's own prohibitions (such as being burned upon grasping a flame) engender fear of instinctual acts. Education is effective not only because of the adult's physical power, but also because of the child's need for affection from the adult. Third, the child thinks animistically and, accordingly, believes that his own instinctual demands are identical with those of his environment. Also, since the child feels that any of his acts might provoke the same response from the environment, he will fear fantastic dangers from the environment in connection with his own instinctual impulses. For example, on meeting a rebuff in his phantasies of devouring the environment, the child may phantasy that he might be eaten by the parents. These are some of the reasons for the development of forces opposing the discharge of instinctual impulses. These forces are known as ego defenses. When successful, the ego defenses are called *sublimations.* The instinctual drives find an adequate discharge in these sublimations. When unsuccessful, however, these defenses are called *pathogenic.* The opposed pregenital impulses do not find discharge but remain in the unconscious and in fact keep on gaining strength, because of the continued functioning of their physiological sources. These warded-off instincts continue to

seek discharge. A state of tension results and a breakthrough may occur. This breakthrough is the basis of neurotic symptoms that express simultaneously both a repressed drive and the defense against it.

Some examples of pathogenic defenses are denial, projection, introjection, repression, reaction formation, undoing, isolation, and regression. In many of these defenses the ego's function of reality-testing has been conspicuously suspended and, in some of them, old archaic modes of thinking, perceiving, and relating to reality have been utilized again.

defense psychoneurosis. See *psychoneurosis, defense.*

defenses, Ur See *Ur-defenses.*

defensive reaction See *defense.*

defiance-based strategy See *therapy, paradoxical.*

deficiency, mental Mental retardation; intellectual inadequacy, feeblemindedness, hypophrenia, oligophrenia, oligergasia. In the 1952 nomenclature (DSM-I), the term denoted intellectual defect existing since birth, without demonstrated organic brain disease or known prenatal cause. As thus used, the term was equivalent to an older term, familial or idiopathic mental deficiency. Mental retardation is the term preferred currently. See *retardation, mental.*

deficiency, moral *Obs.* Moral insanity. Most psychiatrists today prefer to use the term *psychopathic personality* (q.v.) for such cases. See *anethopathy.*

deficit model An explanation that relates disorder to a lack of some element that would be expected to be present. The *alexithymic deficit model* of psychosomatic symptoms, for example, posits that the symptoms result from the direct shunting of arousal into the endocrine and autonomic nervous system, due to absent or diminished psychological processes that would be mobilized in the average person.

deficit symptoms See *symptoms, deficit; symptoms, productive.*

definitive Conclusive; serving to define or separate from others of a class or group. In diagnosis and classification of psychiatric disorders, for example, definitive symptoms are those necessary to distinguish between related disorders.

deformation While in general medicine this term is identical with *disfigurement* or *want* *of harmony,* in the field of constitutional medicine it refers to De Giovanni's particular hypothesis, the "law of deformation," which is basic to his concepts of constitutional types: that individuals having a small trunk tend to assume a *longilinear* body that corresponds to the *phthisic habitus* (see *habitus, phthisicus*). Analogously, individuals having a large trunk are thought to be inclined to assume a *short* body that corresponds to the *habitus apoplecticus* (q.v.), and individuals having a normal trunk are said to be inclined to maintain *normal* proportions of the body.

defusion In psychoanalysis, the separation or detachment of the instincts, so that they operate independently. Normally, the energy of the aggressive or death instinct is fused with the sexual. With regression, however, this unification and organization of part-instincts crumbles; the destructive instincts are freed and often work directly against the sexual instincts. This is the process of defusion, which in severe form will lead to such prepotency of the destructive instincts that negation of life is the result.

degeneration *Deterioration* (q.v.); reduction to a lower type of personal and social conduct as defined by existing moral and organic laws to which the person is expected to conform. Often the term is used in a pejorative sense to imply a sexual offense.

degeneration, cerebromacular See *Tay-Sachs disease.*

degeneration, cortico-striato-spinal Spastic pseudosclerosis; *Creutzfeldt-Jakob's disease* (q.v.).

degeneration, hepatolenticular (he-pa-tō-len-tik-ū-lêr) Tetanoid chorea of Gowers; Westphal's pseudosclerosis; progressive lenticular degeneration; Wilson's disease. An autosomal recessive hereditary disorder of copper metabolism characterized by degeneration of the corpus striatum (especially the putamen) and cirrhosis of the liver, with decreased serum ceruloplasm and increased urinary excretion of copper and amino acids. The disease begins early in life (10 to 25 years of age) and is progressive. The initial symptom is usually tremor, which is increased by voluntary movement. This is followed by rigidity, similar to that seen in parkinsonism, and

including a vacant, expressionless appearance or a vacuous smile. Involuntary laughing and crying may occur and also some degree of mental deterioration.

In a certain number of cases, a zone of golden-brown granular pigmentation (the *Kayser-Fleischer ring*) can be seen in the cornea; some would distinguish these patients from those with Wilson's disease and term the syndrome Westphal-Strümpell's pseudosclerosis. Untreated cases are invariably fatal, half of them within six years from onset of symptoms. Treatment with penicillamine or BAL (British anti-lewisite, dimercaprol) to remove copper from the body has afforded at least temporary amelioration.

degeneration, neuroaxonal Also known as *Seitelberger's disease;* the syndrome consists of spastic paraplegia, equilibrium disturbances, ocular tremor, and mental retardation. Pathology includes eosinophilic spheroid masses throughout the cerebral gray matter, spongiosis of the globus pallidus, and demyelination of the pyramidal tracts.

degeneration psychosis See *psychosis, degeneration.*

degeneration, subacute combined See *sclerosis, posterolateral.*

degeneration, Wallerian (Augustus Volney Waller, English physician, 1816–70) Myelin sheath degeneration of the axon distal to the point of severance from the cell body.

dégénérés superieurs *Obs.* (F. "high-class degenerates") Magnan's term for those sexual deviates whose perversions serve as an inspiration for great achievements in some special field of endeavor—social, artistic, ethical, etc. An example is the sadistic pedophile who built and maintained a home for disadvantaged children.

degenitalization *Desexualization* (q.v.).

deglissando See *glissando.*

degradation, senile *Obs. Senile dementia* (q.v.).

dehypnotize To bring out of the hypnotic state.

deinstitutionalization Discharge from hospital to community, particularly of those chronically mentally ill patients who would otherwise be kept in hospital for long periods of time. Full rehabilitation of the so-called chronic patient requires more than placement in appropriate residential settings, however. Also needed are *mainstreaming*, helping the deinstitutionalized patient to function as a member of the community, and *normalization*, all those interventions whose aim is to eliminate or minimize behavior that would identify the patient as being abnormal in the eyes of his fellows. See *domicile*.

déjà entendu (F. "already heard, perceived") The feeling, not demonstrable in fact, because it never was associated with reality, that one had at some prior time heard or perceived what one is hearing in the present.

déjà eprouvé (F. "already experienced, tested, tried out") The feeling that an act or experience in which the subject has never in fact engaged, has already been carried out by him.

déjà fait (F. "already done") P. Marie's term for a type of paramnesia in which the patient believes that what is happening to him now has happened to him before. Thus one hebephrenic believed he had experienced exactly one year before, everything that was happening to him at the time.

déjà pensé (F. "already thought") A patient's feeling, verging on certainty, that he has already thought of the matter. "The *déjà vu* and *déjà pensé* phenomena that are a part of many psychomotor attacks . . . suggest that many of them are associated with disorders localized to the temporal lobes." (DeJong, R.N. *American Journal of Psychiatry CVII*, 1951)

déjà raconté (F. "already told, recounted") A forgotten experience, particularly one from the distant past, is recalled, and the individual feels as if he had known all the time that the experience had been told to him. The term is also applied to the conviction of the patient in psychoanalysis that he has already related an episode to the analyst, when in fact he has not.

déjà voulu (voo-lü') (F. "already desired") P. Marie's term for a type of paramnesia in which the patient believes that his present desires are exactly the same as the desires he had some time before. See *déjà fait; déjà vu*.

déjà vu (F. "already seen") Feeling of familiarity. Upon perceiving something that he has never seen before, a person has the distinct feeling that he had had the experience some time in the past. It is not uncommon among psychiatric patients, particularly those with hysteria and epilepsy. A patient, for example, while visiting a town for the first time in his life may feel certain that he has been there on some previous occasion.

Freud suggested that déjà vu feelings correspond to the memory of an unconscious phantasy; the experience probably represents a combination of ego defenses in a situation that both symbolizes and stimulates the revival of an anxiety-provoking memory or phantasy. The ego defenses include wish-fulfillment (in the form of "Don't worry; you have been in the same situation before and came out all right") and regressive reanimation of omnipotent feelings (in the form of predicting the future). (Arlow, J.A. *Journal of the American Psychoanalytic Association 7*, 1959)

dejectio animi *Obs.* (L. "depression of spirit") Melancholia.

dejection Melancholy. The word dejection refers to the mood-tone change that is part of a clinical depression and is approximately equivalent to the word depression as used by the layman. In psychiatry, *depression* (q.v.) has a more specific meaning and should not be used when only a lowered mood tone is meant.

Déjérine, Jules-Joseph (1849–1917) Swiss-born French neurologist; described various medullary syndromes, paralyses, muscular dystrophies, and neuropathies.

DeJong, H. Holland (1895–1956) Dutch psychiatrist, in later years in U.S.; production of symptoms of mental illness in animals (especially catatonia).

delahara A culture-specific syndrome in Philippine women similar to amok. See *amuck*.

Delay, Jean (1907–87) French psychiatrist; introduced electroencephalography into France; originated modern psychopharmacotherapy when in 1952, with Pierre Deniker and other colleagues, he reported on the effect of chlorpromazine on psychotic symptoms; introduced the term "neuroleptic."

delay therapy *Response prevention;* a form of behavior therapy for obsessive-compulsive subjects in which the usual ritualistic response is prevented or postponed.

delayed auditory feedback See *feedback*.

delayed sleep phase syndrome See *sleep-wake schedule disorders.*

delayed stress syndrome See *post-traumatic stress disorder.*

deletion Omission; generally used to refer to a chromosomal abnormality in which part of a chromosome breaks off during cell replication and gives rise to a smaller than normal chromosome. The *cri-du-chat syndrome* is associated with deletion of chromosome 5.

deliberate self-harm See *suicide, attempted; syndrome, deliberate self-harm.*

delibidinization Technically, the act of removing libido from an object. In practice, this term is used to refer to an interpersonal relationship that is predicated on spiritual, objective, or nonemotional grounds. In certain Jewish forms of culture, for example, the father's authority rests primarily on his status as an exponent of the religious and scholarly tradition, rather than on the status of comforter, nurse, or donor of material or emotional comforts. Insofar as is possible his personality is delibidinized.

delinquency Behavior by a juvenile that is in violation of the criminal law; behavior that if occurring in an adult would be considered a crime. No uniformly acceptable definition of either delinquency or crime is possible by reason of the fact that the line between what is normal and what is criminal, deviant, immoral, or improper varies from state to state, from country to country, from culture to culture, and from one time to another. Further, the age at which an offense is defined as crime rather than delinquency is by no means fixed; under certain conditions, certain times, in certain regions, it may be as low as 14 years or as high as 21 years. In the case of juvenile offenders, moreover, there has been a tendency to broaden the definition of delinquency to include violations of regulations that would not ordinarily be considered crimes, such as truancy and running away from home.

By reason of the shifting and uncertain definition of what constitutes delinquency, it has been difficult to gather reliable data on its incidence, and it has proved impossible to pinpoint a specific, single cause for delinquent behavior. In any one juvenile offender, it may well be that a genetic, biologic, psychologic, or social factor has been of paramount significance in producing the behavior that is identified as delinquency. Yet even in the individual youth such behavior is much more likely to be the result of many factors, and it is their simultaneous action at a particular period of the offender's life that has been crucial in the evolution of that behavior.

All in all, it is generally agreed that delinquents or juvenile offenders resemble their nondelinquent peers psychologically and psychodynamically more than they differ from them. The number who suffer from a clearcut psychiatric disorder or from mental retardation is small, notwithstanding the many popular misconceptions to the contrary.

delinquent, defective *Obs.* A juvenile offender who is mentally retarded; used more often in a legal than in a medical or clinical context, to give recognition to the special needs of the mental retardate who happens to enter into the criminal justice system.

deliquium animi (dā-lē′kwē-oom à′nē-mē) *Obs.* Mental deficiency.

deliramentum (L. "nonsense, absurdity") *Obs.* Delirium.

deliratio senum (L. "dotage of the old") *Obs.* Senile psychosis.

deliration *Obs.* Delirium.

délire (dā-lēr′) (F. "delirium") A nebulous term, which sometimes refers to *delirium* (q.v.), at other times to *delusion* (q.v.) or to *compulsion* (q.v.). In general, the term could best be described as referring to a complex or system of ideas that forms a prominent part of the patient's mental condition.

délire à quatre (F. "quadruple insanity") A psychiatric constellation, usually consisting of systematized delusions of persecution, involving four people. The delusions are found first in one person, and then are taken over, as in a contagious disease, by a second, third, and fourth person. See *association, psychosis of.*

délire aigu (ā-gü′) (F. "acute delirium") Acute mania.

délire alcoolique (àl-kô-lik′) (F. "alcoholic delirium") Delirium tremens.

délire ambitieux (äN-bē-syē′) (F. "grandiose delirium") Maniacal excitement with grandiosity.

délire chronique In the French nomenclature, *délires chroniques* are paranoid states without deterioration of personality. They are subdivided into *focused,* with a single delusional theme, and *unfocused,* in which several areas of mental activity are affected. See *paranoia completa.*

délire crapuleux (krà-pü-lē′) (F. "dissolute delirium") Delirium tremens.

délire de négation Nihilistic delusion. See *negation, delusion of; syndrome, Cotard's.*

délire de négation généralise Nihilistic delusion. See *nihilism.*

délire de toucher (F. "mania for touching") Compulsion to touch objects. See *touching.*

délire d'emblée (däN-blā′) (F. "delirium at one blow") A delusion that is fully formed and developed at the time of its first appearance, equivalent to the autochthonous or primordial delusion of other systems. See *delusion, autochthonous.*

délire d'énormité (F. "mania of vastness") Delusion of grandeur; *megalomania* (q.v.).

délire ecmnesique (ek-mnā-zēk′) (F. "ecmnesic delirium") See *ecmnesia.* Pitres's term for preoccupation with events that transpired years before. He describes the condition in conjunction with hysteria, pointing out that the patient in this state lives almost entirely in the past.

délire en partie double (F. "double-entry delirium") Induced "insanity"; *folie à deux.* See *association, psychosis of.*

délire onirique (aw-nē-rēk′) (F. "oneiric delirium") See *deliria oneirica.* Dreamlike delirium.

délire terminal See *hysteria.*

délire tremblant (F. "trembling delirium") Delirium tremens.

délire vésanique (F. "insane delirium") *Vesania* (q.v.).

deliria (dā-lē′rē-à) *Obs.* Insanity, in general.

deliria oneirica (ô-nā′rē-kà) *Obs.* "These deliria are constituted of scenes from dreams, changing, varied, and uninterrupted, the subject being as if he were in a somnambulic dream. These occur generally at night, but sometimes they continue after waking. On recovery the patient has no recollection of his delirium." (Bianchi, L. *A Text-Book of Psychiatry,* 1906)

delirious reaction See *syndrome, organic.*

delirium An acute organic reaction consisting of alteration of consciousness and attention (the patient alternates at various times between preoccupation and coma); impaired orientation and (especially recent) memory, which give rise to illusional falsifications and hallucinations of dreamlike scenes; delusions which are fleeting, unsystematized, and illogical because they are often secondary to the hallucinatory experiences; emotional lability and incontinence; and marked restlessness and agitation. The most common causes are intoxicants, drugs, infections, avitaminoses, metabolic disturbances (such as diabetes, uremia, and hyperthyroidism), and trauma; but a delirious reaction can occur in the course of any organic brain disorder.

Delirium at one time was used in a general way to indicate insanity, psychopathy, and almost any psychopathologic manifestation; now obsolete, such usage explains the appellations depressive delirium (melancholia), persecutory delirium (paranoia), touching delirium (compulsive touching), etc.

delirium, abstinence The state of delirium, usually delirium tremens, that follows the immediate withdrawal of alcohol from an alcoholic individual. The syndrome may be observed in any form of drug addiction.

delirium alcoholicum *Obs.* Delirium tremens.

delirium ambitiosum (L. "conceited delirium") *Obs.* Megalomania.

delirium, asthenic *Obs.* Delirium occasioned by fatigue. See *delusion, psychasthenic.*

delirium, collapse Kraepelin's term for a condition, usually associated with high fever, characterized by marked disorientation, illusions, unsystematized delusions, and emotional variability; the condition is marked by physical collapse.

This term is also sometimes used to refer to delirious mania (*Bell's mania*).

delirium e potu (L. "delirium from drinking") Delirium tremens; used by some to refer to pathological intoxication. See *intoxication, alcoholic.*

delirium ebriosorum (L. "delirium of drunkards") Delirium tremens.

delirium, emotional Morel's term for the mental state in which the patient unqualifiedly accepts a false idea.

delirium ferox (L. "wild, savage, fierce") A psychiatric state characterized by violence.

delirium furiosum (L. "furious delirium") *Obs.* Mania.

delirium grave Collapse delirium. Also used by some to refer to delirious mania (*Bell's mania*).

delirium, idiopathic *Obs.* Name for psychiatric states occasioned by brain injury or toxic cerebral conditions.

delirium, initial *Obs.* A delirious reaction of toxic-infectious origin in which delirium appears before the fever is at its height. The term *fever delirium* is similarly used to indicate a delirious reaction occurring at the height of the fever, while *collapse delirium* is sometimes used for delirium following high fever.

delirium, intellectual *Obs.* Hysterical mania.

delirium, metamorphosis *Obs.* The state in which the patient believes that his body is transformed into that of a beast.

delirium, micromaniacal The form of insanity in which the patient believes himself to be a little child or a dwarf with shrunken limbs.

delirium mite (mē′te) (L. "mild, calm, gentle") A mental state characterized by low, delirious muttering. See *delirium, muttering*.

delirium mussitans (moos′-sē-tàns) *Delirium mite* (q.v.). See *delirium, muttering*.

delirium, muttering A severe form of delirium in which movements are reduced to tossing or trembling and speech is disorganized by iteration, perseveration, slurring, and dysarthria.

delirium, occupational See *hyperactivity, purposeless*.

delirium, oneiric Dream delirium. See *deliria oneirica*.

delirium palingnosticum The delusion that what one is experiencing in the present is a repetition of past experiences. See *déjà fait; déjà vu*.

delirium, post-traumatic Organic brain syndrome of the delirious type following injury to the brain.

delirium potatorum *Obs.* Delirium tremens.

delirium, psychasthenic See *delusion, psychasthenic*.

delirium, rhyming A symptom of the manic phase of manic-depressive reaction characterized by utterances in rhyme. See *mania*.

delirium, senile One form of *senile dementia* (q.v.). Onset is usually acute and often follows head injury, infection, or surgical anesthesia. Its principal characteristics are clouded consciousness, hallucinations, marked insomnia, restlessness, resistance,

and wandering. The delirium may be intermittent, or it may be prolonged with only occasional return to clear consciousness. The chief danger to the patient is exhaustion.

delirium, sensorial A mental state characterized by hallucinations and illusions.

delirium, subacute "A syndrome in which incoherence of thought, speech and movement appear together with perplexity, in a setting of clouding of consciousness, fluctuating in degree. The state may follow a typical delirium or appear independently. It may persist over a considerable period, weeks or months, outlasting the signs of the underlying physical illness, but always ending in recovery." (Mayer-Gross, W., et al. *Clinical Psychiatry*, 1960)

delirium, toxic See *brain syndrome associated with systemic infection*.

delirium, traumatic A mental disturbance characterized by a acute delirium occurring immediately after head or brain injury as a result of force directly or indirectly applied to the head. Other patients, following such injury, may show a protracted or chronic delirium with marked disorientation, confabulation, and memory defect, but with apparent superficial alertness. This latter condition may resemble the Korsakoff syndrome. See *organic mental disorders*.

delirium tremens *Alcohol withdrawal delirium; alcohol abstinence delirium;* an acute brain syndrome due to alcohol, characterized by an acute hallucinatory delirium, marked memory impairment, disorientation, and, usually, a coarse, generalized tremor that involves particularly the fingers, face, and tongue. The condition is often precipitated by intercurrent infection or injury.

The syndrome begins suddenly with fever, rapid pulse, leukocytosis, profuse perspiration, headache, anorexia, nausea, weakness, and dehydration. Along with the tremor there are seen ataxia and hyperreflexia, and all these appear to be due to an encephalosis involving mainly the fronto-ponto-cerebellar pathways. Increased cerebrospinal fluid pressure and increased globulin in the cerebrospinal fluid are usual, and in about 50% of cases a mild transitory albuminuria is seen. Epileptiform convulsions may also occur; these *rum fits*, as they are sometimes called, are probably due to pyridoxine (vitamin B$_6$) deficiency.

The delirium itself begins within a few days after onset of the disorder. Persecutory delusions are common and are usually in reference to a gang of the same sex or some obvious castration fear. These delusions may lead to suicide or homicide. Illusions are frequent and are easily suggested. Visual hallucinations are the most common of the hallucinatory elements, and these are typically of animals, such as snakes or rats, which symbolize mainly sexual fears (pink elephants, incidentally, are most uncommon). Haptic hallucinations, of animals crawling over the skin, are also seen, but many of these are probably illusions based on paresthesiae. Auditory hallucinations, when they occur, are usually of a derogatory and/or homosexual nature. In the midst of the delirium, disorientation is marked; there is loss of attention and memory impairment, most marked for recent memory. There is an incontinence of emotions—panic, anxiety, and terror most commonly, although some few show euphoria or indifference to their hallucinations and illusions. Misidentification is common, and patients are highly suggestible and can easily be made to confabulate.

The delirium usually lasts three to six days; the patient usually has amnesia for the delirium and frequently returns to his pattern of heavy drinking and thus there is often an early repetition of the syndrome. Auditory hallucinations usually indicate that the course will be prolonged. In uncomplicated cases, death is rare (3 to 4%). If there is not full recovery, there is usually progression into a Korsakoff syndrome (in about 15% of cases).

The pathological picture consists of nuclear destruction of the nerve cells, with all degrees of granular degeneration and disintegration of the nuclei. In most patients, the cortex is mainly affected, but in those tending clinically to progress into a Korsakoff psychosis, the brain stem is affected to a greater degree.

Terms formerly used for delirium tremens include enomania, oinomania, and the horrors.

delta alcoholism See *alcoholism.*

delta EEG activity See *sleep.*

delta rhythm or wave See *electroencephalogram.*

delusion A false belief that is firmly maintained even though it is contradicted by social reality. While it is true that some superstitions and religious beliefs are held despite the lack of confirmatory evidence, such culturally engendered concepts are not considered delusions. What is characteristic of the delusion is that it is *not* shared by others; rather, it is an idiosyncratic and individual misconception or misinterpretation. Further, it is a thinking disorder of enough import to interfere with the subject's functioning, since in the area of his delusion he no longer shares a consensually validated reality with other people.

Like hallucinations, delusions are condensations of perceptions, thoughts, and memories and can be interpreted much the same as hallucinations and dreams. Delusions are misjudgments of reality based on projection. The sequence of events in the form of delusions is often seen to be as follows: the patients's relationship to objects is an archaic, ambivalent one; he attempts to incorporate the object, which then becomes a part of his own ego; the object is then reprojected into the external world and becomes the persecutor. Persecutory delusions thus represent projections of the patient's bad conscience; since the superego (conscience) is usually an introjected object of the same sex, the struggle against the superego represents also a struggle against the patient's homosexuality. The imagined persecutors, however, not only threaten and punish the patient; often also they are perceived as tempters who lead the patient into sin or weaken his potency. "This can be explained by the fact that . . . the hallucinations and delusions of reference represent not only the superego but also, at the same time, the (ambivalent) loved object; the sexual wish for this object is perceived as a destructive sexual influence that emanates from him." (Fenichel, *PTN*) See *paranoia.*

CLASSIFICATION OF DELUSIONS

Nonexistence: nihilism; nihilistic delusion; délire de négation

   of being dead: necromimesis

of not having a body: Cotard's syndrome; acenesthesia

of memory or orientation being lost: negativistic amnesia

if one stops, so will the world: ergasiophobia

denial of existing body change, illness, defect: anosognosia

Involving one's body: somatopsychic delusion

of being beautiful: callomania

of being physically deformed: dysmorphomania; dysmorphophobia; dismemberment complex

part(s) of one's body are larger: macromania; macrosomatognosia; délire d'enormité

part(s) of one's body are smaller: micromania; micromaniacal delirium; microsomatognosia

that one's penis is small or has shrunken or retreated into one's abdomen: Koro; small-penis complex

of having been changed into a woman: eviration

that one's sex has changed: metamorphosis sexualis paranoia

of infestation: dermatozoic delusion; Ekbom's syndrome; parasitophobia

of animals crawling under the skin: formication

of having a vile or repugnant odor: automysophobia; autodysosmophobia

that one has changed into an animal (or, less common, that one can change others into an animal): delirium of metamorphosis; metamorphosis delusion; melancholia zoanthropia; zoanthropy

into a cat: galeanthropy

into a wolf: lycanthropy; lycomania; insania lupina; melancholia canina

into a horse: hippanthropy

into a dog: cynanthropy; melancholia canina

Involving self or personality: autopsychic delusion

of loss of memory: negativistic amnesia

déjà fait: delirium palingnosticum

of having become another person: appersonation; appersonification

with a religious content: hieromania

of guilt, sinning, having committed some unpardonable sin: enosimania

of grandiose ability (special mission or purpose): delusion of omnipotence; megalomania; ambitious mania; Caesar mania; delirium grandiosum; folie (or délire) ambitieuse; Napoleon complex; cosmic identification; délire d'enormité; delirium ambitiosum; expansive delusion.

when delusion is clearly contradicted by reality: delusion of orientation; double orientation

of grandiose identity:

of being God: theomania

of being the universe: cosmic identification

of being of divine or celestial origin: uranomania

of being of distinquished or royal parentage: Mignon delusion; family romance

of being of superior intelligence: sophomania

of being loved by another: aidoimania; delusional loving; erotomania; Clérambault's complex; phantom lover syndrome

Involving the outside world: allopsychic delusion

of having an imaginary companion: Doppelganger

of one's spouse or sexual partner having been unfaithful: conjugal paranoia; delusion of infidelity; Othello syndrome; virginity scruple

of persecution, harrassment, libel, slander, undue influence, external control: delirium of interpretation; delusional perception; self-referential delusion; misomania; sensitiver Beziehungswahn; Wahnstimmung

of being watched: delusion of observation;

that being wronged warrants legal redress: litigious mania; delirium of revindication; reformist delusion

that one's mind is controlled by an outside agency: Clérambault-Kandinsky complex

that one's thoughts are influenced by others: constraint of thought

of possession by evil spirit, of being poisoned by the devil: cacodaemonomania

that one is to be subjected to homosexual attack: Kempf's disease; homosexual panic

of being influenced by an imposter: delusion of false recognition

that a known person has been replaced by an imposter: Capgras's syndrome; illusion of doubles; illusions of false recognition that a persecutor has adopted the form of a known person: Frégoli's phenomenon; illusion of a negative double; intermetamorphosis syndrome

delusion, allopsychic See *delusion, autopsychic.*

delusion, autochthonous Primary delusion, i.e. one that arises as an immediate experience, out of the blue, with no external or objective cause or explanation, but nonetheless with a strong feeling of conviction. Autochthonous delusions are characteristic of the schizophrenias; unlike delusions seen in other psychiatric disorders, they are not a disturbance of perception in which the subject tries to rationalize changes that he perceives in himself or in the outside world. Neither are they disturbances of apperception or intellect, for the subject can understand what specific objects in external reality are. Rather, autochthonous delusions are disturbances of symbolic meaning: because the legs of a chair are twisted, the world is twisted.

delusion, autopsychic When a delusional concept refers to the person's own personality, it is called an autopsychic delusion; when it relates to the outside world, it is known as an allopsychic delusion; when it has to do with one's own body, it is called a somatopsychic delusion. This classification was suggested by Wernicke.

delusion, expansive See *megalomania.*

delusion, explanatory Bleuler's term for delusions that give reasons for the false belief. A patient who believes that men are persecuting him explains the delusion by "showing" that they open his mail, that they publish photographs of him, that they assemble to discuss methods of injuring him.

delusion, infidelity See *paranoia amorous.*

delusion, interpretation An interpretation or a meaning of a delusion as given by the patient himself.

"Paranoia . . . turns to another source in forming symptoms; the delusions which, by means of a compromise, succeed in becoming conscious (symptoms of the return of the repressed) absorb the thought-processes of the ego until they finally become accepted without contradiction. Since the delusions themselves are not to be influenced, the ego must accommodate itself to them; and thus the combinatory

delusion-formations, such as *interpretation-delusions* ending in a *change within the ego,* correspond to the secondary defense in the obsessional neurosis." (Freud, *CP*)

delusion, isolated See *monosymptomatic hypochondriacal psychosis.*

delusion, Mignon (mē-ñon′) The belief that one is the offspring of some distinguished family (e.g. royalty) rather than one's own parents. This delusion is seen most frequently in the schizophrenias, although it may appear as a more or less disguised wish in almost any psychiatric entity. See *romance, family.*

delusion, nihilistic See *syndrome, Cotard's.*

delusion of grandeur In the *PSE* glossary (see *Examination, Present State*), these delusions are divided into *delusions of grandiose ability* (the subject believes he has been chosen by destiny or some higher power for a special mission or purpose) and *delusions of grandiose identity* (the subject believes he is rich, titled, famous, or related to royalty or prominent people). See *megalomania.*

delusion of observation Delusion of reference; delusion of being watched. See *reference, ideas of.*

delusion, partial A delusion about which the subject has doubts, seen frequently in subjects who are recovering from an acute delusional state in which the false idea was firmly held.

delusion, primordial See *délire d'emblée.*

delusion, psychasthenic Janet's term for delusions occasioned by fatigue.

delusion, reformist A delusion with a religious, philosophical, or political theme, with never-ending criticism of those who resist or oppose the subject's "cause." Reformist delusions may be associated with violence, and some political assassins appear to have reformist delusions.

delusion, secondary With Bleuler this denotes a delusion that is based upon a primary one. "When the patient is convinced that the physician wants to murder him and after taking medicine he feels indisposed, then it is a conclusion, based on logical probability, that the physician has prescribed poison (secondary delusion)." (Bleuler, *TP*)

delusion, somatic The subjective reports and complaints made by patients that their body is perceived, or felt, by them as disturbed or disordered in all, or in individual, organs or parts.

delusion, somatopsychic See *delusion, autopsychic.*

delusional disorders Paranoid disorders. See *paranoia.*

delusional loving *Erotomania* (q.v.).

delusional mood *Wahnstimmung* (q.v.).

delusional syndrome, organic One of the forms of *organic mental disorders* (q.v.), consisting of the appearance of delusions in a state of full wakefulness and alertness. The delusions may be simply formed and poorly sustained, or they may be highly organized and systematized and indistinguishable from schizophrenic or schizophreniform disorders. There have been some reports of brief recurrences of the delusional syndromes even though the toxic agent originally responsible has not been used again—analogous to "flashback" hallucinosis of LSD intoxication. The organic delusional syndrome is seen most often as a form of drug intoxication (amphetamines, cannabis, hallucinogens); it can be seen as an interictal syndrome in temporal lobe epilepsy, and sometimes in Huntington's chorea.

demand See *feeding, demand.*

demand language See *language disability.*

dement A person with an absence or reduction of intellectual faculties in consequence of known organic brain disease. Earlier writers used the term for deteriorated schizophrenics. Thus the paranoid dements of Kraepelin are those with unstable and unorganized delusions, apparent marked reduction in intellectual capacities, and a break in psychic unity.

dementia An acquired, persistent, or irreversible reduction in intellectual functioning that occurs after the brain has matured (around 15 years of age). It is manifested in impaired language, memory, visuospatial skills, emotion or personality, and cognition (e.g. abstraction, judgment, mathematics).

Characteristic is a dysmnesic syndrome progressing to full dementia, with deterioration of previously acquired intellectual abilities of sufficient severity to interfere with social or occupational functioning and to impair the patient's capacity to meet the ordinary demands of living. Intellectual disintegration is manifested in im-

pairment of memory, abstract thinking, or judgment, and defects in counting, calculation, and general knowledge (any or all of which are often termed *cognitive deficits*). In addition, disintegration of feeling and striving as well as personality change or impaired impulse control typically appear at some point in the development of the disorder. See *organic mental disorders.*

In years gone by, the term dementia had various meanings. It was once synonymous with madness, insanity, and lunacy; in the early part of the 17th century it was synonymous with delirium. Nowadays it tends to be limited to primary memory loss on an organic basis, and in the usage of at least some it connotes irreversibility. *Deterioration* also refers to loss of intellectual faculties, but without intimating a specific cause and without stressing the permanency of the change. *Regression,* on the other hand, emphasizes reversibility, and with Freud the term came to refer primarily to emotional disturbances rather than to loss of intellectual ability. See *dementia, schizophrenic; syndrome, organic.*

dementia, abiotrophic atrophic See *dementia, atrophic.*

dementia, acute Anergic stupor, such as seen in catatonic stupor and hysterical trance states. The term is little used today; in the past, however, it was considered a distinct nosological entity.

dementia, affective See *affectivity, disturbances of; hebetude.*

dementia, alcoholic Lack of recovery and progression of *Korsakoff psychosis.* Alcoholic dementia consists of impairment of memory and intellectual capacity, emotional instability, loss of the finer ethical and moral sensibilities, carelessness in dress and personal cleanliness, and, frequently, delusions of marital infidelity. See *syndrome, Wernicke-Korsakoff.*

dementia, Alzheimer type (DAT) See *Alzheimer's disease.*

dementia apoplectica Apoplectic attacks, associated with cerebral arteriosclerosis, may be due to hemorrhage or to softening of brain tissue. Usually there are prodromes of variable duration; they may appear as headache, dizziness, fainting attacks, together with ideational and emotional changes. Depending upon the nature and severity of the arteriosclerotic process, the apoplectic ("stroke") condition may be followed by diffuse cerebral atrophy, giving rise to the organic type of dementia. Clinically the last condition is known as apoplectic dementia. See *accident, cerebrovascular.*

dementia, apperceptive *Obs.* Used by Weygandt to denote a type of dementia induced primarily by disorder in the volitional and intellectual spheres. Weygandt applied the term to dementia praecox (schizophrenia), conceiving the so-called deterioration in the light of "disintegration" of the will, which in turn interrupted the normal train of thought, the final effect appearing as dementia.

dementia, arteriosclerotic See *psychosis, arteriosclerotic.*

dementia, atrophic Atrophic dementia, known also as *abiotrophic atrophic dementia,* refers to the presenile organic reactions or brain syndromes, e.g. *Pick's disease* and *Alzheimer's disease* (qq.v.).

dementia, boxer's One type of chronic cerebral disorder seen in boxers, especially those who have sustained many head blows; also known as dementia pugilistica. Boxer's dementia is a chronic, slowly progressive disorder with pathologic changes similar to those seen in postencephalitic parkinsonism. See *punch-drunk.*

The other common cerebral disorders in boxers include (1) boxer's traumatic encephalopathy, where predominantly neurological defects are directly related to head blows, and (2) paranoid and catatonic psychoses, the nature of whose relationship to oft-repeated brain traumata is incompletely understood.

dementia, chronic *Obs.* Dementia praecox (schizophrenia).

dementia, circular Kraepelin's term for a form of schizophrenia characterized by alternating phases of excitement and depression.

dementia, depressive Kraepelin's designation for a special subdivision of schizophrenia. The syndrome resembles that of *simple depressive dementia,* save that all symptoms are more intense and the course of the illness is protracted. *Rare* in the United States.

dementia dialytica An aluminum-induced encephalopathy, with progressive mental deterioration, paranoid ideas, and psychotic behaviors occurring in patients undergoing dialysis; accompanying neurologic signs include dysarthria, dysnomia, dyspraxia, and seizures. All the foregoing are aggravated during and immediately following dialysis, and within six months of onset of the syndrome most patients have died.

dementia, driveling *Rare.* Kraepelin's term for "the general *decay of mental efficiency*" observed in the terminal states of certain syndromes of schizophrenia.

dementia, epileptic The progressive mental and intellectual deterioration seen in a small number of epileptics (not more than 5%, and there are many famous epileptics who showed no such dementia: Helmholtz, Flaubert, Dostoyevsky). The resultant deterioration is more likely when the attacks have begun early in life. It is probable that both this and the convulsions are expressions of some unknown physiological abnormality, although some believe that the dementia is due to nerve cell degeneration secondary to vascular disturbances during the convulsive episodes.

In a small group of epileptics, more complicated clinical psychiatric syndromes are seen, with mainly depressive or mainly schizophrenic symptoms. It will thus be noted that epilepsy and schizophrenia are not antagonistic, even though a belief to the contrary afforded a rationale for the electroconvulsive treatment of schizophrenic psychoses. See *personality, epileptic.*

dementia, hallucinatory See *dementia paranoides gravis.*

dementia, higher Van Guden's term for inability to apply knowledge or make use of one's intelligence; also known as *parlor dementia* (Hoch) and *relative dementia* (Bleuler).

dementia infantilis *Heller's disease;* disintegrative psychosis of childhood; infantile dementia occurs in children at 3 to 4 years of age. The patient becomes resistive, whining, and anxious, shows a general loss of acquired functions with mutism, dementia, and posturing, but an intelligent facial expression is usually retained. In DSM-III-R, such cases are classified as either autistic disorder or pervasive developmental disorder not otherwise specified.

dementia paralytica (L. "paralytic dementia") See *paresis, general.*

dementia paranoides gravis "Those paranoid morbid states, which, it is true, begin with simple delusions, but which as time goes on terminate in severe so-called deterioration, a *peculiar disintegration of the psychic life.*" (Kraepelin, *DP*)

The *milder* type of paranoid schizophrenia, hallucinatory feeblemindedness, Kraepelin called *dementia paranoides mitis,* when the patient has hallucinations and "the substance of the personality seems to be less seriously damaged." Today Kraepelin's term is used only occasionally and even then not in the diagnostic sense assigned to it by Kraepelin.

dementia paranoides mitis (mē'tes) See *dementia paranoides gravis.*

dementia paratonita progressiva A. Bernstein's term for catatonic schizophrenia, which he also sometimes called *paratonia progressiva.*

dementia, parlor See *dementia, higher.*

dementia, post-traumatic An absence or diminution of intellectual faculties secondary to brain injury. Post-traumatic dementia constitutes 0.6% or more of annual admissions to mental hospitals; approximately 44% of them are secondary to motor vehicle accidents. Less severe disturbances with memory impairment and minor personality changes are more frequent. Psychologic changes following head injury become prominent approximately two months after the injury and generally subside within the next three months. In 50% of cases, symptoms persist for at least six months, and in 15%, for a year or more. There is no correlation between severity of the injury and severity of the post-traumatic psychiatric sequelae. Persons with pretraumatic psychoneurotic personalities, and those with many complicating factors, such as pending litigation, anxiety about compensation, occupational stresses, or associated bodily injuries, are more likely to develop post-traumatic psychiatric sequelae. Traumatic epilepsy develops within two years in about 10% of cases who manifest psychiatric sequelae.

dementia praecocissima (prī-kô-kēs'sē-mà) According to DeSanctis this condition, occurring in young children, sometimes as early as the fourth year, is characterized by a more or less abrupt appearance of catatonia. Stereotypy, fixed postures, negativism, angry outbursts, echolalia, emotional blunting are particularly noticeable. Marked intellectual deterioration is present.

Kanner feels that the case material presented by DeSanctis as dementia praecocissima includes a variety of pathologic conditions. "Some of the cases are indistinguishable from childhood schizophrenia (Bromberg), others represent rapidly progressing brain diseases (Lutz; Schilder). An autopsy performed by Ciampi showed chromatolysis of the pyramidal cortical cells.

"Rapid disorganization after a fairly normal start is encountered in small children on rare occasions and offers baffling problems of diagnosis. Some cases prove to belong to the group of Heller's disease (*dementia infantilis*), some few are cases of Tay-Sachs disease with or without the characteristic eye ground findings, others are instances of even more unusual cerebral disease processes." (Kanner, L. *Child Psychiatry,* 1948)

dementia praecox (dē-men'shē-a prē'koks) A term coined by Morel in 1857 to describe those psychoses ("vesania") with a poor prognosis, i.e. those ending in deterioration (dementia) and incurability. Praecox refers to the fact that the onset of the disorders occurs early in life—typically in adolescence. In the years following the introduction of this term, various symptom complexes were described which later were included in the group, dementia praecox. Thus Kahlbaum described catatonia, Hecker described hebephrenia, Pick and Sommer described simple deterioration, and Zieber described paranoia. In 1896, Kraepelin made the important differentiation between manic-depressive psychosis and dementia praecox, and he included the aforementioned entities as subgroups of dementia praecox. He, too, emphasized the poor prognosis in dementia praecox and believed that those cases that could be cured permanently or arrested for very long periods were really instances of manic-depressive psychosis.

In 1911, Bleuler introduced the term *schizophrenia,* which in present-day psychiatry has largely replaced the term dementia praecox. Bleuler rejected the latter term because, in his experience, dementia is not a constant end product of the disorder (or group of disorders), and because at least 40% of cases did not manifest gross disturbances until after their twenty-fifth year.

Some contemporary authorities, and particularly European psychiatrists, continue to use the term dementia praecox in a fairly restricted sense to refer to "nuclear" or "process" schizophrenia, i.e. unquestionable cases with a high tendency to deterioration and little tendency to remission or recovery. See *schizophrenia*.

dementia praesenilis See *senium praecox*.

dementia pugilistica See *dementia, boxer's*.

dementia, relative See *dementia, higher*.

dementia, schizophrenic One of the fundamental symptoms of the schizophrenias (Bleuler). Schizophrenic patients, despite generally adequate preservation of their intellectual potentialities, are often not able to make use of this potential in a constructive, appropriate, purposeful, goal-directed way. Knowledge, although present, is not always available to them at the moment it is called for. Schizophrenic dementia seems to be the result of disturbances of primary elemental functions, such as associations, affectivity, attention and concentration, and will.

Schizophrenic dementia reveals itself in various forms: stupid, foolish mistakes; senseless generalizations; gullibility; faddism; pseudomotivations; vacuity and banality of thought; an insipid, unintegrated, disconnected quality in thought and speech; difficulty in forming new concepts; ellipsis in thought and speech; treating the concrete as though it were abstract; etc. On psychological testing, probably, the most frequent expression of schizophrenic dementia is *scattering* (q.v.).

dementia, secondary *Obs*. The schizophrenic syndrome that follows what was known as the initial "acute" attack or dementia simplex. In the psychiatry of today no such differentiation is made, the entire course of the illness, whether periodic or continuous, being known merely as schizophrenia.

dementia sejunctiva (sā-yoongk-tē'vȧ) *Obs*. Dementia praecox; schizophrenia.

dementia, semantic The inability to experience or evaluate the meaning of things. In psychiatry this term has been used by Cleckley (*Psychiatric Quarterly 16*, 1942) to refer to the inability of the psychopathic personality to evaluate or experience life as a totally integrated organism. Although the psychopath can react verbally, as though he understood love, pride, grief, shame, or the other emotions, he has no real experience of these human values or connotations. Cleckley believes that failure to function at this level provokes regression, which is expressed in a drive toward failure and folly, a destruction of the self at the personal or cultural level.

dementia senile Simple senile deterioration. See *senile dementia; deterioration, simple senile*.

dementia, sequential *Obs*. Synonymous with *secondary dementia*.

dementia, simple depressive *Stuporous dementia*, one of Kraepelin's subdivisions of schizophrenia.

The syndrome is characterized by depression, resembling that seen in the depressive phase of manic-depressive disorder; the projection mechanism appears to a greater or lesser degree. The condition often leads toward periodicity, but not with the same sharpness that marks clear-cut depressive states.

dementia, simple senile See *deterioration, simple senile; senile dementia*.

dementia, subcortical A type of senile dementia characterized by emotional or personality changes, memory dysfunction, defective ability to manipulate acquired knowledge, and striking slowness in the rate of information processing. It is probable that both cortical and subcortical structures are affected in all the dementias, clinical differences reflecting the imbalance between various neurotransmitter systems. Subcortical dementias may be those in which the dopaminergic system is most impaired, whereas cortical dementias may be those in which the cholinergic system is most impaired. (Albert, M.L., in *Alzheimer's Disease, Senile Dementia and Related Disorders*, ed. R. Katzman, R.D. Terry, and K.L. Bick, 1978)

Less commonly, subcortical dementia is used as a synonym for tardive dysmentia. See *dysmentia, tardive*.

dementia, thalamic Encephalomalacia or other degenerative lesions of the thalami produce a typical form of dementia, characterized by diminution or absence of motor initiative and spontaneity, and ordinarily also some abnormal movements.

dementia, traumatic When dementia, intellectual, affective, or both, is directly or indirectly caused by an injury, usually to the head, the condition is known as traumatic dementia. See *dementia, post-traumatic*.

"Common to most of them are rapid exhaustion, irritability, tendency to spontaneous and reactive moods, up to the most intensive anger, which is in part labile and in part of a more torpid persistent affect. . . . Not rarely epileptic attacks appear in which the typical *epileptic dementia* may occur (traumatic epilepsy). Pictures similar to catatonia can last for a long time." (Bleuler, *TP*)

demissio animi (dā-mēs'sē-ō à'nē-mē) *Obs.* (L. "lowering of the spirit") Melancholy.

demography The statistical study of populations, including births, marriages, mortality, health, geographic distribution, population shifts.

demonolatry A form of mental deviation in which a person worships a demon or devil.

demonomania Morbid dread of demons; entheomania. Freud believes that the original pleasurable affect associated with an act, such as masturbation, is first repressed, then transformed into anxiety, which contains features of punishment in it and brings dread of an evil spirit as the next stage.

demophobia Morbid fear of crowds; ochlophobia. See *agoraphobia*.

demoralization, personal The repudiation by the person in a crisis situation of old habits and restraints without reorganizing his life.

"Demoralization is the decay of the personal life-organization of an individual member of a social group. . . . Prevalent social disorganization, in those periods when the old system which controlled more or less adequately the behavior of the group members is decaying so rapidly that the development of a new social situation cannot keep pace with this process of decadence, is particularly favorable for the growth of individual demoralization." (Thomas, W.I., & Znaniecki, F. *The Polish Peasant in Europe and America,* 1927)

demorphinization The process of gradual or rapid withdrawal of morphine in the treatment of addicts.

demyelination (dē-mī-e-lin-ā'shun) The process of destruction of the myelin sheaths of the nerve fibers. There is a large group of neurologic diseases, the demyelinating diseases of the nervous system, characterized by foci of demyelination. These foci are usually in the white matter and vary in size, shape, distribution, and in the acuteness of the pathological process. Classification of these disorders is unsatisfactory; their etiology is unknown, their differential pathology is indistinct, and clinical forms are often transitional, presenting features common to more than one of the specific diseases recognized. The four major forms, divided on the basis of clinico-pathologic manifestations, are acute disseminated encephalomyelitis (following acute infections); disseminated myelitis with optic neuritis (Devic's disease); multiple sclerosis (disseminated sclerosis); and diffuse sclerosis (Schilder's disease, Baló's disease, etc.).

demyelination, concentric Baló's disease. See *sclerosis, diffuse*.

denarcissism The state of being unselfish, altruistic. In early infancy instinctual energy is incorporated almost completely within the infant. In the very early stages it is bound to the soma. Later, with the development of the psyche, much of the energy is transferred to it. When psychic energy is devoted to one's own psyche, the condition is known as *narcissism* (q.v.) . Still later, for healthy mental growth, a part of the psychic energy must be objectivated, externalized, detached from its very personal value to the individual. When psychic energy exists in what may be called an impersonal state, that is, it exists in something not strictly related to the individual, it is said to be in a state of denarcissism.

dendrite, dendritic zone See *neuron*.

dendrophilia, dendrophily Love of trees, which may often be phallic symbols. M. Hirschfeld defines it as "a sexual obsession for trees." He reports: "A few years ago a man confided in me who was having an 'affair' with an oak tree in Machnow near Berlin. He had, as he said, an idolatrous veneration for it, and often in the darkness, when he felt quite safe from observation, he would press his naked member against the 'vulnerable trunk,' until an ejaculation resulted." (*Sexual Pathology,* 1939)

deneutralization Resexualization or reaggressivization, or both, as a result of which energy that had previously been neutralized and thereby made available to the ego in noninstinctual form for its secondary-process work reappears as overtly sexual or aggressive. Thus what had been an aid to the ego in solving its problems has become, again, a problem that the ego must solve. See *neutralization.*

denial Refusal to admit the reality of, disavowal of the truth of, refusal to acknowledge the presence or existence of. Known also as *negation,* denial is a primitive *defense* (q.v.), consisting of an attempt to disavow the existence of unpleasant reality. Because denial must ignore data presenting themselves to the perceptory system and garnered by the memory apparatus, such a defense can operate only in the undeveloped, infantile psyche, or in persons whose ego is weak or disturbed (as in the psychoses), and even so, denial succeeds best against single internal perceptions of a painful nature. Denial and negation are also used, more loosely, to refer to any form of *resistance* (q.v.).

deniers See *anxiety typology.*

denotation See *connotation.*

deontology A theory of ethics which holds that what is morally right is independent of the ends for judging the means and that it is incorrect to define morality in terms of ends and means. Like utilitarian theories of ethics, deontologic theories may be monistic (holding that there is a single rule or principle from which all others may be derived) or pluralistic (holding that there is more than one basic and irreducible principle), and they may focus on acts or on rules that encompass classes of acts. See *utilitarianism; utilitarianism, act.*

deorality The state in which instinctual activity, formerly connected with the oral region, is expressed through some other agency. It is said by psychoanalysts that the pleasure of suckling at the breast may in later life assume the form of a pleasure in being morally dependent upon a maternal person.

deoxyribonucleic acid See *chromosome.*

depatterning D.E. Cameron used this term almost synonymously with regressive ECT. He used intensive ECT and prolonged sleep with chlorpromazine and barbiturates to treat chronic paranoids.

dependence, drug All clinically significant behaviors that indicate a serious degree of involvement with a psychoactive substance, such as repeated efforts to cut down on intake, inability to fulfill social or occupational obligations because of intoxication, need for increasing amounts of drug to maintain effect, withdrawal symptoms when intake is reduced or eliminated, preoccupation with seeking or taking the drug even to the extent of relinquishing important social or occupational activities, continuation of drug use even after developing a significant illness or social problem (such as job jeopardy) that clearly contraindicates futher use, development of a mental or physical disorder that is typically a complication of prolonged substance use.

As thus defined, drug dependence includes what was formerly labeled drug abuse as well as what was termed drug *addiction* (q.v.). It is classified within the psychoactive substance use disorders.

dependence, oral The unconscious wish for maternal protection, to be encompassed by the mother, to regain the peace, protection, and security of her sheltering arms. This stems from the original intense and forgotten gratifications of the infantile nursing period, when the infant's prehensile mouth anchored it to the mother's nipple and breast. To the child, to be fed means to be loved, i.e. to be protected, ergo, to be secure. The nostalgic urge toward the reinstatement of such security has been found nuclear in asthmatics. (Alexander, F. *Psychosomatic Medicine,* 1950)

dependency State of being reliant on others. Dependency reflects needs for mothering, love, affection, shelter, protection, security, food, warmth, etc.

In Horney's terminology, *morbid dependency* is a form of self-effacement manifested in a compulsive need to surrender to and unite with a stronger person.

dependency, alcohol See *alcoholism.*

dependency, assumption See *group, basic assumptions.*

dependency, drug See *dependence, drug.*

dependency, ontic The existential dependency on the "other" within one's inner family circle. Loyalty is the key linkage between generations and it involves integrity and certain things that are owed. Over time, family members balance their accounts; loyalty ties are real, but there is no objective measure of what is owed by whom, and each family member has a sense of the balance of payments.

depersonalization A nonspecific syndrome in which the subject feels that he has lost his personal identity, that he is different or strange or unreal. Derealization, the feeling that the environment is also strange or unreal, is usually part of the syndrome. Other frequent symptoms are mood changes (e.g. dejection, apathy, bewilderment, or a feeling of emotional emptiness); difficulty in organizing, collecting, and arranging thoughts; and cephalic paresthesiae (e.g. numbness of head or a feeling that the brain has been deadened). Depersonalization has been reported in depression, hysterical and dissociative states, schizoid personality, schizophrenia, toxic psychoses, temporal lobe epilepsy, and in states of fatigue. It most commonly occurs in the third and fourth decades and is more common in women. It may last for one or two years before disappearing spontaneously; it rarely responds to treatment of any sort. See *dissociative disorders*.

M. Roth (*Proceedings, Royal Society of Medicine 52*, 1959) has described a more specific syndrome, the phobic anxiety-depersonalization neurosis (sometimes also called pseudo-schizophrenic neurosis). In this neurosis, phobic anxiety is combined with depersonalization; the patient often complains of giddiness, swaying feelings, and fears of collapse or loss of self-control in public. Roth suggests that the neurosis may be at least in part related to some disorder of the temporal lobes, the limbic system, or the cerebral mechanisms regulating awareness. Others have suggested that it is a variant of endogenous depression and report good response to treatment with imipramine.

G. Langfeldt (*Proceedings, Royal Society of Medicine 53*, 1960) used the terms depersonalization and derealization to describe syndromes characterized by experiences of a particular type of disturbance of volition and the self that are found usually only in schizophrenia. Unlike similar phenomena in neurotic states, those in the schizophrenic are always experienced as originating outside the self, and the patient has no insight into his own condition.

depersonification Loss of, or failure to achieve, individuation and independence. Inability to separate from the parents may reflect distorted family relationships, as when the parent(s) views the child as a parent, or a spouse, or a sibling, or an inanimate object, or a lifelong infant.

D.B. Rinsley (*Psychiatric Quarterly 45*, 1971; *Borderline and Other Self Disorders*, 1982, Chapter 11) uses *appersonation* as equivalent to depersonification.

depopulation Reducing the residents or population of an area, facility, etc.; in psychiatry, used particularly to refer to the shifting of patients from one system (e.g. psychiatric hospitalization) to another (e.g. the criminal justice system). See *chronic mentally ill*.

depot neuroleptic A long-acting form of antipsychotic drug that is administered parenterally, usually by intramuscular or subcutaneous injection, as maintenance therapy. Esterification of fluphenazine, for example, markedly extends the drug's duration of effect, and a single injection of fluphenazine decanoate may be effective in controlling symptoms for two or more weeks. Because the depot form of the drug is released slowly, over so long a period, each dose administered is typically much larger than that required when the drug is given by mouth one or more times a day. In consequence, such maintenance therapy is sometimes termed *megadose* treatment (q.v.).

deprehensio *Obs.* Catalepsy.

depressio apathetica *Obs.* See *anxietas praesenilis*.

depression A clinical syndrome consisting of a lowering of mood tone (feelings of painful dejection or an irritable mood), loss of interest or pleasure in comparison with the subject's premorbid state, psychomotor retardation or agitation, and difficulty in thinking or concentration. Complaints of fatigue or loss of energy and of feelings of worthlessness or guilt are common. The depressed patient often has recurrent thoughts of death, and a significant number of depressed patients attempt suicide or make plans to do so. *Biological symptoms* of depression include sleep disturbance (insomnia or hypersomnia), diurnal variation of mood, loss of appetite, loss of weight, constipation, loss of libido, and, in women, amenorrhea.

As used by the layman, depression typically refers only to the lowering of mood tone (dejection, sadness, gloominess, despair, etc.)

See *affective disorders; depression, psychoneurotic; depression, psychotic; psychosis, involutional; psychosis, manic-depressive.*

depression, acute See *melancholia.*

depression, agitated Any *depression* (q.v.) in which restlessness and increased psychomotor activity are a prominent part of the clinical picture. Sometimes the term is used interchangeably with involutional melancholia, where agitation rather than psychomotor retardation is the rule.

depression, ambivalent Minkowski's term for cases of depression in which ambivalence is a prominent symptom.

depression, anaclitic A term used by Spitz to refer to the syndrome shown by infants who are separated from their mothers for long periods of time. Initially, the infant gives indications of distress, but after three months of separation "the weepiness subsided, and stronger provocation became necessary to provoke it. These children would sit with wide open, expressionless eyes, frozen immobile face, and a faraway expression, as if in a daze, apparently not perceiving what went on in their environment. . . . Contact with children who arrived at this stage became increasingly difficult and finally impossible. At best, screaming was elicited." (*The Psychoanalytic Study of the Child,* 1946)

In Spitz's series, the reaction occurred in children who were 6 to 8 months old at the time of separation, which continued for a practically unbroken period of three months. This reaction was seen in full form only in children who had left a "good" mother-child relationship; those with a "bad" relationship did not develop the syndrome.

Bakwin noted a similar syndrome, with listlessness, emaciation and pallor, relative immobility, quietness, unresponsiveness, indifferent appetite, failure to gain weight despite adequate diet, frequent stools, poor sleep, an appearance of unhappiness, proneness to febrile episodes, and absence of sucking habits. Bakwin and others refer to this syndrome as "hospitalism."

The anaclitic depression is reversible if the mother is restored to the child within three months.

depression, anancastic Lion uses this term to refer to dejection or depression accompanied by tension, perplexity, anxiety, and obsessive and paranoid ideas that occurs in individuals whose premorbid personality was of the rigid, obsessive anancastic type. See *anancasm.*

depression, anxious See *depression, classification of.*

depression, autonomous See *depression, classification of.*

depression, classification of For the DSM-III classification, see *affective disorders.*

In DSM-II, depression was considered in the following groups: (1) involutional melancholia; (2) manic-depressive illness (manic, depressed, and circular types); (3) psychotic depressive reaction; (4) schizophrenia, schizo-affective type; and (5) depressive neurosis.

An older scheme after Kraepelin classified manias and depressions (or melancholias) under the general heading Affective Psychosis, as follows: (A) Manic-Depressive Psychosis: (1) Manic phase; (a) hypomania; (b) acute mania; (c) delirious mania (Bell's mania); (d) chronic mania; (2) Depressive phase; (a) simple depression; (b) acute depression; (c) depressive stupor; (3) Periodical psychoses; (a) recurrent mania; (b) recurrent melancholia; (c) alternating insanity; (4) Mixed states; (a) maniacal stupor; (b) agitated depression; (c) unproductive mania; (d) depressive mania; (e) depression with flight of ideas; (f) akinetic mania; (g) perplexity state; (B) Involutional Melancholia: (1) depressed type (agitated depression); (2) paranoid type

Various authors have suggested other classificatory schemes, but these seem to compound rather than alleviate the difficulties inherent in categorizing disturbances whose etiology is only poorly understood. Thus Gillespie speaks of reactive, autonomous, and involutional depressions. Reactive depression, in this scheme, is characterized by lack of activity and thought; autonomous depression has more activity, restlessness, and self-accusatory tendencies; involutional depression is chiefly distinguished by a hypochondriacal trend.

Mira y Lopez differentiates the following types: (1) physiogenetic or symptomatic depression; (2) simple affective depression; (3) melancholic depression, with self-destructive tendencies; (4) anxious depression; (5) psychogenic depression; (6) depression associated with aboulia or other disturbances of the will; (7) schizophrenic depression.

depression, constitutional See *disposition, constitutional depressive.*

depression, cyclical Recurrent episodes of depression that may or may not alternate with periods of exaltation.

depression, double A condition in which a major depressive episode occurs in a subject with preexisting chronic minor depression (dysthymic disorder) of at least two years' duration.

depression, ictal See *emotions, ictal.*

depression, involutional See *psychosis, involutional.*

depression, major See *depression, unipolar.*

depression, melancholic See *depression, classification of.*

depression, physiogenetic See *depression, classification of.*

depression, postinfectious See *organic mental disorders.*

depression, postschizophrenic *Depression* (q.v.) following an acute schizophrenic episode. According to some, such a depression is a routine development in the course of recuperation from schizophrenic decompensation; others view it as secondary to neuroleptic treatment for the schizophrenic disorder; others consider it to be a manifestation of preexisting mood disturbance that was hidden by the more florid schizophrenic symptoms; and a few ascribe it to intensive psychotherapy that may reveal to the patient his limited ability to establish meaningful interpersonal relationships.

depression, psychoneurotic In the 1952 nomenclature (DSM-I), the diagnosis of psychoneurotic depressive reaction is synonymous with reactive depression (see *depression, reactive*). "The anxiety in this reaction is allayed, and hence partially relieved, by depression and self-depreciation. The reaction is precipitated by a current situation, frequently by some loss sustained by the patient, and is often

associated with a feeling of guilt for past failures or deeds." To be considered in differentiating this group from the corresponding psychotic reaction are the following points: "(1) life history of patient, with special reference to mood swings (suggestive of psychotic reaction), to the personality structure (neurotic or cyclothymic) and to precipitating environmental factors and (2) absence of malignant symptoms (hypochondriacal preoccupation, agitation, delusions, particularly somatic, hallucinations, severe guilt feelings, intractable insomnia, suicidal ruminations, severe psychomotor retardation, profound retardation of thought, stupor)." (Ibid.)

In the 1968 revision of psychiatric nomenclature (DSM-II) this entity is termed *depressive neurosis;* in DSM-III, it is termed *dysthymic disorder.* See *affective disorders.*

It is recognized that attempts to differentiate between psychotic and neurotic depressions, either on phenomenological or on psychodynamic grounds, are inadequate. While it is obvious that severe dejection can be superimposed on any nosologic entity (and is particularly common in phobics and obsessional neuroses), that this should justify a special diagnosis of depression is questionable.

depression, psychotic In the 1968 revision of psychiatric nomenclature (DSM-II) psychotic depressive reaction refers to those severely depressed patients with gross misinterpretation of reality (including delusions and hallucinations) who do not have a history of previous depressions or of marked mood swings, but whose symptoms are reactive (i.e. attributable to some identifiable experience) and of psychotic degree.

In DSM-III, a major depressive episode is more specifically identified as "with psychotic features" when there is gross impairment in reality testing, as manifested by hallucinations, delusions, mutism, or stupor.

depression, reactive A depressive state that is directly occasioned by some external situation and relieved when the external situation is removed. A mother, intensely joyous at the expectation of rejoining her children after a long absence abroad, was held by federal authorities until the legality of her admission to the country was established. She remained acutely depressed until a decision favorable to her was rendered.

Some use this term synonymously with psychoneurotic depressive reaction, depressive neurosis, or dysthymic disorder.

depression, retarded See *melancholia*.

depression, secondary See *depression, unipolar*.

depression, simple affective See *depression, classification of*.

depression, stuporous See *melancholia*.

depression, unipolar Major depression without manic episodes; in Kraepelinian terminology, the recurrent depressive form of manic depressive illness; also known as *unipolar illness* to contrast it with *bipolar illness* (which refers to affective disorder characterized by episodes of both mania and depression). See *affective disorders; psychosis, manic-depressive*.

K. Leonhard challenged Kraepelin's unitary concept, and in 1957 he suggested that bipolar and unipolar forms of affective illness are different disorders. Various studies in both Europe and the United States appeared to confirm Leonhard's view. Yet response patterns to the new psychopharmacologic agents whose development began around 1952–1954 supported Kraepelin's divisions. They separated the so-called functional psychoses into (1) schizophrenia, paranoia, and other disorders of thinking which respond to neuroleptics, and (2) the disorders of affect which respond either to lithium, in the case of manic states, or to tricyclics and other antidepressant agents in the case of depressions.

It now appears that bipolar illness is a more severe and earlier-onset form. This is a return to the view of Kraepelin, who placed both illnesses in the same family of disorders.

Major depression itself is subdivided into primary and secondary. *Secondary depression* and minor depressive illness occur in medical illnesses and in nonaffective psychiatric illnesses such as obsessive-compulsive neurosis, personality disorders, schizophrenia, drug and alcohol dependence, sexual dysfunction, and, particularly, organic mental disorders.

Akiskal and others further subdivide

primary unipolar depression into *Unipolar I*—a pure depressive form with unipolar but no bipolar family history and with a relatively low frequency of episodes, and *Unipolar II*—depressions with a high frequency of episodes and with bipolar family history. Unipolar II, in other words, is considered a phenotypic expression of bipolar genotype.

depressive crash Abrupt onset of severe depression, usually in response to frustration or disappointment, as in acute depressive reaction of the hysteroid dysphoric to abandonment or rejection. See *dysphoria, hysteroid*.

depressive disorders In DSM-III-R, a major subdivision of mood disorders (affective disorders) comprising major depression, dysthymia, and otherwise unclassified depressions.

depressive neurosis See *depression, psychoneurotic*.

depressive position See *position, depressive*.

depressive spectrum disorder *DSD* (q.v.).

deprivation, emotional Inadequate or inappropriate interpersonal and environmental relationships, especially in the early years of development; isolation of an infant from its mother to the degree that identification with the maternal figure is not made, with the result that personality development is impaired. The validity of the general proposition regarding the adverse effects of emotional deprivation has been established by two sets of observations—studies of children who were reared in institutional settings and whose difficulties reflected early distortions in personality development; and studies of infants' reactions to separation from their mothers. See *depression, anaclitic; developmental disorders; object relations theory*.

deprivation, maternal The absence of a positive and continuous relationship between infant and mother or mother surrogate. Many workers in developmental psychology and related fields have maintained that maternal deprivation has important deleterious short-range as well as long-range effects on personality development. See *mother, schizophrenogenic*.

deprivation, perceptual See *deprivation, sensory*.

deprivation, sensory Perceptual deprivation; perceptual or sensory isolation; *in-*

formational underload. These terms are ordinarily used to refer to experimental techniques that either reduce the absolute intensity of stimuli reaching the subject, or reduce the patterning of stimuli or impose a structuring of stimuli upon the subject. One of the methods employed to reduce intensity of stimuli, for example, is to suspend the subject, wearing only a blacked-out head mask for breathing, in a tank of water maintained at a constant temperature of 34.5°C. Such experimental sensory deprivation is considered to be similar to "brainwashing" and the isolation experienced by many explorers and shipwrecked persons, who under conditions of severe environmental stress are known to develop mental abnormalities. The following features are common to the various situations, whether "naturally" or experimentally produced: intense desire for extrinsic sensory stimuli and bodily motion, increased suggestibility, impairment of organized thinking, oppression, depression and, in extreme cases, hallucinations, delusions, and confusion.

It is believed that such abnormalities may be explained as follows: the correspondence between external reality and sensory neuronal activity is not a one-to-one relationship; perception is learned through motor interactions with objects in the environment, and when sleep or other states minimize or eliminate such interactions, percepts based on previous experience will emerge from the brain itself in the form of hallucinations and delusions (e.g. in dreams). This may be because the sensory input from the viscera augments spontaneous neuronal activity, especially in the thalamus, to such an extent that impulses over relay tracts are initiated, giving rise to visceral hallucinations and similar phenomena.

deprivation, thought *Blocking* (q.v.).

deprivational dwarfism See *dwarfism, psychosocial.*

deprogramming All those measures used to counteract the effects of brainwashing; reindoctrination of a subject in the values, customs, beliefs, or philosophy that he has rejected and deserted in favor of a different ideology. The underlying assumption is that the new ideology has been adopted under pressure or undue influence, but

such an assumption raises many ethical questions as to the person's right to decide for himself, the limits of paternalism, etc. See *brainwashing; menticide.*

depth psychology The psychology relating to the realm of the unconscious, in contradistinction to the psychology of the conscious part of the mind. In psychoanalysis (Freud), depth psychology may be represented by the id and superego; in analytical psychology (Jung), by the collective unconscious.

derailment Abnormal deviation or disorganization of psychic processes.

derailment of volition A type of *parabulia,* most commonly seen in schizophrenic disorders, in which tangential, insignificant, and irrelevant impulses replace consistency of aim and purpose. Dependability and deliberation give way to whimsy, and goal-oriented behavior disintegrates into a disorganized flurry of contradictory wishes, ill-sustained passions, and short-lived causes.

derailment, speech A type of *paraphasia,* most commonly seen in schizophrenic disorders, in which speech mannerisms substitute for meaningful content. Whatever message the subject may be trying to communicate is lost in the bellowings, screechings, murmurings, or whispers that replaced modulated, logical, and orderly speech.

derailment, thought A type of thinking disorder, seen most commonly in schizophrenic disorders, in which incomprehensible and disconnected ideas replace logical and orderly thought. The subject jumps from one topic or word to another topic or word for no apparent reason and is seemingly insensitive to the contradictoriness, illogicality, or incomprehensibility of his utterances. Thought derailment has also been called *Knight's move.*

Dercum, Francis Xavier (1856–1931) American neurologist; described neurolipomatosis dolorosa, characterized by painful accumulations of subcutaneous fat.

derealization The feeling of changed reality; the feeling that one's surroundings have changed. The symptom is usually (though not always) indicative of schizophrenia and is based on the sense of passivity toward the environment that is secondary to projection feelings. "Everybody is doing things to me; something has happened to the whole world; the world has changed." If severe enough, this feeling of changed reality may be expressed as a feeling of imminent or actual catastrophe. See *depersonalization; dereism.*

dereism (dē'rē-iz'm) Mental activity that deviates from the laws of logic and experience and fails to take the facts of reality into consideration. In many schizophrenic states, psychic activity is largely expressed without respect to the realities of life. When a patient firmly believes that, as the Redeemer, he cures all illnesses by a simple gesture, his thinking is said to be out of harmony with facts, that is, dereistic.

"The separation of associations from experience naturally facilitates dereistic thinking in its highest degree, which is actually based on the very fact that natural connections are ignored." (Bleuler, *TP*) See *autism; depersonalization.*

derivation, psychological Janet's term for substitute, derivative, conversion actions that occur when the full, desired action cannot be carried out. The worker who dare not vent his rage against an unfair and unyielding employer, for example, may express his feelings in tics, paralyses, somatic symptoms, agitation, etc.

derivative See *substitute formation.*

dermatome The skin area supplied by the dorsal root of a single nerve segment.

dermatophobia Fear of skin(-lesion).

dermatosiophobia Fear of (acquiring a) skin disease.

dermatozoic Of or pertaining to the sensation of animals in the skin. Dermatozoic delusions, also called *formication* (q.v.), are seen in toxic psychosis and in some (usually female) patients with depression.

desaggressivization (des-ag-gres-iv-i-zā'-shun) Neutralization of the aggressive drive (just as desexualization is neutralization of the sexual drive), so that the energy that would ordinarily be discharged is made available to the ego for carrying out its various tasks and wishes according to the secondary process.

desanimania (des-an-i-mā'nē-à) *Obs.* Psychosis with mental deficiency.

descriptive Concerned with the observable and the objective, rather than with the internal forces that may affect or determine overt behavior. Thus *descriptive psy-*chiatry typically refers to any system of psychiatry that is based primarily on the study of symptoms and phenomena; often contrasted with *dynamic psychiatry,* which is primarily concerned with internal, unconscious drives or energies that are presumed to determine behavior.

descriptive ethics See *ethics; ethics, descriptive.*

desensitization Also *systematic desensitization;* a variant of reciprocal inhibition psychotherapy of particular value with some phobic patients. The procedure entails three maneuvers: (1) the subject is trained in relaxation; (2) during those training sessions an *anxiety hierarchy* is constructed, consisting of a list of stimulus situations that provoke anxiety grouped according to themes and then ranked from most to least anxiety-provoking; (3) when the subject is as relaxed as he can be, he is asked to imagine a scene that includes the least anxiety-provoking situation. The scene is presented again and again until the subject can tolerate it without anxiety. The therapist then proceeds to the next rung on the ladder until even the most anxiety-provoking situation can be tolerated in phantasy. Almost always, as it turns out, what the subject can imagine without anxiety he can experience in reality without anxiety. See *behavior theory; therapy, behavior.*

deséquilibrés (dā-zā-kē-lē-brā') (F. "unbalanced persons") A term coined by Magnan for those affected by what was then known as inherited neurasthenia.

desexualization Neutralization of the sexual drive so that the energy that would ordinarily be expended in immediate id discharge (the primary process) is held up and made available to the ego for its various tasks and wishes according to the secondary process.

design, factorial A method of research in which two or more variables are manipulated deliberately to allow study of the interaction between them as well as the main effect of each variable.

designer drug Any version of a regulated drug whose chemical structure has been modified so that it falls outside the restrictions placed on the regulated drug it imitates. Current law requires that the exact chemical structure and name of an individual compound be specified before it can be controlled. Addition of a single fluoride or carbon molecule to a regulated drug, for example, will change a drug enough so that the modification is no longer a controlled substance, even though it may be even more potent than the original regulated compound. It is estimated that the amphetamine series of drugs has between 2,000 and 3,000 variations, many of which are more hazardous than the amphetamines that are already regulated.

desire Until the introduction of modern concepts in psychopathology, the term desire was defined essentially from the standpoint of the conscious part of the mind. It meant, and continues to mean, a wish, a longing for, a craving, an inclination. With the development of fuller knowledge of the unconscious, the term desire was applied to many impulses or tendencies of that part of the psyche. There are forces in the unconscious that strive for expression in reality. To indicate this striving, the terms desire, wish, etc., have been retained, amid great opposition, because it is not conceded in general that there is, for example, a wish to die, a wish for incest, for exhibitionism, etc. That is true, from the standpoint of consciousness; yet in the unconscious are impulses, the antitheses of conscious desires or wishes, that press for overt expression. They may be regarded as biological urges or "wishes" or "desires," in contradistinction to the personal ones. To wish or desire generally carries the idea that it is done wittingly and consciously; we are not in the habit of thinking that we wish also unconsciously. It suits our morality to have unconscious impulses and conscious wishes.

"In other words, the latter (unconscious) consists of thoughts, desires, and wishes of a kind that are highly unacceptable to the conscious personality." (Jones, E. *Papers on Psycho-Analysis,* 1938)

desocialization The process of withdrawing or turning away from interpersonal contacts and relationships, such as seen commonly in schizophrenics, who tend to replace social behavior and language habits with personal, highly individual behavior.

despair Erikson describes *integrity vs. despair* as one of the eight stages of man. See *ontogeny, psychic.*

despeciation (dē-spē-shē-ā'shun) The presence in a person of a number of extreme variants of physical characteristics, such as a scaphoid shoulder blade, a supernumerary breast, a deformed earlobe, an anomalous distribution of hair. The variants, when alone, have little pathogenic value or meaning, but the accumulation of them in a single individual is regarded as a sign of biological inferiority or despeciation (Apert). J. Bauer uses the term *degeneration* to refer to such marked deviations from the type of the species.

destiny, neurosis of Moral masochism; fate neurosis. This type of neurotic ailment afflicts the person who unconsciously arranges all of his life's experiences so that he is in the position of suffering continual reverses, while he consciously holds that destiny or fate brings them. His friends will always remark on his bad luck and continual ill-fortune. Moreover, he invariably tends to blame his fate for his continual reverses, being unaware that he is responsible for them himself. See *masochism; success, failure through.*

As the "all-consuming task of his life" this neurotic has in the first place the "mastery of guilt-feelings," which he hopes to accomplish through his own suffering, and thus ingratiate himself with an implacable superego. Second, the patient turns all of his life's activities into situations where he can experience this suffering. In Fenichel's words, he uses his environment solely as "an arena in which to stage his internal conflicts." All real-life actions "are repetitions of childhood situations or attempts to end infantile conflicts rather than rational undertakings." (*PTN*)

destructive instinct See *instinct, death.*

destrudo E. Weiss coined this term to denote the energy associated with the death or destructive instinct. (*Imago,* 1935) It is the opposite of *libido,* the energy of the instinct Eros. See *Thanatos.*

desynchronosis Temporal disorientation, or feeling out of place or displaced in time relationships. See *circadian desynchronosis.*

detachment Separation; divorce from emotional involvement. See *affect, detached.*

detachment, somnolent Withdrawal into sleep; as used by Sullivan, the infant's reaction of drowsiness and apathy to anxiety in the mother. As the infant withdraws from the situation and sleeps, the mother's anxiety will often subside and thus the cause of the infant's own anxiety is removed. But if such detachments persist, the infant may progress into a *marasmic state* in which he may die unless appropriate nursing care is brought to him.

detector, lie A machine designed to record the various physiological changes that accompany changes in emotional tone, such as changes in respiratory rate, pulse rate, blood pressure, and skin moisture; the original machine was the *Keeler polygraph.* "The lie detector is based upon the fact that the impact of emotionally charged ideas or the conscious suppression of a true recollection and the substitution of a false statement cause detectable physiologic changes through stimulation of the autonomic nervous system, over which one has no voluntary control." (Guttmacher, M.S. *Psychiatry and the Law*, 1952) It appears that accurate diagnosis on the basis of the test is possible in 75–80% of cases, that in 15–20% results may be too indefinite for confident diagnosis, and that the remaining 5% constitute the margin of probable error. Such errors as do occur are usually those on the side of failing to detect a guilty person rather than on the side of mislabeling an innocent person guilty. Overall uncertainty of 25% has made courts increasingly likely to prohibit introduction of results as evidence.

detentio *Obs.* The fixed attitude in catalepsy.

detention Commitment; involuntary hospitalization.

deterioration Worsening of the clinical condition; progressively increasing impairment in functioning. Compare with regression, *dementia* (q.v.).

Intellectual deterioration generally refers to diminution or impairment of the ability to remember, together with disorders attendant upon memory losses. Intellectual deterioration is characteristic of patients with destructive processes in the cerebral cortex.

deterioration, alcoholic A complication of *alcoholism* (q.v.) characterized by emotional blunting, organic memory defect, and deterioration in the moral and ethical spheres.

deterioration, emotional Occurs mainly in patients suffering from schizophrenia: the patient becomes careless and indifferent about the surroundings and people around him and shows no adequate emotional reaction to environmental stimuli.

deterioration, epileptic See *dementia, epileptic.*

deterioration, habit The abandonment of integrated and socialized behavior in favor of disintegrated and personal behavior; regression; a failure of the habits appropriate to the patient's social standing.

deterioration index or quotient An index of the degree of intellectual impairment, based on comparison of scores on those tests of the Wechsler-Bellevue that show little or no decline, with scores on those tests that generally show a steep age decline. The tests that do not decline are often termed "Hold" tests: information, vocabulary, picture completion, and object assembly; those that do decline are often termed "Don't Hold" tests: digit span, arithmetic, block design, digit symbol. The deterioration index, or DI, is computed as follows:

$$DI = Hold - \frac{Don't\ Hold}{Hold}$$

deterioration, post-traumatic mental *Obs.* Organic brain syndrome, usually of the dementia or personality syndrome variety, following injury to the brain.

deterioration scale See *GDS.*

deterioration, simple senile One form of *senile dementia* (q.v.). Symptoms include narrowing of interests, sluggishness of thought, misoneism, recent memory gaps that are filled in with fabrications, defective orientation, hoarding, inattentiveness except to immediate personal wants, apathy or irritability, and sometimes suspiciousness, ideas of persecution, and restless wandering from the home.

determinant See *determinant, dream.*

determinant, dominant See *determinant, dream.*

determinant, dream The real or principal motive or reason responsible for the production of the dream, since it is true that even if "dreams are always abundantly overdetermined, one determinant is invariable in the dreams of neurotics." This invariable factor is called the "dominant determinant" and is in direct connection with the dreamer's most important conflict. To discover the dominant determinant is no easy task: most of the time it is not revealed through association and may be discovered only by the use of the interpreter's intuition. (Stekel, *ID*)

determination, sex See *sex determination*.

determinative idea See *idea, determinative*.

determiner A cause or determinant; in genetics, a *gene* (q.v.).

determining quality See *quality, determining*.

determining tendency See *set*.

determinism "It is the concept which states, first, that our actions can change nothing in the events of life which were firmly established through causal connection, and, second, that man is not free to dispose of his own will and to choose between good and evil in his actions." (Bleuler, *TP*) See *free will*.

determinism, biological A structure of social explanation that uses basic concepts in anatomy, evolutionary theory, genetics, and neurobiology; it posits that biology is destiny, and that the differences among individuals and between sexes, ethnic groups, and races in status, wealth, and power are based on innate biologic differences in temperament and ability. According to Stephen Jay Gould, the major conceptual error of the theory was the determinist's conversion of the abstract idea of intelligence into a thing, a single entity, located in the brain. Once viewed as a unit, methods were developed to measure it and reduce it to a single number for each person through the statistical method. The error is not in the arithmetic but in the supposition that, having gone through the mathematics, one has produced a real object.

In the older mental retardation literature, biosocial determinism referred to the extent to which hereditary or other biologic factors determined the degree of disability.

determinism, biosocial *Obs*. In mental retardation, recognition that the degree of disability is due neither to biologic nor social factors alone, but to their combination.

deterrent therapy See *therapy, aversion*.

detouring, conflict See scapegoating.

detumescence (dē-tū-mes′ens) Subsidence of erection and genital engorgement as a result of emptying of the genital blood vessels. See *contraction; tumescence*.

deuteropathy (dū-tēr-op′a-thē) A secondary disease, disorder, or symptom.

Deutsch, Helen Rosenbach (1884–1982) Polish-born psychoanalyst, first woman to

be analyzed by Freud, founded Vienna Psychoanalytic Institute; to U.S. in 1935; *The Psychology of Women* (1944); "as-if" personality.

devaluation In DSM-III-R, a defense mechanism consisting of attribution of exaggerated negative qualities to self or others when faced with emotional conflicts or stressors.

development, atypical A term used by some (notably Rank, Putnam, and Kaplan) as a diagnostic label for those children whom others would classify as childhood schizophrenia or early infantile autism.

development, genital-psychical A psychoanalytic term that stresses the importance of psychosexual, developmental, emotional maturation as a true basis for genito-sexual potency—in contrast to mechanical, anatomical, physiological, and orgastic criteria that give rise to pseudopotency and the masking of impotence. Genito-sexual potency is characterized by the ability to love in the adult sense and by a free, full, and satisfactory orgasm as well. Genito-sexual pseudopotency is manifested in a masturbatory preoccupation with personal, orgastic, and tactile sensation. Even though orgasm in the pseudopotent may be deceptively satisfactory, it is frequently entirely dependent upon thinly disguised perversion stimuli, and perversion auspices. Genito-sexual pseudopotency is associated with self-love and self-satisfaction; in contrast the genito-sexual potency of the psychosexually mature is strongly marked by love of and consideration for the partner. See *impotence, psychic; sexual disorders*.

developmental Referring to the process of maturation and the changes that occur in an organism or structure over time. Developmental studies attempt to describe the changes that do occur and to determine the causes of developmental differences. See *ontogeny, psychic; psychobiology, developmental*.

Developmental disorders are usually first evident in infancy or childhood; included are mental retardation, pervasive developmental disorders, and specific developmental disorders.

developmental articulation disorder A type of *language retardation*, believed to be due to lag in cerebral maturation (in which heredity may be a significant factor), consisting of deviant production of speech sounds such as distortion, substitution, or omission of one or more sounds (e.g. g, r, s, or th).

developmental disorders Manifestations of the child's struggle for mastery at various stages of development; such manifestations are not disorders per se. Included are such symptoms as nonhunger crying in the baby, stranger anxiety at 6 to 12 months of age, separation anxiety at 18 to 30 months, negativism and tantrums around 2 years of age, and crankiness or transitory fears in children from 3 to 5 years old.

Others use the term in a different sense, to refer to infantilism or slow rate of development, or to a group of childhood conditions including autism, mental retardation, epilepsy, childhood spasticity, speech problems, and some disorders of speech and hearing.

developmental disorders, pervasive A group of childhood disturbances characterized by severe distortions in the timing, rate, and sequence of the psychologic functions basic to the development of language, communications, and social skills in general. In DSM-III-R, autistic disorder is the only specified pervasive developmental disorder. See *autism, early infantile.*

developmental disorders, specific A group of childhood disturbances characterized by a lag, delay, or deviance in the development of a specific function, such as reading, speaking, or arithmetic ability, and not explicable in terms of mental age or inadequate schooling. These disorders frequently coexist with other disorders (e.g. conduct disorders, attention deficit disorders). Included within the group are (1) language and speech disorders (articulation disorder, stuttering, cluttering, expressive language disorder, receptive language disorder); (2) academic skills disorder (reading disorder, expressive writing disorder, arithmetic disorder); and (3) motor skills disorder (coordination disorder).

developmental dysphasia A type of *language retardation,* believed to be due to cerebral damage or lag in cerebral maturation, characterized by defects in expressive language and articulation (*expressive dysphasia*) and also, in the more severe forms, by defects in the comprehension of language (*receptive dysphasia*).

developmental hyperactivity See *learning disability, specific.*

developmental levels Divisions of the life span in terms of chronological age; the following levels are generally recognized: (1) neonatal period, from birth to 1 month; (2) *infancy* (q.v.) from birth to 1 year; (3) early (preschool) childhood, from 1 to 6 years; (4) midchildhood, 6 to 10 years; (5) late childhood or preadolescence, 10 to 12 years; (6) *adolescence* (q.v.), 12 to 21 years; (7) adulthood or maturity, beginning at 21 years and ending with old age according to some, but with others ending at (8) the involutional period or climacterium, 40 to 55 years for women, 50 to 65 years for men; (9) old age or the senium, beginning at 65 or 70 years. See *ontogeny, psychic.*

developmental psychobiology See *psychobiology, developmental.*

developmental psychology Study of the processes of maturation of the intellectual, emotional, attitudinal, and social aspects of the organism with particular emphasis, in the human, on the childhood and adolescent years. Jean Piaget's theories recognized the importance of cognitive learning processes and concept formation in the young child, and he described the regular stages of intellectual development. In the period of *sensorimotor intelligence* (the first two years of life), the child learns to use senses and muscles to deal with external events, and he begins to symbolize, i.e. to represent things by word or gesture. In the period of representative intelligence (2 to 7 or 8 years), words and other symbols are used to represent the outer world and inner feelings. He begins to understand relationships—spatial, temporal, and mathematical (grouping, sizes, qualities, etc.). Although Piaget emphasized the internal processes of development, he also noted their dependence on an environment conducive to learning the necessary skills.

developmentalism The genetic, longitudinal view of human behavior. The term is used to describe Gesell's emphasis on maturation as a biological process in a cultural setting. Each level of development of children's behavior is determined and standardized on the basis of long-term studies; there is little concern with interpretation of the inner life of the child.

deviance, communication See *communication deviance.*

deviant, deviate Any person differing markedly from what is accepted as the norm, the average, or the usual. Probably the most common use of the term is in relation to the sexual form. See *deviation, sexual.*

deviation, average See *deviation, mean.*

deviation, conjugate See *nerve, oculomotor.*

deviation, ego See *children, ego deviant.*

deviation, mean (MD) A description of the variability of a frequency distribution; also called *average deviation* (or AD). The mean deviation from the mean is computed by tabulating the amount by which each individual score in distribution differs from the mean score, considering all these deviations as positive, and then computing their mean.

The *standard deviation* (SD, also called σ) is similar to the mean deviation, except that each deviation from the mean is squared, the squared deviations are totaled and averaged, and the square root of the average is then extracted. This gives a more reliable measure of variability than the mean deviation and is in wider use because other statistical measures are calculated on the basis of the SD. In any distribution that approximates the normal curve in form, about 65% of the measures will lie within one SD of the mean, and about 95% will lie within two SD's of the mean. When used as a measure of variability the SD is known as the *standard error.*

deviation, median A description of the variability of a frequency distribution; also called probable deviation or probable error (PE) The median deviation from the mean is computed by tabulating the amount by which each individual score in a distribution differs from the mean score, considering all these deviations as positive, and then computing their median. The median deviation is the absolute amount of deviations from the mean that is exceeded by half the measures in a distribution.

deviation, probable See *deviation, median.*

deviation, sexual In the 1968 revision of psychiatric nomenclature, sexual deviation

is a major category of personality disorders and includes:

302.0 *homosexuality* (q.v.)
302.1 fetishism (see *fetish*)
302.2 *pedophilia* (q.v.)
302.3 *transvestitism* (q.v.)
302.4 *exhibitionism* (q.v.)
302.5 *voyeurism* (q.v.)
302.6 *sadism* (q.v.)
302.7 *masochism* (q.v.)
302.8 other sexual deviation

In DSM-III, all of the above are included within the subgroups of *sexual disorders* (q.v.).

deviation, skew Skew deviation (Hertwig-Magendie phenomenon) is a rare cerebellar or collicular sign, characterized by downward and inward rotation of the eyeball on the same side of the lesion and upward and outward rotation of the eyeball on the opposite side.

deviation, standard (SD, σ) The standard deviation is a summary of the variation of the items in a frequency distribution. It is the square root of the mean square of the deviation of each variable in the series from the mean of the series. See *deviation, mean.*

device, safety Karen Horney's term for any means of protecting the self from threat, especially the hostility of the environment; although a more general term, safety device is approximately equivalent to defense mechanism.

Devic's disease Neuromyelitis optica; ophthalmoneuromyelitis; disseminated myelitis with optic neuritis. An acute demyelinating disease that is sometimes self-limited but which in 50% of cases is relapsing, progressive, and fatal. It consists of massive foci of demyelination in the optic nerves and chiasma and spinal cord, which may undergo softening and cavitation. Etiology is unknown and there is no definitive treatment.

Devil's Pact See *compliance, strategic.*

devolution Hughlings Jackson's term, approximately equivalent to *regression* (q.v.).

dexamethasone See *DST.*

dextrality-sinistrality See *dominance, cerebral; laterality.*

dextrophobia Fear of objects to the right.

DFP See *psychotomimetic.*

DI *Deterioration index* (q.v.).

di Rorschach scoring symbol for inside detail.

diabetic exophthalmic dysostosis (ek-sof-thal-am'ik dis-os-tō'sis) *Xanthomatosis* (q.v.).

diaboleptics Maudsley's term for those who claim to have supernatural communications.

diagnosis, negative Diagnosis by means of exclusion; "wastebasket" diagnosis.

diagnosis, social Psychiatric social workers thus denote the conditions prevailing in the environment of the patient.

diagnosis, structural See *structural.*

diagnostic confidence See *sensitivity.*

diamine Any substance that contains two amine groups. Such substances may be of etiologic significance in the production of endogenously occurring psychoses. See *amine; epinephrine; ergotropic; serotonin.*

diaphragma sellae (dē-à-fràg'mà sel'lē) See *meninges.*

diaschisis (dī-as'ki-sis) A term introduced by Monakow to indicate that when one "center" of the brain is affected another distant "center," which has a definite relationship to the affected one, becomes functionally disordered.

diastematomyelia (dī-as-tem-à-tō-mī-ē'lē-à) Partial duplication of the spinal cord, usually in the thoracolumbar segments, with a column of connective tissue that sometimes contains bone or cartilage in the cleft between the two halves of the cord. Myelography shows a filling defect and dilatation of the vertebral canal, and also congenital deformity of two or more vertebrae.

diathesis (dī-ath'ē-sis) Constitutional disposition, or predisposition, to some anomalous or morbid condition "which no longer belongs within the confines of the normal variability, but already begins to represent a potential disease condition." These various *diathetic* conditions are distinguished by the fact that diathetic individuals respond with abnormal or truly pathological reactions to physiological stimuli, such as foods, or other ordinary conditions of life, such as sunlight, that are borne by the majority of individuals without injury. (Pende, N. *Constitutional Inadequacies,* 1928) See *defense, character; structure, character;* and the multiple listings under *character; constitution; diathesis; disposition; personality; temperament.*

diathesis, arthritic Constitutional morbid condition that according to the Italian school, includes the closely related exudative and hypersecretory diathesis as well as arthritism and is said to occur especially in the *megalosplanchnic* (q.v.) hypervegetative constitution.

Arthritic subjects are prone to syndromes grouped by the French school under the heading of diseases of *bradytrophism* (q.v.). Their organs have a tendency to sclerosis (fibroplastic diathesis) due to the special primary hyperplasia and irritability of the visceral connective tissue.

Czerny's exudative diathesis readily becomes engrafted upon the overnourished megalosplanchnic constitution, inclined as it is to anomalies of metabolism. This condition occurs in growing children and is so similar to the arthritic diathesis of adults that it has been called infantile arthritism. Skin and mucosae are very delicate, fragile, and soft, and there is a tendency to infection of the connective-lymphatic tissue.

diathesis, colloidoclastic A morbid condition in children that results from an imperfect albuminoid metabolism and leads to an unstable colloidoplasmatic equilibrium (colloidoclasia). The condition is believed to belong to the syndrome of infantile arthritism which is an arthritic (exudative) diathesis in children. See *diathesis, exudative.*

diathesis, eosinophilic A subtype of the *arthritic diathesis.* The condition is characterized by various degrees of eosinophila, which may range from 8 to 30% and seems to reflect anaphylactic crises.

diathesis, explosive A clinical subdivision of the traumatic psychoses characterized by intense irritability, particularly after the ingestion of alcohol; the irritability sometimes leads to acts of violence that appear unmotivated, that is, automatic. See *dyscontrol, episodic; neurosis, traumatic; psychosis, traumatic.*

diathesis, exudative (eks-ū'dà-tiv) This term, introduced by Czerny, designates a form of *arthritic diathesis* occurring in growing children and characterized by a constitutional condition called *colloidoclastic diathesis* by Widal.

diathesis, fibroplastic A constitutional anomaly characterized by a sclerotic degeneration of various organs, due to a primary hyperplasia and irritability of the visceral connective tissue, and occurring in the course of a general *arthritic diathesis*.

diathesis, glial (glēal) A constitutional condition characterized by a hyperplastic or neoplastic tendency of primitive or more differentiated glial cells. The condition is believed to underlie a series of "heredo-familial nervous diseases that usually develop on the soil of the lymphatic or hypoplastic constitution, and which include cerebral tuberous sclerosis and gliomatous cerebral hypertrophy, spinal gliosis and syringomyelia, glioma, neurofibromatosis, progressive lenticular degeneration, and other degenerative scleroses of the corpora striata." (Pende, N. *Constitutional Inadequacies,* 1928)

diathesis, hypersecretory See *diathesis, arthritic*.

diathesis, lithic A constitutional condition characterized by uricemia and a tendency to form urinary calculi. It is often combined in the same family or subject with an oxalic acid diathesis, in which case it alternates with gout, oxaluria, and oxalic lithiasis.

diathesis, neoplastic Tendency of certain constitutional types to develop neoplastic conditions, especially carcinoma. Some typologists assign the equivalent of the pyknic or megalosplanchnic constitutions to persons with this tendency, while others postulate an association of the arthritic and the neoplastic diathesis, or an association between the cancerous and the *exudative diathesis*.

diathesis, neuroarthritic Practically identical with *arthritic diathesis*.

diathesis, neuropathic *Obs.* Neurasthenia.

diathesis, oxalic acid See *diathesis, lithic*.

diathesis-stress model See *model, diathesis-stress*.

diathesis, traumatophilic A predisposition to accidents, sometimes referred to as *accident proneness*. Fenichel considers this to be a manifestation of Freud's repetition compulsion. "The repetition is desired to relieve a painful tension; but because the repetition is also painful, the person is afraid of it and tends to avoid it. Usually, therefore, a compromise is sought: a repetition on a smaller scale or under more encouraging circumstances. The ambivalence toward this repetition shows itself in the phenomena of traumatophilia and

traumatophobia, in the fact that whatever these persons [of traumatophilic diathesis] undertake turns into a trauma; they fear this, and nevertheless they strive for it." (*PTN*) See *proneness, accident; recidivism*.

diathesis, uric acid See *diathesis, lithic*.

DIB Diagnostic Interview for Borderlines (see *borderline personality; borderline psychosis*). A semistructured interview that includes a systematic review of social adaptation, impulse/action patterns, affects, psychotic episodes and experiences, and interpersonal relationships described by John Gunderson, Jonathan Kolb, and Virginia Austin (*American Journal of Psychiatry 138,* 1981)

didactic Fitted or intended to teach; used often to refer to formal teaching lessons, such as lectures, in contrast to discussion groups or seminars. Didactic psychoanalysis is also known as training or tuitional analysis. See *analysis, orthodox; analysis, tuitional*.

diecious, dioecious (dī-ē'shus) Sexually distinct, that is, being of one or the other sex and not hermaphroditic.

diencephalon See *forebrain*.

diencephalosis A term used to refer to any of the many possible disturbances or functional alterations of the diencephalon and/or its interconnections. The following symptom groups are included: (1) lack of restraint and inhibition, (2) paradoxical coexistence of opposed functional disturbances, (3) alterations of biological rhythm, (4) various endocrine dysfunctions, (5) abnormalities of growth and development, (6) certain forms of psychopathy, (7) vascular lability, (8) dysthermia, (9) electroencephalograph abnormalities, and (10) cranioradiographic abnormalities. (Pende, N. *Medicina 6,* 1957)

dietary chaos syndrome See *restricters*.

differential fertility See *fertility, differential*.

differentiation, sex See *sex differentiation*.

diffuse sclerosis See *sclerosis, diffuse*.

dihybrid (dī-hī'brid) A hybrid individual differing in two hereditary characters, or hereditary traits based on two pairs of genes. See *hybrid*.

diisopropyl fluorophosphate (dī-ī-sō-prō-pil) See *psychotomimetic*.

dikephobia Fear of justice.

dilapidation *Deterioration; dementia* (qq.v.).

dilemma, Scull's The dilemma highlighted by sociologist Andrew Scull, consisting of claims that it is wrong both to get patients out of mental hospitals and to keep them in. Because both commitment to mental hospital and release of a patient from mental hospital often depend on a prediction of that patient's future behavior, there can never be absolute certainty about the decision either to admit or discharge. As in most such situations, positions have been taken at each extreme, and a small number of people oppose involuntary hospitalization under any conditions. One extreme is expressed by those sociologists who, critical of the entire existing organization of mental health care, sometimes label community care *decarceration,* just as they speak of *social control* instead of care and treatment.

dilution, transference The diminution of the intensive transference toward the therapist owing to the presence of sibling and identification transferences to other members of a group.

dim-out *Blackout* (q.v.).

DIMS Disorders of initiating and maintaining sleep; the insomnias. See *sleep disorders.*

dinomania Dancing mania; *choreomania* (q.v.).

Diogenes syndrome *Hoarding* (q.v.).

dionism Heterosexuality. See *uranism.*

diplegia Bilateral paralysis of corresponding parts of the body.

diplegia, congenital spastic *Little's disease* (q.v.).

diploid The original stage in the maturation of a reproductive cell, in which the number of chromosomes is full, that is, not yet halved by the reduction division following the first or equation division. See *chromosome; maturation.*

diploid mode The normal number of chromosomes—in humans, 46.

diploidy (dip'loid-ē) In the meiotic process of cell division the genetic term diploidy signifies the original quota of chromosomes, that is, the *full* number resulting from the duplicating equation division, prior to their reduction to the halved or haploid number through the reduction division. See *haploidy.*

diplopia (di-plō'-pē-à) Double vision; due to paralysis of the ocular muscles, which causes the image of an object to fall upon noncorresponding portions of the two retinae. See *nerve, oculomotor.*

diplopia, monocular A condition in which two images are seen with one eye. The existence of true monocular diplopia is questioned and when present is regarded as a sign of hysteria.

dippoldism Flogging of (school) children. The German schoolteacher Dippold was tried and convicted of manslaughter for flogging a child to death. Thereafter the act of flagellation came to be known as dippoldism. See *flagellation.*

dipsomania Enomania; oinomania; a type of *alcoholism* (q.v.) characterized mentally by a variety of responses peculiar to the drinker. Some become shy and retiring; others quite boisterous and pugnacious; still others exhibit paranoid reactions. The alcoholic bout and its results last as a rule for several days, rarely for several weeks. "In the intervals, that may last several weeks but also many months, most of these patients are temperate, and some are abstinent." (Bleuler, *TP*) Dipsomania is usually regarded as a symptom or a syndrome of some more fundamental disorder, such as psychopathic personality, epilepsy, or schizophrenia. Bleuler includes dipsomania among the acute syndromes in the schizophrenias.

dipsosis avens (dēp-sō'zēs àv'ens) *Obs.* Excessive craving for alcohol.

directive In psychiatry, and particularly in the areas of psychotherapy and counseling, directive refers to an active and often authoritarian approach in which the therapist gives advice, suggests or demands that the patient follow certain courses of action, etc. See *D-O psychiatrist.*

directive, genetic Determination of form, structure, behavior, function, etc., by genes or heredity, basically a description of the *genotype* as opposed to the *phenotype* (qq.v.).

dirty urine See *urine, dirty.*

DIS Diagnostic Interview Schedule; see *NIMH-DIS.*

disability A handicap, defect, or lack, especially when such defect interferes with adequate or normal functioning; current popular term is "physically challenged." Disability refers to what the patient does not do and is defined in terms of the relationship of the patient to his environment; *handicap* refers to what the person cannot do and is something that is a part of the patient.

A lack of ability is an *inability* rather than a disability if it is either characteristic of a species until a certain developmental or maturational level is reached or due to lack of specialized training. See *disease*.

disadvantaged Lacking assets; a social psychiatry neologism of the 1970s denoting persons or groups who are economically poor and/or members of minority groups. Disadvantages typically include deprivations in housing, education, work opportunity, and medical (and particularly prenatal) care and are associated with family disruption, faulty identity formation or malignant identity diffusion, and excessively high rates of juvenile offenses and of admissions to state mental hospitals.

disaggregation, mental According to Janet, "a special form of weakness owing to which an elementary idea is left in isolation, and is not combined with others to form a higher unity. . . . It is a condition of natural and perpetual distraction, which prevents these persons from appreciating any other idea than the one which actually occupies their mind." (*PH*)

disaster Sudden and unexpected loss, reversal, injury; catastrophe or *trauma* (q.v.). Three stages of early reaction are recognized: (1) initial shock and disorganization because of immobilizing and overpowering anxiety; (2) dependency and suggestibility with passive and almost blind acceptance of direction from others; (3) reorganization and recovery, with a return of control and independence often accompanied by apprehensiveness and repetitive descriptions of the incident and the rescue efforts. See *neurosis, traumatic; post-traumatic stress disorder*.

disattach See *attachment, liquidation of*.

discharge An unloading, release, dismissal. In neurophysiology, synonymous with *firing*, the delivery of excitation from one neuron to the next. In mental hospital statistics, the dropping of a patient from the rolls because of termination of services (patients transferred to other facilities and patients who die are not usually counted as discharges).

discharge, affective Release of emotion, usually an energetic reaction including the whole range of voluntary and involuntary reflexes, by which, according to experience, the emotions—from weeping up

to a clear act of revenge—are habitually worked off.

"If this reaction occurs with sufficient intensity a great part of the affect disappears; common speech bears witness to these facts of everyday observation in the expressions 'to cry out,' 'to storm oneself out.' " (Freud, *CP*)

discriminanda See *intelligence*.

disease Many words have been used to refer to conditions whose definitions to date have been generally unsatisfactory; among them are *abnormality, affliction, condition, defect, deviation, disability, disfigurement, disorder, disturbance, dysfunction, illness, injury, lesion, reaction, variant, wound*.

"Illness and disease are closely related, but diseases are more robust ontologically than illnesses. They are regarded as entities having characteristic signs and symptoms with known or discoverable underlying 'mechanisms' and, ultimately, known or discoverable etiologies." C. Culver and B. Gert (*Philosophy in Medicine*, 1982) suggest instead the term *malady* to designate any condition in which there is something wrong with the person. "A person has a malady if and only if he has a condition, other than his rational beliefs and desires, such that he is suffering, or at increased risk of suffering, an evil (death, pain, disability, loss of freedom or opportunity, or loss of pleasure) in the absense of a distinct sustaining cause." See *abnormality*.

disease, Allan-Dent *Argininosuccinic aciduria* (q.v.).

disease, association 1. Coexisting myoclonia and epilepsy; see *epilepsy, myoclonus*. 2. Schizophrenia; see *associations, disturbances of*.

disease, Baló's (Jozsef Matthias Baló, Hungarian neurologist, b. 1895) Concentric demyelination. See *sclerosis, diffuse*.

disease, Bamberger's (Eugen Bamberger, Austrian physician, 1858–1921) A neuromuscular disorder consisting of clonic spasms of the leg muscles which produce jumping motions.

disease, barbed wire Vischer's term for any reactive mental disturbance of prisoners, who are often held in barbed wire camps. See *psychosis, prison*.

disease, Beard's (George M. Beard, American physician, 1839–83) An old term for *neurasthenia* (q.v.); named after the physician who introduced the name neurasthenia in 1869.

disease, Bell's Collapse delirium, delirious mania; the most severe of the manic type of manic-depressive psychosis. See *Bell's mania; psychosis, manic-depressive.*

disease, Binswanger's See *lacuna.*

disease, caisson Caisson disease (*diver's paralysis, the bends, tunnel disease*) is a circulatory disturbance occurring in the nervous system, observed when a person, subjected to high air pressure (e.g. in diving or working under compressed air in a caisson) returns too suddenly to normal atmosphere. There is a question as to whether the sudden release of pressure causes air emboli in the brain and spinal cord or whether the blood vessels dilate, giving rise to congestion and stasis. Pathologically, the spinal cord shows softening and necrosis.

The symptoms are acute in onset with headache, pains in the epigastrium, limbs, and back, sufficient to double the patient up (the bends), dizziness, dyspnea, nausea, vomiting, coughing, and partial or complete paralysis, usually of both lower extremities. Cerebral symptoms may occur, such as aphasia, double vision, confusion, coma, and convulsions.

disease, demyelinating (dē-mī'e-lin-ā-ting) See *demyelination.*

disease, Fahr's Idiopathic nonarteriosclerotic symmetrical calcification of cerebral vessels; a slowly progressive disorder, with onset between the ages of 30 to 50 years, manifested by organic dementia and extrapyramidal motor dysfunction; first described by T. Fahr, a German neurologist, in 1930.

disease, flight into "By means of *flight into the disease* one achieves definite aims through the disease; by an attack of rage one achieves a yielding; by a fainting spell, a new hat; and by the more protracted disease one gets a pleasant sojourn in a sanatorium. By means of all these one can at the same time compel consideration, secure care and tenderness, obtain power over others who have to adjust themselves to the disease, extort an allowance, evade tasks from the simple household duties up to the terrors of the trenches." (Bleuler, *TP*) See *gain, epinosic; gain, morbid.*

disease, Friedmann's (Max Friedmann, German physician, 1858–1925) *Narcolepsy* (q.v.).

disease, Gaucher's (gō-shā') (Philippe Gaucher, French physician, 1854–1918) A familial disorder of lipoid metabolism (lipid histiocytosis) characterized by the deposition of keratin in the reticuloendothelial cells of the liver and spleen and in the ganglion cells of the cerebral cortex, basal ganglia, and cerebellum. Onset of the disorder is usually between the ages of 6 and 12 months, typically in females. Symptoms include listlessness, apathy, head retraction, hypertonicity, bulbar signs, and sometimes mental retardation. Associated typical findings are hepatosplenomegaly, pancytopenias, and bone lesions. Diagnosis is relatively simple by measuring the activity of leukocyte acid beta-glucosidase, which is greatly decreased. Clinical manifestations vary widely, probably because some of the different mutations of the beta-glucosidase locus produce very mild forms of the disease.

disease, genetotrophic A disease "in which the genetic pattern of the afflicted individual calls for an augmented supply of a particular nutrient (or nutrients) for which there develops, as a result, a nutritional deficiency." (Williams, R.J., et al. in *Management of Addictions*, ed. E. Podolsky, 1955) "On the basis of our studies with rats it seems likely that the basic etiologic factor in human alcoholism is genetotropic, and that the sociological and psychological factors so generally considered as fundamental factors are only precipitating factors for the development of the clinical syndrome." (Ibid.) The factor described is believed to depend on one or more partial genetic blocks: "Briefly described, such a block involves a heritable trait that is characterized not by a complete inability to carry out a specific enzymatic transformation, but by a diminished potentiality for producing the biochemical change. This in turn leads to an augmented requirement for some specific nutritional factor or factors." (Ibid.)

disease, Hakim's See *hydrocephalus, normal-pressure.*

disease, Heller's See *dementia infantilis.*

disease, Jakob-Creutzfeldt's See *Creutzfeldt-Jakob's disease.*

disease, Janet's (zhȧ-nāz') *Psychasthenia* (q.v.).

disease, Leber's (Theodor Leber, German ophthalmologist, 1840–1917) Hereditary familial primary optic atrophy, occurring between the ages of 18 and 30, more common in the male progeny, but transmitted from the female. It is a bilateral, slowly progressive condition, often remaining stationary or even regressing. There is a central scotoma and a normal peripheral field. See *atrophy, optic.*

disease, Lindau's (Arvid Lindau, Swedish pathologist, b. 1892) An angioma of the brain occurring in connection with angiomatosis of the retina, occasionally familial and hereditary. See *angiomatosis, trigeminal cerebral.*

disease, Little's (William John Little, English surgeon, 1810–94) Includes the spastic diplegias, presumably due to bilateral congenital brain defects, involving especially the pyramidal motor system, or to lesions acquired at birth. Walking is retarded, the gait is spastic, and the child walks on its toes (pes equinovarus). The thighs are adducted, the knees rub together, and the legs cross in progression (*scissors gait*). This spastic paralysis may involve both upper extremities as well. Frequently present are various grades of mental disturbance, ranging from hyperexcitability and irritability to severe retardation. Typical epileptic convulsions may occur. Strabismus, dysarthria, drooling, and abnormal involuntary and associated movements may be observed.

disease, Niemann-Pick A familial disturbance in phospholipid metabolism (a lipid histiocytosis) characterized by mental deterioration, progressive blindness, hepatosplenomegaly, and brownish discoloration of the skin. The disease is rapidly progressive and leads to death within two years of onset.

The disease is due to a deficiency of the spingomyelin-cleaving enzyme, sphingomyelinase, and is manifested by accumulation of sphingomyelin in the reticuloendothelial cells of the liver, spleen, bone marrow, and lymph nodes. Diagnosis is confirmed by demonstration of vacuolation and degeneration of ganglion cells in biopsies of the rectal wall.

disease, Norrie's (Gordon Norrie, Danish ophthalmologist, 1855–1941) Atrophia bulborum hereditaria; an X-linked recessive syndrome consisting of retinal malformation, mental retardation, and deafness; often misdiagnosed as retrolental fibroplasia, retinoblastoma, retinal pseudoglioma, or congenital toxoplasmosis. The eye pathology consists of bilateral gliomalike masses of tissue arising from the retina, with subsequent atrophy of the iris, lens, and corneal opacities and shrinking of the eyes, usually in the preschool years. No chromosomal or biochemical abnormalities have yet been identified as being responsible for the disease. Female carriers do not demonstrate ocular or hearing defects. (Holmes, L.B., *New England Journal of Medicine 284*, 1971)

disease, Pick's See *Pick's disease.*

disease, pink *Acrodynia* (q.v.).

disease, Saint Dymphna's (St. Dymphna, patron saint of the insane, a British noblewoman, murdered by her insane father, in Gheel, Belgium) Any mental disease; insanity.

disease, Saint Mathurin's (St. Mathurin, patron saint of idiots and fools) Epileptic psychosis.

disease, Saint Valentine's Epilepsy.

disease, sanatorium *Hospitalism; hospitalitis* (qq.v.).

disease, Schilder's (Paul Schilder, American neurologist, 1886–1940) Schilder's disease, or encephalitis periaxialis diffusa, is a slowly progressive degenerative disease of the brain occurring mainly in children and young people; it is characterized essentially by slowly advancing cerebral blindness and progressive mental deterioration terminating usually in complete amentia. See *sclerosis, diffuse.*

disease, Simmonds' (Morris Simmonds, Hamburg physician, 1855–1925) See *cachexia, hypophysial.*

disease, Tay-Sachs See *Tay-Sachs disease.*

disease, tunnel *Disease, caisson* (q.v.).

disease, Urbach-Wiethe (Eric Urbach, U.S. dermatologist, 1893–1946) An autosomal recessive trait involving storage of protein and lipid and manifested clinically by (1) cutaneous and mucosal lesions—papillomatous deposits of protein-lipid complex in the eyelids, labial mucosa, and sublingual areas; (2) bilateral intracranial calcifications in the caudate nucleus, globus pallidus, and amygdala; (3) seizures (grand mal and/or psychomotor), rage attacks, and recent memory loss but otherwise intact intellect; (4) short stature; (5) alopecia; and (6) photosensitivity.

disengagement Detachment, breaking free from involvement or commitment; most often used to refer to the disengagement theory of old age, which holds that acceptance of the inevitability of diminishing social and personal interactions with increasing age is associated with a higher degree of satisfaction and better adjustment. This is in contrast to the *activity theory*, which holds that continued activity and involvement are essential for maintaining satisfaction, self-esteem, and health in old age. See *continuity theory of aging.*

disfigurement See *disease.*

dishabituation According to A.K. Nyman of Lund University, a phenomenon characteristic of borderline ("nonregressive") schizophrenia consisting of hypersensitivity, overreactions to, and intense, unpleasant feelings aroused by involuntary scratching, sounds, gestures, etc.

disharmony, affective Lack of conformity of the emotional reaction and the ideational content characteristic of schizophrenic disorders.

disinhibition Removal of an inhibition. The inhibitory function of the cerebral cortex can be reduced by various agents—for instance, alcohol. If such a cortical function is impaired or reduced in its activity, the inhibitory influences of the cortex are diminished or removed and then a disinhibition takes place, indicating that without the high cortical control, lower vegetative or emotional functions are manifested.

disintegration Disorganization of psychic processes. "We may therefore expect that a weakening or annihilation of the influence which general conceptions, higher emotions, and the permanent general trend of volition exercise on our thinking, feeling, and acting, must draw after it that inner *disintegration*, those 'schizophrenic' disorders, which we meet with in dementia praecox." (Kraepelin, *DP*) See *integration; disruption.*

disintegrative psychoses In ICD-9 (see *International Classification of Diseases*), disorders in which normal development for the first few years is followed over a period of a few months by loss of social skills and speech and severely disordered emotions,

behavior, and relationships. Most such psychoses are organic in origin. In DSM-III they would be classified as dementia, with an indication on Axis III of the specific organic basis, such as lipoidosis or leukodystrophy.

disk, choked See *papilledema.*

disk, herniated lumbar intervertebral Protrusion of the central portion of the intervertebral disk (the nucleus pulposus) through the surrounding annulus fibrosus, which holds the bodies of the vertebrae together. Such herniation is usually due to trauma, induced typically by lifting a heavy object in a bent-forward position or by a fall in a similar posture. Almost half of the cases begin in the fourth decade, and approximately three-quarters of the cases are male. Most herniations are between the fourth and fifth lumbar bodies, or betwen the fifth lumbar and first sacral bodies. Herniation of the disk results in compression of the spinal nerve running to the foramen one segment below; the clinical result is *sciatica*, i.e. pain beginning in the lumbar region and spreading down the back of one lower limb to the ankle, usually intensified by coughing or sneezing.

Four symptom-phases are recognized: (1) back pain, muscle spasm, and trunk tilt; (2) compression of the spinal nerve resulting in sciatica, with paresthesiae in the lateral calf and foot, muscle spasm, focal tenderness, and diminution of the ankle jerk; (3) paresis of the lower extremity and muscle atrophy; (4) paralysis of the affected extremity, marked sensory loss, and bladder and bowel disturbances.

In most cases, conservative treatment with analgesics and mobilization is adequate; in about 10% of cases, interlaminar operation is indicated.

dismemberment, fear of A patient's fear that he is losing part of his body is called the dismemberment complex, or fear of dismemberment. It is most often seen in the involutional psychoses and in the schizophrenias. In some cases described by Schilder, the patient develops a strong feeling of persecution. This is explained in the following manner: Through the process of fear of dismemberment the individual projects to the outside world parts of his body, and then the endangered parts of the body regain their relation to the individual by coming back in the form of persecutors. Such a mechanism is clearly illustrated in the example of the depressive menopausal woman who feared she was going to cut off all her fingers every time she held a knife in her hand. She later developed a persecution complex in which five different enemies were following her. (Schilder, P. *Psycho-therapy*, 1938)

disorder See *disease*.

disorder, affective determined An expression used by Adolf Meyer as equivalent with manic-depressive psychosis.

disorder, behavior See *behavior disorders*.

disorder, neurotic In DSM-III, a mental disorder in which the predominant feature is one or more symptoms that are a source of distress and are recognized as alien to the personality (ego-dystonic); without treatment, the condition is relatively enduring or recurrent, and although it may be severely disabling it does not lead to gross violation of social norms or to loss of reality testing. Further, the condition is not a mild transitory reaction to stress nor is there any demonstrable organic factor in its etiology. Instead, it is believed, the specific etiology is the *neurotic process*, consisting of the following sequence: (1) unconscious conflicts between opposing wishes, prohibitions, etc., leading to (2) unconscious perception of potential danger, or dysphoria, leading to (3) defense mechanisms, leading to (4) symptoms and/or personality disturbance. Neurotic disorders are manifested in diverse ways and are included among the affective, anxiety, somatoform, dissociative, and psychosexual disorders of DSM-III. See *neurosis*.

disorder, personality See *personality disorders*.

disordered behavior, classification of Rado (*American Journal of Psychiatry 110*, 1953) offered the following provisional classification of disordered behavior, based mainly on the psychodynamic phase of etiology: (A) Overreactive disorders: (1) Emergency dyscontrol; (2) Descending dyscontrol; (3) Sexual disorders; (4) Social overdependence; (5) Common maladaptation or combination of sexual disorder with social overdependence; (6) Expressive pattern; (7) Obsessive pattern; (8) Paranoid pattern; (B) Mood cyclic disorders; (C)

Schizotypal disorders: (1) Compensated schizo-adaptation; (2) Decompensated schizo-adaptation; (3) Schizotypal disintegration marked by adaptive incompetence; (D) Extractive disorders; (E) Lesional disorders; (F) Narcotic disorders; (G) Disorders of war adaptation.

disorders, episodic Any precipitous interruption in the lifestyle of the subject, with the appearance of behavior that is out of character for the person himself and usually out of context or inappropriate to the situation at hand. Such bursts of impulsivity or *acting-out* (q.v.) may be the first sign of personality change in an organic psychosyndrome, or they may represent dyscontrol on a more purely psychologic-motivational basis. See *dyscontrol, episodic*.

disorders, extractive See *psychodynamics, adaptational*.

disorders, genetic See *counseling, genetic*.

disorders, moodcyclic See *psychodynamics, adaptational*.

disorders of impulse control Impulse disorders (q.v.) ; in DSM-III, the following are included: (1) *pathologic gambling*—characterized by chronic preoccupation with urges to gamble and gambling behavior that interferes with personal, family, or vocational responsibilities and pursuits (e.g. arrests for attempts to obtain money illegally, defaulting on debts, absenteeism); (2) *kleptomania* (q.v.) ; (3) *pyromania* (q.v.) ; (4) *trichotillomania*, or repetitive *hair pulling* (q.v.).

disorders, overreactive See *psychodynamics, adaptational*.

disorganization Loss or reduction in the usual or expected degree of organization, structure, or systematization, or evenness of performance. Disorganization may be indicative of structural damage to any organ whose ability to function is thereby compromised. Disorganization of movement, a type of dyssynergia that is also known as *decomposition of movement*, indicates cerebellar dysfunction and is characterized by a jerky, broken, "by the numbers" quality of movements that are ordinarily performed smoothly and easily. Mental or *personal disorganization* usually refers to a significant inability of the person to organize and maintain his living in a reasonably orderly, predictable, and integrated fashion. Such disorganization is

characteristic of many patients with organic mental disorders or with schizophrenia or acute manic episodes, although the
term is sometimes applied loosely to any
person who does not meet the standards of
the observer's desire for organization and
orderliness.

disorientation Impairment in the understanding of temporal, spatial, or personal
relationships. See *syndrome, organic.*

disorientation, autopsychic Synonymous
with impairment of insight. See *orientation,
autopsychic.*

disparagement, mania for A term used by
Janet, who says that "one who feels himself
to be a weakling and has a terrible dread
of effort, has a different idea of competition. His aim is to triumph, not by raising
himself, but by lowering his rival. Thus it
is that the psychasthenic secures a partial
and thrifty success by preventing others
from acting.... In many instances, an
additional factor is his dread of others'
success." (*PH*)

dispersion, semantic See *dissociation, semantic.*

displaced child syndrome See *syndrome, displaced child.*

displacement 1. Transference of the emotions (affective cathexis) from the original
ideas to which they are attached—to other
ideas. It is assumed in psychoanalysis that
psychic energy may exist as an entity, such
as "free-floating" libido, that is, that it possesses a certain autonomy. It is sufficiently
mobile to leave one set of ideas and go to
another. By such an arrangement the affects may be able to gain the realm of consciousness, attaching themselves to ideas to
which the patient is ordinarily indifferent.
By such an arrangement the patient is
spared the pain of knowing the original
source of the affects. A patient had a morbid fear that illuminating gas was issuing
from the jet in his room. The fear was not
allayed in any way by logic. The patient
recognized how ridiculous it was to let such
an idea control his life. Upon analysis it was
found that the fear was associated with the
repressed wish for his father's death.

Schizophrenic patients exhibit displacement of affects to a remarkable degree.
What are seemingly the most inconsequential thoughts may be heavily emotion-
alized. One schizophrenic patient used to
get into a state of uncontrollable rage over

his shoestrings. Another was ecstatic over
the word "there."

The displacement of affects presupposes also the displacement of ideas.

2. Shifting of id impulses from one
pathway to another. When, for instance,
aggression cannot express itself through
direct motor discharge, as in fisticuffs, it
may take the pathway of verbalization.

Displacement manifests itself also with
regard to organic zones. The instincts
shift, for example, from the oral to the
anal, to the genital zones, or to any other
erotogenic zone. In conversion hysteria a
psychic complex may be displaced upon
any potentially acceptable organic structure. Or all the issues connected with
genitality may be displaced to the oral
zone. Displacement "from below upward"
is a common phenomenon.

Dreams afford notable examples of displacement. See *dream.*

displacement of affect See *affect, transposition
of.*

displacement, retroactive Unconscious displacement that reaches back into the patient's early life. When we begin to investigate how far memory can go back into life,
we find that quite often memories are
concealed. "If the content of the concealed
memory belongs to the first years of childhood, but the ideas it represents belong to
a later period of the individual's life, we
speak with Freud about a retroactive displacement." (Brill, A.A. *Basic Principles of
Psychoanalysis,* 1949)

disposing mind and memory *Obs.* "A sound
mind, capable of making a will; remembering the property to be disposed of and the
persons who are the natural objects of
bounty, and comprehending the manner
in which the property is to be distributed."
(Singer, H.D., & Krohn, W.C. *Insanity and
Law,* 1924)

disposition 1. Susceptibility to a disease,
vulnerability. 2. *Temperament* (q.v.); relatively consistent qualities of mood or behavior characteristic of a person that allow
a degree of predictability of his reactions
to particular situations. 3. Prevailing humor or mood.

disposition, brain See *neurogram.*

disposition, constitutional depressive That
type of person who is more or less consistently depressed throughout life. Such per-

sons are retarded in thinking and acting, show a protracted pessimism, and as regards all life experiences, have difficulty in making and completing decisions and lack self-confidence. Bleuler says they display the *melancholic mood*.

The term constitutional depression is used by some to indicate endogenous depression, i.e. one in which precipitating factors are not clear or definite.

disposition, constitutional manic This denotes the type of personality that is more or less of a "manic" disposition throughout life.

"The manic temperament of such people disposes to over-hasty acts and to a thoughtless manner of living in general, when it is not restrained by a particularly sound understanding and a particularly good morality. For that reason we find here on the one hand snobbish, inconsiderate, quarrelsome and cranky ne'er-do-wells, who have no staying powers in their transactions, but on the other hand 'sunny dispositions,' and people endowed with great ability, amounting sometimes to genius, and not rarely gifted with artistic ability who possess a tireless energy." (Bleuler, *TP*) Bleuler says these people have the *manic mood*.

The term constitutional mania is used by some as an equivalent to "endogenous mania," or mania without clear-cut precipitating factors.

disposition, personal See *Allport, Gordon Willard*.

disposition, polymorphous-perverse See *perverse, polymorphous*.

disposition system See *complex, systematized*.

dispositional attribution See *attribution*.

disruption Sudden loss of organization; although disruption is often used synonymously with *disintegration* (q.v.), the latter term more properly is reserved for slow or gradual loss of organization.

disruptive behavior disorders In DSM-III-R, this category includes attention deficit-hyperactivity disorder, oppositional-defiant disorder, and conduct disorder (with aggresive and delinquent subtypes).

disseminated sclerosis See *sclerosis, multiple*.

dissimilation See *assimilation*.

dissimulation The act of pretending or feigning; *denial* (q.v.).

dissimulator One who dissimulates, dissembles, or pretends.

dissociate To split off some part or component of mental activity, which component then acts as an independent unit of mental life. See *dissociation*.

dissociation Segregation of any group of mental processes from the rest of the psychic apparatus; dissociation generally means a loss of the usual interrelationships between various groups of mental processes with resultant almost independent functioning of the one group that has been separated from the rest. As so defined, dissociation and "splitting" are approximately equivalent (for a discussion of differences between splitting in hysterical dissociative states and splitting in the schizophrenias, see *personality, multiple*); the mental mechanism of *isolation* (q.v.) can also be considered a type of dissociation.

" 'Double' and 'multiple' personality are the terms applied when the same individual at different times appears to be in possession of entirely different mental content, disposition and character, and when one of the different phases shows complete ignorance of the other, an ignorance which may be reciprocal. Each 'sub-personality' (for the personality in these conditions at least is compounded of a series of sub- or partial personalities or 'monads,' as McDougall calls them) is said to be 'dissociated' from the total personality, and from the other sub-personalities, on each occasion when its activities are fully conscious and control the motor apparatus of the individual." (Henderson, D.K., & Gillespie, R.D. *A Text-Book of Psychiatry*, 1936) See *multiple personality disorder*.

Another form of dissociation is included in the definition framed by E.A. Strecker and F.G. Ebaugh: "In effect, *dissociation is the separation of the mind or consciousness by a splitting off of one (sometimes more) component or system of ideas, the personality or remainder of the mind being unable to exert any control over the split-off portion*. This phenomenon of dissociation may be witnessed in the automatic writing of hysteria, in somnambulism, in double personality and in the many delusions of patients." (*Practical Clinical Psychiatry*, 1935)

Another expression of dissociation has to do with the separation of ideas from their consonant affects. For example, a schizophrenic patient laughed heartily while discussing his delusion that he was cut into millions of pieces.

dissociation, semantic The distortion between symbol and meaning that is characteristic of the thought disorder of many schizophrenics. The term includes (1) *enlargement of the semantic halo*—language becomes ambiguous, vague, indeterminate (schizophrenic systematic abstractionism), but is comprehensible and coherent; (2) *semantic distortion*—transfer of meaning to a new symbol (neologism) or to another word (paralogism); (3) *semantic dispersion*—meaning is lost or reduced; language becomes incoherent, agrammatical, asyntactic; and (4) *semantic dissolution*—complete loss of meaning and of communication ability; language is used as a game, or automatically. See *associations, disturbances of.*

dissociative disorders A group of disorders characterized by alterations, typically sudden in onset and of temporary duration, of the normally integrated functions of consciousness or identity; in older classifications usually called hysterical neurosis of the dissociative type or conversion hysteria with predominantly mental symptoms. Included are multiple personality disorder, psychogenic fugue, psychogenic amnesia, and depersonalization disorder. See *depersonalization; dissociation; fugue; hysteria; multiple personality disorder.*

dissolution, semantic See *dissociation, semantic.*

dissonance, cognitive In information theory, *incongruity* (q.v.).

distinct sustaining cause See *sustaining cause, distinct.*

distortion The process of disguising, hiding, or otherwise modifying unconscious mental elements so that they are allowed to enter consciousness, whose censoring mechanisms would not allow them access to consciousness in undisguised form.

There are many ways in which distortion may be effected, e.g. dropping out (repression) of associative links between conscious content and unconscious impulse, displacement of activity onto a substitute object, replacement of objectionable impulse with another one that is associatively connected. "It is the task of the analyst's interpretative work to undo and make retroactive the distortion caused by resistances." (Fenichel, *PTN*)

distortion, apperceptive A subjective interpretation of a perception that is dynamically meaningful in that perception of the contemporary stimulus is influenced by memories of previous percepts. The various projective tests (Rorschach, TAT, etc.) deal with apperceptive distortions of different degrees.

distortion by transference Misperceptions of the analyst or analytic situation based on *transference* (q.v.). The accusation that the analyst is bored or uninterested may be an expression of the childhood wish for more love and attention from mother rather than an accurate appraisal of the analyst's current attitude toward the patient.

distortion, compromise See *compromise-distortion.*

distortion, ego An inexact, general term that is approximately equivalent to "ego impoverishment," "ego deviation," or "ego immaturity." Some writers, however, use "ego distortion" in a more specific sense to refer to an inability to use the usual ego functions of defense in adapting to painful reality. Thus S. Nacht (*International Journal of Psycho-Analysis 39,* 1958) differentiates between (1) the classical disturbances of ego function, which stem primarily from memory falsifications of past experiences that are distorted by unconscious phantasies of the patient, and (2) ego distortion, where the ego is injured by objectively harmful events that occurred in reality rather than in phantasy.

distortion, memory See *displacement.*

distortion, parataxic Any attitude toward any other person that is based on a phantasized or distorted evaluation of that person or on an identification of that person with other figures from past life.

Freud defined *transference* (q.v.) as a repetition of the attitude toward the parents at the time of the Oedipus complex. Almost invariably in the course of analysis, the patient begins to concern himself with the analyst in terms of these transferred attitudes. Some classical analysts would confine the term transference to this original meaning. Others, however, accept character attitudes also as a part of transference, for these, too, are reaction patterns from the past that are applied indiscriminately to the analytic situation, where they are not suitable. In an attempt to avoid confusion, Sullivan has used the term parataxic distortion to include this whole picture. "Sullivan uses neither the libido concept nor the repetition compulsion as formulated by Freud. Parataxic distortions, according to Sullivan, develop from early but essentially nonsexual integrations with significant people. One develops ways of coping with these people and then tends to apply these ways in later interpersonal integrations. However, the need to repeat is by no means as rigid a compulsion as Freud formulated in the repetition compulsion. Later experiences can modify the pattern consciously and unconsciously. In fact, the process of cure is an example of such a modification. The analyst, by his objectivity and insight, fails to conform to the patient's expectations and this, when the patient realizes it, constitutes a new interpersonal situation which helps to make clear the irrational nature of his own behavior." (Thompson, C. *Psychoanalysis: Evolution and Development*, 1950) One way to learn what is true and what is parataxic in thinking or feelings about another is to compare one's evaluations with those of others. Sullivan calls this comparison *consensual validation*.

distortion, semantic See *dissociation, semantic*.

distractibility See *mania*.

distributed processing See *connectionism*.

distributive analysis and synthesis See *psychobiology*.

disulfiram See *Antabuse*.

ditention Burrow's term, used to indicate the intrusion of affect or bias into the process of attention. In his view, ditention now characterizes human interrelational behavior throughout. Contrasted with cotention. See *attention*.

diurnal Occurring each day, or in the daytime, as opposed to occurring at night (nocturnal).

divagation (dī-và-gā'shun) Rambling thought and speech.

division, cell Process by which new cells originate from old ones, following a definite order. The division of ordinary body cells takes place by *mitosis* and is initiated by the nucleus.

In the nucleus of a resting cell the chromatin is scattered and appears like a fine network. At the first indication of imminent division, however, it is formed in a long thread that breaks up into separate pieces, the *chromosomes*. The mitotic *prophase* is finished when each of the chromosomes splits longitudinally into two and the centrosome has also divided into two halves, which migrate to opposite poles of the nucleus.

In the *metaphase* of mitosis, the nuclear membrane breaks down, and a spindle-shaped mass of fiberlike structures accumulates beside the nucleus, converging toward two opposite poles. The split chromosomes arrange themselves in a plane across the equator of the cell, in such a manner that a spindle fiber is attached to each half-chromosome, apparently connecting it with the adjacent pole.

The next stage, known as the *anaphase*, is characterized by a polar migration of the separated two halves of each chromosome. "The result of this activity is the aggregation at each pole of a group of chromosomes, similar in number and all other visible respects to the single set of mother cell chromosomes from which they arose." (Sinnot, E.W., & Dunn, L.D. *Principles of Genetics*, 1939)

The last stage of division, the *telophase*, completes the replacement of one old cell by two new ones. The chromosomes of each polar group become surrounded by new nuclear membranes and reorganize daughter nuclei exactly like those of the mother cells. Finally, the cytoplasmic cell body is divided between the new nuclei, in animals by a cleavage furrow going inward from the periphery, and in most plants by a row of pellets forming a wall across the middle of the cell.

divorce See *marriage, psychiatric aspects of*.

divorce, emotional A type of marital relationship in which the partners live in separate worlds; contrasted with *mutuality*, which refers to normal interaction between the partners and a give-and-take relationship. Emotional divorce appears to be much more frequent in parents of schizophrenics than in other parents. See *psychotherapy, family*.

divorce, stations of As described by Bohannan (1973), the various issues that confront a divorcing couple: (1) *emotional divorce*—the loss of face and involvement preceding separation; (2) *legal divorce*—one person leaves the house and legal proceedings are initiated; (3) *economic divorce*—reduction in income for each of the couple, property settlement, and other economic entanglements; (4) *coparental divorce*—negotiating the transition to remaining parents while no longer being spouses; (5) *community divorce*—reorganization of friendship networks; (6) *psychic divorce*—reestablishing autonomy as a single person.

divorce therapy A subspecialty of marriage and family therapy consisting of counseling and support for partners who are in the process of terminating their formal, contractual relationship. Major forms are (1) individual treatment for a divorcing person; (2) family counseling with focus on parenting and separation, or counseling each parent separately with the children concerning establishment of separate households; (3) divorce groups, consisting of task- or information-oriented sessions with same-sex persons at various stages in the separating process; and (4) divorce mediation, consisting of helping the couple deal with practical issues such as property settlement and visitation rights; this proffers a therapy model as an alternative to the more usual legal adversary model.

Dix, Dorothea Lynde (1802–87) American reformer in the care of psychiatric patients.

dizygotic (dī-zī-got′ik) Pertaining to a twin pair produced by two eggs; preferable to the synonymous *fraternal, nonidentical.*

DMPEA See *pink spot.*

DNA Deoxyribonucleic acid. See *chromosome.*

DNA probe See *probe.*

Do In Rorschach scoring, an "oligophrenic" response; according to Piotrowski, the *Do* indicates excessive intellectual caution and anxiety, rather than feeblemindedness.

dodge, insanity Fictitious defense of insanity designed to evade punishment for a criminal act.

DOES Disorders of excessive somnolence. See *sleep disorders.*

Dolè-Nyswander program See *methadone.*

dolichocephaly (dol-i-kō-sef′a-lē) See *index, cephalic.*

dolichomorphic (dol-i-kō-mor′fik) Relating to long, thin stature. Dolichomorphic is equivalent to *microsplanchnic* of Viola and corresponds closely to Kretschmer's *asthenic.* See *type, asthenic.*

doll, amputation A doll that can readily be taken apart; used in play therapy with children; introduced by David Levy, who used the doll in a specific situation, where it represented the mother. "It is suggested that breasts be made of clay and attached to the mother doll. A baby doll may then be put to the breast. A brother or sister doll representing the child under investigation or treatment is added to the play setup. The child is encouraged to destroy the baby at the breast, the breasts, and also the mother. The patient may also punish the brother or sister doll." (Bender, L. *Child Psychiatric Techniques,* 1952)

domatophobia Fear of being confined in a house.

domicile Dwelling; residence. *Domiciliary care* is a generic term referring to a spectrum of housing or residential settings ranging from a highly structured, intensively supervised facility to a loosely organized living arrangement that provides patients maximal independence and minimal supervision. Successful *deinstitutionalization* of long-term, chronic mental patients depends upon a combination of continuing medical supervision and regulation of psychopharmacological treatment with the organization technology to ensure ready access to whatever level of psychiatric care their changing needs may require.

Included within the spectrum of settings are (1) *chronic care hospitals,* which provide a high level of continuous nuring care and/or rehabilitation as well as immediately available medical attention (2) *skilled nursing facilities* or *therapeutic residential centers,* which provide 24-hour nursing care or supervision in a community-based facility; (3) *health-related facilities,* most often operated in association with a skilled nursing facility, to provide institutional care less extensive than available in a skilled nursing facility or chronic care hospital; (4) *intermediate care facilities* or *community treatment houses,* which provide 24-hour nursing care or supervision on a temporary basis, typically in a converted residence or similar homelike setting; (5) *halfway houses,* nonmedical facilities that promote socialization and provide patients with a place to stay until a suitable residence is available; (6) *residential facilities, residential care homes,* or *board and care homes,* which provide room and board and limited personal assistance in a group or family setting within the community; (7) *social rehabilitation facilities,* which provide 24-hour services in a group setting to persons who need temporary assistance, guidance or counseling; (8) *satellite housing,* apartments or single-family houses that do not provide live-in staff but do offer some professional supervision and access to assistance in emergencies. Variants of satellite housing are landlord-supervised apartments and *Fairweather lodges.* The latter are operated by patients themselves, with only occasional visits by professionals. (Fairweather, G., et al. *Community Life for the Mentally Ill,* 1969) Other experimental settings include *Soteria House,* a residence for first admission, unmarried schizophrenic patients between 15 and 30 years of age; the setting is usually drug-free (including antipsychotic agents) and the staff is nonprofessional. The Missouri Foster Community Program is patterned after the Gheel Colony in Belgium and provides full integration of former patients into the community.

dominance The genetic mechanism by which one member of an allelic pair of hereditary factors is endowed with the capacity of expressing itself so strongly that it prevails in the hybrids over the contrasting factor and determines the visible appearance of a hybridized individual either completely or, at least, predominantly. The phenotype of any hybrid inheriting a *completely dominant* character from one of the parents exhibits no manifestations of the suppressed, or *recessive,* factor and is thus enabled to appear as a pure-bred organism in spite of its heterozygosity (see *recessiveness*).

In this dominant or *direct* mode of inheritance we observe as a rule that the phenotypically healthy children are also germinally healthy. Once a descending stock is free of a dominant anomaly, it is free forever. A diseased carrier of a dominant trait must always have one diseased parent and, on the average, 50% diseased siblings and children.

Some genetic disorders (e.g. phenylketonuria) are recessive with respect to the occurrence of overt disease but dominant with respect to the chemical abnormality. It will accordingly be seen that the terms dominance and recessiveness are relative rather than precise and exact terms, and

different authorities use the terms in different ways. Some, for example, define a dominant gene as one that causes expression of the disease when present in one parent, and a recessive gene as one that causes expression only when present in both. Genes that always cause the disease are termed fully penetrant, while those that cause it only irregularly are termed partially penetrant.

Since the heterozygotic hybrids of a dominant character appear phenotypically like the homozygotes, homozygosity of a trait-carrier can be assumed only if *both* parents are affected by the same trait. Such cases, of course, are very rare.

If a spontaneous interruption of the direct transmission of a dominant trait is found in some affected families, it must be concluded that the clinical pathology of the trait was not diagnosed, or was inhibited by certain antagonistic factors, or could not be manifested because of the early death of the ordinary trait-carriers.

dominance, cerebral The tendency for certain functions of the brain to be concentrated on a single side of the brain. In right-handed persons, such functions tend to be concentrated in the left cerebral hemisphere; this is spoken of as "left cerebral dominance" or "left hemispheric dominance." The dominant hemisphere is the one that is organized to express language and handle other symbolic functions; it processes information in a sequential, logical, rational, analytic, linear fashion. The nondominant hemisphere processes information in a holistic, parallel, simultaneous fashion; it deals with relational perception, visuospatial information, and orientation. Cerebral or hemisphere dominance is also referred to as *lateralization* or *bimodality.*

There is a relation between hemisphere dominance and handedness, but the two are not identical. Approximately 90% of humans are right-handed (*dextral*), and in 99% of these the left hemisphere is dominant. In 60% of left-handed (*sinistral*) people, the left hemisphere is dominant for language; in 40%, dominance is mixed or language is organized in the right hemisphere.

dominance test See *test, Wada dominance.*

dominant In a strictly genetic sense, this term describes the particular faculty of a hereditary factor, transmitted to a hybrid by one of the parents, to constitute the only expressible member of a given pair of contrasting characters and thus to appear in the hybrid to the exclusion of the contrasted character transmitted by the other parent. See *dominance.*

dominant determinant See *determinant, dream.*

dominant mentality See *group tension, common.*

Don Juan (The Chronicle of Seville relates that Don Juan Tenorio killed Comendador Ulloa at night and carried off his daughter. The father was buried in the family chapel and his statue was erected there. The statue and chapel were destroyed by fire. To end the profligate's debauchery the Franciscan monks lured and killed him and spread the rumor that Don Juan had insulted the Comendador on his tomb and that the new statue had dragged the Don to hell.)

In psychiatry the term Don Juan refers to a type of male *hypersexuality* (q.v.). Sexual activities are aimed toward contradicting inferiority feelings by proof of erotic successes. The Don Juan type is little interested in his woman partner of the moment; for having proved that he can excite her sexually, he must then allay his doubts about his ability to excite other women and so moves on to another conquest. The condition depends on intense narcissistic needs and fears of loss of love, with a pregenital and sadistic coloring of the total sexuality. The Don Juan type of erotomania is frequently a defense against unconscious homosexual impulses.

"Don Juans of achievement" are also recognized; these are people who must pile one success upon another in an attempt to undo previous failures and allay guilt.

donatism Donato (professional name of the Belgian "magnetizer" Alfred d'Hont, 1845–1900) demonstrated the role of imitation in hypnosis; the term donatism was given to that form of hypnosis in which imitation forms an important part.

door, revolving See *readmission.*

dopamine A catecholamine. See *epinephrine.*

dopamine hypothesis The theory that relative overactivity of mesolimbic, mesocortical, or nigrostrial dopaminergic neurons may be present, in at least some schizophrenics. The increase may be responsible for specific symptoms, such as delusions or hallucinations, or for specific mechanisms, such as attentional impairment. This formulation is based largely on the clinical evidence that effective antipsychotic drugs such as the neuroleptics block dopamine (DA) receptors or, as with α-methyltyrosine (AMPT), inhibit DA synthesis, and that indirect DA agonists such as amphetamine and phencyclidine can produce or exacerbate psychotic symptoms.

Doppelganger (dop'el-geNg-ger) A reduplicative paramnesia consisting of the delusion that a double of a person or place exists elsewhere. The phenomenon suggests nondominant parietal lobe pathology and is related to other disturbances of recognition. See *nonrecognition; prosopagnosia; syndrome, Capgras's.*

Dora The subject of a case history written by Freud in 1901 and published in 1905 as "Fragment of an Analysis of a Case of Hysteria." Freud's writings include four other extensive case histories: Little Hans (see *Hans*), the *Rat-Man, Schreber,* and the *Wolf-Man* (qq.v.). The case of Dora was used to illustrate how Freud interpreted dreams and how symptoms could be understood in terms of the repressed parts of mental life.

Dora had been referred to Freud by her father when she was 19. She was subject to fits of depression, irritability, suicidal ideas, and vengeful outbursts. During the 11-week treatment period, it became evident that Dora felt she had been handed over to Herr K, her middle-aged admirer, in return for his toleration of the sexual relationship between her father and Herr K's wife. Beginning at the time Dora was 14, Herr K had made sexual overtures to her. She was both excited and disgusted by his advances and rejected them. Thereafter, however, she began to suffer a loss of appetite, she became fearful of passing any man engaged in affectionate conversation with a lady, and she found any form of kissing disgusting. In addition, she developed a feeling of pressure in the upper part of her body, and fits of coughing accompanied by aphonia or mutism, which sometimes persisted for weeks.

As it turned out, Dora's attacks of coughing and aphonia/mutism coincided with

Herr K's absence, suggesting that speech had no value for her since her loved one was not there to hear it. The pressure in the upper body was interpreted as a displacement from below of feelings of genital engorgement. Dora broke away from treatment before the meaning of all her symptoms was understood and in the transference took revenge on the lover she could not allow herself to have.

doraphobia Fear of the skin of animals.

Dorian love See *love, Dorian.*

doromania Cumpulsive gift giving.

dose dependence, therapeutic Development of physical and psychologic dependence on a prescribed drug even though the patient has never exceeded the prescribed dose. Seen most frequently with sedative-hypnotic drugs after long-term use, therapeutic dose dependence is related to rebound of REM sleep and deterioration of sleep patterns that occur when the drug is withdrawn.

dotage *Senile dementia* (q.v.).

double-agentry See *consent, informed.*

double bind See *bind, double.*

double bind, therapeutic See *therapy, paradoxical.*

double blind Referring to a research method, used primarily in drug investigations, in which neither subject-patient nor rater-evaluator knows whether the drug being studied or a placebo is being administered.

Use of the double-blind method, advantageous as it may be from a research point of view, raises certain ethical questions when the subjects of the study are humans. The physician who permits his patient to be a subject, for example, has to some degree abrogated responsibility for the care of the patient by relinquishing control over selection of the particular treatment modality. For another thing, conventional treatment is being withheld from those subjects who are in the experimental group, while those in the control group are not given the opportunity to receive what may turn out to be a therapeutic breakthrough in the treatment of their condition. Double-blind experiments, in other words, put the experimenter into a double bind, the only solution to which would appear to revolve about obtaining fully informed consent from the subjects of the experiment. See *consent, informed.*

double heterozygousness See *heterozygousness.*

double personality See *personality, multiple.*

double simultaneous tactile sensation See *tactile sensation, double simultaneous.*

doubles, illusion of See *syndrome, Capgras's.*

doubt See *ontogeny, psychic.*

doubt, obsessive An uncertainty that persistently forces itself on the mind of the person and cannot be banished or reasoned away. Obsessive brooding and doubt may represent sexualization of thought, and their unconscious content is the same as in other symptoms of the obsessive-compulsive: bisexuality, ambivalence (love vs. hate), and id impulses vs. superego demands. See *obsession.*

doubting spells See *brooding spells.*

down-regulation Progressive desensitization, usually used to refer to the effects of neurohormones and pharmacologic agents on brain cell receptors. The therapeutic effects of antidepressants, for example, may be achieved by down-regulation of central β-adrenergic receptors that occurs as a result of increased concentration of norepinephrine at the synapse. See *up-regulation.*

Down's disease (John Langdon-Down, English geneticist, 1828–96) Mongolism. See *syndrome, Down.*

doxogenic Induced by one's own ideas, opinion, or belief about what should happen.

Dr In Rorschach scoring, a rare version of a normal or large detail such as one that includes more of the blot than is used in the usual detail response, or one that combines two or more detail responses.

dr Rorschach scoring symbol for an unusual (rare) detail.

dram shop laws Legislation that regulates the selling or serving of alcohol (from dram, meaning a small drink or draft of spirits), including attachment of legal liability to anyone who serves alcoholic beverages.

dramatism Flamboyant or histrionic behavior.

dramatization The part of the manifest dream that appears as an action or situation.

dramatogenic J.L. Moreno's term to denote people "especially sensitive for collective experiences and able to dramatize them easily ... Just as there are some people who are photogenic, there are some individuals who are dramatogenic. . ." (*Sociometry VI*, 1947)

drapetomania Uncontrollable impulse to wander; dromomania. See *deterioration, simple senile.*

drauci Males who adopt the passive role in homosexual activity. See *active.*

drawing, automatic The execution of drawings without a person's conscious volition, but often after being directed to do so in a hypnotic trance. Automatic drawing constitutes an important aid and method in hypnoanalytical technique: "Drawing is both a form of motor expressiveness and a means by which the individual can reveal inner problems, wishes, and fears. It is an excellent method of gaining access to deep material where the patient is unable or unwilling to associate freely. Drawings have many of the characteristics of dreams. They provide symbolic ways of representing unconscious impulses." Automatic drawing can be done in a hypnotic trance (hypnotic drawing), or after awakening if the person has previously, during the state of hypnosis, been instructed to do so. (Wolberg, L.R. *Hypnoanalysis*, 1945)

drawing, Goodenough See *test, Goodenough.*

dread Anxiety related to a specific danger situation. In his analysis of the nature of anxiety, Freud points out that it originates as the reaction to helplessness in a traumatic situation. Later on, as the ego develops, it anticipates that a situation of helplessness will occur or it is reminded of a previous traumatic experience by the present situation. The situation that is the cause of this anticipation or reminder is called the danger situation. And the ego will now react with anxiety in this danger situation. Thus anxiety has become an expectation of trauma in a danger situation.

However, the affect of anxiety "is endowed with a certain character of indefiniteness and objectlessness." This objectlessness and indefiniteness pertain "to the traumatic situation of helplessness which is anticipated in the danger-situation." Freud states that in proper usage the term anxiety should be reserved for the original reaction of helplessness in a traumatic situation where no specific danger situation is expected. The term dread should be used for the anxiety that relates to a specific danger, i.e. "when it

has found an object." Therefore, "dread in an individual is provoked either by the greatness of a danger or by the cessation of emotional ties (libidinal cathexes); the latter is the case of neurotic dread." (Freud, S. *The Problem of Anxiety*, 1936; *Group Psychology and the Analysis of the Ego*, 1922)

dread, talion A fear of "retaliation in kind" as punishment for forbidden acts or impulses. A vivid example is seen in the Oedipus situation, wherein the boy fears loss of his penis, i.e. castration by his father, as punishment for his misuse of it (in incestual relationship with his mother). Another example is to be seen in the neurotic's fear of death and in the hysterical attacks during which he feels he is dying. The talion relationship of these phenomena with unconscious wishes for the death of another will readily be seen.

dream A psychic phenomenon occurring during *sleep* (q.v.) in which thoughts, images, emotions, etc., present themselves to the dreamer, usually with a definite sense of reality. Dreams are not random psychic productions, for they fulfill a vital purpose in the mental economy. They safeguard sleep; they foster solution in phantasy of needs and conflicts too dangerous for solution in reality; they provide an outlet for the discharge of instinctual tension; they allow a working through of destructive and traumatic experiences that defy the coping capacities of the waking state. Dreaming is a universal psychic function, typical of the human mind. It is one of the vehicles by which impulses from the unconscious reach the level of consciousness.

Studies by Dement, Kleitman, Jouvet, and others, have demonstrated that dreaming is an essential psychobiologic function, suppression of which may produce serious psychic disturbances.

Because sleep includes a shutting out of sensory receptors and progressive cortical inhibition, the dream itself works in the manner of the primitive mental apparatus. Visual images tend to replace words, thinking becomes archaic, prelogical and distorted, and there is a tendency toward a universal language.

The recollected dream emerges as the "manifest dream content," which tends to be constructed out of events in the recent past. The "latent dream content" is uncovered by analysis of the manifest content, usually by means of free association. Freud considered the dream a detour by means of which repression could be avoided. The day's residues (events of the waking day) establish contact with repressed, unconsious impulse(s), which attempt to find fulfillment in the material of the latent thoughts. Thus the latent content will include some or all of the following: early memories and experiences, attitudes and phantasies, present-day wishes (both acceptable and nonacceptable), and conflicts and defenses against these, habitual character strivings and character defenses, attitudes to therapy and attitudes toward the therapist. The unrecognizability, strangeness, and absurdity of the manifest dream are partly the result of translation of thought into archaic modes of expression and partly the result of the restrictive and disapproving dream censorship of events in the dream.

Dream research has cast doubt on some of the teleological explanations that have traditionally been used in psychological theories. Dreaming does not appear to be a unique response to a specific psychological experiential factor; instead, it serves to maintain or reestablish homeostasis on a neurophysiologic-biologic level as well as on a psychologic one. It is not an unconscious wish that determines dreaming; rather, neurophysiologic changes in the sleep-wakefulness apparatus provide opportunities for representation of unconscious wishes, which "ride along on" the waves of neurophysiologic disequilibrium, as it were, but which can hardly be credited with primary responsibility for dream production itself. Furthermore, it seems unlikely that repression is a major factor in producing amnesia for dreams, the majority of which are followed by a period of deep sleep that inhibits or prevents memory consolidation.

The processes that transform the latent into the manifest content are called the *dream work:* condensation, displacement, symbolization, dramatization, and secondary elaboration.

The *condensation* of latent thoughts, memories, and phantasies in a dream operates like a magnet gathering together out of the whole reservoir of past and present-day experiences all those pertinent to the magnet. *Displacement* is achieved by giving high interest in the manifest content to an element that will have little significance when the latent thoughts are evoked, or by representing an important latent thought as an insignificant detail in the manifest content. Similarly, the affective accompaniment may be very strong with the least important dream thought, but feeble with the most important thought. Displacement may also be achieved by reversal; e.g. representing the inside as the outside, the bottom as the top, etc.

Symbolism is the chief method of distorting the latent content. Psychoanalytic experience has shown that the ideas symbolized concern the fundamental factors of existence—our bodies, life, death, procreation—in relation to ourselves and our families. Dream symbolism has many mechanisms in common with formation of figures of speech. The simplest figure of speech is *simile,* i.e. the equation of two dissimilar things by means of a common attribute, the similarity being indicated by "as" or "like." When these words are omitted, the compressed simile is known as *metaphor.* These devices also occur in dreams. Personal metaphor involves the transference of human activities to the nonhuman, such as "sighing oak." A flowing stream in a dream will suggest a stream of urine or a flow of talk; or a particular type of tree may have special significance such as "pine" tree meaning someone longed for, etc. Through *metonymy,* a name that has a usual or accidental connection with a thing is used for the thing itself, such as the "bar" for the profession of law. *Synecdoche* employs a part to represent the whole, such as a factory accommodating so many "hands." When the sounds of the words echo the sense, the term is *onomatopoeia. Antithesis* appears in dreams in the form of opposition in position, as in sitting. Parallels are used to convey similarity of position, such as sitting alongside a person. The repetition of a dream element is similar to the repetition of phrases in diction to secure emphasis. Through the implied metaphor abstract ideas are expressed in terms of the concrete; e.g. "food for thought," "hot temper." Although words acquire a second meaning and convey abstract ideas, they do not lose their original concrete significance in the unconscious; language itself, therefore, may yield significant information. Thus, "She is her mother's spoiled darling" may mean she is pampered; but to the unconscious, spoiled also means dirty or ruined.

Dramatization is the representation in the manifest dream of an action or situation evolved from the latent thoughts by the dream mechanisms. It is the subjective attempt within the psyche to project anxiety and control stimuli. The mechanisms may attempt to draw a unity from the conflicting forces of many years, balancing and neutralizing affects. Different persons may represent conflicting parts of the psyche. If a balance is not achieved, the dream may leave a disagreeable affect or anxiety. *Secondary elaboration* molds the latent thoughts and wishes, disguised by the processes of condensation, displacement, and symbolization, into the semblance of a logical story. Ernest Jones considers it as being closely allied to rationalization. (Sharpe, E.F. *Dream Analysis,* 1938)

Every dream is capable of many meanings, on many different psychic levels, and not all of them will necessarily be interpreted by the analyst. There are several choices possible in the technique of dream interpretation: to proceed chronologically and in order, to start with one particular element, to ask the dreamer what events of the previous day are associated with the dream, or to let the dreamer begin where he will to free associate. L. Wolberg (*The Technique of Psychotherapy*, 1954) lists the following techniques of interpretation: (1) summarizing for the patient the basic trends in the dream; (2) asking the patient for spontaneous associations; (3) tentative, unverbalized formulation of the dynamics based on therapist's knowledge of the patient (which formulation will take account of the setting of the dream, the characters in the dream, underlying wish or need, personality traits disclosed in the dream, mechanisms of defense, conflicts expressed in the dream, the movement and outcome of the dream, and the resistance and transference manifestations expressed); and (4) encouraging further associations by focusing the patient's attention on particular problems or conflicts as they seem to be expressed in the dream.

According to Adler, the dream has an anticipatory, prescient function. It foreshadows the preparations developed in connection with actual difficulties encountered by the dreamer's life-plan and the safeguarding purpose is never lost sight of. In other words, the dream attempts to influence the future complexion of things. It is an attempt to solve a problem and has no sexual connotation. It is an indication of power, a sign and a proof that both body and mind are making an attempt at anticipatory thinking and at anticipatory groping in order to justify the personality of the dreamer in connection with some approaching difficulty. It provides a glimpse of the dreamer's unconscious life-plan by means of which he strives to dominate the pressure of life and his own feeling of uncertainty. In dreams all the transitional phases of anticipatory thinking occur as if directed by some previously determined goal and by the utilization of personal experiences.

"The main function of dreams consists of simplified early trials and of warnings and encouragements favorable to the life-plan; and to have as their object the solution of some future problem." (Adler, A. *The Practice and Theory of Individual Psychology*, 1924)

dream anxiety disorder Nightmare (q.v.).

dream, artificial Any dream that is apparently induced by sensory stimulation. Freud cites from Maury, who, when his neck was lightly pinched during sleep, dreamed that a blister was being applied. Freud holds that sensory stimuli may instigate a dream, but they cannot be held responsible for the content of the dream.

dream censorship See *censorship, dream.*

dream, color in The specific report of having dreamed in color suggests that the color has analyzable and significant meaning, including any or all of the following: to camouflage or to identify specific portions or excretions of the body; representation of a specific affect system; synaesthetic representation of other sensory systems; to serve as a screen for traumatic experiences. Dreaming in color may also reflect some kind of neurophysiologic disturbance, for such dreams have been reported frequently in patients with epilepsy, migraine, and drug intoxication.

dream, compensatory nature of Jung says: "It is an assured finding of scientific experience that dreams, for example, almost invariably have a content which can act as an essential corrective to the conscious attitude. Hence our justification for speaking of a compensatory function of the unconscious." (*CAP*)

dream, consolation A dream that contains an encouraging note.

dream content The material of which the dream is composed. Dreams have a latent dream content, made up of dream thoughts and manifest dream content, usually presented in a highly symbolic form. "The dream-content is, as it were, presented in hieroglyphics, whose symbols must be translated, one by one, into the language of dream-thoughts." (Freud, *ID*)

dream, convalescent Dreams can and do occur in *any* convalescence, but in no other period than the convalescence of traumatic neurosis is it true that convalescent dreams are of a specific type and *only* of that type. The nature and content of the dreams of a traumatic neurotic are characteristic of this particular disorder, so much so in fact that they may be taken as pathognomonic of the illness.

The traumatic neurotic exhibits a stereotyped dream life. The most common content of the dream is the threat of annihilation, usually a representation of the original trauma. See *neurosis, traumatic; post-traumatic stress disorder.*

dream, counterwish According to Freud certain dreams seem not to be associated with a wish; in fact they seem to be of the opposite character, that is to convey a counterwish. The wish may be concealed behind its opposite. An impotent patient dreamed he had syphilis. He said that if he had syphilis it would signalize potency to him. A second motive for a counterwish dream is seen in dream-distortion. A patient, who had often punished his brother, dreamed that the brother had foreclosed his (the patient's) mortgage on a house highly prized by the dreamer. Under analysis it was evident that the dreamer, out of a sense of guilt, was expressing a hidden wish for punishment.

dream, examination Examination dreams (Freud), or matriculation dreams (Stekel), are dreams connected with examinations. See *anxiety, examination.*

dream, exhibition A dream of nakedness.

dream function According to Freud, "the dream is the (disguised) fulfilment of a (suppressed, repressed) wish." (*ID*)

Jung holds that the general function of dreams is to reflect "certain fundamental tendencies of the personality, either those whose meaning extends over the whole life, or those that are momentarily of most importance. The dream gives an objective statement of these tendencies, a statement which does not trouble itself about conscious wishes and convictions." (*CAP*)

While referring to Freud's dream theory Adler says: "In reality these infantile wishes already stand under the compulsion of the imaginary goal and themselves usually bear the character of a guiding thought suitably arrayed, and adapt themselves to symbolic expression purely for reasons of thought economy." (*The Neurotic Constitution*, 1917)

dream illusion A dream may be precipitated by an objective sensory stimulus. A ringing alarm clock may set a dream in motion that has nothing to do with ringing or an alarm clock. The ringing stimulated a patient to dream of a locomotive swiftly passing by him. He was panic-stricken lest he be drawn into the path of the locomotive. The ringing of the clock had aroused a painful complex in him, that of castration. In this case, the locomotive was the illusory symbol.

Dream illusions may come about as a consequence of organic, visceral stimulation. Thus an organ, activated by disease or by any physiological urge, may stimulate memory images that superficially have nothing in common with the source of the stimulus.

dream, made-to-order A dream that the patient seems to produce at the analyst's direct suggestion, as if the patient dreams in response to the urgent demands of the psychiatrist. Of course, determined as they are by the relationship between the patient and the analyst, such dreams are often extremely distorted and usually express a derisive attitude toward the physician.

dream, manifest The name given by Freud to the dream itself, as reported by the dreamer. The dream text or manifest dream in itself is not intelligible as far as gaining new information about the patient is concerned. In the process of analysis of the manifest dream, however, information concerning the patient, which would otherwise be inaccessible, is obtained. This information that lies behind the dream is termed the latent dream thoughts. The technique by which the latent dream thoughts are derived from the manifest dream is called dream interpretation. This technique utilizes the associations of the patient to the various parts of the manifest dreams and the meaning of certain symbols with which the patient often is unable to associate. The process by which the latent dream thoughts become the manifest dream in the dreamer's mental life is called the dream work. The two major techniques by which the dream work is accomplished are condensation and displacement. (Freud, S. *New Introductory Lectures on Psycho-analysis,* 1933)

dream pain Hypnalgia; pain occurring during the dream state.

dream, perennial A dream that, being first dreamt in childhood, recurs again and again in adult years.

dream, prophetic Stekel considers it justifiable to use the term "prophetic" for describing those dreams that seem to forecast a wish of the dreamer and later on come true. To illustrate a dream of this type Stekel gives the example of the patient who was attached to his mother and his family with unduly strong ties and expressed symbolically, in a dream, his wish to break these bonds. After the meaning of the dream was explained to him, he was able to fulfill his wish and become engaged to a girl with whom he had been in love for a long time. (*ID*)

dream, reconstruction In M. Levin's terminology, a dream in which a succession of events culminate, seemingly by chance, in a stimulus coinciding with an external stimulus of like nature that wakes the dreamer. Thus a dream that ends with a bell ringing when the ringing of an alarm clock wakes the sleeper is a reconstruction dream. It is probable that such dreams are mainly instances of the dynamic and "economizing" purpose of dreams to protect the sleeper from disturbances. There seems to be no

reason to doubt that reconstruction dreams are further utilized, as is any other dream, in the symbolic expression of unconscious conflicts: that is, reconstruction dreams are subject to psychoanalytic interpretation. (*Psychoanalytic Quarterly 10,* 1941)

dream, secondary elaboration of The account of a dream given by the dreamer upon awakening, insofar as it differs from the original content, is referred to as secondary elaboration of the dream.

dream, Sisyphus Frustration dream. See *neurosis, traumatic.*

dream stimulus The exciting cause of a dream. It may be (1) an external sensory stimulus, (2) an internal (subjective) sensory stimulus, (3) an internal (organic) physical stimulus, or (4) a stimulus from the psyche itself.

dream within a dream Sometimes part of a dream is regarded during the dream state as having been dreamed; the dreamer therefore does not consider that the dream within a dream belongs to the dream. He continues to dream, looking upon the continuation only as the real dream.

"The inclusion of a certain content in 'a dream within a dream' is therefore equivalent to the wish that what has been characterized as a dream had never occurred." (Freud, *ID*) The attitude that the dreamer assumes toward it constitutes a repudiation of it.

dreams, paired Alexander's term for dreams based upon the concepts of punishment and gratification, in the sense that one is allowed to indulge in a forbidden act, if he has already paid the penalty for it. During the same night the subject may first dream that he is being punished; later he dreams that he is engaging in a forbidden act.

DRG Diagnosis-related group, a type of case mix for prospective reimbursement purposes based on the diagnosis of patients treated.

drift, genetic A change in succeeding generation of the frequency of certain genes, due to chance rather than to selection.

drift hypothesis See *breeder hypothesis.*

drinker, problem See *alcoholism.*

drinking behaviors The conditions under which alcohol is ingested (e.g. how much, what type, how often, under what circumstances) and the effects (health, familial, social, occupational, etc.) associated with particular patterns of ingestion.

Under *alcoholism* (q.v.), DSM-II differentiated *episodic excessive drinking* (episodes of intoxication, with clear-cut alteration in behavior or impairment of coordination or speech, occurring at least four times a year), *habitual excessive drinking* (more than 12 episodes of intoxication a year), and alcohol addiction.

drive A genetically determined mental element that generates tension or need, which in turn propels toward activity that will produce gratification or cessation of tension. In psychoanalytic psychology, two drives are distinguished, the sexual or erotic and the aggressive or destructive.

drive, internal See *instinct.*

drive reduction theory See *reductionism.*

drivel Drooling or, by extension, uncontrollable flow of foolish or silly speech. Drooling of saliva is frequent in parkinsonism, including the form induced by neuroleptic drugs.

driveling Fluent jargon-filled speech, a characteristic of Wernicke's receptive aphasia. See *aphasia, jargon; aphasia, Wernicke's.*

drivenness, organic Kahn and Cohen's term for the overactivity of the brain-damaged individual, which is attributed to defective brain stem organization. See *syndrome, organic.*

driving, photic See *electroencephalogram.*

driving, psychic Continuously repeated playback of psychodynamically significant material that has been recorded on a device such as a tape recorder.

If the psychic driving is in response to the patient's own verbal cues, it is termed "autopsychic"; if it is in response to cues verbalized by others but based on his known psychodynamics, it is termed "heteropsychic." The values of psychic driving are said to include penetration of defenses, elicitation of hitherto inaccessible material, and the setting up of a dynamic implant. See *implant, dynamic.*

dromolepsy A short spurt of running occurring just prior to and generally ending in an epileptic attack. By many it is believed to be the beginning of the attack. It is known also as *procursive epilepsy.*

dromomania An abnormal impulse to travel; used by Hirschfeld to denote the desire to escape from a disagreeable sex-

ual situation. It is also known as *vagabond neurosis.*

dromophobia Fear of (running across) a street.

dropout A student who leaves school before completing a grade or before graduation; a patient who withdraws from and terminates treatment. In the latter case, the term generally implies that the therapist has not concurred in the patient's decision to terminate.

drug, abreactive Any of the preparations, usually barbiturates, used in narcocatharsis. See *narcotherapy.*

drug abuse See *dependence, drug.*

drug, addicting See *addiction.*

drug defaulter See *defaulter.*

drug interactions See *interactions, drug.*

drug, orphan See *orphan drug.*

drunkards, acute hallucinosis of Wernicke's name for alcoholic hallucinosis. See *hallucinosis, alcoholic.*

drunkenness, maudlin Intoxicated state characterized by mawkish, silly, and blissful behavior. Bleuler regarded it as an abnormal reaction, but he did not consider it a psychosis.

drunkenness, pathological See *intoxication, alcoholic.*

drunkenness, sleep See *sleep drunkenness.*

Ds Rorschach scoring symbol for an associative response to a white space on the card.

DSA Digital subtraction angiography. See *NMR.*

DSD 1. *Depressive spectrum disorder,* a subtype of unipolar primary depressive illness characterized by alcoholism or antisocial disorder, or both, in first-degree relatives of the depressed subject. 2. *Depression sine depression,* or *masked depression,* when the affect disorder is hidden or disguised by symptoms suggesting other disorders such as psychosomatic illnesses or conversion hysteria.

DSH Deliberate self-harm. See *suicide, attempted.*

DSIP Delta sleep-inducing peptide; may be involved in the regulation of sleep.

DSM-I *Diagnostic and Statistical Manual of Mental Disorders,* 1st edition (1952); the official nomenclature of the American Psychiatric Association. It included, for the first time, experience that did not derive solely from mental hospital data, such as World War II military experience and data from clinics and private practice. In labeling most of the categories "reactions" it moved away from the concepts of constitutional and assumed organic factors, stressing instead the psychosocial and adaptational aspects and the transitory nature of many of the functional disorders.

DSM-II *Diagnostic and Statistical Manual of Mental Disorders,* 2nd edition; the 1968 revision of the nomenclature of mental disorders, prepared by the Committee on Nomenclature and Statistics of the American Psychiatric Association. See *nomenclature, 1968 revision.*

DSM-III *Diagnostic and Statistical Manual of Mental Disorders,* 3rd edition (1980), prepared by the Task Force on Nomenclature and Statistics of the American Psychiatric Association. The aim of this classificatory system is to provide clear descriptions of diagnostic categories while avoiding insofar as possible bias in favor of any particular theory of etiology. The manual suggests criteria that would warrant inclusion in each of the categories; most of the proposed criteria are based on clinical judgment and have yet to be validated in terms of other correlates, such as prognosis and response to particular forms of treatment. Although in a general way modeled after *ICD-9-CM* (International Classification of Diseases, 9th edition, 1978, clinical modification for use in the United States), DSM-III is not compatible with it in every instance because it is of greater detail or reflective of more recent evidence than was included in ICD-9-CM. Further, DSM-III employs a *multiaxial classification* that calls for data to be coded on each of the axes, on the assumption that attention to more than one clinically relevant parameter of a disorder will provide greater specificity and objectivity and a firmer basis for identifying subtypes.

DSM-III-R Revision of DSM-III, 1987. Most of the changes from *DSM-III* (q.v.) have been indicated in appropriate entries, and the aim and format of the revision remain essentially as described for DSM-III itself. The five axes of DSM-III-R are:

Axis I—Clinical Syndromes and V Codes (conditions not attributable to a mental disorder that are a focus of attention or treatment

Axis II—Developmental Disorders and Personality Disorders, which generally begin in childhood or adolescence and persist without remissions or exacerbations into adult life

Axis III—Physical Disorders and Conditions

Axis IV—Severity of Psychosocial Stressors

Axis V—Global Assessment of Functioning on a nine-point scale

DST *Dexamethasone suppression test;* a measure of the degree to which cortisol suppression is overcome. Dexamethasone is a glucocorticoid that ordinarily suppresses or inhibits the hypothalamic-pituitary system, as manifested in a lowered cortisol (ACTH) level for up to 48 hours. Some patients with a clinical depression overcome the usual inhibiting effect of cortisol; in such *nonsuppressors,* the cortisol level quickly returns to pretest levels. Nonsuppression is a positive DST, and it may reflect a relative lack of norepinephrine or a relative excess of serotonin in the central nervous system.

The test shows highest sensitivity in very severe, especially psychotic, affective disorders; it is less sensitive and less consistent in other affect disorders. Its clinical utility therefore is limited—a positive test is no guarantee of significant response to antidepressant treatment, and a negative response is certainly no reason for withholding treatment.

dual leadership See *psychotherapy, multiple.*

dual personality See *multiple personality disorder.*

dual transference therapy See *therapy, dual transference.*

dualism, psychic Coexistence of double consciousness or of two fairly distinctly formed superego streams (double conscience) as in *multiple personality,* where one personality may alternate with a second with complete amnesia of the active personality for the behavior of the inactive one, or where the two personalities live side by side, one or the other being predominant periodically but still influenced by the inactive one. But such co-conscious mentation may also be a normal phenomenon, as when one writes a letter and at the same time listens to the radio. Usually, however, when the co-conscious thinking is pathological, each of the co-conscious organizations strives to drive the ego in a different direction. Psychic dualism is perhaps responsible for critical self-observation, the ability of one conscious stream to observe the remainder of the personality. See *personality, alternating; multiple personality disorder.*

Dubois, Paul-Charles (1848–1918) French psychiatrist; psychotherapy.

dullard See *moron.*

dulling Obnubilation, clouding of consciousness, hampered ability to concentrate or think; productive of intellectual or affective depression.

dullness, mental *Obs.* Used to refer to children who, at about the middle of their school career, are behind the normal average of their age to the extent of two years or two classes. This corresponds to a retardation of between 15 and 20% of their age, or to about twice the standard deviation, and roughly to an IQ of between 80 and 85.

dumbness, word See *aphasia, motor.*

dummy *Placebo* (q.v.).

Dunham, H. Warren (1906–85) Sociologist; epidemiology of mental disorders; *Mental Disorders in Urban Areas* (with Robert E.L. Farris, 1939), *Community and Schizophrenia* (1965).

duplicative reaction See *reaction, duplicative.*

dura mater See *meninges.*

Durham decision, Durham test See *responsibility, criminal.*

duty, prima facie In some systems of moral ethics, a duty that is binding unless overridden by a stronger prima facie duty. Truth-telling, for instance, is a prima facie duty, although under certain circumstances it may conflict with a stronger prima facie duty to which it would give way.

duty to warn See *warn, duty to.*

DW In Rorschach scoring, a confabulated whole response in which a portion of the inkblot is used as the basis for interpretation of the whole picture. Such untenable extensions of percepts indicate an insistence that reality conform to the subject's wishes; they are seen most in the records of psychotics and psychopaths.

dwarfism Extreme deficiency in stature; *microsomia;* usually divided into the following three special forms:

1. Dwarfs with regular physical proportions and normal psychic development, going under such names as *nanosomia primordialis, heredo-familial essential microsomia,* and *pygmeism.*

2. Dwarfs with a serious hypogenesis of the skeleton except for a very large skull, falling under the heading of Paltauf's *nanism.*

3. Dwarfs with a combination of infantilism and premature senility, known as Gilford's *progeria* or the *senile nanism* of Variot and Pirronneau.

In addition to these specific forms, there is a heterogeneous group of *infantilistic* dwarfisms, or nanisms, of endocrine origin, which assume different clinical forms according to the gland principally attacked by dysfunction. (Pende, N. *Constitutional Inadequacies,* 1928)

dwarfism, psychosocial *Deprivation(al) dwarfism;* a syndrome of decelerating linear growth and such behavior disturbances as sleep disorder and bizarre eating habits, due to inadequate physiologic, emotional, or intellectual stimulation. In general, symptoms are reversible with a change in the psychosocial environment. See *failure to thrive.*

dwindles *Failure to thrive* (q.v.) in the older person, sometimes manifested as the "tea and toast syndrome." See *syndrome, tea and toast.*

dyad In social psychiatry, a two-person relationship.

dying, stages of E. Kubler-Ross (*On Death and Dying,* 1969) posits five: (1) denial; (2) anger ("Why me?"); (3) bargaining; (4) depression; (5) acceptance and increasing detachment.

dymorphins Endogenous opioid peptides which, like the enkephalins and β-endorphins, appear to be part of a signaling system that relates to pain perception, mood regulation, and learning.

dynamic Relating to the operation of mental forces or energy.

dynamic psychiatry See *descriptive.*

dynamics Used interchangeably with *dynamism(s)* (q.v.). See *psychodynamics.*

dynamism The action of psychic structures and the forces behind the action; "a specific force operating in a specific manner or direction." (Healy et al., *SMP*) While the authors cited prefer *dynamism* to *mechanism,* the latter is more commonly used. See *defense; mechanism.*

dynamophany The expression of psychic force (P. Dubois).

dynamopsychism G. Geley's theory of libido or energy. The unconscious is the seat of both lower and higher functions, but the latter are purposely kept in abeyance during normal life in order to maintain the sense of limitation and deficiency necessary for ambition and progress. Thus a person forgets, because too much knowledge would remove the spurring to further efforts. But with impending death, the sense of limitation and deficiency is no longer necessary, so that the higher faculties are allowed to appear. The mind then becomes clearer and sharper, and certain manifestations such as clairvoyance and telepathy may occur. (*From the Unconscious to the Conscious*, 1921)

dysapocatastasis (dis-ap-ō-kȧ-tas'tȧ-sis) *Obs.* Restless discontent.

dysarthria Difficulty in articulation; partial impairment of articulatory speech.

dysautonomia Dysfunction of the autonomic or vegetative nervous system, as a result of brain abnormality. Dysautonomia is often familial and bears many resemblances to childhood schizophrenia; the affected child is tense, irritable, subject to recurrent physical crises, defective in organizing complex behavior and adapting to change, and as a result typically develops any number of emotional disturbances.

dysbasia (dis-bā'zhē-ȧ) Any form of difficult or distorted walking, whether organically or psychically determined.

dysbulia, dysboulia (dis-boo'lē-ȧ) Disturbance in the will or in the volitional aspects of the personality. See *will, disturbances of the.*

dyscalculia See *acalculia.*

dyschezia Inadequate evacuation of the stool from the rectum, commonly found in children who suffer from constipation on what is presumed to be an emotional basis.

dyscontrol, descending See *disordered behavior, classification of; psychodynamics, adaptational.*

dyscontrol, emergency See *disordered behavior, classification of.*

dyscontrol, episodic A syndrome first described by Bach y Rita et al. (1971) consisting of violent outbursts with loss of control over aggressive behavior upon minimal provocation, often related to alcohol ingestion or occurring in a setting of alcoholism, and frequently with a history of hyperkinesis and truancy in childhood. Aurae and postictal states are seen in some cases,

and aggressive use of automobiles is a frequent manifestation. Functional abnormalities of amygdalar or other limbic regions are suspected in such cases but often cannot be demonstrated. Psychotherapy and treatment with tranquilizers have generally been ineffective; many patients, however, respond well to diphenylhydantoin or other anticonvulsants. See *disorders of impulse control.*

dyseneia (dis-e-nē'ȧ) Defective articulation secondary to deafness.

dysergasia Adolf Meyer's term for those psychiatric syndromes that are presumably associated with disordered physiology of the brain. The dysergasias are generally known as toxic psychoses, one of the chief symptoms of which is delirium.

dysesthesia (dis-es-thē'zhē-a) Distortion of the sense of touch. It may be organically or psychically determined.

dysesthesia interna *Obs.* Amnesia.

dysfunction, minimal brain See *impulse disorder, hyperkinetic.*

dysgenesis 1. Faulty development and infertility in general. 2. More specifically, a condition in which hybrids are sterile among themselves, but fertile with members of either parent stock.

dysgenic This term, specifically genetic, applies to various biological conditions that have a detrimental effect on the hereditary qualities of a stock or tend to counteract improvement of a species through influences bearing on reproduction. In a more general sense, the term denotes any factor that is in contrast with *eugenic* principles by tending to impair the qualities of future generations. See *eugenics.*

dysgeusia (dis-gū'sē-ȧ) Impairment or perversion of the sense of taste; any aberration of the appetite.

dysglucosis Any disturbance in the blood sugar level, and particularly those disturbances in which the central nervous system (cortex, diencephalon, hypothalamus, or hypophysis) plays some role.

dysgnosia (disg-nō'sē-ȧ) *Obs.* Intellectual impairment or anomaly.

dysgraphia Defective ability to write. As seen clinically, the dysgraphia is often dissociated in that the patient is unable to write spontaneously but is able to copy from printed material to script or vice versa. Dissociated dysgraphia is an almost constant finding in patients with primary reading retardation and in the Gerstmann syndrome. See *reading disabilities; syndrome, Gerstmann; legasthenia.*

dysidentity A term suggested by Rabinovitch to refer to what he considers the characteristic and basic problem of childhood schizophrenia: the child's inability to experience a clear-cut self-percept and to appreciate identities, their boundaries and limits. See *image, body.*

dysimmune response See *myasthenia gravis.*

dyskinesia Distortion of voluntary movements; involuntary muscular activity such as a tic, spasm, or myoclonus.

dyskinesia, orofacial A syndrome appearing in the elderly and associated with edentulousness (toothlessness), dementia, and chronic institutionalization. Symptoms include chewing, mouthing, and tongue movements; the condition is difficult to differentiate from tardive dyskinesia except the latter often includes choreoathetoid movements of the extremities. See *dyskinesia, tardive.*

dyskinesia, tardive Late-appearing dyskinesia, consisting of slow, rhythmical, automatic, stereotyped movements in a single muscle group or more universally, occurring as an undesirable side effect in some patients treated with psychopharmacologic agents (especially the phenothiazines and other neuroleptics). Tardive dyskinesia was first described in the late 1950s. (Schonecker, M. *Nervenartzt 28,* 1957; Sigwald, J., Bouthier, D., Raymond, C. et al. *Revue Neurologie 100,* 1959)

Because tardive dyskinesia is characterized by repetitive involuntary movements of the tongue, lips, and mouth it is often called *oral-lingual dyskinesia,* or *buccal-lingual-masticatory dyskinesia (BLM syndrome);* particularly in younger patients choreoathetoid movements of the trunk and limbs are also a part of the clinical picture.

The mechanism of neuroleptic-induced dyskinesias is unclear but appears to be related to some kind of dopaminergic-cholinergic imbalance. While neuroleptic agents may be the most likely drugs to be associated with the syndrome, it is known to be induced or worsened also by the tricyclic antidepressants, antihistamines, and sympathomimetic drugs.

Tardive dyskinesia typically appears late in treatment, often after several years; it is more common in patients over the age of 50 than in younger patients, in patients who have had previous ECT than in those who have not, and in females than in males.

Acute dystonia is another type of neurologic side effect of tranquilizer therapy and consists of spasmodic movements of the limbs, torticollis, opisthotonus, oculogyric crises, swelling and protrusion of the tongue, and stridorous respiration. This complication typically begins after only a few doses of the drug have been administered, and it occurs more frequently in males than in females.

dyskinesis, professional See *neurasthenia, professional; neurosis, occupational.*

dyslalia Impairment of, partial disorder in, or specific inability for uttering (speaking).

dyslexia A specific developmental disorder, in DSM-III terminology, consisting of impaired ability in reading; initially it is seen as difficulty in learning to read and later as erratic spelling and lack of facility in manipulating written as opposed to spoken words. Affected subjects have problems with perception of shapes of words. Letters may seem to weave on the page, transposing themselves or dancing off the edge. Most often, the condition is genetically determined. It is not caused by intellectual inadequacy, lack of sociocultural opportunity, faults in the teaching technique, emotional factors, or any known structural brain defect. It probably represents a specific maturational defect. Some studies suggest that the basis is an overdevelopment of the right hemisphere, which then rivals the left hemisphere for control of the language function. It is possible that an abnormal alignment of brain cells occurs during the second trimester of pregnancy, when the outer cerebral cortex is formed. Dyslexia tends to moderate as the child grows older, and considerable improvement is possible, especially if appropriate training is provided. (Critchley, A., & Critchley, M. *Dyslexia Defined,* 1978)

dyslexia, literal The inability to distinguish individual letters within a word which itself can be read; often a letter surrounded by numbers can be read more easily than if surrounded by other letters.

dyslogia Incoherence of speech.

dyslysimelia (dis-lī-si-mē′lē-à) A condition consisting of localized muscle contractions, which may be painful, occurring in both lower limbs during relaxation or sleep. The term is commonly shortened to dyslysis.

dyslysis (dis-lī′sis) *Dyslysimelia* (q.v.).

dysmegalopsia Illusory change in the size or shape of an object that is perceived visually; sometimes called the *Alice in Wonderland effect*. When the object is perceived as smaller than it actually is, the illusion is termed *micropsia;* if the object appears to be enlarged, it is termed *macropsia*.

dysmentia Pseudoretardation; impaired performance on psychological tests secondary to psychological factors rather than to primary or constitutional mental retardation.

dysmentia, tardive A behavior disorder involving changes in affect, activation level, and interpersonal interaction that is hypothesized to be the limbic system counterpart to tardive dyskinesia. It has been described in patients under long-term treatment with neuroleptic drugs. Symptoms include loquaciousness, intrusively loud voice, disconnected, aimless, and often inappropriate thoughts, a generally euphoric mood with occasional unpredictable explosions of hostility or petulance, and social withdrawal or autistic preoccupation broken by episodes of overactivity that is often blatantly invasive of others' privacy. (Wilson, I.C., et al. *Schizophrenia Bulletin 9,* 1983) It has also been termed *iatrogenic schizophrenia, tardive psychosis,* and *subcortical dementia*. See *dementia, subcortical*.

The symptoms as described are not highly correlated with manifestations of cognitive impairment, but they do closely resemble frontal lobe syndromes (and there is evidence that frontal lobe abnormalities are characteristic of at least some subgroups of schizophrenia. On these grounds, many object to the term dysmentia—since cognitive impairment has not been demonstrated—and to the implication of "tardive" that the syndrome is related to treatment with neuroleptic agents.

dysmetria Inability to gauge distance for bodily movements; elicited by asking patient to raise both arms and bring them quickly to a stop at the horizontal level;

when one arm sinks below the horizontal level, correction is required for the dysmetria. See *cerebellum*.

dysmimia Inappropriate mimicry.

dysmnesia (-nē′sē-à) Impaired memory. See *memory; syndrome, organic*.

The term is sometimes used, either by itself or in the form of "the dysmnesic syndrome," to refer to reversible Korsakoff-like syndromes that may be seen after a delirium, especially in the middle-aged and older. The patient has amnesia for the acute delirious episode but in addition has difficulty in retaining recent events and a faulty orientation. Generally the syndrome clears rapidly within a few days, but occasionally it may abate only slowly, over a period of weeks or months.

dysmorphic delusion *Dysmorphic somatoform disorder; dysmorphophobia* (qq.v.); a fixed, false belief that some part of one's body is defective—nose, eye, ear, etc. See *monosymptomatic hypochondriacal psychosis*.

dysmorphic somatoform disorder Preoccupation, but not of delusional degree, with some imagined defect in one's physical appearance. See *dysmorphophobia*.

dysmorphomania *Dysmorphophobia* (q.v.).

dysmorphophobia Obsessive fear or, more commonly, delusional conviction that one is physically deformed or otherwise abnormal; sometimes used loosely to refer to any hypochondriacal complaint of delusional intensity. When the patient presents with a single complaint, the condition is sometimes called *monosymptomatic psychosis* and is generally found to lie somewhere along the paranoia/paraphrenia/paranoid schizophrenia axis. In general, the more exposed to full view is the area of supposed deformity, the worse is the prognosis. See *paranoia, hypochondriacal*.

dysneuria *Obs.* Mental weakness.

dysnisophrenia Psychopathy; *psychopathic personality* (q.v.); a general term for the heterogeneous psychopathic disorders.

dysnomia See *aphasia, amnestic*.

dysnusia *Obs.* Mental enfeeblement.

dysorexia Impaired or perverted appetite.

dysorthography *Dysgraphia* (q.v.).

dysostosis, diabetic exophthalmic (eks-of-thal′mik) *Xanthomatosis* (q.v.).

dysostosis multiplex See *syndrome, Hurler's*.

dyspareunia A sexual pain disorder characterized by persistent genital pain before, during, or after intercourse. It is much more frequently described in females, but it can occur in males.

dysperception Any difficulty, impairment, or abnormality of *perception* (q.v.).

dysperception, metabolic A term suggested by Bella Kowalson (1967) as a substitute for dementia praecox or schizophrenia to emphasize the wide variety of perceptual changes that have been observed in schizophrenic patients and the probable metabolic basis for such changes.

dysphagia (-fā′jē-à) Difficulty in eating; it may be organically or psychically determined, but the term generally implies an organic etiology.

dysphagia globosa *Globus hystericus* (q.v.).

dysphasia See *developmental disorders, specific; developmental dysphasia.*

dysphemia Stuttering; stammering.

dysphoria Dejection; disaffection; unhappiness; dissatisfaction with life or self, often manifested as underestimation of self on any or every level; dysthymia.

dysphoria, hysteroid According to M. Leibowitz and D. Klein (*Psychiatric Clinics of North America 4*, 1981) a chronic, nonpsychotic disturbance characterized by repeated episodes of abruptly depressed mood in response to feeling rejected; the acutely depressed period is typically associated with overeating, marihuana use, and consumption of sedatives and/or alcohol. Some workers consider hysteroid dysphoria to be part of a subaffective spectrum of disorders; others classify it as a type of borderline disorder.

dysphoria nervosa Fidgets.

dysphrasia Impaired speaking due to intellectual defects.

dysphrasia, imitative Echolalia; echophrasia.

dysphrenia *Obs.* General term for mental disorder. Wolff used the term synonymously with dementia praecox (schizophrenia).

dysplasia Abnormal tissue development. The term came into prominence in psychiatry particularly through the studies of Kretschmer on body configuration. According to him, there are three basic types of physique among psychiatric patients: the asthenic, athletic, and pyknic. The fourth, called the dysplastic, is a heterogeneous group, "varying much among themselves, of which any one group contains only a few members." Among the types

described under this heading may be mentioned elongated eunuchoids, those with polyglandular syndromes, infantilism, and hypoplasia.

dysplastic See *type, dysplastic; dysplasia.*

dyspraxia Partial impairment of the ability to perform skilled movement, with no associated defect in the motor apparatus.

dysprosody Disordered rhythm, accent, or melody; clinically, used especially to refer to a cortical dysarthria, basically dyspraxic in nature and due to a frontal lesion, that makes the patient's speech sound foreign. See *aprosodia.*

dysrhaphic Dysontogenetic; referring to disturbances of development and particularly to developmental disorders of the central nervous system such as the *Arnold-Chiari malformation.*

dysrhythmia, dart and dome See *pyknolepsy.*

dysrhythmia, major See *hypsarrhythmia.*

dysrhythmia, paroxysmal cerebral (pa-rok′sis-mal) *Epilepsy* (q.v.).

dyssocial See *sociopathic personality disturbance.*

dyssocial drinking See *alcoholism.*

dyssomnia Insomnia; a nonspecific term for any disorder of sleep, sometimes used in a more limited sense to denote dysfunctions associated with sleep stages or partial arousals (parasomnias). See *sleep disorders.*

dyssymbiosis A pathological type of symbiosis between mother and child in which the child uses psychotic defenses to control the degree of closeness to the mother. He must maintain a symbiotic relationship since the separation from the mother is experienced as annihilation; but he must also maintain control over the relationship, which, if it becomes too close, will result in engulfment by the mother. See *psychosis, symbiotic infantile.*

dyssymbole A state of mind characterized by the inability to formulate conceptual thoughts upon personal topics or to discriminate the gradations of personal emotions in language intelligible to others. Dyssymbole is certainly apparent in some schizophrenics, but many physicians believe that it is present in all schizophrenics. Whether dyssymbole represents a defect in the patient's semantic power or is indicative of a more basic emotional deficiency is not known.

dyssynergia A failure to work in unison or harmony, such as is seen in the motor and gait disturbances that follow cerebellar lesions. See *disorganization*.

dyssynergia cerebellaris myoclonica See *syndrome, Hunt's*.

dysthymia 1. In DSM-III-R one of the *depressive disorders*, consisting of a chronic (over two years) pattern of "down" or "low" days outnumbering symptom-free days; in addition to dejected mood, the most frequent symptoms are altered eating and sleeping habits (loss of appetite or overeating, insomnia or hypersomnia), lowered energy and self-esteem, difficulty in concentrating, and ideas of suicide or wishing to be dead. In time, major depressive episodes may be superimposed on the chronic condition. The DSM-III-R definition is similar to a usage that had approached obsolescence, applying dysthymia to depression of less intense degree than that found in manic-depressive psychosis and associated in addition with neurasthenic and hypochondriacal symptoms.

2. Eysenck's term for the group of symptoms found in patients with a high degree of neuroticism and a high degree of introversion.

dysthymic (-thim′ik, -thī′mik) Pertaining to certain cyclothymic reactions that have the appearance of neurasthenia.

dysthymic disorder Depressive neurosis. See *affective disorders; depression, psychoneurotic*.

dystonia Abnormal muscle tone, including both excessive or exaggerated tone, as in muscle spasm, and deficient or absent tone. See *dyskinesia, tardive*.

dystonia musculorum deformans See *dystonia, torsion*.

dystonia, tardive Persistent dystonia that appears as a complication of treatment with antipsychotic drugs, usually developing insidiously and progressing over months or years after the initiation of treatment. When it appears in younger patients, the dystonia is often generalized; in older patients, it is more frequently segmental or focal. Like tardive dyskinesia, tardive dystonia is resistant to treatment.

dystonia, torsion Oppenheim's dystonia musculorum deformans. Torsion dystonia is usually familial and is particularly common among Jews of Russian descent. The characteristic lesion is *status marmoratus* (a disorder of glial formation leading to hy-

permyelination and giving a marble slab appearance), particularly in the caudate nucleus and putamen. The disease has its onset in childhood or adolescence and consists of involuntary movements that produce a torsion spasm of the limbs and spine. There is no muscular wasting, sensory loss, or reflex changes, and no mental deterioration. It appears that torsion dystonia is a symptom complex rather than a specific disease, for it may occur in a number of disorders.

dystonic Relating to abnormal (muscular) tension. The psyche or personality is said to be dystonic when it is not in harmony either with itself or with its environment.

dystrophia myotonica (mī-ō-ton′i-kà) Myotonia atrophica; a hereditary disorder characterized by atrophy of the sterno-cleido-mastoid muscles and the muscles of the face (leading to a "hatchet-face" appearance), shoulder, forearm, and hand and of the quadriceps muscles. There is also myotonia and, usually, other dystrophic disturbances such as cataract and gonadal atrophy. Males are more commonly affected, between the ages of 20 and 30 years. Affected patients usually succumb to intercurrent illness in late middle life. The disease was first described by Déléage in 1890.

dystrophy, pseudohypertrophic muscular The most common form of muscular dystrophy, first described by Duchenne in 1868. It is inherited as a sex-linked recessive and affects males six times as often as females. Onset is gradual, beginning at about 5 years of age. The child is noted to be clumsy and falls frequently. There is pseudohypertrophy, but weakness, of the muscles of the calves, the glutei, quadriceps, and deltoids; the face and hands always escape. The patient adopts a waddling gait and an attitude of lordosis when standing; characteristically, he rises from the ground by climbing up on his own legs. Further progression of the disease leads to contractures in the muscles and death within 10 to 15 years.

dystropy (dis′trō-pē) A term used by Adolf Meyer, meaning abnormality of behavior.

dystychia (-tik′ē-á) See *euphoria*.

DZ *Dizygotic* (q.v.).

E

Earle, Pliny (1809–92) American psychiatrist; hospital administration; in 1877 published statistical study entitled *The Curability of Insanity.*

early infantile autism See *autism, early infantile.*

eaten, fear of being Whether conscious or unconscious, the fear of being eaten originates early in the development of the infant's ego during what is termed the oral stage. During this stage the infant develops the normal aim of pleasure or satisfaction through eating and, in a more general sense, through the incorporation of objects. Frustrations of this erotic aim of eating or incorporating and fears of such frustration are of frequent occurrence. These anxieties take the form of a fear of being eaten, because of infantile animistic thinking which assumes that what the infant feels and does will also take place in the world around it. Clinically, it has been found that the archaic fear of being eaten may have another function—it may be used as a cover for castration anxiety, disguised by being distorted through regression into the older fear of being eaten.

eaten, phantasy of being The phantasy of being eaten or incorporated frequently occurs as part of a certain type of relationship to a love object. In this relationship the patient's only aim is "to become part of a more powerful personality" whom he overestimates to an enormous degree, though having at the same time no interest in or idea about the partner's real personality. Those who have this sort of aim, attitude, and phantasy are characterized by an overwhelming feeling of inadequacy and inordinate need for self-esteem. As a result they can never give love but have an extreme need to feel loved, and this they achieve in the way described above.

eating disorders *Limosis;* in DSM-III-R, this category includes *anorexia nervosa, bulimia nervosa, pica,* and *rumination* (qq.v.). Changes in eating habits occur as symptoms in many disorders, including bereavement, drug abuse, and mood disorders. See *syndrome, night-eating.*

eating without saturation See *syndrome, night-eating.*

ebriecation *Obs.* Paracelsus's term to denote mental disorder associated with alcoholism.

ébriécation celeste *Obs.* (F. "heavenly intoxication") A Paracelsian term, meaning religious excitement and enthusiasm in psychiatric patients.

ecdemomania, ecdemonomania Morbid impulse to travel or wander about. See *deterioration, simple senile.*

ecdysiasm (ek-di'si-az'm) A morbid tendency to disrobe in order to provoke useless erotic stimulation in the opposite sex. See *exhibitionism.*

écho des pensées (F. "echo of thoughts") The imagined sound reproduction of the patient's thoughts; audible thoughts (see *symptoms, first-rank*). A special form of auditory hallucinations in which the acoustic verbal images of the thought itself are projected outside in such a way that whatever the subject thinks, he hears repeated in speech. See *Gedankenlautwerden.*

echo phenomena Kraepelin's term for *echolalia* and *echopraxia* (qq.v.).

echo sign See *sign, echo.*

echo speech *Echolalia* (q.v.).

echoencephalography A technique of neurodiagnosis in which ultrasound is transmitted to the brain and its echo is recorded on an oscilloscope. A shift in echo may indicate the presence of a space-occupying mass.

echoing, thought *Écho des pensées* (q.v.).

echokinesis *Echopraxia* (q.v.).

echolalia The pathological repetition by imitation of the speech of another, seen in some patients with the catatonic form of schizophrenia and also in Alzheimer's disease and other cerebral degenerative disorders.

echomatism *Echopraxia* (q.v.).

echomimia *Echopraxia* (q.v.).

echopalilalia The morbid repetition (reechoing) of words spoken by another person.

echopathy (ē-kop'à-thē) Pathological repetition through imitation of the actions or speech of another. It occurs most frequently in the catatonic phase of schizophrenia, when the patient assumes the postures, gestures, and speech of another in "mirror" form, so to speak. See *echopraxia; echolalia*.

echophrasia *Echolalia* (q.v.).

echopraxia Repetition, by imitation, of the movements of another; the action is not a willed or voluntary one, and it has a semiautomatic, compulsive, and uncontrollable quality. A catatonic patient acted as the "mirror image" of his physician, assuming every posture and gesture of the physician while he was in the room with him.

"Contrasting with negativism is the so-called *automatic obedience,* showing itself in echopraxia (repetition of actions seen), echolalia (repetition of words heard), and flexibilitas cerea (the maintenance of imposed postures)." (Henderson, D.K., & Gillespie, R.D. *A Text-Book of Psychiatry,* 1936)

echul A culture-specific syndrome described in Native Americans in southern California consisting of sexual anxiety and convulsions related to severe stress, such as death of a child or spouse.

eclactisma A synonym for epilepsy, in part descriptive of the movements of the lower limbs during the grand mal seizure.

eclecticism In psychiatry, the selection of compatible features from diverse (and, often, superficially incompatible) systems of metapsychology in an attempt to combine whatever is valid in any theory or doctrine into an integrated, harmonious whole.

eclimia *Bulimia* (q.v.).

eclipse, cerebral Short-lived loss of consciousness, or loss of perception and motor power, in chronic cerebral circulatory insufficiency. Such episodes are not syncopal, nor do they give evidence of cardiac arrest, lowered blood pressure, or the neurovegetative manifestations characteristic of carotid sinus syncope.

eclipse, mental Janet's term for the "stealing" of ideas from patients, particularly from patients with schizophrenia, who claim that whenever they have an idea, someone takes it away.

ECM External chemical messenger; *pheromone* (q.v.).

ecmnesia *Rare.* Anterograde amnesia. See *amnesia, retrograde; délire ecmnesique.*

ecnoea *Obs.* Mental disorder or disease.

ecnoia A type of fear reaction seen in children consisting of a prolongation of what began as a normally motivated sudden fright; for days or weeks the child is startled by everything and sheds tears at the slightest provocation. During this period, sleep, appetite, and excretory functions may be affected.

ecological systems model See *psychiatry, community.*

ecology Study of the mutual relationships between living things and their environment. One of its basic principles is that no form of life can continue to multiply indefinitely without eventually coming to terms with the limitations imposed by its environment. Ecology includes such studies as the differential incidence of mental disorder in various populations and the distribution of crime and delinquency within a specified geographical area. The psychiatric ecologist (or *social psychiatrist*) is particularly interested in why one person falls ill while his neighbor (or sibling, parent, etc.) maintains good health. "The responses to stress vary from case to case between the widest extremes. The reasons for the variation lie in *genetical and constitutional differences* between individuals as well as in *developmental and psychological ones*. Genetical data are among the few solid facts we have, and hypotheses about the role of social factors in mental disease which take account of them are bound to be more fruitful than those which ignore them." (Mayer-Gross, W. *Clinical Psychiatry,* 1960)

Ecology is also known as *bionomics;* psychiatric ecology is often called *social psychiatry*. See *psychiatry, community; psychiatry, comparative*.

Behavioral ecology is the study of the interactions between the organism and its environment that determine the actions of the organism contributing to its survival and reproduction; included are such behaviors as habitat selection, social grouping, competition for mates, dominance and territoriality claims, food seeking, and antipredator activity.

ecomania *Obs.* Morbid attitude toward the members of one's family. Also *oik(i)omania*.

economic divorce See *divorce, stations of*.

Economo's disease (Konstantin von Economo, Austrian neuropathologist, 1876–1931) See *encephalitis, epidemic*.

economy, token See *token economy*.

ecophobia See *oikophobia*.

ecosystem The balance attained within a society, population, or group between competing and mixed components, variation in any one of which requires commensurate change in all other components.

écouteur (ā-koo-tĕr′) One who obtains gratification through listening to sexual accounts; eavesdropper; the audible counterpart of a *voyeur* (q.v.).

écouteurism Sexual pleasure obtained from sounds or listening to the sexual or toilet activities of others. F.M. Mai (*Australia and New Zealand Journal of Psychiatry 2*, 1968) described a 32-year-old male who derived sexual satisfaction from secretly recording and playing back the sounds emanating from a toilet used by women. See *voyeurism*.

ecphoria Evocation of an engram by a memory or by an experience similar to the one stored in the engram.

ecphronia *Obs.* Mason Good made the order *Phrenetica*, in the class *Neurotica*, and subdivided it into *ecphronia (mania and melancholia), empathema* (ungovernable passion), *alusia* (illusion), *aphelxia* (reverie), *paroniria* (sleep disturbance), and *moria* (fatuity). (Mann, E.C. *A Manual of Psychological Medicine and Allied Nervous Diseases*, 1883)

ecplexis *Obs.* Galen's term for stupor.

ecstasy Trance states in which religious ideation or similar ideas of dedication and complete surrender occupy almost the entire field of consciousness; it was also known as *contemplatio* or *ébriécation celeste*.

ECT Electroconvulsive therapy. See *therapy, electric convulsion*.

ECT, regressive See *therapy, regressive electroshock*.

ectoderm The first, or outer, germ layer.

The ectoderm is early differentiated into a thickened axial *neural plate* and thinner lateral portions. When the neural canal has become closed, the surface ectoderm forms a continuous layer which gives rise to the *epidermis*, while the entire nervous system originates in the thickened walls of the dorsally situated axial groove, which is subsequently converted into a canal (see *cephalogenesis*).

In addition to the epidermis, with hair and nails, and all neurons and neuroglia of the nervous system, the ectodermal tissue derivatives include the epithelium of mouth, anus, nostrils, conjunctiva, and lacrimal glands; the lens of the eye and the epithelium of the membranous ear labyrinth; the epithelium lining the central canal of the spinal cord and the ventricles of the brain; certain ductless glands such as the pineal, the nervous portion of hypophysis, and the adrenal medulla.

ectomorphic In Sheldon's system of constitutional types this means characterized by a predominance of its third component (linearity); that is, the physical structures developed from the *ectodermal* layer of the embryo. Persons of this type are contrasted with the *endomorphic* and *mesomorphic* types and correspond roughly to Kretschmer's *asthenic* type.

ectopia pupillae Displacement of pupil

ectype Outstanding or unusual type; types of physical or mental constitution that vary considerably from the average. From the physical point of view two ectypes are recognized, the megalosplanchnic (brevilineal, brachymorphic) and the microsplanchnic (longineal, dolichomorphic). There are likewise two personality ectypes, the introverted and the extraverted.

edema, angioneurotic *Quincke disease;* angioedema; giant urticaria; a chronic condition consisting of recurrent episodes of localized, painless swellings of the subcutaneous tissue or submucosa of various parts of the body. The disease may be fatal if the edema involves the glottis and larynx. It appears as a rare hereditary form due to a lack of inhibitor of complement (C_1 esterase inhibitor deficiency), and as a sporadic form which is often an allergic or anaphylactic reaction to infectious, toxic, or autotoxic processes. Despite its name, angioneurotic edema is not considered to be primarily of psychologic origin, although emotional upsets may sometimes trigger the reaction in the sporadic form.

Edinger-Westphal nucleus See *accommodation*.

edipism (ed'i-piz'm) (From Oedipus, who beat out his own eyes) *Rare.* Self-inflicted injury to the eyes.

EDR Electrodermal response. See *reflex, psychogalvanic.*

education, compensatory Any program designed to enrich intellectual and social skills in disadvantaged children as early in their lives as possible; probably the best known example of such early intervention is the *Head Start Program,* begun in 1965 by Julius B. Richmond, M.D. Despite early reports that cast doubt upon the value of the program, most long-term studies have found that the program did in fact increase the social competence of disadvantaged children and raised their IQ scores.

education, progressive A movement within the field of education, founded by John Dewey, that emphasizes the needs of the individual and the individual's capacity for self-expression and self-direction.

educational-socialization model See *psychiatry, community.*

eduction Sullivan's term for central processes, i.e. whatever lies between receptor functions and effector functions.

EE *Expressed emotions* (q.v.).

EEG *Electroencephalogram* (q.v.).

effect, Matthew A semihumorous term for the phenomenon of those already enjoying an abundance of professional or scientific recognition being likely to receive more recognition than relatively unknown writers or investigators, even though they both publish similar material. Their articles are cited frequently by other authors, and they "have established reputations, are likely to serve on editorial boards in their areas, are more likely to receive research grants, etc." (Blashfield, R.K., et al., *Schizophrenia Bulletin 8, 1982)*

effect, placebo See *placebo.*

effeminated man See *man, effeminated.*

efferent See *afferent; reflex.*

efficiency, sleep See *sleep efficiency.*

effort syndrome A type of anxiety neurosis or anxiety reaction, approximately equivalent to soldier's heart, neurocirculatory asthenia, or, in current terminology, hyperventilation syndrome. See *asthenia, neurocirculatory; syndrome, hyperventilation.*

egersis (ē-gĕr'sis) *Obs.* Intense wakefulness.

ego In psychoanalytic psychology, the ego is that part of the psychic apparatus that is the mediator between the person and reality. Its prime function is the perception of reality and adaptation to it. The ego is the executive organ of the reality principle and is ruled by the secondary process. The various tasks of the ego include perception, including self-perception and self-awareness; motor control (action); adaptation to reality; use of the reality principle and the mechanism of anxiety to ensure safety and self-preservation; replacement of the primary process of the id by the secondary process; memory; affects; thinking; and a general synthetic function manifested in assimilation of external and internal elements, in reconciling conflicting ideas, in uniting contrasts, and in activating mental creativity. Unlike the id, the ego has an organization (i.e. it is not chaotic), it can generate coordinated action, and it is ruled by the secondary rather than the primary process. Its functions develop gradually, dependent upon physical maturation (and particularly, the genetically determined growth of the central nervous system) and upon experiential factors.

Ego strength, essentially, is the degree to which the ego's functions are maintained, even in the face of wide variations in the supply of instinctual energy to the ego.

In studies of ego function patterns in schizophrenic, neurotic, and normal subjects, Bellak and his co-workers assess ego function in the following areas: reality testing, judgment, sense of reality, regulation and control of drives, object relations, thought processes, adaptive regression in the service of the ego, defensive functions, stimulus barrier, autonomous functions, synthetic functions, and mastery-competence.

Beginning at birth, stimuli from the external world act upon the organism. Over the ensuing months and years, with the accumulation of more and more experiences, certain mental events have a peculiar intimacy and a new psychic structure, the ego, is formed. The ego mediates between the person and reality; it is a clearinghouse for stimuli from both the unconscious and from conscious reality. It develops on the basis of unsatisfied demands (thus if there were always to be satisfaction, there would be no development of reality). Birth floods the infant with excitation, and this becomes the model for all later anxiety. But the infant is still in the primary undifferentiated phase of consciousness; he is ignorant of any sources of pleasure other than himself and there is, at this stage of objectivation, no differentiation of the mother, or other objects, from himself. The breast is thought of as a part of his own body, and his slightest gestures are followed by satisfaction of his instinctive nutritional needs. This gives rise to the autarchic fiction of false omnipotence, and this is the stage of primary narcissism. The infantile ego only unwillingly orients itself to objects, which at this stage are seen only as ego substance that satisfies instinctual demands. Thus there is only ego and non-ego. Soon, however, reality makes increasing demands. Perceptions and memory system are differentiated, and the ego defends itself against stimulation by shutting off the perceptive system, by mastery through "fascination" (empathy), or by mastery through swallowing and introjection. The infant develops the attitude that objects exist only for the ego's satisfaction, and the purified pleasure ego perceives anything unpleasant as non-ego. The ego believes itself to be omnipotent, but this is disproved by experience and frustration. The ego then comes to believe that the parents are omnipotent and partakes of their omnipotence by introjection. This is the primary identification: the putting into the mouth results in perception, and the ego imitates what is perceived in order to master the object. The imitation of the external world by oral incorporation is the basis for that primitive mode of thinking called magic. Even though reality destroys the feeling of omnipotence, the longing for this primary narcissism remains—the narcissistic needs—and self-esteem is the

awareness of how close the ego is to the original omnipotence. The desire to partake of the parental omnipotence, even though it arose originally from the basic desire for the satisfaction of hunger, soon becomes differentiated from the hunger itself, and the ego craves affection in a passive way (passive object love), being willing to renounce other satisfactions if rewards of affection are promised.

By substituting actions for mere discharge reactions, the ego achieves the stage of active mastery. This is achieved through the interposing of time, the development of a tension tolerance, and the development of judgment (the ability to anticipate the future in the imagination by testing reality). Primary anxiety is the passive experiencing of excitation that cannot be mastered but that must be endured; with judgment, the ego declares that a certain situation might give rise to this primary anxiety; and instead of the original panic itself being experienced, a moderated, tamed fear is experienced that is anxiety in anticipation of what might happen.

The first fear is of a recurrence of the primal anxiety, and from this develops the fear that the child's own instinctual demands, which gave rise to the overwhelming excitation beyond his capacity to master, are dangerous in themselves. This fear is complicated by animistic thinking (the belief that the external environment has the same instincts as the self), for if the desire to recapture the primary narcissism is to be achieved by eating the parents, the child feels that the deed will be undone by his being devoured himself (talion principle). This is how anxieties of physical destruction originate; the most important representative of this group is castration anxiety.

The development of speech initiates a further decisive step in the development of reality testing, since connecting words and ideas makes thinking possible. Thinking is an anticipatory acting out done with reduced energy. The faculty of speech changes archaic prelogical thinking (*primary process*) into logical and orderly (*secondary process*) thinking. With the arrival of speech and logical thinking, a final differentiation of conscious and unconscious is made. Now prelogical thinking will be used as a substitute for logical thinking only when the latter cannot master unpleasant reality.

The maturing ego must not only postpone action, but on occasion it must inhibit action completely. Thus the ego develops reactions of defense against instinctual demands (countercathexis). There are various reasons for the development of these defenses: (1) instinctual demands that cannot be satisfied become traumatic in themselves; (2) prohibitions from the outside world, through education, experience, etc.; (3) the danger is phantasied because of a projective misunderstanding of the world; (4) the ego becomes dependent upon the superego (which has meanwhile developed), and anxiety is transformed into guilt. See *stress, ego.*

The above paragraphs outline the gradual development of the ego as theorized by the psychoanalytic school of psychology. Others conceive of the ego in somewhat different ways.

Jung says that the ego "consists of record-images from the sense functions that transmit stimuli both from within and from without, and, furthermore, of an immense accumulation of images of past processes." The record-images are innumerable. "Therefore, I speak not merely of the ego, but of an ego-complex, on the established presupposition that the ego, having a fluctuating composition, is changeable, and therefore cannot be just simply *the* ego." (*CAP*)

From the standpoint of analytical psychology (Jung), the ego is "a complex of representations which constitutes the centrum of my field of consciousness and appears to possess a very high degree of continuity and identity." The ego "is not identical with the totality of my psyche, being merely a complex among other complexes. Hence, I discriminate between the ego and the Self, since the ego is only the subject of my consciousness, while the Self is the subject of my totality: hence it also includes the unconscious psyche. In this sense the Self would be an (ideal) factor which embraces and includes the ego. In unconscious phantasy the Self often appears as a super-ordinated or ideal personality." (Jung, *PT*)

According to E. J. Kempf the ego "is constituted of the inherent segmental functions that have become *conditioned* to seek stimuli in a manner that not only obtains gratification but also wins social justification and esteem. Hence, this egoistic unity must keep the asocial segments under control. . . . This general, incessant, autonomic compensation becomes essentially integrated into a unity to prevent any division from jeopardizing the unity. *This unity, having the capacity of reacting so as to be conscious or aware of any segment's activities constitutes the ego, and learns to speak of itself, as 'I,' 'me,' 'myself,' 'I am,' 'I wish,' etc.*" (*PP*)

In Parsons's *social role theory,* the ego is the subject in any process of interaction. The object with whom the ego interacts is the *alter.*

ego-alien *Ego-dystonic* (q.v.).

ego alteration, reactive A type of anticathexis—that is, expenditure of energy in maintaining the repression of libidinal or aggressive impulses—in which the ego is altered by a reaction formation against the particular libidinal impulses. Freud gives the example of the compulsion neurosis in which an exaggeration of the normal character traits of pity, conscientiousness, and cleanliness is found. These character traits are the antithesis of the anal-sadistic impulses repressed by the compulsion neurosis. Thus the ego is altered through an exaggeraton of the abovementioned character traits, which are a reaction against the repressed impulses; that is, some of the energy spent in repressing these anal impulses is spent in reactive ego alteration.

Another type of reactive ego alteration occurs in hysteria, illustrated by the hysterical woman who treats with an excess of tenderness the children she really hates, but who is more tender neither in general nor toward other children. Freud contrasts the two types of reactive ego alteration as follows: "The reaction-formation of hysteria adheres tenaciously to a specific object and is not elevated to the status of a general disposition of the ego. Of compulsion-neurosis it is precisely this universalization, the looseness of object relationships, the displaceability marking object choice, which are characteristic." (*The Problem of Anxiety,* 1936)

ego analysis See *analysis, ego.*

ego, auxiliary The auxiliary ego is an individual who identifies himself consciously with all the subject's expressions and purposes as far as organic limitations permit, thus strengthening the ego of the subject. The auxiliary ego, acting in the subject's behalf, is a genuine prolongation or extension of the subject's ego. "An auxiliary ego operating upon the instinctive level is a function known as an 'alter-ego.' Illustrations of an alter-ego are the mother to her child, the lover, or the friend. . . . In the case of an interpersonal difficulty, the consulting psychiatrist becomes an auxiliary ego of two or more persons involved. . . . In the psychodrama the function of the auxiliary ego is to enact such roles which the patient may require for presenting his situation adequately. Such roles may be upon the private level or the auxiliary ego may have to assist in embodying concrete persons in the patient's milieu, such as a specific father, wife or child. Or, the role may be upon a symbolic level, such as God, Judge, or Satan. Finally, the auxiliary ego may embody delusionary roles or peculiar symbolic combinations characteristic for the patient's world." (Moreno, J.L. *Sociometry 1*, 1937)

ego, body That part of the perceiving portion of the ego around which all concepts of one's own ego are grouped. The body ego consists of the psychic representations of one's body and self—the memories and ideas connected with the body along with their cathexes. At first the various parts of the body, and eventually the body as a whole, occupy a particularly important place in the psyche throughout life.

The ego perceives not only external stimuli but also inner, mental processes (ideas, wishes, thoughts, strivings, sensations, and fantasies). External stimuli are intercepted by the sense organs and led to the central nervous system. Here they leave traces in the form of memories and ideas whose nature depends upon the particular sense organ that has received the stimulus (sight, hearing, touch). These precipitates in the psyche of external experiences, together with the internal processes, such as thinking, imagination, feelings, emotions, and visceral sensations, form what we call the psychic body scheme or image. The nucleus around which all concepts of one's own ego are grouped is the *body ego*, whose main function is perception." (Nunberg, H. *Principles of Psychoanalysis*, 1955)

Federn used the term "bodily ego-feeling" to refer to the body ego. See *image, body; limb, phantom.*

ego boundary See *boundary, ego*

ego cathexis See *cathexis.*

ego center P. Schilder's term for the nucleus, or inner part of the ego, surrounded by a peripheral part of the ego in the same manner that the nucleus of a cell is enclosed by the protoplasm.

According to Schilder, the various experiences of our life are at different distances from the center of the ego, some being closer than others. Some sensations are particularly close to this hypothetical nucleus, and specifically pain, sexual excitement, and anxiety seem to be in the very center of the personality. Certain parts of the body are nearer than others to this center, and the importance of surgical operations varies in accordance with the part of the body operated upon: operations on genitals, breasts, or eye threaten the body parts that are nearer than others to the center of the ego. (*Psychotherapy*, 1938)

ego, collective The ego is not only a product of the individual, but it also reflects the group and its concepts. See *collective unconscious.*

ego, decomposition of In the dream the ego appears divided into its various tendencies, and represented by different persons, actions, things, or localities.

ego deviation See *children, ego deviant.*

ego distortion See *distortion, ego.*

ego, dream With this expression Jung (analytical psychology) designates "a mere fragment of the conscious ego" that is active during the dream stage. "In a dream, consciousness is neither fully awake nor fully extinguished; there is still a small remnant of consciousness. There is, for instance, nearly always some consciousness of the ego, but rarely of the ego as it appears to the consciousness of waking life. It is rather a limited ego, sometimes peculiarly transformed or distorted. The psychic contents of the dream appear to the ego very like those external phenomena which appear to it in the waking state.

Hence it happens that we find ourselves in situations like those in real life, but rarely exercise thought or reason about them." (*CAP*)

ego drive Impulse toward self-preservation, ego maximation, and group conformance, the development of which is deeply rooted in biological constitution and markedly influenced by the social nature of man's existence. Also called *ego instinct* (q.v.).

ego, duplication of See *personality, multiplication of.*

ego-dystonic Anything that is unacceptable to the ego. Stimuli from any source that are rejected by the ego or that are prevented from reaching the ego for its consideration are called ego-dystonic. Its opposite is *ego-syntonic* (q.v.).

ego-dystonic homosexuality A seldom-used term, listed for a short time in the official American Psychiatric Association nomenclature but deleted in 1987 because there was no evidence of its scientific validity. The term was applied to a sustained pattern of overt homosexual arousal in a person who explicitly complains that such responses are unwanted and a source of distress. Further, such a person desires to acquire or increase heterosexual responsivity so that heterosexual relations can be intitiated or maintained. If there are persons who fit such a description they must be few, since a five-year literature search (1981–1986) uncovered only 13 references to the term. Any such case would be classified as sexual disorder not otherwise specified.

ego, effective The ego that has learned how to adapt itself to the environment and deal with it *effectively*, as differentiated from the infantile ego—helpless at birth and therefore *ineffective* in this respect.

ego erotism Narcissism. See *ego libido.*

ego, escape from the A phenomenon of psychic displacement by which the compulsive-neurotic shifts the goals of his own ego to another person by way of identification or differentiation. This is, for instance, the case of the rich man, suffering from a compulsion, who "identifies himself with the man who sweeps the streets every day. This may go so far that the compulsive does not permit himself to enjoy a good meal at a restaurant, because the street-cleaner can afford only a modest

one. For this identification, the compulsive is rewarded with the pleasure that he does not have to restrain himself in certain other aspects: he may swear, curse, or tell vulgar stories, in public, since it is the street-cleaner talking, not he." (Stekel, *CD*) For another, and far more prevalent, mechanism of escape from the ego, see *ego, negation of the.*

ego, extinction of A psychoanalytic term referring to the relationship between a punitive superego and a guilt-ridden ego. The guilt of the ego stems from the strength of denied and repressed unconscious hostility (or sexuality) of an infantile and primitive nature. The obsessional neurotic, for example, must constantly neutralize his infantile omnipotent destructive powers through equally omnipotent magical means, so that he can protect his loved objects from his repressed hostility. In this way he attains the right, or justification, for his own ego to continue to exist. When these ritualistic and magical processes fail, extreme guilt with deep inhibition, feelings of painful dejection, apathy, and nihilistic unworthiness overwhelm the ego (individual). It is this state that is tantamount to extinction of the ego through the wrath of the superego.

ego, fragmentation of See *dedifferentiation.*

ego function See *ego.*

ego, ideal The ideal ego is the ego that feels as one with the id, as is the case with the unorganized ego of the child. This ideal condition begins to disappear with the first opposition to the gratification of his needs, and while all people presumably strive to recapture this state, it is for the most part only in certain psychoses (e.g. manic and catatonic episodes) that the patient grants himself everything pleasurable and rejects everything unpleasurable. The phantasy of a return to the womb is an expression of the desire to return to the state of the ideal ego.

ego-ideal In psychoanalysis ego refers to a psychic structure that undergoes gradual evolution from the time that it makes its embryonic appearance as a modification of a part of the id until it acquires more or less final form late in life. As the ego expands, as it develops new structures and functions, its limits extend from the id to reality. The person is constantly identifying himself with others. The first important identifications are connected with the parents; hence a part of the developing ego is set aside, so to speak, to contain the mental images of the parents. Later the composite image, constituting the superego, occupies a position in the unconscious, where it continues to act as the "inner conscience" and controlling agency of the id. "During the course of its growth, the super-ego also takes over the influence of those persons who have taken the place of the parents, that is to say of persons who have been concerned in the child's upbringing and whom it has regarded as ideal models. Normally the super-ego is constantly becoming more and more remote from the original parents, becoming as it were more impersonal." That part of the ego devoted to the development of parental substitutes (parental imagos) and in which the parental imagos are laid down is called the ego-ideal. "Identifications take place with these later editions of the parents as well, and regularly provide important contributions to the formation of character; but these only affect the ego, they have no influence on the superego, which has been determined by the earliest parental imagos." (Freud, S. *New Introductory Lectures on Psycho-Analysis*, 1933) The ego-ideal is a precipitation of the superego.

The ego-ideal may change from time to time as newer identifications are made. When the person's own narcissism is threatened, it is usually withdrawn from the ego-ideal of later development and regresses to what is called the narcissistic ego-ideal, namely, the mental image of perfection that the child constructs of himself. See *ego; superego*.

ego-ideal, narcissistic See *ego-ideal*.

ego instinct Defined by Jones as all the nonsexual instincts. See *ego drive*.

ego libido The libido when attached to the ego; generally used in contradistinction to the expression *object libido*. It is synonymous with ego cathexis. K. Abraham defines ego libido as "that stage in the development of the libido in which the child is himself the center of his own narrow world and in which he receives proofs of love from other persons without himself giving any return." (*SP*) See *libido, mobility; narcissism*.

ego, loss of boundaries of Often, as in schizophrenia, the usual sharp delineation of the ego is lost, the ego merging with that of another or with the entire world (cosmic identity). "We often found ourselves confronted by experiences in which the discrimination between the consciousness of self and the consciousness of the object were entirely suspended, the ego being no longer separated from the nonego; the subject no longer distinct from the object; the self and the world were fused in an inseparable total complex." (Storch, A. *The Primitive Archaic Forms in Schizophrenia*, 1924)

ego maximation Ego drives to maintain feelings of personal adequacy in competitive situations. See *self-maximation*.

ego, mental See *ego, body*.

ego, motor control of the The control exerted by the ego over one's motor activities. The mastery of the motor apparatus is a task gradually learned by the human infant. It learns to substitute "actions for mere discharge reactions" by acquiring a tolerance for the tension that arises from stimuli and results in immediate reaction impulses. In addition, the infant must develop the function of judgment as a "prerequisite for an action. . . . This means the ability to anticipate the future in the imagination." According to Fenichel, learning to walk, to control the sphincter, and to speak "are the main steps in the development of the mastery of physical motor functions." See *ego*.

Disturbances in the ego's motor control can be seen in certain types of symptoms. One example of this type of symptom is psychogenic dystonia. The patient suffers from either localized or general muscular spasms or hypotonic muscular attitudes. In some cases hypertonic and hypotonic states alternate. Whichever is the case, there is "a partial weakening of the voluntary mastery of motility." (These symptoms are a defense aimed at "barring warded-off impulses from motility.") Another example is the tic. (*PTN*)

ego narcissism *Narcissism* (q.v.).

ego, negation of the A mental mechanism through which the compulsive-neurotic avoids the responsibilities of his own ego by putting himself in the place of another person (identification) and then trying with all his might to differentiate himself from the chosen person (differentiation). The object in this case may be called a "negative ruler of the soul." The patient achieves the negation of his own ego through a negative and antagonistic attitude toward the person chosen as object. He will tell himself: "I have no free will. I must do the opposite of what my object does. My actions are determined by his, but in such a manner that I become his opposite."

ego neurosis See *neurosis, ego.*

ego nuclei The smaller component elements of the ego. "According to Edward Glover, . . . in the first place an oral ego-nucleus and later an anal ego-nucleus predominates over the others." (Klein, M. *Contributions to Psycho-analysis 1921–1945*, 1948)

ego, perception P. Schilder's term for the censoring forces emanating from the ego and preventing certain psychic material from becoming conscious: "The repressive forces originating from the ego are the representatives of the social functions of perception, action, and reality testing." (*Psychotherapy,* 1938)

ego, pleasure The part of the ego made up of components agreeable with instinctual impulses. See *ego, reality.*

ego, preschizophrenic The prepsychotic personality of the schizophrenic, characterized by impairment of ego synthesis; that is, the patient does not give the impression of a personal oneness that the normal person gives. The preschizophrenic child daydreams excessively, and the phantasies here have the aim of withdrawal from reality; in the normal child, phantasies have the goal of experimentation and preparation for mastery of reality. Often, during sleep, the preschizophrenic child has dreams of its own death; there is a predominance of regressive (even prenatal) phantasies; exaggerated conscience, bizarre somatic sensations, frequent severe temper tantrums, and a pervasive aggressiveness are typical. "The boundaries of the prepsychotic ego are progressively constricted by aimless aggressiveness. . . . The inability adequately to test reality is closely connected with the limitation of the boundaries of the ego, a basic disturbance in schizophrenia." (Bychowski, G. *Psychoanalytic Quarterly 16,* 1947)

ego psychology Psychoanalytic development psychology. See *object relations theory.*

ego, purified pleasure That stage in the development of the *ego* (q.v.) in which anything unpleasant is considered non-ego, anything pleasant is considered ego. The purified pleasure ego strives to reverse the separation of ego from non-ego, thus expressing a longing for the original objectless state of affairs. By swallowing anything pleasant, the infant adjoins pleasurable stimuli to the ego and attempts to make parts of the external world flow into the ego. By "spitting out" anything painful, the infant adjoins unpleasant stimuli to the non-ego and puts unpleasant sensations into the external world.

These mechanisms of the state of the purified pleasure ego may be used by the ego for defensive purposes. For example, projection is a derivative of the first negation of unpleasurable stimuli described above. Psychotics show the use of this mechanism most clearly, for, by narcissistic regression, the reality testing of their egos has been severely damaged. The boundaries between ego and non-ego are no longer clear. The psychotic perceives emotions or excitements that are unpleasant to him as being outside the ego. The offensive impulse is perceived in another person instead of in one's own ego.

ego, reality That part of the ego formed by the introjection of external objects. When the objects of reality are pleasurable they are absorbed by (introjected into) the ego. Hence an object of reality, incorporated into the ego, helps to constitute that part of the ego known as reality ego.

The ego absorbs both painful and pleasurable objects, but it separates them, retaining the pleasurable to form the *pleasure ego* and projecting the painful back into the outer world as a hostile object.

ego, reality life of A psychoanalytic concept referring to the practical everyday life of the patient with all its reality problems, in contrast to the goals and aims of the psychoanalytic procedure, as confined to the analyst's office. In the analyst's office, the patient's relationship to the analyst per se (i.e. the transference situation) is of paramount concern. The main task of the analyst is directed not at helping the patient with his reality problems but at assisting the patient in acquiring the courage to face the truth about himself. This is achieved mainly through the analysis of what are called defensive resistances. In this way, insuperable conflicts between powerful and primitive instinctual forces on the one hand, and horror-filled guilt-feelings on the other, stemming from childhood conscience pressures, can eventually be resolved. When this resolution has been brought about, symptomatic improvement in the reality life of the ego will usually ensue.

ego, reasonable "Lack of a reasonable ego" is discussed by Fenichel as a major factor to be considered in deciding whether or not psychoanalysis should be tried with a given patient. A part of the ego must be split off into a reasonable, cooperative, judging portion. And "this cleavage is accomplished by utilizing positive transference and transitory identifications with the analyst."

ego resistance See *resistance, ego.*

ego retrenchment The act of diminishing or removing the need for a given function of the ego. Thus inhibitions may make it unnecessary for the ego to form symptoms in order to appease an unconscious impulse.

ego, safety of A psychoanalytic term that refers to the function of conscious and unconscious ego defense mechanisms in allaying or fending off anxiety. The ego is more or less constantly threatened from three different directions: (1) the objective reality of the outer world; (2) the severity of an archaic and infantile conscience (superego); (3) the urgent impulsive and compulsive power of instinctual drives.

ego, split in the A psychoanalytic term designating the phenomenon in which the ego may develop several divergent yet coexisting attitudes toward the same thing. This situation exists (1) in the normal personality; (2) in neuroses; and (3) in psychoses.

In the normal person, "The ego can take itself as object, observe itself, criticize itself." In particular, Freud describes that faculty of the ego that serves and criticizes the ego, which he names *superego.* This is one example of a split in the ego, and the self-observation and self-criticism demonstrate the existence of two attitudes toward whatever is being done by the person at the time.

In neuroses, two contrary and independent attitudes are always present as regards some particular behavior, for the ego's defensive efforts to ward off danger are never completely successful and the weaker attitude that is repressed nevertheless leads to "psychological complications," such as the neurotic symptoms. This split in the ego is most vividly demonstrated when an effort is made to deny certain perceptions of the external world that represent painful demands of the external world on the person. The detachment from reality is always incomplete and the rejection is coupled with an acceptance. For example, the fetishist is trying to reject his perception of the fact that women have no penis, because then he must admit the fact that he, too, could be castrated. The fetish, a symbolic penis, is usually something that was seen at the same moment the woman's genitals were seen or it is something suitable as a symbol for a penis. But many fetishists have a dread of castration. Thus these patients must also recognize the fact that women have no penis. The coexistence of fetishism and a dread of castration may be classified as a split in the ego.

In psychotic episodes, the patients may describe how, even during acute hallucinatory and delusional states, one part of their mind was watching in an objective way the remainder of the patient and his feelings, behavior, and thoughts. This is particularly clear in those catatonic patients who, after the attack has ended, can report coherently on all their behavior and upon all that was going on about them during a catatonic episode in which they appeared to be completely out of contact. Here one attitude, the stronger one, arising from instincts, has detached the patient from reality, represented by a now weaker attitude. When the psychosis has been cured, the normal attitude that takes account of reality has become stronger and the attitude represented by the psychosis has become weaker and is now unconscious. (Freud, S. *An Outline of Psychoanalysis,* 1949; *New Introductory Lectures on Psychoanalysis,* 1933)

ego, stability of Health, strength, maturity, or normality of the ego. The usual differentiating criteria of the more normal ego, in contrast to the neurotic one, are the following: (1) less severe primitive or infantile hostility (id); (2) less severe self-punitive archaic conscience drive (super-ego); (3) fewer magical defensive systems; (4) less infantile omnipotent (wishful) thinking; (5) enhanced object reality functioning.

ego state, adult In transactional analysis, the analyzing, deciding, computerlike aspects of the ego which emphasize the objective and the rational. The child ego state creates the wanting part of the person, but the adult ego state decides whether the want can be fulfilled, and how that fulfillment can be achieved.

ego strength The effectiveness with which the ego discharges its various functions. A strong ego will not only mediate between id, superego, and reality, and integrate these various functions, but further it will do so with enough flexibility so that energy will remain for creativity and other needs. This is in contrast to the rigid personality in which ego functions are maintained, but only at the cost of impoverishment of the personality.

ego subject When the ego is the object of its own instincts (ego instincts), the ego is called the ego subject. "Originally, at the very beginning of mental life, the ego's instincts are directed to itself and it is to some extent capable of deriving satisfaction from them on itself. This condition is known as narcissism and this potentiality for satisfaction is termed autoerotic. The outside world is at this time, generally speaking, not cathected with any interest and is indifferent for purposes of satisfaction. At this period, therefore, the ego-subject coincides with what is pleasurable and the outside world with what is indifferent (or even painful as being a source of stimulation)." (Freud, *CP*)

ego suffering Guilt feelings and/or any of their substitute expressions such as attempts at atonement, punishment, or remorse. See *guilt.* While present in many psychiatric syndromes, including the character disorders, ego suffering is most evident in depressive states.

ego, supportive This term was first introduced by Slavson (*IGT*) to denote one who is dynamic in activity group psychotherapy. In therapy groups it refers to the relation in which one member—because of his greater strength or maturity—helps a fellow member to gain status in a group or to work out his intrapsychic problems. It has been observed that supportive-ego relations are temporary and progressive in nature. A weak child may attach himself to another weak child in order to forward his own adaptation to a group, but, growing stronger and less fearful, he makes friends with the stronger members of the group. Finally, the child functions on his own, without support from any one of the group members.

ego-syntonic Referring to the acceptability of ideas or impulses to the ego, which receives the impulses as consonant and compatible with its principles. Its opposite is *ego-dystonic* (q.v.).

egocentrism 1. Piaget's term for a type of thinking in which no distinction is made between subjective and objective components of experience, and the world is seen only from the subject's point of view. As a developmental stage, this is approximately equivalent to Freud's stage of primary narcissism (see *ego*), but it can be observed also in later periods of life.

2. Term proposed by Healy, Bronner, and Bowers (*SMP*) as clearer and less confusing than *egoism* (q.v.).

egoism Selfishness; the condition of evaluating things in terms of oneself and of one's personal interests. When the self-centeredness is heavily laden with a sense of self-importance, it is called *egotism.*

egoity (ē-gō′i-tē) Egohood; personality; individuality.

egology A term devised by S. Rado to mean study of the ego, the "I."

egomania Exaggerated self-centeredness.

egomorphism The attributing of one's own needs, desires, motives, etc., to someone else; the tendency to build a system of thought and interpret the reactions of others in terms of one's own ego needs—*projection* (q.v.). It has been suggested that the interpretations a psychiatrist makes to a patient are based on the egomorphism of the physician. This is one factor that has led psychoanalytic training institutes to require their students to undergo psychoanalysis. See *analysis, orthodox; analysis, tuitional.*

egopathy (ē-gop′ȧ-thē) Hostile behavior due to a psychopathically exaggerated sense of self-importance. Egopathic patients are characterized by a strong egocentric trend that compels them to deprecate others in their constant aggressive and unconceding attitude.

egotheism Self-deification.

egotism See *egoism.*

egotistic suicide See *anomie.*

egotropy Adolf Meyer's term for egocentricity or *narcissism* (q.v.).

egregorsis Egersis; intense wakefulness.

egrimony *Obs.* Sadness, sorrow.

egritude *Obs.* Mental sickness.

eidetic Pertaining to or characterized by clear visualization (even by a voluntary act) of objects previously seen. Eidetic images (also known as primary memory images) are clearer and richer in detail than the usual memory images and are also more intense and of better quality. Except that the subject recognizes the eidetic image as a memory experience, the phenomenon is analogous to a hallucination. Visual eidetic imagery is more common than auditory. Such imagery is rare in adults. See *imagery, eidetic.*

eidetic personification In Sullivan's terminology, any holdover or representation of previous experiences that influences current behavior.

Eigengrau *Phosphene* (q.v.).

eight stages of man See *ontogeny, psychic.*

Einheitspsychose Unitary psychosis, a concept held by Griesinger (and others) that all psychiatric symptoms are manifestations of a single psychosis and that it is impossible to separate them or classify them into specific entities.

eisoptrophobia Fear of mirrors.

ejaculato deficiens *Obs.* Absence or diminution of ejaculation; ejaculatory impotence. See *impotence, psychic.*

ejaculatio praecox The ejaculation of semen and seminal fluid during the act of preparation for sexual intercourse, i.e. before there is penetration; classified as an orgasm disorder within the group of sexual dysfunctions.

Psychoanalysis views ejaculatio praecox (premature ejaculation) as usually based on a feminine orientation and/or a sadistic desire to soil the woman and/or intense urethral eroticism. Typically, such patients have marked masturbatory guilt. The sexual partner is identified with the mother,

and the patient aims to have his genitals touched by the woman and then to ejaculate as though he were passing urine. This is in part determined by infantile narcissism, in that the penis and urinary activities are thought to exercise an irresistible charm over the woman. The praecox patient can only receive love, and his exhibitionism is a hostile attitude of contempt for the woman. In ejaculatio praecox there is a defiant relapse into the infantile uncontrolled emptying of the bladder; in this way, the person takes revenge on every woman for the disappointments in love he suffered as a child at the hands of his mother.

ejaculatio retardata When ejaculation during sexual intercourse is unduly delayed. It is a type of sexual dysfunction that is often based on narcissistic and sadomasochistic object relations.

ejaculation From the sexual point of view ejaculation is the expulsion of semen and seminal fluid from the urethra; to be differentiated from *orgasm* (q.v.).

ejaculatory impotence See *impotence, psychic.*

Ekbom's syndrome 1. Restless legs syndrome, consisting of irregular, intermittent paresthesiae of the legs and a need to move the legs for relief. Etiology is unknown. 2. Dermatozoic delusions. See *dermatozoic.*

elaboration, secondary One of the four mechanisms of dream-making, which are (1) condensation, (2) displacement, (3) dramatization, (4) and secondary elaboration. The psychic material from which the dream is derived is transformed by these four mechanisms into the picture of the dream as it appears to the dreamer. In the process of transformation the psychic material undergoes great distortion. "This [secondary elaboration] is the product of consciousness, and is brought about by the alteration undergone by the dream processes during their apprehension in consciousness. To it is due whatever degree of order and consistency there may be found in a dream. It particularly affects those parts of the dream that have been insufficiently distorted during the dream-making; its action continues after waking, so that a memory of a dream becomes more altered the greater is the period that has elapsed since it was experienced." (Jones, E.J. *Papers on Psycho-Analysis,* 1949)

élan vital Bergson's term for the creative life-force or life-impulse, the basis of evolutionary progress.

elation An affect consisting of feelings of euphoria, triumph, intense self-satisfaction, optimism, etc.; an elated, though unstable, mood is characteristic of *mania* (q.v.).

elective mutism See *mutism, elective.*

electric convulsion therapy See *therapy, electroconvulsive.*

electrodermal response See *reflex, psychogalvanic.*

electroencephalogram (EEG) The graphic record of the electrical activity of the brain, usually obtained by means of electrodes attached to the scalp. The regular, spontaneous oscillations of the electrical potential of the brain are amplified and recorded on an oscillograph. Characteristic changes in type, frequency, and potential of the brain waves occur in various intracranial lesions.

The alpha wave or rhythm (also known as the Berger wave) is the most common wave form of the adult cortex. It is found mainly in the parietooccipital area when the subject is at rest and consists of smooth, regular oscillations at a frequency of 8 to 12 cps. It is usually diminished ("blocked") by sensory stimulation and mental activity.

The beta rhythm has a frequency of 18 to 30 cps and is associated with alertness. The delta rhythm is an abnormal rhythm with a frequency slower than 4 cps; it is often found when the subject is in light sleep. The theta rhythm is 4 to 7 cps rhythm, seen not uncommonly in the temporal region.

Various techniques are used to accentuate abnormal waves or to bring out latent abnormalities, among them overventilation, natural or drug-induced sleep, photic driving (rhythmic optic stimulation with a stroboscope), chemical stimulation (especially with Metrazol, and often combined with photic driving), and hydration induced by Pitressin, alcohol, hypoglycemia, or oxygen lack. Such activated EEGs, however, often give false positives and are therefore even more difficult to interpret than the standard record. See *neurometrics.*

electroencephalograph The apparatus used in making a graphic record of the electrical activity of the brain.

electroencephalography The process of recording the electrical activity of the brain; the recording itself is the electroencephalogram (EEG). Electrodes are applied to the scalp (or directly to the brain), and eight or more matched channels simultaneously record the amplified brain potentials on graph paper as it passes beneath galvanometer pens. Usually the EEG is recorded under conditions of nonattentive wakefulness, overbreathing, and natural sleep. Deviations from normal or usual brain wave patterns (*dysrhythmias*) may be correlated with underlying disease such as epilepsy, cerebrovascular abnormalities, neoplasm, and infection. See *potential, evoked; tomography.*

electronarcosis Electric narcosis; "subconvulsive" electroshock therapy consisting of an initial tonic phase similar to that of conventional ECT and a clonic phase whose development is limited or prevented by continued electrical stimulation (usually for a period of 7 minutes). Most clinical reports indicate that electronarcosis is less effective and produces more undesirable side effects than conventional ECT. See *therapy, electric convulsive.*

electronic media See *media.*

electro-oculograph (EOG) See *polysomnogram.*

electrophobia Fear of electricity.

electrophysiological battery See *Battery, Quantitative Electrophysiological.*

electroplexy Electroconvulsive treatment (ECT). See *therapy, electroconvulsive.*

electrosleep Electrical transcranial stimulation (ETS) developed in Russia in the 1940s and reported to be effective in the treatment of chronic anxiety, depression, and insomnia. A relaxed state is induced by means of transcranial application of a low-intensity electric current.

electrostimulation Electric shock, usually of painful intensity, used as a technique of negative conditioning in aversion therapy. See *therapy, aversion.*

elemental anxiety See *panic, primordial.*

elementary process See *process, elementary.*

Elgin checklist A list of behavioral activities that occur frequently in a psychotic population but rarely in a normal one.

elimination disorders In DSM-III-R, this category includes functional *enuresis* and functional *encopresis*.

ellipsis Omission of one or more words or ideas, leaving the whole to be understood or completed by the reader or listener. Ellipsis is frequent in dreams, symptom formation, and other types of primary process thinking. Much of the effort in psychoanalytic treatment is directed toward uncovering the omitted ideas as a way of understanding the symptoms. See *process, primary psychic.*

Ellis, Henry Havelock (1859–1939) British sexologist.

elopement In psychiatry, escape; absenting oneself from a mental hospital without permission.

emanative Indirect but often powerful effects of psychopharmacologic agents on self-concept and social interactions.

emancipated Free, independent. In legal language, emancipation is the legal process by which minors are released from the custody, control, and authority of their parents. An *emancipated minor* is a person below the age of majority who exercises general control over his or her life and as a result is able to claim the legal rights of an adult.

emancipation Detachment of instinctual qualities with particular reference to the Oedipus complex as it reappears at puberty. According to psychoanalysis the Oedipus situation loses many of its original manifestations at the close of the period of infantile sexuality and remains dormant during the latency period. At puberty it is reanimated and to it "there is added a powerful current of unmistakable sensuality, which always at first attaches itself in the unconscious to the early incestuous objects of affection." (Jones, E. *Papers on Psycho-Analysis,* 1938) The child is obliged to relive the earlier complex, following which in normal instinctual growth he frees himself from the libidinal attachment to the parents and from dependence upon parental authority. The emancipation leads to heterosexual object-choice.

emancipation disorder A disorder of late adolescence or early adulthood characterized by symptomatic suggestions of a conflict over independence in situations where the subject has moved to what he considers a position of desirable freedom from parental control. The symptomatic suggestions include indecisiveness, paradoxical overdependence on the advice of the parents he wants to break away from, excessive dependence on peers, homesickness that contradicts the desire to be free, etc.

emasculation Castration; physical eviration; eunuchism.

embarrassment psychosis *Sensitiver Beziehungswahn* (q.v.).

embolism, cerebral Brain obstruction; emboli (i.e. plugs or stoppers, usually detached clots) arising from the pulmonary circulation, from thrombosis of the arteries of the neck and head, or from vegetations on the heart valves, may interfere with cerebral circulation, causing cerebral softening and neurological or psychotic symptoms. Stupor or coma may be present with focal signs of hemiplegia or paralysis. Irritability and anger, dulling of general intelligence, and memory defects may occasionally be observed. See *accident, cerebrovascular; multi-infarct dementia.*

embololalia, embolalia A type of speech disorder, frequently associated with stuttering, in which the patient interpolates short sounds or words that are out of place in the structure of the sentence.

embolophrasia *Obs.* "A melancholic subject in my clinique became quite oppressive, because he interlarded his speech with 'really, now.' 'Really now, you cannot understand, really now, how much I suffer, really now. . . .' This dysphrasic disorder goes under the name of *embolophrasia.*" (Bianchi, L. *A Textbook of Psychiatry,* 1906)

emboloplasia *Embolophrasia* (q.v.).

embrujo See *curanderismo.*

emergence *Epigenesis* (q.v.); the theory that mind or consciousness arises from living matter that has reached a certain state of complexity; the term emergence is used to indicate that such an end result is not predictable from a consideration or knowledge of its constituent parts. Emergence is antireductionistic and emphasizes that although the different parts are essential, the final whole that is constructed from them is qualitatively much more than a mere summation of the individual components.

emetomania *Obs.* Morbid desire to vomit, usually a hysterical symptom. See *anorexia nervosa.*

emetophobia Morbid dread of vomiting, not uncommon in hysteria. See *anorexia nervosa*.

EMG Electromyograph. See *polysomnogram*.

emic Referring to socially unique, intracultural phenomena such as amok, koro, and lata. See *etic; syndromes, culture-specific*.

emission, nocturnal See *ejaculation; wet dream*.

emotion Feeling; mood; *affect* (q.v.). In current usage, emotion and affect are used interchangeably, although some use *emotion* to refer primarily to the consciously perceived feelings and their objective manifestations, and *affect* to include also the drive energies that are presumed to generate both conscious and unconscious feelings.

Developmental psychobiology views emotions as behavioral adaptations that have occurred during evolutionary development as attempts to achieve control over survival-related problems such as predators, food, reproduction, and communication. They are genetically programmed responses that have been maintained because they have increased the chances of the organism's survival.

For Adler, emotions do not determine goals and hence are never the cause of undesirable or antisocial behavior; rather, goals are set in accord with cognitive processes (even though the subject may not be consciously aware of these). Emotions are generated secondarily to suit those goals, and to permit and support what the subject intends to do. "People are not emotionally disturbed; they are deficient in their social movement, in their goals, in their form of social integration, because they have wrong concepts about themselves." (Dreikurs, R. in *Contemporary Psychotherapies*, ed. M. Stein, 1961)

"The usual way of thinking about the emotional experiences and their facial or other bodily manifestations is that the emotional experience is excited by the perception of some object, and that the emotional feeling then expresses itself in the bodily manifestations in question." (*Encyclopaedia Britannica*, 14th ed.) See *Cannon hypothalamic theory of emotion; emotion, Papez's theory of; ergotropic*.

The James-Lange Theory of Emotions states that the so-called expressions or bodily changes are the direct results of the perception of the exciting object, and that the emotion is just the feeling of these bodily changes as they occur.

emotion, conversion of The psychosomatic process through which an unconscious emotional conflict concerning the function of one organ is displaced upon and expressed, vicariously, through the energizing of the functional disturbance of another organ. In this process symbolic representation of organ function plays a major role.

Blushing is a good example of the displacement of the erotic functions of congestion, tumescence, and erection from their primary phallic (clitoral or penile) glans, or head, onto the head (caput) of the body as a whole. In this process the body, as a whole, functions symbolically and unconsciously as a phallus, and is utilized to express and carry out conflicts that relate primarily to the genital area, and not primarily to the organ involved. (Weiss, E., & English, O.S. *Psychosomatic Medicine*, 1949)

emotion, Papez's theory of A modification of Cannon's hypothalamic theory: the hippocampus, fornix, mammillary bodies of the hypothalamus, anterior thalamic nuclei, and gyrus cinguli form a circle ("Papez's circle") that elaborates the functions of central emotion and participates in emotional experience. The midbrain reticular formation is connected indirectly to Papez's circle by means of the olfactory tubercle and the amygdaloid and septal nuclei.

emotional divorce See *divorce, stations of*.

emotionality, pathologic A variety of emotional responses characterizing one type of *psychopathic personality* (q.v.), which are usually held under control in the presence of superior strength or police force. The commonest pathologic emotion is pugnacity. A person afflicted with this type of malady is uncivil and bullying, and scorns the rights of others. Pathologic emotionality is also shown by inordinate bragging, by the person's acting the part of a beggar in order to gain money or favors, or by his enacting sadness for purposes of attention. In all these instances there is a certain slyness or cunning.

emotionally handicapped See *handicap, emotional*.

emotionally unstable personality See *personality trait disturbance.*

emotions, Cannon-Bard theory of See *Cannon hypothalamic theory of emotion.*

emotions, emergency See *psychodynamics, adaptational.*

emotions, ictal Any suddenly occurring and quickly disappearing emotional reactions, but especially depression and anxiety. While affective disturbances may accompany almost any organic cerebral disorder, they are most frequently associated with disorders of the temporal lobe. A. A. Weil (*American Journal of Psychiatry 113,* 1956) suggests that such disturbances may be due to subclinical hippocampal-amygdaloid-temporal lobe epilepsy and/or after-discharge from these areas following manifest seizure activation.

emotions, welfare See *psychodynamics, adaptional.*

empacho See *curanderismo.*

empathema *Obs.* Ungovernable passion.

empathema atonicum *Obs.* Good's term for melancholy.

empathema entonicum *Obs.* Good's expression for what is now known as the manic phase of manic-depressive psychosis. See *mania.*

empathetic Relating to intellectual, in contrast to emotional, identification.

empathic In Burrow's phylobiology the organism's primary feeling-motivation and response. Contrasted with affects or projective feeling. See *empathy.*

empathize To diagnose; to recognize and identify the feelings, emotions, passions, sufferings, torments through observing their symptoms is to *realize intellectually, to understand* them, in a remote way to identify oneself with the patient, without ever having personally experienced those feelings.

On the other hand, to place oneself in the position of the patient, to get into his skin, so to speak, to be able to duplicate, live through, *experience* those feelings in a vicarious way, is closely to identify oneself with another, to *share his feelings with him,* to *sympathize,* from the Greek *syn,* together with, and *páthos,* suffering, passion. See *sympathy.*

empathy Putting oneself into the psychological frame of reference of another, so that the other person's thinking, feeling, and acting are understood and, to some ex-

tent, predictable. Carl Rogers defines empathy as the ability to accompany another to wherever the other person's feelings lead him, no matter how strong, deep, destructive, or abnormal they may seem.

Although communication and empathy are related, empathy is not primarily aimed at exchanging information or altering another's belief or action systems. On the contrary, empathy is concerned rather with aligning one's state of mind with another's in order to commune rather than communicate, and in order to expand the interactive repertoire between the participants rather than to transmit the knowledge of one to another.

empirical Depending or based on experience and observation rather than on hypothesis, intuition, or theory. An empirical problem is one that can be solved by the collection and analysis of appropriate data through the use of relevant statistical techniques.

empirical self See *self.*

empiricism A school of philosophic thought that claims that the only source of knowledge is observable fact or objective experience. Watson's behaviorism is a form of empirical psychology.

empresiomania *Obs.* Pyromania (q.v.).

emprosthotonos (em-pros-thot′ō-nos) A forward bending of the body. It is the opposite of opisthotonos. See *arc de cercle; camptocormia.*

EMR Educable mentally retarded.

emulation Conscious, willful copying or imitating of another. Emulation is to be differentiated from *identification* (q.v.), which is an unconscious process.

enabler 1. A mental health paraprofessional, indigenous to the community, who assists the mental patient in adjusting to life within his community. The enabler may take a patient into his home, or may help the patient to manage his own apartment and routine of living. See *caregiver.* 2. Any person, organization, or institution whose actions or policies have the effect of facilitating the continuation of abuse or dependence.

enantiodromia "Enantiodromia means 'a running counter to.' In the philosophy of Heraclitus this concept is used to designate the play of opposites in the course of events, namely, the view which maintains that everything that exists goes over into its opposite." Jung quotes from Zeller (*History of Greek Philosophy*): "From the living comes death, and from the dead, life; from the young, old age; and from the old, youth; from waking, sleep; and from sleep, waking; the stream of creation and decay never stand still." (Jung, *CAP*)

enantiopathic Tending to induce an opposite passion.

encapsulation Enclosure in a capsule or sheath; the process of walling off from surrounding areas, as in encapsulation of a brain abscess. Used in clinical psychiatry to refer particularly to the ability of some schizophrenic patients to keep their delusional life almost completely separated from their routine life in the real, external world. See *orientation, double.*

encatalepsis Hippocratic term for catalepsy.

encephalasthenia Mental exhaustion; *Obs.* for *psychasthenia.*

encephalitis Any inflammatory process involving the brain.

encephalitis, epidemic Encephalitis lethargica; von Economo's encephalitis; popularly known as sleeping sickness. First described by von Economo in Vienna in 1917; by 1918 the epidemic had reached Germany and Great Britain, and by 1920 the whole world. There was another peak incidence in 1924, but if the virus that is presumed to have been the etiologic agent now exists at all, it is not known to have produced an epidemic since 1927. The major reason for continued interest in this type of encephalitis is the discovery that it tended to persist in diverse chronic forms for many years after initial infection. Among the chronic stage syndromes are:

1. Parkinsonism, with rigidity of posture and movement, and subsequent appearance of tremor (in idiopathic Parkinson's disease, the sequence of symptoms is the reverse);

2. Sleep disturbances, including lethargy, insomnia, narcolepsy, or inversion of the sleep pattern;

3. Disturbances of vision, including misty vision, slight inequality of pupils, some impairment to accommodation, weakness of conjugate conversion, or oculogyral spasm;

4. Involuntary movements, such as tor-

sion spasms, tremors, and tics, many of which were commonly misinterpreted as being primarily of psychologic origin;

5. Disturbances of respiratory rate and rhythm;

6. Rarely, metabolic and endocrine disorders, probably due to hypothalamic involvement; among these are obesity, polyuria and polydipsia, and hyperthyroidism;

7. Mental disturbances, particularly depression and, in children, behavior disorders of a restless and aggressive kind. See *impulse disorder, hyperkinetic.*

encephalitis, Japanese B A virus infection of the brain that occurs most often in summer epidemics. The brain stem, basal ganglia, and white matter of the cerebral hemispheres are mainly involved. Mortality is high (50–60%) but recovery, when it does occur, is rapid (10–14 days) and ordinarily complete. Mosquitoes are the vector for the virus.

encephalitis, myoclonic See *hypsarrhythmia.*

encephalitis, paraneoplastic limbic An inflammatory involvement of the limbic cortex associated with visceral neoplasm (e.g. bronchial or renal carcinoma). Typically the patient manifests severe memory disturbance and confusion that progress steadily over an average period of one year; the visceral cancer is often detected only at autopsy, which shows inflammatory involvement of the limbic cortex, but no evidence of metastases to brain.

encephalitis periaxialis diffusa Schilder's disease. See *sclerosis, diffuse.*

encephalitis, purulent Brain abscess.

encephalitis, sclerosing See *panencephalitis, subacute sclerosing.*

encephalitis, St. Louis A virus infection of the brain that occurs most often in summer epidemics, spread through mosquito vectors. The brain stem, basal ganglia, and white matter of the cerebral hemispheres are mainly involved. Mortality probably does not exceed 20%; in the remainder, recovery is rapid (10–14 days) and ordinarily complete.

encephalitis, traumatic A term suggested by Osnato and Giliberti (1927) to replace *postconcussion neurosis*, because of actual cerebral injury in cases of concussion. In current usage, the term *traumatic encephalopathy* has superseded both older terms. See *encephalopathy, traumatic.*

encephalization In higher mammals the cerebral cortex has taken over more and more the task of controlling and exerting a regulative function on bodily processes and on emotions. In the human being this process of encephalization has reached its highest degree. In humans, the cerebral cortex governs not the somatic system alone, but all systems involved in emotional expression, psychological tensions, fears, and phobias. The lower animals are regulated by the hypothalamus and other centers. In the human, the lower centers cooperate in directing the behavior but are themselves increasingly dominated by the cortex.

encephalocele Hernia of the brain. A developmental anomaly of cerebral substance protruding through a cleft in the skull.

encephalogram An X-ray of the skull following replacement of cerebrospinal fluid by air by means of lumbar puncture.

encephalography, radioisotopic A measurement of brain function that depends upon the uptake of radioisotopes by different structures in the brain. The isotope is injected at a specific time before the examination, which consists of a *scanning* of the brain by an isotope-sensitive probe whose intensity of reaction is recorded in graphic form and compared with normal patterns. Positive brain scans (increased focal uptake) are found with some neoplasms, subdural hemotoma, arteriovenous malformation, brain abscess, and cerebral infarct.

In addition to the static scan, serial imaging is used to increase accuracy of detection. The dynamic study of arterial, capillary, and venous phases is said to be more specific and more sensitive than the static image. *Nuclear imaging* or *cerebral dynamic imaging* is typically performed as serial 1- to 2-second interval exposures taken for 16 seconds following administration of the radiopharmaceutical. See *tomography*.

encephaloleukopathia scleroticans See *sclerosis, diffuse*.

encephalomalacia Softening of the brain.

encephalomyelitis, acute disseminated Acute perivascular myelinoclasis; an acute demyelinating disease occurring in the course of infection with the causal virus of one of the exanthemata (e.g. measles, mumps, smallpox, chickenpox, vaccination, antirabic inoculation).

encephalomyelitis, equine A virus infection of the central nervous system transmitted by mosquitoes from bird and wood-tic reservoirs. Two types are recognized and are immunologically distinct: (1) western, with lower mortality (c. 10% and more complete recovery, usually within one or two weeks) and (2) eastern with higher mortality (c. 65%) and severe sequelae in those who do recover (e.g. mental defect, epilepsy, spastic palsies).

encephalomyelomalacia chronica diffusa See *sclerosis, diffuse*.

encephalomyelopathy, subacute necrotizing (SNE) A rare, progressive, hereditary disorder of thiamine metabolism due to an abnormal protein that inhibits an enzyme essential to thiamine synthesis. Symptoms usually appear before one year of age, and death typically ensues within one year of onset. Symptoms include ataxia, nystagmus, seizures, mental retardation, peripheral neuropathy, difficulty in swallowing, and cessation of growth. Successful treatment has been reported with replacement therapy, using massive doses of thiamine or thiamine propyl disulfide.

encephalopathy Disease of the brain.

encephalopathy, AIDS See *syndrome, acquired immune deficiency*.

encephalopathy, boxer's See *dementia, boxer's*.

encephalopathy, hypertensive A diffuse, usually transient, cerebral disturbance that may complicate the course of arterial hypertension (as in glomerulonephritis, malignant or essential hypertension, and eclampsia). Increased intracranial pressure is evidenced by papilledema, raised cerebrospinal pressure, headaches, vomiting, convulsions, coma, etc. Onset is usually subacute, with focal signs (e.g. visual disturbances, aphasia, or hemiplegia), but in some cases onset is chronic and characterized by personality changes, poor judgment, and anxiety.

encephalopathy, lead Diffuse brain disease due to *lead poisoning* (q.v.). Abnormal ingestion of lead-based paint (pica) is the most common cause of lead poisoning, and as a preventive measure many states have enacted laws limiting the use of such paints. Lead encephalopathy is much less frequent in adults, in whom ingestion of illicit whiskey is the most frequent source.

In adults, seizures and polyneuropathy are the most frequent neurologic manifestations. In children, early symptoms are apathy, irritability, headache, vomiting, emotional lability, incoordination, memory lapses, and sleep disturbance. With continued exposure disorientation, psychosis, ataxia, lethargy, and focal neurologic signs develop, sometimes progressing to stupor, siezures, and coma.

Chelating agents (dimercaprol, calcium disodium edetate, and penicillamine), which bind lead and promote tissue excretion, have reduced mortality to 5%. Neuropsychiatric symptoms are slow to respond, especially in children. If treatment does not begin before encephalopathy develops, between 25 and 50% of survivors show permanent sequelae such as siezures or mental retardation.

encephalopathy, progressive degenerative subcortical See *sclerosis, diffuse.*

encephalopathy, subcortical arteriosclerotic Also known as *Binswanger's disease;* one of the presenile dementias, not as clearly defined as *Alzheimer's disease* or *Pick's disease* (qq.v.).

encephalopathy, traumatic A diffuse organic brain disease due to injury to the brain. Clinical symptoms are persistent headache, dizziness, spots before the eyes, poverty of memory, general mental and physical fatigability, poor concentration, loss of energy, irritability, outbursts of anger, and either drowsiness or insomnia; personality changes are commonly a part of the syndrome. See *constitution, post-traumatic; post-traumatic and postencephalitic syndromes, classification of.*

encephalopsychosis Southard's term for psychosis associated with cerebral lesions.

encephalopyosis Brain abscess.

encephalosis A degenerative brain process produced by infectious disease. Clinically, it is characterized by headache, irritability, apathy, stupor, and convulsions. Pathologically, there occur petechial hemorrhages, anemic infarcts, endarteritis of small vessels, degeneration of ganglion cells, and brain hydration.

encoding In communications, the process of translating data (i.e. a message) into signals (a code) that can be carried by a communication channel.

In studies of memory, encoding refers to the processes that heighten or favor retrieval. Encoding may be shallow (such as no more than reading the word to be remembered) or deep (thinking of the meanings of the word and of its emotional significance), simple or elaborate. The deeper the level of encoding, and the more elaborate the encoding, the greater the success of retrieval. The *encoding specificity principle* states that the retrieval cue and the memory trace must have something in common if retrieval is to occur; that is, the retrieval cue must to some extent reinstate the original conditions of encoding.

encopresis (en-kop-rē′sis) Involuntary defecation not due to organic defect or illness. Encopresis in a child over 2 years old is a result of faulty training, mental retardation, or regression on a psychogenic basis.

encounter group *T-group* (q.v.).

end plate, motor That part of a nerve fiber making functional contact with the muscle spindle of an effector organ.

end pleasure In psychoanalysis, the culmination of the sexual act in the mature, genital stage of psychosexual development. The term emphasizes the subservience of pregenital satisfactions to adult genitality. At puberty "the excitations . . . that gave satisfaction to the child's desires now come to contain a disagreeable component (*Unlust*) due to the feeling of tension experienced. Thus they constitute merely a 'fore-pleasure' (*Vorlust*), which impels to further activities destined to produce the 'end-pleasure' (*Endlust*) that relief of tension brings about." (Jones, E. *Papers on Psycho-Analysis,* 1938)

ending, act Termination of an act, such as eating, that was begun in order to relieve tension, once tension release or drive satiation has been reached; also termed "completion of the act." Childhood schizophrenics often show impairment of such act ending and will continue to eat, for example, without evidence of satiation.

endoderm See *entoderm.*

endogamy Restriction of marriage to members of one's own social, religious, or cultural group.

endogenous, endogenic, endogenetic In psychiatry, referring to conditions that are based primarily on special heredito-constitutional factors, thus originating predominantly *within* the organism itself and affecting the nervous system *directly.*

Schizophrenic and manic-depressive psychoses are the most characteristic types of endogenous disorders, while the so-called *symptomatic* psychoses that arise—as a secondary symptom of organic diseases in part of the body other than the nervous system—from causes *outside* of the nervous system, even though *within* the body, are quite reasonably classified today as exogenous.

When used with depression, endogenous (or autogenic, autonomous, endogenic, or endomorphogenic) denotes a biological, somatic, or nonreactive condition (termed *melancholia* in DSM-III). See *exogeny.*

endogeny, endogenism, endogenesis The term, relating in biology to any process of "growing from within," used in medicine to denote physical and mental conditions that are known or suspected to arise predominantly from causes *within* the body, and more specifically, from causes inherent in that system of the body that is the seat of the morbid character in question.

endomorphic Sheldon's term for the type characterized by a predominance of its first component (circularity), that is, the physical structures developed from the *endodermal* layer of the embryo. Persons of this type are contrasted with the *mesomorphic* and *ectomorphic* (qq.v.) types and correspond roughly to Kretschmer's *pyknic* type. See *type, pyknic.*

endomusia Silent recall of a melody; often appears as a type of obsessive thought.

endonuclease See *recombinant DNA.*

endopsychic Characterizing something as being within the mind or psyche; those mental mechanisms that occur completely within the mind; thus *psychic suicide* is determined by the same processes that determine physical suicide, but in the case of the former the processes work endopsychically. Endopsychic structure refers to the structure of the psyche itself: the conscious, the preconscious, and the unconscious, the ego, the superego, and the id are all parts of the endopsychic structure.

endoreactive Endogenous; not related to external events. An unfortunate term in that the internal events to which he is supposedly reacting are usually unknown

to the patient, in which case use of "reactive" would seem to be inappropriate.

endorphins One of the major families of endogenous opioids, the other being the *enkephalins* (q.v.). The endorphins are components of β-lipotropin, a pituitary factor, and in addition to modulating pain perception they may be involved in modulating mood and responses to stressful stimuli. See *peptide, brain.*

enduring In DSM-III-R, a duration of stressful events of six months or more; acute stressors are those which last less than six months.

enelicomorphism (en-el-i-kō) *Adultomorphism* (q.v.).

energizer See *psychotropics.*

energy lack Fatigue, a nonspecific symptom; among psychiatric disorders, it is most frequent in alcohol or substance abuse, bereavement, depression, schizophrenia, and sleep disorders.

enforced treatment See *forced treatment.*

enfrenzy *Rare.* To madden, to make frenzied.

engineering Manipulation of knowledge for practical uses. *Genetic engineering* refers to alteration of genetic information for practical uses.

engineering, behavioral See *behaviorism.*

engineering, microsocial See *therapy, contract.*

engineering, social See *social policy planning.*

engram In neurology, a neuronal pattern of an acquired skilled act. The term has been used somewhat loosely in psychiatry to refer to the persisting psychical traces (usually in the form of an unconscious or latent memory) of any experience.

engram, function See *function engram.*

engrossment The involvement of the father with his newborn; the developing bond between them is characterized by perception of the newborn as attractive or even perfect, a desire to touch and hold the baby, elation following the birth of the child, and an increased sense of self-esteem and worth within the family.

enkephalins One of the major families of endogenous opioids, the other being the *endorphins* (q.v.). The enkephalins are pentapeptides; their two natural forms (met- and leu-) differ from each other only in the terminal amino acid. The amino acid sequence for met-enkephalin is contained within the β-endorphin molecule, but enkephalins are not the result of degradation of β-endorphin. See *peptide, brain.*

enlightenment effect The result of knowing a theory, as when a theory's predictions come true because the people to whom the theory applies have learned about the theory. That particular enlightenment effect is termed *self-fulfilling prophecy.*

enmeshment A form of faulty family functioning consisting of overinvolvement of family members in one another's lives.

enomania *Oinomania* (q.v.).

enosimania *Obs.* Obsessional belief of the patient that he has committed an unpardonable sin.

enosiophobia *Obs.* A morbid dread of having committed an unpardonable sin.

entatic Invigorating, aphrodisiac.

enteroptosis See *habitus, ptotic.*

entheomania *Obs.* Demonomania.

entitlement 1. The rights granted to a person or group by law or regulation. 2. The special privileges that a narcissistic person feels are owed him, such as expecting to be treated as a *VIP* (q.v.). See *type, "the exceptions."*

entoderm The second primitive germ layer that develops during gastrulation, and the tissues derived from that layer. The entoderm subserves chiefly trophic functions. Its tissue derivatives consist of the epithelium of the digestive tract and associated glands, including pancreas, liver, and gall bladder; epithelium of the respiratory system, thyroid, middle ear, and auditory tube; epithelium of the urinary bladder, female urethra, proximal part of the male urethra, and the prostatic and bulbourethral glands. See *ectoderm; mesoderm.*

entomophobia Pathologic fear of insects.

entrainment See *rhythms, biologic.*

entrance events See *event, life.*

entropy A measure of the unavailable energy in a thermodynamic system; a measure of the unavailable information in an information system, usually "in terms of the number of a priori equiprobable states compatible with the macroscopic description of the state—that is, it corresponds to the amount of microscopic information missing in the macroscopic description." (Goldstine, H.H. *Science 133,* 1961)

The term is used more loosely in psychoanalytic theory to refer to the affective cathexis unavailable for displacement in a psychodynamic system. Freud pointed out that as one grows older there is a "striking diminution" in the movements of "mental cathexes." Some people lose mental plasticity prematurely, whereas others retain it far beyond the usual age limit. "So that in considering the conversion of psychical energy no less than of physical, we must make use of the concept of an *entropy,* which opposes the undoing of what has aleady occurred." (Freud, *CP*)

enuresis (en-ū-rē′sis) Involuntary passage of urine after the age by which full control of urinary excretion (bladder control) should have been attained. It may be organic in origin (e.g. neurologic or urologic disorders), or it may be functional.

Functional enuresis may be nocturnal (bedwetting), diurnal, or both. (See *sleep disorders.*) It is considered primary if it is not preceded by a period of at least one year during which bladder control has been maintained; by definition, then, primary functional enuresis has its onset by the age of 5. Secondary functional enuresis, which appears after bladder control has been established, usually has its onset between the ages of 5 and 8. Enuresis is about twice as common in males as in females and tends to abate with time and finally disappear. By the age of 18 years, only about one of every 100 males is enuretic, while the condition is almost nonexistent by that time in females.

Despite its name, that even functional enuresis may often be on an organic basis is suggested by the findings that approximately 75% of enuretics have a first-degree relative with a history of the disorder, and that concordance for enuresis is significantly higher in monozygotic than in dizygotic twins.

According to psychoanalysis, enuresis may represent nocturnal masturbation (Jones), exhibitionistic impulses (Abraham), or penis envy. Freud and Ferenczi noted a relationship between bedwetting and fire-setting and considered enuresis as a urethral-erotic trait.

enuresis nocturna Bed-wetting; nocturnal enuresis; technically, urinary incontinence at night. Enuresis nocturna is more often psychic than physical in origin, although it may be secondary to urinary tract pathology, spina bifida, or other spinal cord anomalies. See *enuresis.*

environment Everything surrounding a person; the aggregate of external elements that stimulate and influence an organism, including physical, biologic, social, and cultural factors.

environment, neutral A physical and social environment that aims to impose no specific or rigid limitations or make demands upon the patient. "Psychological determinants for what appear to be the same maladjustments may be quite different, and because of that, they require different situations. Since a therapy group supplies a neutral environment, each member can take from it whatever his needs may be. The aggressive child finds relief from his anxiety . . . while the shy and withdrawn one overcomes his fears." (Slavson, *IGT*)

environment, permissive A social and physical environment in which acting out and verbalization are allowed but not necessarily sanctioned or approved.

envy, penis In psychoanalysis, the girl's desire for a penis; a part of the castration complex.

Freud says that when the little girl realizes she has no penis, she reacts either by hoping that some day she will have one or by denying that she does not have one. In the latter case she may be "compelled to behave as though she were a man."

Penis envy is responsible for "a loosening of the girl's relation with her mother as a love-object," because the girl blames her mother for the alleged loss. At this stage the girl is prepared for the further development of the Oedipus situation. The wish for the penis is transformed into the wish for a child. "With this object in view, she takes her father as a love-object. Her mother becomes the object of jealousy."

The concept of penis envy has been criticized for its androcentric bias and for ignoring the effects of familial, social, and cultural input. The concept is embedded in Freud's insistence on a framework of biologically unfolding psychosexual stages. By reducing mental processes to biology, the influences of experience and learning are minimized. His strictly instinctual frame of reference leaves no room for understanding the influences on female development of early object relations, the prephallic development of personality, or the subordinate societal role of women. Others have viewed his approach as the acceptance of an evolutionary value system: nature has its procreative plan and it is better for people to be "natural" and not defy "natural order." See *unnatural.*

enzygotic Of the same egg; usually the term refers to identical (homozygotic) twins.

enzyme See *chromosome.*

enzymes, restriction See *recombinant DNA.*

EOG Electro-oculograph. See *polysomnogram; sleep.*

eonism The adoption of the female role by a male. See *transsexualism.*

eosophobia Fear of dawn.

EP Evoked potential. See *neurometrics.*

ephebiatrics The branch of medicine that treats the development and pathology of adolescence; the specialty of diseases of adolescents.

ephialtes *Obs.* Nightmare.

ephialtes vigilantium (L. "nightmare of those awake") Daymare.

EPI Extrapyramidal involvement; generally used to refer to drug-induced symptoms. Also Eysenck Personality Inventory.

epicritic sensibility The ability to appreciate light touch and its localization; point discrimination; discrimination of moderate variations; distinguished from protopathic.

epidemiology In psychiatry, the study of mental disorders in specified populations, including study of variations in the distribution of specific disorders and of the factors that influence that distribution. The findings are usually expressed in terms of (1) *incidence:* the number of new cases that appear during a specified time period, such as the number of first admissions to mental hospitals during one year; and (2) *prevalence:* the number of cases of any mental disorder that exist currently within the population. *Point prevalence* is the number of cases that exist at a specific point in time, such as the number of schizophrenics in a population on 1 January 1990; *period prevalence* is the number of cases that exist within a defined period of time, such as a month or a year; *lifetime prevalence* is the number of persons who have had a mental disorder in their lifetimes.

Knowledge of the magnitude of a disorder (i.e. its prevalence and the incidence rates) and the patterns of risk for the occurrence of a disorder may suggest ways in which that disorder can be prevented.

epigenesis Those genetically determined processes that give direction and stability to the organism in its development of species-specific end states. In the case of the nervous system, epigenetic processes ultimately determine the integrative power of the brain. See *emergence*. Epigenesis also refers to any process or factors added to or interacting with the heritable genotype (i.e. to the process of gene-environment interaction during development). Epigenic rules are the neurobiologic constraints imposed, for example, on cognitive processing of information, resulting in a channeling of mental development in specific directions.

Epigenetic also describes phenomena that are a result rather than a cause of illness.

epilempsis Hippocratic term for epilepsy.

epilepsia corticalis continua See *epilepsy, continuous.*

epilepsia cursiva *Obs.* A symptom of epilepsy with apparently aimless running about.

epilepsia dromica *Obs.* Semmola's term denoting a syndrome of epilepsy resembling chorea.

epilepsia partialis continua (L. "partial continuous epilepsy") Kozhevnikoff originally described this doubtless somewhat rare motor variant of epilepsy: "It differs from the general myoclonic type in that the twitching is limited to one segment of the body, nearly always a peripheral part such as the wrist and fingers, is practically continuous between the paroxysmal fits, and on the whole partakes of the form less of movements than of irregular, individual muscular contractions." (Wilson, S.A.K. *Modern Problems in Neurology,* 1929) See *epilepsy, continuous; virus infections.*

epilepsy A paroxysmal, transitory disturbance of brain function which develops suddenly, ceases spontaneously, and exhibits a conspicuous tendency to recurrence. The typical epileptic attack, or fit, or convulsion, consists of the sudden onset of loss of consciousness, with or without tonic spasm and clonic contractions of the muscles. There are many forms of epilepsy, which vary depending upon the site of origin, the extent of the area involved, and the nature of the etiological factors; at the present time the term also includes transient episodes of sensory or psychic disturbances. Epilepsy, in short, is not a disease but a symptom, consisting of recurrent episodes of changes in the state of consciousness, with or without accompanying motor or sensory phenomena. Epilepsy has also been called paroxysmal cerebral dysrhythmia.

Among the many older terms for epilepsy are caduca passio, cadiva insania, caducus morbus, cataptosis, decidentia, eclactisma, epilempsis, St. Valentine's disease, St. John's evil, faunorum ludibria, grande nevrose, Herculeus morbus, hieronosus, hylephobias, insania cadiva, lues divina, magnus morbus, malum caducum, morbus astralis, morbus sacer.

The average frequency or expectancy of epilepsy in the general population is 1 in 200; but persons with one epileptic parent have a higher expectancy (1 in 35), and those with both parents epileptic have a much higher expectancy (1 in 10). For each person who develops seizures during his lifetime, it is said that there are 20 more with a predisposition to the affliction. There is no difference in incidence between the sexes, although epilepsy tends to begin earlier in the female.

Today it is customary to divide epilepsy into two major groups on the basis of etiology: (1) *genuine* or *idiopathic* or *cryptogenic epilepsy,* in which there is no known local, general, or psychologic cause; and (2) *symptomatic epilepsy,* in which an organic basis is demonstrable. Approximately 25% of all epileptics fall clearly within the symptomatic group. But as the horizons of neurology widen to include the more recent pathological, physiological, and biochemical advances, it can be anticipated that specific etiologic agents will be demonstrable in an increasing number of cases. Electroencephalograph studies, for example, show that epilepsy is an uncontrolled discharge of cortical and/or subcortical neurons, i.e. an abnormal conversion of the potential energy of the neurons into kinetic energy. Epilepsy can thus be considered a physiochemical disturbance, which could be produced by any number of agents.

Within the *symptomatic* group of epilepsies are those due to (1) local causes—intracranial infection, brain trauma, congenital abnormalities, degenerative diseases such as Pick's disease, various circulatory disturbances of the brain, etc.; (2) general causes—exogenous poisons, anoxemia, endocrine disorders, metabolic disorders (uremia, hypoglycemia, alkalosis, eclampsia, and hypertension of pregnancy), etc.; and (3) psychogenic causes.

In regard to the psychogenic group; there is little evidence that epileptic seizures, as distinct from hysterical fits, are ever purely psychogenic, but it is well recognized that the individual attack may be precipitated by fear, excitement, or other strong emotions. In his article "Dostoevsky and Parricide" (1928), Freud suggested that epilepsy was an organic discharge mechanism that could be brought into play by any number of factors, and that hysteroepilepsy represented an instance of the mechanism being called into play for impulse discharge in hysteria. See also *personality, epileptic; dementia, epileptic.*

The *idiopathic epilepsies* have no known local, general, or psychologic cause; this is a large and heterogeneous group that suffers from a predisposition to convulsions, the nature of which is not yet understood. This predisposition in some cases seems to be largely hereditary in origin, but not all workers would subscribe to the view that idiopathic epilepsy is essentially a hereditary disorder. What is inherited is not epilepsy itself, but rather a predisposition to the development of convulsions under certain conditions, i.e. the physical basis of a cortical dysrhythmia. And only a small proportion of those with this cortical dysrhythmia become epileptic.

The onset of epilepsy is often difficult to determine, for minor attacks may not be recognized, and major attacks (25%) may be only nocturnal, especially in children. The first seizure occurs before the age of 20 in 75% of cases.

Epilepsy is divided into types on the basis of etiology, as discussed above; it may also be subdivided on the basis of physical manifestations. The International League Against Epilepsy has proposed an elaborate scheme that avoids many traditional terms, such as petit mal and grand mal.

The basis of the proposal, now generally accepted, is a tripartite division into:
A. Partial seizures, with focal onset
  1. Elementary: motor or sensory, consciousness not impaired; includes Jacksonian motor seizures, a variety of sensory fits.
  2. Complex: includes psychomotor seizures, temporal lobe epilepsy; consciousness usually impaired; automatisms may occur during ictal or post-ictal phase; ictus usually preceded by an aura, one of the most frequent of which is the epigastric aura.
B. Generalized seizures, without focal onset
  1. Tonic-clonic convulsion (formerly *grand mal*).
  2. Myoclonic, atonic, or akinetic.
  3. Absences (formerly *petit mal*).
C. Unclassified.

In *grand mal epilepsy*, the convulsion or fit consists of a tonic spasm of all the limbs, rarely lasting longer than 30 seconds. This is followed by the clonic phase—a series of sharp, short, interrupted jerks that result from a series of interruptions of the tonic phase. Following cessation of these spasms, the patient may pass into a heavy sleep lasting for hours; some patients, in this *postictal phase*, evidence postepileptic automatism in which they wander, completely amnesic and disoriented, from the scene of attack (this may last for hours or days). Other patients become psychotic, maniacal, or even homicidal.

Petit mal epilepsy may be associated with major seizures or may occur without them. Laymen know them as faints, sensations, or spells. They consist of one or more of the following: mild attacks of dizziness, faintness, queer sensations, dazed states, hot flashes, pallor, vomiting, belching, temper tantrums, sudden relaxation of musculature (so that the patient drops anything in his hand and stops speaking for a moment), momentary confusion and change of color, dreamy sensations, sudden visual or auditory or gustatory sensations, peculiar rushing sensations through the body, sudden jerks and starts. Petit mal attacks are usually extremely brief in duration and often there is no memory of the loss of consciousness so that the patient is only dimly aware of the occurrence of a spell. These minor spells sometimes take the form of the patient's aura preceding his major attacks, as if the attack were incomplete; patients will often spontaneously label them their frustrated or incomplete spells. Petit mal epilepsy occurs typically in young people and only rarely begins after the second decade. Associated psychiatric symptoms are rare and there is almost never an aura. Usually there is immobility during an attack, and the patient is mentally clear immediately after the attack. Incontinence is infrequent in petit mal epilepsy.

Petit mal epilepsy associated with a spike and wave complex (also known as dart and dome complex) in the electroencephalogram, usually at a frequency of 3 cps. Some workers use the term *pyknolepsy* (q.v.) synonymously with petit mal.

The group called *complex partial seizures* or *psychomotor epilepsy* includes a bewildering variety of recurrent periodical disturbances, which usually take the form of some mental disturbance during which the patient carries out movements of a highly organized but semiautomatic character. These seizures are rare in children, the attack itself is marked by confusion rather than loss of consciousness, and there is later amnesia. Psychomotor attacks last longer than petit mal attacks, with which they are easily confused; but incontinence and postictal confusion, which do not occur in petit mal, are seen frequently in psychomotor epilepsy. About two-thirds of the psychomotor group also have grand mal seizures, but only about 3% also have petit mal attacks. There is general agreement that the great majority of psychomotor seizures are the epileptic manifestations of temporal lobe lesions.

epilepsy, acousticomotor See *epilepsy, reflex.*

epilepsy, affective Bratz's term to designate a form of epilepsy characterized by exaggerated emotional responses, which generally culminate in an epileptiform seizure. Bonhoeffer referred to such states as *reactive epilepsies* and Kraepelin classified many of them as *epileptic swindlers.*

epilepsy, akinetic A type of petit mal epilepsy. See *epilepsy.*

epilepsy, alcoholic This is an ill-defined clinical disorder, including a variety of manifestations associated with alcoholism and so-called epilepsy.

An alcoholic may experience an epileptiform seizure; or a person with the epileptoid personality may try to solve his personality difficulties through alcohol; or the alcoholism and epilepsy may be more or less independent of each other.

epilepsy, autonomic Diencephalic epilepsy; sympathetic epilepsy; parasympathetic epilepsy. Autonomic epilepsy refers to symptoms of sudden, diffuse discharge of the autonomic nervous system in otherwise normal individuals. In some, symptoms are primarily of sympathetic discharge; in others, symptoms are primarily of parasympathetic discharge. Usually, however, symptoms are mixed.

Penfield in 1929 described predominantly sympathetic seizures consisting of fever, flushing, tearing, sweating, salivation, hiccupping, and shivering, which he termed "diencephalic autonomic epilepsy." In this case a ball valve tumor of the third ventricle had resulted in compression of adjacent hypothalamic nuclei. Cushing in 1932 reported on parasympathetic outbursts occurring in response to intraventricular injections of pituitrin and pilocarpine. Symptoms included profuse sweating, flushing, fall in blood pressure, lowering of temperature and basal metabolic rate, and increased peristalsis in the stomach and intestines.

epilepsy, centrencephalic Generalized (in contrast to focal) epilepsy, in which extensive areas of both hemispheres are simultaneously activated by epileptic discharge from some midline center (probably the thalamus). See *system, centrencephalic.*

epilepsy, continuous This is a form of epilepsy including the polyclonia epileptoides continua of Choroschko, the epilepsia corticalis continua of Kozhevnikoff, and the epilepsia partialis continua of Wilson, characterized by myoclonic attacks in single muscular groups; it is limited to one side of the body and consciousness is retained during the attacks.

epilepsy, coordinated A type of focal seizure in which the movements seem purposive and voluntary but are repeated aimlessly without accomplishing what appears to be their goal.

epilepsy, cryptogenic Epilepsy without known etiology and pathology.

epilepsy, diencephalic See *epilepsy, autonomic.*

epilepsy, digestive The commonest form of visceral epilepsy, manifested in gastrointestinal symptoms such as colic, eructation, nausea, vomiting, epigastric distention, meteorism, diarrhea, and tenesmus.

epilepsy, erotic A type of epileptiform focal seizure in which the patient experiences spells of intense erotic sensation; first reported by T.C. Erickson (*Archives of Neurology & Psychiatry* 53, 1945) in a 43-year-old housewife, in whom a small vascular tumor was later disclosed on the medial surface of the cerebral hemisphere, impinging upon the motor and sensory representation of the genitalia.

epilepsy, essential Idiopathic epilepsy. See *epilepsy.*

epilepsy, gelastic A form of epilepsy in which laughter is a part of the seizure pattern, usually due to a lesion in the left temporal region.

epilepsy, genuine Idiopathic epilepsy. See *epilepsy.*

epilepsy, gestational Seizures that appear only during pregnancy. The incidence of gestational epilepsy is relatively low, but it highlights the problems of management of the pregnant epileptic. Anticonvulsants appear to increase by two or three times the risk of congenital malformations in the fetus (especially cleft palate, cleft lip, and septal or other cardiac defects). *Fetal hydantoin syndrome* includes craniofacial abnormalities, limb defects, growth abnormalities, and mental retardation. *Fetal trimethadione syndrome* includes epicanthal folds, low-set ears, V-shaped eyebrows, ocular defects, short stature, developmental delays, and speech disturbances.

epilepsy, hallucinatory A type of focal epilepsy in which complex hallucinations are the main part of the attack. The hallucinations are short-lived, paroxysmal, and irresistible in quality; they tend to be identical in each attack.

epilepsy, inhibition of See *epilepsy, reflex.*

epilepsy, inhibitory A rare form of petit mal epilepsy in which transitory loss of power occurs in a limb or on one side of the body without preceding tonic spasm or clonic

movements; there may be an associated impairment of consciousness.

epilepsy, Jacksonian A variant of grand mal epilepsy described by J.H. Jackson. The convulsion begins with clonic movements, which increase in severity and spread (the "cortical march") to involve large segments of the limb, then the other limb on the same side, then the face, and finally sometimes the other side, at which point consciousness is usually lost. The spread is along anatomical and/or physiological lines, and this type of epilepsy almost always indicates organic disease of the precentral cortex. Jacksonian epilepsy usually begins in one of three foci: thumb and index finger; angle of the mouth; or the great toe.

epilepsy, larvated Epileptic equivalent.

epilepsy, major Grand mal epilepsy.

epilepsy, masked Epileptic equivalent.

epilepsy, minor Petit mal epilepsy. See *epilepsy.*

epilepsy, musicogenic See *epilepsy, reflex.*

epilepsy, myoclonic A type of petit mal epilepsy. See *epilepsy.*

epilepsy, myoclonus A variant of grand mal epilepsy first described by Unverricht in 1891. This type of epilepsy is usually familial and occurs in several siblings. Symptoms usually begin between 6 and 16 years. Generalized epileptiform attacks with loss of consciousness appear first, often only at night. After several years, the characteristic myoclonic contractions develop; they involve simultaneously the symmetrical muscles on both sides of the body and are strong enough to produce movements of limb segments. The face, trunk, and upper and lower limbs are most commonly involved. The contractions disappear during sleep and are intensified by emotional excitement. They tend to increase in severity before a generalized epileptic attack; sudden contraction of the lower limbs may throw the patient to the ground. For a period of years, myoclonic contractions and epileptic attacks are associated; during this time, a progressive dementia develops and there is a passing into a third stage, where the grand mal attacks tend to disappear. Then dysarthria and dysphagia increase and death often follows progressive cachexia.

epilepsy, nocturnal Jelliffe and White (*DNS*) state that "the possibility of exclusively nocturnal attacks—*nocturnal epilepsy*—should be borne in mind. It is suspicious if the patient awakens tired and lame, as if his muscles had been beaten, particularly if he shows conjunctival ecchymoses, a wounded tongue and flecks of blood on the pillow. A localized muscular weakness that passes off promptly would add certainty to the diagnosis."

Exclusively nocturnal attacks occur in approximately 25% of known epileptics; both day and night attacks occur in another 25% of patients. Exclusively nocturnal attacks are more common in children.

epilepsy, parasympathetic See *epilepsy, autonomic.*

epilepsy, photic See *epilepsy, reflex.*

epilepsy, post-traumatic Convulsions following brain trauma, i.e. a type of symptomatic epilepsy. Post-traumatic epilepsy develops in 3–5% of cases with closed head injury and in 30–50% of cases with open head injury. Convulsions tend to occur (1) within a few seconds of injury; (2) within a day or two; or (3) within the first two years following injury. About half of early-appearing epilepsy disappears; in late-appearing epilepsy, there is a tendency to abatement of attacks within two years of onset, and in 30%, convulsions disappear completely.

epilepsy, procursive An epileptic symptom, characterized by sudden, impulsive running forward.

epilepsy, psychic Epileptic equivalent, such as automatisms, dream states, and affective states. See *equivalent, epileptic.*

epilepsy, psychomotor See *epilepsy.*

epilepsy, psychopathology of See *personality, epileptic.*

epilepsy, reactive Bleuler (*TP*) speaks of "the rare 'reflex epilepsy,' whose attacks are set free by the irritation of a scar or some other pathological focus."

epilepsy, reading A type of reflex epilepsy in which the affected person has the sensation of his jaw snapping or opening when he reads; if he continues to read once the myoclonic jaw movements appear, a generalized convulsion is likely to occur. See *epilepsy, reflex.*

epilepsy, reflex Epileptic convulsions precipitated by some external stimulus, such as a sudden loud noise (*acousticomotor epilepsy*), music (*musicogenic epilepsy*), visual (*photic epilepsy*), or cutaneous stimuli. Reflex inhibition of the fit is an allied phenomenon: if, for example, a focal convulsion begins with movement in one limb, a strong stimulus such as a firm grip applied to the limb will often abort the attack if this is begun immediately after onset of the attack.

epilepsy, reflex inhibition of See *epilepsy, reflex.*

epilepsy, regional See *epilepsy, myoclonic.*

epilepsy, retropulsive An epileptic symptom, characterized by sudden, impulsive running backward.

epilepsy, sensory A type of petit mal epilepsy consisting of paresthesiae involving part or the whole of one side of the body, often without loss of consciousness. Sensory epilepsy is usually due to a contralateral lesion in the parietal lobe.

epilepsy, short stare A type of petit mal epilepsy. See *epilepsy.*

epilepsy, sleep *Obs.* Narcolepsy.

epilepsy, sympathetic See *epilepsy, autonomic.*

epilepsy, symptomatic A condition in which the convulsions represent a symptom of an underlying organic disease process. This may occur in such conditions as congenital defects of the brain, intracranial hemorrhages, meningitis, brain abscess, senile degeneration, carbon monoxide poisoning.

epilepsy, tetanoid Pritchard's term for epilepsy in which the spasm is tonic only.

epilepsy, tonic Epileptic fits exhibiting only tonic contractions, to the exclusion of clonic contractions.

epilepsy, traumatic See *epilepsy, post-traumatic.*

epilepsy, true Idiopathic epilepsy. See *epilepsy.*

epilepsy, vertiginous A rare type of seizure pattern precipitated by vestibular stimuli, characterized by recurrent attacks of vertigo (of the rotatory type); associated often with short lapses of consciousness.

epilepsy, visceral A form of focal epilepsy in which the fit is manifested as visceral sensations, usually referable to the gastrointestinal tract, the cardiorespiratory system, or the genitourinary system. The principal loci of lesions in such cases have been found to be in the frontotemporal and mid-frontal parasagittal regions, indicating that the visceral sensations arise from some central location, probably the amygdalohippocampal portion of the temporal lobe.

epileptic character See *personality, epileptic.*

epileptic clouded states Psychotic reactions occurring in epileptics. At times, either preceding or following a convulsive attack, the epileptic may manifest a dazed reaction with deep confusion or excitement, anxiety, and bewilderment. Associated with this, there may be violent outbreaks, hallucinations, fears, or ecstatic moods with religious exaltation.

epileptic cry See *cry, epileptic.*

epileptic deterioration See *dementia, epileptic.*

epileptic equivalent See *equivalent, epileptic.*

epileptic psychopathic constitution See *personality, epileptic.*

epileptic psychoses See *dementia, epileptic.*

epileptic, pyknic An epileptic with the pyknic type of body build. According to Westphal most epileptics are dysplastic, athletic, or asthenic, and less than 10% are pyknic.

epilepticism *Obs.* Status epilepticus.

epileptoid Resembling epilepsy.

epileptoid, orthostatic *Obs.* Children who have fainting spells and occasional convulsions when forced to stand for a long time or after getting up in the morning were referred to as *orthostatic epileptoids* by J. Husler.

epileptosis Southard's term for the various manifestations of epileptic psychoses.

epiloia See *sclerosis, tuberous.*

epinephrine (e-pin-e′frin) The active hormone of the medullary portion of the adrenal glands, $C_9H_{13}NO_3$, often referred to by its proprietary name, Adrenalin. Epinephrine is a potent vasopressor drug; it increases blood pressure, stimulates heart muscle, accelerates heart rate, and increases cardiac output.

Stimulation of sympathetic nerve fibers releases a substance similar to epinephrine known as *sympathin.* Sympathin is the chemical mediator of the excitatory processes initiated by sympathetic nerve impulses at neuroeffector junctions. Like epinephrine, sympathin has both excitatory and inhibitory effects; that released when excitatory responses are stimulated is sympathin E, and that released when inhibitory responses are stimulated is sympathin I.

It has been suggested that epinephrine or products in its metabolism may be in-

volved in the natural occurrence of mental disorders. Some doubt is cast on this by the fact that epinephrine itself is present in the brain only in small quantities. A closely related substance, norepinephrine (noradrenaline, arterenol), which is also present in the adrenal medulla, is known to occur in significant amounts in the brain, particularly in the hypothalamus, and derivatives of this substance might therefore be more likely as possible precursors of clinical psychoses. For these same reasons, it seems more likely that norepinephrine is the central sympathetic neurohumor. See *catecholamine hypothesis; dopamine hypothesis.*

More recent evidence suggests that it is *dopamine* rather than norepinephrine that is involved in schizophrenic disorders. The antischizophrenic activity of phenothiazines is directly related to their ability to block postsynaptic receptors in the brain to the transmitter actions of dopamine, rather than norepinephrine. It may be that such blocking action is exerted by inhibition of the dopamine-sensitive, cyclic AMP-forming enzyme adenylase cyclase.

Both epinephrine and norepinephrine are normally present in the blood only in low concentration, but in response to stress both increase markedly. When the stess agent is removed, the circulating blood level of these *catecholamines* falls quickly back to normal. This rapid disappearance might be achieved by storage in tissues or by enzymatic destruction, and evidence to date favors the latter mechanism. It is possible that one mechanism for in vivo inactivation of these catecholamines is breakdown by the particular enzyme monoamine oxidase (MAO, amine oxidase). See *ergotropic.*

epinosic, epinosis See *gain, epinosic.*

episodic disorders Impulse disorders. See *disorders, episodic; dyscontrol, episodic.*

episodic dyscontrol syndrome See *dyscontrol, episodic.*

epistasis A genetic mechanism by which the phenotypical expression of one hereditary factor masks, or prevents, the manifestation of another factor that concerns the same organ, although it is not allelic to the factor with the greater expressivity. The factor exercising the masking effect is called *epistatic,* while the hidden factor is said to be *hypostatic.*

The result of *epistasis* is similar to that produced by a *dominant* character. However, there is a significant difference between the phenomena of dominance and epistasis. While a dominant and a recessive factor are always alleles of each other, an epistatic and a hypostatic factor are merely related to the same trait or organ, but they are not the two members of an allelic pair. See *dominance*.

epistemic Relating to the need to know, considered by many to be one of the basic motives of human behavior.

epistemophilia The love of knowledge or the impulsion to inquire into things; said by psychoanalysts to receive its earliest important stimulation during the phallic phase, although preliminary preparation is gained through interests in other and earlier erotogenic zones, particularly the o: al and the anal. The many subsequent manifestations of the impulse to learn are regarded as sublimations of the several varieties of infantile sexuality.

epithalamus A zone of brain tissue above the thalamus composed of (1) *habenular ganglion* or *trigone*, a depressed triangular area anterior to the superior colliculus; (2) *pineal body*, which lies between the superior colliculi; (3) *posterior commissure*, some of whose fibers connect the two superior colliculi.

EPSDT Early and periodic screening, diagnosis, and treatment. Often an essential element in any *prospective* study of disorder, but increasingly subject to stringent limitations because of ethical issues involved. Subjects must be told what is being done to and for them as part of informed consent; but such action may become a self-fulfilling prophecy, as labeling theory would predict. See *consent, informed*.

epsilon alcoholism See *alcoholism*.

equilibrium, homeostatic See *instinct, aim of*.

equilibrium, narcissistic A state of harmony between the demands of the superego and the capabilities of the ego; derived from the original harmony between the obedient child and its loving parents. The superego does not demand of the ego more than it can produce. The ego is not terrified by the threat of the superego severity.

equinophobia Pathologic fear of or aversion to horses.

equivalent, anxiety See *anxiety attack, equivalent of*.

equivalent, epileptic The manifestations of genuine epilepsy are many. When an epileptic patient has an "attack" that is neither of the grand or petit mal type, he is said to have an *equivalent* or a "substitutive" attack. For example, a twilight state may take the place of a grand mal attack. A patient about to have a major seizure developed a condition in which he believed that he was in heaven, curing all the ailments of the universe.

Some authors use this term to refer to psychomotor epilepsy. See *epilepsy*.

equivalent, psychic Psychomotor epilepsy. See *epilepsy*.

Equus-Laingian view Romanticization or eroticization of madness, ranging from a tendency to overvalue the positive aspects of bipolar illness while minimizing the negative, painful ones to a conviction that all psychopharmacologic interventions in such illnesses are oppressive, intrusive, and contraindicated. The term was suggested by K.R. Jamison and F.K. Goodwin (in *Psychiatry Update II*, ed. L. Grinspoon, 1983).

erbfest *Inheritable* (q.v.).

Erdheim's tumor Craniopharyngioma. See *tumor, intracranial*.

erective impotence See *impotence, psychic*.

eremiophobia Fear of a lonely place or solitude.

eremophilia *Obs*. Morbid desire to be alone.

eremophobia Fear of being alone.

erethism *Obs*. Pathologic irritability, sensitivity, excitability, or overactivity; often used to denote sexual erethism, which may be manifested as erotomania, nymphomania, satyriasis, etc.

erethistic Erethismic. See *erethism*.

erethizophrenia Exaggerated cortical excitability.

erethizophrenic Pertaining to or suffering from erethizophrenia. J.R. Hunt's term equivalent to *cycloid*.

ereuthophobia *Erythrophobia* (q.v.).

erg R.B. Cattell proposed this term to replace *instinct* and defined it as "an innate psychophysical disposition which permits its possessor to acquire reactivity to certain classes of objects more readily than others, to experience a specific emotion in regard to them, and to start on a course of action which ceases more completely at a specific goal activity than at any other." Erg is also used as a general term for a unit of work, functioning, or activity.

ergasia This term, introduced into psychiatry by Adolf Meyer, is designed to express the total of functions and reactions of an individual, in contradistinction to the functions of individual organs or parts of the human organism. It embraces the concept known as *the personality as a whole* and refers to those responses of a person that represent the results of the activity of many of his parts. It stands for the action of the total organism.

ergasiatry Adolf Meyer's term for psychiatry.

ergasiology Adolf Meyer's term for psychology.

ergasionomania *Obs.* A morbid impulse to work, to keep busy. It is observed in pronounced form in the manic state of manic-depressive psychosis.

ergasiophobia Fear of functioning or acting generally associated with an underlying dread that if movement takes place something disastrous will happen; related to the magical feeling that what happens to oneself also happens to the environment. A patient may believe that if he stops functioning or moving, the world will do the same.

ergasthenia *Obs.* A condition of fatigue or debility due to overwork or excessive functioning.

ergastic See *ergasia*.

ergodialeipsis Action that ceases before it is completely carried out. It occurs most commonly in schizophrenia and appears to be a type of *blocking* (q.v.).

ergomania Compulsion to work, "workaholism."

ergonomics The science and engineering of human factors involved in adapting to work conditions or to the general environment. The field is limited because tools and measures for quantification of ergonomic qualities thus far are lacking.

ergonomics, cognitive The study of information exchange between humans and computers (or other machines).

ergotherapy *Praxitherapeutics* (q.v.).

ergotism Chronic poisoning with ergot alkaloids, one of the most powerful of which is isoergine (lysergic acid amide). In the 17th and 18th centuries, ergotism was a common condition in Europe and the United States, resulting from eating contaminated rye bread. As seen at that time, ergotism was of two types: (1) gangrenous—dry gangrene of the extremities, the affected portions of which finally fall away; and (2) convulsive—with paresthesiae of skin and extremities, vertigo, tinnitus, headaches, vomiting, diarrhea, painful muscular contractions, epileptiform convulsions, and hallucinations.

ergotropic Having the quality of turning to, predisposing toward, or preparing for action. Hess and others applied this term to that portion of the diencephalic subcortical system that integrates sympathetic with somatomotor activities and prepares the body for positive action. The other division of this system is called the trophotropic; the latter integrates parasympathetic with somatomotor activities and promotes protective and recuperative behavior patterns.

Much of the work of experimental psychiatry in the mid-20th century has been devoted to attempts to define more specifically the neurophysiological bases of emotion in the belief that this will open the way to a better understanding of emotional disorders. Hess's proposal that the reactions of the organism to environmental change are effected by a subcortical system coordinating visceral, somatic, and psychic functions is an example of one way in which the general problem has been attacked.

The significance of Hess's hypothesis depends upon recognition of the brain as a communication system, whose functional integrity is maintained by neural excitation and transmission, which in turn depend upon metabolic production of energy and its transformation into neural activity. If disordered or abnormal behavior is considered to be due, possibly, to some fault in this communication system, either because of defective transmission of the impulse or because of abnormal response of the nerve cells involved, the problem becomes one essentially of production and/or destruction of metabolites and the enzyme systems involved.

Emotions and emotional behavior depend upon the functional integrity of a subcortical coordinating system, which in turn depends on the balance and interaction of two opposing functional systems—the ergotropic, whose neurohumor may be *norepinephrine* (q.v.), and the trophotropic, whose neurohumor may be *serotonin* (q.v.). The "functional" psychoses may be due to a shift in equilibrium, to one side or the other, by any number of possible mechanisms. Thus one neurohormone might be underproduced, or overproduced, or faultily stored, or inadequately released; or metabolic breakdown of neurohormone might be aberrant, and/or abnormal intermediary metabolites might be formed in the course of neurohormone breakdown.

Erikson, Erik H. (b. 1902) Psychoanalyst; psychosocial development of the ego, cross-cultural analysis, child analysis; eight stages of man (see *ontogeny, psychic*); *Children and Society* (1950), *Identity and the Life Cycle* (1959), *Youth: Change and Challenge* (1963), *Insight and Responsibility* (1964).

Erklären Jasper's term for the type of etiologic statement about a psychiatric condition that is based on an objectively verifiable conclusion, such as "This paranoid syndrome is due to amphetamine intoxication." Jaspers contrasted Erklären, "explanation," with *Verstehen*, an "understanding" of the dynamics based on an intuitive grasp of the connection between the psychiatric manifestations and the subject's life, such as "This paranoid syndrome is based on the patient's doubts about his masculinity after being rejected by his love object."

erogeneity The state or quality of being erogenous. See *anality; orality.*

Eros (Gr. *Eros*, the god of love) The life instinct or drive. See *instinct; instinct, death.*

erotic seizure See *epilepsy, erotic.*

eroticism See *erotism.*

eroticism, olfactory Pleasurable sensation associated wth smelling; in psychoanalysis, considered a part of anal eroticism.

eroticize To charge with libidinal or erotic energy. Any part of an object or person may be invested with the erotic instinct, that is, eroticized (libidinized).

erotism (eroticism) A condition characterized by the instinctual quality called "love" or Eros. Thus one speaks of erotism relating to body zones, such as anal, oral, and genital erotism; or to psychic structures, such as ego-erotism (narcissism); or to objects outside of the body or mind such as alloerotism.

erotism, ego See *narcissism; ego libido.*

erotism, oral The pleasure and gratification derived from using the mouth for other than the utility value of taking in food and drink. In the child it means the pleasure experienced when close to the mother's warm body, when sucking her breast or the nipple of the bottle and thus feeling secure and protected.

erotization Libidinization; the act of erotizing or state of being erotized. During infancy the body becomes erotized, notably those parts of the body called erotogenic zones. All forms of activity subsequent to the stage of infantile sexuality may and usually do undergo erotization. Character traits, ideas, actions of all sorts, hobbies, recreations, etc. are erotized.

erotocrat A person of powerful sexuality.

erotodromomania *Obs.* Hirschfeld's term to denote the morbid impulse to travel as an escape from some painful sexual situation.

erotogenesis The springing or origination of libidinal or erotic impulses. In *Three Contributions to the Theory of Sex,* Freud shows that the sexual instincts in humans are complex and result from impulses coming from several sources, among them the oral, anal, and phallic zones.

erotogenetic *Erotogenic* (q.v.).

erotogenic Relating to or having its origin in the libidinal or erotic instinct; commonly applied to libidinal impulses that are expressed through special body areas or erotogenic zones (genitals, mouth, anus, urethra).

erotographomania A morbid impulse to write love letters. The letters are generally written anonymously.

erotolalia Sexually obscene speech, especially in reference to the use of such speech during sexual intercourse as a means of enhancing gratification. This term emphasizes the sexual content of speech in contrast to the obscene or socially tabu speech of coprolalia, which term is more properly limited to verbal expression of excretory processes.

erotomania A syndrome that occurs almost exclusively in females, consisting of the delusional belief that a man, usually older and of higher social status, is deeply in love with the patient; described in 1922 by G. G. de Clérambault. Some authors regard the syndrome as a denial of unconscious homosexual impulses; most, however, interpret it as a grandiose phantasy constructed as a defense against a narcissistic injury that has made the patient feel unloved or unloveable.

Mary V. Seeman (*Archives of General Psychiatry 35*, 1978) distinguishes two types of *delusional loving*: (1) *phantom lover syndrome*, a fixed and unshakeable conviction that one is loved, usually by an "ordinary" person; the syndrome is found most often in poorly integrated, schizophrenic women and survives repeated confrontations with reality; (2) erotomania proper or *De Clérambault's syndrome*, which occurs in healthier, sexually active, aggressive women who develop intense but short-lived delusions about a man whom they admire for his wealth, power, or position. As time brings more denials of the reality of their beliefs, such women give up the man in question and move on to another with whom they repeat the cycle.

Sometimes erotomania is used as an equivalent of *hypersexuality* (q.v.).

erotopathy (ē-ro-top′ă-thē) Any abnormality of the sexual impulse; *paraphilia* (q.v.).

erotophobia Aversion to sex, including avoidance or denial of sexual feelings; in DSM-III-R, *sexual aversion disorder*.

ERP *Event-related potential;* a brain wave response to external events such as auditory stimuli. Both adult schizophrenics and children at risk for schizophrenia show a reduction in late positive amplitude in comparison with ERPs in controls. See *neurometrics.*

error Errors of memory are distinguished from forgetting and false recollections through one feature only, namely, that the error (false recollection) is not recognized as such but finds credence. Back of every error is a repression. More accurately stated: the error conceals a falsehood, a disfigurement which is ultimately based on repressed material. (Freud, *BW*)

error attribution See *attribution.*

error, beta Also known as *Type II error*—failure to find a statistically significant difference when an actual difference exists.

error, logical A mistake in thinking, such as basing a conclusion on insufficient evidence. Cognitive therapy emphasizes the importance of typical logical errors that are based on negatively biased thinking: drawing arbitrary inferences from inadequate data, overgeneralization, personalization (giving personal meaning to a neutral event), magnification, selective attention (ignoring any positive aspects of an experience), etc. See *therapy, cognitive.*

error, Type I The rejection of the *null hypothesis* (q.v.) when it is true; the experimenter falsely concludes that a relationship exists when, in fact, there is none.

error, Type II *Beta error;* acceptance of the *null hypothesis* (q.v.) when it is false; the experimenter fails to find a significant difference when a difference in fact exists.

erythema multiforme See *syndrome, Stevens-Johnson.*

erythrism (ē-rith′ris′m) In medicine and anthropology, a condition characterized by the presence of red hair in certain regions of the body, notably in the beard and pubic zone, where it contrasts with the color of the remainder of the body hair. This condition attains its significance for constitutional medicine from the theory that in analogy to *flavism* (q.v.) it constitutes a stigma of the *asthenic, microsplanchnic* physique and its tendency to tuberculosis. See *type, asthenic.*

erythroblastosis fetalis See *icterus gravis neonatorum.*

erythroedema polyneuritis *Acrodynia* (q.v.).

erythrophobia Fear of red. This is most commonly associated with blood, although, as with other fears, anything identified with the original fear may act as a substitute for it. For example, the fear of blood may be expressed as the fear of red, of anything that is red; the fear may then spread to all colors; the fear of colors may then give way to that of certain localities in which colors are prominent. Fears amass with great facility; moreover, as fears grow they tend to appear less associated with the original one, until finally the fear seems thoroughly illogical and unrelated to any previous experiences.

The conscious fear is often symbolic of an unconscious and antithetic impulse. Thus the fear of blood may be related unconsciously to a wish for it. The wish may be a sadistic expression connected with the castration phantasy or one of its many subsequent symbolic expressions.

Not infrequently erythrophobia appears as a fear of blushing. It is said that the latter is related to exhibitionism and that it means genitalization of the face or head. The individual fears the red face as if it were the penis.

escape drinking See *alcoholism*.

escapism In psychoanalytic therapy, the tendency to escape from reality functioning to the relative security of childhood, a tendency often manifested by an accentuation of neurotic symptoms. It is a form of resistance.

ESL 1. "English is their second language," used particularly to refer to children whose parents' native tongue is a language other than English, in consequence of which the children are reared speaking the other language even though when they go to school they will be expected to be familiar with English. 2. "English as a second language," a specialized field of education.

ESN Educationally subnormal.

esophoria See *heterophoria*.

ESP Extrasensory perception. See *perception, extrasensory*.

espiritismo A form of *folk healing* (q.v.) culture-specific to Puero Ricans, based on the belief that the world is inhabited by spirits that require one or more incarnations in human bodies before they can finally accomplish their mission of union with God. Some spirits (*causas*) have trouble reaching that goal and intrude on people during their dreams or enter their bodies, causing physical and psychiatric illness. The affected person consults an *espiritista* (medium or spiritualist) either in a private session (*consulta*) or at regularly held meetings (reuniones). Several seances may be needed to convince the spirit of its wrongdoing and to get it back on track. Herbal medicines, prayers, and consultation with physicians may all be advised by the espiritista. See *folk medicine*.

Esquirol, Jean Etienne Dominique (1772–1840) French physician who specialized in treatment of the mentally ill. He was Pinel's favorite pupil. In 1817 at the Salpétrière he inaugurated the first offi-cial course on mental disease; his textbook, *Des Maladies Mentales*, was published in 1837.

EST Electroshock therapy. See *therapy, electroconvulsive*.

est Erhard Seminar Training, a consciousness-expanding technique developed by Werner Erhard; usually given as a 60-hour seminar that takes place on two consecutive weekends. Est is an eclectic integration of Eastern and Western philosophies, of various psychological theories and practices, and of motivation techniques from the business world; in the 1970s it was one of the most popular of the human-potential movements.

esthesia Sensibility; capacity for sensation. Used frequently as a combining form.

esthesiogenesis The production of a reaction in a sensory zone.

estrangement, inner Federn's term to refer to the feeling that external objects, even though well perceived, have a strange, unfamiliar or unreal quality. He considered estrangement to be characteristic, nosologically and clinically, of the depressive psychoses (while depersonalization is characteristic of the schizophrenias). Federn ascribed estrangement to a failure of cathexis of the external ego boundary, one of whose functions is to identify non-ego (external objects) as real and familiar. This failure is due to a primary disturbance in the bodily ego feeling, which is derived from the narcissistic libido (the sexual energy investing the ego).

estromania *Obs.* Oestromania; *nymphomania* (q.v.).

état marbré Status marmoratus. See *dystonia, torsion*.

eternity, fear of By this term Fenichel designates one in the group of fears of "surroundings that imply the loss of the usual means of orientation," such as fear of cessation of customary routine, fear of death, fear of uniform noises, etc. The patient who has such fears is particularly afraid of a loss of control over infantile sexual and aggressive impulses, and then projects onto the outside world his own fears of losing control. A concept such as eternity, in which the normal assessment of time loses its significance, is seen as a great threat to him, for it means a loss of the forces protecting him against his own unconscious unmastered sexual and aggressive impulses. (*PTN*)

etheromania Ether-drinking; ether was drunk as an inebriant in many parts of the world in the early 13th century and in some European peasant communities rivaled alcohol in popularity. This form of inebriety is now rare.

ethics That branch of philosophy concerned with the moral life and consisting of consideration of one's ordinary actions, judgments, and justifications as a means of discovering what one ought to do and of determining what actions are morally good, acceptable, or right, and what actions are unacceptable or wrong. Ethics is more than *morality*, which refers to any system of beliefs and values against which behavior is judged. Ethics comes into being when morality itself is problematic, and when conflicts arise between opposing moral systems or sets of values. (Pellegrino, E. *Bulletin, New York Academy of Medicine 54*, 1978)

Codes of professional ethics, despite their names, more often address themselves to matters of professional etiquette than to questions of morals. They typically enjoin the physician to do what he deems best for the patient and ignore the possibility of conflict between the value systems of the patient and the physician.

Some writers differentiate between *general normative ethics*, or ethical theories, and *applied normative ethics*, the attempt to apply the principles to specific problems that call for concrete decisions. Normative ethics is concerned with what ought to be. *Nonnormative ethics*, on the other hand, is concerned with what attitudes and codes do operate in fact. The study of how moral codes differ from one society to another, termed *descriptive ethics*, is one nonnormative approach. Another is *metaethics*, which is concerned with the logic of moral reasoning and the meanings of the fundamental concepts of ethics such as rights, obligations, and responsibilities.

ethics, applied The use of ethical theory in the solution of practical, moral, and social problems such as capital punishment, genetic research, racism, and warfare. The premise of such applications of ethics is that moral problems are the cause rather than merely a significant aspect of the social conditions under study. Applied moral philosophy strives for greater clarity, avoidance of logical fallacies, consideration and understanding of the appropriate moral concepts, and critical examination of the arguments propounded in attempting to find solutions to moral problems.

ethics, biomedical *Bioethics;* a form of applied ethics, consisting of the application of general ethical theories and principles to the problems actually encountered in medical practice, delivery of health care, medical and biological research, and public policy determinations affecting health and illness. Because it is applied ethics, biomedical ethics cannot be confined to a systematic analysis of moral principles but must instead be continuously subject to scrutiny and revision in terms of the applicability of provisional principles to actual cases.

ethics, community Focus on an ethic of community obligation in which individual interests must be submerged. Professional and ethical codes are forms of community ethics.

ethics, descriptive A history of different ethical theories or concepts, usually including illustrations of different aspects of ethics from which students or readers are expected to select those views that are applicable to the conditions or dilemmas that confront them.

ethics, situation A monistic form of act-utilitarianism ethical theory which holds that there is one fundamental or basic principle, and that what one must do is determine the meaning of that principle in the situation at hand. The right or morally correct action is whatever will, all in all, cause the most good or prevent the most evil. To a situation ethicist, rules are summarizations of the wisdom of the past rather than determinants of a specific course or action that one must take. See *utilitarianism, negative.*

ethnology The branch of *anthropology* that deals with the division of humankind into races and studies the origin, history, customs, and the institutions of the various racial groups.

ethnopsychology See *psychiatry, comparative.*

ethnoscience Also known as *componential analysis, ethnosemantics,* and *cognitive anthropology,* ethnoscience comprises the organized study of the thought systems of people in other cultures and sometimes in our own. Ethnoscientists search for the ways in which knowledge of a culture's rules is reflected in the behavior of natives, and especially in their speech. An ethnoscientific description attempts to write a set of rules for a culture so complete that an outsider could use them to behave appropriately in that culture.

ethnosemantics *Ethnoscience* (q.v.).

ethology 1. The study of group behavior as it is reflected in the mores and customs of a human group. 2. More commonly, the study of the behavior of animals in their natural habitat. Some of the key concepts of ethology are *instinct* (q.v.), *imprinting,* and *social releaser.* See *releaser, social.*

etic Referring to phenomena that, if not universal, at least are not culture-bound. See *emic.*

etiology The division of medical science relating to the cause of disease. The cause of general paresis is the germ of syphilis; not all patients with syphilis develop general paresis. Etiologic studies involve also investigations into the nature and response of the tissues of the host as well as of the response of the total personality to the results of the disease.

ETS Electrical transcranial stimulation; *electrosleep* (q.v.).

eu- Combining form meaning good, well, advantageous.

EUCD Emotionally unstable character disorder. See *personality trait disturbance.*

eudemonia, affective Flight into mental illness as an escape from frustrating or frightening reality. The *Ganser syndrome,* certain cases of *hypochondriasis,* and *Faxenpsychosis* (qq.v.) are instances of affective eudemonia. This term emphasizes secondary gains, which are particularly prominent in these cases.

euergasia (ū-ēr-gas'ē-à) Adolf Meyer's term for wholesome or normal mental functioning.

eugenic Used in its original sense, the ideology or methods of preventive medicine in *applying* genetic principles to human health conditions as postulated by eugenics.

eugenics This term was coined by Francis Galton, in 1883 to denote the systematically organized efforts of preventive medicine to improve average human qualities through the observation of *heredity.* Galton's introduction of the word "study" into his final definition—"the study of agencies under social control that may improve or impair the racial qualities of future generations, either physically or mentally"— makes it clear that he was thinking of such studies as would be the foundation of plans. Eugenics is thus complementary to *euthenics,* which aims at the betterment of the human race by studying the *environmental* conditions of human beings and differs from *genetics,* which is the branch of natural science that studies the origin, transmission, and manifestation of hereditary characters.

Eugenic measures are (1) *positive,* to encourage reproduction by persons biologically most highly qualified (*aristogenic*), or (2) *negative,* for the reduction or stoppage of parenthood among those least qualified physically and mentally (*cacogenic*).

Society has long tried to control heritable disorders. In 1757 Sweden passed a law forbidding epileptics to marry on eugenic grounds. During the early 1900s, many laws calling for sterilization of the mentally retarded were passed in various states in this country. More recently, other nations have used the same argument of eliminating alleles that produce undesirable phenotypes in what have been viewed by others as genocidal efforts. Such misuses of medical knowledge have highlighted the dangers of uncontrolled application of genetic principles as well as the ethical issues involved.

Many heritable disorders can be detected prenatally, and most people would not fault a program of voluntary detection (by means of amniocentesis, for example) followed by voluntary abortion of genetically defective fetuses. Such programs, however, have not been notably successful.

In the case of severe illnesses, for which there exists no cure or effective treatment and whose victims must be supported by public funds, the question inevitably arises as to the advisability of mandating a program for prenatal detection and then of mandating abortion of those fetuses found to be defective. There are many objections to such a program concerning who will decide what disorders are severe enough to warrant such action, who has the right over the body of the fetus and the body of the woman who carries it, what is an acceptable quality of life, and what the rights to procreational privacy are.

eumorphic According to the classification of constitutional types by the Italian school, this term means "built along normal lines" and refers to a type intermediate between *dolichomorphic* and *brachymorphic* and is equivalent to Viola's *normosplanchnic* type.

Etymologically the term eumorphic is derived from the structure or shape of the body, as a whole, whereas normosplanchnic is derived from the size of the viscera and their effect on the contour of the body.

eunuch A man *castrated before puberty* and subsequently developing the secondary sexual characteristics of a female. See *castration.*

eunuchoid In constitutional medicine this term describes the physical appearance of a male whose secondary sexual characteristics resemble those of a female. See *type, hypogenital.*

eunuchoidism In the classificatory system of constitutional medicine, a male resembling a *eunuch;* that is, a man who develops after castration the secondary sexual characteristics of a female: large hips, narrow sloping shoulders, absence of beard and body hair, and high-pitched voice.

Eunuchoidism sometimes results from early derangement of the sex glands without operative castration before puberty. It may even occur in mature men, especially in old age, following drastic changes in their glandular balance, and is easily recognizable by high-pitched voice. See *castration.*

euphoria In psychiatry, a morbid or abnormal sense of well-being. See *mania.*

Various terms have been suggested for varying degrees of feelings of happiness and unhappiness: euphoria, a feeling of physical well-being, relaxation, and happiness; *eutychia*, a state of general satisfaction; *hypertychia*, an excited elation with acceleration of physical and mental activity; *ecstasy*, a state of exaltation, exhilaration, or trance; *cacophoria*, a generalized feeling of unhappiness; *apathy*, a lack of interest and feeling; and *dystychia* or *anhedonia*, a loss of the ability to enjoy. See *depression; dysphoria; dysthymia.*

euphoria, indifferent Elation and cheerfulness that lack emotional depth. Bleuler applies this term to apparent euphoria in the schizophrenic, where seemingly marked euphoria is often expressed in the same sentence, side by side with marked depression or indifferent expressions. Indifferent euphoria is an instance of the lack of homogeneity of mood and of the dissociation between mood and verbal expression, which are almost pathognomonic of schizophrenia.

euphoriants See *psycholeptica.*

eupraxia Normal ability to perform coordinated movements.

eurotophobia Fear of female genitals.

euryplastic A type described by Bounak, corresponding to the *pyknic* type in Kretschmer's system and the *megalosplanchnic hypervegetative* constitution of Pende.

eurythmia In constitutional medicine, harmonious body relationships.

eusthenic In comparison with the *oligosthenic* and *phthinoid* divisions of the *asthenic* type in Kretschmer's system of constitutional types, this denotes the asthenic variety, which is relatively the most vigorous and the closest to the *athletic.*

eustress Any kind of stress with a beneficial effect on the subject, such as stress that promotes learning.

eutelegenesis In genetics, synonymous with *artificial insemination,* denoting the technical process of artificially impregnating a female with the sperm of a male without any contact between the two.

euthanasia Applies mainly to the measures by which physicians alleviate, or seek to remove, the distress attending the approach of death in the course of a chronic disease. According to this concept, the removal of pain is regarded as essential for an "easy death."

In a more specific sense, the term implies not only an easy, painless death, but also the means of bringing one on by legally putting to immediate death every sufferer from an incurable disease who prefers this kind of death to being tormented for a lengthy period before an eventual, painful death. This particular procedure is commonly known as "mercy killing" and is legal in some countries. In the United States it has been advocated by small groups of physicians subscribing to the belief that, with adequate safeguards, euthanasia should be legalized "to allow incurable sufferers to choose immediate death rather than await it in agony." These advocates of euthanasia hold that most of the legal and religious arguments against mercy killing are founded on emotion rather than on reason.

Within the province of eugenics, it is the method of *infanticide*—that is, the destruction of infants with marked congenital defects—which has at certain times been practiced as a form of euthanasia that seemed advisable for the particular purposes of race betterment. It was in Plato's Republic and in ancient Sparta—whose population was essentially military and had become accustomed to looking at marriage chiefly as a means of supplying new soldiers—that infanticide was urged for the first time and actually practiced, upon the decision of the ephors, when a child was unlikely to turn out a vigorous citizen (soldier). Following the pattern of Sparta, numerous tribes and nations contrived, at one time or another, to destroy their unfit, in order to prevent them from becoming a burden to themselves and to society.

euthenics In contrast to *eugenics,* which aims at improving the biological qualities of future human generations with the aid of data gained from the observation of heredity, euthenics relates to the study of environmental conditions tending to improve the human race. See *peristasis.*

euthymia (ū-thīm'ē-à) Joyfulness or mental tranquility; bienaise.

eutonia sclerotica A feeling of intense physical well-being experienced by some patients with multiple sclerosis, even when the disease itself is far advanced. See *sclerosis, multiple.*

eutychia (ū-tik'ē-à) See *euphoria.*

evaluated time See *time, evaluated.*

evaluation Measurement of worth or value; assessment of the degree of success in achieving a predetermined objective. Evaluation requires that concrete objectives or achievement tasks be set, that the measures and indices for assessing success be specified, that degrees of success be defined in terms of output expected within stated periods of time, and that the information obtained be fed back into the system so that the program can be altered as indicated. Evaluation aims to determine the effectiveness, efficiency, and scope of the system under investigation, to define its strengths and weaknesses and thereby to provide a basis for informed decision-making.

evaluation, false A. Adler's term for underevaluation of other persons or objects and overevaluation of personal achievement or aims.

As an example of underevaluation, Adler presents the story of the "fox and the sour grapes." He states that "instead of realizing his own inferiority the fox deprives the grapes of their inherent value— and thus *retains his high spirits*. He is prepared for his *megalomania*. These types of psychical procedure primarily serve the maintenance of 'free will' and of personal worth. The same purpose is served by the over-evaluation of *personal achievements* and aims caused by the individual's flight from the pessimistic feeling of his own inferiority. They are thus 'arranged' and arise out of an *exaggerated safety-tendency* directed against the feeling of 'being below.' " (*The Practice and Theory of Individual Psychology,* 1924)

evaluation, family See *family evaluation.*

evasion See *paralogia.*

event, life Any specific happening, rather than life change in general, that is associated temporally and perhaps causally as well with the onset or occurrence of psychiatric disorder, such as depression. Changes in a person's social milieu, such as in one's marriage, work or neighborhood, or in parenting, if they are undesirable or demand out of the ordinary adaptational maneuvers or attempts at coping, constitute *social stressors.*

Many studies have found a positive relationship between current social stressors and the development of symptoms of depression. Marital stressors have the highest correlation with depressive symptoms, followed by parental stressors for women and job stressors for men.

Some investigators report that depressed patients experience significantly more markedly life-threatening events, more *exit events* (i.e. loss of a significant person from the social field), and more undesirable events than the general population or schizophrenic patients. In contrast, more desirable events and *entrance events* (i.e. appearance of a significant person into one's social field) occur with approximately equal frequency in depressives, schizophrenics, and normals. Recurrence of depression has been found to be associated with the occurrence of undesirable events. (Paykel, E.S., & Tanner, J. *Psychological Medicine 6*, 1976)

event-related potential *ERP* (q.v.).

event, traumatic See *trauma*.

eversion theory See *aging, theories of*.

evil, St. John's *Obs.* Epilepsy.

eviration Emasculation; feminization; sometimes used also to indicate a delusion in a male that he has become a woman.

evocative memory See *memory; object constancy*.

evoked potential See *potential, evoked*.

evolutility The capability of an organism to exhibit change in growth and other aspects of the physical structure as a result of nutrition.

evolution Development; unfolding. In biology, the process by which living things have acquired their present form. The theory of evolution proposed by the British naturalist Charles Darwin (and independently but almost simultaneously by A. R. Wallace), that the more complex forms of life are descended from more primitive forms, provided much of the basis of modern biology (see *Darwinism*). In *On the Origin of Species by means of Natural Selection or the Preservation of Favored Races in the Struggle for Life,* published in 1859, Darwin argued that progress was a result of natural selection, exercised through competition. Although Darwin implied that acquired characteristics, if helpful to survival of a species, would be transmitted by inheritance to succeeding generations, modern genetics has recognized that mutations, and not acquired characteristics, are transmitted genetically and are subject to the same processes of natural selection as are all other inherited traits. See *mutation*.

By extension, Darwin's theory was interpreted by some to mean that the key to social progress was control of the unfit and not of their environment, which they would only recreate in any event. Such control, perhaps through sterilization or other ways of limiting reproduction, would provide the answers to crime, poverty, mental illness, etc. Many laws mandating sterilization of mental retardates, epileptics, and others believed to be carriers of defective or undesirable genes, were an outgrowth of such interpretations, which are generally disavowed nowadays because of their ethical implications. See *psychopolitics*.

exaltation, reactive See *mania, reactive*.

examination, mental See *mental status*.

Examination, Present State (PSE) An instrument developed by J.K. Wing, J.E. Cooper, and N. Sartorius (*The Measurement and Classification of Psychiatric Symptoms,* 1974) for use in the WHO-supported International Pilot Study of Schizophrenia. The PSE is a structured interview containing almost 400 items that include a wide range of symptoms likely to be present during an acute episode of one of the "functional" neuroses or psychoses. See *Schizophrenia, International Pilot Study*.

examinations, psychometric Various psychological tests that are administered to the subject in order to test one, several, or all of the following factors in his mental make-up: intelligence, special abilities and disabilities, manual skill, vocational aptitudes, interests, and personality characteristics.

exanthropia *Obs.* What was called the third stage of melancholia, namely, dislike for society.

excandescentia furibunda *Obs.* (L. "furious irascibility") Plattner's term for psychosis characterized by violent reactions.

exceptions See *type, "the exceptions."*

excessive daytime sleepiness Difficulty in staying awake that occurs daily for at least three weeks, or for recurrent periods of shorter duration. See *sleep disorders*.

excitation, subliminal See *summation*.

excitatory state, central See *summation*.

excitement, anniversary Bleuler's term for episodes of agitation that appear on specific calendar dates and usually disappear after a few repetitions. He included anniversary excitements among the acute syndromes of the schizophrenias. On analysis it is found that the anniversary excitement is related to something that had happened to the patient on a certain day having some connection with his complex or complexes.

excitement, catatonic See *schizophrenia, catatonic*.

excitement, constitutional *Obs.* Kraepelin's term for *manic temperament.* See *temperament, manic.*

exclusion criteria See *SADS.*

executive information system See *information system, executive.*

exercises, intergroup See *Conferences, A.K. Rice Group Relations.*

exhaustion, combat See *shell shock.*

exhaustion death See *Bell's mania.*

exhaustion psychosis See *psychosis, infective-exhaustive.*

exhaustion, stage of See *syndrome, general adaptation.*

exhibitionism A paraphilia, within the group of *sexual disorders* (q.v.), consisting of repeated exposure of the genitals to strangers; the exposure itself gives sexual excitement and no further contact is sought with the victim. Exhibitionism is believed to be limited to males, and the victim is usually a female adult or child. See *ecdysiasm; flasher.*

During the infancy period the sexual instinct consists of several "component" or partial impulses, one of which is exhibitionism. This impulse, manifested early in the form of genital exhibitionism, is later subject to all the modification that may take place with any of the instincts. It may be progressively displaced from the genital zone to the body as a whole, to the oral zone (the pleasure of speaking), to clothes, to dramatics, to the possession of material assets, etc. Or, it may be expressed in terms of reaction-formation; that is, there may be aversion of display of any kind.

"The *turning around* of an instinct *upon the subject* is suggested to us by the reflection that masochism is actually sadism turned round upon the subject's own ego, and that exhibitionism includes the love of gazing at the subject's own body." (Freud, *CP*)

existentialism A system of philosophy particularly associated with Jean-Paul Sartre, Martin Heidegger, Karl Jaspers, and Søren Kierkegaard. Existential philosophy is essentially of European origin and is a reaction to the realization that technology and a belief in pure rationalism, logical positivism, or similar philosophies have only alienated man from society and from himself. Existentialism rejects the Hellenic view of man as a man of detached, logical reason and instead emphasizes the Hebraic view of man as a man of faith and a concrete, individual doer. See *humanistic psychology.*

Philosophy in the Western world before the time of Kierkegaard tacitly accepted Parmenides's belief that if a thing cannot be thought, it cannot be real. Yet existence cannot be thought, it can only be lived; thus reason must ignore existence completely or reduce it to nothingness. For Kierkegaard, existence was not a matter of speculation but a reality in which the individual is personally and passionately involved; the decisive encounter with the Self is in the Either/Or of choice. For Heidegger, existence is a Being spread over a field or region that is the world of its care and concern. This field of being is called *Dasein* (q.v.). In the everyday world, none of us is a private Self confronting a world of external objects; we are simply one among many—"the One," a fallen state in that we have not yet become a Self and recognized our mortal, feeble, impotent nature. Sartre and his followers, representing a small part of existential philosophy, emphasize the despair of a world from which God has departed, and their themes include "Alienation and estrangement; a sense of the basic fragility and contingency of human life; the impotence of reason confronted with the depths of existence; the threat of Nothingness, and the solitary and unsheltered condition of the individual before this threat." (Barrett, W. *Irrational Man,* 1958)

In psychiatry, existentialism forms the philosophic background for "existential analysis," which in the main is represented by Europeans trained originally as psychoanalysts. The existential group does not consider itself divorced from the body of orthodox psychoanalytic theory and method, but it looks to existentialism rather as a more extensive and practicable approach to the patient and his world. Existential analysis is considered to have appeared in reaction to existing inadequacies in the various schools of thought in psychopathology.

Existential analysis places more emphasis on conscious experience than does classical psychoanalysis and is more confrontational than person-centered counseling. It assumes that a person's decisions about life give meaning to life, and the therapist is active in asking difficult questions to highlight the subject's decision-making process. Decisions can be seen as choosing the unknown future or the familiar past (the status quo). Choosing the future is anxiety-provoking but nonetheless desirable, for by giving meaning to life it promotes continued growth. To tolerate the anxiety associated with choosing the future, it is necessary to develop *hardiness*, an attitude of commitment, confidence in the ability to control, and a perception of the new as challenging rather than threatening.

Choosing the past, on the other hand, brings guilt and the feeling of missed opportunity. It narrows perspectives, obstructs learning, enforces conformity, and ultimately leads to boredom, stagnation, meaninglessness, and despair.

exit events See *event, life.*

exogenous, exogenetic, exogenic In modern medical classification, physical or mental disorders which are caused predominantly by factors acting either from outside of the body or from another part of the body (outside of the system) which is the very seat of the morbid condition in question. See *endogenous.*

exogeny, exogenism, exogenesis In medicine, originally the pathogenetic process of only those morbid conditions caused by factors acting from *outside* of the body; in psychiatry it is used in a more specific sense. The psychiatric classification includes disorders which are at least predominantly due to influences of pathological processes outside of the nervous system, and are not inherent in its particular genetic constitution.

According to this definition, a *symptomatic* psychosis that originates within the body, but arises primarily from morbid factors outside of the nervous system, thus constituting merely a secondary symptom of an organic disease affecting parts of the body other than the nervous system itself, must similarly be classified as exogenous, as are the more obvious cases of traumatic psychosis, alcoholic hallucinosis, or reactive depression. See *endogeny.*

exophoria See *heterophoria.*

exophthalmic dysostosis *Xanthomatosis* (q.v.).

exophthalmic goiter *Thyrotoxicosis* (q.v.).

exotic psychosis *Obs.* Culture-specific syndrome. See *syndromes, culture-specific.*

expansiveness Lack of restraint in feelings and actions and especially overvaluation of one's own work. Sometimes used to refer to megalomaniacal trends; thus delusions of grandeur and omnipotence are called expansive delusions. Horney uses the term to refer to a type of neurotic solution of inner conflicts based on identification with the idealized self and expressed in the form of narcissism, perfectionism, arrogance, and vindictiveness, or as other qualities consistent with mastery.

expectation, anxious "A lurking sense of apprehension. This 'anxious expectation' shows itself most intensely on all occasions that depart from what is usual, in regard to anything that involves something novel, unexpected, unexplained, uncanny." (Freud, *CP*) See *neurosis, expectation.*

expediter In social psychiatry and psychiatric ecology, a person (or mechanism) who routes a patient through the network of social subsystems with which he articulates and effects linkages between those systems, as part of the total treatment and rehabilitation plan. See *ecology; psychiatry, community.*

experience, accidental See *accidental.*

experience, corrective emotional One of the briefer and more direct techniques advocated by Alexander to expedite psychotherapy. In this technique, the therapist temporarily assumes some particular role to bring the patient more quickly to an awareness of transference relationships and to other personal insights and reorientations.

experimental neurosis See *neurosis, experimental.*

expiation The act of atoning for, or making complete satisfaction for, a misdeed. Expiatory behavior (especially expiatory self-punishment) has been emphasized by Rado in his writings on obsessive behavior. According to him, obsessive attacks are derived from the temper (rage) tantrums of childhood, but in the obsessive patient the discharge of rage is slow and incomplete since it is always opposed by guilty fear. The latter, in turn, must be followed by expiatory behavior, just as in the child the mother's punishment and threats led to fearful obedience.

Such expiatory behavior would be considered by some an expression of moral masochism. See *masochism.*

explicit role See *role.*

exploiting type See *assimilation.*

explosion-readiness See *readiness, explosion.*

explosive disorder One or more serious aggressive outbursts that are grossly out of proportion to any identifiable stressors; there may be associated nonspecific EEG abnormalities suggestive of subcortical or limbic system involvement, and some observers have reported a familial trend. See *dyscontrol, episodic.* When classified among the disorders of impulse control, explosive disorder was subdivided into the intermittent type (several discrete episodes) and the isolated type (single episode, sometimes referred to as *catathymic crisis*).

exposure in vivo See *therapy, behavior.*

exposure, indecent See *exhibitionism.*

exposure, self-directed In treatment of phobia, the homework tasks required of the patient outside therapy sessions: entering into and remaining in phobic situations hitherto avoided. Some workers enhance instructions to the patient with manuals describing the rationale for self-directed exposure (also called *programmed practice*).

expressed emotions (EE) In studies of schizophrenics and their families, high relapse rate was found to be related to frequency and quality of EE, defined as criticism, hostility, and overinvolvement expressed by the family toward the patient. Relapse was particularly high (79%) in high-EE–high-contact families (i.e. families in which patients spent 35 hours a week or more with their families) as compared with a relapse rate of 29% in high-EE–low-contact families. (Brown, G.W., Birley, J.L.T., & Wing, J.K., *British Journal of Psychiatry 121,* 1972)

expressible Penetrant. See *penetrance.*

expressive dysphasia See *developmental dysphasia.*

expressive pattern See *psychodynamics, adaptational.*

expressivity See *chromosome; penetrance.*

extended stay review Concurrent review of a continuous hospital stay that equals or exceeds the period defined in that hospital's utilization review plan.

extender, physician A generic term that includes physician's assistant, nurse clinician, nurse practitioner, and medex, all of whom perform various medical services as authorized by state laws and under the direction and supervision of a doctor of medicine or osteopathy who is licensed within the state.

exteriorization The act of objectivizing one's interests and affects.

externalization In discussing the Thematic Apperception Test, Bellak (in Abt, L.E., & Bellak, L. *Projective Psychology,* 1950) defines externalization as "those apperceptive processes which function on a preconscious level and can therefore readily be made conscious." The writer thereby differentiates between, on the one hand, projection as an unconscious defense mechanism that leads to extreme and pathological distortion of reality, and, on the other, the apperceptive distortions that make up the subject's responses in "projective" tests.

R.D. Chessick (*Archives of General Psychiatry 27,* 1972) defines externalization as a dual process, consisting first of projecting and second of manipulating, perceiving, and selectively reporting on external reality so that it will conform to and thus validate the subject's projections.

Horney uses the term to refer to the experiencing of any intrapsychic process as occurring between oneself and others. In active externalization, the feelings toward oneself are experienced as feelings toward others; in passive externalization, feelings toward others are experienced as being directed by others toward oneself. (In Horney's system, projection is the shifting of responsibility or blame for one's own undesirable qualities onto others.) See *projection.*

externalizing/internalizing A classification used by T.M. Achenbach (*Psychological Monographs 80,* 1966) to classify children on the basis of the psychiatric symptoms that manifest at the time of referral. *Externalizing* symptoms include acting-out and antisocial behavior and a turning against others; *internalizing* symptoms include excessive inhibition, anxiety, somatization, and depression. Some studies suggest that externalizers are likely to be more disturbed in adulthood (as measured by global mental health ratings) and have a higher incidence of schizophrenia than internalizers.

extinction In neurophysiology, disappearance of excitability to a previously adequate stimulus. Immediately after application of a stimulus to a nerve, there occurs a progressive depression of excitability of that nerve; at the point at which the nerve or focus becomes completely inexcitable, extinction is said to have occurred.

Extinction for visual and tactile stimuli is found in occipitoparietal lesions; it is a defect of visual and tactile attention (and hence is also termed *inattention*). The subject is able to perceive stimulation in the affected sensory area when this is the only area stimulated; but if stimulated in some other area of the visual or tactile field he cannot recognize the stimulus object in the affected area.

In operant conditioning, extinction refers to the weakening and ultimate disappearance of the conditioned response when it is not reinforced or rewarded.

For the meaning of extinction in psychoanalysis, see *ego, extinction of*.

extinction, order of In genetic family studies, the statistical estimate of families dying out in a certain generation because of lack of reproduction.

extractive disorders See *psychodynamics, adaptational*.

extrapunitive See *intropunitive*.

extrapyramidal system A functional system of nerve tracts whose main action is concerned with automatic movements involved in postural adjustments and with autonomic regulation. It is usually considered to include three layers of integration: cortical, basal ganglia, and midbrain (tegmental). Parkinsonism, athetosis, chorea, and torsion spasms are all possible results of extrapyramidal dysfunction. The mechanisms involved in the production of these syndromes are only poorly understood, but many believe that they are a result of release from suppressor action. There is also evidence that extrapyramidal disorders both naturally occurring and secondary to medication with phenothiazine compounds are due to a deficiency of dopamine.

extrasensory perception See *perception, extrasensory*.

extraversion Disposition to turn one's interests upon or find pleasure in external things. Jung speaks of *active* extraversion, when the libido is "deliberately willed," and *passive* extraversion, "when the object compels it, i.e. attracts the interest of the subject of its own accord, even against the latter's intention." (*PT*)

The act or process of extraverting is *exteriorization* (q.v.).

extremity, phantom See *limb, phantom*.

extroversion, extrovert Less correct, but equally frequent spellings of *extraversion, extravert*.

eye movement, rapid See *dream*.

eye movements, pursuit Eye tracking; deviant smooth pursuit eye movements may be an indicator of genetic susceptibility to schizophrenia. Eye tracking impairment has been reported in 65 to 85% of schizophrenic patients and in 45 to 50% of their first-degree relatives, as compared with an incidence of 15% in other psychiatric populations and 6% of normal subjects. See *saccade*.

eye tracking See *eye movements, pursuit*.

eyelash sign See *sign, eyelash*.

eyes, dancing A characteristic feature of myoclonic encephalopathy of infants, whose other typical symptoms are somatic myoclonic ataxia and irritability.

F

F In Rorschach scoring, a form response, i.e. a response determined solely by the shape or outline of the area in the blot to which it refers. The *F* responses indicate what is most conventional and socialized in the subject and are a measure of the capacity for consistent thinking. When the form response is of good quality, i.e. when it fits its area at least as well as the popular responses fit their respective areas, it is scored as *F+*. When the form response is of poor quality, i.e. when it is vaguely perceived and/or it corresponds only indefinitely to the area of the blot selected for interpretation, it is scored as *F−*. The *F+* is a measure of the tenacity with which a task is pursued, the evenness of performance, the consistency of thinking, and the adequacy of reality testing. *F−* responses, on the other hand, indicate indecision and inability due to perceptual vagueness; they occur primarily in schizophrenia and in organic brain disorders.

f Frequency.

F− Rorschach scoring symbol for a form response (see *F*) of poor quality.

F+ Rorschach scoring symbol for a good form response.

fabrication See *confabulation; psychosis, Korsakoff*.

Fabry's disease An inborn error of glycosphingolipid metabolism, transmitted by an X-linked gene, characterized by the systemic accumulation of glycolipids and by deficiency of the enzyme ceramide trihexosidase. (Other inborn errors of glycosphingolipid metabolism are metachromatic leukodystrophy, Gaucher's disease, and Tay-Sachs disease.)

fabulation Meyer's term for *confabulation* or *fabrication*. He spoke of "forms of protracted deliria usually with numerous fabulations." (*American Journal of Insanity LX*, 1904)

facial hemiatrophy See *hemiatrophy, facial*.

facies, ironed-out (fā′shē-ēz) This expression is usually applied to the facial expression of patients with general paresis. The loss of tone of the muscles of expression gives the face the appearance as if it has been "ironed-out," flattened.

facilitation In neurophysiology, shortening of the central reflex time (the synaptic delay, i.e. that portion of the total latent period of a reflex that is due to passage of impulse through internuncial neurons) either by giving a second stimulus soon after the first, or by increasing the strength of the stimulus. Facilitation is to be differentiated from *summation* (q.v.).

The above definition refers to local facilitation. It is known that facilitation (or suppression) from a distance may also occur, especially in motor areas of the cortex. The existence of bands of facilitation and suppression in the cortex has been established by Dusser de Barenne et al.

In genetics, facilitation refers to that form of interaction between hereditary and environmental factors in which a genetic tendency to a particular malformation or abnormality becomes manifest only under conditions of gestational stress.

factitial Factitious; artificial. A factitial disease, such as hypoglycemia factitia, is any symptom, syndrome, injury, or illness that is self-inflicted. See *syndrome, Munchhausen*.

factitious disorders A group of disorders whose physical or psychologic symptoms are produced by the subject and are under his voluntary control; *pathomimicry*. In contrast to *malingering* (q.v.), there is no apparent goal other than to assume the role of patient.

Factitious disorder with psychologic symptoms formerly included the Ganser syndrome, which is now classified as a dissociative disorder.

Chronic factitious disorder with physical symptoms (Munchhausen syndrome) is also known as *hospital addiction syndrome,* and patients are called *hospital hoboes.* Physical symptoms, presented so convincingly that multiple hospitalizations are the rule, may include acute abdominal and neurologic complaints, hemorrhage, skin rashes and abscesses, or involvement of any organ system. See *syndrome, Munchhausen.*

factor In genetics, practically identical with *gene.*

factor, Frankenstein See *Frankenstein factor.*

factor, intrinsic See *sclerosis, posterolateral.*

factor, risk See *risk factor.*

factorial Pertaining to a genetic factor or a combination of factors.

factorial design See *design, factorial.*

facultative Having the power to live or operate under other conditions; that is, nonobligatory. In psychiatry, most commonly applied to homosexuality, *faute de mieux* (q.v.), and to other cases in which homosexuality is symptomatic of specific neurotic conflicts. See *homosexuality; homosexuality, female; homosexuality, male.*

Fahr's disease (Theodor Fahr, German neurologist, 1877–1945) *Cerebral calcinosis; idiopathic calcification of the basal ganglia;* a rare hereditary disorder consisting of calcification of the basal ganglia, motor symptoms, and neuropsychiatric symptoms. Motor symptoms include choreoathetosis, a Parkinson-like syndrome, cerebellar ataxia, and paralysis. Neuropsychiatric symptoms include schizophreniform or depressive psychosis and dementia. Cases with relative early onset (30 years) often present with psychotic symptoms and progress to dementia. Cases with later onset (50 years) usually present with dementia.

failure through success See *success, failure through.*

failure to thrive Also nonorganic failure to thrive (*NFTT*) and *attachment disorder of infancy* (qq.v.); a nonorganic disorder of the first two years of life characterized by marked deceleration of weight gain and growth and slowed acquisition of developmental milestones. Several subtypes have been described: Type I, in which the caregiver both undernourishes and understimulates the infant; Type II, in which the caregiver provides adequate stimulation but, because of misinformation or lack of resources, fails to provide adequate nutrition; and Type III, in which the mother reacts with anger or depression to the infant's struggle for autonomy, which is then typically expressed in behavioral disturbance based on food refusal but not in any developmental abnormalities.

At least in Types I and II, such distortions in early life experience bespeak a poor prognosis in the long run; persisting defects in physical or intellectual development and behavior problems or conduct disturbances are the rule rather than the exception.

failure to warn See *warn, duty to.*

Fairweather lodges See *domicile.*

faith cure Improvement (much less frequently, cure) as a result of faith or confidence of the patient in the therapist and/or the therapeutic method. Usually faith cures occur in favorable responses to the supportive type of psychotherapy, and particularly in the types known as prestige suggestion and persuasion.

faith healing A form of *folk healing* (q.v.) found in many fundamentalist Christian denominations in the United States, with an emphasis on personal testimonials of successful healing, coming forth in a group meeting with the complaint(s) and being prayed over by the healer and the elders of the church. See *folk medicine.*

fallacia (fal-lä′kē-ä) *Obs.* An illusion or hallucination.

fallectomy See *salpingectomy.*

fallen fontanel syndrome *Susto* (q.v.).

falling out A culture-specific syndrome, reported among black Americans and black Caribbeans, consisting of sudden collapse and inability to move, see, or speak. See *syndromes, culture-specific.*

Falret, Jean-Pierre (făl-rā′) (1794–1870) French psychiatrist; in 1854, Falret and Baillarger independently described recurring attacks of mania and melancholia in the same patient.

Falret, Jules Ph.J. (1824–1902) French psychiatrist; in 1879 described "folie circulaire" and "mixed states," which he considered to be transitory stages between attacks of mania and depression.

false recognition, illusions of See *syndrome, Capgras's*.

falsehood, unconscious A false or untrue statement made by a person without intention or without his being aware of its false nature.

falsification, memory See *confabulation; psychosis, Korsakoff*.

falsification, retrospective The addition of false details and meanings to a true memory; especially common in paranoid schizophrenia, where past experiences may be related to conform with the delusional system.

falx cerebelli See *meninges*.

falx cerebri See *meninges*.

fames canina *Obs.* Bulimia.

familial A normal or morbid trait tending, or observed, "to run in families." As the hereditary origin of such a trait is not proved by the mere observation of its occurrence in several members of the same family, the use of the expression "familial" is to be interpreted in the sense that in the particular case of a disease or another trait the genetic basis is either not to be stressed or as yet unknown. See *heredity*.

familianism A sociological and psychological term emphasizing the tendency to maintain strong intrafamilial bonds, ties, and demands, culturally transmitted and inherited, and making for intensely compact family life and solidarity.

famille névropathique (F. "neuropathic family") A group of degenerative diseases in which Charcot included hysteria, since heredity, he felt, was the unique originating cause.

family, artificial Used in research especially in schizophrenia; introduced by N.E. Waxler (*Family Process 13*, 1974). She created artificial families composed of parents of normal or schizophrenic children paired with normal and then schizophrenic offspring from other families. She found that the schizophrenic child gave only minimal disruption to normal parents; that schizophrenic parents have little effect on normal children; but that schizophrenic children showed significant improvement in cognitive performance after working on a task together with normal parents.

family care The boarding out of chronic patients (usually schizophrenics, tractable mental retardates, or senile cases) with relatives or, more commonly, with unrelated guardians. The patient is absorbed not only into the guardian's home but into the life of the local community as well. Perhaps the best known organized system of family care is the *Gheel Colony* (q.v.) in Antwerp, Belgium.

family culture, indigenous The structure of a family such as its belief about itself, its conceptions about its relation to the social world in which it lives, its hierarchy of power and influences, and the openness of its boundaries to outsiders. Various objective measures of different aspects of such structures have been developed, among them *coordination* and *configuration* (qq.v.).

family evaluation "One or more family interviews conducted to assess the structure and process of family interactions, to determine how the family influences and is influenced by the behavior and symptoms of its individual members, and to gather the data necessary to decide whether family treatment is possible and indicated." (Grunebaum, H., & Glick, I.D. in *Psychiatry Update II*, ed. L. Grinspoon, 1983)

family, extended See *conjugal unit, isolated*.

family group intake See *intake, family group*.

family group therapy See *therapy, family group*.

family identity A family's experience of itself as a group, including its distance from or closeness to the outside world, its traditions and feelings of continuity with the past, and its feelings of internal cohesion.

family pattern The style of living within a family, and particularly the quality of the relationship between parents and child. Among the different family patterns described are *symbiotic unions*, where parent and child form an inseparable bond; *family sacrifice*, where the child is rejected and excluded from the family; *open*, when the family has friends, entertains, and is active in the community; and *closed*, when the family shuns contact with the outside. Some workers have found that families of schizophrenics are often symbiotic unions and/or are closed, and that more demonstrate family sacrifice than do families of nonschizophrenics.

family romance See *romance, family*.

family social work See *social work, family*.

family studies 1. In family therapy, the formal, quantitative investigations of family process and clinical descriptions of family life and family therapy. 2. In genetics and epidemiology, case-controlled investigations of illness in the relatives of patients or in normal controls.

family systems interview A diagnostic-therapeutic interview conducted over one or two sessions very early in the treatment process as a way of understanding the contexts in which the symptomatic behavior is distinctively present or absent, and as an opportunity to observe the reactions of the family as various subjects are discussed.

family therapy A professionally organized attempt to ameliorate disturbances in the marital or family unit, primarily through nonpharmacologic means with an emphasis on relationships and behavior patterns rather than on individual pathology. The goal is more satisfying ways of living for the entire family and not just for one family member.

family therapy, psychoeducational See *psychoeducation.*

family therapy, strategic A form of communication therapy (rather than a medical model therapy) for disturbances of late adolescence, which are viewed as failures of separation-individuation that have produced a hierarchical incongruity in the family: the adolescent has gained dominance through symptoms or intimidation or both. Therapy is directed toward restoring dominance to the parents, who must then demand normal role functioning.

family therapy, systematic A form of communication therapy (rather than a medical model therapy) in which the family system is redefined in various ways as working for its own best interests in its apparent dysfunction. As an example, the dysfunction is recognized as a way to avoid change that would be even more threatening to the family than the dysfunction is. Characteristic of systematic family therapy is a radical neutrality of therapeutic attitude. It is associated with Selvini-Palazzoli, Boscolo, Cecchin, and Prata.

family types Alanen of Helsinki University (Finland) reports that two general types of families can be distinguished in the group of schizophrenics: chaotic and rigid. Intru-

sive parent-child relationships are found in both, but in rigid families possessive and restrictive parental attitudes predominate, whereas in chaotic families the parents are unable to separate themselves psychologically from their children and, in addition, often hold unusually fanatical or deviant norms and are excessively inconsistent.

fanaticism Excessive, unreasonable zeal on any subject, such as religion; fanaticism, like litigiousness, is extremely frequent in paranoids, whose zealotry in the espousing of causes may approach the delusional.

fantasy See *phantasy.*

fantasy, autistic See *autistic fantasy.*

fantasying, active A psychotherapeutic procedure in which the patient is asked to relate his spontaneous imagery. An analysis of these fantasied images enables the physician to find out the roots of the patient's conflicts. If it becomes possible to show the patient these unconscious connections, he is in a position to recognize the source of his conflicts and is able to bring the conflict within the sphere of conscious insight and control. (Baynes, H.G. *Mythology of the Soul,* 1940)

FAP Fixed action pattern. See *instinct.*

far-field evoked potential See *neurometrics.*

fasciculation See *tremor.*

fasciculus cuneatus Tract of Burdach, located in the posterior white column of the spinal cord between the fasciculus gracilis and the posterior gray column. The fasciculus cuneatus carries proprioception and vibratory sensation fibers from the upper limbs. These fibers terminate in the nucleus cuneatus at the medulla, whence arise internal arcuate fibers, some of which proceed to the homolateral restiform body and most of which cross to form the medial lemniscus of the opposite side.

fasciculus gracilis Tract of Goll, located in the posterior white column of the spinal cord next to the posterior (dorsal) median septum. The fasciculus gracilis carries proprioception and vibratory sensation fibers mainly from the lower limbs. These fibers terminate in the nucleus gracilis at the medulla, whence arise internal arcuate fibers, some of which proceed to the homolateral restiform body and most of which cross to form the medial lemniscus of the opposite side.

fascination When a desire for mastery of some factor in the environment cannot be gratified, a partial mastery of it is sometimes achieved by means of identification with it. This reaction is called *fascination.* For example, if an infant is seen paying rapt attention to a rattle which the mother waves before it, a phase preliminary to mastery can be assumed. But if mastery is not possible because the rattle is beyond reach, or perhaps because the knack of reaching has not yet been learned, there still remains the rapt attention, which becomes greatly intensified. The infant, so to say, loses itself in the sight and sound of the rattle and thus becomes one with it, and through identification, a partial mastery is achieved by way of fascination.

fascinum (fàs'kē-noom) (L. "witchcraft") An ancient belief that certain people possess "the evil eye," because of which they are capable of fascinating and injuring others by looking at them.

fashion Fashion refers to changes in dress, manners, the arts, literature, and philosophy based fundamentally on differentiation and emulation.

FAST See *GDS.*

fastidium cibi Loathing of food.

fastidium potus Loathing of drink.

father fixation Inordinate attachment to the father. See *complex, Oedipus; fixation.*

father-ideal A psychoanalytic term for the father component of the ego-ideal. Jones writes: "If we inquire into the matter and origin of the ego-ideal, we discover that it is compounded of two constituents, derived from the Father and the Self respectively—the original (primal) narcissism of the infant becomes in the course of development distributed in four directions, the actual proportion in each of these varying enormously with different individuals. *One* portion remains in an unaltered state attached to the real ego; that is probably the one concerned in the genesis of hypochondria. A *second* portion is deflected from any direct sexual goal and becomes attached to the ideal of the parent, leading to adoration, devotion, and general over-estimation. It is important to bear in mind that to begin with this process is much more a matter of narcissistic identification than of any form of object-love. A *third* is transferred on to an ideal ego, and is one of the constituents of the 'ego-ideal.' The *fourth* is gradually transformed into object-love. Now the second and third of these commonly fuse during the latency period of childhood or even earlier. The form assumed by the resulting ego-ideal is largely derived from the ideas and mental attitudes of the father, the bond being effected through the second portion of the narcissistic libido mentioned above—that attached to what may be called the *father-ideal.* On the other hand, the energy that gives the ego-ideal its significance is wholly derived ultimately from narcissistic libido. There are three routes for this: (1) directly from the original narcissism of the primary ego (third portion mentioned above); (2) via the attachment to the *father-ideal* (second portion); (3) via the regression of narcissistic identification with the father that often takes place after a disappointment at the lack of gratification of object-love (fourth portion)." (Jones, E.J. *Papers on Psycho-Analysis,* 1949) See *ego-ideal; super-ego.*

father-imago (ē-mä'gō) See *image.*

father substitute See *surrogate.*

father surrogate See *surrogate.*

father, vaginal A motherly, unaggressive feminine kind of husband or father, who typically has significant conflicts revolving about unconscious identification with his own mother.

fatigue, battle See *shell shock.*

fatigue, combat See *shell shock.*

fatigue state See *hypoglycemia.*

fatuity Feeblemindedness; sometimes used synonymously with dementia of any kind.

fault, basic Balint's term for impairment of narcissism based on inadequate mother-infant bonding and expressed as a feeling that one is defective or damaged. See *partialism, persistent.*

faunorum ludibria *Obs.* Sometimes meaning nightmare, at other times referring to epilepsy.

faute de mieux (fōt dē mew) (F. "for want of anything better") In psychiatry, this term is ordinarily used to refer to so-called accidental homosexuality, in which a person chooses a same-sexed person as a sexual object when no other-sexed person is available.

Faxenpsychosis The German psychiatric term, literally in its English equivalent, *buffoonery psychosis*. See *psychosis, buffoonery.*

FC Rorschach scoring symbol for a form response determined by the colored areas of the card.

Fc In Rorschach scoring, a shading response to the black areas of the blots that is to some degree influenced by the form of the blot area. See *ShR.*

Fc′ In Rorschach scoring, a shading response to the light gray areas of the blots that is to some degree influenced by the form of the blot area. See *ShR.*

fear See *anxiety.*

fear, guilty Rado's term for the fear that dire consequences are in store for one because of a misdeed (or forbidden impulse). Guilty fear is thus a derivative of the dread of conscience. It is a prominent feature of the obsessive syndrome where it opposes the patient's defiant rage and leads, ultimately, to repression of the latter. See *attack, obsessive.*

fear hypnosis See *hypnosis, father.*

fear, impulse A fear that arises within the individual, more or less directly from an instinctual source. It is contrasted with real fear, which is associated with some real object in the environment. The fear of being in a dark place is a real or a "reality" fear. The fear of imminent collapse and death, while in excellent health, is an impulse fear.

fear of:
  air: aerophobia
  animals: zoophobia
  anything new: kaino(to)phobia; neophobia
  bacilli: bacillophobia
  bad men: pavor sceleris; scelerophobia
  barren space: cenophobia; kenophobia
  bearing a monster: teratophobia
  bees: apiphobia; melissophobia
  being alone: autophobia; eremiophobia; monophobia
  being beaten: mastigophobia
  being buried alive: taphephobia
  being enclosed: clithrophobia
  being laughed at: catagelophobia
  being locked in: claustrophobia; clithrophobia
  being looked at: scopophobia
  being touched: (h)aphephobia; haptephobia
  birds: ornithophobia
  blood: hematophobia; hemophobia
  blushing: ereuthophobia; erythrophobia
  brain disease: meningitophobia
  burglars: scelerophobia
  cats: ailurophobia; geleophobia; gatophobia
  change: kainophobia; kainotophobia; neophobia
  childbirth: maieusiophobia
  choking: anginophobia; pnigophobia
  cold: cheimaphobia; psychropophobia
  color(s): chromatophobia; chromophobia
  comets: cometophobia
  confinement: claustrophobia
  contamination: coprophobia; molysmophobia; mysophobia; scatophobia
  corpses: necrophobia
  (crossing a) bridge or river: gephyrophobia
  (crossing a) street: dromophobia
  crowds: demophobia; ochlophobia
  cumbersome pseudoscientific terms: hellenologophobia
  dampness: hygrophobia
  darkness: achluphobia; nyctophobia; scotophobia
  dawn: eosophobia
  daylight: phengophobia
  death: necrophobia; thanatophobia
  definite disease: monopathophobia
  deformity: dysmorphophobia
  demons: demonia; demonomania; entheomania
  depths: bathophobia
  devils: demonophobia; satanophobia
  dirt: mysophobia; rhypophobia; rupophobia
  disease: nosophobia; pathophobia
  dogs: cynophobia
  dolls: pediophobia
  dust: amathophobia
  eating: cibophobia; phagophobia; sitophobia
  electricity: electrophobia
  emptiness: kenophobia
  everything: pamphobia (*obs.*); panphobia; panophobia; pantophobia
  examination: examination phobia
  excrement: coprophobia; scatophobia
  eyes: ommatophobia
  failure: kakorrhaphiophobia
  fatigue: kopophobia
  fearing: phobophobia
  feathers: pteronophobia
  female genitals: eurotophobia
  fever: fibriphobia; pyrexiophobia

filth: mysophobia; rhypophobia; rupophobia

filth (personal): automysophobia

fire: pyrophobia

fish: ichthyophobia

flash of lightning: selaphobia

flogging: mastigophobia

floods: antlophobia

flutes: aulophobia

flying: aviophobia

fog: homichlophobia

food: cibophobia; phagophobia; sit(i)ophobia

forests: hylophobia

frogs: batrachophobia

functioning: ergasiophobia

ghosts: phasmophobia

girls: parthenophobia

glass: crystallophobia; hyelophobia

God: theophobia

gravity: barophobia

hair: trichopathophobia; trichophobia

heat: thermophobia

heaven: siderophobia; uranophobia

heights: acrophobia; hyposophobia

hell: hadephobia; stygiophobia

heredity: patroiophobia

high objects: batophobia

horses: equinophobia

houses: domatophobia; oikophobia

humiliation: catagelophobia

ideas: ideophobia

impending death: meditatio mortis; thanatophobia

infinity: apeirophobia

injury: traumatophobia

innovation: neophobia

insanity: lyssophobia; maniaphobia

insects: acarophobia; entomophobia

jealousy: zelophobia

justice: dikephobia

knives: aichmophobia

large objects: megalophobia

left: levophobia; sinistrophobia

light: photophobia

lightning: astraphobia; astrapophobia; keraunophobia

loneliness: erem(i)ophobia; monophobia

machinery: mechanophobia

many things: polyphobia

marriage: gamophobia

materialism: hylephobia

medicine(s): pharmacophobia

men: androphobia

metals: metallophobia

meteors: meteorophobia

mice: musophobia

mind: psychophobia

mirrors: eisoptrophobia; spectrophobia

missiles: ballistophobia

moisture: hygrophobia

money: chrematophobia

motion: kinesophobia

myths: mythophobia

naked body: gymnophobia

naming, being named: onomatophobia

needles: belonephobia

neglecting duty: paralipophobia

Negro(es): negrophobia

night: noctiphobia; nyctophobia

northern lights: auroraphobia

novelty: kainophobia; kainotophobia; neophobia

odor (personal): bromidrosiphobia

odor(s): olfactophobia; osmophobia; osphresiophobia

open space(s): agoraphobia; agyiophobia

pain: algophobia; odynophobia

parasites: parasitophobia

people: anthropophobia; phobanthropy

places: topophobia

pleasure: hedonophobia

points: aichmophobia

poison: iophobia; toxi(co)phobia

poverty: peniaphobia

precipices: cremnophobia

public places: agoraphobia

punishment: poinephobia

rabies: cynophobia

railroads or trains: siderodromophobia

rain, rainstorms: ombrophobia

rectal excreta: coprophobia

rectum: proctophobia

red: erythrophobia

responsibility: hypengyophobia

ridicule: catagelophobia

right: dextrophobia

rivers: potamophobia

robbers: harpaxophobia

(the) rod: rhabdophobia

ruin: atephobia

sacred things: hierophobia

scabies: scabiophobia

(receiving a) scratch: amychophobia

(the) sea: nautophobia; thalassophobia

self: autophobia

semen: spermatophobia

sex: genophobia

sexual intercourse: coitophobia; cypri(do)phobia

shock: hormephobia
ships: nautophobia
sin: hamartophobia
sinning: enosiophobia; peccatiphobia; scrupulosity
sitting: thaasophobia
sitting down: kathisophobia
skin disease: dermatosiophobia
skin lesion: dermatophobia
skin (of animals): doraphobia
sleep: hypnophobia
small objects or animals: microbiophobia; microphobia
smothering: pnigerophobia
snakes: ophidiophobia
snow: chionophobia
solitude: erem(i)ophobia; monophobia
sounds: acousticophobia; phonophobia
sourness: acerophobia
speaking: lal(i)ophobia
speaking aloud: phonophobia
spiders: arachneophobia
stairs: climacophobia
standing up: stasiphobia
standing up and walking: stasibasiphobia
stars: siderophobia
stealing: kleptophobia
stillness: eremiophobia
stories: mythophobia
strangers: xenophobia
streets: agoraphobia; agyiophobia
string: linonophobia
success: polycratism
sunlight: heliophobia
symbolism: symbolophobia
syphilis: syphilophobia
talking: lal(i)ophobia
tapeworms: taeniophobia
taste: geumaphobia
teeth: odontophobia
thinking: phronemophobia
thirteen: triskaidekaphobia
thunder: astra(po)phobia; brontophobia; tonitrophobia
time: chronophobia
travel: hodophobia
trembling: tremophobia
trichinosis: trichinophobia
tuberculosis: phthisiophobia; tuberculophobia
vaccination: vaccinophobia
vehicles: amaxophobia
venereal disease: cypridoophobia; cypriphobia
voids: kenophobia

vomiting: emetophobia
walking: basiphobia
water: hydrophobia; nautophobia
weakness: asthenophobia
wind: anemophobia
women: gynophobia; horror feminae
work: ponophobia
writing: graphophobia

fear, real See *fear, impulse; anxiety.*

febriphobia Pyrexeophobia; fear of fever.

feces-child-penis concept See *concept, feces-child-penis.*

Fechner, Gustav Theodor (fek'nēr) (1801–87) German physicist, psychologist, philosopher.

feeblemindedness Mental deficiency; oligophrenia; hypophrenia. See *retardation, mental.*

feeblemindedness, affective Ferenczi's term for pseudodementia, diminution in intellectual capacities secondary to anxiety, depression, or other emotional states.

feeblemindedness, epileptic Often during the course of epilepsy there is a steady decline of intelligence that may result in a greater or lesser degree of feeblemindedness. See *dementia, epileptic.*

feeblemindedness, hallucinatory See *dementia paranoides gravis.*

feedback In psychiatry, information given to patients about the nature and effects of their behavior, in the form of direct comments, videotape replays, role playing, etc. Also, communication to the sender of the effect his original message had on those to whom it was relayed. Feedback may alter or reinforce the original idea; it is a function that is basic to correction and self-correction.

Feedback is positive when it increases the level or probability of future behavior ("the more you eat the more you want" phenomenon), negative when it decreases the level of future behavior (e.g., the usual consequence of food intake, which is to decrease the likelihood of eating in the near future).

Auditory feedback is the hearing of one's own speech. When this is delayed (as by transmitting the subject's voice to him through special headphones after a temporal delay of 200 to 300 milliseconds), the normal person shows dramatic changes in speech. He begins to stutter, vocal intensity increases, words become slurred, pitch is distorted, speech slows, and various emotional disturbances and other psychophysiological changes occur. In contrast, *delayed auditory feedback (DAF)* often has no adverse effect on the speech of schizophrenic children, a finding that has been interpreted to mean that the schizophrenic child excludes hearing as a basis for continued monitoring of his speech.

feedback, alpha See *alpha wave training.*

feedback, deviation-amplifying Positive feedback; a process whereby the output of a system is fed back into the system with the effect of increasing or decreasing the output of the system. The vicious circle—and its opposite, the virtuous circle—are examples of deviation-amplifying feedback. *DAF,* as it is sometimes abbreviated, is a mechanism wherein a small and relatively insignificant variation leads to consequences of major proportions. It may be the mechanism at work in brief therapy, where small therapeutic interventions can foster behavioral alterations of appreciable magnitude.

feedback, information See *therapy, behavior.*

feeding, demand. See *feeding, self-demand.*

feeding, forced See *alimentation, forced.*

feeding problem A common type of behavior disorder in which the child will not eat at all, or only under certain conditions, or shows any number of untoward and unusual reactions if and when he does eat.

feeding, self-demand In infant feeding, the modern concept that the infant is a reacting human being and should be fed whenever he is hungry. Everything else being equal, the child will cry when hungry and at the time he should be fed. This is opposed to the Spartan attitude which requires that the infant be fed every four hours, regardless of his physiological needs, and that, even when hungry, he should be made to wait until the scheduled feeding time. During the first two or three weeks of life, hunger stimuli make themselves apparent at rather irregular intervals, but thereafter the normal infant settles gradually into a time schedule of his own.

feeding, tube Feeding through a nasal catheter that terminates in the stomach.

feeling Sensation; affect; emotion; empathic reaction. Contrasted with cognition and conation.

feeling-apperception Jung says: "The nature of feeling-valuation may be compared with intellectual apperception as an *apperception of value.* An *active* and a *passive* feeling-apperception can be distinguished. The passive feeling-act is characterized by the fact that a content excites or attracts the feeling; it compels a feeling-participation on the part of the subject. The active feeling-act, on the contrary, confers value from the subject—it is a deliberate evaluation of contents in accordance with feeling and not in accordance with intellectual intention. Hence active feeling is a *directed* function, an act of will, as for instance, loving as opposed to being in love. This latter state would be *undirected,* passive feeling, as, indeed, the ordinary colloquial term suggests, since it describes the former as activity and the latter as a condition. Undirected feeling is *feeling-intuition.*" (Jung, *PT*)

feeling, ataxic See *ataxia, intrapsychic.*

feeling, bodily ego See *ego, body.*

feeling, directed See *feeling-apperception.*

feeling, discharge of See *abreaction; discharge, affective.*

feeling-into A literal translation of the German *Einfühlung;* empathy.

feeling-intuition See *feeling-apperception.*

feeling, oceanic See *omnipotence; nautomania.*

feeling-sensation "Ordinary 'simple' feeling is *concrete,* i.e., it is mixed up with other function-elements, frequently with sensation for instance. In this particular case we might term it *affective,* or ... *feeling-sensation,* by which a well-nigh inseparable blending of feeling with sensation elements is to be understood." (Jung, *PT*)

feeling, superiority The boy's feeling that he is superior to a girl in the domain of sex. "The amalgamation of the desire for a child with the epistemophilic impulse enables a boy to effect a displacement on to the intellectual plane; his sense of being at a disadvantage is then concealed and overcompensated by the superiority he deduces from his possession of a penis, which is also acknowledged by girls." (Klein, M. *Contributions to Psycho-analysis, 1921–45,* 1948) See *envy, penis.*

feeling, undirected See *feeling-apperception.*

feelings analysis See *transactional analysis.*

feelings, made See *symptoms, first-rank.*

feigned bereavement See *bereavement, feigned.*

fellatio Oral stimulation of the penis. The original object of the lips and mouth is the nipple. "It then needs very little creative power to substitute the sexual object of the moment (the penis) for the original object (the nipple) or for the finger which did duty for it later on, and to place the current sexual object in the situation in which gratification was originally obtained." (Freud, *CP*)

fellation See *fellatio.*

fellator, self- See *autofellatio.*

fellatrice (fel-là-trēs') A female who performs fellatio.

felt needs See *need.*

femaleness See *feminine.*

feminine Referring to a set of sex-specific social role behaviors, unrelated to procreative or nurturant biologic function, that identify the person as being a girl or woman. Contrast with *femaleness,* which refers to anatomic and physiologic features relating to the female's procreative and nurturant functions. See *gender identity.*

feminine traits in male See *traits, feminine, in male.*

femininity In contrast to the concept of *femaleness,* which is primarily related to the proper sex chromosome structure of XX individuals, *femininity* preferably means a female individual's possession of the typical and well-developed *secondary* sex characteristics of a woman. See *sex determination.*

feminism 1. The social system or viewpoint that assigns equality to the sexes, an orientation espoused by the feminist movement. 2. Based on the assumption that the word is formed in the same way as *racism* and *sexism* (qq.v.), feminism is used by some in a directly opposite way to refer to the social system that assigns to women the status of inferior, undesirable, etc.

In most cultures, gender is the primary element of social classification and social relationships, but since the 1960s it has become increasingly evident that both cultural and scientific conceptions of masculinity and femininity are grossly inadequate.

While social classifications reduce complexity and provide simple models for self-definition, sex stereotyping can lead to conflicts for both sexes and particularly for females. Current emphasis is on integrative conceptualizations that focus on the ways in which the sexes are alike more than they are different, and on dualistic conceptualizations that recognize the important differences between the sexes but emphasize the feminine as a valid alternative to the masculine.

Féré phenomenon See *reflex, psychogalvanic.*

Ferenczi, Sandor (fe'ren-sē) (1873–1933) Hungarian psychoanalyst; "active" analysis.

Ferri, Enrico (far'rē) (1856–1929) Italian forensic psychiatrist.

fertility, differential A degree of reproductiveness that differs from that of the normal population; used in genetics to refer to the effect on fertility of subjects with a hereditary disorder. Their effective fertility may be lowered by biologic, psychologic, or sociologic factors; the degree of lowering is a measure of the selective disadvantage associated with the disorder in question.

fertility, net The number of children of carriers of a hereditary trait who reach the age group that corresponds to the manifestation period of the trait in question.

fertilization That creative process in sexual reproduction that brings a sperm and an egg into union and enables them to form one single cell, the fertilized egg or *zygote.* By a series of cell divisions, this new cell develops into an embryo and finally into an adult organism (see *reproduction*). The essential feature in fertilization is the fusion of the nuclei of the gametes.

festination Involuntary inclination to hurry one's gait; typical of Parkinsonism. See *paralysis agitans; Parkinson's disease.*

fetal alcohol syndrome See *syndrome, fetal alcohol.*

fetal screening See *screening, genetic.*

fetalism Penrose's term for the signs of *mongolism* (*Down's syndrome*), many of which appear to be remnants of fetal existence.

fetish A fetish is a material object of any kind (idol, charm, talisman) that embodies mysterious and awesome qualities and from which supernatural aid may be expected.

In psychiatry, the love object of the person who suffers from the paraphilia called fetishism—usually a part of the body or some object belonging to or associated with the love object. See *perversion; sexual disorders.* The fetish replaces and substitutes for the love object, and although sexual activity with the love object may occur, gratification is possible only if the fetish is present or at least fantasied during such activity. Typical also is the ability of the fetishist to obtain gratification from the fetish alone, in the absence of the love object. The most common fetishes—shoes, long hair, earrings, undergarments, feet—are penis symbols or serve to avoid complete nudity of the female, and fetishism is thus considered to be a means of denying castration fears. Such denial of the woman's lack of a penis in the adult male (and almost all fetishists are male) presupposes a degree of splitting in the person's ego that ordinarily is found only in cases with a defective or severely limited ego. The term is also loosely used to refer to current rules and conventions that are misapplied or unduly revered.

fetishism, adherent Hirschfeld uses this expression to refer to the form of fetishism in which clothing is donned by the fetishist. See *fetishism, coherent.*

fetishism, beast A paraphilia in which "touching furs or animal skins produces peculiar and lustful emotions (analogous to hair-, braid-, velvet-, and silk-fetishism)." (Krafft-Ebing, R. v. *Psychopathia Sexualis,* 1908)

fetishism, coherent Hirschfeld's term for "the attraction which is exercised, for many people far more than is normal, by stuffs, and objects which are not donned or thrown over the body as clothing, but are brought into immediate contact with the body surface." (1939)

fetishism, foot See *retifism.*

fetishism, transvestic *Transvestitism* (q.v.).

Feuchtersleben, Ernst von (1806–49) German psychiatrist; author of *Lehrbuch der aerztlichen Seelenkunde.*

fever, machine See *machine fever.*

Fiamberti hypothesis (A. M. Fiamberti, 20th-century Italian psychiatrist) The theory that schizophrenia is due to a deficiency of acetylcholine (which Fiamberti believes to be essential for normal psychic activity), perhaps secondary to toxic-infectious influences.

fibrillation Slow, vermicular twitchings of individual muscle fibers or bundles, occurring anywhere in the body, without producing movements of muscles or joints; the condition is mainly indicative of slow degeneration of anterior horn cells (nuclear masses of motor cells).

fibriophobia Pathologic fear of developing a fever.

fiction, autarchic The false belief of the child in its own omnipotence. At the beginning of extrauterine life the infant is ignorant of any sources of pleasure other than those within itself: the infant even thinks of the breast as a part of its body. Ferenczi called this the period of unconditional omnipotence. The infant tries to cling to this feeling of omnipotence and only unwillingly orients itself to objects. This is the basis for the frequency of masturbation in children when they are weaned: they turn to themselves for pleasure rather than recognize their dependency upon the environment.

fiction, directive This term is used by Adler to describe the phantasy or idea of superiority that a person originally conceives as a subjective compensation for a feeling of inferiority. This phantasy or idea he utilizes and reacts to as if it were an absolute truth.

fictional finalism See *psychology, individual.*

fictions, guiding Adler's term for the principles by which one understands, categorizes, and evaluates his experiences.

fidgetiness Fidgety state. Increased motor activity, more frequently used in reference to children than to adults. Winnicott distinguishes three causes of fidgetiness: anxiety, tics, and chorea.

fidgets Vague uneasiness, usually accompanied by restless movements. Fidgets or creeps were colloquial terms for the disease or morbid symptom called *dysphoria* (q.v.).

fiduciary relation In law, the trust between patient and physician, including the expectation of confidentiality and undivided loyalty on the part of the physician.

field defect The field of vision is the limit of peripheral vision, the area within which an object can be seen while the eye remains fixed on some one point. The normal visual field has a definite contour, any change in which from the normal constitutes a field defect.

The various visual field defects (with their common causes) are (1) *circumferential blindness* or *tubular vision* (hysteria, optic or retrobulbar neuritis), consisting of a concentric contraction of the visual fields;

(2) *total blindness* in one eye (complete lesion of optic nerve on same side); (3) *hemianopia* or hemianopsia, loss of one-half of the visual field, which may be (a) homonymous, i.e. loss of vision in the temporal half-field on the same side as the lesion and loss of vision in the nasal half-field of the other eye (lesions posterior to optic radiation); or (b) heteronymous with loss of vision in the same half-field (usually the temporal) of both eyes (chiasmal lesion); or (c) unilateral hemianopia with loss of vision in the nasal or temporal half-field of one eye (perichiasmal lesion); (4) *quadrantic hemianopia* or *quadrantanopia* (partial involvement of optic radiation), with loss of vision in one quadrant of the visual field, usually homonymous. See *lobe, occipital; lobe, temporal.*

field dependence An expression of the degree of reliance on the environment to provide a definition of the self. The field-dependent person uses the visual context to establish spatial orientation, whereas the field-independent person relies more on postural and gravitational cues. Females in general are more field dependent than males, and field dependence tends to decrease with age in both sexes.

field, phenomenal Adler's term for one's constructed representation of objective reality, the meaning given to the profusion of stimuli that bombard and are organized and conceptualized on the basis of individual and personal prior experiences.

fields of Forel See *subthalamus.*

fifth pathway See *pathway, fifth.*

fight-flight assumption See *group, basic assumptions.*

figure In psychoanalytic psychology particularly, this term, in combination with other nouns denoting familial or close interpersonal relationships (e.g. father figure, mother figure, authority figure), is approximately equivalent to substitute, replacement, representative, or surrogate.

figure ground See *ground.*

figure, helpful In the child's world of phantasy, a male or female fairy-creature with so much love, understanding, and sympathy that the child could turn to it for help in any need.

filicide Murder of one's child; if the child is less than 24 hours old, the term *neonaticide* is used.

finding, object The process of transferring and finally placing libido upon environmental objects. The libido, formerly invested in erotogenic zones, may exhibit externalization in various forms.

"Adult object-finding is frequently determined by fetishism; the love-object must possess certain colored hair, wear certain clothing, or perhaps have certain physical blemishes." (Healy et al., *SMP*) See *fetish.*

finger agnosia See *agnosia.*

fingerpainting See *painting, finger.*

fingers, insane Inflammation at the end of a finger or toe (called a whitlow) seen in residents of psychiatric hospitals, usually a reflection of poor hygiene and a low level of care.

firesetting See *pyromania* (q.v.).

firing Discharge (q.v.).

first admission See *admission, first.*

first attack See *attack, first.*

first-pass effect In pharmacokinetics, binding of a drug and metabolism by the liver before it reaches the systemic circulation for distribution throughout the body.

first-rank symptoms See *symptoms, first-rank.*

fit, cerebellar Tonic or cerebellar fits were originally described by Hughlings Jackson in connection with tumors of the vermis. The patient suddenly loses consciousness, falls to the ground, develops cyanosis; the pupils are immobile and dilated. There is no tongue biting or incontinence. The head is retracted, the back arched, upper extremities extended and adducted with forearm pronated, the wrist and hand flexed and everted. The lower extremities are extended and the toes plantar flexed. There is no clonic phase; the phenomenon is one of decerebrate rigidity.

fit, tonic See *fit, cerebellar.*

fit, uncinate A subjective disturbance (hallucination) of smell and taste, characteristic of deep, mesial lesions involving the tip of the temporal lobe, at times accompanied by champing movements of the jaw; due to lesion of uncinate gyrus. See *absent state; lobe, temporal.*

fits of horrific temptation See *temptation, horrific.*

fixate In psychoanalysis, to retain excessive amounts of libidinal or aggressive energy in one or more of the infantile structures to which they were originally attached. See *ontogeny, psychic.*

fixatio mononoea *Obs.* Melancholia.

fixation In psychoanalysis, persistence of the libidinal or aggressive cathexis of an object of infancy or childhood into later life. Fixation generally implies pathology and this connotes that the amount of energy retained at the infantile level is greater than is seen in the normal person, who never fully abandons an object or mode of gratification that was strongly connected with psychic energy. In the normal, even though earlier levels persist along with or under higher levels of psychic development, most psychic energy is concentrated in the higher levels. When the energy retained at lower levels exceeds the amount to be expected in the normal, the term "fixation" is applicable, and in a general way fixation is indicative of a weak spot in psychic structure that may predispose to neurosis. See *inertia, psychic; ontogeny, psychic.*

Closely related to fixation is *regression* (q.v.), for when the latter occurs it is typically to an object or mode of gratification on which he was fixated that the patient regresses.

In social work, fixation is "a form of aberrancy of affection in which there is exaggerated devotion to someone, usually, in the parental role; as mother fixation." (Hamilton, G. *A Medical Social Terminology,* 1930)

fixation, cannibalistic The fixation of the libido and/or aggressive energy at the late oral or biting phase. This may lead to later cannibalistic impulses, such as the phantasy of biting and eating, swallowing, and incorporating a hated object.

fixation, mother Inordinate attachment to the mother. See *complex, Oedipus; fixation.*

fixation point It is the opinion of psychoanalysts that the different neuroses and psychoses are reflections of a fixation of psychic energy at given foci or *fixation points.* Schizophrenia, for example, is believed to have its fixation point at the autoerotic stage of development; paranoia signifies fixation at the narcissistic and homosexual levels; melancholia at the oral sadistic phase; hysteria at the early genital level; obsessional neurosis at the anal stage.

fixity, social The social plan in which the role and status of each individual are rigidly fixed or defined, as in feudal and caste societies. Social fixity also appears in modern society and in social and other groups where the place of members is defined and fixed. See *mobility, social.*

flagellantism Erotic pleasure or stimulation derived from whipping or being whipped.

flagellation The act of whipping as a sexual excitant. "As for erotic flagellation, pure and simple, we know that it has existed from a remote antiquity, and that it was a recognized part of the love ritual of the ancients, a preparation for the rites of Eros, and as such, known to every debauchee." (Putnam, S. in *Encyclopaedia Sexualis,* ed. V. Robinson, 1936) See *dippoldism.*

A patient was capable of sexual excitation only when his wife whipped him to the point of bleeding. He owned a unique collection of whips, each of which was given a proper name by him. See *masochism; sadism.*

flagellomania *Flagellantism* (q.v.).

flapping tremor *Asterixis* (q.v.).

flare, histamine See *histamine.*

flashback Sudden recurrence of a memory, feeling, or other perceptual experience from the past even though no adequate stimulus for its recurrence is readily identifiable. The organic flashback syndrome (in DSM-III-R termed *posthallucinogen perception disorder*) is a psychoactive substance-induced organic mental disorder in which one or more of the perceptual disturbances experienced during past episodes of intoxication with a psychoactive substance recur. The hallucinations, illusions, feelings of derealization, macropsia, micropsia, or other perceptual disturbances are markedly distressing to the subject. Because they occur without warning and during a period when he is not under the influence of the drug that produced such experiences in the past, he feels he is out of control and typically worries that he is losing his mind.

Flashback phenomena are also seen in post-traumatic stress disorders.

flasher Exhibitionist; so called because of the way in which the genitals are exposed—many exhibitionists clothe themselves solely with a topcoat, and when they chance upon their victim open the coat quickly to display their genitalia. See *exhibitionism.*

flattening In psychiatry, a disturbance of affectivity. Flattening of affect (or "flat affect") is rarely seen outside the schizophrenic group, although affect-block, which is seen also in obsessive-compulsive patients, may be difficult to distinguish from flattening. Flattening of the affect consists of a general impoverishment of emotional reactivity or failure to react appropriately to affect-tinged stimuli. The affect-flattened patient is often described as emotionally bleak or dull, colorless, flat, unresponsive, cold, removed, apart, uninvolved, or unconvincing. The patient himself may complain that reality seems far away, that nothing has meaning for him, or that his emotional responses seem forced, false, and unreal.

flavism The presence of yellow hair in certain regions of the body in contrast with the stronger, darker hair on other parts of the body. This condition attains its significance for constitutional classification from the theory that, like the phenomenon of *erythrism,* it constitutes a stigma of the *asthenic, microsplanchnic* physique and its tendency to tuberculosis.

fletcherism (Horace Fletcher, 1849–1919, American dietitian) The doctrine, or the carrying out of the belief, that each bite of food must be masticated thoroughly before it is swallowed, and that liquids should be ingested only in small sips; often includes an injunction as to the specific number of times each mouthful should be chewed.

flexibility, waxy See *catalepsy.*

flicker Flutter; rapid change in frequency of stimulation (usually auditory or visual) producing corresponding periodic change in the visual or auditory perception. In the case of vision, for example, a flickering light will be perceived as such until brightness of the light and/or frequency of the flicker is increased to a certain point (critical flicker frequency); at this point, the stimulus will be perceived as a single, continuing stimulus (fusion).

flight Act of fleeing or running away, as to escape danger. See *fugue.*

flight into disease *Conversion;* the flight away from threatening reality by means of the conversion symptoms represents the paranosic or primary gain of the illness.

flight into health *Transference cure* or *improvement* (see *transference*); a relinquishing of symptoms that occurs not because the patient has resolved his neurosis, but

rather as a defense against further probing by the analyst into painful, unconscious material. In many instances, the flight into health depends upon the patient's passive-dependent relationship to the analyst, whom he endows with magical power and omnipotence.

flight of ideas A near-continuous flow of speech that is not disjointed or bizarre, but that jumps rapidly from one topic to another, each topic being more or less obviously related to the preceding or to adventitious environmental stimuli. Flight of ideas is characteristic of acute manic states; consequently, it is seen most commonly in the manic phase of manic-depressive psychosis but can also be seen in the acute manic syndrome of schizophrenia. N. Cameron terms flight of ideas "topical flight": "The manic makes rapid shifts from topic to topic, but the alert, attentive listener can keep up with the changes because they do not differ fundamentally from the changes in subject a normal elated person might make. The shifts in schizophrenic talk . . . are confused by the indiscriminate overinclusion of material belonging to both shared social and private fantasy contexts. The manic in his talk keeps to social trails of communication, even though he may change his direction on them at every moment; the schizophrenic does not keep to social paths, but makes his own trail as he goes." (*The Psychology of Behavior Disorders,* 1947)

flight, topical Cameron's term for *flight of ideas* (q.v.).

floccillation *Carphology* (q.v.); aimless picking or plucking.

flogger One who whips; flagellator.

flooding *Implosion* (q.v.).

flow chart See *algorithm, clinical.*

fluctuating ego states See *dedifferentiation.*

fluency, intermodal Ability to transfer knowledge from one sensory channel to another, as in feeling an object while blindfolded and being able subsequently to pick that object from a group on the basis of its visual appearance. Infant research has shown that the infant is intermodally fluent and that such ability is inherent in how the organism perceives.

fluent aphasia See *aphasia, fluent.*

fluidity Mobility; in Kurt Lewin's theory of personality, fluidity refers to the permeability of boundaries between the different regions or subsystems of the person. Lewin uses the term *accessibility* for the permeability of the personality boundaries to external stimulation.

FM In Rorschach scoring, a nonhuman (i.e. animal) movement response, characterized by movement or tension that is unnatural or physically impossible for a human being. According to Z. Piotrowski, the *FM* reflect the action and behavioral potentials of the subject when he is in a state of diminished consciousness and/or self-control. (*Perceptanalysis*, 1957)

focal suicide See *syndrome, deliberate self-harm.*

focused delirium See *délire chronique.*

focusing disturbance A disturbance of adaptability that may occur in patients with organic brain disease: some tasks can be performed when approached one way, but not if they are approached in any other way.

folie (F. "insanity") The French distinguished *mental alienation* and insanity (*folie*), considering the former in a generic sense, while they used *folie* to denote a psychiatric condition acquired by a person who had previously been in good mental health.

folie à deux (F. "double insanity") Folie à deux has been known by a number of names: shared paranoid disorder (DSM-III), induced psychotic disorder (DSM-III-R), communicated insanity, induced insanity, double insanity (Tuke), folie simultanée (Régis), folie imposée (Lasègue and Falret), folie induite (Lehmann). See *association, psychosis of.*

"Suggestibility plays a part, among other factors, in the genesis of folie à deux ' . . . when two persons closely associated with one another suffer a psychosis simultaneously, and when one member of the pair appears to have influenced the other. The condition is not of course necessarily confined to two persons, and may involve three or even more (*folie à trois*, etc.).' " (Henderson, D.K., & Gillespie, R.D. *A Text-book of Psychiatry*, 1936)

"It happens that paranoid or paranoiac and rarely hypomanic patients not only can make those with whom they live close together believe in their delusions, but they so infect them that the latter under

conditions themselves continue to build on the delusion." (Bleuler, *TP*)

folie à double forme *Obs.* (F. "insanity in double form") Manic-depressive psychosis.

folie à quatre (F. "quadruple insanity") The appearance of the same delusions in four members of a family. Bleuler cites the following case: "At one time we had in Burghölzli four siblings (two brothers and two sisters) who all had the same persecutory and religious delusions. It turned out that one sister, the most intelligent of the four, was the first to become ill; she imposed her delusions on the others. She deteriorated severely and later developed catatonic symptoms. The second sister could eventually be released, but had to be readmitted later. The two brothers managed to maintain themselves outside the hospital. There was no doubt that the two sisters were really schizophrenic; and we had excellent reasons for believing that the two brothers were also schizophrenic, not only because they never recovered completely afterwards, but also because of their peculiar modes of life already before the acute attack." (*Dementia Praecox or the Group of Schizophrenias*, 1950) Bleuler considers this a form of *induced schizophrenia.* See *association, psychosis of.*

folie à trois (F. "triple insanity") The appearance of the same delusions in three members of a family. See *association, psychosis of; schizophrenia, induced.*

folie circulaire (F. "cyclic insanity") Falret's term for manic-depressive psychosis, circular or alternating type.

folie communiquée (F. "infectious insanity") *Folie à deux* (q.v.).

folie d'action (F. "madness of movement, action") Brierre de Boismont's term for moral and emotional insanity.

folie démonomaniaque (F. "demonomaniacal insanity") *Demonomania* (q.v.).

folie des grandeurs (F. "insanity of greatness") *Megalomania* (q.v.).

folie des persécutions (F. "insanity of persecutions") Paranoid psychosis.

folie du doute (F. "insanity of doubt") *Doubting mania*, today usually subsumed under the heading of anxiety neurosis or obsessive-compulsive reaction.

"The fear of responsibility expresses itself in the compulsion to examine repeatedly whether a match thrown away no longer burns, whether the doors of closets are locked, whether letters are sealed, or whether a mistake was made in calculating (doubting mania, *folie du doute*)." (Bleuler, *TP*)

Falret introduced the expression as a nosological entity, calling it *la maladie du doute*. At an earlier date Esquirol termed the same condition *monomanie raisonnante;* Baillarger referred to it as *monomanie avec conscience;* at other times it was known as *alienation partielle;* Oscar Berger named the condition *Grübelsücht.*

folie du pourquoi (F. "craze of 'why'") Question-asking insanity. This is a manifestation of the compulsive-obsessive form of psychoneurosis, in which the patient has the morbid urge to ask questions.

folie gémellaire (F. "twin-insanity") Psychoses in twins occurring simultaneously.

folie hypocondriaque (F. "hypochondriacal insanity") Neurasthenia.

folie imitative (F. "imitative insanity") *Folie à deux* (q.v.).

folie imposée (F. "imposed insanity") See *association, psychosis of; folie à deux.*

folie induite (F. "induced insanity") See *folie à deux.*

folie instantanée (F. "momentary insanity") *Mania transitoria* (q.v.).

folie morale (F. "moral insanity") See *insanity, moral.*

folie morale, acquired Kraepelin's term for antisocial behavior that masks an underlying schizophrenic disorder, which breaks through in the form of acute psychotic states with delusions, auditory hallucinations, and agitation or stupor.

folie paralytique (F. "paralytic insanity") *General paresis* (q.v.).

folie pénitentiare (F. "penitentiary insanity") Prison psychosis. See *syndrome, Ganser.*

folie raisonnante (F. "reasoning insanity") *Folie du doute* (q.v.).

folie raisonnante mélancolique *Obs.* (F. "melancholic reasoning insanity") Griesinger's expression for what was called in his time hypochondriacal melancholia.

folie simulée (F. "feigned insanity") Feigned psychosis.

folie simultanèe (F. "simultaneous insanity") See *folie à deux.*

folie systématisée *Obs.* (F. "systematized insanity") *Paranoia; primary delusional insanity.*

folie utérine *Obs.* (F. "uterine insanity") A general term, denoting psychiatric conditions supposedly associated with uterine disorders; also *nymphomania* (q.v.).

folie vaniteuse (F. "conceited insanity") *Megalomania* (q.v.).

folk healing *Folk medicine* (q.v.).

folk medicine *Folk healing;* the interrelated beliefs, behaviors, treatment techniques, and medicines that have evolved indigenously within specific cultural settings to cope with illness and injury. Folk medicine includes unorthodox forms of medical care that, by conventional medical standards, seem pointless or even harmful; among them are the *voodoo* of the Haitians, *santeria* of the Cubans, *espiritismo* of the Puerto Ricans, *curanderismo* of Spanish-speaking people, folk healing, charismatic faith healers, and rootworkers. Lately folk healing has been treated more respectfully as evidence grows that a patient's belief in a treatment may be an important factor in effecting the cure.

folk soul See *soul, folk.*

folklore Folk wisdom or folk learning; suggested by Thoms in 1846. In the present-day life of civilized peoples, folklore is the sum-total of meager, often fragmentary relics (which have survived, through tradition, from earlier primitive-culture stages) of cultural monuments in word and art: historical accounts, legends and myths, adages and sayings, beliefs, customs, magic practices, folk remedies, household prescripts, fairy tales, fables, and songs (words, music, dances).

folkways Group habits or customs; the whole system of behavior patterns characteristic of a group; the accepted or expected ways of performing the nearly infinite number of minor rituals of normal social living.

Fölling test See *phenylketonuria.*

follow-back See *follow-through.*

follow-through A type of follow-up technique in research in which the investigator examines his subjects (both experimental and control) in childhood and then reevaluates them at intervals until they reach the age at which he measures the outcomes in which he is interested.

Particularly when they are used to monitor the development of children or others at risk, such follow-up studies have disadvantages, such as the period of time required, changing concepts of nosology over time, development of different diagnostic or treatment techniques over time, and the ethical questions of how the researcher can maintain a role of uninvolved, objective observer if a treatable condition is detected or if a new treatment is developed that will alter the natural course of the condition under study. See *risk; vulnerability factor.*

Follow-back approaches the problem from the other end of the temporal spectrum. The experimental group is formed by persons diagnosed as suffering currently from the disease under study. Their development is then traced retrospectively—by the examination of birth records, school performance, and medical history, for example—in an attempt to identify the significant factors in the development of the disorder. This method also has drawbacks, including the unavailability of some of the records considered crucial in at least some of the subjects.

follow-up Pursuing or repeating an earlier action, including assessment of the effects of an earlier action. To the clinician, the term generally means aftercare and monitoring of the patient's response to initial and subsequent interventions. To the researcher, the term is likely to mean periodic evaluation or *follow-through* (q.v.).

folly The clinical syndrome known in the early part of the 19th century as *folly* was roughly the equivalent of what is today known as *schizophrenia;* Guislain (early 19th century) used the terms *folly* and *paraphrenia* interchangeably.

fomes ventriculi (L. "foreign body as 'contagium-carrier of the stomach'") Hypochondriasis.

force, anti-instinctual See *anticathexis.*

force, central "The central force out of which at one time the individual psyche has been differentiated. This central force goes through all further differentiations and isolations, lives in them all, cuts through them to the individual psyche, as the only one that goes absolutely unchanged and undivided through all layers." (Jacobi, J. *The Psychology of C.G. Jung,* 1942) This central force (which Jung calls primal libido) lies at the very bottom of the whole structure of an individual's total

psychic system. It is synonymous with undifferentiated energy, is psychical in nature, and has the general meaning of a life force.

force, psychic Mental power, a force generated by thought or mental action, apart from energy or physical force.

forced feeding See *alimentation, forced.*

forced impulses See *symptoms, first-rank.*

forced treatment *Coercive* or *enforced treatment;* imposition of a treatment procedure or therapeutic regimen on a patient against his will. Standard 9 of the *Wyatt v. Stickney* decision (1972) states that patients have a right not to be subjected to unusual or *hazardous treatment* procedures without their expressed and informed consent, after consultation with counsel or an interested party of the patient's choice. Specified as high risk or as less commonly used treatments were lobotomy, electroconvulsive therapy, and adversive reinforcement conditioning—treatments considered by the courts to be *invasive* or *intrusive.* Since then, the concept has been broadened to the *right to refuse treatment* as part of the growing concern over the potentiality of misuse of psychotechnology to achieve *behavior control* or *social control.* See *consumerism.*

forebrain Prosencephalon, from which develop the telencephalon (which forms the cerebral cortex, striate bodies, rhinencephalon, lateral ventricles, and the anterior portion of the third ventricle) and the diencephalon (which forms the epithalamus, thalamus, metathalamus, hypothalamus, optic chiasm, tuber cinereum, posterior lobe of hypophysis, mammillary bodies, and most of the third ventricle). See *ergotropic.*

foreconscious, *Preconscious* (q.v.).

Forel, fields of (Auguste Forel, Swiss psychiatrist, 1848–1931) See *subthalamus.*

forensic Relating to public policy, especially that formulated in judicial decisions. *Forensic psychiatry* (*legal psychiatry*) refers to the application of psychiatry in the courts of law. See *advocacy; consumerism; forced treatment.*

forensic proof See *proof, forensic.*

forepleasure In psychoanalysis, the pleasure that precedes final genital pleasure or end-pleasure. During the phase of infancy libido is invested in many erotogenic zones, the mouth, anus, skin, muscles, eyes, nose, etc. During the so-called pregenital stage, stimulation of these zones constitutes an end-pleasure, but with the advent of genital stimulation which will eventually culminate in adult genital behavior, the pregenital zones are subordinated to the genital; hence they later become a fore-pleasure. The many physical and psychical antecedents to final genital action are called forepleasure. "The increment of pleasure which is offered us in order to release yet greater pleasure arising from deeper sources in the mind is called an 'incitement premium' or technically 'fore-pleasure.'" (Freud, *CP*)

forgetfulness, organic Memory disturbances based on organic disorders.

forgetting, motivated Forgetting that is motivated by the desire to avoid painful memories. There are many cases of forgetting in which the subject feels that the impression or experience is so well known that it should not have been forgotten at all. In these and other cases the thing forgotten is often one that would be painful to the person if remembered. As a defense against experiencing this pain, he forgets the experience in question. The capacity for forgetting disagreeable things is differently developed in different persons: the individual will therefore often find it impossible to rid himself of painful memories or emotions, hard as he might strive to do so. On the other hand, things that have associative connection with the disagreeable material may frequently be forgotten. (Freud, *BW*)

format treatment The specifics of how treatment will be delivered: duration, intensity, focus, identification of subsystems involved (e.g. individual, marital, or family), relationship to concurrent therapies or position in a sequence of planned interventions, who is included in therapy, where it takes place, etc.

formation, character See *formation, personality.*

formation, habit See *training, habit.*

formation, inhibition The organization of inhibiting or restraining influences. Inhibition formation is one type of mental activity that serves to restrain the appearance in consciousness of impulses unacceptable to it. Symptom formation is a method by which the unacceptable impulses gain the level of consciousness, but in symbolic form.

formation, personality The structure or arrangement of the constituents of the personality. Psychoanalysts use *personality formation* and *character formation* synonymously.

formation, replacement An idea or set of ideas that substitute for another or other ideas. "The generalization can be safely hazarded that all members of the family group, from brother to grandfather, from sister to aunt, are all replacement-formations of the image of the original trinity of father, mother and child." (Jones, E. *Papers on Psycho-Analysis*, 1938)

formation, reticular The primitive, diffuse system of interlacing fibers and nerve cells that forms the central core of the brain stem; also called the bulbotegmental reticular formation. The reticular formation projects to the thalamic intralaminar nuclei via the reticulothalamic, tegmentothalamic, and tectothalamic tracts. From the reticular nucleus of the thalamus, nonspecific fibers project to all parts of the cerebral cortex. It is believed that these fibers can activate the cortex independently of specific sensory or other neural systems, and the reticular formation is thus considered a part of the "reticular activating system" (RAS) or *alerting system,* which also includes subthalamus, hypothalamus, and medial thalamus. The RAS seems to be essential for the initiation and maintenance of alert wakefulness, for alerting or focusing of attention, perceptual association, and directed introspection. Impaired fucntion of the RAS may be associated with anesthesia and comatose states.

formes frustes (F. "defaced, worn, blurred forms") Indefinite or less significant or atypical symptoms or types of a disease.

formication An abnormal subjective sensation of ants (or other small insects) creeping in or under a given skin area; while the condition may occur in the so-termed psychogenic mental states, it is perhaps most commonly seen in those patients in whom there is some organic agent, usually in the form of narcotic drugs (alcohol, cocaine, morphine, etc.). Also known as the *signe de Magnan* and cocaine bug.

formula, Jellinek's See *Jellinek's formula.*

fornication Sexual intercourse on the part of an unmarried person.

fornix An arched white fiber tract lying beneath the corpus callosum, extending from the hippocampus and terminating in the mammillary body. See *emotion, Papez's theory of.*

Foster Kennedy syndrome (Foster Kennedy, New York neurologist, 1884–1955) See *nerve, olfactory.*

Fothergill's neuralgia (Samuel Fothergill, English physician, 19th century) See *tic douloureux.*

fouetteuse A female flogger or flagellator.

Fournier tests (Jean Alfred Fournier, French dermatologist, 1832–1914) Occasionally an ataxic gait may be absent in normal walking; to overcome this, the Fournier tests may be utilized to verify the presence of equilibratory ataxia in walking; the patient is commanded to rise quickly from a sitting position; he is asked to rise and walk, then stop quickly on command; he is requested to walk and turn about quickly on sharp command.

Foville's syndrome (Achille L. Foville, French neurologist, 1799–1878) A form of *hemiplegia alternans* (q.v.) with contralateral hemiplegia and homolateral paralysis of the abducens and facial nerves.

FPDD Familial pure depressive disease (in Winokur's terminology).

Fragesucht (frä′ge-sookt) Compulsion to ask irrelevant questions even though not particularly interested in the answers.

fragging The use of explosives (typically, the fragmentation grenade—hence the name for the action) in an assault on a superior officer. Such assaults are said to have been more frequent in the Vietnam war than in previous wars. The hypothesized relationship between fragging and disinhibition of aggressive impulses by a variety of drugs has not been firmly established.

fragile X chromosome See *syndrome, fragile X.*

fragmentation See *thinking, fragmentation of.*

fragmented communications See *communication, disordered.*

Frankenstein factor *Antitechnology bias;* specifically, the fear that advances in macromolecular chemistry, immunology, etc., will make possible the creation of a monster or threat that can easily escape the control of its originator.

free-running See *rhythms, biologic.*

free will The concept that people are free to dispose of their own will; that they can choose between alternatives in such manner that the choice is entirely uninfluenced by factors not consciously controlled by them.

Discussing the subject of free will and its opposite, determinism, E. Jones writes: "One of the psychological arguments against the belief in a complete mental determinism is the intense feeling of conviction that we have a perfectly free choice in the performance of many acts. This feeling of conviction must be justified by something, but at the same time it is entirely compatible with a complete determinism. It is curious that it is not often prominent with important and weighty decisions. On these occasions one has much more the feeling of being irresistibly impelled in a given direction (compare Luther's 'Hier stehe ich, ich kann nicht andres' [Here I stand, I cannot do otherwise]). On the contrary, it is with trivial and indifferent resolutions that one is most sure that one could just as well have acted otherwise, that one has acted from non-motivated free will. From the psychoanalytical point of view, the right of this feeling of conviction is not contested. It only means that the person is not aware of any conscious motive. When, however, conscious motivation is distinguished from unconscious motivation, this feeling of conviction teaches us that the former does not extend over all our motor resolutions. What is left free from the one side receives its motive from the other—from the unconscious—and so the physical determinism is flawlessly carried through. A knowledge of unconscious motivation is indispensable, even for philosophical discussion of determinism." (*Papers on Psycho-Analysis,* 1949) The interrelation of conscious and unconscious mental processes provides the key to the problem of psychological *determinism* (q.v.).

freebasing Increasing the potency of cocaine by extracting pure cocaine alkaloid, the free base, and then inhaling the heated vapors through a cigarette or water pipe. Extraction is simple and requires only baking soda and a source of heat, but many cocaine abusers extract the alkaloid by mixing it with ether and acetone. This is an extremely dangerous form of cocaine abuse because the mixture is explosive and highly flammable. See *crack*.

freedom to choose See *coercion*.

Freeman, Walter J. (1895–1972) American psychiatrist and neurologist; psychosurgery.

Fregoli's phenomenon See *syndrome, Capgras's*.

frenetic See *phrenetic*.

frenzy *Obs.* Extreme excitement and mental agitation; sometimes considered synonymous with *mania*.

frequency The number of subjects with a given character (e.g. the number of persons aged 20–24 years). See *table, frequency*.

frequency, flicker (fusion) See *flicker*.

Freud, Anna (1895–1982) Vienna-born lay analyst, daughter of Sigmund Freud; *The Ego and the Mechanisms of Defence* (1936); play therapy; psychoanalysis of children and adolescents.

Freud, Sigmund (1856–1939) Austrian neurologist and psychoanalyst; founder of psychoanalysis; concepts of the libido, regression, transference, repression, sublimation, id, ego, superego, Oedipus complex, etc.; psychopathology of dreams; evaluation of infantile experiences and impressions.

Freudian slip See *slip*.

friction In social work, "conflicts arising out of unlike temperaments or emotional needs which, instead of resolving themselves in a constructive manner, continue on a level of chafing and irritation. *Family Friction*—a generalized tension or irritation in any combination of family life, excepting when otherwise distinguished; *Marital Friction*—the spouse being the patient; *Parental Friction*—between the parents of a minor child, the child being the patient; *Parent-Child Friction*—between parent and child, either being the patient." (Hamilton, G. *A Medical Social Terminology*, 1930)

Friedmann's complex (Max Friedmann, German neurologist, 1858–1925) See *constitution, post-traumatic*.

Friedreich's ataxia See *ataxia, Friedreich's*.

friendly In computer language, relatively easy to use by those not versed in computer science. It takes a great many circuits (*VLSIC*, very large scale integrated circuits) to make a system easy to learn and friendly to use, and the *person-machine interface* may remain a barrier to effective use of the computer that is not friendly.

fright The reaction to an unexpected danger. According to Freud, "Fright is the name of the condition to which one is reduced if one encounters a danger without being prepared for it; it lays stress on the element of surprise." This element of surprise distinguishes fright from both fear and apprehension. "Apprehension denotes a certain condition of expecting a danger and preparation for it, even though it be an unknown one; fear requires a definite object, of which one is afraid."

Also, the element of surprise appears to be the essential causal factor in the traumatic neurosis. Apprehension cannot produce a traumatic neurosis: "In apprehension there is something which protects against fright and therefore against the fright-neurosis." Apprehension prepares the organism for "oncoming masses of excitation" and it can therefore defend itself, whereas in fright the organism, taken unawares, is overwhelmed by the excitation. (*Beyond the Pleasure Principle*, 1922)

fright, magic *Susto* (q.v.).

frigidity, sexual Inability of the woman to achieve orgasm through coitus; *psychosexual dysfunction with inhibited sexual excitement;* the analogous condition in the male is termed impotence. See *impotence, psychic; orgasm*. "Frigidity may be total or partial, but whatever its degree it is not a disease entity in itself; rather, it is a symptom or manifestation of underlying neurotic conflict and, as such, can be traced to any number of psychological mechanisms. It is difficult to say how common frigidity is; some estimate that it affects as many as 90% of women . . . while others would put it closer to 50%. . . . But whatever the actual incidence, all agree that it is high, and certainly that frigidity is more common than impotence in the male, even though the symptom itself may be less commonly complained of because it does not interfere so directly or so disastrously with the mechanics of intercourse or with reproduction." (Campbell, R.J. in *Mar-*

riage: A Psychological and Moral Approach, ed. W. Bier, 1964)

Total frigidity includes complete anesthesia; absence of sexual interest; vaginismus, with or without dyspareunia—and women so afflicted will generally tolerate intercourse only if forced.

More common than total frigidity is some type of *relative frigidity,* among the more frequent of which are the following: (1) *vaginal hypoesthesia,* with sensitivity limited to the clitoral area; (2) sudden abrupt cessation of excitement before orgasm, even though there has been pleasure during intercourse, during both clitoral stimulation and vaginal friction; some women of this group, in their search for satisfaction, appear insatiable in their sexual demands and may go from one partner to another hoping that each new experience will bring orgasm; (3) vaginal orgasm achieved, but only under certain conditions—such as concurrent beating or rape phantasies—or only with certain men; (4) whatever the degree of satisfaction obtained during intercourse, the sexual act is followed by anxiety, tension, insomnia, guilt feelings and depression, physical complaints, or any other kind of symptom, all of which point to some kind of unconscious conflict about sexuality, usually revolving about unsatisfied infantile wishes.

fringe Used by M. Prince, generally in *fringe of consciousness;* approximately equivalent to *preconscious* (q.v.).

fringe, subliminal See *summation.*

Fröhlich's syndrome (Alfred Fröhlich, Viennese neurologist, 1871–1953) Fröhlich's syndrome or *dystrophia adiposogenitalis* described in 1901 is caused by a chromophobe adenoma that destroys the anterior lobe of the pituitary gland occurring mainly in individuals in the pre- or post-adolescent period. It is characterized by eunuchoidal obesity, alteration of the secondary sex characters, metabolic disturbances, and change in bodily growth—gigantism, hypoplastic genitals, polyuria, polydipsia, and increased sugar tolerance.

Frohman Factor A protein factor found in the serum of schizophrenics isolated by C.E. Frohman and his colleagues at the Lafayette Clinic. The factor alters the anaerobic metabolism of chicken red blood cells. It has been suggested that the Frohman Factor is the same as *Bergen's fraction* (q.v.).

Froin's syndrome (George Froin, Viennese physician, b. 1874) High protein content of the cerebrospinal fluid (0.5% or more) associated with xanthochromia, massive coagulation, and pleocytosis. Froin's syndrome is seen mainly in chronic meningitis, especially syphilitic, in obstruction of the spinal subarachnoid space by cord tumor or epidural abscess, and in cases of polyneuritis and Landry's paralysis.

Fromm-Reichmann, Frieda (1890–1957) German-born psychoanalyst; director of psychotherapy, Chestnut Lodge Sanitarium; Washington School of Psychiatry and Psychoanalysis; psychotherapy of schizophrenia.

frottage Sexual perversion in which orgasm is induced by rubbing against the clothing of the sexual object as occurs when the subject is pressed close to others in a throng or crowded public transportation. A person so afflicted is a *frotteur* (q.v.).

frotteur (F. "one who rubs") One who gains sexual excitement through the sense of touch by rubbing up against somebody. The term usually implies that the act of touching or being touched is not directly or overtly of a genital character, or at least that there is some measure of disguise. For example, some individuals are sexually stimulated when they are pressed closely by others as often happens when they are in a crowd. Some authorities use the term to mean direct genital or sexual activity, not including the union of the genital organs.

frotteurism *Frottage* (q.v.). The DSM definition of this paraphilia emphasizes that the frotteur's sexual object is nonconsenting.

frozen watchfulness An alert but inhibited appearance observed in many children who have suffered abuse.

frustration From the standpoint of instinctual psychology (psychoanalysis), frustration generally refers to the denial of gratification by reality. Sometimes it is spoken of as external frustration to distinguish it from the thwarting of impulses by forces in the unconscious or also in consciousness.

When in a mentally healthy person the environment is not prepared for the acceptance of a libidinal urge, the latter may be held in suspension until reality is suitably arranged or until some form of substitutive gratification may present itself. Frustration may be eluded by means of sublimation.

When the instinctual urge cannot be handled normally by the subject, he may summon all his energies to the satisfaction of the urge, disregarding the mores of his surroundings. Or he may regress; that is, the frustrated libido may be withdrawn from objects in reality and take "refuge in the life of phantasy where it creates new wish-formations and reanimates the vestiges of earlier forgotten ones." (Freud, *CP*)

Internal frustration means the checking of instinctual impulses by forces in the unconscious, chiefly by the superego. E. Jones says: "The ego defends itself against external danger by repressing [in this case] the genital impulses directed towards the love-object. Regression to the anal-sadistic level ensues, but the relation of this process to the frustration and to the influence of the ego-instincts is not clear." (*Papers on Psycho-Analysis*, 1938)

frustration tolerance The ability to withstand tension arising from a buildup in instinctual demand that is not immediately relieved or gratified. Development of tension or frustration tolerance is essential for achieving active mastery by the ego; low frustration tolerance and/or the need for immediate instinctual gratification are indicative of severe ego weakness.

FTA-ABS The fluorescent treponemal antibody absorption test for syphilis; the test is extremely sensitive and highly specific, with less than a 1% incidence of false-positive reactions.

fugue A condition in which the patient suddenly leaves his previous activity and begins to wander or goes on a journey that has no apparent relation to what he has just been doing, and for which he has amnesia afterwards. In fugues of short duration, the patient is generally agitated and confused, but in those of long duration he may often appear completely normal to the observer. Fugues may occur as one type of epileptic twilight state, as a form of catatonic excitement, or as a form of conversion hysteria (dissociative reaction). As a psychogenic reaction, they appear often to be precipitated by a need

to escape an intolerable situation; such fugues are typically "orderly," while epileptic fugues are typically disorderly.

fulfillment, punishment Freudian term for self-punishment.

Fulton, John Farquhar (1899–1960) American physician; neurophysiology (especially hypothalamus, cerebellum, autonomic nervous system); history of science and medicine.

function The operation of the structure (or organization) of the psyche. The ego, as a structure of the psyche, has capacities for working or functioning.

Functioning is "a certain form of psychic activity that remains theoretically the same under varying circumstances. From the energic standpoint a function is a phenomenal form of libido, which theoretically remains constant, in much the same way as physical force can be considered as the form or momentary manifestation of physical energy." (Jung, *PT*)

function, auxiliary See *function, principal*.

function complex See *complex, function*.

function, directed See *intellect*.

function, dream See *dream-function*.

function engram For Jung, an inherited, archaic residue. "The symbol is always derived from archaic residues, or imprints engraven in the very stem of the race, about whose age and origin one can speculate much, although nothing definite can be determined. It would certainly be quite wrong to look to personal sources for the source of the symbol, as for instance repressed sexuality. At best such a repression could only furnish the libido-sum which activates the anchaic imprint. The imprint (engram) corresponds with a functional inheritance whose existence is not contingent upon ordinary sexual repression, but proceeds from instinct differentiation in general." (*PT*)

function, Gestalt See *psychology, gestalt*.

function, inferior See *function, superior*.

function, irrational See *irrational*.

function pleasure See *pleasure, function*.

function, principal Among the many aspects of *function*, Jung speaks of the *principal* and *auxiliary* functions. "For all the types appearing in practice, the principle holds good that besides the conscious main function there is also a relatively unconscious, auxiliary function which is in every respect different from the nature of the main function. From these combinations well-known pictures arise, the practical intellect for instance paired with sensation, the speculative intellect breaking through with intuition, the artistic intuition, which selects and presents its images by means of feeling judgment, the philosophical intuition which, in league with a vigorous intellect, translates its vision into the sphere of comprehensible thought, and so forth." (*PT*) See *analytic psychology*.

function, rational See *rational*.

function, superior In Jung's analytical psychology, there are four basic psychological types—thinking, feeling, intuitive, and sensational. Any one of the functional types may predominate as the means by which the person adjusts himself to the problems of living. The predominating is called the *superior* function, while the remaining three functions are *inferior* in varying degrees. See *analytic psychology*.

function type The generic name for Jung's various types: feeling, thinking, intuitive, and sensation. The characters of introversion and extraversion are ways of regarding reality rather than methods of adaptation to reality; hence they are called attitude types. See *analytic psychology*.

function-way, archaic In analytical psychology, thinking, acting, and feeling characteristic of the primitive type of mind. While discussing *regression* Jung says: "The draining of libido involves their gradual relapse below the threshold of consciousness, their associative connection with consciousness gets loosened, until they sink by degrees into the unconscious. This is synonymous with a regressive development; namely, a recession of the relatively developed function to an infantile and eventually archaic level. But, since man has spent relatively only a few thousand years in a cultivated state, as opposed to many hundred thousand years in a state of savagery, the archaic function-ways are correspondingly extraordinarily vigorous and easily reanimated. Hence, when certain functions become disintegrated through deprivation of libido, their archaic foundations begin to operate in the unconscious." (*PT*)

functional Relating to performance or execution; in psychiatry, refers to disorders that are without known organic basis, thus often (incorrectly) equated with "psychogenic" or emotional. A functional disturbance is one in which the performance or operation of an organ or organ system is abnormal, but not as a result of known changes in structure. Although psychogenic disorders are functional, in that their symptoms are not based upon any detectable alterations in the structure of the brain or psyche, it is not true that all functional disorders of the psyche are of emotional origin—no more so than functional heart murmurs are based on emotional conflict. A drug-induced, temporary disturbance in synaptic transmission, for example, may produce many alterations in thinking, affect, and behavior. Since such a disturbance does not depend upon structural changes in the brain, it is properly termed "functional"; yet it can hardly be considered to be of psychogenic origin.

functional assessment stages See *GDS*.

functional budgeting In this system of resource allocation and control, the budget is not constructed according to line items (*inputs*), but instead according to functions or activities carried out by the departments or components of an organization (*outputs*). Resources are then assigned for the accomplishment of the organization's objectives. Thus the budget focus is where it should be, on the programs of the organization designed to achieve its goals. Functional budgeting is an essential element of *strategic planning* (q.v.).

functional inferiority See *inferiority, functional*.

functions, seriatim Organization or synthesis of skilled acts or thoughts into an orderly series; such organization requires ability to anticipate a goal and ability for temporal organization. The seriatim functions are generally disturbed in the schizophrenias.

Funkenstein test (Daniel Hertz Funkenstein, American psychiatrist, b. 1910) See *test, Adrenalin-Mecholyl*.

fureur génitale *Obs.* Bruisson's term for nymphomania and satyriasis.

furibundus *Obs.* Maniacal, mad, raging.

furiosi (L. "those full of madness, raging, fury") This is one of the the two subdivisions of the insane recorded in the old Roman laws. Those who were violent and maniacal were called *furiosi;* those exhibiting dementia or feeblemindedness were termed *mente capti.*

fusion In psychoanalysis, the union of the instincts. Normally during the early infantile months the two primal instincts, life and death, are separated from one another, each operating alone. Later the two fuse to a greater or lesser extent. In psychiatric conditions there is often some defusion of the instincts.

For example, when the ego is threatened by an external danger associated with a genital impulse, the latter is repressed and regression to the anal-sadistic level follows. Several possibilities then occur regarding the redistribution of libido. "A part regresses and fuses with the hate instincts to constitute sadism." (Jones, E. *Papers on Psycho-Analysis,* 1938) See *instinct.*

fusion See *flicker.*

G

G Rorschach scoring symbol for a response that includes the entire inkblot. See *W*.

GABA Gamma-aminobutyric acid; a *neurotransmitter* (q.v.).

GABA-receptor complex See *receptor complex, supramolecular*.

Gabob The hydroxyl derivative of GABA (gamma-aminobutyric acid). Both GABA and Gabob are chemical mediators with an important role in cerebral metabolism, but their relationship to psychiatric disorders is unclear.

GAD Generalized *anxiety disorders* (q.v.).

GAI *Guided affective imagery* (q.v.).

gain, epinosic Secondary advantages accruing from an illness, such as gratification of dependency yearnings or attention seeking. "In the traumatic neuroses, *secondary gains* play an even more important role than in the psychoneuroses; there are certain uses the patient can make of his illness which have nothing to do with the origin of neurosis but which may attain the utmost practical importance. . . . Obtaining financial compensation or fighting for one creates a poor atmosphere for psychotherapy, the more so if the compensation brings not only rational advantages but has acquired the unconscious meaning of love and protecting security as well. . . . Perhaps the idea of giving one single compensation at the right time may be the best way out." (Fenichel, *PTN*)

gain, morbid Synonymous with *gain, epinosic; illness, advantage by* (qq.v.).

gain, secondary See *gain, epinosic*.

gain, tertiary A term suggested for benefits accruing to someone other than the patient from the illness of the patient, including other family members, others from the patient's social system, the physician, etc.

gait, ataxic Tabetic gait, due to loss of proprioceptive sense in the extremities as a result of posterior column disease. The patient walks on a wide base, slapping his feet, and typically watching his legs and feet so he will know where they are.

gait, cerebellar In diseases of the cerebellum, the patient walks unsteadily with a "drunken," wobbly gait. There is lack of association between the movements of the legs and body, so that in walking, the body either lags behind, or is abruptly brought forward, and there is a tendency to reel to one side.

gait, clumsy See *gait, waddling*.

gait, drunken Staggering gait, seen not only in acute alcoholic intoxication but also in other drug intoxications, polyneuritis, multiple sclerosis, general paresis, and brain tumors.

gait, festination See *gait, propulsion*.

gait, foot-drop See *gait, steppage*.

gait, hemiplegic In patients with hemiplegia, the lower extremity is held stiffly and circumducted in walking, and the patient leans to the affected side.

gait, myopathic A waddling gait is characteristic of the myopathies. See *gait, waddling*.

gait, propulsion *Festination* gait, *marche à petits pas*; characteristic of Parkinson's disease. The patient leans forward and takes short, shuffling steps that begin slowly but accelerate as he continues to walk; he looks as though he must run to keep up with his head.

gait, scissors In patients with bilateral spastic limbs, there is crossed progression in the process of walking; the legs cross in scissors fashion. See *disease, Little's*.

gait, spastic The patient walks stiffly with legs extended and feet shuffling.

gait steppage Foot-drop gait due to paralysis of the anterior tibial group of muscles, as in alcoholic neuritis, peroneal nerve injuries, poliomyelitis, and progressive muscular atrophy. The patient raises his affected knee high, and the foot flops with the toe usually dragging along the floor.

gait, stuttering A disorder in walking, usually, though not necessarily, psychogenic. It is characterized by a hesitancy in walking analogous to that observed in speech stuttering. It is sometimes seen in hysterical and in schizophrenic subjects.

gait, tabetic See *gait, ataxic.*

gait, waddling Clumsy gait, seen in dislocation of the hip and in muscular dystrophies with hip weakness. The weakness necessitates use of the trunk muscles in walking, so that the patient rolls from side to side as he walks.

galactosemia An autosomal recessive disorder (in which the patient is homozygous for the gene) consisting of an absence of the enzyme galactose-1-phosphate uridyl transferase, which is essential for the conversion of galactose-1-phosphate to glucose-1-phosphate. Galactose-1-phosphate accumulates in erythrocytes, liver and kidney tissue, brain, and lens, with resultant impairment of tissue metabolism. Mental retardation may in large part be prevented by early administration of a galactose-free diet.

galeanthropy The delusion that one is a cat.

galeophobia Fear of cats; also *ailurophobia, gatophobia.*

Galgenhumor See *humor, gallows.*

gallows humor See *humor, gallows.*

Galt, John Minson 2nd (1819–62) American psychiatrist; forensic psychiatry, psychiatric records research.

galvanic skin response See *reflex, psychogalvanic.*

gambling See *disorders of impulse control.*

game, hallucinatory In children, the same factors that are responsible for illusions may produce reactions A. Stern called hallucinatory games. (*Psychologies der frühen Kindheit,* 1928) These hallucinations differ from real hallucinations in their being actively created by the child instead of being felt as something foreign and externally induced. The infant literally makes a game of creating objects out of phantasy and amusing itself thereby. It is at all times fully aware of the unreality of these self-created objects and can easily banish them when tiring of them. A very young child's play store is largely a hallucinatory game: the business of the "store" is playfully transacted through pantomime and the use of hallucinated merchandise and money. See *companion, imaginary.*

game, middle The period in psychoanalytic treatment following establishment of a stable transference in which the analyst maintains a neutral stance and focuses on interpretation of intrapsychic processes as a way of encouraging the patient's regression and thereby facilitating the analysis of instinctual vicissitudes. The name is derived from Freud's analogy of the analytic process to a chess game.

games See *transactional analysis.*

gamete In genetics, a specialized sexual cell that unites with another germ cell to form a zygote. Among animals the male gametes are known as spermatozoa and the female gametes as *eggs* or *ova.*

Gametes are always haploid and genetically pure, because they contain only one member of a given factor pair. Since the formation of a gamete involves a reduction of 50% in the amount of genetic material carried, each gamete has only half of the factorial equipment of an ordinary body cell and never shows the hybrid character of the individual producing it. See *chromosome.*

gamma alcoholism See *alcoholism.*

gammacism Common speech defect (the "baby talk") of young children who replace the *velars (g,k)* with corresponding *dentals (d,t).*

gamo- (gam′ō-) Combining form meaning marriage, (sexual) union, from Gr. *gámos.*

gamonomania Morbid desire to marry.

gamophobia Fear of marriage.

gang An intimate social group characterized by a high degree of close personal contact among its members, who share common values or standards of behavior. Largely an urban phenomenon, the gang is a subculture whose interests and attitudes are typically different from, and sometimes even in direct conflict with, those of the larger society. The usual gang comprises male youths. A gang of adult men is often organized around criminal activity; delinquents are more often members of gangs than are nondeliquents, but not all youth gangs are overtly antisocial by any means.

ganglia, basal See *basal ganglia*.

gangliosidosis, G$_{M2}$ *Tay-Sachs disease* (q.v.).

Ganser syndrome See *syndrome, Ganser*.

Ganymede In medieval Europe, gay. In Greek mythology, Ganymede was a youth raped by Zeus, and some scholars trace the derivation of the Latin word *catamitus* (used by first-century Romans to refer to a male prostitute who took the "active" roll in homosexual activity) to Ganymede.

gargalesthesia Sensation of tickling.

gargoylism See *mucopolysaccharidosis*.

GAS General adaptation syndrome. See *syndrome, general adaptation*.

gastropaths, false Déjérine and Gauckler so designate those who express *food phobias*.

gastrulation In embryological development of a human organism, the stage characterized by the conversion of the monodermic *blastula* into a didermic *gastrula*. The gastrulating process is effected by the invagination, in the form of a blind tube, of the vegetal pole into the segmentation cavity. The wall of this tubular invagination is constituted by the primitive *entoderm* while its opening, or primitive mouth, is known as the *blastopore*.

gatekeeper In community psychiatry, an extramural, nonprofessional person whose role in the community (e.g. bartender, policeman, playground worker) is such as to allow him to observe segments of population for signs of stress, disharmony, disaffection, and discord. He may receive specialized training from the Community Health Center (at orientation sessions) so that he can function as a liaison worker between the Center and the community.

gatekeeper variables See *recidivism*.

gateway drugs Those substances of abuse—alcohol and marihuana—which provide the major portals of entry into abuse of other drugs. They are considered particularly dangerous because they are believed by so many to be relatively harmless.

gating Inhibiting, suppressant. The *gating theory* of schizophrenia proposes that schizophrenics are characterized by a deficit in inhibiting (gating) irrelevant sensory input; in comparison with normal persons, they respond more to irrelevant features of situations or tasks and less to the central or significant issues. See *gating, spinal*.

gating, spinal A theory of how pain impulses are conducted within the central nervous system; according to this theory, afferent fibers exert an inhibitory action on pain perception, and an analyzer or coordinating mechanism in cells of the substantia gelatinosa (the *spinal gate* or *gating mechanism*) transmits the sum of the net stimulus from both excitatory and inhibitory signals to the brain, and also modifies the pain signals themselves in accordance with messages coming to the core from higher centers. Such a theory provides a way of explaining the influence of personality, memory of past experiences, emotional factors, etc., on the total experience of pain, and it further suggests that relief of pain may be achieved not only by interrupting excitatory fibers but also by stimulating inhibitory pain fibers.

gatophobia Fear of cats; also *ailurophobia, galeophobia*.

Gaucher's disease See *disease, Gaucher's*.

Gault decision A 1967 decision by the U.S. Supreme Court mandating fair and accurate fact-finding procedures for juveniles when serious punishment could be inflicted should they be found guilty. The rights thereby guaranteed the juvenile include the right to notification of the specific charges, the right to counsel, the right against self-incrimination, and the right to confront and cross-examine the accusers. The decision stemmed from the case of an Arizona adolescent, Gerald Gault, who had been accused of making an indecent telephone call. Under the law of that state he could have been committed to a state industrial school for six years.

gay A person whose erotic contacts are limited to another person of his or her own gender. Many whose romantic attachments are to members of their own gender object to the term "homosexual" to describe themselves because it seems to refer solely to sexuality, whereas their orientation means far more to them than sexual behavior. Further, homosexual was coined (in the late 19th century) in the context of pathology. Gay, in contrast, antedates homosexual by at least several centuries, it is more precise in that it describes persons who are conscious of their orientation, and it is applicable to both men and women. If the term homosexual is used at all, the current tendency is to use it to refer to gay men, and to use "lesbian" to refer to gay women.

Gayet-Wernicke's encephalopathy *Wernicke's encephalopathy* (q.v.).

gaze, fascinating In hypnosis this term refers to the fixation of the eyes of the hypnotist upon the subject.

gazing, crystal A technique used in hypnoanalysis consisting of having the hypnotized subject observe a glass ball or a mirror and then produce associations. The subject is instructed to look at the glass and told that he will see in it things that he will describe to the analyst afterward.

GDS *Global Deterioration Scale,* a description of seven levels of cognitive performance for use in assessing the extent of mental deterioration in the elderly person. In addition to a general description of changes, the scale includes objective changes in behavior that are expressed as *functional assessment stages (FAST).* The FAST stages proceed in ordinal fashion in uncomplicated Alzheimer's disease (primary degenerative dementia), and any deviation from that pattern suggests that something other than Alzheimer's disease is a complicating factor or is the primary cause of the subject's cognitive impairment. Decreased ability to perform complex tasks, such as planning dinner for guests, handling finances, or shopping, is characteristic of Stage 4 (late confusional stage, with moderate cognitive decline); having problems in choosing the proper clothing to wear, or needing coaxing to bathe properly, is characteristic of Stage 5 (early dementia with moderately severe cognitive decline). In uncomplicated Alzheimer's disease, Stage 5 manifestations always occur after Stage 4 manifestations, and should the subject demonstrate Stage 5 deficits but retain Stage 4 functions, some other complicating condition should be suspected.

Gedankenlautwerden Auditory hallucination consisting of hearing voices that speak the subject's thoughts as he is thinking them. If the thoughts are repeated immediately after the subject thinks them, the phenomenon is termed *écho de la pensée.*

Gegenhalten See *paratonia.*

gelasmus (jĕ-laz-'mus) Spasmodic laughter, observed in hysteria and the schizophrenias, and in some organic (especially bulbar) diseases of the brain.

gelatio *Obs.* Rigid state of the body in catalepsy, as though it were frozen.

Gélineau's syndrome (Jean Baptiste Edouard Gélineau, French neurologist, 1828–1906) Idiopathic *narcolepsy* (q.v.).

gender identity The inner conviction that one is male, female, ambivalent, or neutral. *Gender role* is the outward appearance or image that one gives, through behavior and manner, that indicates he or she is to be classed as male or female. Both gender identity and gender role are established in accordance with the sex of assignment and rearing; they are clearly evident by 18 months of age and for the most part irreversible after 30 months of age. Ordinarily, both are the same, although *transvestitism* or *cross-dressing* is a notable exception. Gender role and gender identity are to be distinguished from *sexual identity,* which is biologically determined.

In DSM-III-R, gender identity disorders include transsexualism, non-transsexual cross-gender disorder, and gender identity disorder of childhood.

gender identity disorder of childhood In a child, persistent and intense distress about being his or her anatomical sex and intense desire to be of the opposite sex; usually there is more or less overt repudiation of the child's anatomic sexuality and a rejection of the clothing, games, etc., that are culturally appropriate for the child of the given sex.

gender role The behavior and appearance that one presents in terms of what the culture considers to be "masculine" or "feminine." That the gender role and sexual identity are not wholly determined by genetic constitution is demonstrated by pseudohermaphrodites who were reared contrary to their chromosomal sex; in all such cases, the gender role and orientation are congruent with the assigned sex and rearing, rather than with the biological sex. See *gender identity.*

gene Morphologically a gene is best understood as a particular state of organization of the chromatin at a particular point in the length of a particular *chromosome* (q.v.). This state of organization is to be regarded as the physical basis explaining how a hereditary character passes as a unit from parent to offspring, while it is the parallelism between the behavior of chromosomes and genes that supports the assignment of a physical basis in the chromosomes to the Mendelian units.

Both chromosomes and genes behave in inheritance as though they were individual units, and the principles of segregation and independent assortment apply to chromosomes in precisely the same way as they have been demonstrated to apply to genes. It is assumed that the genes always occur in pairs, and that one member of each pair is contributed by one parent and the other by the other parent. Owing to the phenomenon of *crossing over* it has even been possible not only to map each chromosome in certain organisms, but also to assign the genes to their relative positions on the chromosome, and to establish the fact of the *linear order* of the genes.

In accordance with these experimental findings, Morgan's *theory of the gene* is formulated as follows:

1. The hereditary characters of the individual are referable to paired elements (the genes) in the germinal material (the chromosomes) that are held together in a definite number of linkage groups.

2. In accordance with Mendel's first law, the members of each pair of genes separate when the germ cells mature and in consequence each ripe germ cell comes to contain one set only.

3. The members of different linkage groups assort independently in accordance with Mendel's second law.

4. An orderly interchange, or crossing over, also takes place between the elements in corresponding linkage groups.

5. The frequency of crossing over furnishes evidence of the linear order of the genes in each linkage group and of the relative position of genes with respect to each other.

genealogy Although in a sense identical with the actual pedigree of an individual or with the demonstration of such a pedigree in the form of a genealogical family tree, the term applies to the scientific study, or the proper historical account, of the biological descent of persons, or a group of persons, from a certain number of ancestors. These studies aim to provide a complete list of ancestors for as many generations as possible and to clarify the relationship of a person with the families of a given population group, rather than to investigate either the biological qualities of these families or the variations of certain hereditary family traits in successive generations.

general paralysis See *paresis, general.*

general paresis See *paresis, general.*

general paresis, juvenile See *neurosyphilis, congenital.*

general systems theory "A set of related definitions, assumptions, and propositions which deal with reality as an integrated hierarchy of organizations of matter and energy. General systems behavior theory is concerned with a special subset of all systems, the living ones." (Miller, J.G. *Behavioral Science 10,* 1965) General systems behavior theory is an attempt to develop an embracing general theory of the behavior of man by identifying the organized, interacting components that make up the system; by defining the controls that keep those subsystems or fields stable and in equilibrium; and by establishing the roles, relationships, inputs, outputs, and routes of flow within the hierarchy of subsystems that make up the whole. General systems theory thus provides a holistic approach to the study of human behavior and attempts to integrate the different conceptions of how each subsystem operates from a wide variety of disciplines and specialties in a search for the general truth inherent in all. See *emergence.*

generalization Applying to a whole group or class of conclusions, ideas, judgments, etc., based upon experience with a limited number of the class. While generalization is an essential element of conceptualization in the processes of normal thought, it attains particular significance in psychiatry in that one of the many thought disorders in schizophrenia is the tendency to overgeneralize and to treat the concrete as though it were abstract.

generation Even in the field of biology, this term has several meanings. It denotes the act of producing offspring, or the biological process by which reproduction is accomplished, or a group of offspring produced. In the last sense the term may mean that the given offspring are (1) of the same genealogical rank, as a stage in the succession of natural descent; (2) a series of siblings within one family as the offspring of the same parents; (3) a particular group of persons within the general population, living at the same time; or (4) people of the same period.

As a statistical concept the term refers to the average duration of life in a species or group.

generativity The general impulse for procreation in the human race. "Generativity is primarily the interest in establishing and guiding the next generation or whatever in a given case may become the absorbing object of a parental kind of responsibility." (Erikson, E. *Childhood and Society,* 1950) *Generativity vs. self-absorption* is the seventh of Erikson's eight stages of man. See *ontogeny, psychic.*

generic *Biol.* Pertaining to a *genus,* as compared with *specific.*

genes, modifying All those genes that have some influence on the effect of any particular gene; for all practical purposes, the modifying genes are all the genes other than the one under specific study, for even genes which produce a single large effect are subject to modification and qualification by the entire remainder of the genetic constitution.

genetic, genetical Whereas *genetical* is used exclusively in the sense of pertaining to the province of genetics, the term *genetic* has two meanings: (1) it is synonymous with *genetical;* and (2) produced or predetermined by a gene or a combination of genes—practically identical to *hereditary.*

genetic block See *disease, genetotrophic.*

genetic directive See *directive, genetic.*

genetic drift See *drift, genetic.*

genetic loading See *model, diathesis-stress.*

genetic marker See *marker, genetic*

genetic redundancy See *aging, theories of.*

genetic screening See *screening, genetic.*

genetic vulnerability See *vulnerability, genetic.*

genetics Bateson introduced this term to designate the portion of biology that seeks to account for the resemblances and the differences in organisms related by descent. It is the science that simply *studies* in living organisms such genetic phenomena as heredity and evolution, development

and variation, whereas the doctrinal movement that tries to anticipate or enforce the practical utilization of the scientific principles studied is eugenics.

Genetic investigation seeks the cause, the material basis, and the manners of maintenance of the specificity of the germinal substance: it strives to clarify the problems of how the characters of parents and offspring are related, how those of the adult, latent in the egg, become patent as development proceeds.

Population genetics is the study of hereditary traits and the distribution of genes in normal and abnormal populations. *Biogenetics* is the study of the biochemical and biophysical aspects of heredity; included herein is *cytogenetics* or *chromosomal genetics,* the study of anomalies in the number and structure of chromosomes. *Behavioral genetics* is the study of the effects of gene action on behavior. Since most elements of behavior—including intelligence and personality characteristics—are affected by many genes, it is rarely possible to identify the role that any one gene plays in determining the trait or pattern under study. Further, it is always difficult to separate gene action from environmental effect.

genetics, political Applications of genetic concepts to social processes through political action; the incorporation of genetic theory into political dogma or national policy. See *eugenics.*

genetophobia Stigmatization of and fear of the effect of a genetic disorder on the subject discovered to have an abnormal gene or chromosome. Often the significance of a discovered defect is impossible to predict, but the mere fact that it is discovered may influence those who know about it to treat the subject in such a way that the diagnosis becomes a self-fulfilling prophecy.

genetotrophic disease See *disease, genetotrophic.*

genial *Biol.* Pertaining to or having the particular genetic quality or the individual manifestations of a *genus.*

genic drift See *drift, genetic.*

geniculate bodies (jen-ik′ū-lät) The medial and lateral geniculate bodies are part of the posterior nuclei of the thalamus. The medial geniculate body receives auditory fibers from the cochlear nuclei (via the lateral lemniscus) and from the inferior colliculus. It sends fibers to the temporal cortex (Heschl's gyrus) via the auditory radiation, which ascends through the internal capsule. The lateral geniculate body receives most of the fibers of the optic tract; it sends fibers to the visual cortex (around the calcarine fissure) via the optic or geniculocalcarine radiation, which ascends through the internal capsule.

genidentic Having identical genes.

genital Pertaining to the organs of reproduction.

genital love See *love, genital.*

genitality A general term referring to the genital components of sexuality, and sometimes used to refer to adult sexuality; but genitality is evident before genital primacy is complete, as in childhood and adolescent genital masturbation. "Infantile sexuality differs from adult sexuality in several respects. The most impressive difference lies in the fact that the highest excitation is not necessarily located at the genitals, but that the genitals, rather, play the part of *primus inter pares* among many erogenous zones. The aims, too, are different; they do not necessarily lead toward sexual intercourse, but linger at activities that later play a role in forepleasure.... In time, however, the genitals begin to function as a special discharge apparatus, which concentrates all excitation upon itself and discharges it all no matter in which erogenous zone it originated. It is called genital primacy when this function of the genitals has become dominant over the extragenital erogenous zones, and all sexual excitations become finally genitally oriented and climatically discharged." (Fenichel, *PTN*) Unlike orality and anality, genitality probably cannot be sublimated, for the genitals represent an apparatus for achievement of a full unsublimated orgastic discharge. See *character, genital; primacy, complete genital; ontogeny, psychic.*

genitalize To displace genital libido, as onto a nonsexual (but predisposed) organ in hysteria, where libido is discharged, but inadequately and incompletely.

genius A generic, nonspecific term used loosely to denote an individual child or adult of markedly superior intellectual, emotional, volitional, affective, or creative abilities.

genocopy A genetic imitator, such as all those genetic disorders that can present a clinical picture of schizophrenia.

genogram Graphic representation of the history and the relationship structure of the family, emphasizing the connection between events and patterns; the genealogy of a family; family tree. In family therapy, the genogram frames the generational context in which present difficulties are embedded and of which they are often an expression. It is a means of identifying intergeneration continuities and the ways in which the past determined both the expressed and the unexpressed expectation that family members have of one another.

genophobia Fear of sex.

genotropism Szondi's hypothesis that latent recessive genes determine instinctive or spontaneous choice reactions. This is manifested in one way of attraction of libido between persons possessing similar gene stock. The Szondi test (see *test, Szondi*) was constructed to demonstrate this hypothesis experimentally, and it is Szondi's belief that the test subject chooses a particular picture because the corresponding need system within himself is in a state of tension.

genotype The term was coined by the Danish botanist Johannsen in connection with his pure-line theory, in order to distinguish the factorial structure of an organism from its manifested *phenotype* (q.v.). According to this theory, all individuals descended from a common ancestor by asexual reproduction have an identical genotype and will continue to breed true, regardless of environmental differences, forming lines genetically pure for all their characters.

Although originally the term meant the sum of all inherited predispositional characters of an individual, it has become customary to use it now in the sense of a particular *predisposition* (q.v.) underlying an individual morbid condition.

genotypical Pertaining to the *genotype.*

genus In biology this term signifies a group of related *species* and classifies the group as ranking above a species and next below a subfamily. See *species.*

geography, psychological "Psychological geography is the mapping of a whole community in which the interrelations of its inhabitants and the interrelations of its collectives or groups are depicted in respect to (a) its locality and (b) the psychological currents between them." (Moreno, J.L. *Who Shall Survive?* 1934)

geophagia, geophagy Dirt eating; a form of *pica* (q.v.).

gephyrophobia Fear of crossing a bridge or river.

geriatrics The science of curing or healing disorders and ailments of old age. See *psychiatry, geriatric.*

geriopsychosis A term suggested by Southard for psychoses of the senescent period; senile psychoses.

germ cell See *cell, germ.*

germ plasm See *plasm, germ.*

germinally affected See *affected, germinally.*

gerocomy The belief, or practice, that an older man absorbs virtue and youth from younger women.

gerontology The study of old age.

gerontophilia Love for old persons.

gerontophobia See *ageism.*

gerophilia Same as *gerontophilia.*

Gerstmann syndrome See *syndrome, Gerstmann.*

Gesell, Arnold L. (1881–1961) Founder and director (for 37 years) of Yale Clinic of Child Development.

Gestalt See *psychology, gestalt.*

Gestalt theory See *therapy, Gestalt.*

gesticulation, involuntary A parakinesis, suggestive of a posterior or posteromedial frontal lobe lesion on the contralateral side; often observed in conjunction with a grasp reflex.

geumaphobia (gū-mȧ-fō′bē-ȧ) Fear of taste.

Gheel Colony A boarding-out type of domiciliary care in Gheel, Belgium, that has existed since the 13th century for the treatment of a large number of psychotic patients who reside in private homes in the community. See *domicile; family care.*

gibberish Unintelligible and incoherent language such as is seen in some patients with schizophrenia, who, as Storch and others have shown, often regress to the stage in which language is founded on the principles of primitive mentality. The language of the patient is gibberish to those who cannot understand it, in much the same sense that dreams are gibberish, or that any mode of communication foreign to one is gibberish. The term was appropri-

ate when the "language" of the patient was undecipherable; it is not in use today because the language of schizophrenia is often recognizable and translatable.

gifted As used in child psychiatry, this term is meant to refer to a child whose intelligence is in the upper 2% of the total population of his age. Often, however, the term is used more loosely to refer to a child who shows outstanding ability in any single area. See *child, bright.*

gigantism (jī-gan′tiz'm) A constitutional anomaly characterized by a stature greatly above the average (any height above 205 cm in white population groups) and by a corresponding excess of body mass. It is due either to a heredito-constitutional hyperplasia of the entire endocrine system or to a particular form of hyperfunction in the anterior lobe of the hypophysis during the period of growth of the person affected. This condition of hyperpituitarism may be primary or it may be secondary to genital hypofunction. Only in rare cases, glands other than the pituitary may be primarily implicated, for instance, the adrenal cortex or the pineal gland.

Among the various forms of gigantism are Berlinger's *gigantosomia primordialis,* Pellizzi's *precocious macrogenitosomia,* and *eunuchoid small gigantism.* The latter consists of excessive growth, especially of the lower extremities, which takes place just before puberty and is associated with a hypogenesis of the secondary sexual characteristics. It is often found in the phthisic or dolichomorphic types of constitution and may correct itself in later years, unless it is complicated by active pulmonary tuberculosis. The syndrome has also been reported as a residuum of rheumatic encephalitis.

gigantism, eurythmic *Gigantosomia primordialis* (q.v.).

gigantosomia primordialis Berlinger introduced this term for the extremely rare syndrome best described as a well-proportioned form of *gigantism* with normal sex development. Some authors attribute this condition to the effect of an excessive idiopathic energy in the development of the entire organism, while others consider it as a special form of gigantism with similar etiology.

Gilles de la Tourette syndrome See *syndrome, Gilles de la Tourette.*

girl, phallus The unconscious symbolic equivalent of girl with phallus. Such a situation arises most frequently in a paraphilia, such as *transvestitism* (q.v.). The male transvestite has phantasied that the woman has a penis. Having thus overcome his castration anxiety, he identifies with this phallic woman. He himself represents the phallic woman under whose clothes a penis is hidden. Moreover, the female identification frequently represents an identification not with the mother but with a "little girl," for example, with a little sister. On the other hand, on a deeper level, the identification is with one's own penis. "At deeper levels, fantasies of introjections are found in which the penis is equated with an introjected woman." Thus, occasionally in these cases, "girl" comes to have the symbolic meaning "penis."

Another example in which "girl" has the symbolic significance of "penis" occurs in *urophilia* (q.v.), in which men have a sexual interest in female urination. As always in paraphilias, the interest in female urination is used to achieve reassurance against castration fears. In one case that was analyzed, "The perversion meant primarily an intense rejection of any idea of a penis." As a child the patient had thought women had only one opening and urinated from the anus. "The perversion was conditioned by a simultaneous prohibition against looking which enabled the patient to cling to the fantasy of women urinating through the anus and thus avoid again being reminded of castration by the sight of a urinating woman." On a deeper level, moreover, "The interest in watching urinating women meant the hope of finding out that they, too, have a penis. The 'urinating girl' herself had the significance of a 'urinating penis.' "

This equation may also occur in heterosexuals who are not overtly perverse. Certain narcissistic men who in childhood liked to think of themselves as girls may fall in love with more or less boyish "little girls," in whom they see the reincarnation of themselves. They treat these girls with the tenderness with which they would like to have been treated by their own mothers. They love them not for themselves but they love in them the feminine parts of their own ego. As a result of "a castration anxiety, similar to that in cases of homosexuality . . . the narcissistically chosen girl 'may represent' not only one's own person in adolescence but specifically one's own penis." Here again we see the unconscious symbolic equation of girl with penis. (Fenichel, *PTN*)

Gjessing's syndrome See *syndrome, Gjessing's.*

glia (glē-à) *Neuroglia* (q.v.).

Glick effect Positive correlation between dropping out of school and subsequent marital instability ("marriage drop-out"); not observed in all studies.

glioma (glē-ō′mà) The generic name for one of the commonest types of brain tumor. The gliomata (gliomas) account for approximately 50% of all intracranial tumors. They arise from glial cells and are composed predominantly of astrocytes or their embryonal precursors (medulloblasts, spongioblasts, astroblasts). By common usage, nearly all tumors of neuroepithelial origin are included in this term. In general, prognosis is unfavorable because gliomata tend to grow deep into the neural tissue; the more adult cell types (astrocytoma, oligodendroglioma, ependymoma) grow more slowly and are relatively benign, while the more immature cell types (medulloblastoma, spongioblastoma, or glioblastoma) tend to grow more rapidly, are more invasive, and are more malignant.

glissando Originally, sliding up and down the musical scale; in neurology as *glissando/ deglissando* to refer to a gait disturbance: the subject walks with a shuffling gait but as he moves from one point to another he accelerates to a near run and then gradually slows down to a stop. Such a gait is seen in Parkinson's disease and also in the frontal lobe convexity syndrome. See *syndrome, convexity.*

Global Deterioration Scale *GDS* (q.v.).

globus hystericus A term for the sensation of a ball or globe that arises in the stomach area and progresses upward, being finally felt in the throat where it produces the feeling of strangulation.

Although the term suggests that the symptom is usually psychogenic in origin, the complaint is also frequent in patients with diaphragmatic hernia and esophageal reflux. In those cases in whom the etiology is primarily psychogenic, globus hystericus and other esophageal neuroses are often based on an unconscious rejection of incorporation secondary to aggressive impulses, which are often of a sexual nature (such as castration wishes) and which are connected with eating and swallowing. Disgust plays an important role and is probably a combination of temptation and rejection along with an ambivalent attitude toward incorporation. See *anorexia nervosa; eating disorders; neurosis, esophageal.*

globus pallidus See *basal ganglia.*

glorified self *Idealized self* (q.v.).

gloss, metallic Tschisch's term for what he believed to be a characteristic facial expression in patients suffering from essential epilepsy.

glosso- Combining form meaning tongue, language, from Gr. *glōssa.*

glossodynia An itching, burning sensation in the tongue and buccal mucous membranes.

glossolalia Neologisms that simulate coherent speech; despite the fact that they are expressed as unintelligible conglomerations of sounds, or written as series of unintelligible letters, such neologisms mimic normal speech by maintaining the distinctions of words, sentences, and even paragraphs. Glossolalia is most often seen in ecstatic and somnambulistic states, and, somewhat less commonly, in schizophrenia. If completely devoid of content, glossolalia is termed psittacistic, although certain writers use glossolalia and psittacism interchangeably. See *neophasia, polyglot.*

glossospasm Rapid protrusion and retraction of the tongue; the spasm generally lasts for several minutes.

glossosynthesis *Neologism* (q.v.).

glucagon A hyperglycemic-glycogenolytic factor excreted by the alpha cells of the pancreas in response to hypoglycemia or stimulation by growth hormone of the anterior pituitary. Glucagon hydrochloride is a pharmacological preparation used to treat hypoglycemia (including the hypoglycemia of insulin coma therapy); it acts by mobilizing glycogen from the liver.

glucocorticoid See *syndrome, general adaptation.*

glucogenosis *Von Gierke's disease;* mental retardation due to a deficiency of glycogen-metabolizing enzymes, so that glycogen is deposited in the brain and other organs.

glucoprivation Decrease in level of circulating glucose, once believed to be the physiologic reason for hunger.

glue-sniffing Inhalation, through the mouth or nose or both, of the aliphatic and aromatic hydrocarbons in glue (such as the glue used in making model airplanes). Glue-sniffing is one of the psychoactive substance use disorders, and it is often practiced by very young children (9 to 12 years of age). Most inhalant abusers use other psychoactive substances as well. See *inhalant intoxication.*

Glueck, Eleanor Touroff (1898–1972) Criminologist; with her husband, Sheldon Glueck, developed social prediction tables for early identification of delinquents.

Glueck, Sheldon (1896–1980) Lawyer, criminologist; juvenile delinquency; with his wife, Eleanor Glueck, developed controversial prediction tables based on 40 decisive factors in forecasting the appearance and level of criminal behavior.

glutamate A *neurotransmitter* (q.v.).

gnostic A term applied by the Dutch school of neurologists (Brouwer and Kappers) to designate the deep and epicritic sensations in contradistinction to the protopathic sensations that are considered as vital or *paleosensations.*

goal, life This term is used by Adler to describe the *secret* strivings of the individual, implicit in everything he thinks and does, for a superiority that compensates for the chief inferiority. This phantasy of what he thinks he could be acts as a striving from "below" (ideas of his own disadvantages) to "above" (ideas of how to gain advantages).

gold curve See *Lange's colloidal gold reaction.*

Goldstein, Kurt (1878–1965) German psychiatrist and neurologist; aphasia.

Goll, column of (Friedrich Goll, Swiss anatomist, 1829–1904) *Fasciculus gracilis* (q.v.).

gonad A germ-gland; sexual gland.

gonadocentric Relating to the genitals as focal points. At puberty the sex urge becomes fully gonadocentric, with masturbation at the threshold and fringe of object love.

good and evil test See *responsibility, criminal.*

good object See *position, paranoid-schizoid.*

Goodenough test See *test, Goodenough.*

Gordon Holmes, rebound phenomenon of (Gordon Holmes, British physician, 1876–

1965) A test for ataxia, specifically illustrating the loss of cerebellar "check" on coordinated movement; if an attempt is made to extend the flexed forearm against resistance and suddenly let go, the hand or fist flies unchecked against the mouth or shoulder.

Gordon reflex (Alfred Gordon, American neurologist, 1874–1953) Dorsal extension of the great toe, induced by compression of the calf muscle.

gorger-vomiter A person with a form of *bulimia* (q.v.) in which the eating binges end in spontaneous or self-induced vomiting, followed by guilt and shame over loss of control, and depression. The depression is often severe, with suicidal ideas, starvation, and self-mutilation.

government, patient See *patient-government.*

Gowers' tetanoid chorea (Sir William R. Gowers, English neurologist, 1845–1915) See *degeneration, hepatolenticular.*

GPI General paralysis of the insane. See *paresis, general.*

Graefe's disease (Albrecht von Graefe, German ophthalmologist, 1828–70) See *nerve, oculomotor.*

Graftschizophrenia *Propfschizophrenia* (q.v.).

grand mal (F. "great malady") See *epilepsy.*

grande attaque hysterique See *hysteria.*

grande nevrose *Obs.* French term for epilepsy.

grandiosity See *delusion of grandeur; megalomania.*

Grantham lobotomy See *lobotomy, Grantham.*

grapevine Rumor spread through underground channels; informal communication channels by which information is disseminated among persons and groups belonging to formal organizations.

graphanesthesia A disturbance of graphesthesia (a function of the contralateral nondominant parietal lobe), consisting of the inability to recognize letters that are traced one at a time on the palm of the hand while the subject's eyes are closed.

grapho- Combining form meaning to write, from Gr. *graphein.*

graphology The study of handwriting, especially in the sense of deducing some of the personality traits of the writer from a handwriting sample.

graphomania Pressured writing or a compulsive need to write, often without regard to the worth of what is being written.

graphophobia Pathologic fear of writing, a common form of which is severe anxiety or tremulousness if forced to sign one's name while being observed by others.

graphorrhea Inordinate, uncontrolled, senseless writing, whose purpose seems to be to fill pages rather than to record or transmit a message.

grasping, forced See *lobe, frontal.*

gratification Satisfaction; in psychiatry, usually satisfaction of a person's needs or desires.

Grave's disease *Thyrotoxicosis* (q.v.).

gray-out A relatively mild or partial loss of consciousness due to anemia of the brain or anoxemia such as occurs in high-altitude flying. A more complete or total loss of consciousness is known as a *blackout* (q.v.).

Great Mother See *analytic psychology.*

Greenacre, Phyllis (b. 1894) U.S. psychoanalyst; *Trauma, Growth and Personality*, 1952; biography in depth.

Greenfield's disease Infantile metachromatic leukodystrophy. See *sclerosis, diffuse.*

gregariousness See *instinct, herd.*

grief Sorrow or pain secondary to bereavement; sadness or remorse; normal mourning, as contrasted with *depression* (q.v.). See *melancholia.*

Grieg's disease *Hypertelorism* (q.v.).

Griesinger, Wilhelm (1817–68) German psychiatrist; *Mental Pathology and Therapeutics* (1845); described mental disorders as brain diseases, combined psychiatric and neurological clinics into a single department.

grimace A distorted facial expression or facial tic, often a result of organic neurological disorder; in psychiatric syndromes, grimacing is most frequently seen in the catatonic group of the schizophrenias.

grisi siknis A culture-specific syndrome, reported among the Miskito of Nicaragua, consisting of headache, anxiety, unprovoked anger toward people in the immediate environment, aimless running, and falling down. See *syndromes, culture-specific.*

groping, forced Same as forced grasping, grasp reflex or instinctive grasp reaction. See *lobe, frontal.*

ground Background; the scenery, area, etc., on which the figures or objects in a picture appear to be superimposed. The figure is generally the part attended to, although the relationship of figure to ground may be reversed. Defective differentiation of figure and ground is common in the patient with organic brain disease, who as a result is almost always experiencing the uncertainty and instability that a normal person experiences only when confronted with ambiguous figures.

group Groups have been variously classified as (1) *primary*, characterized by intimate face-to-face associations, and *secondary*, where the members, typically without presence, are formally and impersonally associated; (2) *in-groups*, of which the person is a member and *out-groups*, to which he does not belong and with which his group is often in conflict; (3) *homogeneous* and *heterogeneous*; (4) *conflict* groups, e.g. nationalities, parties, labor unions, and gangs, and *accommodation* groups, e.g. classes, castes, vocations, denominations.

group analysis See *analysis, group; psychotherapy, group.*

group, basic assumptions In group therapy, a small group of 7 to 12 members in which the leader refuses to participate in group decision making or structuring. The name emphasizes the major regressive processes that characterize such a group.

The first is a *dependency assumption:* the leader, who is perceived as omnipotent, fails to live up to that demand; the group first denies and then devalues the leader; finally the group seeks a substitute.

The second is the *fight-flight assumption:* the leader is expected to protect the group from infighting by helping it deny intragroup hostility and project aggression onto external enemies.

The third operates under a *pairing assumption:* a focal couple in the group symbolizes the group's hope that the couple will reproduce itself and thereby preserve the group's threatened identity.

group, blanket See *group, structured.*

group, closed A therapy group to which no new patients are added in the course of treatment or after treatment has proceeded for a time. See *group, open.*

group, continuous Same as *open group.*

group feeling Same as *instinct, herd.*

group marriage See *marriage, group.*

group, open A therapy group to which new patients are added at any time during the course of treatment. Sometimes this is referred to as a *continuous group.*

group, structured A term introduced by S.R. Slavson to emphasize the fact that the selection and combining of patients is essential for group psychotherapy, though some group psychotherapists pay little or no attention to it. Since in group psychotherapy the group is an important factor and the major therapeutic agency, it must be planned in such a way that, according to Slavson, the patients, individually and as a group, would have a therapeutic effect upon every other constituent member. He has described some of the criteria for selection and grouping in his *Analytic Group Psychotherapy* (1950). This term is opposed to *blanket group*, in which no criteria for grouping are employed.

group tension, common In psychoanalytically oriented treatment of a group, the predisposition at any point of individual members to participate in a certain group theme. The theme may be a dominant *required relationship*, a defense against *avoided relationship*, which, because of his phantasies, the subject fears will be another disastrous or *calamitous relationship*. Common group tension, Ezriel's term, is approximately equivalent to the *dominant group mentality* of Bion. (Ezriel, H. *Journal of Mental Science 96*, 1950)

group, transitional A therapy group devised for children (in latency period and puberty) who do not require intensive group psychotherapy but are unable to participate with confidence in ordinary social clubs. A form of "protective groups" has been developed for these young patients. (Slavson, *IGT*)

group work, social A kind of guided group experience in which individuals are helped to meet their needs and develop their interests along socially acceptable lines, with the assistance of a group leader. (Coyle, G.L. in *Social Work Year Book 1939*, ed. R.H. Kurtz)

groups, divorce See *divorce therapy.*

Grübelsucht (grü'bel-sookt) Brooding over trifles; seen most commonly in obsessive-compulsive psychoneurosis and in depressive psychoses.

Gruhle, Hans W. (groo'le) (1880–1958) German psychiatrist and psychologist; phenomenology (especially schizophrenia and delusions) and social psychiatry.

grumbling mania See *mania, grumbling.*

Grundsymptoma Basic or fundamental symptoms. Bleuler used this term to refer to the primary or fundamental symptoms of *schizophrenia* (q.v.)

GSR Galvanic skin response. See *reflex, psychogalvanic.*

guidance A form of supportive psychotherapy in which the patient is counseled and instructed in ways to set and achieve specific goals and in ways to recognize and avoid areas of conflict and anxiety-provoking situations. Educational guidance refers particularly to helping the patient find the school or courses best suited to him on the basis of his intelligence, aptitudes, preferences, and available opportunities. Vocational guidance refers particularly to helping the patient find a job that is realistically suited to his capacities.

Guidance is a relatively superficial type of psychotherapy and makes little attempt to deal with the unconscious motivants of behavior. It is based upon an authoritarian relationship in which the patient often overvalues the therapist and in which he must suppress any doubts or hostility against the therapist.

guidance, child See *child guidance.*

guided affective imagery (GAI) A waking dream technique in psychotherapy, used particularly in brief therapy and group therapy. See *phantasy, forced.*

Guillain-Barré syndrome (gē-yaN′ bàr-rā′) (Georges Guillain, French neurologist, 1876–1961, and Jean Alexander Barré, French neurologist, b. 1880) Acute infective polyneuritis; acute toxic polyneuritis; rheumatic polyneuritis; polyradiculoneuritis. An acute, diffuse disease of the nervous system, probably due to a virus, consisting of chromatolysis of the anterior horn cells and the posterior roots and of myelin degeneration of the peripheral nerves. Most cases occur in males between the ages of 20 and 50 years. Initial symptoms are headache, vomiting, fever, and pain in the back and legs. These are followed by sudden paralysis of the limbs, in all segments, and of the facial muscles. The paralysis is flaccid in type and the deep reflexes are lost. There is pain, numbness, and tingling in the limbs. Cerebrospinal fluid protein is markedly elevated, but there are few or no cells. In sporadic cases the prognosis is good, but in some epidemics the mortality (usually from respiratory paralysis) is high. No specific treatment is known.

guilt, guilt feelings Realization that one has done wrong by violating some ethical, moral, or religious principle. Associated with such realization typically are lowered self-esteem and a feeling that one should expiate or make retribution for the wrong that has been done. See *proof, forensic; shame.*

As used in psychoanalytic writings, the term usually refers to neurotic, unreasonable, or pathologic guilt feelings that do not appear to be justified by the reasons adduced for the guilt. Such guilt is indicative of a conflict between the ego and the *superego* (q.v.); the latter acts as an internal authority that stands between ego and id, compelling the person on his own to renounce certain pleasures, and imposing punishment (loss of self-esteem, guilt feelings, etc.) for violations of its orders. Often, of course, the superego's prohibitions are directed against impulses (and especially hostile and destructive ones) of which the subject is not consciously aware; but because the unconscious impulses have incurred the superego's wrath, the end result is guilt. It is because the reasons for the guilt feelings are unconscious that the incorrect term "unconscious" feelings of guilt has come into being; Freud suggested that the phrase "unconscious need for punishment" would be a more correct substitute.

Guilt feelings are thus seen to be topically defined anxiety, the anxiety of ego toward superego. What is feared by the ego is that something terrible will happen within the personality (food, affection, love, and/or narcissistic supplies will be cut off) and that there will be a loss of certain pleasurable feelings, such as of well-being and security. In its most severe form, the loss of self-esteem characteristic of guilt feelings becomes a feeling of complete annihilation, such as is seen in depression.

In Adlerian psychodynamics, guilt feelings are the demonstration of good intentions that one does not have (or at least that one is unable to effect or exercise). They occur when past transgressions are blamed for a present unwillingness to behave as one feels he should.

Erikson describes *initiative vs. guilt* as one of the eight stages of man. See *ontogeny, psychic.*

Guislain, Joseph (gē-lâN´) (1797–1860) Belgian physician; introduced work therapy in his institution for the mentally ill in Ghent.

gull wing pattern An MMPI profile said to be characteristic of pseudoneurotic schizophrenia.

gumma, intracranial A rare form of cerebral syphilis. The predominating pathological process is the gumma or syphiloma. This is an irregular or round granulomatous nodular growth, varying in size from that of a pinhead to a walnut; it is generally multiple. Occasionally when single and of large size, it may produce symptoms of intracranial pressure with or without focal signs. The mental symptoms include the acute organic type of reaction, and consist of delirium, with a memory defect for recent events, and emotional lability. When there is evidence of increased intracranial pressure, a dull, stuporous state is common, with a loss of sphincter control. The blood and spinal fluid findings may be similar to those observed in cerebral syphilis, and response to antisyphilic treatment is fairly successful. See *syphilis, cerebral.*

Gunn's synkinetic syndrome See *synkinesia.*

Gunther-Waldenstrom syndrome *Porphyria, acute intermittent* (q.v.).

gustatism See *sensation, secondary.*

Guthrie test See *phenylketonuria.*

gymnophobia Fear of a naked body.

gynander, gynandromorph (ji-nan´dēr, drō-morf) An individual of a bisexual species, exhibiting a "sexual mosaic" of male and female characters as a result of the development of both types of sex tissue in the same organism.

Most specimens are *lateral* or *bilateral* gynandromorphs, male on one side of the midline of the body, and female on the other, with a sharp demarcation between the two kinds of tissue. In some instances, the distribution is in a ratio of about 1:3, or the head may be female and the rest of the body male.

It is assumed that on the male side there appear the sex-linked characters received from either the mother or the father; while the characters of the female parts show the presence in these parts of both the maternal and paternal X chromosomes, as though one of the X chromosomes had been eliminated from the male parts, leaving them XO, while the female parts are XX. "Such a gynander appears to have begun development as an XX female and at some early cell division to have lost one of the X chromosomes from part of the tissues." (Sinnott, E.W., & Dunn, L.D. *Principles of Genetics,* 1939)

gynecomania Morbid desire for women; *satyriasis* (q.v.).

gynephobia Fear of women.

gyno- (jinō´-, jīnō-) Combining form meaning woman, female, from Gr. *gyne.*

gynomonoecism (jin-ō-mō-nē´siz'm) A genetic female's capacity for developing spermatozoa in the ovary, at certain times. See *hermaphroditism.*

gynophobia Morbid fear of women.

gyrectomy One of the several surgical operations on the brain performed as a therapeutic measure in certain cases of mental illness. In the gyrectomy procedure bilateral symmetrical removals of frontal cortex are carried out along fissure lines in order to leave the normally functioning gyri. For a more detailed discussion of psychosurgical operations see *topectomy.*

gyrus, angular The posterior portion of the lower parietal region; the left angular gyrus is associated with speech function.

gyrus cinguli *Cingulate gyrus* (q.v.).

gyrus, postcentral See *lobe, parietal.*

gyrus, precentral See *lobe, frontal.*

H

h In Rorschach scoring, human response, a measure of the subject's interest in the psychology of other people.

habeas corpus (L. "you must have the body") In forensic psychiatry, a writ or order for a person being held in a hospital or other institution to appear before the court, so that a determination of the appropriateness or necessity for the confinement can be made.

habenular ganglion See *epithalamus*.

habilitation Producing or improving fitness through training, applied particularly to congenital disorders and disorders of early infancy.

habit, accident See *proneness, accident*.

habit, act See *act-habit*.

habit, complaint Kanner's term for hypochondriasis in children. At various times and in connection with a variety of situations children are known to complain of various aches and pains that clearly are emotionally rather than physically caused. For example, one child may complain of severe headache the morning of a day on which a severe test is to be given at school; another may complain of stomachache when some particularly disliked kind of food is served, but these are *isolated*, not habitual, complaints.

The complaint habit refers to a *habitual* way of reacting by means of complaints of bmdily disorder, according to definite patterns. In some instances the pattern has been set by the child himself, out of certain material from his own experience. If a real stomachache or a real cough has kept the child from school, which he happens to dislike, and has brought all sorts of kindly attentions, comforts, and privileges not ordinarily forthcoming, it may be found thereafter that a great desire for all this as

a relief from some stress or other will be heralded by a stomachache or cough which, though felt and complained about, is *not* real. More often the pattern is suggested to the child by observation of his environment. If he notices that mother or father seems always to be relieved of this or that chore by reason of the complaint of headache or backache, the child, too, will be found feeling and complaining of headache or backache when the performance of some hated task is expected. (*Child Psychiatry*, 1948)

habit deterioration See *deterioration, habit*.

habit disorder Also stereotypy/habit disorder; repetitive, nonfunctional behavior (such as hand waving, body rocking, head banging, nail biting, picking at face) that is injurious to the child or interferes markedly with normal activities. See *behavior disorders*.

habit formation See *training, habit*.

habit-forming As a description of a drug, incidence of psychologic craving or dependency in its users. The likelihood of psychologic craving is generally independent of proneness to physiologic craving, or *addiction* (q.v.).

habit, hysterical Kretschmer distinguishes two kinds of hysteria, *reflex hysteria* and *hysterical habit*. The latter is a hysterical reaction that begins as a conscious, voluntary process and gradually becomes automatic by repetition. See *hysteria, reflex*.

habit-residual, hysterical Kretschmer's expression for a reflex hysteria that continues because of the patient's lack of desire to get well. It is distinguished from simple reflex hysteria in that the latter usually occurs upon occasions when there is something to be gained by the reaction.

habit-training See *training, habit*.

habituation The process of becoming accustomed to or familiar with an object, situation, etc.; in neurophysiology, a decrement in response magnitude resulting from repetitive stimulation. Habituation in this sense is *tolerance* (q.v.). It is characteristic of many drugs and is a significant factor in substance abuse, since increasing dosage of the substance is required in order to obtain the same effect(s) produced by the initial dosage. See *addiction*.

habitus In general medicine, constitutional disposition or tendency to some specific disease, in the sense of the *habitus phthisicus* and *habitus apoplecticus* as described by Hippocrates.

Later extended also to the type of physique associated with such tendencies by different typological schools of constitutional medicine and to the general characteristic appearance of the human body.

habitus apoplecticus (L. "apoplectic constitution") A thick-set, rounded physique, corresponding to Kretschmer's *pyknic type* and its equivalent in other systems.

habitus, asthenic See *type, asthenic*.

habitus phthisicus (L. "consumptive constitution") Hippocrates's term for the tendency of certain persons to *pulmonary tuberculosis*. He ascribed a slender, flat-chested physique to such persons, and the term is used in a derived sense to indicate the type of physique corresponding approximately to Kretschmer's *asthenic type* and its equivalents in other systems.

habitus, ptotic (tō′tik) In constitutional medicine, a special body type described by Stiller as associated with the constitutional anomaly *enteroptosis*—a sagging or a dropped condition of the intestines.

According to Pende, enteroptosis exerts secondary effects on the digestive functions and also—through lack of diaphragmatic support—on the respiratory and circulatory systems and on the configuration of the thorax, thus contributing to the production of the "general *dolichomorphic-asthenic* constitution." (*Constitutional Inadequacies*, 1928)

habromania *Obs.* General term for morbid gaiety.

HACS Hyperactive child syndrome. See *impulse disorder, hyperkinetic*.

hadephobia Fear of hell.

Haeckel's biogenetic law (Ernst Heinrich Haeckel, German naturalist, 1834–1919) According to this formula, "The child is on a lower developmental level of mankind than the adult." In the child all the criminal drives of humanity are latent. In other words, the child is "universally criminal." Following Haeckel's conception, Stekel asserts that "phrases about purity and innocence in the child are empty." Compulsive acts are protective measures against the evil of one's self. A neurosis arises when the instinctual criminal drives are too powerfully developed. (*CD*) See *law, biogenetic mental; perverse, polymorphous*.

haem(at)o- See *hem(at)o-*.

hair pulling *Trichotillomania;* the hair is usually pulled from the head, less often from the pubic area, in an almost compulsive fashion. Hair pulling may be a masturbatory substitute, and/or it may be an expression of aggressive and exhibitionistic impulses, and a denial of castration.

half-life $T_{1/2}$; the time necessary for the concentration of a drug in the blood to decrease by half after absorption and distribution are complete. A drug's half-life is a function of drug binding to tissue other than plasma or blood constituents and the clearance of the free or unbound drug.

"half-show" A modification of the puppet show technique in psychotherapy of children in which the patient sees only that part of the puppet show that presents or states a problem in dramatic fashion. When the conflict is at its height, the show is stopped with the promise that it will be continued later. Then the subject or group is asked what should happen. The solutions suggested, of course, are colored by the child's own problems, and the child will try to unravel the conflict in terms of his own constitution, background, emotional involvement, and general level of maturity.

halfway children R. Geist's term for chronically ill children and adolescents who are neither well nor so sick as to require continuous, intensive inpatient care. Instead, their course is characterized by repeated in-and-out hospital stays and dependence on a complex system of hospital care, pharmacologic treatments, surgical procedures, and artificial devices. (*American Journal of Orthopsychiatry 49,* 1979)

halfway house A specialized residence for mental patients who are not sick enough to require full hospitalization, but not well enough to function completely within the community without some degree of professional supervision, protection, and support. See *domicile; family care.*

Hall, G(ranville) Stanley (1844–1924) American psychologist and sexologist.

Halloween effect Hyperactivity and other behavioral and cognitive dysfunctions in response to ingestion of sugar, such as the candy given to children in the "trick-or-treat" ritual of Halloween. Although many claims of such reactions have been made, all attempts to replicate them have failed. What few changes in activity have been found in response to sucrose and fructose challenges have, in fact, tended to be in the direction of decreased, rather than increased, activity. See *attention deficit disorder.*

hallucinate To have a sense perception for which there is no external reality (i.e. sensory stimulus). See *hallucination.*

hallucinatio hypochondriasis *Obs. Hypochondriasis* (q.v.).

hallucination An apparent perception of an external object when no such object is present. A paranoid patient, sitting alone in a quiet room, complains that his persecutors, who are miles away, speak directly to him in derogatory terms; moreover, he believes implicitly that he feels electrical stimuli over the entire body, the stimuli coming, he alleges, from a machine operated by his persecutors. The auditory and tactile stimuli have no source in the environment; rather they are sensations arising within the patient himself. A hallucination is a *sense perception* to which there is no external stimulus. The *false beliefs* regarding persecutors are *delusions;* a delusion is a *belief* that is obviously contrary to demonstrable fact.

When the same paranoid patient, sitting alone in an otherwise quiet room, upon hearing the crackling of the floorboards, is firmly convinced that the crackling sounds like those of a telegraph ticker are messages from the persecutors to him (the patient), he misinterprets actual stimuli from the environment. An *illusion* is a false impression from a real stimulus. But the text he thereupon reads into these messages is a *delusion.* See *illusion; delusion. Obs.* Fallacia.

hallucination, auditory See *hallucination, haptic.*

hallucination, auditory peripheric An auditory illusion (mainly of voices) experienced as a result of auditory sensory stimulation, as the pouring of water, rumpling of paper, or a person's walking.

hallucination, autoscopic The experience of seeing one's body appear for a moment or two, usually in front of the subject.

hallucination, blank A general term that includes the *Isakower phenomenon,* the *dream screen* of Lewin, and the *abstract perceptions* of Deutsch and Murphy; it refers to certain uncanny experiences of sensations of equilibrium and space, such as unclear rotating objects, rhythmically approaching and receding objects, sensations of crescendo and decrescendo, typically localized in the mouth, skin, and hands and at the same time in the space immediately surrounding the body. Most often such feelings occur in stress situations, when falling asleep, and in dreams. They are believed to be defensive repetitions of responses to early oral deprivation and to reflect the infant's subjective experience of being overwhelmed by excitation in the early traumatic situation. Their appearance in an analytic session suggests that primal scene material is approaching.

hallucination, diminutive visual *Hallucination, Lilliputian* (q.v.).

hallucination, elementary "As *elementary hallucinations* in the optic field we designate such unformed visions as lighting, sparks, and cloudlike partial darkening of the visual field, and in the acoustic field, the simple noises such as murmurs, knocks, and shooting." (Bleuler, *TP*)

hallucination, extracampine "Hallucinations which are localized outside of the sensory field in question. In the nature of the thing one deals mostly with visions, the patient sees with perfect sensory distinctness the devil behind his head, but it may also concern the sense of touch; thus the patient feels how streams of water come out from a definite point of his hand." (Bleuler, *TP*)

hallucination, gustatory See *hallucination, haptic.*

hallucination, haptic Hallucination associated with the sensation of touch. A paranoid patient complained that his persecutors, operating an electrical apparatus hidden in the walls of the building, induced very disagreeable sensations over his body through the machine.

Alleged persecutors reach the patient's body through many avenues, among which are the sensory zones. In clear-cut cases of schizophrenia the persecutors aspire to tempt the patient to engage in homosexual practices. Indeed, they constantly stimulate him sexually through the several sense areas. "He operates a machine that masturbates me" is a common expression among paranoid schizophrenic patients. The persecutors are said also to surround the patient with "bad sexual odors" (*olfactory hallucination*); they put "scum" (seminal fluid) in his food (*gustatory* or *taste hallucination*); they call him a sexual pervert with men (*auditory hallucination*); they grimace at him, meaning he is homosexual (*visual hallucination*).

hallucination, hypnagogic Hypnagogic imagery. See *imagery, hypnagogic.*

hallucination, induced A hallucination aroused in one person by another, such as may occur during hypnosis. See *association, psychosis of.*

hallucination, Lilliputian (From the six-inch-tall inhabitants of the island of Lilliput, in Swift's *Gulliver's Travels*) When hallucinated objects, generally persons, appear greatly reduced in size, it is said that the patient has Lilliputian or microptic hallucinations. The term should be used only when true hallucination is present, that is, when there is no object in the environment that stimulates the perception. When a real object is misinterpreted by a patient, the condition is called an illusion. Certain patients, notably those with idiopathic epilepsy, while actually looking at objects, may believe them to be extremely diminutive; this constitutes an illusion. See *Lilliputian; micropsia.*

As a rule Lilliputian hallucinations occur in psychiatric states associated with febrile or intoxicating conditions. They may be observed in the absence of recognizable organic disorders.

hallucination, macroptic See *macropsia.*

hallucination, memory Freud's term for the return of unconscious, repressed material as a visual image.

hallucination, microptic See *hallucination, Lilliputian.*

hallucination, motor *Obs.* Hallucination, psychomotor (q.v.).

hallucination, negative Not a hallucination at all, but refers to the condition in which the subject fails to see an object while apparently looking at it. It is a phenomenon that can be induced through hypnosis.

hallucination of conception See *hallucination of perception.*

hallucination of perception An auditory hallucination in which the patient hears the sound or noise as coming from outside himself, in contrast to *hallucination of conception* (or, in Baillarger's terminology, *psychic hallucination*), in which inner voices are heard.

hallucination, olfactory See *hallucination, haptic.*

hallucination, psychic See *hallucination of perception.*

hallucination, psychomotor A patient's sensation that certain parts of his body are being transferred to body regions distant from their natural location.

hallucination, psychosensorial Baillarger distinguished two kinds of hallucinations—psychosensorial and psychic. He said that the first are the result of the combined action of the imagination and of the organs of sense, while the second are the result of the imagination without the interposition of a sensory stimulus.

hallucination, reflex *Obs.* A sensory impression induced through stimulation of a distant and different sensory area. "An auditory sensation may in this way arise from irritation in the region of the inferior alveolar nerve (carious tooth)." (Henderson, D.K., & Gillespie, R.D. *A Text-Book of Psychiatry,* 1936)

hallucination, retroactive Hallucination, memory (q.v.).

hallucination, teleologic A hallucination advising a patient about what course he should take.

hallucination, vestibular (L. *vestibulum,* "forecourt"; in *Anat.* the approach to the cochlea of the internal ear) False sensory perceptions that come from irritation of the vestibular apparatus. This form of hallucination is referred mainly to visual and tactile organs. Visual images (real or imaginary) are affected by vestibular function. Under vestibular irritation these images show changes such as occur when the subject is submitted to passive rotating movement. In such experimental circumstances, there are certain typical movements, or deviations of the optic image. In one experiment, related by Bibring-Lehner, the subject, while turning, imagines a child; this image seems to turn in the same direction as the subject under experiment. Sometimes half of the image disappears and often the colors become gray during the turning, but the most remarkable features are the multiplication of the image and its reduction in size. According to P. Schilder, this is very important, "because it shows that turning induces the same changes in optic images as in optic vision." In alcoholic hallucinations one may also observe vestibular phenomena. Indeed, Schilder describes the case of a patient who said: "Sometimes I saw three or four people on the street instead of one. I saw three faces in glaring white; faces of Negroes and whites. They moved forwards and backwards and when I saw them they started to chase me. I felt them behind me." In psychosis the vestibular influences are not related exclusively to the visual sphere, but one also encounters marked changes in the feelings that the patient has about his own body, particularly sensations of the body's lightness or heaviness. (*Mind Perception and Thought,* 1942)

hallucination, visual See *hallucination, haptic.*

hallucinogen Any substance capable of producing hallucinations in an experimental subject. See *psychotomimetic; psychotropics.*

Hallucinogen abuse is characterized by continuous or episodic use for one month or more; impaired social, occupational, or academic functioning; and psychological dependence or a pathologic pattern of use. Because no withdrawal syndrome has been demonstrated, no category of hallucinogen dependence or hallucinogen addiction is recognized. Hallucinogen abuse is, however, associated with several organic mental disorders: hallucinosis, delusional

syndrome (persisting more than 24 hours after cessation of hallucinogen use), and organic affective syndrome (with depression, anxiety, and preoccupation with tormenting thoughts that the abuser has destroyed his brain and can never regain his sanity).

hallucinosis Persistent or recurrent appearance of hallucinations, usually in a clear intellectual field, without confusion or intellectual impairment; most commonly due to intoxication with alcohol or drugs, or following traumata such as surgical procedures and childbirth. Usually there is a slow return to normal within a period of weeks; if symptoms persist, the condition is generally considered to be a schizophrenic reaction. The most common form of acute hallucinosis is alcoholic hallucinosis. See *hallucinosis, alcoholic; organic mental disorders.*

hallucinosis, alcoholic *Alcoholic withdrawal hallucinosis;* a form of acute hallucinosis seen in alcoholics following an unusual excess of alcohol intake. The condition is relatively rare in the female. It consists of auditory hallucinations, and sometimes also paranoid delusions, usually of a derogatory or persecutory nature, that appear in a clear intellectual field without confusion or intellectual impairment. The hallucinations persist even when all other symptoms of withdrawal have disappeared. During the period of acute hallucinosis the patient may commit crimes of violence in response to the delusions. There is a slow return to normal within a period of weeks; recurrence is frequent, however. If the condition becomes chronic, it is considered to be a schizophrenic disorder.

halo, semantic See *dissociation, semantic.*

hamartophobia Fear of error or sin. Commonly misspelled harmatophobia.

Hand-Christian-Schüller's syndrome *Xanthomatosis* (q.v.).

hand-to-mouth reaction See *reaction, hand-to-mouth.*

handedness *Laterality* (q.v.). See *dominance, cerebral.*

handicap See *disability.*

handicap, collective life *Obs.* In social work, "Any disability (physical, mental, or emotional) which limits or threatens the patient's normal range of social intercourse, association, and enjoyment of fellowship."

(Hamilton, G. *A Medical Social Terminology,* 1930)

handicap, emotional In educational psychology, a learning disability or behavioral disturbance of enough severity to render the affected child unable to function in the regular classroom. The emotionally handicapped child is of average or superior intellect, demonstrates no gross neurological disorder, but nonetheless is unable to learn and/or to maintain satisfactory interpersonal relationships with peers and teachers. In addition, the child may overreact to what appears to the observer to be minimal stress, or he may develop any number of somatic or psychic symptoms in relation to ordinary school pressures, or he may show generalized unhappiness and disenchantment with living. See *impulse disorder, hyperkinetic.*

handicap, family life *Obs.* In social work, "Any disability (physical, mental, or emotional) which definitely interferes with or limits either one's capacities for home making or for marriage." (Hamilton, G. *A Medical Social Terminology,* 1930)

handicap, mental Mental retardation; see *retardation, mental.*

hangings, erotized repetitive Accidental death by hanging, which is initiated in order to produce neck constriction and cerebral hypoxia as a way of heightening sexual excitation. H. Resnik (*American Journal of Psychotherapy 26,* 1972) presents evidence of at least 50 such deaths each year in the United States. The subjects, usually teenagers or young adults, are nude or partially clothed; nearby sexually exciting materials or literature suggests that the hanging has been part of a masturbatory act.

hangover The aftereffect ("morning after") syndrome following ingestion of alcohol or other sedatives, such as barbiturates. Symptoms include a bad taste, nausea, vomiting, polypnoea, pallor, irritability, sweating, conjunctival injection. The syndrome may be a direct result of ethanol intoxication or due to effects of acetaldehyde, an intermediate metabolite that develops in the course of alcohol oxidation, and/or a result of toxic congeners contained in most forms of commercially available alcohol that extend and amplify the effects of alcohol itself.

Hans The patient on whom Freud reported in a 1909 paper, "Analysis of a Phobia in a Five-Year-Old Boy." The initial phobia of little Hans was directed to horses, and analysis revealed that the phobia represented the father, against whom Hans nourished jealous and hostile wishes because of rivalry for the mother. One interesting feature of this case is that the analytic treatment was carried out by the father, who corresponded with Freud and received the latter's suggestions about interpretation and technique by mail.

haphalgesia See *aphalgesia.*

haphephobia See *haptephobia.*

haploidy The genetic process of reduction by division of reproductive cells results in haploidy as the stage of meiosis at which the number of chromosomes per cell is reduced to half. Consequently, the haploid number of chromosomes in all daughter cells is just half as large as their original or *diploid* number in the cells from which they are derived. See *diploidy.*

haplology Omission of syllables in words because of speed in speech; seen often in mania and in schizophrenic syndromes in which there is pressure on speech.

haptephobia Fear of being touched.

haptophonia The hearing of noises or voices in response to tactile or haptic stimulation. One patient, for example, complained of hearing voices coming from his forearm, where there was the scar of an old injury.

hardiness See *existentialism.*

harm, weighted See *principle, weighted harm.*

harmine (har′mēn) See *psychotomimetic.*

harpaxophobia Fear of robbers.

Harris's syndrome Hypoglycemic syndrome. See *hypoglycemia.*

Hartmann, Heinz (1894–1970) Viennese-born U.S. psychoanalyst; *Ego Psychology and the Problem of Adaptation* (1939).

Hartnup disease A pellagralike disorder caused by a genetic abnormality of tryptophan metabolism: instead of conversion into nicotinamid, tryptophan is converted into indican. A variety of mental symptoms may result, including anxiety, feelings of depersonalization, depression, delusions, hallucinations, delirium, confusion, irritability, apathy, emotional lability, and in many cases mental retardation. See *nicotinic acid deficiency.*

hashish (Arabic, "grass") See *marihuana*.

hate See *aggression*.

hate, fetish *Antifetishism* (q.v.).

haut mal (ō mȧl′) Major epileptic attack; grand mal.

hazard, moral In insurance terminology, a demand for services that is created by their being offered in the first place or determined to a significant degree by the relatively low cost of the insurance premium as compared with the cost to the beneficiary of the service provided by the policy. The term moral is applied because, at least to some degree, the benefit is used even though the service is not essential or would not have been sought had not the policy provided it as a benefit.

hazardous treatment See *forced treatment*.

HCA Heterocyclic antidepressant drug.

HD Huntington's disease. See *chorea, Huntington's*.

Hd Rorschach scoring symbol for a response of parts of the human figure.

headache, cluster Migrainous neuralgia; a syndrome characterized by paroxysms of severe pain, usually located in the fronto-temporal region and eye, lasting for as long as 2 hours and occurring several times during a 24-hour period. Each bout of headaches tends to last a few weeks and then recur after a free interval of several months or even a year. Etiology is unknown; treatment is symptomatic, with oral ergotamine. Some writers use the term to refer to any atypical facial neuralgia that is not *migraine* (q.v.), including histamine cephalalgia, ciliary neuralgia, and sphenopalatine neuralgia (vidian neuralgia, Sluder's syndrome).

headache, histamine See *histamine*.

headache, lead-cap Neurasthenic symptom; a sensation as if the head were splitting or the skull lifting; a terrible weight or a severe constriction about the head.

head-banging One of the many typical physical exertions commonly observed during a temper tantrum in small children. The child works up to a pitch of excitement and by almost every conceivable physical or muscular movement literally throws himself or herself all over the place. See *stereotyped movement disorders*.

head-knocking A habit developed by some infants that consists of bumping the head against the crib sides or other objects.

head-rolling Rhythmical, semicircular movements of the head exhibited by some children before going to sleep. When sufficiently constant, this movement may be considered similar to tics in its nature. In some instances, the rolling of the head may be attributed to restraint of movement in the crib and, in other instances, to absence of play material (monotony). It seems that in other cases it may have as its origin the passivity of the fetus during intrauterine life. In these cases the rolling of the head will represent a hyperactive function which serves as a balance for the intrauterine inactivity.

Head Start See *education, compensatory*.

head trauma See *compression, cerebral; concussion; contusion, brain; neurosis, traumatic*.

health, flight into See *flight into health*.

health law The body of rules governing the provision of medical care, including not only the legislation formally enacted but also the regulations that have been devised to implement what is perceived as the intent of the legislation. Health law includes *forensic medicine* and *medical jurisprudence*, which refer to a relatively limited area involving proof of such facts as paternity, competence, insanity, guilt, and responsibility. Health law extends into a broad area and includes as well all laws governing the relationships among health professionals, other health care providers, third-party payers, and patients.

health maintenance organization *HMO* (q.v.).

health, mental 1. Mental hygiene, in which sense mental health is a field based on the *behavioral sciences* (q.v.) and amplified with scientific, professional, and social applications. See *hygiene, mental*. 2. Psychologic well-being or adequate adjustment, particularly as such adjustment conforms to the community-accepted standards of human relations. Some characteristics of mental health are reasonable independence; self-reliance; self-direction; ability to do a job; ability to take responsibility and make needed efforts; reliability; persistence; ability to get along with others and work with others; cooperation; ability to work under authority, rules, and difficulties; ability to show friendliness and love; ability to give and take; tolerance of others and of frustrations; ability to contribute; a sense of humor; a devotion beyond oneself; ability to find recreation, as in hobbies. (Appel, K.E. *Journal of the American Medical Association 172*, 1960) See *norm, psychic.*

health policy The many roles of governmental and nongovernmental organizations in the prevention and treatment of illness, including planning for the directions that will be taken in promoting health and eliminating disease. See *policy, public.*

health-related facilities See *domicile.*

hearing, color Usually believed to be a hallucinatory disturbance, characterized by a sensation of color when sounds are heard. A schizophrenic patient said that people talked to him in colors, meaning that colors occurred to him when he heard voices.

heart, soldier's See *neurasthenia, war.*

hebephrenia A symptom complex now considered a chronic form of schizophrenia. In 1871 Hecker described hebephrenia and the heboid, and in 1896 Kraepelin included hebephrenia in the group dementia praecox. See *schizophrenia.*

hebephrenia, depressive Some patients with the hebephrenic form of schizophrenia run, for some time, a course that resembles the periodic changes observed in manic-depressive psychosis. When the constituents of a depression appear in hebephrenia, the state is known as *depressive hebephrenia.* When there is similarity to a manic phase, it is known as *manic hebephrenia.*

hebephrenia, insurance Maier's term for schizophrenia manifested initially as a compensation neurosis; in time, the patient's claims become increasingly absurd, illogical, and bizarre.

hebephrenia, manic See *hebephrenia, depressive.*

hebephrenic schizophrenia See *schizophrenia, hebephrenic.*

hebetude Emotional dullness or lack of interest. It is most characteristically expressed in schizophrenia in which the pronounced withdrawal of interest from the environment and apparently, in late cases, from the patient himself causes the patient to appear thoroughly listless, unemotional, uninterested, and apathetic. See *affectivity, disturbances of.*

"In the severer forms of schizophrenia the '*affective dementia*' is the most striking

symptom. In the sanatoria there are patients sitting around who for decades show no affect no matter what happens to them or to those about them. They are indifferent to maltreatment; left to themselves they lie in wet and frozen beds, do not bother about hunger and thirst. They have to be taken care of in all respects. Toward their own delusions they are often strikingly indifferent." (Bleuler, *TP*)

An older meaning of hebetude included listlessness or apathy from any cause, physical or mental. It is still sometimes used in this sense.

hebetudo animi (L. "dullness of spirit") *Obs.* Imbecility.

heboidophrenia *Rare.* Kahlbaum's term for the simple form of schizophrenia.

Hecker, Ewald (1843–1909) German psychiatrist; known from his studies in hebephrenia (a term he coined.)

hedoni- Combining form meaning, delight, enjoyment, pleasure, from Gr. *hēdonē.*

hedonic level See *psychodynamics, adaptational.*

hedonism 1. A philosophic doctrine in which pleasure or happiness is presented as the supreme good. In psychiatry, it refers to the seeking of certain goals because they afford some type of gratification. Hedonism, then, is in opposition to the doctrine that goals may be sought as ends in themselves, irrespective of the pleasure or gratification they give the individual. See *hormism.* 2. A form of social cohesion that is based on reward, in contrast to *agonic social cohesion,* which is based on avoidance of punishment.

hedonistic utilitarianism See *utilitarianism, hedonistic.*

hedonophobia Fear of pleasure.

heel-to-knee test See *test, heel-to-knee.*

Heidenheim's disease *Jakob-Creutzfeldt's disease* (q.v.).

Heine-Medin disease (Jacob Heine, German physician, 1800–79, and Karl Oskar Medin, Swedish physician, 1847–1928) *Poliomyelitis* (q.v.).

Heinroth, Johann Christian (1773–1843) Leipzig physician who was the first to propose that psychiatry be acknowledged as a discrete medical discipline; beginning in 1811 he occupied the first chair in psychiatry at Leipzig.

heir of the Oedipus complex See *superego.*

heliophobia Fear of sunlight.

hellenomania Impulse or tendency to use complicated, cumbersome terms, frequently Greek or Latin, instead of readily understandable English words. The impulse is rampant in the field of psychiatric writing, as witness the list of (generally undesirable) terms under *fear of.*

Interestingly enough, hellenomania is itself a pseudoerudite misnomer since literally it means a pathologic love of Greeks or their country. The correct term for what is defined above is *hellenologomania.* In like fashion, *hellenophobia* is a fear of Greeks (a subtype of xenophobia), while *hellenologophobia* would denote a fear or avoidance of Greek terms.

Heller's disease (Theodore Heller, German neuropsychiatrist, early 20th century) See *dementia infantilis.*

helmet, neurasthenic A feeling of pressure over the entire cranium in certain cases of neurasthenia, as if from a tight-pressing helmet. See *headache, lead-cap.*

Helmholtz See *accommodation.*

helper, magic Fromm's term describing a particular form of interpersonal relationship. Man has today become aware of himself as a separate entity. The growing realization of his separateness gives him a sense of isolation and a longing to return to the earlier feeling of solidarity with others. So he uses certain irrational methods of relating back to the group, and these are termed mechanisms of escape. One method is to seek to lean on another for support. The other person represents a power or authority who can be used for that purpose. Sometimes the individual expects the other person to solve all his problems for him and endows the person with almost magical omnipotence. This other person is then termed the magic helper. It is obvious that the person so endowed with magical power must himself be affected by it and to a degree be dependent on it. The power he has illustrates a form of *irrational authority,* which is based not on competence but on a neurotic need for power. See *authority, irrational.*

helping relationship A type of relationship, as defined by Carl Rogers, in which one of the participants intends that there should come about, in one or both parties, more appreciation, expression, or functional use of latent inner responses. Examples include mother and child, and teacher and student, as well as therapist and patient.

helplessness, learned A state of apathy that occurs as a type of experimental neurosis in animals who cannot escape an aversive stimulus. It has been suggested that depression in the human may be similar and based on repeated experiences of being unable either to achieve a desired outcome or to avoid physical or emotional pain.

helplessness, psychic The state that occasions the first expression of anxiety in early infancy. Freud describes anxiety as a state of unpleasure in which there is an increase of excitation relieved through physiologic discharge phenomena such as an increase in the respiratory and pulse rates or rise in blood pressure. The prototype of this experience of anxiety is seen as the experience of birth, in which the above-described sensations and responses first occur. All later anxiety states are reproductions of this earliest experience. Anxiety as experienced in later life, however, is clearly a response to a danger situation. Thus some type of danger is understood to be associated with the production of anxiety from the time of its earliest appearance.

hematidrosis Bloody perspiration.

hem(at)o- Combining form meaning blood, from Gr. *haîma, -atos.*

hematoencephalic barrier See *barrier, blood-brain.*

hematophobia See *hemophobia.*

hemeralopia Day-blindness; vision is poor by day, in bright light, and good in dim light; the opposite of *nyctalopia.*

hemeraphonia Voicelessness during daytime, usually a symptom of hysteria.

hemi- Combining form meaning half, from Gr. *hemi-.*

hemiakinesia See *neglect, sensory.*

hemianopic, hemianopsia See *field defect.*

hemianopsia, heteronymous Bitemporal or binasal loss of vision.

hemianopsia, homonymous Loss of vision in the similarly situated (both right or both left) halves of one's eyes, i.e. in the nasal half of one eye and in the temporal half of the other. See *field defect.*

hemianthropia *Obs.* Insanity.

hemiasomatognosia, hemisomatagnosia Defective or lack of awareness of one side of the body, as in the subject's denial of hemiplegia (*Babinski's syndrome*) or blindness (*Anton's syndrome*).

hemiatrophy, facial *Parry-Romberg's syndrome.* A trophic disorder, perhaps due to disturbance of the sympathetic nervous system, in which there is progressive wasting of some or all of the tissues of one side of the face, which as a result looks old and wrinkled. The disorder usually begins during the second decade; it causes no disability.

hemiballism Violent, uncontrollable shaking, twisting, and rolling movements involving one side of the body, occurring as a result of hemorrhage into the subthalamic body.

hemichorea Chorea affecting one side of the body only.

hemichorea, preparalytic A condition in which unilateral choreic movements precede an attack of hemiplegia.

hemicrania *Migraine* (q.v.).

hemidepersonalization Hemisomatognosis (q.v.).

hemiopia Hemianopia. See *field defect.*

hemiparesis Slight paralysis or weakness of only one side of the body.

hemiplegia A symptom complex and not a disease, characterized by paralysis of one side of the body.

hemiplegia alternans Crossed paralysis; paralysis of one or more cranial nerves and paralysis of the arm and leg of the opposite side. Hypoglossal hemiplegia alternans involves the twelfth cranial nerve; *Weber's syndrome* involves the oculomotor (third cranial) nerve.

hemiplegia cruciata (Mod. L. "crossed hemiplegia") Paralysis of an upper extremity and of the lower extremity on the side opposite to that of the upper extremity.

hemiplegia, nocturnal See *paralysis, sleep.*

hemisomatognosis *Hemidepersonalization;* a disorder of body image in which the subject feels that one limb is missing, usually the left arm or leg. It often occurs in combination with hemiparesis and unilateral spatial agnosia.

hemispatial neglect See *neglect, sensory.*

hemisphericity Cerebral dominance and/or the hypothesis that some types of emotion or affective behavior are mediated through one hemisphere of the brain rather than the other. Some studies, for example, have found dysfunction of the right, nondomi-

nant hemisphere to be associated with affective disorders; others have found hysterical repression to be consistent with the right hemisphericity and obsessive compulsive traits to be consistent with the left hemisphericity. See *dominance, cerebral.*

hemo- *Hem(at)o-* (q.v.).

hemophobia, hematophobia Fear of blood.

hemorrhage, cerebral See *accident, cerebrovascular.*

hemothymia Passion for blood; morbid impulse to murder.

hepatolenticular degeneration Wilson's disease. See *degeneration, hepatolenticular.*

herbalist Witch doctor.

herbivorous In zoology, animals (herbivora) subsisting on herbaceous plants or vegetables; in constitutional medicine, a type described by Bryant and corresponding roughly to Kretschmer's *athletic* type and its equivalents in other systems.

Herculeus morbus *Obs.* Epilepsy, supposedly because of the epileptic's Herculean violence and strength.

herd See *instinct, herd.*

hereditary (hereditarial) Referring both to the Mendelian mechanism by which physical or mental attributes are transmitted from one generation to another and to the inherited attributes to which an organism is predisposed by the presence of a certain gene or combination of genes.

"We usually call what is programmed in the chromosomes hereditary or genetic. The sum of what is biologically given (whether determined by genetics or intrauterine environment) is referred to as constitutional. . . . The unfolding of biologically given factors and their manifestation at critical periods in the life history are referred to as maturation, a somatically programmed schedule. The opposite of maturation is involution." (Redlich, F.C., & Freedman, D.X. *The Theory and Practice of Psychiatry,* 1966)

hereditary cerebellar ataxia of Marie See *ataxia, Marie's hereditary cerebellar.*

hereditary spastic paraplegia See *paraplegia, hereditary spastic.*

heredity As it has become customary to use the terms *inheritance* and *transmission* for designating the actual genetic process by which physical or mental traits are transmitted from parents to offspring, *heredity* has a more general and abstract sense—of classifying the process of inheritance as a biological phenomenon and identifying it with the forces responsible for the resemblance between an individual and his ancestors, insofar as this resemblance is due to the operation of predisposing gene units rather than to the similarity of environmental influences.

The morphological equivalent of heredity is the *Mendelian* mechanism based on the integrity of the chromosomes and their continuity from one cell generation to the next, while the science dealing with the study of heredity is usually called *genetics*. See *Mendelism.*

heredo-familial essential microsomia See *dwarfism.*

heritable *Inheritable* (q.v.).

hermaphrodism *Hermaphroditism* (q.v.).

hermaphrodism, psychical Adler's term for the constant striving of the person to free himself from feelings of weakness, inferiority, and futility to attain self-confidence, superiority, and self-gratification. It is the conflict between the masculine and feminine components.

hermaphroditism State of being a hermaphrodite; bisexuality; the biological phenomenon of *bixexuality* (q.v.) occurring either synchronously or heterochronously and originating in the production of both male and female gametes by the same organism. There are two types of hermaphroditism.

In *nonfunctional hermaphroditism,* both male and female germ cells are provided transiently or permanently, yet only one kind of germ cell functions. Of this type there are three forms:

1. *Accessory,* when, in addition to the testis there is a *rudimentary ovary,* which, however, does not reproduce ova.

2. *Accidental,* with sporadic occurrence of ova in the testis or of spermatic tissues in the ovary.

3. *Teratological* (common in birds and mammals), when the reproductive system presents an intimate mixture of male and female structures.

In *functional hermaphroditism,* both male and female gametes, produced by one and the same individual, are functioning. Of this type, which is characterized by *monoecism,* there are also three forms :

1. *Unisexual monoecism,* when at certain times a genetic female develops spermato-

zoa in the ovary (*gynomonoecism*) or a genetic male develops ova in the testis (*andromonoecism,* less common), so that one sex becomes hermaphroditic, i.e. the individual previously functioning as female (or male) now functions as male (or female).

2. *Consecutive monoecism,* when a male later functions as a female, or (less commonly) a female later becomes a male. Genetically these organisms are either males or neutrals.

3. *Spatial monoecism,* manifesting real functional hermaphroditism, is characterized by the presence of both male and female reproductive organs.

hermeneutics The principles or methods of interpreting the meaning of the Bible, or the study of those principles; sometimes applied to the study of psychotherapy, in which case *hermeneutic theory* denotes the study of the rules or methods governing interpretation of the patient's productions (associations, dreams, etc.) during analytic treatment.

herniation, lumbar disk See *disk, herniated lumbar intervertebral.*

hero-birth, primordial image of The source of the pregnancy dream in the unconscious; the hero to be born represents the dreamer's individuality. "We can be certain only that, when a man is identical with his persona, the individual qualities are associated with the soul. It is this association which gives rise to the symbol, so often appearing in dreams, of the soul's pregnancy; this symbol has its source in the primordial image of the hero-birth. The child that is to be born signifies the individuality, which, though existing, is not yet conscious. Hence in the same way as the persona, which expresses one's adaptation to the milieu, is as a rule strongly influenced and shaped by the milieu, so the soul is just as profoundly moulded by the unconscious and its qualities." (Jung, *PT*) See *image, primordial.*

hero worship From the psychoanalytic point of view, a product of the need of the great majority of people "for authority which they can admire, to which they can submit, and which dominates and sometimes even ill-treats them." The need for such an authority is simply the longing of each person for the ideal or perfect father. As a result of this need it is possible for a great man to rise to extraordinary significance in the lives of large masses of people so that he is regarded as a hero. "The decisiveness of thought, the strength of will, the forcefulness of his deeds, belong to the picture of the father; above all other things, however, the self-reliance and independence of the great man, his divine conviction of doing the right thing, which may pass into ruthlessness. He must be admired, he may be trusted, but one cannot help also being afraid of him." (Freud, S. *Moses and Monotheism*, 1939)

heroin See *opium*.

heroinomania Morbid craving for heroin. See *addiction; dependency, drug; opium*.

Herrick, Charles Judson (1868–1960) American neurologist; comparative neurology; *The Evolution of Human Behavior*.

Herstedvester A town in Denmark, of importance in psychiatry because of the rehabilitation program in use in its Institution for Criminal Psychopaths. The program was a combination of group and individual treatment that provided a therapeutic community for the inmates. See *community, therapeutic*.

Hertwig-Magendie phenomenon (Oscar Hertwig, German physiologist, 1849–1922, and François Magendie, French physiologist, 1783–1855) See *deviation, skew*.

Herxheimer reaction See *Jarisch-Herxheimer reaction*.

hetero- Combining form meaning other, different, from Gr. *heteros*, the other, one of two.

heterocentric Directed away from oneself; opposed to autocentric.

heteroclite A person who deviates from the common rule, as opposed to *homoclite*, a person who follows the common rule and is ordinary, normal, healthy, etc.

heteroerotism The attachment (cathexis) of the energy of the libidinal drive to objects outside of oneself, and specifically to objects of the opposite sex. If one uses the term *libido* synonymously with *Eros*, then heteroerotism is heterolibido or object-libido.

Heteroeroticism is a phase in the development of object relationships (see *ontogeny, psychic*); its achievement constitutes the chief task of adolescence. At puberty, libidinal strivings that have been dormant during the period of *latency* (q.v.) reappear because of biological intensification of sexuality. In childhood, the person had come to recognize his sexual impulses as dangerous; at puberty, he returns to just that point in his sexual development where he had abandoned it earlier, and the fears and guilt connected with the Oedipus complex reappear. But overt sexuality now has a physiologically mature genital discharge apparatus, and finally, at about 16 or 17, the adolescent desexualizes his relationship with all but one person of the opposite sex and the stage of heterosexuality is reached.

heterogamous Relating to the structural and functional differences between the male and female gametes, as they appear in most animals and plants. See *syngamy*.

heterogeneity, heterogeny Dissimilarity in the genotypical structure of individuals originating through sexual reproduction. See *homogeneity*.

heterohypnosis Hypnosis induced by another, as opposed to autohypnosis.

heterolalia The substitution of meaningless or inappropriate words for those meant or intended; malapropism.

heteronymous hemianopia See *field defect*.

heterophasia *Heterolalia* (q.v.).

heterophemy The saying of one thing when another is meant.

heterophonia *Heterolalia* (q.v.).

heterophoria Deviation of one eye because of muscular imbalance. Inward deviation is known as *esophoria;* outward deviation is *exophoria;* downward deviation is *hypophoria;* upward deviation is *hyperphoria*.

heterorexia Alibert's term for morbid appetite; dysorexia. See *eating disorders*.

heterosexuality Sexuality (in all its manifestations, normal and morbid) directed to the opposite sex. See *character, genital; genitality*.

"There is no conceivable way of quantifying the homosexual vs. heterosexual.... If, for instance, Alexander the Great had sexual relations with hundreds of women and only two men, but one of the men (Bagoas) was unquestionably the erotic center of his life, the statistics would give us a highly misleading picture.... At best these categories group together according to one arbitrarily chosen aspect of sexual actions—the genders of the parties involved—varieties of sexual behavior which may be more dissimilar than similar." (Boswell, J. *Christianity, Social Tolerance, and Homosexuality,* 1980)

heterosis The favorable influence of crossing on growth and other developmental properties of animals and plants, as exercised by an increase in heterozygocity in contrast to the decrease in vigor following inbreeding. In genetics, the beneficial effect of heterosis is observed and utilized by breeders of animals and plants all over the world. It is best evidenced in the generation immediately following the cross, by greater size, larger parts, increased longevity, and higher resistance to disease. Equally significant is the fact that any form of hybrid vigor disappears rapidly under inbreeding.

The mule is commonly cited as a hybrid animal whose vigor, hardiness, and resistance to disease are due to heterosis.

heterosociality Social relationship between members of the opposite sex.

heterosome The sex chromosome, as distinguished from all other chromosomes (autosomes). See *chromosome; sex determination.*

heterosuggestibility The state of influencing another; the opposite of auto- or self-suggestibility.

heterosuggestion See *autosuggestion.*

heterotopia Congenital displacement of gray matter of the spinal cord into the white substance.

heterotropia *Strabismus* (q.v.); squint.

heterozygosis *Heterozygousness* (q.v.).

heterozygousness *Obs. Heterozygosity, heterozygocity;* relates to the genetic condition of an organism whose two genes of a given factor pair are *different.*

Only dominant characters can appear in the state of heterozygousness, while the heterozygotic condition of a recessive trait affects the organism merely "germinally." A heterozygotic individual transmits the trait to the offspring but is not able to manifest the trait in his own phenotype. See *heterosis; inbreeding.*

Double heterozygousness refers to the individual who has both dominant and recessive alleles for two linked genes. See *linkage.*

hexafluorodiethyl ether A convulsant agent used in psychiatric treatment in the same capacity as ECT. The trade name is Indoklon.

hexing See *rootwork.*

HHHO See *syndrome, Prader-Labhart-Willi.*

HI Hyperglycemic index. See *index, hyperglycemic.*

HIAA Hydroxyindoleacetic acid. See *depression, unipolar.*

hibernation Prolonged sleep therapy, especially when accompanied by a lowering of the body temperature. High dosages of chlorpromazine, for instance, were used to keep patients in a continuous semisomnolent state with a lowered body temperature; such treatment was called hibernation therapy.

hiccup, hiccough A spasmodic myoclonous of the diaphragm producing a sudden inhalation of air that is interrupted by a spasmodic closure of the glottis, thus producing a sound that may simulate an ordinary cry or an unpleasant crow; also known as *singultus.*

hidden self See *personality, multiple.*

hidrosis Perspiration.

hieromania *Obs.* Religious insanity.

hieronosus *Obs.* Linnaeus's term for epilepsy.

hierophobia Fear of sacred or religious things.

HIF Higher intellectual function.

high utilizer See *selection, adverse.*

high-volume hospital See *volume sensitive.*

hindbrain Rhombencephalon, from which develop the metencephalon (cerebellum, pons, part of the fourth ventricle) and the myelencephalon (medulla oblongata and part of the fourth ventricle).

Hinkemann Term generally used in Germany for a castrated male. Hinkemann, the principal character of a play by the same name, written by Toller, lost his genitals as a result of injury sustained in World War I.

hippanthropy A symptom in which a patient imagines he is a horse.

hippocampus See *memory; rhinencephalon.*

hippus A condition in which the pupil alternately contracts and dilates on stimulation with light.

Hirschfeld, Magnus (1868–1935) German sexologist.

histamine An amine occurring in all animal and vegetable tissues. Histamine dilates capillaries and arterioles, constricts the bronchioles, stimulates the smooth muscles of the uterus, and stimulates many glands of external secretion, expecially the gastric glands. Intracutaneous injection of histamine produces focal erythema within 1 to 5 seconds, within 30 to 50 seconds a spreading flush (the *histamine flare*) and, later, a wheal. The flare reaction is dependent upon an intact arteriolar circulation and an intact axon reflex; hence it has been used in diagnosis of peripheral nerve lesions. Histamine has also been used in the determination of circulation time, in various gastric function tests, and in the diagnosis of histamine headache (histaminic cephalalgia, *Horton's syndrome*). The latter is a unilateral headache associated with redness of the eye, lacrimation, rhinorrhea or stuffiness of the nostril, swelling of the temporal vessels of the affected side, and dilatation of the vessels of the pain area (usually the orbital area).

Histamine has been used in the treatment of peripheral vascular disease, rheumatoid arthritis and Ménière's disease.

histiocytosis, lipid See *disease, Gaucher's; disease, Niemann-Pick.*

histrionic personality *Hysterical personality* (q.v.).

HIV Human immunodeficiency virus, proposed (1986) by the International Committee on the Taxonomy of Viruses as a replacement for the more cumbersome dual terminology of human T-cell lymphotropic virus type-III/lymphadenopathy-associated virus (HTLV-III/LAV). See *syndrome, acquired immune deficiency.*

HMO Health maintenance organization; an organized health care delivery system combining health care services with a prepaid fixed group rate. The HMO contracts to provide its enrolled members with comprehensive health care services for a fixed period (usually one year), in return for fixed premiums (usually payable monthly).

hoarding The practice of collecting any number of objects, generally of limited size and of no practical use. Hoarding is seen most commonly in deteriorated schizophrenics and in other organic cerebral disorders. Hoarding is one of the behavioral manifestations on which an opinion of *incompetency* (q.v.) may be based.

When hoarding leads to neglect of one's home or environment, it is sometimes referred to as the *Diogenes syndrome.* See *mania, collecting.*

hoarding type See *assimilation.*

Hoch, August (1868–1919) American psychiatrist; described shut-in personality.

Hoch, Paul Henry (1902–64) Hungarian-born neuropsychiatrist, to U.S. in 1942; somatic treatment, mental hospital administration, community psychiatry.

Hoche, Alfred (1865–1945) German psychiatrist; Hoche's tract, or fasciculus septomarginalis: the myelinated descending axons in the lumbar dorsal column near the posterior septum; in the sacral cord they form a superficial, median triangular zone, the fasciculus triangularis.

hockey stick strategy See *strategy, hockey stick.*

hodophobia Fear of travel.

Hoffer, Willi (1897–1967) Austrian psychoanalyst; fled to London with S. Freud in 1938.

Hoffmann (or Tromner's) sign (Johann Hoffmann, German neurologist, 1857–1919) In hemiplegia, due to organic brain disease, snapping of the index or ring finger produces flexion of the thumb.

holergasia A psychiatric disorder of such a nature as to involve the *whole* person. For example, schizophrenia and manic-depressive psychosis ordinarily are associated with a disorganization of the entire personality and the syndromes are therefore known as holergastic reactions.

holism *Gestalt totality;* the thesis that the study of parts cannot explain the whole, because the whole is something different from the simple summation of its parts. The application of the holistic principle to the study of human beings has far-reaching implications. There are several sciences *relating to* the person, but no science *of* the person in its totality. From a holistic point of view the human being is more than a mere aggregation of physiological, psychological, and social functions: the person as a whole has attributes that cannot be explained by the attributes of its constituent parts.

Adler particularly emphasized the need for the holistic approach in the understanding of personality; recognizing that the whole person cannot be understood by an analysis or dissection of his parts, he emphasized that he could be understood in terms of the goals he sets for himself and toward which he moves.

holistic healing A system of health care based upon the theory that health is the result of the body, mind, and spirit in harmony and that stress—whether from physical agents or social or psychological pressures—is the enemy of good health. Since a person's reaction to stress depends upon his perception of the world, which in turn is determined by his belief system, healing efforts must be directed toward eliminating the patient's self-limiting thoughts, distorted ideas, negative self-images, and other programmed attitudes that have disturbed the balance and harmony requisite for normal functioning. Self-direction, self-regulation, and self-actualization are important elements in achieving the inner balance essential for health. See *therapy, cognitive.*

holistic psychology *Humanistic psychology* (q.v.).

Holmes, Gordon, rebound phenomenon of See *rebound phenomenon of Gordon Holmes.*

holophrastic Expressing a complex of ideas in a single word, as in some primitive languages that require a completely new word for any slight change in the total situation. Schizophrenics, who typically demonstrate a reduction in their connotation ability and a relative overemphasis on denotation, can be described as manifesting holophrastic association defects. See *connotation.*

Homburger, August (1873–1930) German psychiatrist; psychopathology of children.

home, loveless From the standpoint of mental hygiene, those homes in which an inharmonious atmosphere is prevalent as the result of constant discord among the members of the family, and where the children are made buffers between quarreling parents who have "fallen out of love." This is the type of surrounding that breeds delinquency. In these loveless homes the children are constantly exposed to traumatic experiences that have a definite influence in the development of neuroses and other mental disturbances. Furthermore, it is an established fact that such loveless homes have a much more deleterious effect upon the children's mental development than have the so-called broken homes, which seem to play a rather secondary role in this respect. (Seliger, R.V., et al. *Contemporary Criminal Hygiene,* 1946)

homebound See *agoraphobia.*

homeostasis The status quo; the tendency of an organism to maintain a constancy and stability of its internal environment; the result of the various autonomic mechanisms that adjust and adapt the body as a whole to changes in the external or internal environment. Homeostasis is Cannon's term for a steady, balanced, internal constitution; Claude Bernard's term was "milieu interieur." "Autonomic adjustments, while allowing for necessary responses of the organism, must maintain a physiological state adequate for the needs of the tissues. . . . The physiological requirements of any tissue must be balanced against those of all others, and with minor fluctuations, a steady 'internal constitution' maintained. . . . Forces pulling in opposite directions are equilibrated so as to give an appearance of rest." (Fulton, J.F. *Physiology of the Nervous System,* 1949) In general, rapid adjustments are made by the autonomic nervous system while slower adjustments occur through chemical and hormonal influences.

homeostenosis Inflexibility or narrowed range of homeostatic ranges available to an organism, characteristic of the aged and one of the factors that predisposes them to multiple disorders and to prolongation of any disorder they develop as compared with younger people.

homesickness An acute separation syndrome appearing in dependent persons when for any reasons they are removed from their usual sources of dependency gratification. See *separation; separation anxiety.*

homichlophobia Fear of fog.

homicidomania See *mania, homicidal.*

homilopathy Kraepelin's term for disease due to mental induction and persecution mania of the deaf.

homilophobia Fear of sermons; also, fear that in a group of people the others in the group might find something wrong with one's appearance, attire, or demeanor. See *agoraphobia.*

homo- Combining form meaning one and the same, common, from Gr. *hómos;* opposed to *hetero-.*

homoclite See *heteroclite.*

homocystinuria An inborn error of metabolism, transmitted as an autosomal recessive, associated with mental retardation and characterized by excretion of moderate amounts of the essential amino acid methionine and of an abnormal amino acid, L-homocystine, in the urine. The syndrome was first reported in 1962.

Clinical features include skeletal abnormalities similar to Marfan's syndrome (pigeon breast or chicken breast), joint enlargement, fine and fair hair, and ectopia lentia. It may be associated with thrombo-embolic episodes.

homoerotic Relating to or manifesting the erotic or libidinal instinct toward one of the same sex.

homoerotism, homeroticism A general term for the objectivation of erotic or libidinal interests upon a member of the same sex. The impulse is subject to all the modifications of erotic impulses. It may be directly expressed (homogenitality); it may be sublimated (homoerotism or homosexuality); it may be severely repressed; if so, the impulses may be subjected to reaction-formation, that is, they may appear as aversions against the homerotism; or they may be transferred into reality in symbolic form (delusions, hallucinations, etc.).

Homoeroticism is a phase in the development of object relationships (see *ontogeny, psychic)* and the term is generally applied to that period following the Oedipal phase and lasting until adolescence, when libidinal energies are repressed and aggressive energies are redirected into elaborating a more effective web of defenses, including the superego, and into increasing mastery in the social sphere, in socially condoned and desirable competitiveness, conquest, and domination. See *latency.*

homogamy In contrast to *panmixia,* this genetic term applies to the *inbreeding* conditions in isolated population groups composed of organisms with the same hereditary characteristics.

homogeneity, homogeny Identical genotypical structure of two or more organisms of common descent, as found in the case of pure lines or in monozygotic sets of twins.

homogenic love Homosexuality. See *gay.*

homogenitality Interest in the genitals of one's own sex. See *homosexuality.*

homologous Referring to gene units that belong to the same pairs of *homologues.* See *allelic.*

Homologous indicates similarity on the basis of shared ancestry, whereas analogous indicates similarity that is not genetically determined but has occurred by chance or through other mechanisms. The Schnauzkrampf of the catatonic is analogous to the snout of a pig, not homologous.

homologue If one form or condition of a genetic character is contrasted with another form or condition of the same character, such as two eye colors or two color patterns, the genes that are responsible for these two conditions are said to belong to the same pair of *homologues.* See *chromosome.*

homology In comparative biology, similarity based on common descent. See *allometry; analogy.*

homonym A word that has same sound as another, even though the two words differ in meaning and often in spelling as well; *agnomenatio, homophone,* and *paranomasia* are approximate equivalents. Examples are here and hear, there and their. Ordinarily the listener is able to grasp the intended meaning of what is said because of the context in which it occurs. In various conditions that interfere with attention and concentration, including manic states and organic confusional states, the subject fails to grasp the intended meaning, however, and any misinterpretation of the environment may be based on the more familiar meaning of the homonym. Thus the delirious child may believe that the Lord's prayer includes the phrase "Harold be thy name" rather than "hallowed be thy name." See *association, clang.*

homonymous hemianopsia See *field defect.*

homonymous quadrantic field defect See *field defect.*

homophile A lover of one's own kind; a gay person; specifically, a homosexual, and a term used especially by organizations that purport or attempt to represent homosexuals as a group.

homophobia Negative attitudes to homosexuals and homosexuality, reflecting both conscious and unconscious fears and reactions. Homophobia includes not only irrational and persistent fear of homosexuality (often manifested in extreme rage reactions to homosexuals), but also the self-hatred experienced by gay men and women because of their homosexuality.

Religious and other cultural taboos against homosexuality are a part of early learning and are reinforced by experience. They may be used unconsciously in denying one's own impulses, and successful denial, reaction formation, and other defenses are often rewarded by the environment. This in turn tends to perpetuate and intensify the defense so that the prejudice and discrimination against persons perceived to be of a homosexual orientation become increasingly entrenched or even ineradicable. As with sexism and racism, homophobia is frequently expressed in humor based on negative stereotypes (e.g. the effeminate male hairdresser or ballet dancer, the masculine female athlete or executive). The homophobic attitudes of gay people themselves may perpetuate such negative stereotypes.

homophone See *homonym.*

homosexual Relating to or directed toward one of the same sex.

homosexual panic An acute, severe episode of anxiety related to the fear (or the delusional conviction) that the subject is about to be attacked sexually by another person of the same sex, or that he is thought to be a homosexual by fellow workers, etc. First described by Kempf in 1920 and hence sometimes known as *Kempf's disease;* symptoms include agitation, ideas or delusions of reference, conscious guilt over homosexual activity, hallucinations, ideas and threats of suicide, depression, and often perplexity. The panic state is typically precipitated by loss or separation from a member of the same sex to whom the subject is emotionally attached, or by fatigue, illness, fears of impotence, failures in sex performance, homesickness, etc. It may appear as the first acute episode in schizophrenic disorders, and it is more frequent in males than in females.

Sometimes, instead of overt sexual material, the anxiety is related to fears of undue malignant influence, physical violence, or impending death. Such an episode is termed *acute aggression panic.* (Glick, B.S. *Journal of Nervous and Mental Disease 129,* 1959)

homosexuality Sexual orientation characterized by erotic attraction to others of the same sex; feelings of love, emotional attachment, or sexual attraction to persons of one's own gender and/or sexual behavior with a person of the same sex. Homosexuality usually appears first in childhood and develops in adolescence and throughout adulthood.

Homosexuality is considered a nonpathologic variant of human sexuality. DSM-III-R does not include the category *ego-dystonic homosexuality,* which was used in DSM-III to denote a sustained pattern of overt sexual arousal in a person who complained explicitly that such responses were unwanted and a source of distress. Further, the person so diagnosed wanted to acquire or increase heterosexual responsivity so that heterosexual relations could be initiated or maintained. In clinical practice, the term was almost never used, and it was therefore deleted from the 1987 revision.

Although most homosexuals engage in sexual activity, genital sexual behavior is by no means an absolute predictor or sign of sexual orientation. Sexual behavior is not always congruent with sexual desire, patterns of sexual behavior fluctuate during a person's life, and behavior may be inhibited by intrapsychic conflict, societal pressures, or both. Heterosexuality and homosexuality are not dichotomous. For both heterosexual and homosexual persons, early sexual behavior (in childhood or adolescence) may be congruent or incongruent with the direction of adult sexual expression.

The term itself is compounded of a Greek prefix and a Latin root; it means, literally, of one sex. It was coined in the late 19th century by German psychologists to refer to preference for erotic contact with one's own gender.

Some authors differentiate between *overt* homosexuality (physical sexual contact) and *latent* homosexuality (unrecognized or unconscious attraction, or recognized ideas and impulses not openly expressed). A less frequent subdivision is into *homogenitality* (genital sexuality), homosexuality (preference, phantasies, impulses without genital activity with another of the same sex), and *homoerotism* ("well-sublimated" attraction or preference expressed in other than specifically genital or sexual activities).

In general, the term "inversion" is equivalent to homosexuality. When "sex-role inversion" is used, however, it must be differentiated from homosexuality. Homosexuality refers to sexual desires and/or activity between members of the same sex, whereas sex-role inversion refers to adoption of the sex role and introjection of the psychologic identity of the opposite sex. Occasionally the two may coexist, but more frequently one or the other is present alone.

homosexuality, female A female's sexual orientation characterized by erotic attraction for, or behavior with, one or more other females, including emotional attachments, phantasies, desires, impulses, and sexual or genital contact. Female homosexuality is often referred to as *lesbian* or *sapphic*, after the isle of Lesbos, home of the classic Greek poet Sappho, who wrote of her erotic attachments to women. See *homosexuality*.

Data on the frequency of female homosexuality vary considerably and are marred by problems of definition as well as by the social stigma that prevents many subjects from identifying themselves in research samples. Kinsey et al. (1953) reported that between 2 and 6% of unmarried women, but less than 1% of married women, had been more or less exclusively homosexual between the ages of 20 and 35. Cross-cultural studies have found female homosexuality in all world regions, in all types of economies, settlement patterns, family and household types, and economic exchange systems. Female homosexuals are diverse in age, education, occupation, religion, lifestyle, race, and interests.

homosexuality, latent Sometimes used interchangeably with *unconscious homosexuality*. See *homosexuality*.

homosexuality, male A male's sexual orientation characterized by erotic attraction for, or behavior with, one or more other males; a male whose sexual phantasies are exclusively or nearly exclusively of others of the same sex. There may be men who are homosexual but unaware of their sexual orientation because of repression or denial of their phantasies. There are also some homosexual men who are conscious of their phantasies and sexual arousal patterns but cannot acknowledge their homosexuality because of social pressures or intrapsychic conflict.

Data on the frequency of male homosexuality are difficult to obtain. Havelock Ellis (1936) estimated its incidence as between 2 and 5%, Hirschfeld (1920) at 2 to 3%. Most estimates are biased by the belief that to be considered a homosexual the subject must be exclusively homosexual and must behave homosexually. Kinsey's data are based on sexual contact resulting in orgasm and thus exclude those who engage in sexual activity without coming to a climax and those who are erotically aroused by homosexual stimuli but never have overt relations. As thus defined, however, Kinsey (1948) reported that 37% of the male population has some homosexual experience between the beginning of adolescence and old age; of unmarried men who are 35 years of age or over, almost 50% have had a homosexual experience since the beginning of adolescence. Kinsey found that 4% of the white male population is exclusively homosexual throughout their lives. Current estimates are that 10% of the population is exclusively or predominantly homosexual, including married and celibate men.

Homosexuality has been reported in all cultures studied, and most men are capable of homosexual behavior. Incidental homosexuality, the choice of another man as sexual object when no women are available (*faute de mieux*), may occur in same-sex schools, the military, and prisons, even though homosexuality may not be the primary sexual orientation of the participants.

Since the late 1960s, homosexual males have often preferred to be identified as *gay* (q.v.), considering it less pejorative and judgmental than "homosexual."

Freud hypothesized at one time or another that fear of castration, intense oedipal attachment to the mother, narcissism, narcissistic object choice, and sibling rivalry with overcompensatory love for the rival were significant etiologic factors in male homosexuality. None of these hypotheses, however, proved to be of much value in the therapy of gay men. There is increasing suggestive evidence that male homosexuality, like heterosexuality, has a genetic or constitutional basis. F.J. Kallmann (*Heredity in Health and Menal Disorder,* 1953) long ago presented evidence of a genetic basis of homosexuality based on twin studies. Although these studies were flawed by methodological error, more recent reports support his conclusion and find (1) a significantly greater concordance of homosexual behavior in monozygotic than in dizygotic twins and (2) a significantly higher percentage of homosexual or bisexual brothers of gay men than of heterosexual men.

The view that homosexual object choice is determined by conflict evolving from faulty parenting (such as a close binding mother or a distant father) is not supported by recent observation, nor do psychological tests support the view that homosexuals are more disturbed psychologically than heterosexuals.

A clinical approach based on the theory that homosexuals must change their sexual orientation in order to live healthy and productive lives has proved to be harmful to the psychological well-being of homosexual men. Current approaches to gay men with concerns about sexual orientation are directed to internalized *homophobia* (q.v.), supporting a positive view of the self, and exploring other issues that affect self-esteem. (Cabaj, R.P. *Journal of Homosexuality 15*, 1987; Isay, R.A. in *Contemporary Perspectives on Psychotherapy with Lesbians and Gay Men*, ed. T. Stein & C.J. Cohen, 1986)

homosexuality, masked Unconscious homosexual impulses. For example, a married man, complaining that his wife was frigid, insisted on having solely anal intercourse with her, since this was much more gratifying to him than genital relations. The unique pleasure found exclusively in anal contact represented his masked homosexuality.

homosexuality, unconscious See *homosexuality, latent.*

homosociality A term coined by J.C. Fluegel to denote social relationship between members of the same sex.

homozygocity *Homozygousness* (q.v.).

homozygote A zygotic organism produced by the union of two similar gametes and therefore possessing two like genes of a given factor pair. In the case of *recessive* Mendelian inheritance, a hereditary character can be manifested only by those offspring who have inherited its predispos-

ing factor from both parents and thus are homozygous for the character in question.

homozygousness *Obs. Homozygosity; homozygocity;* the "germinally pure" condition of a person who inherits the same gene factor from each parent, so that in his organism the two genes of the given pair are *alike.*

Homozygousness of a dominant anomaly is very rare, as it can be assumed only when both parents of a diseased person are also patients. In the case of a recessive anomaly that can only appear in the phenotype of a homozygote, all trait-carriers must be homozygotes. Consequently, the occurrence of such a recessive anomaly is not possible, unless *both* parents are either homozygotes or heterozygotes for the anomaly in question. See *recessiveness.*

Certain deleterious effects of inbreeding are now assumed to be due chiefly to the attainment of homozygousness rather than merely to the process of inbreeding itself. The frequent mating of persons closely related in descent must automatically result in a reduction of *heterozygosity* unless new mutations occur in these inbred lines. If the mutation rate is high, this may defer or prevent the attainment of homozygousness. See *heterosis; inbreeding.*

Hooton, Ernest Albert (1887–1954) American anthropologist; anthropometry; *Up from the Ape* (1931).

Hoover's sign (Charles F. Hoover, American physician, 1865–1927) Observed in organic hemiplegia and used for differentiating organic from hysteric hemiplegia; if the patient, lying on his back, attempts to raise the paretic leg, he unconsciously presses down forcibly the heel of the healthy leg; this accentuation does not occur in hysteria.

horizontal transmission See *transmission, vertical.*

horme *Libido* (q.v.).

hormephobia Fear of shock.

hormism Used by the school of psychology that holds that goals are sought for their own sake because of some intrinsic value, regardless of any pleasure attendant upon their attainment. McDougall believes that in humans and animals there are certain tendencies or urges that account for all forms of behavior, including abstract mental processes. Each tendency leads to a definite end, or purpose. Hormism is thus opposed to hedonism, which states that goals are sought only because they give pleasure or gratification to the person. See *hedonism*.

hormone A chemical messenger produced by a tissue or organ which regulates or modulates the activity of another tissue or organ. See *neurohormone*.

Horner's syndrome See *syndrome, Horner's*.

Horney, Karen (1885–1952) American psychoanalyst; the Horney school emphasizes environmental and cultural factors in the genesis of neurosis. Horney and H.S. Sullivan represent the two chief branches within the "dynamic-cultural" school of psychoanalysis.

horror feminae *Obs.* "The essential feature of this strange manifestation of the sexual life is the want of sexual sensibility for the opposite sex, even to the extent of horror, while sexual inclination and impulse toward the same sex are present." (Krafft-Ebing, R. v. *Psychopathia Sexualis*, 1908)

hospice A program of care for the dying, a place where such care is provided, or both. The hospice movement has developed in recognition of the fact that there comes a point in medical care when cure is no longer a real possibility and attention must be directed toward comforting patients and families.

horrors *Delirium tremens* (q.v.).

hospital, day or night See *day hospital*.

hospitalism See *depression, anaclitic*.

hospitalitis A humorous term coined to emphasize the complete hospital conditioning (or dependency on the hospital) of a patient who is usually an utterly helpless or incompetent person before his admission to the hospital. It may be difficult for him to leave the hospital, and each attempt to prepare the patient for discharge results in an aggravation of symptoms. Also called *sanatorium disease*.

host mother See *surrogate mother*.

hostel Lodging place, such as an inn; in psychiatry the term includes short-stay hostels, such as *halfway houses* and other rehabilitation units, and long-stay hostels, for patients who are unlikely to improve further but who do not require the intensive level of care provided in a hospital or nursing home.

housebound Unable to leave one's residence, most often due to *agoraphobia* (q.v.), but

sometimes found in paranoid self-referential patients and in severely withdrawn depressed patients.

housewife's syndrome See *neurosis, housewife's*.

HSCL The Hopkins Symptom Checklist, a self-report inventory consisting of 58 items that are representative of the symptom patterns commonly observed in outpatients, including somatization, obsessive-compulsive, interpersonal sensitivity, anxiety, and depressive symptoms.

Hsieh-Ping (sē-ping′) A culture-specific trancelike state, seen in Taiwan, characterized by tremor, disorientation, delirium, and ancestor identification, and often accompanied by visual or auditory hallucinations. The seizure may last from 30 minutes to several hours.

HTLV-III Human T-cell leukemia virus, type III. See *syndrome, acquired immune deficiency*.

HTP See *test, House-Tree-Person*.

Hübner, Arthur (1878–1949) German forensic psychiatrist.

huffing Deliberate inhalation of organic solvents to achieve a euphoric sensation or *high*. Like glue-sniffing, the procedure is habituating and is typically repeated at 5- to 15-minute intervals for hours. Also like glue sniffing, the habit may produce severe damage to the nervous system, most commonly in the form of peripheral neuropathy.

human potential See *humanistic psychology*.

human relations group *T-group* (q.v.).

human surrogate See *surrogate, human*.

humanistic psychology An orientation that rejects both the quantitative reductionism of behaviorism and the psychoanalytic emphasis on unconscious forces in favor of a view of man as uniquely creative and controlled by his own values and choices. Through experiential means, each person can develop his greatest potential, or *self-actualization*. Humanistic psychology is related to the *human potential* movement and its encounter groups, growth centers, sensitivity training, etc.

Humanistic psychology is related to and draws from group dynamics, *existentialism* (q.v.), the person-centered approach in counseling (with its emphasis on expressing the self and also taking responsibility for one's actions), Jung's individuation as a process of achieving selfhood, and oriental philosophies with emphasis on meditation, body awareness, and peak experiences.

humiliation Feeling of being disgraced, shamed, debased, or ignominiously dishonored; it may represent a frustration of narcissistic aspirations and disapproval or punishment by the superego. Such feelings are frequent concomitants to the dejection of clinically depressed patients (loss of self-esteem). Provocation of others into actions that appear to warrant feelings of humiliation is seen often in *masochism* (q.v.).

humor In DSM-III-R, humor is recognized as a defense mechanism used by some to cope with stress or conflict; it consists of emphasizing the amusing or ironic aspects of the conflict.

humor, gallows Galgenhumor; humorous and comical behavior in the face of disaster or death. Gallows humor is seen most frequently in the organic psychoses, and particularly in delirium tremens cases.

hunger, affect Indiscriminate and insatiable demand for attention and affection, seen often in children who have suffered *emotional deprivation*. Affect hunger frequently takes the form of aggressive, hostile, antisocial behavior with an inability to accept limitations or recognize the needs of others. See *deprivation, emotional.*

hunger, nervous Urge to eat (orally incorporate) as a method of allaying anxiety or tension and of gratifying frustrated pleasure cravings. Obesity is frequently the secondary symptomatic result of such chronic and intense nervous hunger. Nervous hunger is an expression of intense dependence and stems back to the oral incorporative stage of infantile development.

Food addiction and cigarette addiction are closely related phenomena. Thumbsucking, which is closely related to the use of pacifiers in infancy, with the thumb replacing the pacifier, is an early infantile prototype of nervous hunger. See *eating disorders.*

hunger, social The desire to be accepted by the group; the major incentive for improvement in a therapy group.

hunger strike, neurotic Adler thus denotes the fear of eating, occurring mainly in females at about age of 17. There follows

usually a rapid decrease in weight. The goal, to be inferred from the whole attitude of the patient, is the rejection of the female role.

"In other words, it is an attempt by means of an exaggerated abstinence—as is so generally the case—to retard the development of the female bodily form." (Adler, A. *The Practice and Theory of Individual Psychology,* 1924) See *anorexia nervosa.*

Hunter's syndrome See *mucopolysaccharidosis.*

Huntington, George (1850–1916) American neurologist; hereditary chorea was first described by C. Waters in 1841 and again by Huntington, whose name it was given, in 1872.

Huntington's disease (HD) *Huntington's chorea;* a heritable neuropsychiatric disorder transmitted as an autosomal dominant trait, characterized by progressive chorea, impairment of voluntary movement, dementia, and depression or other emotional symptoms. Onset is typically in middle adult life, with death on the average 15 years after onset usually from subdural hematoma secondary to head trauma or from suffocation secondary to aspiration of food. Affected children of affected fathers have an earlier onset than do affected children of affected mothers. Offspring of affected parents have a 50% likelihood of developing the disorder.

Hurler's disease *Gargoylism.* See *mucopolysaccharidosis.*

hybrid The inbred offspring of two parents who differ with respect to one gene factor or a combination of factors or even belong to different species. In genetics, used also as an adjective. The hybrids that constitute the first filial generation are heterozygotic individuals originating from the cross of parents who carry a given hereditary stock in a pure, unmixed form. When such hybrids differ with respect to only *one* character, they are called *monohybrid.* When they differ in two characters, they are *dihybrid;* analogously, other hybrids are *trihybrid* or *polyhybrid.*

"It is not always, not even usually, possible to cross species, for there is a strong tendency for species to be interimsterile. Some of them will not mate, or their germ cells will not unite, or the hybrid does not reach maturity. Other species leap all these hurdles, cross, and yield offspring, but the hybrids are sterile. There are, however, many grades of interfertility between species, and some such crosses are as fruitful as matings within species." (Shull, A.F. *Heredity,* 1938)

hybridization Genetic term for the process of increasing the variability in a species or group of plants or animals through the production of *hybrids.*

hydro- Combining form meaning water, hydrogen, from Gr. *hydor.*

hydrocephalus An increase in the volume of cerebrospinal fluid within the skull. If cerebrospinal fluid pressure is normal, the condition is termed *compensatory hydrocephalus,* since the excess fluid compensates for brain atrophy, as in congenital cerebral hypoplasia and in acquired cerebral atrophy due to diffuse sclerosis, general paralysis, and senile or presenile degeneration. If pressure is increased, the condition is termed *hypertensive hydrocephalus,* which may be (1) obstructive, when an obstruction to the circulation of cerebrospinal fluid within the ventricles or at the outlet from the fourth ventricle prevents free communication between the ventricles and the subarachnoid space; or (2) communicating, when communication between ventricles and subarachnoid space is free and hydrocephalus is due to increased fluid formation (as in meningitis, certain toxic states, and after head injury), decreased absorption (as in compression of venous sinuses by tumor, products of infection, etc., or in impaired venous drainage secondary to increased intrathoracic pressure in cases of pulmonary neoplasm, aneurysm of the aorta, or severe emphysema) or to obstruction within the subarachnoid space (as in the case of tumor, adhesions following trauma, inflammation or hemorrhage, or congenital abnormalities such as platybasia or the Arnold-Chiari malformation).

Hypertensive hydrocephalus may be congenital or acquired. In congenital hydrocephalus, the most conspicuous symptom is enlargement of the head, which usually is slowly progressive. The cranial sutures are widely separated and the anterior fontanelle is greatly enlarged. Convulsions are common, as is optic atrophy due to pressure on the optic nerves. Mental deficiency is seen in severe cases. Most cases die by the age of 4; in the survivors,

mental deficiency, epilepsy, and blindness are the usual sequelae.

In acquired obstructive hydrocephalus, increased intracranial pressure causes headache, vomiting, and papilledema. In time, there is usually some mental deterioration, often with emotional lability, hallucinations, and delusions. Cranial nerve palsies may occur.

hydrocephalus, normal-pressure *Hakim's disease;* often abbreviated NPH; a syndrome consisting of mild dementia, apraxia of gait, urinary incontinence, and enlarged ventricles in the presence of normal cerebrospinal fluid pressure, first described by S. Hakim and R.D. Adams (*Journal of Neurological Sciences 2,* 1965). The original patients described benefited remarkably from ventricle shunting. The procedure is a serious one, however, and complications may occur in as many as 20% of patients.

hydrocephalus, toxic See *pseudotumor cerebri.*

hydrodipsomania Periodic attacks of uncontrollable thirst often found in epileptic patients.

hydroencephalocele A developmental anomaly of the brain in which the brain protruding through the skull contains a cavity that communicates with the cerebral ventricles.

hydromania *Obs.* Impulse to commit suicide by drowning.

hydromyelia (-mī-ē'lē-à) An increase of fluid in the dilated central canal of the spinal cord or elsewhere in the cord substance where congenital cavities may be present.

hydromyelocele (-mi'el-ō-sēl) The protrusion of a portion of the spinal cord, thinned out into a sac that is distended with cerebrospinal fluid, through a spina bifida.

hydrophobia 1. Fear of water. 2. Rabies. The symptoms of rabies are (1) in the premonitory stage, irritability, general malaise, anorexia, headache, insomnia; tingling, numbness, or pain in the course of the nerves radiating from the site of the wound; spasms of the muscles of the larynx and pharynx; huskiness; difficulty in swallowing; (2) in the stage of excitement there is exaggeration of the premonitory symptoms; intense excitement with terror; intense thirst, but every effort to drink is forthwith followed by choking and dyspnea; elevation of temperature and pulse. As the disease progresses, convulsions become generalized; (3) in the stage of paralysis, restlessness abates, convulsions cease, the musculature becomes limp and paralytic.

hydrophobophobia Fear of rabies; in severe cases, the symptoms of rabies are actually paralleled.

hyelophobia Fear of glass.

hygiene, criminal The branch of mental hygiene of which the object is the "study and investigation related to the causes, prevention and treatment of the social-medico-psychological illness known for centuries as crime."

In taking into consideration the complexity of this problem in modern society, the science aiming at the study of crime has necessarily to deal with many aspects of the offender: heredity, environment, home, social, economical, and political factors, legal aspects, emotional and physical development, psychiatric investigation, etc. (Seliger, R.V., et al. *Contemporary Criminal Hygiene*, 1946)

hygiene, mental The science and practice of maintaining mental health and efficiency— for a twofold purpose: first, to develop optimal modes of personal and social conduct in order to produce the happiest utilization of inborn endowments and capacities; and second, to prevent mental disorders. See *health, mental; orthopsychiatry.*

hygrophobia Fear of moisture or dampness.

hylephobia *Obs.* Epilepsy.

hylophobia Fear of forests.

hypacusia, hypoacusia Partial deafness.

hypalgia, hysterical A psychogenically induced decrease in the normal sensitivity to pain in any body area. The psychogenic basis has two elements:

1. As in all hysterical symptoms, the hypalgia is a defense against unconscious instinctual demands. Sexual or aggressive sensations that would be painful—that is, would cause anxiety—are repressed. These anxiety-causing impulses are often linked to specific memories. Hypalgia helps suppress these memories by decreasing the sensitiveness to pain in the body areas connected with these particular memories.

2. The decrease in painful sensation permits this body area to be used for unconscious phantasies and thus the re-

pressed material can be expressed without concomitant painful anxiety. (Fenichel, *PTN*)

hypapoplexia A mild form of apoplexy.

hypengyophobia Fear of responsibility.

hyper- Combining form meaning over, beyond, from Gr. *hypér.*

hyperactivity Excessive muscular activity; *hyperkinesis* (q.v.). In psychiatry, manifestations of disturbed child behavior, indicating the child whose movements and actions are performed at a higher than normal rate of speed and/or the child who is constantly restless and in motion. Hyperactivity may be (1) physiologic, i.e. not integrally associated with any other pathology although it may secondarily produce disturbances in living; (2) based on organic brain damage or dysfunction, and typically showing additional symptoms such as educational deficits, short attention span, perceptual difficulties, perseverative tendencies, and sleep disturbances (see *attention deficit disorder*); (3) associated with mental retardation without evident brain damage; (4) a symptom of reaction or neurotic behavior disorder, usually with more or less devious motivational character as part of an attempt to cope with environmental stress and/or neurotic conflicts within the child; or (5) a symptom of childhood schizophrenia. (Chess, S. *New York State Journal of Medicine 60*, 1960)

hyperactivity, developmental See *learning disability, specific.*

hyperactivity, purposeless A symptom seen often in organic brain disease: stimulation of a great enough intensity to provoke any reaction evokes an exaggerated emotional response or a prolonged bout of excessive activity that fulfills no purpose. Also known as *occupational delirium.* See *syndrome, organic.*

hyperacusia, hyperacusis Inordinate acuteness of the sense of hearing.

hyperadrenocorticism Cushing's syndrome. See *adenoma, basophile.*

hyperaldosternism *Aldosteronism* (q.v.).

hyperalgesia Inordinate sensitiveness to pain.

hypercathexis See *cathexis.*

hypercedemonia *Obs.* Excessive grief or anxiety.

hypercenesthesia A feeling of exaggerated well-being.

hyperdynamic β-adrenergic circulatory state See *circulatory state, hyperdynamic β-adrenergic.*

hyperechema (-ē-kē'mà) Auditory magnification or exaggeration.

hyperephidrosis Excessive sweating; *hyperhidrosis.*

hyperepidosis An abnormal or excessive growth of any part of the body.

hyperepithymia Inordinate desire.

hyperergasia The manic form of manic-depressive psychosis (Meyer).

hyperericdic Characterized by excessive strife or violence. The term *hyperericdic state* has been used to refer to attempted suicide triggered by acute interpersonal conflict that produced impulsive, uncontrolled rage.

hyperesthesia Inordinate sensitiveness to a tactile stimulus.

hyperesthesia psychica *Obs.* Hypochondriasis (q.v.).

hyperevolutism In constitutional medicine, excessive morphological, physiological, and psychological development.

hyperfunction Activity or functioning above the subject's own or a standard group's average.

hypergenitalism Overdevelopment of the genital system.

hyperglycemic index See *index, hyperglycemic.*

hypergnosis Exaggerated perception, such as the expansion of an isolated thought into a philosophical system that is seen in some paranoids.

hyperhidrosis Excessive sweating; *hyperephidrosis.*

hyperindependence In social work: "Exaggerated desire to live one's own life in one's own way; extreme individualism and disregard for the advice of others or limitations imposed by the situation." (Hamilton, G. A. *Medical Social Terminology*, 1930)

hyperinsulinism, functional See *hypoglycemia.*

hyperkalemia Excessive blood potassium; hyperpotassemia.

hyperkinesia, axial Thrusting pelvic movements such as sometimes occur in tardive dyskinesia and other extrapyramidal disorders, in barbiturate and other drug intoxications, and as conversion symptoms.

hyperkinesis Excessive muscular activity, observed in many disordered states, physical and psychical. For example, in epidemic en-

cephalitis, due to definite organic changes, exaggerated motility is often observed. Excessive activity is likewise associated with functional disorders, such as manic-depressive and schizophrenic psychoses.

hyperkinetic impulse disorder See *attention deficit disorder.*

hyperlogia Morbid loquacity.

hypermanic See *mania.*

hypermetamorphosis An excessive tendency to attend and react to every visual stimulus; noted in monkeys by Bucy and Klüver following bilateral removal of the temporal lobes.

hypermimia Excessive mimetic movements.

hypermnesia Exaggerated memory; ability to recall material that is not ordinarily available to the memory process. Hypermnesia as a psychopathologic phenomenon has been reported in the following conditions: (1) manic phase of manic-depressive psychosis; (2) schizophrenic disorders, where the remembered material is sometimes woven into the patient's hallucinations; (3) organic brain disorders, and particularly the acute confusional deliria; (4) hypnosis; (5) psychoanalytic reactivation; (6) during the seconds of shock and fright in situations that endanger life; (7) fever; (8) as an effect of certain drugs, and particularly amphetamines and other stimulants, and hallucinogenic agents; (9) during neurosurgery, especially when this involves stimulation of the temporal lobes; and (10) following some brain injuries.

hypernea, hypernoia *Obs.* Exaggerated mental activity; hyperpsychosis. See *apsychosis.*

hyperontomorph One of the two constitutional types distinguished by Beu, characterized by long, lanky bodies with short intestines, in contrast to the *mesontomorph;* corresponds roughly to Kretschmer's *asthenic type.*

hyperopia Far-sightedness, long-sightedness. As a result of an error in refraction or flattening of the globe of the eye, parallel rays are focused behind the retina. See *myopia.*

hyperorexia *Bulimia* (q.v.); excessive hunger. See *eating disorders.*

hyperosmia Exaggerated sensitiveness to odors.

hyperpathia Sensation of pain in a hypesthetic zone as may be observed in association with lesions of the thalamus.

hyperpathia, thalamic See *thalamus.*

hyperphoria See *heterophoria.*

hyperphrasia Hyperlogia; polyphrasia; excessive loquacity.

hyperphrenia 1. Excessive mental activity, such as occurs in the manic phase of manic-depressive psychosis or in the severe preoccupations associated with the psychoneuroses. 2. Intellectual capacity far above the average. See *phrenalgia.*

hyperpituitary constitution See *constitution, hyperpituitary.*

hyperplasia Increase in the bulk of a part or organ of the body, due to an increase in the number of the individual tissue elements, excluding tumor formation.

Some pathologists make this increase in *number* the criterion for sharply distinguishing *hyperplasia* from *hypertrophy* (q.v.), which is defined by them as an increase in bulk due to the increase in *size* of the individual tissue elements. Others restrict the usage of the concept of hyperplasia to cases in which the proliferative changes mentioned are not occurring to meet a demand for increased functional activity or to compensate for an organic inferiority elsewhere, which would fall under their definition of hypertrophy.

hyperponesis Increased invisible motor activity, measurable electromyographically, presumed to be due to hyperactivity of neurons of the motor portion of the nervous system. Hyperponesis is seen in patients with clinical depressions; increased invisible motor activity is also seen with increasing age.

hyperpragia Excessive mentation; the type of mental activity commonly observed during the manic phase of manic-depressive psychosis, namely, an excess of thinking and feeling.

hyperpragic Relating to or characterized by excessive mental activity; in constitutional medicine, by excessive or increased activity of various systems and organs of the body, with a *miopragic* type.

hyperprosessis, hyperprosexia Exaggerated attention. Diminished attention is called *hypoprosessis.*

hyperpselaphesia Eulenburg's term for tactile oversensitiveness.

hyperpsychosis See *apsychosis.*

hypersexuality A disturbance of sexuality in which there is a greatly or morbidly increased sexual activity. Since all neurotics are unable to attain complete sexual satisfaction, any neurotic may show this symptom. He might try to gain satisfaction through persistent repetition of the sexual act, yet never achieve that quelling of desire that comes with complete orgasm. Also he may boast about the frequency with which he can perform the sexual act, or behave in an "oversexed" way, giving sexual connotations to many of his relationships or activities. This occurs for two reasons: (1) the dammed-up sexuality will come out in unsuitable places at inconvenient times, just because it cannot be satisfied with orgasm; (2) there is a narcissistic need to prove through such activity that the subject is not impotent or frigid.

When the symptom of hypersexuality is so marked as to dominate the clinical picture, additional factors are at work. The genital apparatus is being used to discharge some nongenital, warded-off, and dammed-up need. These needs might stem from different sources. The primary purpose of the sexual activity might be to obtain self-esteem by contradicting an inner feeling of inferiority with erotic "successes." Whether the person is a *Don Juan* or a *nymphomaniac* (qq.v.), "Analysis shows that the condition depends on a marked narcissistic attitude, on a dependency on narcissistic supplies, on an intense fear over loss of love, and a corresponding pregenital and sadistic coloration of the total sexuality. . . . The sadistic attitude is manifest in the attempt to coerce the partner by violence into 'giving' complete sexual satisfaction and therewith a re-establishment of self-esteem." As soon as the sexual act has been performed, the patient is no longer interested in his partner, but must find another, both because his narcissistic needs demand that he continually prove his ability to excite other partners, and because this partner has failed to satisfy him completely. Another source of hypersexuality which can be traced to nongenital needs is an unconscious homosexual inclination. Though aroused, the patient cannot, through increased heterosexual activity, obtain the satisfaction he seeks. Still another source, operative in women, might be an intense penis envy.

Through nymphomanic activities the patient seeks to fulfill the wish phantasy of depriving the man of his penis. (Fenichel, *PTN*) See *erotomania*.

hypersomnia Sleep of excessive duration as in lethargic encephalitis; sometimes used to refer to coma vigil. See *mutism, akinetic; sleep disorders*.

hypersomnolence disorder Idiopathic central nervous system hypersomnolence consists of excessive daytime sleepiness and persistently prolonged major sleep periods (nine hours or longer). Unlike narcolepsy, this disorder has no attacks of refreshing sleep during the day. See *sleep disorders*.

hypersthenic In constitutional medicine, excessive tension and strength or a hyperfunction of the lymphatic elements and organs, in contrast to an *asthenic lymphatic* condition.

In Pende's constitutional system, the term is used in connection with the *hypertonic* type to designate a subgroup of both the *megalosplanchnic hypervegetative* constitution and the *microsplanchnic hypovegetative* constitution.

In Mills's system, the term has a sense that corresponds roughly to the characteristics of the *pyknic* type of Kretschmer.

hypertelorism Excessive distance between two parts or organs. D.M. Greig's term denotes a form of mental deficiency characterized by general mental and physical retardation, not very dissimilar to the essential features of Down's syndrome.

hypertension, essential Abnormally high blood pressure without known cause. In psychiatry, many consider this to be a psychophysiologic (psychosomatic) cardiovascular disorder. Alexander believes that the specific dynamic pattern is the repression of all hostile, competitive tendencies, which are intimidating because of fears of retaliation and failure; this general readiness for aggression is combined with a passive-receptive, dependent longing to be rid of the aggression. But these dependent longings arouse inferiority feelings and thereby reactivate the hostile competitiveness; this leads to anxiety and the need for further inhibition of aggressive, hostile impulses. This vicious circle is the basis for arterial hypertension, but the syndrome probably occurs only in those whose vaso-motor system (and/or kidneys and/or endocrine constitution) is predisposed to instability, perhaps by virtue of inherited factors. Essential hypertension is probably so frequent in the American business executive because in business a great amount of aggression seems necessary.

"A fully consummated aggressive attack has three phases. At first there is the preparation of the attack in phantasy, its planning and its mental visualization. This is the conceptual phase. Second, there is the vegetative preparation of the body for concentrated activity: changes in metabolism and blood distribution. . . . Finally there is the neuromuscular phase, the consummation of the aggressive act itself through muscular activity. . . . If the inhibition takes place as early as the psychological preparation for an aggressive attack, a migraine attack develops. If the second phase, the vegetative preparation for the attack, develops but the process does not progress further, hypertension follows. And finally if the voluntary act is inhibited only in the third phase, an inclination toward arthritic symptoms or vasomotor syncope may develop." (Alexander, F. *Psychosomatic Medicine, Its Principles and Applications,* 1950) See *encephalopathy, hypertensive.*

hyperthermia, malignant A rare and potentially fatal hypermetabolic disorder, susceptibility to which is transmitted as an autosomal dominant trait. Episodes of malignant hyperthermia are usually triggered by some pharmacologic agent, such as succinylcholine (the one most frequently reported), anesthetics, haloperidol, tricyclic antidepressants, and monoamine oxidase inhibitors.

Clinical manifestations include unexplained tachycardia, cardiac dysrhythmias, spasm of the masseter with administration of succinylcholine, fulminant increase in temperature (e.g. a rise of 1°C every 5 minutes), increased respiratory rate, metabolic acidosis, and increased tissue utilization of oxygen with peripheral cyanosis.

Treatment includes hyperventilation with 100% oxygen and intravenous dantrolene sodium, a hydantoin derivative which is a direct-acting skeletal muscle relaxant. Since dantrolene therapy was introduced in 1979, mortality of episodes has fallen from approximately 60% to less than 30%.

hyperthymia State of overactivity, greater than average but less than the overactivity of the manic stage of manic-depressive psychosis.

Hyperthymia is a subdivision of *cyclothymia* (q.v.). It is probably very close to hypomania, but occupies a position between normal overactivity and hypomania.

hypertonia Extreme tension of the muscles; spasticity or rigidity.

hypertrophic obesity See *obesity, hyperplastic.*

hypertrophy The process of overgrowth, or the kind of increase in the bulk of an organ or part of the body which is not due to tumor formation.

Some pathologists restrict usage of the term to denote greater bulk through increase in *size,* but not in *number,* of the individual tissue elements; it is then contrasted with *hyperplasia.*

Other pathologists limit the term to those cases in which the increase in size meets a demand for increased functional activity or compensates for an organic inferiority elsewhere. The other cases fall under their definition of hyperplasia.

In the field of constitutional medicine, the term is used by some typologists to indicate undue size of a body area relative to other parts of the body.

hypertropia A type of strabismus in which the affected eye deviates upward.

hypertychia (-tik′ē-á) See *euphoria.*

hyperuricemia Abnormally high blood content of uric acid; seen typically in gout, but it occurs also as an inborn metabolic disorder in children. In the latter case, symptoms include severe mental retardation, spastic cerebral palsy, choreoathetosis, and bizarre self-destructive behavior such as biting of the flesh—sometimes so deeply that the bones themselves are gnawed.

hyperuricosuria See *syndrome, Lesch-Nyhan.*

hypervegetative See *hypovegetative; type, hypervegetative.*

hyperventilation Overbreathing. See *syndrome, hyperventilation*

hypesthesia Subnormal sensitiveness to a tactile stimulus.

hyphedonia A state in which the subject experiences slight pleasure from what normally gives great pleasure.

hypn- Combining form meaning sleep, from Gr. *hýpnos.*

hypnagogic Inducing sleep; hypnotic. See *imagery, hypnagogic.*

hypnagogic intoxication See *intoxication, hypnogogic.*

hypnalgia Dream-pain.

hypnenergia *Obs.* Somnambulism. Other obsolete terms include *hypnobadicus, hypnobadisis, hypnobasis, hypnobatesis,* and *hypnonergia.*

hypnic Relating to or causing sleep; hypnotic.

hypnoanalysis In psychoanalytic therapy, an aid to removing resistances that prevent awareness of unconscious material. Regression and revivication under hypnosis may open up pathways to memories that are not available to the patient at an adult, waking level. It is obvious, however, that no matter what material is elicited in the trance state, in order to be effective it must be integrated and incorporated into the more conscious layers of the psyche.

hypnobades, hypnobat (hip-nob′á-dēz) *Obs.* Somnambulist.

hypnobat (hip′nō-bat) A sleep walker; somnambulist.

hypnobatia *Obs.* The performance, during sleep, of actions that take place in the waking stage.

hypnocatharsis "Essentially, this method consists of hypnotizing the patient and having the patient free-associate while in this state. Often memories will flow more easily under such circumstances. The difficulties, however, lie in the fact that all patients are not hypnotizable and that hypnosis casts a shroud of mystery about the process, making a 'mystic' affair of that which one desires the patient to be very clear about." (Kraines, S.H. *The Therapy of the Neuroses and Psychoses,* 1948)

hypnodia *Obs.* Somnolence.

hypnogenic spot See *spot, hypnogenic.*

hypnograph An instrument to measure sleep. The basic hypnograph consists of a recording pen attached to a coil of the sleeper's bed so that any movement is communicated to the instrument and traced in a graph. This gives a measure of the amount of gross motor activity during sleep. In the same manner other functions may be tested during sleep, and there are modifications of the hypnograph that will measure any or all of the following: blood pressure, pulse, temperature, respiration, metabolic rate, muscle tone, reflexes, urine volume, sweating, gastric secretion, lacrimal and salivary secretion, etc.

hypnolepsy *Obs. Narcolepsy* (q.v.).

hypnology The science of sleep and hypnotism.

hypnonarcosis A state of deep sleep induced through hypnosis.

hypnopathy Hypnolepsy.

hypnophobia Fear of falling asleep.

hypnophrenosis A general term, introduced by C.H. Schutze, for various forms of *sleep disorders* (q.v.).

hypnopompic Sleep-dispelling. Relating to or ushering out the semiconscious state between the stages of sleep and awakening.

hypnosigenesis Induction of hypnosis.

hypnosis The state or condition induced through hypnotism. The subject to be hypnotized is commanded to fix his attention, usually by staring at an object, while the hypnotist keeps repeating in a monotonous manner that the subject is growing tired, drowsy, and sleepy.

Stephen Black (in *Modern Perspectives in World Psychiatry,* ed. J.G. Howells, 1971) defines hypnosis as "a sleepless state of decreased consciousness which occurs in most animal phyla as a result of constrictive or rhythmic stimuli usually imparted by another organism and which may be distinguished from sleep by the presence of catatonia, relative awareness or increased suggestibility and in which direct contact is made with the unconscious mind in man."

As defined by the British Medical Association (1965): "A temporary condition of altered attention in the subject which may be induced by another person and in which a variety of phenomena may appear spontaneously or in response to verbal or other stimuli. These phenomena include alterations in consciousness and memory, increased susceptibility to suggestion, and the production in the subject of responses and ideas unfamiliar to him in his usual state of mind. Further, phenomena such as anesthesia, paralysis and muscle rigidity, and vaso-motor changes can be produced and removed in the hypnotic state."

"Hypnosis may be applied therapeutically in many ways. We shall distinguish for the present between three such applications:

"1. The hypnotically induced sleep is used directly as a healing factor.

"2. The suggestion given in hypnosis is directed outright against the psychic or physical symptom which is to be eliminated.

"3. Forgotten experiences are brought back to memory in hypnosis and are made accessible to the consciousness (cathartic hypnosis)." (Schilder, P., & Kauders, O. *Hypnosis,* 1927)

hypnosis, cathartic See *hypnotism.*

hypnosis, coaxing See *hypnosis, father.*

hypnosis, dependency in The patient under hypnosis may establish an exaggerated transference to the analyst based upon an overvaluation of the power and authority of the hypnotist. This exaggerated identification is called dependency in hypnosis. The patient plunges himself into a subordinate position in order to achieve his objectives, but such a position is incompatible with normal self-esteem. "It tends to destroy assertiveness, to sap independence, and to vitiate activity and creative self-fulfillment. It may render the patient progressively more helpless—an automaton who lives without a self and is secure and confident only insofar as the omniscient hypnotist can shield him from harm and gratify his needs for him. Unable to achieve his goals through his own efforts, the patient may become increasingly hostile and finally may interrupt the therapy with a return to his neurotic symptoms." (Wolberg, L.R. *Hypnoanalysis,* 1945)

hypnosis, father "We could maintain that hypnotic submission is to be traced back to blind obedience, but this again to the transference of paternal fixation. There are only two kinds of hypnosis: father-hypnosis (that might also be called fear-hypnosis) and mother-hypnosis (in other words, coaxing-hypnosis)." (Ferenczi, FCT)

hypnotic See *sedation.*

hypnotism The theory and practice of inducing hypnosis or a state resembling sleep induced by psychical means. It is also known as braidism (or Braidism) and induced somnambulism.

hypnotization, collective Simultaneous hypnosis of several subjects.

hypo-, hyp- Combining form meaning under, below, less than (the normal), from Gr. *hypó.*

hypoaffective type See *type, hypoaffective.*

hypoalgesia Lessened sensibility to painful stimuli.

hypoboulia, hypobulia Deficiency or inadequacy of the will or will power, seen primarily in schizophrenic patients. See *unforthcomingness; will, disturbances of the.*

hypocathexis See *cathexis.*

hypochondria *Hypochondriasis* (q.v.).

hypochondriac language See *speech, organ.*

hypochondriacal psychosis See *monosymptomatic hypochondriacal psychosis.*

hypochondriasis Hypochondria; hypochondriacal neurosis; somatic overconcern; morbid attention to the details of body functioning and/or exaggeration of any symptom, no matter how insignificant. One of the *somatoform disorders* (q.v.), characterized by preoccupation with the fear or belief of having a physical disease for which there are no demonstrable organic findings or known physiologic mechanisms. The affected person interprets any number of physical signs or symptoms unrealistically as indicative of serious disease. Despite reassurance by physicians that no illness exists and continuing failure on examination to uncover evidence of underlying organic pathology, the persisting fear or belief of illness colors the person's entire life and interferes with social and occupational functioning. See *sick role.*

Hypochondriasis is rare as a primary disorder, and most cases are secondary to a depressive illness or some other disorder.

Although hypochondriasis may appear in the form of a specific neurosis, it may also occur in association with such disorders as anxiety neurosis, obsessive-compulsive neurosis, and most often with the initial states of any psychosis. The hypochondriacal patient is typically self-centered, seclusive, and sometimes almost monomaniacal in his attention to his body; his major environmental contacts are somatically colored and he seeks one consultation after another with his family physician or with as many specialists as will agree to reexamine him. In other cases, preoccupation with his own health leads the hypochondriac to seek a career in medicine; similarly, he may become a health faddist. If he uses reaction formation as a defense, hypochondriacal concern may ultimately be expressed in a total neglect of his health and well-being.

Psychodynamically, hypochondriacal anxiety is seen often to represent castration anxiety; further it may represent an attempt to expiate guilt feelings by the turning of hostility and sadism onto the self.

"Hypochondriasis is a chronic complaint habit. It may arise from a variety of sources. Imitation of observed adult patterns, the desire to retain privileges derived during a period of actual illness, unhappiness at home or at school, ill-treatment, overwork with no recreational outlets, solitary life, parental oversolicitude, feeling of insecurity, medical mismanagement, and fear of punishment may all contribute to the development of somatic complaint on a psychogenic basis." (Strecker, E.A., & Ebaugh, F.G. *Practical Clinical Psychiatry,* 1935)

Freud regarded hypochondriasis as an *actual neurosis,* as he does *neurasthenia* and *anxiety neurosis.* "Hypochondria, like organic disease, manifests itself in distressing and painful bodily sensations and also concurs with organic disease in its effect upon the distribution of the libido. The hypochondriac withdraws both interest and libido—the latter specially marked—from the objects of the outer world and concentrates both upon the organ which engages his attention. A difference between hypochondria and organic disease now becomes evident: in the latter, the distressing sensations are based upon demonstrable organic changes; in the former, this is not so. But it would be entirely in keeping with our general conception of the processes of neurosis if we decide to say that hypochondria must be right; organic changes cannot be absent in it either." (*CP*)

hypochondrophthisis (-kon-drof'this-sis) *Obs.* The wasting away of the body in hypochondriasis.

hypochoresis Defecation.

hypodepression Simple depression, i.e. mild depression occurring as an episode in manic-depressive psychosis. This form of depressive episode may be difficult to distinguish from normal grief and from so-called psychoneurotic depressive reaction. As in all clinical depressions, however, lowering of the self-esteem and self-depreciatory, self-accusatory thought content are seen in hypodepression but do not occur in normal grief (mourning). For differentiation of hypodepression from psychoneurotic depression, see *depression, psychoneurotic; depression, reactive.*

hypoergasia The depressed type of manic-depressive psychosis.

hypoesthesia, vaginal See *frigidity, sexual.*

hypoevolutism Deficient morphological, physiological, and psychological development; applicable to the body as a whole, to particular systems, organs, and tissues, as well as to the psyche and aspects thereof. One usually distinguishes between *ontogenetic* and *phylogenetic* hypoevolutism.

hypofrontality hypothesis The theory that early developmental abnormalities of the frontal lobe and, in particular, of the dorsolateral prefrontal cortex may produce the syndrome of schizophrenia. Consistent with such a hypothesis are the following: (1) frontal lobe signs such as lack of initiative, poor insight, social withdrawal, flat affect, and poor judgment resemble the negative symptoms of schizophrenia; (2) some studies have found a relative decrease in cerebral blood flow in the frontal lobes of schizophrenics; (3) some positive emission tomography studies have demonstrated a relative decrease in glucose metabolism in the frontal lobe in schizophrenics; (4) slow frontal EEG activity has been reported in schizophrenics; (5) eyetracking dysfunction, one of the most consistent findings of different research groups, may be due to disinhibition of frontal eye field mechanisms.

The posited frontal lobe development abnormality might be genetic in origin, but it could also be a result of other factors such as maternal nutritional disorders or maternal alcohol consumption during pregnancy, difficulties during delivery, or adverse enviroment during the first two years of life (e.g. nutritional deficiencies, emotional deprivation or lack of appropriate stimulation, viral and other infections).

hypofunction Reduced action or function.

hypoglossal hemiplegia alternans See *hemiplegia alternans.*

hypoglycemia Concentrations of blood sugar below the normal range. In psychiatry, hypoglycemia is of interest (1) in insulin coma treatment, where the blood sugar is deliberately lowered by injection of insulin; and (2) in functional hypoglycemia (functional hyperinsulinism), which is believed by some to be the psychophysiologic disturbance at the basis of many fatigue states. Franz Alexander (*Psychosomatic Medicine, Its Principles and Applications,* 1950) believes that under the influence of emotional protest and regression, the vegetative functions may regress toward a state of passivity and relaxation characterized by a preponderance of parasympathetic tonus. The organism is then forced either by external pressure or by the internal voice of conscience to undertake activity, even though the person is physiologically in a state of relaxation. Alexander calls this "vegetative retreat." The specific psychodynamic constellation is the conflict between passive, dependent wishes and reactive aggressive ambition—a conflict, to be sure, almost universal in our civilization, but in fatigue states the following factors are more specific: little hope of success in a struggle against insuperable odds; no genuine incentive; the inconstancy of anxiety; and in many male cases, a feminine identification, which opposes aggressive, ambitious attitudes.

hypokinesis Slow or diminished movement. It may be physically or psychically determined. Depressed patients are generally hypokinetic.

hypolepsiomania A general term, coined by Andral, to denote the various forms of monomania.

hypologia Reduction in speech, used usually to refer to cases of organic origin in which capacity for speech is limited.

hypomania See *mania.*

hypomelancholia Mild case of the depressed form of manic-depressive psychosis.

hypomotility Diminished or slowed-down movement.

hyponoia *Rare.* Deficient mental activity; hypopsychosis. See *apsychosis.*

hyponoic Kretschmer's term for hysterical reactions that stem from the deeper psychic layers. "If the stimulation of the experience is overstrong or the personality, as a result of degeneration, is dissociable with abnormal ease, the deeper psychic layers, which we have already begun to study in hysterical volitional processes, are not always laid bare by simple repression, but through a splitting of the personality. These deeper layers, now working separately, in the field of ideational content furnish us with *hyponoic formations* belonging to an early ontogenetic functional type. We recognize these hyponoic formations in mythology and the art of primitives; in the modern normal adult person, we can study them, above all in the dream, and, aside from hysteria, very frequently in the schizophrenias." (*HS*)

hypophoria See *heterophoria.*

hypophrasia Bradyphrasia; slowness of speech, such as is seen as a part of the generalized psychomotor retardation of depressed patients.

hypophrenosis Southard's term for mental retardation.

hypophysial cachexia See *cachexia, hypophysial.*

hypoplasia In pathology, the underdevelopment of a tissue or organ, whether due to deficient number or deficient size of the cells that constitute the body structure in question.

The usage of the term in constitutional medicine is somewhat different, and varies. Kretschmer applies it to underdevelopment of certain body areas; for instance, to a hypoplastic condition of the midface. Other typologists distinguish between relative and absolute hypoplasia.

When hypoplasia is *uniform* and relates to an organism as a whole, it results in a dwarf. However, it occurs more frequently as a *selective* condition, and in this case it implies *dysplasia.*

hypoplastic Pertaining to the condition of hypoplasia or, in constitutional medicine, to a type characterized by Bartel's *status hypoplasticus* and equivalent to Rokitansky-Benecke's *habitus phthisicus* (qq.v.).

hypoprosessis See *hyperprosessis.*

hypopsychosis Hyponoia. See *apsychosis.*

hyposomnia Lack of sleep; sleeping for shorter periods than usual. See *sleep disorders.*

hypostasis (hī-pos'tà-sis) The obstructive mechanism by which one hereditary factor is prevented by the manifestation of another factor from being phenotypically expressible. The masking effect itself is known as *epistasis,* (q.v.) while the factor that is hidden is called *hypostatic.*

hyposthenia Deficient strength.

hyposthenic Pertaining to or suffering from hyposthenia. In the systems of constitutional types described by Mills and by Pende, the term contrasts the *hyposthenic* with the *hypersthenic* variety of constitution and corresponds roughly to the characteristics of Kretschmer's *asthenic* type.

hypotaxia Durand introduced this term for the emotional rapport existing between the subject and the operator in a hypnotic setting. E. Jones refers to the relationship as *affective suggestion.*

hypotaxis Light, hypnotic sleep.

hypothalamotomy A psychosurgical procedure, employing the same technique as in *thalamotomy* (q.v.) and producing partial ablation of the hypothalamic area—performed subsequently in the thalamotomy cases that have not responded to the original operation.

hypothalamus A phylogenetically old constellation of nuclei lying in the ventral part of the diencephalon just above the optic chiasm and sella turcica. "It is the principal centre in the forebrain for integration of visceral functions involving the autonomic nervous system. The constituent nuclei may be divided into four groups: (1) anterior including the paraventricular and the supraoptic nuclei, (2) the middle including the tuber, dorsomedial and ventromedial hypothalamic nuclei, (3) the lateral area, and (4) the posterior group including the posterior hypothalamic nucleus and mammillary bodies. Pervading the whole area are ill-defined neurons, grouped under the general heading of 'substantia grisea centralis.' " (Fulton, J.F. *Physiology of the Nervous System,* 1949)

Functions of the hypothalamus include regulation of sexual activity, water, fat, and carbohydrate metabolism, and heat regulation. The posterior hypothalamus is concerned primarily with the sympathetic system, the middle and anterior nuclei with the parasympathetic system; but all levels of the structure are subject to regulation from thalamic, striatal, and cortical levels.

The following hypothalamic syndromes are recognized: hypothermia, hypersomnia, the adiposogenital syndrome, diabetes insipidus, and autonomic epilepsy.

hypothermia, accidental The loss of thermoregulatory ability, found most often in older patients being treated with phenothiazines. Exposure to cold in such persons requires prompt treatment to prevent widespread physical deterioration or possibly death.

hypothesis, antagonism The theory that the development of one specific disorder generally precludes the development of a specific second disorder, as in the belief that there is a mutual antagonism between epilepsy and schizophrenia. The *affinity hypothesis* is the opposite: the development of one specific illness puts the subject at higher than normal risk for the development of a second specific illness.

hypothesis, biogenic amine *Catecholamine hypothesis* (q.v.).

hypothesis, dopamine The theory that schizophrenic disorders are related to or caused by some abnormality in the metabolism of dopamine in the brain. See *epinephrine.*

hypothesis, Fiamberti See *Fiamberti hypothesis.*

hypothesis, hypofrontality See *hypofrontality hypothesis.*

hypothesis, mediumistic Baynes's hypothesis that the schizophrenic patient is closer than others to the *collective unconscious* and is strategically in a position to recognize forthwith the early signs of his own disintegration; therefore he is able to foresee the unconscious trend of events better than can those whose firm clinging to existing forms and conditions renders them insensible to such signs.

hypothesis, structural See *id; structural.*

hypothesis, topographic See *id.*

hypothesis, transmethylation See *transmethylation.*

hypothymia Diminution in the intensity of the affective or emotional state.

hypothyroidism Deficiency or absence of thyroid hormone secretion, in the adult resulting in lethargy, sluggishness, lowered basal metabolic rate, reduced oxygen consumption, loss of hair, a relatively hard edema of the tissues (myxedema), obesity, and mental changes. Psychomotor retardation and generalized sluggishness of mentation are almost universal, and depression is frequent. Also seen are paranoid ideas, although the general intellectual dulling tends to minimize self-criticism. When paranoid ideas are prominent or systematized, the condition may be termed *myxedema madness.* Thyroid failure in the infant produces *cretinism* (q.v.).

hypotonia Subnormal tension of the muscles; flaccidity.

hypovegetative In contradistinction to the *hypervegetative* biotype of Viola and Pende, the constitutional type in which the animal system (muscular, nervous, and skeletal systems) predominates in forming contact with the external world, over the organs in the trunk, which represent the nutritional system and are associated with the vegetative life of an individual.

The biotype thus described corresponds exactly to the *dolichomorphic* and *microsplanchnic* types and approximately to Kretschmer's *asthenic.* See *type, hypervegetative.*

hypovigility Pathological subnormal awareness or response, or complete lack of it, to external stimuli. Hypovigility is the opposite of exaggerated distractibility. Although exaggerated distractibility sometimes occurs in catatonic excitement, hypovigility is more characteristic of the schizophrenic group as a whole. "The [schizophrenic] patients converse only rarely with those around them even when they are talking a great deal. The incitement to speech as well as its content originates for the most part autistically from inner sources." (Bleuler, E. *Dementia Praecox or the Group of Schizophrenias,* 1950) Bleuler considers this an important point in the differential diagnosis of manic schizophrenia and true mania.

hypoxyphilia A paraphilia in which oxygen deprivation is a necessary condition for full sexual satisfaction.

hypsarrhythmia An EEG pattern associated with certain infantile spasms of epileptic origin; also known as *major dysrhythmia* and *myoclonic encephalitis.* It affects children, usually under the age of 1 year, and appears in the form of generalized, symmetrical flexion spasms lasting a few seconds. Between attacks, the EEG shows a diffuse dysrhythmia of the delta-wave type. Psychomotor regression with loss of motor skills and mental deterioration is typical; complete recovery is unusual.

hypsophobia Fear of a high place.

hysteria Currently, the term is used in several ways: (1) to describe a pattern of behavior, the *hysterical personality* (q.v.); (2) to refer to a conversion symptom, such as hysterical paralysis (see *dissociative disorders*); (3) to refer to a psychoneurotic disorder, such as conversion hysteria or *anxiety hysteria* (q.v.); (4) to refer to a specific psychopathologic pattern in which repression is the major defense; and (5) loosely, as a term of opprobrium.

Conversion hysteria appears clinically as (1) a physical manifestation without accompanying structural lesion, or as a peripheral physiologic dysfunction; (2) a calm mental attitude (called "la belle indifference" by Janet) that is specifically limited to the physical symptom and not generalized to include the entire life of the patient; and (3) episodic mental states, in which a limited but homogeneous group of functions occupies the field of consciousness, often to the complete exclusion of the usual contents of consciousness—fugues, somnambulisms, dream states, hypnotic states, etc. There is, in other words, a dissociation of the mental or bodily functions, and the dissociated functions may operate in coexistence with normal consciousness, or they may operate to the exclusion of the other functions. In conversion hysteria, the split-off function is ordinarily a unity and the splitting is seldom into more than two parts; thus it is commonly said that in schizophrenia the splitting is molecular or fragmentary, whereas in hysteria it is molar or massive.

Hysteria has usually been found to occur more frequently in women, with an estimated lifetime prevalence of 3 to 6/1,000. Onset is usually before the age of 35 years, although hysterical symptoms may occur as part of some other disorder in later years.

M.H. Hollender (*Archives of General Psychiatry 26,* 1972) views conversion hysteria as a dramatized message, expressed in nonverbal and usually pantomimic form when more conventional forms of expression are blocked. The message typically involves a forbidden wish or impulse, its prohibition, or some compromise between the two.

There are no physical symptoms in hysteria that cannot be produced by volition or by emotion, although it may ordinarily be possible to maintain these symptoms for only a short time. Further, the physical symptoms correspond strikingly with the usual lay concepts of disease. Thus hysterical paralysis shows an exact delimitation and an excessive intensity, and it is more frequently accompanied by sensory disturbances than organic paralysis.

The *motor symptoms* include paralysis with or without contracture, tics, tremors, etc. The *sensory symptoms* include anesthesiae, paresthesiae, and hyperesthesiae; their distribution is rarely according to anatomical lines; they vary at different examinations; and they are susceptible to suggestions. Blindness and deafness are also seen. The *visceral symptoms* include anorexia, bulimia, vomiting, hiccup or respiratory tic, various abdominal complaints, flatulence.

The *mental symptoms* include amnesiae, somnambulisms, fugues, trances, dreamstates, hysterical fits or attacks. The amnesia is commonly for a circumscribed series of events, and occasionally is for the entire period of life up to a certain recent point. In a fugue, the patient suddenly leaves one activity and goes on a journey that has no apparent relation to it and for which she has amnesia afterward. Somnambulisms are fugues that begin during sleep and are usually of shorter duration than fugues. The movements of the somnambulist are in response to the manifest or latent content of the dream; the meaning may be an escape from the temptation of the bed, or a movement toward a positive goal that represents gratification or reassurance. In double or multiple personalities, there is further elaboration so that the groups of dissociated functions when fully conscious and in charge of the motor apparatus can at least superficially appear as a complete personality. Hysterical spells are a pantomimic expression of (mainly oedipal) phantasies; in them can be seen condensation, displacement, representation by the opposite, exaggeration of details that represent the whole, reversal of the sequence of events, multiple identifications, and suitability for plastic representation. Dreamstates are similar to these but here the pantomimic discharge is lacking; dreamstates may represent repression, orgasm, death wishes turned against the ego, or the blocking of any hostile impulse.

Until Freud advanced his theory of hysteria, there had been few attempts at explanation. Charcot had described the "grande attaque hysterique" with its four phases: (1) epileptoid phase; (2) large movement phase; (3) phase of "attitudes passionelles"; (4) the "délire terminal." Janet's theories of restriction of the field of consciousness and the hereditary tendency to dissociate at moments of great emotion did not explain what it was that brought the dissociation to pass. Freud's earlier theory was that the hysterical attack was a symbolic representation of a repressed sexual trauma. He believed that the patient had undergone a passive sexual experience in childhood, but that this psychical experience could not find adequate discharge because the nervous system was incapable of dealing with it at that time; the experience was forgotten, but with puberty the memory of it was reawakened. But adequate discharge (*abreaction*) was still not possible, because the memory conflicted with the conscious strivings of the personality and/or culture. Instead, the strong affect associated with the memory is diverted into the wrong somatic channels (*conversion*) and the hysterical symptom results. Freud and Breuer found that *catharsis*—reactivation of the childhood memory, at that time by means of hypnosis, and allowing abreaction—removed the hysterical symptom. This theory was later revised when it was discovered that the sexual traumata uncovered in hysterical patients were really fictitious memories designed to mask the autoerotic activities of childhood.

The hysterical attack itself may be aroused (1) associatively, if the content of the complex is stirred by a conscious occurrence; (2) organically, if for any reason the libidinal cathexis exceeds a certain amount; (3) in the service of the primary tendency (paranosic gain) as an expression of *flight into illness* if reality becomes painful or frightening; (4) in the service of the epinosic gain, to achieve some end through an attack. To the hysterical patient, all sexuality represents infantile incestuous love, so she cannot love fully if the genitals are present because of the oedipal fears. The conversion symptom is a distorted substitute for sexual (and/or aggressive) gratification; but because of the effectiveness of repression, the symptom leads to suffering rather than gratificatory pleasure.

The choice of the afflicted region is determined by (1) the unconscious sexual phantasies and the corresponding erogeneity of the area; (2) somatic compliance (*locus minori resistentiae*); (3) the situation in which the decisive repression occurred; (4) the ability of the organ to symbolize the unconscious drive in question.

Since Freud, many investigators have stressed pregenital determinants of conversion hysteria, and particularly oral conflicts arising from intense frustration of oral-receptive needs or excessive gratification of those needs by one or both parents.

Conversion symptoms have also been viewed as unconsciously simulated illnesses, with the patient enacting a sick role as a way to reduce, mask, avoid, or deny a variety of other psychological disturbances (such as anxiety from any cause, identity problems, depression, and incipient schizophrenia). The disorder may be monosymptomatic or may involve many symptoms; these will sometimes be crude and transparent imitations, but equally often they can be accurate simulations of disease or exaggerations of symptoms of genuine physical problems. (Ziegler, F.J., Imboden, J.B., & Rodgers, D.A. *Journal of the American Medical Association 186*, 1963)

hysteria, anxiety See *anxiety hysteria.*

hysteria, combat See *shell shock.*

hysteria, degenerative See *psychosis, degenerative.*

hysteria, epidemic Hysteria or hysteroid disturbances apparently acquired by association with hysterical patients.

hysteria, fixation That form of conversion hysteria in which the area or function affected is one that had previously been, or is presently, the site of some organic disorder. An example is conversion paralysis of an area that had been wounded in an accident. Closely allied to fixation hysteria is *pathohysteria*, wherein a chronic disease process is itself productive of hysterical symptoms. A more general term for the latter phenomenon is *pathoneurosis.*

hysteria, major Grand hystérie; a clinical syndrome of hysteria, perhaps first described at length by Charcot, later by Richer. It is characterized by several stages: (1) the aural stage; (2) the stage of epileptoid convulsions; (3) the phase of tonic, then clonic spasms; (4) the phase of intense and dramatic emotional expressions; (5) the stage of delirium. The total attack lasts from several minutes up to half an hour. There are many modifications in the form and order of the above states.

Some authorities use the expression *major hysteria* synonymously with *hysteroepilepsy* (q.v.).

hysteria, masked *Obs.* A form of hysteria in which the symptoms resemble those of organic disease.

hysteria, reflex Kretschmer's term for a hysterical sign in which an automatic nervous process, that is, a reflex, plays a dominant part, while the will plays a minor role. Examples of reflex hysteria are simple spasm, tremors, and tics.

hysteria, retention Hysteria resulting not from splitting of consciousness or dissociation, but rather from failure to react to the traumatic situation when it occurred; the dammed-up or retained emotions may later be discharged through *abreaction* (q.v.).

hysteria, traumatic A neurotic illness developing in consequence of an injury (a traumatic neurosis). "The traumatic or accident neuroses rarely occur when the victim of the injury must bear the brunt of the financial responsibility for the accident, as in the case of injuries in sports. There is usually an incubation period between the injury, which may be quite slight, and the appearance of the mentally determined symptoms. This interval before the development of the chronic disabilities is of value in excluding an organic source. It is usually occupied with vague ruminations which tend to be of an imaginative, affective, wish-determined and suggestive nature." (Noyes, A.P. *Modern Clinical Psychiatry,* 1940)

hysterical personality Also known as *histrionic personality;* includes any or all of the following: vain, egocentric, attention-seeking, dramatic description of past symptoms and illnesses with a multiplicity of vaguely described complaints and overtalkativeness during the psychiatric interview; suggestibility; soft, coquettish, graceful, and sexually provocative, although frigid and anxious when close to attaining a sexual goal; easily disappointed, excitable, emotionally labile, and often unaware of inner feelings; dependently demanding in interpersonal

situations; history of excessive operations and hospitalizations.

Such a manipulative adaptational pattern occurs in those with a tendency toward rigid repression of dysphoric emotion and a denial of threatening stimuli; hence it has also been termed *repressive personality.* Conflicts in such patients are often centered around genital incest strivings and/or oral disappointments. See *defense, character.*

hysterical psychosis In current usage, an acute situational reaction consisting of sudden onset of hallucinations, delusions, depersonalization, bizarre behavior, and volatile affect. It rarely lasts beyond three weeks and is sealed off without residua; such reactions typically occur in those of the hysterical or histrionic personality type. Hysterical psychosis includes such entities as *amok,* Imu, *lata, miryachit,* olonism, pibloktoq (Arctic hysteria), Puerto Rican psychosis, *Wihtiko psychosis* (qq.v.).

hysteriform Resembling or having the character of hysteria.

hysteriosis Used mainly by Russian investigators to refer to greatly exaggerated responses of the organism to various stimuli if the latter follow prolonged (and, presumably, exhausting) stimulation of some other part of the organism. When, for example, the tibial nerve of an experimental animal is tetanized for several hours and loses its capacity to respond, mild inflation of a segment of intestine (which ordinarily has little effect on blood pressure, pulse, etc.) may prove fatal to the animal, so exaggerated is the response. The conclusion that has been drawn from such data is that the effects of internal stimuli are highly dependent upon the current functional state of the brain that receives the signals.

hysteroepilepsy *Obs.* "The clumsy name *hystero-epilepsy* originated at a period when epileptiform attacks were still looked upon as neuroses, and when they could not be differentiated. Besides the ordinary epilepsies with lesser striking hysterical symptoms, there are such who in addition show hysteroid attacks. Furthermore, there are hysteriacs, though they are extremely rare, who can imitate or produce an epileptiform attack. . . . *What is usually called hystero-epilepsy is hysteria with severe* *motor attacks,* which were falsely added to the side of epilepsy." (Bleuler, *TP*)

hysterofrenic, hysterofrenatory Aborting or arresting a hysterical attack. For example, when digital pressure is applied to some part of the body to check a hysterical episode, the pressure is called hysterofrenic.

hysterogenic spot See *zone, hysterogenic.*

hysteroid dysphoria See *dysphoria, hysteroid.*

hysteromania *Obs.* Sometimes used synonymously with nymphomania and metromania; it has also been used to describe states of psychomotor overactivity in hysteria.

hysteropathy *Obs.* Hysteria.

hysterophilia Lewandowsky's term for certain clinical conditions resembling hysteria, such as migraine, epileptiform attacks, asthma, membranous enteritis, and occupational cramps.

hysteropnix *Obs. Globus hystericus* (q.v.).

hysterosyntonic A special personality type that represents a mixture of the hysterical personality type and the syntonic personality type. See *syntone.*

5HT 5-Hydroxytryptamine, serotonin.

I

I-boundary In gestalt psychology, the limits defining the range of permissible contact with the outside world, including actions, ideas, people, values, settings, and images with which the subject is willing and free to engage.

I cell disease Mucolipidosis II; a type of mental retardation, probably an autosomal recessive trait, characterized by early onset of retardation, short stature, cytoplasmic inclusions (of cells) in fibroblasts (which also are deficient in lysosomal hydralases and have excessive lipids and mucopolysaccharides), and progressive course leading to death (usually from pneumonia and congestive heart failure) before puberty.

I-complex See *I-persona.*

I-persona By this term Burrow denotes the identity or personality constellation that represents the systematized sum of the organism's cortical, partitive, or symbolic processes. With the attempt, by means of the cephalic segment, to symbolize or project feelings and sensations that are intrinsic to the organism as a whole, there has resulted the artificial conversion of these total sensations into partitive and divisive "feelings" or affects. It is through this mechanism that the I-persona has become a purely partitive, affective identity throughout human interrelations. Contrasted with organic persona. Synonyms: social substantive "I," pseudo-persona. (*The Biology of Human Conflict,* 1937)

I-R specificity See *specificity, individual-response.*

"I," social substantive See *I-persona.*

iatrogeny (ē-à-troj′e-nē) Production or inducement of any harmful change in the somatic or psychic condition of a patient by means of the words or actions of the doctor. The physician may tell the patient that he has an enlarged heart, for example, or low blood pressure, or a glandular disturbance, and such information may provide a nucleus around which the patient builds a neurosis or psychosis.

IB See *body build, index of.*

ICD *International Classification of Diseases* (q.v.).

iceblock theory Kurt Lewin's theory of behavior change in relation to group dynamics, as seen in sensitivity training or T-groups: (1) existing attitudes and behavior must be unfrozen; (2) group members are encouraged to consider and explore new attitudes and behavior in a supporting climate; and (3) the new attitudes and behavior are frozen into habit patterns.

ichthyophobia (ik-thē-ō-fō′bē-à) Fear of or aversion to fish.

iconic storage The registration of sensory information, a step in the memory process that precedes short-term memory. See *memory.*

iconomania Morbid impulse to worship and/ or collect images.

ICS Intracranial self-stimulation.

ictal emotions See *emotions, ictal.*

icterus gravis neonatorum *Kernikterus;* a manifestation of erythroblastosis fetalis in which the infant becomes jaundiced two or three days after birth and, if untreated, develops convulsions, rigidity, and coma. Mortality is high (75%) in untreated cases, and those who survive manifest residua such as mental defect, epilepsy, chorea, or athetosis (*bilirubin encephalopathy*). Treatment is exchange transfusion with Rh-negative whole blood. Those in whom jaundice is severe, however, even when so treated show some degree of mental deficiency; follow-up studies indicate that such children have an IQ that averages 23 points below that of their siblings. (Day, R., & Haines, M.S. *Pediatrics 13,* 1954)

ictus An acute apoplectic stroke; epileptic seizure.

id In psychoanalytic psychology, one of the three divisions of the psyche in the so-called *structural hypothesis* of mental functioning; the other two are the ego and the superego. (In Freud's earlier theory, usually referred to as the *topographic hypothesis,* the psyche was divided into the three systems—conscious, pre-conscious, and unconscious.) The id is completely unconscious and hence partakes of the same processes that characterize the latter; viz., the pleasure principle and the primary process (see *process, primary psychic*). It is the reservoir of the psychic representatives of the drives and of all the phylogenic acquisitions. Freud assumed that the id comprised the total psychic apparatus at birth, and that the ego and superego were later differentiated from what had originally been id. At present, however, many psychoanalysts believe that the id itself is differentiated from the totally undifferentiated psychic apparatus and does not give rise to the ego and superego; but all agree that the id precedes, chronologically, the ego and the superego.

"It is the obscure inaccessible part of our personality; the little we know about it we have learned from the study of dreamwork and the formation of neurotic symptoms, and most of that is of a negative character, and can only be described as being all that the ego is not. We can come nearer to the id with images, and call it chaos, a cauldron of seething excitement. We suppose that it is somewhere in direct contact with somatic processes, and takes over from them instinctual needs and gives them mental expression, but we cannot say in what substratum this contact is made. These instincts fill it with energy, but it has no organization and no unified will, only an impulsion to obtain satisfaction for the instinctual needs, in accordance with the pleasure-principle." (Freud, S. *New Introductory Lectures on PsychoAnalysis,* 1933) "Instinctual cathexes seeking discharge,—that, in our view, is all that the id contains." (ibid.)

idea Any mental content, especially imagining or thinking; often the term connotes a mental process that originates endogenously, rather than in response to any specific external stimulus. In psychoanalytic psychology, an idea is conceived of as existing in two parts, the mental representation of the thing being thought about and an accompanying affective charge; the latter, especially when the idea is "painful," may be split off or dissociated from the mental representation and attached to another idea (whose affective charge then appears inappropriate or excessive).

idea, autochthonous (aw-tok′thō-nus) A psychic disturbance of a delusional character in the sphere of judgment, characterized by the existence of a persistent idea, which the patient believes is put into his mind by an influence foreign to him. The idea seems to exist by itself, beyond the control of the patient, who, most of the time, attributes the existence of such ideas to some malevolent cause. See *delusion, autochthonous.*

idea, by See *by-idea.*

idea-chase *Flight of ideas* (q.v.).

idea, co-conscious See *unconscious,* Prince's definition.

idea, determinative The goal or end result toward which thoughts progress. One of the schizophrenic's disturbances of associations is an inability to keep to the determinative idea or to focus his attention on a central goal. See *associations, disturbances of.*

idea, fixed See *idée fixe.*

idea, imperative Obsession.

idea, obtrusive An obsessive idea that persistently repeats itself in the patient's mind and disturbs the normal flow of his thoughts. The patient considers the obtrusive idea as foreign to his ego and vainly attempts to renounce it.

idea of reference A morbid impression that the conversation, smiling, or other actions of other persons have reference to oneself.

idea, overcharged A dreamer's central idea or conflict that has been exceptionally endowed with inner repressed psychic energy and consequently appears in the dream in the form of various symbols and several identifications.

ideal ego See *ego, ideal.*

ideales *Obs.* Linnaeus formulated three subdivisions of mental disorders, one of which he termed the ideales—disturbances of the intellectual faculties.

idealization Process or act of idealizing. Freud says that idealization is "sexual over-estimation" of the love object. It is "the origin of the peculiar state of being in love." Emphasis is placed upon the object rather than the aim. As Freud maintains, the love object "is aggrandized and exalted in the mind."

Idealization is to be distinguished from *sublimation* and *identification*. The process of sublimation involves the *deflection* of the sexual *aim*, whereas idealization concerns the *object*, not the aim. Identification necessitates a partial alteration of the ego, in the sense that the ego is patterned after the love object, whereas idealization constitutes "an impoverishment of the Ego in respect of libido" in favor of the love object.

Idealization may be related to object libido, as stated above, or to ego libido. In the latter case "some of the self-love which in childhood is directed to the Ego (primary narcism) is transferred or displaced onto a substitute [ego-ideal, superego] which now instead of the infantile Ego is looked upon as 'the possessor of all perfections.' " (Healy et al., *SMP*)

idealize In psychoanalysis, to transfer an inordinate quantity of libido from the ego to a love object. The latter is hypercathected, overevaluated.

idealized image See *idealized self*.

idealized self In Horney's terminology, grandiose overestimation of the self based on identification with the idealized image. The identification is a defense against recognition of the gap between the person as he really is and the person that his neurotic pride says he should be (*idealized image*).

ideas, complex of "The elemental ideas which make up the experiences of any given moment tend to become organized (i.e. synthesized and conserved) into a system or complex of ideas, linked with emotions, feelings and other innate dispositions, so that when one of the ideas belonging to the experience comes to mind the experience as a whole is recalled. We may conveniently term such a system, when in a state of conservation, an *unconscious complex or neurogram, or system of neurograms*." (Prince, M. *The Unconscious*, 1916)

ideas, concatenated Interconnected or interdependent ideas.

ideas, flight of See *flight of ideas*.

ideas, insanity of irrepressible Kraepelin's expression for what is now called the compulsive-obsessive form of psychoneurosis.

ideas, overproductive See *mania*.

idée fixe (ē-dā′ fēks′) A delusion; an unfounded or unreasonable idea that is staunchly maintained despite evidence to the contrary. In contrast is an *imperative idea*, an obsessive thought that is recognized as unreasonable but cannot be resisted. An *autochthonous idea*, on the other hand, is an imperative idea that is attributed to some malevolent influence. See *delusion, autochthonous; idea, autochthonous*.

identical In genetics, *monozygotic*, arising from one egg, as opposed to *dizygotic* or *fraternal*, twin pairs arising from two eggs. It is incorrect, therefore, to speak of "almost identical" twins.

identification Literally, the process of making (or considering to be) the same. In psychoanalysis it carries a similar connotation. When a person incorporates within himself a mental picture of an object and then thinks, feels, and acts as he conceives the object to think, feel, and act, the process is called identification, but the process is largely an unconscious one.

It is a common misconception that conscious emulation can somehow lead to unconscious identification. That this is not primarily true can easily be seen from a consideration of the events that lead to identification in the first place. In the beginning of extrauterine life, the infant is ignorant of any sources of pleasure other than in himself. The mother's breast is thought of as a part of the child's body. This is probably the first identification and represents no emulation of a pleasure-giving object but a reluctant admission of frustrating reality. When hungry the infant is not fond of the mother's breast but angry with it because the breast has allowed him to become hungry. Frustration at the hands of this object is mastered by identification with the object. "Identification is the most primitive method of recognizing external reality; it is, in fact, nothing less than mental mimicry. Its necessary preconditions are an unbroken narcissism, which cannot bear that anything should exist outside itself, and the weakness of the individual, which makes him unable either to annihilate his environment or to take flight from it." (Balint, A. *The Yearbook of Psychoanalysis I,* 1945) The child, then, uses identifications to transform what is strange and frightening in the external world into what is familiar and enjoyable. The same process holds true in identification at the oedipal stage. Balint says: "According to the schematic formula of the Oedipus complex, a small boy should love his mother and identify himself with his father. And in general, this is the case. The boy's mother is after all the source of gratification and his father is the powerful rival against whom he cannot defend himself successfully either by attack or by flight, so that he is eventually obliged to resort to identification . . . What I have said applies also, *mutatis mutandis,* to little girls." In other words, the male identifies with his father not because he emulates him, but because his father is to him a source of frustration in reality. And later in life, the sensitive person protects his self-esteem and can continue to love himself by identification with his frustrating and humiliating environment. This is the basis for the well-known mechanism of "identification with the aggressor." Identification, then, operates in the interest of and clings to the defense of narcissism.

According to Balint: "After we have taken mental possession of a portion of the external world by means of identification, mental material which has thus been assimilated can itself serve as a basis for further identifications. So there would seem to be no essential distinction between ego-identification (i.e. identification of the ego with an object) and object-identification (i.e. identification of one object with another). For it is only objects which have already been identified with ourselves that can become the starting-point for further identifications."

From the psychoanalytic point of view there are two forms of identification, *primary* and *secondary.* The *primary* form, arising during the oral phase, represents "oral mastery of the object." (Freud) It is first associated with the erogenous zones. Thus the child identifies itself with the parent on the oral, then the anal, and still later on the genital basis, depending upon the area in which reality frustrations operate. Subsequently the child identifies itself with the character traits of the parents, and this leads to the formation of the superego. These early identifications with the parent or parents are called primary identifications. The energy of the child flows out to the real object. It is a manifestation of object cathexis, of object identification. Balint says: "The outcome of the struggle round an individual's narcissism is one of the most important events of his development. As a result of identification with the various commands and prohibitions, his ego undergoes a decisive transformation. Since obedience takes place not through understanding but through identification, the command becomes a part of the child's ego, which he defends henceforward just as much as his own will. . . . The consequence is a splitting of the ego into two parts, of which one is the vehicle of the original instinctual wishes, while the other is the vehicle of the wishes that have been incorporated by means of identification. This second, transformed part of the ego, is called by Freud the 'super-ego.' "

Secondary identification is the consequence of incorporating the object within the psyche of oneself. The psychic energy now becomes attached to the object as it is represented in the mind of the person. The libido (psychic energy) is withdrawn from the object as it exists in reality. "The Ego itself becomes the Id's libidinal-object." (Healy et al., *SMP*) It is as if the instinctual impulses were asked to take a substitute (namely, the introjected object) for the real object. Secondary identification serves the purpose of detaching libido from an object outside of oneself; it makes it easier for an object to be given up.

It seems that *secondary identification* and *introjection* are synonymous in psychoanalysis; Freud himself interchanges them. During the early stages of introjection, however, an introjected object is apparently recognized by the person as foreign to his ego, whereas an object of identification is regarded as an original, not a borrowed, expression of his ego. Prolonged introjection, as in depressed states, may eventually bring about the quality of identification. It would be technically more correct to say that introjection (incorporation) is the mechanism whereby identification takes place; but this distinction is often not carefully drawn in present-day writings. See *incorporation*.

identification, cosmic Belief that one is the universe; a failure, on the part of the patient (usually a schizophrenic), to differentiate between himself and the outside world.

identification, multiple Identification with more than one model or object, seen most commonly in hysterical seizures wherein the patient simultaneously or serially plays the part of various persons with whom he has identified. Such seizures may even represent the enactment of a whole drama. Multiple identification is also seen in cases of multiple personality.

identification, projective Attribution to another of an introjected part of the self which is repressed or repudiated. In couples, it requires that the partner, because of his or her own needs, collude consciously or unconsciously in accepting the projection.

identify To incorporate an object into one's ego system and to act toward the object as if it were originally one's own self and not something borrowed from the environment. See *identification*.

identity A person's image, concept, or inner conviction, held as a whole or in relation to particular functions or roles, as in body identity, gender identity, mental or psychological identity, social identity.

Core *gender identity* (q.v.) refers to the subject's self-concept: "I am female/male"; gender identity refers to femininity/masculinity as expressed behaviorally. Gender identity disorders include disturbances in both.

identity, body See *image, body*.

identity crisis Social role conflict as perceived by a person; loss of the sense of personal sameness and historical continuity, and/or inability to accept or adopt the role the person believes is expected by society. Identity crises are frequent in adolescence, when they appear to be triggered by the combination of sudden increase in the strength of drives with sudden changes in the role the adolescent is expected to adopt socially, educationally, or vocationally.

identity diffusion 1. Instability of the view of the self, as. seen in severe borderline personality disorders when split-off contradictory self-images are acted out in rapid chaotic succession. See *splitting; structural*.

2. Lack of stability and consistency of the personality as seen in some borderline personality disorders whose pseudocompliance and passivity cover their motives, goals, feelings, etc. Bleuler termed this a disturbance in the person in describing fundamental symptoms of the schizophrenias. See *person, disturbances in the; personality, "as if"*.

3. Identification with inadequate or pathologic models, as seen in some antisocial or psychopathic personalities. See *crime and mental disorder*.

identity disorder of childhood Exhibited by the child or adolescent who is abnormally uncertain and concerned about long-term goals or career choice, patterns of friendship, sexual preference, religious affiliation, moral value system, etc., when the concern is of sufficient depth and extent to interfere with academic or social functioning.

identity, ego That sense of identity which "provides the ability to experience one's self as something that has continuity and sameness, and to act accordingly." (Erikson, E. *Childhood and Society*, 1950) The term refers particularly to the degree to which the boundaries of the physical and the mental self are clearly delineated; those whose ego identity is confused are believed by many to be especially vulnerable to schizophrenia.

"Identity is the unconscious directional pattern or sensing apparatus whereby the individual orients himself to others and to his environment. In part it consists of identifications and representations of relationships with primary love-objects. . . . Ultimately it must represent a temporally persistent, coordinate system whereby the self is located. *Identification*, by contrast, should probably be used to describe the process whereby external objects and the exchanges with them are partially or totally represented in the psychic apparatus, and subsequently subjectified or equated or correlated with the representations of the self." (Suslick, A. *Archives of General Psychiatry 8*, 1963)

identity, family See *family identity.*

identity, gender See *gender identity.*

identity integration See *structural.*

identity, organic See *persona, organic.*

identity, sexual See *gender identity.*

identity vs. role confusion One of Erikson's eight stages of man. See *ontogeny, psychic.*

ideogenetic Relating to mental processes in which images of sense-impressions are employed, rather than ideas that have reached the form or stage of being ready for verbal expression.

ideoglandular Relating to the effect of mental impression on glandular functions.

ideographic See *nomothetic.*

ideokinetic praxis See *praxis, ideokinetic.*

ideology A systematic scheme of ideas that forms the characteristic perspective of a social group.

ideophobia Fear of ideas.

ideophrenia Guislain's term for delirium, characterized by ideational disorders.

ideoplastic See *stage, ideoplastic.*

ideoplasty Durand's term for the process of molding, making plastic, the subject's mind by means of ideas suggested by the hypnotist; called *verbal suggestion* by Ernest Jones.

ideosynchysia (-sin-kis′ē-à) *Obs.* Delirium.

idio- Combining form meaning one's own, private, personal, from Gr. *idios.*

idioctonia *Obs.* Suicide.

idiocy, amaurotic family See *amaurotic family idiocy.*

idiocy, Kalmuk (Kalmuk, member of a nomad Tartar tribe) Mongolism. See *syndrome, Down's.*

idiocy, moral See *insanity, moral.*

idiogamist "One who is capable of coitus only with his own wife, or with a few individual women, but is impotent with women in general." (*Encyclopaedia Sexualis,* ed. V. Robinson, 1936)

idioglossia *Idiolalia* (q.v.).

idiogram See *karyotype.*

idiokinesis *Obs.* The "spontaneous" origin of a new hereditary character by means of *mutation* (q.v.), or more specifically, by mutation that takes place without determinable cause.

idiolalia Development of one's own language, such as is seen with some children who suffer from auditory aphasia (word-deafness).

idioneurosis *Obs.* Neurosis.

idiopathic When the etiology of a disease or disorder is undetermined, but its *functional* phenomena are known, it is said that the condition is idiopathic. The National Conference on Nomenclature of Disease refers to "diseases due to unknown or uncertain causes, the functional reaction to which is alone manifest." For example, the syndrome called *narcolepsy* is well known, but its etiology is unknown; hence the symptom complex is named *idiopathic narcolepsy.*

idiophrenia *Obs.* A psychiatric disorder associated with an organic brain disease.

idiophrenic Originating in one's own mind, psychogenic.

idioplasm, idioplasma Introduced into biology by Naegeli to distinguish from the nutritive parts of the protoplasmic substance that portion of a cell upon which its specific qualities depend. Genetically it corresponds closely to the *germ plasm* of a germ cell while its more general meaning embraces all the special hereditary equipment of an organism. See *plasm, germ.*

From the genetic standpoint, the transmission of hereditary characters from parents to offspring depends on the fact that the latter have, entirely or partially, the same idioplasmic structure as the parents, while all the genetic variations among adult individuals must be primarily the outcome of structural or chemical differences in the idioplasm. Minute idioplasmic differences between two ova may produce, in the course of their individual processes of development, a whole series of differences in various parts of the adult organism.

idiosome The idioplasmic unit as the theoretically ultimate element of living matter carrying hereditary characteristics. See *idioplasm.*

idiosyncrasia olfactoria Perversion of the sense of smell.

idiot In ancient times, the differentiation between mental illness and mental retardation was not clear-cut, and often not made at all. For the ancients, *idiot* referred to any person who lived as a recluse in a private world; the term thus included all exceptional children (such as those who nowadays would be termed *autistic*) who were unable to adapt themselves satisfactorily to the community. See *amentia; retardation, mental.*

idiot savant (F. "learned idiot") "These are rare cases, who, although idiots, still have some special faculty wonderfully developed. It may be music, calculation, memory for some certain variety of facts, etc.

"The calculators can name the answer to mathematical problems almost instantly; the musical prodigies often play well and even improvise; one of my cases could instantly name the day of the week for any date for years back." (White, W.A. *Outlines of Psychiatry*, 1929)

idiotism State of being an idiot. Pinel divided insanity into four subdivisions, namely, mania, melancholia, dementia, and idiotism (advanced dementia).

idiotropic Introspective; egocentric.

idiovariation In biology the genetic phenomenon of *mutation,* implying a constant change in the genotypical structure of an organism. Mutated genes necessarily lead to the appearance of new hereditary characters and thus to the origin of hereditarily distinct new groups of a species and new races. See *mutation.*

idolism, sexual Sexual fetishism. See *fetish.*

idolum *Obs.* A false idea, illusion, or hallucination.

Ilg, Francis L. (1903–81) Pediatrician, pioneer in child development; coauthor (with Arnold Gesell) of *Infant and Child in the Culture of Today* (1943); cofounder of Gesell Institute of Child Development.

Illinois Test of Psycholinguistic Abilities (ITPA) A diagnostic test of language abilities that yields language ages for nine specific psycholinguistic areas; precise areas of disability can thereby be identified and an appropriate remedial program can be planned that provides special training in the problem areas.

illness See *disease.*

illness, advantage by Epinosic gain. "Psycho-analysis recognized early that every neurotic symptom owes its existence to a compromise. Every symptom must therefore in some way comply with the demands of the ego which regulates repression, must offer some advantage, admit of some profitable utilization, or it would undergo the same fate as the original impulse itself which is being kept in check." (Freud, *CP*) See *gain, epinosic.*

illness as self-punishment See *resistance, superego.*

illness, unipolar See *depression, unipolar.*

illuminism A state of mental exaltation in which the subject's hallucinations generally assume the form of conversations with imaginary, especially supernatural, beings.

illusion An erroneous perception, a false response to a sense-stimulation; but in a normal person this false belief usually brings the desire to check or verify its correctness, and often another sense or other senses may come to the rescue and satisfy him that it is merely an illusion.

If a straight glass tube is lowered into a tumbler of water, we have the visual illusion that the submerged portion of the tube has bent and forms an angle with its free upper part. This unexpected sight impels us to pull the tube out and convince ourselves that there is nothing the matter with the tube, but our eyes have misinterpreted the situation into an illusion: it merely looks, but actually is not bent. See *kinephantom.*

In all such illusions the stimulus and the illusion (i.e. the reaction) involve the identical sense and can be disproven, making it much harder to realize that it is not an illusion when, sitting alone in a room, we suddenly start because we have "heard" somebody else in the room, only to convince ourselves that we are still alone in the room and that no sound had actually been heard.

This absence of a sense stimulus places the reaction in a different class from those cited above—it is a *hallucination* (q.v.). *Obs.* Fallacia.

illusion, memory Ascribing to oneself the experiences of others and believing implicitly that the experiences are one's own.

"Whoever considers himself Christ, believes that he had been crucified, and, under certain conditions can delude himself into remembering the details of it with perceptible acuteness" shows memory illusions. (Bleuler, *TP*) See *appersonification.*

illusion, necessary A literary term used in psychoanalytic literature in reference to a person's special character defenses as they make for healthy and effective adjustment in the practical and real-life world. In their functioning in relation to the real world these character defenses will make for illusional, private evaluations of what is important and unimportant, what is of great value and of little value—evaluations that represent private predilections in private lives. It is important that an analyst be free of the tendency to confuse his private predilections, and his own unconsciously determined illusions, with the aims and goals of his patient's needs.

E.F. Sharpe (*Collected Papers on Psychoanalysis*, 1950) says: "We may privately prefer beech trees to cedars, that type of character to this, and have our private evaluations of what a worthy life really is . . . . But these things, eminently useful as they are to us as individuals and to our necessary illusions, are of small importance to the world outside us, and most assuredly they are of no use in the consulting-room."

illusion of doubles See *syndrome, Capgras's*.

illusion, proofreader's Failure to detect an error in spelling, punctuation, construction, etc., because of familiarity with the subject matter; a tendency to see things "as they ought to be" rather than as they are.

image (imago [i-mā′gō]**)** In psychoanalysis, the image or likeness of someone, usually not of the subject himself, constructed in the unconscious and remaining therein. The commonest imagos are those of the parents and of those who stand for the parents. E. Jones defines *imago* as "an image preserved indefinitely with persons other than the original one." (*Papers on Psycho-Analysis*, 1938)

"The mother-child relation is certainly the deepest and most penetrating one we know; the child in fact for a long time, so to speak, is a part of the maternal body! Later it is really a continuum of the psychic atmosphere of the mother for years, and in this way, all that is primordial in the child, so to speak, is indissolubly fused with the mother image." (Jung, *PT*)

Jung speaks of *primordial images*. "Thus there naturally exists in the archetype, in the collectively inherited mother-image, that extraordinary intensity of relationship which first impels the child instinctively to cling to its mother." (Ibid.)

"Her inclination towards elderly married men (always platonic) is also traceable to her father *Imago*." (Stekel, W. *Frigidity in Women*, 1926)

Sometimes the person whose image is mirrored in the unconscious is spoken of

as the *imago*. This use of the word is not encouraged.

image agglutinations See *agglutinations, image*.

image, body The concept that each person has of his own body as an object in space, independently and apart from all other objects. The body is always in space and experiences are not possible without this conception of our body, or body image, since we live as human beings with a body. See *ego, body*.

The body image or *body identity* is the conceptualization of the body's structure and functions that grows out of the awareness of the self and one's body in intended action. Schizophrenic children are often deficient in the ability to localize, discriminate, or give pattern and meaning to body perceptions. "Thus, they lack body images that are integrated, stable in time, and clear in form. One child walked about all day feeling her body. Another observed the motions of her hand in fascination and addressed it as a baby." (Goldfarb, W. *International Psychiatry Clinics 1*, 1964) See *limb, phantom*.

L.C. Kolb (in *Schizophrenia, An Integrated Approach*, ed. A. Auerback, 1959) distinguishes between *body percept* (or *body schema*) and the *body concept*. The body percept is the postural image one has of one's body as it functions outside of central consciousness; it is organized over the years, mainly on the basis of incoming kinesthetic and tactile perceptions. The body concept, or conceptual image, includes the perceptions, thoughts, and feelings which the ego has in reference to viewing its own body.

image, conceptual See *image, body*.

image, idealized The defense of having a false picture of one's virtues and assets. The more unrealistic (idealized) this image is, the more vulnerable is the person amid the vicissitudes of life.

The term was introduced by Horney, who was among the first to give a detailed description of the role of cultural pressures in producing neurosis. Though constituting the base from which attitudes toward authority in general develop, the early attitude toward the father is added to and modified by subsequent experiences with father figures. In the relationship to the father, or to subsequent father figures, difficulties often arise, and to circumvent them, neurotic defenses may be developed. For instance, if the patient adjusts to a difficult father by becoming submissive, submissiveness itself becomes a problem. Thereupon, some sort of periodic aggressiveness may be developed to circumvent the problem of submissiveness. This new difficulty, in turn, produces new defenses and the adult patient now presents a complicated defensive system. Thus the patient is sick because of what happened to him and also because, in coping with it, he establishes goals that lead him to pursue false values.

image, memory Anticipation of the recurrence of a past experience, immediately before its recurrence, as in conditioning experiments when the subject anticipates a repetition of the electric shock. According to Reid, "the past situation returns in the service of the present," and it can even be reproduced with hallucinatory vividness. In such cases the memory image may be said to be a part of the conditioned reflex in Pavlov's sense, that is, the memory image is an ingredient of the inner preparedness for the stimulus, and is part and parcel of the individual's total reaction.

image, percept See *percept image.*

image, personal "A *personal* image has neither archaic character nor collective significance, but expresses contents of the personal unconscious and a personally conditioned, conscious situation." (Jung, *PT*)

In contrast is a *primordial image:* "I speak of its archaic character when the image is in striking unison with familiar mythological motives. In this case it expresses material primarily derived from the collective unconscious, while, at the same time, it indicates that the momentary conscious situation is influenced not so much from the side of the personal as from the collective." (Ibid.)

image, primary memory Eidetic image. See *imagery, eidetic.*

image, primary mental See *eidetic; imagery, eidetic.*

image, primordial "The primordial image is a mnemonic deposit, an *imprint* ('engram'—Semon), which has arisen through a condensation of innumerable, similar processes. It is primarily a precipitate or deposit, and therefore a typical basic form of a certain ever-recurring psychic experience. As a mythological motive, therefore, it is a constantly effective and continually recurring expression which is either awakened, or appropriately formulated, by certain psychic experiences." (Jung, *PT*) Also known as *archetype.* See *image.*

"The most immediate primordial image is the mother, for she is in every way the nearest and most powerful experience; and the one, moreover, that occurs in the most impressionable period of a [person's] life. Since the conscious is as yet only weakly developed in childhood, one cannot speak of an 'individual' experience at all. The mother, however, is an archetypal experience; she is known by the more or less unconscious child not as a definite, individual feminine personality, but as the mother, an archetype loaded with significant possibilities. As life proceeds the primordial image fades, and is replaced by a conscious, relatively individual image, which is assumed to be the only mother-image we have." (Jung, *CAP*)

image, social Trigant Burrow's term for an affective impression representing crystallized opinions, beliefs, and prejudices that are deeply ingrained in the individual and in society but for which there is no objective, demonstrable correspondence in actuality. These emotionally toned impressions have no direct relation to the object or situation upon which they are projected. The social image is wishfully determined and is not based upon demonstrable reality. (*Journal of Abnormal and Social Psychology XIX*, 1924) See *I-persona; semiopathic.*

imaged pseudohallucination See *pseudohallucination.*

image, unconscious See *memory, unconscious.*

imagery, eidetic Generally, a psychological phenomenon intermediate between the ordinary visual memory image and the afterimage. This phenomenon attains its significance for constitutional medicine from the observation of E.R. Jaensch that although it occurs in 60% of children under 12, it persists after adolescence only in two types, the *Basedow* type and the *tetany* type, or, as they are usually called, the B type and the T type.

The eidetic image differs from the ordinary memory image by the following details: (1) it possesses a pseudo-perceptual quality; (2) it is superior in clearness and richness of detail, and this clearness is less dependent upon the organization of its content; (3) it is more accurate (mimetic) in its reproduction of detail; (4) it is more brilliant in coloration; (5) it requires more rigid fixation for its arousal; and (6) it shows a greater degree of coherence with the projection ground. It differs from the afterimage by the following characteristics: (1) it may be aroused by a more complicated and detailed object; (2) it is superior in clearness and continues longer in the visual field; (3) it is subject to voluntary recall, even after the lapse of considerable time, as well as to voluntary control; (4) it requires a shorter length of exposure and less rigid fixation for its arousal; and (5) it is more dependent upon factors of interest.

The B type is nearer to the memory image and has been observed only in persons with Basedow's disease or the tendency to it. The T type, in which the imagery approaches the afterimage, has been found in subjects whose blood calcium and potassium show either definite evidence of tetany or changes in the direction of it. These differences in imagery, referable to the different biochemical conditions in Basedow's disease and tetany, are thought to be symptomatic of two contrasting types of mind, the integrated and the disintegrated, respectively. According to the studies of W. Jaensch, characteristic capillary loops of the nail beds are an additional item of difference in these two distinctive psychosomatic types.

imagery, guided See *guided affective imagery.*

imagery, hypnagogic Imagery occurring during the stage between wakefulness and sleep; that is, just before sleep has set in.

imagery, hypnopompic The visions or mental pictures that occur just after the sleeping state and before full wakefulness. The phenomenon is analogous to hypnagogic imagery, differing only in the time at which the images occur.

imagery, spontaneous Jellinek's term for visual images that can be produced at will when the eyes are closed. Spontaneous imagery is not a pathological phenomenon and is seen more commonly in children,

probably because most children have a positive eidetic disposition. Spontaneous imagery is sometimes misinterpreted as visual hallucinations.

imaginarii *Obs.* One of Linnaeus's three subdivisions of mental disorders, characterized by disturbances of the sensory faculties.

imagination Synthesis of mental images into new ideas; the process of forming a *"mental representation* of an *absent* object, an affect, a body function, or an instinctual drive," the results of which process are images, symbols, phantasies, dreams, ideas, thoughts, and/or concepts. Imagination is not, then, the obverse of reality, but affords, rather, a means of adaptation to reality. "Only with the development of the imaginative process, the capacity to create a mental representation of the absent object, does the child progress from the syncretic sensori-motor-affective immediate response to the delayed abstract, conceptualized response that is characteristically human." (Beres, D. *International Journal of Psycho-Analysis XLI,* 1960)

imagination, creative The terms *creative imagination* and *creative work* designate the process in which dormant, unrelated contents of the unconscious become associated with the organized labor of consciousness and accomplish something new.

imaging See *encephalography, radioisotopic; NMR.*

imago See *image.*

imbalance, intellectual "The state of an individual with special abilities or disabilities, markedly competent in some respects and deficient in others, but not well integrated or compensated." (Hamilton, G. *A Medical Social Terminology,* 1930)

imbalance, sibling A situation in which "the number or distribution of children in a family contributes to a problem of spoiling, or economic insufficiency; e.g., only boy in female setting, hyper-large family, etc." (Hamilton, G. *A Medical Social Terminology,* 1930)

imbalance, structural In family therapy, deviations in family patterns that interfere with the family's functioning. Among the most frequent imbalances are *role reversal, alliance and splitting,* and *scapegoating* (qq.v.). See *family culture, indigenous.*

imbecile See *amentia; retardation, mental.*

imbecility, moral See *insanity, moral; psychopathic personality.*

imbecillitas *Obs.* Weakness, feebleness, imbecility, arrhostia.

imitation The tendency to assume certain attitudes, lifestyles, or manners that are valued by one's society.

imitation, hysterical The ability of a hysterical patient to imitate all the symptoms that impress him when they occur in others. The psychological mechanism at work in hysterical imitation is identification: the patient (unconsciously) identifies himself with a person who has the same uncopscious needs as he, who is "just like" him. As a result, the patient reproduces the symptom shown by the person with whom he identifies. Through this hysterical imitation "patients are enabled to express in their symptoms not merely their own experiences, but the experiences of quite a number of other persons; they can suffer, as it were, for a whole mass of people, and fill all the parts of a drama with their own personalities." For example, one girl in a school may react to a love letter with a fainting spell. Some of the other girls then may also get fainting spells. Unconsciously the other girls also wanted love letters, and having had the same unconscious wish they had to suffer the same consequence— they, too, had fainting spells through hysterical identification. (Freud, *ID*)

immediate memory See *amnestic syndrome.*

immobilization-paralysis See *paralysis, immobilization.*

immorality, maniacal *Rare.* The preponderance of overt and uncontrollable sexuality in cases of simple mania.

immune deficiency syndrome See *syndrome, acquired immune deficiency.*

impairment index In neuropsychological assessment, a measure of the degree of brain damage or deterioration in higher intellectual functioning, used to differentiate between organic neurologic disorders and other conditions that mimic them.

impediment, speech Any disorder of speech, but especially stammering or *stuttering* (q.v.). See *speech disorders.*

imperative, authoritative The pressing directives emanating from the superego that subconsciously direct behavior; the commanding voice of parental or social rule in the subconscious mind. According to

Stekel, a compulsion is always a substitute for an imperative. The current (adult) imperative is always a resonance of infantile imperatives. "One may say that neurotics run after their infantile imperatives. The imperative apparently leads to an action which, however, in reality consists only of an inhibition." (Stekel, *CD*)

imperative, categorical In psychoanalysis, the equivalent of *blanket demand.* The superego, for instance, is said to exercise its duties by the rigid "yes" or "no" rule, by the "all or none" law.

imperative, ethical The inexorable disciplinary power of moral principles exerted upon one's mental life and behavior. It represents "the wish of the moral self, the endeavor of the nobler side of man leading the ego to higher and better things in life." One may also speak in terms of "the upward aspiration of man," which in fact constitutes the admonitions of the moral consciousness in the life of an individual. (Stekel, *ID*)

imperative, immoral The antisocial unconscious impulses that compel the person to desire the occurrence of events, or the performance of actions, considered unethical or antimoral. This mental mechanism is often observed in the compulsive-neurotic. It is a compulsion to act against the rules of society, an impulsive subconscious rebellion against moral principles. The destructive aims of the immoral imperative are often directed against religious principles, precisely because religion is one of the most powerful barriers controlling man's instinctual life. (Stekel, *CD*)

impersistence, motor See *persistence, motor.*

impetus In psychoanalysis, one of the parameters defining a *drive* (q.v.). The impetus of a drive is its force, strength, or energy, and in all likelihood is genetically determined. The other parameters by which a drive (or, in older terminology, an instinct) is customarily defined are source (the physiological disequilibrium or organ system through which the drive becomes manifest), and the *aim* and *object* (qq.v.) of the drive.

implant, dynamic Introduction or instillation of a significant idea into consciousness; used mainly in connection with *psychic driving,* one of whose values is said to be long-lasting action on the part of the patient as a result of one or more dynamic implants. The latter bring the patient to focus on specific behavior or action tendencies; this usually leads to intensified activity in the form of tension and anxiety and thus to greater efforts to free himself of such intensification. As a result, the patient tends to ruminate over and to reorganize his reactions to the material in question. This would appear to be a mechanistic description of one type of insight. See *driving, psychic; menticide.*

implicit role See *role.*

implosion *Flooding;* reduction of avoidance behavior by prolonged exposure of the patient to the feared object or situation, thereby demonstrating that the feared situation causes him no harm. Some workers use implosion to refer to imagined exposure to the feared situation and flooding to refer to real-life exposure.

Originally described by Stampfl, implosion did not prove to be more effective than other less unpleasant techniques. In consequence, it has largely been replaced by real-life exposure to the feared object.

impostor A type of pathological liar who seeks to gain some advantage by means of imposing on others fabrications of his attainments, position, or worldly possessions. P. Greenacre (*Psychoanalytical Quarterly 27,* 1958) noted the compulsive, pressured aspect to the impostor's urge to seek the limelight and "put something over" on his audience. She outlines the following features, which appear to be of psychodynamic significance: the typically ambivalent and overpossessive mother creates so intense a maternal attachment in the child that he is unable to develop a full sense of separate identity. At the same time his ability to assume an uncontested supersedence over the father as far as the mother is concerned intensifies infantile narcissism and favors a reliance on omnipotent phantasy to the exclusion of reality testing. Imposture is an outgrowth of the oedipal conflict and represents an attempt to kill the father and/or to rob him of his more adequate penis. Success of this mechanism as evidenced by belief in the impostor by his audience (the mother) furnishes a powerful incentive for endless repetition of the fraudulent behavior. See *factitial.*

impotence (impotency) A *psychosexual* (q.v.) dysfunction consisting of the male's inability to perform sexual intercourse; the corresponding condition in the female is termed frigidity. See *frigidity, sexual; impotence, psychic; tumescence, penile.*

impotence, anal Constipation in which the analogy to cases of neurotic genital sexual impotence in males is emphasized. In this type of constipation, anxiety concerning the injurious or filthy aspect of the fecal mass to be ejected or parted with is of central importance. This is analogous to the anxiety of many orgastically impotent men concerning the poisonous or sullying effect of the seminal ejaculation.

At military induction centers it is a frequent experience that many candidates cannot void (produce a urine specimen) in the presence of others. These symptoms can be thought of as the adult neurotic residues of conflicts between desires for cooperative regularity, giving, and cleanliness on the one hand, and desire for the maintenance of continued stubborn autonomy, spite, defiance, soiling, and direct stool pleasure on the other. (Weiss, E., & English, O.S. *Psychosomatic Medicine,* 1949)

impotence, cerebral M. Hirschfeld postulates four types of impotence: (1) cerebral, due to cerebral causes; (2) spinal, associated with difficulties of erection and ejaculation, of spinal origin; (3) genital, connected with genital defects; and (4) germinal. (*Sexual Pathology,* 1939)

impotence, genital See *impotence, cerebral.*

impotence, germinal See *impotence, cerebral.*

impotence, orgastic A *psychosexual* (q.v.) dysfunction consisting of inability to achieve orgasm or acme of satisfaction in the sexual act. Many neurotics cannot achieve adequate discharge of their sexual energy through the sexual act. For example, the neurotic may attempt to achieve satisfaction by persistent repetitions of the sexual act. Although he thus gives the impression of being very vigorous genitally, in reality he never achieves genuine satisfaction and cannot lose his desire. Also, as a result of their inability to attain genuine end-pleasure, many neurotics lay more stress on the forepleasure mechanisms. The sexual behavior is rigid and, although a certain narcissistic functional pleasure is felt, this is not the complete relaxation of a full orgasm. In this "pseudo-sexuality," narcissistic aims are disturbing the true sexuality.

Finally, in the neurotic there may be a diminution of conscious sexual interest. This reflects his constant struggle with his repressed sexuality, which "diminishes his disposable sexual energy." In some cases, however, the amount lacking is rather small, so that the patient's sexual life appears superficially undisturbed and he feels subjectively as if his sexuality were satisfactory.

According to Fenichel, an important concomitant of orgastic impotence is that such patients are incapable of love. Their need for self-love, for self-esteem, over-shadows their capacity for object love. In further elucidating the mechanism of orgastic impotence, Fenichel quotes Reich's analysis of the course of sexual excitement. According to Reich, in order to obtain an "economically sufficient discharge in orgasm, the full development of the latter part or 'second phase' of sexual excitement in which there are involuntary convulsions of the muscles of the floor of the pelvis is necessary. The climax of pleasure occurs at the climax of sexual excitement in this second phase and coincides with a loss of ego. In orgastically impotent egos this climax of pleasure does not occur. Indeed it is at this very point that the pleasure turns into anxiety and loss of ego control." (*PTN*)

impotence, psychic A *psychosexual* (q.v.) dysfunction consisting of inability of the male to perform sexual intercourse in spite of sexual desire and the presence of intact genital organs. There may be *erective impotence* (inability to achieve or maintain erection), *ejaculatory impotence* (inability to expel seminal fluid), or *orgastic impotence* (inability to achieve full orgasm). Premature ejaculation, *ejaculatio retardata*, the separation of the tender and sensual components of the sexual act so that intercourse is possible only with prostitutes, and the need for fixed and specific conditions to be operative before sexual intercourse can be performed are all types of psychic impotence. Depression following the sexual act (*postcoitum triste*) is a type of orgastic impotence.

E. Bergler (*Psychiatric Quarterly 19,* 1945) classified psychic impotence on the basis of etiology in three main groups: (1) potency disturbance arising from phallic (hysterical) mechanisms; (2) potency disturbance arising from anal mechanisms (obsessional, hypochondriacal, and masochistic types); (3) disturbance arising from oral mechanisms. Impotence based on phallic mechanisms results from an unresolved attachment to the mother of the oedipal period; castration fears lead to subsequent repression of sexual desire for the mother, but finally all sexual objects become identified with her. Persistence of castration fears leads to potency disturbances. In the second group, in an obsessional neurotic, potency disturbances result from the association of sexuality with dirt and filth, which must be avoided at all costs, and from the need to ward off the aggressive and sadistic impulses which are aroused by the sexual act. Erective impotence is rare in the obsessional group, but *ejaculatio retardata* is common. The latter has the significance of anal retention pleasure combined with sadistic pleasure in harming the woman through prolonged intercourse. Potency disturbance arising from oral mechanisms is commonly expressed as either premature ejaculation or *psychogenic aspermia*. The former signifies: "I do not want to refuse the woman anything; indeed, I give immediately." Psychogenic aspermia (ejaculatory impotence) signifies: "I deny you my semen just as mother denied me her milk."

impotence, spinal See *impotence, cerebral.*

impotentia coeundi Inability to cohabit.

imprinting Called *Prägung* by the German ethologists who originally described the phenomenon, imprinting is "the process by which certain stimuli become capable of eliciting certain 'innate' behavior patterns during a critical period of the animal's behavioral development." (Jaynes, J. *Journal of Comparative and Physiological Psychology 49,* 1956) In the mallard duck, for instance, the first moving object the duckling sees during a critical period shortly after hatching is thereafter reacted to as ducklings usually behave toward the mother duck. The degree to which imprinting determines or affects learning and behavioral patterning in the human has not been established, although it has been hypothesized that some forms of mental retardation are due to lack of appropriate stimulation or opportunity when the child is in a critical or sensitive period for the acquisition of specific skills. See *instinct; releaser, social; retardation, mental.*

The concept has also been used to explain psychosexual disorders such as pedophilia and transsexuality. Considering the lack of objective data on the phases of childhood sexuality, the lack of evidence for any critical periods in sexual and attitudinal development, the uncertainty as to whether re-imprinting or partial imprinting can occur, and the time lag of years between hypothesized imprinting and the appearance of behavior that has presumably been learned through the process, such theories appear at least to be premature, if not totally without foundation.

improvement, transference Amelioration of neurotic symptoms on the basis of *transference* (q.v.). The physician is perceived unconsciously as a reincarnation of the parents and as such is thought of as providing love and protection, or as threatening with punishments. So-called *flight into health* is an instance of transference improvement.

impuberism The state of not having reached the age or stage of puberty. While strictly speaking it denotes the life period before puberty and thus embraces the stages of infantilism and childhood, generally it means that the mental and physical characteristics of childhood or occasionally of infancy run into and continue during the chronologically later and distinct adolescent or even adult life.

impulse A stimulus that sets the mind in action. The stimulus may originate in (1) the objective world, or (2) the subject himself: (a) his soma—within any part of the body; (b) his psyche—its conscious or its unconscious part. In psychoanalysis it most commonly refers to the instincts; a basic impulse is an instinct, the source of which is a "somatic process in an organ or part of the body." (Freud, *CP*) See *drive.*

impulse, component Partial impulse; any of the various pregenital or preadult manifestations of drive and particularly, in the case of the libidinal drive, those infantile activities and impulses that will later become subordinate to the adult genital organization. Among the component impulses are

sucking, biting, touching, defecating, urinating, looking (voyeurism), exhibiting, sadism, masochism—all of which, although they may be detectable in adulthood, will generally be expressed as forepleasure activities and will remain subservient to genital primacy. See *genitality; impulse, sexual component; libido, displaceability of; organization, pregenital.*

impulse, cross An impulse that crosses the path of another impulse and in so doing checks the further development of the latter. See *impulse, side.*

impulse disorder, hyperkinetic In DSM-III-R terminology, attention deficit-hyperactivity disorder. See *attention deficit disorder.*

impulse disorders A varied group of personality disorders with the following characteristics: (1) the impulse or symptom is ego-syntonic; (2) there is a pleasurable component; (3) there is minimal distortion of the original impulse, and (4) the impulse possesses a quality of irresistibility. See *disorders of impulse control.*

J. Frosch and J. Wortis (*American Journal of Psychiatry 3,* 1954) differentiate two groups of impulse disorders, the discrete symptom type (including what others call the impulse neuroses, perversions, and catathymic crises) and the diffuse character type, with low frustration tolerance and a tendency to explosive reactions to deprivation.

Some of these patients show rather typical epileptoid records on encephalography, often with indications of pathologic discharge in the temporal lobe. See *personality, epileptic.*

impulse, epistemophilic *Epistemophilia* (q.v.).

impulse, forced See *symptoms, first-rank.*

impulse, fundamental social Desire to check the sprouting manifestations of evil. Influenced by Jung's investigations, Baynes thinks that this impulse expresses itself in various social rituals (such as coronation, marriage, ordination of priests, and other forms of social rites) brought into being by this single fundamental necessity, all of them merely elaborations of the same pattern, their symbolic elements remaining relatively constant with both savage and civilized people all over the world. (*Mythology of the Soul,* 1940)

impulse life The instinctual life. See *drive; impulse.*

impulse, made See *symptoms, first-rank.*

impulse, partial See *impulse, component.*

impulse, sexual component "The sexual instinct is not at first a unit. It consists of various components, emanating from manifold organic sources. These components at first function quite independently of one another, each as it were blindly seeking for organic pleasure and satisfaction, and it is only later that they combine in the function of reproduction." (Jones, E.J. *Papers on Psycho-Analysis,* 1949)

"The small child is . . . full of a still undifferentiated total sexuality which contains all the later 'partial instincts' in one. . . . Every kind of excitation in the child can become a source of sexual excitement: mechanical and muscular stimuli, affects, intellectual activity, and even pain. In infantile sexuality, excitement and satisfaction are not sharply differentiated, although there are already orgasm-like phenomena, that is, pleasureful sensations that bring relaxation and the end of sexual excitation. In time, however, the genitals begin to function as a special discharge apparatus, which concentrates all excitation upon itself and discharges it no matter in which erogenous zone it originated.

"It is called genital primacy when this function of the genitals has become dominant over the extragenital erogenous zones, and all sexual excitations become finally genitally oriented and climactically discharged." (Fenichel, *PTN*)

impulse, side An impulse that exists by the side of another impulse. Kraepelin says that the condition is common in schizophrenia. Often the side or secondary impulse interrupts the primary one, producing irrelevant action or speech. See *impulse, cross.*

impulse, wandering Drapetomania; dromomania; ecdemomania; *wanderlust* (q.v.).

impulse, wish See *wish.*

impulsion Blind obedience to internal drives, such as is seen typically in children, whose interpersonal relations and superego have not yet formed an organized defense against the drives. Impulsion is seen in adults whose defensive organization is weak; the obsessive-compulsive patient, for example, may be a miser, a hoarder, or a cruel moralizer, yet he considers his impulses right and follows them openly. In adults, impulsion tends to be much more symbolic than in children.

impulsive Relating to or characterized by impulse. In psychoanalysis, *impulsive* and *instinctive* are generally used interchangeably. In general psychiatry, impulsive usually applies to swift action without forethought or conscious judgment. See *crisis, catathymic; disorders of impulse control; impulse disorders,*

"In most cases this word refers to the impulses for actions, which are accomplished unexpectedly, without real reflection, or with inconsistent reflection, or without the assent of the whole personality." (Bleuler, *TP*)

impulsiveness See *impulsive.*

Imu A psychoreactive phenomenon seen among the Ainu, consisting of hyperkinesia, catalepsy, echolalia, echopraxia, and command automatism. Imu occurs almost exclusively in adult females. See *hysterical psychosis.*

in-between A literal translation of Hirschfeld's *Zwischenstufe,* meaning an in-between stage or homosexuality.

in vivo exposure See *implosion; therapy, behavior.*

inability See *disability.*

inaccessibility Inability to be reached; unresponsiveness. Used most commonly to refer to the autism and withdrawal of the schizophrenic.

inadequacy, constitutional Any inborn defect; the term, which is vague, often implies some hereditary defect and/or some physical or mental abnormality that is largely unmodifiable. In constitutional medicine, the term refers to anatomical and physiological imbalance between two or more of the systems (physical and mental).

inadequacy, intellectual See *retardation, mental.*

inadequate personality See *personality pattern disturbance.*

inappetence Absence of appetite or desire.

inattention See *extinction.*

inattention, selective Ignoring or disregarding attitudes, traits, values, etc., because they are given no special value by the significant people in the developing child's milieu.

According to Sullivan, the self is finally formed out of a great number of potentialities. The child tends to develop and enhance those of his traits that are pleasing or acceptable to the significant adults, and to block out of awareness and disassociate those attributes that meet with their disapproval. Obviously there are some attributes that are neutral in the estimation of the significant people. Since no special attention is paid to these attributes, the child may or may not be aware of them, and it may be said that "selective inattention" has been at work. Unlike disassociated material, disavowed because it has been disapproved by the significant adults, the material on which selective inattention acts can, without great difficulty, be incorporated into the *self-system* (q.v.) if such behavioral attributes should later become important in the eyes of others. The difference between selective inattention and disassociation is not clear-cut, however, and is merely one of degree.

inbred Produced by inbreeding. Pertaining to the descent and biological conditions of individuals descended from common ancestors; that is, from ancestors who frequently or persistently intermarried among themselves, thus creating a particular population group. See *intermarriage.*

inbreeding In genetics, the special form of reproductive conditions that prevail in a rather isolated and relatively homogeneous group of individuals, exclusively and persistently selecting their marriage partners from their own group. Such selective reproduction gradually leads to the formation of more or less pure-bred stocks and counteracts the normal effects of propagation, consisting of the continuous creation of new combinations of hereditary or nonhereditary differences. See *variation.*

In the reproduction of a species in which *hybridization,* or even *panmixia,* has been the rule, the results of inbreeding are almost invariably disadvantageous. The worst effects are caused by the increased production of homozygotic carriers of *recessive* traits, which under normal reproductive conditions would appear only rarely.

A doubtful kind of dysgenic inbreeding effect may be due to the fact that inbreeding, when of a marked degree, tends to make mutations more frequent. It must be taken into consideration, however, that the majority of mutations are recessive, so that inbreeding may only facilitate their easier discovery.

incendiarism *Pyromania* (q.v.).

incest Sexual congress between male and female who are blood related, such as between mother and son, father and daughter, brother and sister, or among cousins. See *syndrome, battered child.*

incest barrier See *barrier, incest.*

incidence The number of new cases of any disorder that develop in a given population in a given period of time. Incidence rates are usually expressed per year, per 100,000 population:

$$\begin{array}{l}\text{incidence}\\\text{rate of}\\\text{illness}\end{array} = \dfrac{\text{new cases in 1 yr}}{\begin{array}{l}\text{persons exposed,}\\\text{in 1 yr, to}\\\text{the risk of disease}\end{array}} \times 100,000$$

The exposed population may be the entire population or, particularly when the illness in question begins only during a limited period of years or is confined to one sex, it may be specifically limited to an age group or sex within the total population. See *epidemiology; prevalence; rate.*

incipient Beginning, inchoate, threatening, not fully formed; used often to modify the word schizophrenia by those reluctant to make such a diagnosis in the absence of secondary or accessory symptoms.

inclusion criteria See *SADS.*

incoherence Disorganization; used most commonly to refer to speech that is disconnected and unintelligible.

incompetence, incompetency A legal term referring primarily to defects in intellectual functioning such that comprehension of the nature of a transaction is interfered with or otherwise inadequate. It thus refers to intellectual capacity and takes no note of temperament, emotions, or the like, which may also interfere with a person's capacity to function. Ordinarily, incompetence implies an interference with thinking that gives rise to defects in judgment and leads to behavioral abnormalities such as squandering, hoarding, or gullibility. Competence bears little or no relationship to underlying psychiatric diagnosis and will vary in degree according to the magnitude or significance of the action under consideration. Thus a person of low intelligence might be considered competent to handle and manage a weekly allowance of $20, but considered incompetent to manage a trust fund of $20,000.

According to C. Culver and B. Gert (*Philosophy in Medicine*, 1982), "A person is incompetent to do *x* if it is reasonably expected that any person in his position, or any normal adult human being, can do *x*, and this person cannot (and his inability to do *x* is not due to a physical disability)." The term is ordinarily used to characterize people, whereas the word *irrational* typically refers to actions, even though both words relate to the ability of a person to perform certain kinds of action.

incongruity Lack of consistency or appropriateness; used most commonly to refer to the disharmony between speech and affect so characteristic of the schizophrenic. (See *mood-congruent*.) Also applied to inconsistency in the informational interaction between the organism and environmental circumstances; i.e., the discrepancy between incoming information of the moment and information already stored and coded within the brain in the course of previous encounters with the category of circumstances concerned. There appears to be an optimal amount of incongruity (or *novelty, uncertainty, cognitive dissonance,* etc.) for each organism at any given moment, in all probability determined largely by experience. When a situation is too incongruous, the organism withdraws; where it offers too little incongruity, boredom results and the organism seeks another situation offering more incongruity, stimulus change, novelty, dissonance, or uncertainty.

inconstancy, object See *object constancy*.

incoordination Ataxia.

incorporation The earliest instinctual aim directed toward objects and the most primitive method of recognizing external reality by assimilating external objects. Everything that is pleasurable is something to swallow and becomes ego; thus incorporation is the prototype of instinctual satisfaction, and all sexual aims are derivative of incorporation aims. Incorporation is also the prototype of regaining the omnipotence previously projected onto adults. But what is incorporated and taken in is also destroyed, so that the ego later uses incorporation in a hostile way to execute destructive impulses. Any instinctual aim may regress to incorporation or introjection.

Some writers use incorporation synonymously with *identification* and *introjection* (qq.v.); others equate incorporation with introjection and define both as the mechanism by which identification takes place. Others differentiate between them on the basis of the phase or level of psychic organization and development at which the assimilation of the object takes place. Thus incorporation refers to assimilation of external objects at the phase of primary narcissism, when there is no distinction between subject and object; introjection takes place during the phase of differentiation between the I and the not-I; while identification can occur only when the distinction between subject and object is solidly established. Unlike introjection, identification is a purely intrapsychic process.

incubus *Obs.* Nightmare; specifically, a woman's nightmare that a man or evil demon has entered her bed during the night to have intercourse with her. See *succubus*.

incubus, family In social work, a family member who, "because of mental or physical incapacity or difficult personality creates a problem distinctly burdensome or depressing to others." (Hamilton, G. *A Medical Social Terminology*, 1930)

index case In genetics, a person disclosing clinical evidence of the trait under investigation.

index, cephalic A measure of head size obtained by dividing the maximal breadth of the head by its maximal length and multiplying by 100. Medium heads (*mesocephaly*) have an index number from 76.0 to 80.9 cm. Long heads (*dolichocephaly*) have an index below 76.0 cm. Broad or short heads (*brachycephaly*) have an index of 81.0 cm or over.

index, homeostatic Any measure of the capacity to resist alteration of the status quo; the higher the homeostatic index, the more rapidly will an organism recover from any disturbing situation and return to normal balance.

index, hyperglycemic (HI) Measurement used by McGowan as a prognostic indicator in various psychoses.

The index is computed as follows:

$$HI = \frac{\text{2-hr blood sugar level} - \text{fasting blood sugar}}{\text{maximal blood sugar level} - \text{fasting blood sugar}} \times 100$$

A high index is considered unfavorable and is seen in melancholia and in catatonic and depressive stupors, but HI is usually low in mania. McGowan considers the hyperglycemic index to be a measure of the emotional tension under which a patient labors.

index of body build See *body build, index of.*

index of sexuality (IS) An index proposed by Linhares and De Oliveira:

$$IS = \frac{\text{urine 17 ketosteroids (mg)} \times 10}{\text{urine phenol} - \text{steroids (µg)}}$$

Normal values are 2.6 to 4.3 for men, 0.6 to 1.0 for women. The index is low in hypogenital men and high in climacteric women.

index, skelic A measurement used in anthropometry; the ratio between the length of the legs and the length of the trunk.

indexical communication See *communication, nonverbal.*

indicator, complex Any stimulus that arouses an emotion because it has touched off some unconscious complex. "In group therapy . . . it is significant how often 'complex indicators' are uncovered concerning which the patients will evidence far more comprehension than they might be credited with." (Klapman, J.W. *Group Psychotherapy,* 1946)

indigenous family culture See *family culture, indigenous.*

indigenous worker See *caregiver.*

indirect method of therapy See *therapy, client-centered.*

individual Jung defines the psychological individual as "unique-being" and as characterized by its peculiar, and in certain respects unique psychology. The peculiar character of the individual psyche appears less in its elements than in its complex formations.

"Everything is individual that is not collective, everything in fact that pertains only to one and not to a larger group of individuals. Individuality can hardly be described as belonging to the psychologi-cal elements, but rather to their peculiar and unique grouping and combination." (*PT*)

individual psychology See *psychology, individual.*

individual response See *popular response.*

individual-response specificity See *specificity, individual-response.*

individuation "The process of forming and specializing the individual nature; in particular, it is the development of the psychological individual as a differentiated being from the general, collective psychology. Individuation, therefore, is a *process of differentiation,* having for its goal the development of the individual personality." (Jung, *PT*)

"The process of individuation is an intense analytical effort which concentrates, with strictest integrity and under the direction of consciousness, upon the internal psychological process, eases the tension in the pairs of opposites by means of highest activation of the contents of the unconscious, acquires a working knowledge of their structure, and leads through all the distresses of a psyche that has lost its equilibrium, hacking through layer upon layer, to that center which is the source and ultimate ground of our psychic existence—to the inner core, the Self." (Jacobi, J. *The Psychology of C.G. Jung,* 1942)

"The course of individuation has been roughly plotted and exhibits a certain formal regularity. Its sign posts and milestones are various archetypal symbols, whose form and manifestation vary according to the individual." (Ibid.) There exist, however, certain archetypes that seem to be universally identified with and characteristic of the four principal stages of the individuation process. They are, in chronological order: (1) the archetype of the shadow; (2) the archetype of the soul-image; (3) the archetype (in men) of the old wise man or of the Magna Mater (in women); (4) the archetype of the self.

individuation stage See *separation-individuation.*

Indoklon (in′dō-klon) Trade name for hexa-fluorodiethyl ether, which has been used as a form of convulsant therapy in psychiatric patients.

indole A class of biogenic amines that includes lysergic acid (LSD), bufotenin, dimethyltryptamine, and *serotonin* (q.v.). The indole amines derive from the essential amino acid trytophan; monoamine oxidase inhibitors elevate the levels of indole amines by delaying their breakdown. See *amine.*

induced psychotic disorder Shared paranoid disorder. See *association, psychosis of; folie à deux; paranoia.*

induction, dream The production of a dream through hypnotic stimulation. Such dreams may be "artificially stimulated on command during hypnosis or they may be posthypnotically suggested, to appear later during spontaneous sleep." Both the induction and the interpretation of this type of dream play an important part in the technique of hypnoanalysis. (Wolberg, L.R. *Hypnoanalysis,* 1945)

induction, psychological A psychological charging; psychological irradiation. See *infection, psychic.*

industrial psychiatry See *psychiatry, industrial.*

industry vs. inferiority One of Erikson's eight stages of man. See *ontogeny, psychic.*

inertia, motor See *perseveration.*

inertia, psychic Fixation; resistance. Jung says that a peculiar psychic inertia that opposes any change and progress is a basic condition of a neurosis. Freud holds that "this inertia is in fact most peculiar; it is not a general one, but is highly specialized; it is not even all-powerful within its own scope, but fights against tendencies towards progress and reconstruction which remain active even after the formation of neurotic symptoms." He adds: "This specialized 'psychic inertia' is only a different term, though hardly a better one, for what in psychoanalysis we are accustomed to call a *fixation.*" (*CP*)

infancy The period from birth until the beginning of the sixth year.

"This period of life, during which a certain degree of directly sexual pleasure is produced by the stimulation of various cutaneous areas (erotogenic zones), by the activity of certain biological impulses and as an accompanying excitation during many affective states, is designated by an expression introduced by Havelock Ellis as the period of auto-erotism." (Freud, *CP*)

infancy research Study of early development through direct child observation, be-

gun in the 1960s. Many of the findings of such research were incompatible with theories developed on the basis of reconstruction of infantile development through the psychoanalytic approach. In consequence, some of those earlier psychoanalytic theories have been extensively revised.

infant psychiatry See *psychiatry, infant.*

infanticide The killing of an infant or child. See *euthanasia.*

infantile Of or belonging to the period of *infancy* (q.v.); used particularly in reference to those who are adults chronologically but whose behavior, or psychic organization, betrays more of its childhood background than is ordinarily accepted as "normal." See *infantilism.*

infantile amnesia See *memory, affect.*

infantile hyperkinetic syndrome *Attention deficit disorder* (q.v.).

infantile paralysis *Poliomyelitis* (q.v.).

infantilism In psychoanalysis, the state of infancy.

In constitutional medicine, the term means anomalous type of hypoevolute constitution characterized by the persistence of certain constitutional (psychological, physiological, morphological) features of childhood up to an age that is no longer infantile. This anomaly may concern the body mass as well as the proportions, the soma as well as the psyche (although in different degrees), and cause the individual who has either reached or passed the puberal crisis to be left in the psychosomatic condition of an infant or child.

According to Pende, the ordinary form of infantilism is to be differentiated from other forms of *hypoevolutism* such as *hypogenitalism, juvenilism,* and *persistent puberism* (qq.v.).

infantilistic Referring to or characterized by *infantilism* or a particular form of *dwarfism* (q.v.).

infantilization Continuation, by a child, of activities no longer appropriate to his age.

infection, familial mental Séguin's term for psychosis of association. See *association, psychosis of.*

infection, psychic The "induction" of a mental syndrome in another person. "It happens that paranoid or paranoiac and rarely hypomanic patients not only can make those with whom they live close together believe in their delusions, but they so infect them that the latter under conditions themselves continue to build on the delusions." (Bleuler, *TP*) See *folie à deux; association, psychosis of.*

inferences, logical See *KIPS.*

inferiority In general, any type of adaptation of a lower order than normally expected.

Adler is known chiefly for the stress he placed upon feelings of inferiority. He believed that everyone is born with an inferiority—organic or psychical—and that the manner in which the inferiority is handled determines the "style of life" led by the individual. Psychiatric states are the result of faulty management of the inferiority characterizing the individual.

In psychoanalysis, perhaps the most important contribution to what is called the *inferiority complex* stems from the early Oedipus situation. "The irreconcilability of these [oedipal] wishes with reality and the inadequacy of the childhood stage of development lead to a narcistic scar that constitutes the basis of the inferiority feeling." (Healy et al., *SMP*)

Erikson describes *industry vs. inferiority* as one of the eight stages of man. See *ontogeny, psychic.*

inferiority, constitutional psychopathic *Rare.* Psychopathic inferiority; psychopathy; *psychopathic personality* (q.v.).

inferiority, feeling of By this term Adler indicates that through the whole period of development, the child possesses a feeling of inadequacy in its relation both to parents and to the world at large. See *psychology, individual.*

inferiority, functional Adler includes this as a subgroup of organ inferiority; "A quantity or quality of work insufficient to satisfy a standard of required effectiveness." (*Study of Organ Inferiority and Its Psychical Compensation,* 1917)

inferiority, morphologic As used by Adler, a subgroup of organ inferiority characterized by a deficiency in the shape of an organ, or in its size, its individual portions of tissue, its individual cell complexes, of the whole apparatus or of limited parts of it.

inferiority, organ Adler maintained that "inherited inferiorities" of glands or organs, if they made themselves felt psychically, were conducive to a neurotic disposition,

i.e. they caused a child with some "inherited stigma" to feel a sense of inferiority in relation to his environment. This feeling of humiliation and inferiority induced by some constitutional or organ defect produces psychic compensatory and hypercompensatory strivings.

inferiority, psychic constitutional Healy's term for a state of permanent abnormal social and mental reaction to the usual conditions of living on the part of those who are called borderline cases. See *borderline psychosis.*

inferiority, psychopathic *Obs. Psychopathic personality* (q.v.).

inferiority, simultaneous coordinate Adler's term for simultaneous manifold inferiority of organs due to reciprocal embryonic influence, or embryonic connection of many organs. As an example, he cites gastrointestinal affections in diseases of the lungs, in emphysema, and particularly in tuberculosis. He does not feel that these gastrointestinal affections are dependent upon a primary lung disease, but are due to simultaneous inferiority of both systems.

infestation delusions *Parasitophobia* (q.v.).

infidelity delusion See *jealousy, morbid; paranoia, conjugal.*

information feedback See *therapy, behavior.*

information processing See *KIPS.*

information system, executive *Decision support system;* any mechanism that allows an executive to bypass the usual intelligence channels and gain access directly to the data about the operation of his or her organization that ordinarily is filtered through one or more intermediate organizational levels before it is presented. To most people within an organization, power resides in the ability to influence the chief executive officer's perceptions. Staff people who collect, interpret, and analyze executive information therefore tend to be very powerful, as are operating executives who set plans, budgets, and strategies. Executive information systems can render the executive independent of such middle management levels and can thus be powerful tools in exposing the weaknesses of an organization, identifying levels of incompetence, and providing other data that often highlight the advisability of restructuring the organization.

information theory Study of the transmission of messages or the communication of information. Information science and technology are concerned with the structure and properties of scientific information and the techniques for information handling, the characteristics of information processing devices, and the design and operation of information handling systems. See *communication unit; cybernetics.*

informational underload See *deprivation, sensory.*

infradian See *rhythms, biologic.*

inhalant intoxication An organic disorder induced by the use of inhalants such as glue, paint or paint thinners, and gasoline (see *glue-sniffing*). The substance may be inhaled directly from its container, or a rag soaked in the substance may be held over the mouth and nose. Inhalant abuse and inhalant dependence include repeated episodes of intoxication characterized by behavior changes, such as belligerence, assaultiveness, or apathy, and physical signs of central nervous system involvement such as dizziness, nystagmus, ataxia, dysarthria, tremor, psychomotor retardation, stupor, or coma.

inhalation, carbon dioxide See *therapy, carbon dioxide inhalation.*

inheritable Capable of being transmitted from parents to offspring; applied to a physical or mental trait. In genetics, the English term most closely approximating the German term *Erbfest,* "fixed in heredity," and contrasting the hereditary qualities of an individual with those that are acquired by the phenotype during its own lifetime and do not become transmissible by heredity. See *Mendelism.*

inheritance This specifically genetic term has two meanings: (1) the *process* of transmission of inheritable attributes from parent to offspring—being then equivalent to *hereditary transmission;* (2) more commonly, the *trait* transmitted. In the second sense it is frequently modified by an adjective or phrase, as *Mendelian* inheritance, *cytoplasmic* inheritance, inheritance of *acquired characters.* See *chromosome; cytoplasm.*

Among the various modes of inheritance are the *multifactorial (MF) model* and the *single-major-locus (SML) model.* The latter postulates that only two alleles are involved in manifestation of the trait in question—the normal one and the abnormal one responsible for the trait. The multifactorial model assumes that the genetic and environmental causes of the trait constitute a single continuous variable, the *liability,* and that those whose liability exceeds a threshold will manifest the trait. In the MF model, genetic effects are assumed to be due to the additive effects of many genes, each of which contributes only a small part to the final result; similarly, environmental effects are exerted through many minor events that are additive throughout the life of the person.

inheritance, archaic The realization of racial influences operating in the development of the individual psyche. See *phylogenesis.*

As a figurative concept, archaic inheritance rests upon the old theory that "morbid mental conditions presenting themselves as a reflection of a disease of the organism, are rendered more comprehensible, if we look upon them as the reappearance of a peculiar form of life which is normal for a lower level of organic development." On this theory, propounded by Carus early in the 19th century, Jung based and built his doctrines of the "racial unconscious" and "archetypes," but he makes it clear that the archetypes are *literally* inherited.

Dreams are believed to give best evidence of the primitive elements in the individual minds of modern man. According to Freud, they "preserve for us an example of the manner in which the primitive apparatus worked, a mode that has now been abandoned as useless."

inhibition 1. In psychoanalysis, an unconscious confining, hemming in, checking, or restraining of an instinctual impulse or some manifestation of it. The force of the superego inhibits the impulse, prevents it from crossing the boundary line between the id and the ego.

2. In Pavlovian conditioned-reflex psychology, inhibition refers to the active restraining of response by the experimental subject during the latent period of delayed reaction. Inhibition can itself be inhibited by any extraneous stimulus administered during the latent period, and the result will be a release of the response from its original inhibition (disinhibition).

inhibition, competitive See *antagonist, narcotic.*

inhibition formation See *formation, inhibition.*

inhibition, occupational An inhibition in the field of work or vocation of a person, evidenced in diminished pleasure in work, or in its poor execution or in such reactive manifestations as fatigue (vertigo or vomiting), if the subject forces himself to go on working. See *neurosis, occupational.*

According to Freud inhibitions in general, "represent a limitation and restriction of ego functions, either precautionary or resulting from an impoverishment of energy." In some cases, there is a widespread impoverishment of energy, a general inhibition in all the ego functions, of which occupation is only one. This occurs when the ego must use all of its energy for some particularly difficult task such as mourning or the suppression of rage. As a result of concentrating all its energies on this particular task the ego is unable to perform many of its other usual functions such as the sexual function, eating, work.

In other cases of occupational inhibition, there is a specific inhibition, that is, a precautionary limitation of the work function. The inhibition is carried out in order to prevent a conflict with the superego. The strict superego has forbidden that any advantage or success accrue to the patient. Thus the patient must insure inadequate functioning in the work area, i.e. he inhibits his behavior in this area. In Freud's words, occupational inhibitions "subserve a desire for self-punishment." (*The Problem of Anxiety,* 1936)

inhibition, prenefarious In the development of guilt, the initial generalized diminution in activity that accompanies fear; such inhibition is nonspecifically protective, whereas the avoidances of the later stage of guilt proper protect against specific external dangers that come to be recognized as guilt provoking.

inhibition, specific An inhibition in some particular function of the ego, e.g. eating, sexual function, locomotion. An inhibition of eating would most frequently be expressed as anorexia; sexual inhibition as various forms of impotency or frigidity; inhibitions of locomotion as an antipathy to and weakness in walking. These specific inhibitions are renunciations of

functions that if exercised would give rise to severe anxiety or guilt. Under analysis an inhibition such as writing—that is, of functions involving the use of the fingers—reveals an excessive erotization of the fingers. Writing acquires the significance of a sexual activity; and allowing fluid to flow out from a tube upon a piece of white paper might have the symbolic meaning of coitus.

initiation, individual and collective An individual initiation is a ritual that takes place "under the command of heaven." It indicates a dedication to an individual goal that demands the utmost intensity of purpose and unreserved lifelong devotion. In such cases the libido is transformed from its original objective into a cultural one, usually in the framework of a religious idea. The coronation of a king and the ordination of a priest illustrate such an initiation. Initiation also takes place in some ethnic groups in a collective way, where, for instance, adolescents are initiated into adulthood with appropriate ceremonies. The purpose of these ceremonies is to direct the infantile libido into mature objectives. (Baynes, H.G. *Mythology of the Soul,* 1940)

initiative vs. guilt One of Erikson's eight stages of man. See *ontogeny, psychic.*

injury See *disease.*

inner language See *test, Lichtheim's.*

innervation, antagonistic inversion of the In his general remarks on hysterical attacks, Freud states: "A particularly effective form of distortion is *antagonistic inversion of the innervation,* which is analogous to the very usual changing of an element into its opposite by dream-work. For instance, in an hysterical attack an embrace may be represented by the arms being drawn back convulsively until the hands meet above the spinal column. Possibly the well-known *arc de cercle* of major hysterical attacks is nothing but an energetic disavowal of this kind, by antagonistic innervation of the position suitable for sexual intercourse." (*CP*)

innervation, expressive The nervous pathways of emotional behavior such as weeping, laughing, and sexual excitement. The expressive innervations are involuntary, even though they can be influenced, up to a point, by volition.

inputs See *functional budgeting.*

inquiry Questioning or asking about; in Rorschach testing, a review of the subject's responses to the inkblots in order to define as accurately as possible the exact nature of each response and thus facilitate scoring, and also to collect additional data such as elaborations on the original responses and/or further responses that were not given during the performance proper.

insane Of or pertaining to one who is of unsound mind. See *insanity.*

insane, criminally See *crime and mental disorder.*

insania cadiva *Obs.* Epilepsy.

insania lupina *Lycanthropy* (q.v.).

insaniola *Obs.* Eccentricity.

insanity A legal rather than a medical term, referring to mental disorder or defect of such nature or degree as to interfere with the capacity to discharge one's legal responsibilities. If it is determined that insanity is present, various legal consequences may follow, such as commitment to an institution, appointment of a guardian, dissolution of a contract; or certain expected consequences may be altered, as when an accused person is found not guilty by reason of insanity. See *responsibility, criminal.*

insanity, adolescent *Obs.* Hebephrenia. See *schizophrenia.*

insanity, affective *Psychosis, affective* (q.v.).

insanity, alternating See *psychosis, manic-depressive.*

insanity, circular See *psychosis, manic-depressive.*

insanity, collective Ireland's term for psychosis of association. See *association, psychosis of.*

insanity, communicated See *association, psychosis of; folie à deux.*

insanity, constitutional An early 19th-century term referring specifically to a concept of etiology or causation of certain mental disorders. It seemed then that these disorders were of an inborn nature, predetermined by congenital, hereditary, or "constitutional" peculiarities, defects, or deviant trends. Now, "constitutional insanity" would be equated with mental disorders with outstanding phylogenetic or genotypic hereditary etiological factors, in contrast to the ontogenetic, postnatal, environmental, experiential causes.

insanity, cyclic See *psychosis, manic-depressive.*

insanity defense See *responsibility, criminal.*

insanity, deuteropathic *Obs.* Organic mental disorders other than the primary degenerative dementias, i.e. those disorders whose primary etiology is outside the central nervous system itself.

insanity, double Tuke's term for folie à deux. See *association, psychosis of.*

insanity, hysterical *Rare.* General term for "severe" forms of hysteria.

"It is possible that sometimes through a certain treatment the affective relation to the environment may resemble an insanity." (Bleuler, *TP*) See *hysterical psychosis.*

insanity, induced See *association, psychosis of; folie à deux.*

insanity, infectious Ideler's term for psychosis of association. See *association, psychosis of.*

insanity, intellectual *Obs.* Prichard's term for the forms of insanity known in the 19th century as monomania, mania, and dementia.

insanity, intelligential *Obs.* Noble and Mones's (19th century) term for the class of mental disorders known today as *organic dementias.*

insanity, intermittent Manic-depressive psychosis.

insanity, interpretational See *interpretation, delirium of.*

insanity, involute *Obs.* *Feeblemindedness* (q.v.).

insanity, moral The condition of those "in whom the feeling tone of all ideas concerned in the weals and woes of others is stunted (*moral imbeciles*) or is entirely absent (*moral idiots*); both groups together would be designated as moral oligophrenics. Sympathy with others, instinctive feelings of the rights of others (not one's own) is absent, or is inadequately developed. At the same time the other kinds of emotional feelings can be perfectly retained."(Bleuler, *TP*)

Prichard stated that patients of this group showed uncontrollable violence and depravity of the instincts and emotions, without any impairment of the intellectual faculties. See *psychopathic personality.*

insanity, notional *Obs.* A 19th-century term suggested by Noble and Mones; it included roughly what today are known as the schizophrenias and the psychoneuroses.

insanity of negation Psychosis with nihilistic delusions. See *Cotard's syndrome.*

insanity panic, neurotic Severe anxiety arising from the fear of becoming insane.

insanity, partial This expression, usually of medicolegal import, is sometimes synonymous with *monomania;* it was so regarded in the M'Naghten case. It is also defined as a borderline type of mental unsoundness.

Partial insanity "means a mental impairment which is not so complete as to render its victim irresponsible for his criminal acts." The law speaks of "limited responsibility." "There are, as we have seen, two types of cases in which this concept of 'limited responsibility' may be called into play: (1) cases in which, though there is evidence of mental disorder which probably was a contributing cause in the criminal conduct, the disorder is not of such a type as to come within the legal test, so as to render the person irresponsible; (2) cases in which, by reason of mental disorder, the person was incapable of deliberation, premeditation, malice, or other mental state usually made a requisite for first degree offenses, and in which, therefore, a lesser offense than that charged was in fact committed." (Weihofen, H. *Insanity as a Defense in Criminal Law,* 1933)

insanity, primary delusional *Obs.* Folie systématisée, or *paranoia* (q.v.).

insanity, protopathic J.C. Bucknill and D.H. Tuke speak of protopathic insanity as "Insanity or Mental Deficiency caused by Primary Disease or Defective Development of the Encephalic Centres." They subsumed *congenital or infantile deficiency, traumatic insanity, general paresis, paralytic insanity, epileptic insanity,* and *senile insanity* as protopathic forms. (*Manual of Psychological Medicine,* 1874)

insanity, reciprocal Parsons's term for psychosis of association. See *association, psychosis of.*

insanity, saturnine *Obs.* Chronic encephalopathy due to *lead poisoning* (q.v.).

insanity, stuporous *Obs.* Anergic stupor.

insanity, sympathetic *Obs.* Insanity for which the primary cause or seat was believed to be an organic part of the body biologically unconnected with the cerebrum.

insanity, symptomatic *Obs. Organic psychosis* in contradistinction to psychogenic syndromes, termed *idiopathic insanity* by Mercier.

insanity, toxic Bucknill and Tuke classified insanity into three groups: (1) protopathic; (2) deuteropathic; and (3) toxic; examples included alcoholic insanity, pellagrous insanity, and cretinism.

insanity, volitional *Obs. Obsessive-compulsive psychoneurosis* (q.v.).

insecurity A feeling of unprotectedness and helplessness against manifold anxieties arising from a sort of all-encompassing uncertainty about oneself: uncertainty regarding one's goals and ideals, one's abilities, one's relations to others, and the attitude one should take toward them. The insecure person does not or dares not have friendly feelings in what seems to him an unfriendly world. He lives in an atmosphere of anticipated disapproval. He has no confidence today in yesterday's belief, no faith tomorrow in today's truth.

"Children are unable to form the certainties which arise from *consistent* patterns, if they experience unpredictable fluctuations in which there is no cohesion. Frequent changes of residence and schools break constantly into any attempt at forming friendships, belonging to a neighborhood group, cementing the concept of 'home,' getting accustomed to a method of instruction. The child's need of *consistency* rests chiefly for its gratification on parental attitudes and parental behavior. If you can predict what you can do tomorrow from what you have been permitted to do through a series of yesterdays, you acquire confidence in foresight and faith in your ability to 'get along.' If what you are permitted to do today depends, not on what you were permitted to do yesterday, but on parental indigestion, the stock market, the number of last night's highballs, or the latest article on child training published in the Sunday paper, then, as long as you live, you may never know where you stand in relation to any other human being." (Kanner, L. *Child Psychiatry,* 1948)

insemination The act of impregnating or fertilizing. The technical expression for *artificial insemination* is *eutelegenesis* (q.v.). See *surrogate, mother.*

insertion, thought See *symptoms, first-rank.*

insight The patient's knowledge that the symptoms of his illness are abnormalities or morbid phenomena. For example, when a patient who fears crowds realizes that the fear is a symptom of abnormality within his own mind but is unfounded in reality, he is said to have insight. When, on the other hand, a patient affirms that his body is composed of many other human beings, that God, Napoleon, Mithras, and others are actually within his organs, he is described as having no insight.

Insight is further defined from the standpoint of knowledge of the factors operating to produce the symptoms. When a patient says he understands the explanation regarding the origin and development of his symptoms, it is said that he possesses insight.

Intellectual insight is knowledge of the objective reality of a situation, but without the ability to utilize that knowledge in the mastery of or successful adaptation to that situation. It is generally conceded that intellectual insight alone is ineffective in producing therapeutic change, and that the quest for it may even constitute a resistance to the therapeutic process.

insight, derivative Insight arrived at by the patient himself without interpretation by the therapist—characteristic of activity therapy groups.

insipientia *Obs.* Dementia (q.v.).

insolation Sunstroke.

insomnia Sleeplessness. In DSM-III-R, insomnia disorder consists of difficulty in initiating or maintaining sleep at least three times a week for at least a month. The loss of sleep produces significant daytime fatigue or impaired occupational or social functioning. In typical cases, sleep latency exceeds 30 minutes or sleep efficiency is less than 85%. See *sleep disorders.*

insomnia, childhood-onset idiopathic *Insomnia* (q.v.) beginning before puberty and persisting into adulthood. The subject is never without insomnia for more than three months at a time. See *sleep disorders.*

insomnia, learned Difficulty initiating or maintaining sleep based on psychological reasons, such as insomnia that begins during a period of stress but continues after the stress itself has disappeared. Typical of this type of insomnia is daytime preoccupation over possible inability to fall asleep, or increasing efforts to fall asleep are unsuccessful, or paradoxical improvement in sleep when away from the usual sleep environment. See *sleep disorders.*

insomnia, rebound Worsening of sleep beyond the baseline level of insomnia following immediately upon discontinuation of medication that was used to treat the insomnia in the first place. The rebound period is usually brief—sometimes no more than one night—but when it occurs, patients typically misinterpret it as an indication for continuing or increasing medication.

instigator Any member in a therapy group who stimulates others toward activity or verbalization. See *agent, catalytic; isolate; neutralizer.*

instinct "An organized and relatively complex mode of response, characteristic of a given species, that has been phylogenetically adapted to a specific type of environmental situation." (Warren, H.C. *Dictionary of Psychology,* 1934)

"An instinct may be described as having a source, an object, and an aim. The source is a state of excitation within the body, and its aim is to remove that excitation; in the course of its path from its source to the attainment of its aim the instinct becomes operative mentally. We picture it as a certain sum of energy forcing its way in a certain direction." (Freud, S. *New Introductory Lectures on Psycho-Analysis,* 1933)

An instinct, according to Freud, is a primal trend or urge that cannot be further resolved. Jealousy can be resolved into love and hate; therefore, it is not an instinct; it is a "part-instinct" or an "instinct-component." From the Freudian standpoint there are two primal instincts, those of *life* and *death.*

In present-day psychoanalytic psychology, the term *drive* (q.v.) is generally preferred to what Freud termed "instinct." An "instinct" is considered to be an innate capacity or necessity to react in a stereotyped way to a particular set of stimuli; it is a lower-level, automatic response (such as the reflexes). The term "drive," on the other hand, ordinarily does not refer to the organism's response but instead emphasizes the state of central excitation; unlike the instinct, the response to the drive is not automatic but requires the functioning of the ego and depends on learning and experience.

In *ethology* (q.v.), an "instinct" is an inherited system of coordination, made up of an internal drive, which builds up as specific action potential until it is released, and one or more inherited releasing mechanisms (IRM) which release the specific action potential and produce the instinctive act or fixed action pattern (FAP). The specific action patterns are species-specific, uniform, and generally rigid, although (especially as one goes up the vertebrate scale) some links of the instinctual action are subject to modification by learning. Such learning, when it occurs, can be conceived of as a replacement of innate, instinctual links by learned behavior patterns—a phenomenon called "instinct-training interlocking." In man, instinctive behavior patterns are rudimentary, and most genetically determined, instinctual behavior is replaced by learned, plastic, purposive, adaptive behavior—that is, by the ego. (Schur, M. *International Journal of Psycho-Analysis XLI*, 1960) See *imprinting; releaser, social.*

The two instincts are constant psychic forces, arising from the organism itself; their sources are in the soma and represent the biological needs of the body. Somatic processes create the need, which acts through the psyche in order to secure specific forms of motor discharge for the relief of the "tension" set up in the original source. Successful gratification of the instinctual needs can be attained only through contact with the outer world.

The first of the two primal instincts is Eros, or life instinct, the function of which is to maintain life; its aim is constructive. It is composed of three principal manifestations; (1) the uninhibited sexual or organ-gratifying impulses; (2) sublimated impulses derived from those originally associated with organ satisfaction; and (3) self-preservative impulses, which strive to protect and preserve the body and the mind.

The second primal instinct is Thanatos, the death or destruction instinct. Freud says that the tendency of the instinct is to reestablish a state of things which was disturbed by the emergence of life. The death instinct is said to be composed of (1) impulses that tend toward regression, that is, toward a reinstatement of an earlier level of personality development; (2) im-

pulses that aim to injure or destroy the person himself, and (3) those that possess the aim of (2) with regard, however, to objects outside of oneself. Freud emphasized that the death instinct does not exist literally as such in the unconscious; rather it is expressed as complete passivity toward which the organism instinctively strives. See *instinct, death.*

One of the basic theses upon which psychoanalysis rests assumes that the process of life is a conflict and a compromise between the two primal instincts.

Jung says that the collective unconscious consists of the sum of the instincts and their correlates, the archetypes.

instinct, aggressive See *instinct, death.*

instinct, aim of In all cases, the aim of an instinct is the reestablishment of that state of relative total organismal balance that existed before the instinct was aroused, through either external or internal stimulation. The state of instinct arousal in an organism is a state of tension or unpleasure in that organism driving the organism, as a whole, in the direction of finding and applying the appropriate means for relieving the arousal tension—or dissatisfaction through gratification. The Boston physiologist Cannon coined the phrase *homeostatic equilibrium* for this state of relative harmony and balance, and used the term *homeostasis* for the multiplicity of forces that interact within the organism and react to internal or external stimulation in the directional trend of equilibrium.

The *aim* of an instinct must be sharply discriminated from the *object* of that instinct. Water is the object of the instinct of thirst, while the aim of thirst is gratified through the imbibition and absorption of water by the tissues—namely, the disappearance of the unpleasurable state of thirstiness or "thirst." The process of gratifying the instinctual aims is heralded in consciousness by the sensation of pleasure. (Sterba, R. *Introduction to the Psycho-analytic Theory of the Libido*, 1942)

instinct, antipathic sexual "Great diminution or complete absence of sexual feeling for the opposite sex, with substitution of sexual feeling and instinct for the same sex (homosexuality, or antipathic sexual instinct)." (Krafft-Ebing, R. v. *Psychopathia Sexualis*, 1908)

instinct, complementary The tendency of all infantile sexual instincts with an active aim to be integrally associated with, or accompanied by, the antithetical instinct drive with a passive aim. In infancy and childhood, the separation or *defusion* (q.v.) of these equal and opposite active and passive instinctual aims is marked. On the other hand, in adult life, with the achievement of emotional maturity at the so-called genital level, this persistence of antagonistic instinctual trends toward the same object tends to drop out or disappear. In childhood, side by side with the wish to beat, there exists the wish to be beaten; the wish to eat coexists with the wish to be eaten, etc. In adult life one frequently finds, as an infantile remnant, the wish to be loved by a person and, simultaneously, the wish to love that person. See *ambivalence.*

instinct component *Part instinct* (q.v.). See *impulse, component.*

instinct, curiosity *Epistemophilia* (q.v.).

instinct, death The destructive or aggressive or ego instinct(s). In psychoanalytic psychology, two basic instincts or drives are recognized: those under the control of the pleasure-unpleasure principle (the life instincts, the sexual instincts, Eros); and those instincts under the control of the repetition-compulsion principle (the death instincts, destructive instincts, ego instincts, aggressive instincts, destrudo, Thanatos).

It was not until 1920, in *Beyond the Pleasure Principle*, that Freud first recognized the death instincts as an independent drive. During the earlier years of psychoanalysis Freud occupied himself largely with the libidinal or erotic instinct and later conceived of an aggressive or destructive instinct, which in its primary form he considered to be nonsexual. He came to believe that not all mental processes were subject to the pleasure-pain (pleasure-unpleasure) principle, and that there was a phylogenetically older principle, the repetition-compulsion principle. The latter operates to restore a previous condition of pleasure and harmony, whenever noxious stimuli cannot adequately be handled by the pleasure-pain principle. Since the repetition-compulsion tends to restore the status quo, Freud reasoned

that it must ultimately tend to return the organism to the earliest state of all, namely that of inanimate existence; thus the manifestations of the repetition-compulsion principle were called the death instinct, and it was presumed that deflection of the death instinct onto objects in the external world constituted the aggressive instinct.

Because Freud's consideration of the death or destructive drives came relatively late in the development of his psychology, the term *libido*, which technically refers only to the energy of the sexual instinct, is often used as a general term to refer also to the energy of the death instinct. The term *destrudo* was suggested for the energy of the death instinct, but this has not been widely accepted.

The death instinct strives for a state of complete and eternal rest, is averse to new experiences, seeks to return to the past, and is essentially conservative in nature. As a rule, neither the life nor the death instinct is seen in pure and completely independent form; rather, there is fusion of the two. The death instinct goes through approximately the same ontogenetic development as does the sexual instinct, but the death instinct is not as intimately related to the erogenous body zones as is the sexual. It is not known if the discharge of destructive or aggressive drives brings pleasure; Freud believed that it did not, but many contemporary psychoanalytic writers believe that it does.

The death instinct is a biological tendency to self-destruction that, although always operative, is ordinarily deeply hidden; in its earliest developmental stage it is known as *primal masochism*. By union with the narcissistic libido (that part of the sexual libido that has the ego as its object, as is seen in purest form in the narcissistic phase of development, when the libido has not yet come to know or cathect objects in the external world) the death instinct acquires an erotic tinge and becomes pleasurable; it is then known as *actual masochism*. The aggressive or death instinct aims at destroying the outside world, which is the source of disturbing stimuli; but disturbing stimuli may also come from within by means of an increase in (sexual) libido. As the sexual instincts develop, this increase in libido is accompanied by a transformation of narcissistic libido into object libido. The primal masochism, directed originally against the narcissistic libido, is now projected onto the objects of the libido in the outside world as *sadism*.

Just as the genital is the executive organ of the sexual instinct, so is the musculature (both striated and smooth) the executive organ of the death instinct.

The death instinct operates in the oral phase, which thus is often termed the cannibalistic stage; for gratification of hunger also destroys the object. In the anal phase, the destructive instinct appears as soiling, retention, and other means of defiant rejection of the disturbing external world. In the phallic phase, phantasies of piercing, penetration, or dissolution of the object betray the operation of the destructive instinct. Genital sadism appears in the form of hatred, which normally is restricted by love and persists only as the activity involved in taking possession of the love object. In the genital phase, there is fusion of the destructive instinct with the sexual instinct, and the destructive instincts, if not completely paralyzed by the sexual instincts, are at least restrained by them. In certain psychiatric conditions, however, there is a greater or lesser defusion of the instincts; this is seen particularly in depressive psychoses and in certain forms of schizophrenia.

Freud's hypotheses about the death instinct have by no means achieved universal acceptance in psychoanalytic circles, and many feel that although destructiveness may accompany any response pattern, it is not an instinct or drive in itself but is rather a "maladaptive or misdirected expression of the single instinct to live. The only aim of instinct is to reduce the physiological stimulus or disequilibrium, and maintain optimal tension, i.e. life.

"Drives, on the other hand, arise only with the development and operation of psychic structure. They should be conceptualized as a psychological rather than a biological phenomenon—the product of a highly specialized bodily system which is a different level of organization from biological instinctual activity patterns." (Pleune, F.G. *International Journal of Psycho-Analysis XLII*, 1961)

instinct, destruction See *instinct, death.*

instinct eruption See *crisis, catathymic.*

instinct, herd Group feeling; group formation; the desire to be with others and to take part in social activities; gregariousness. From the psychoanalytic point of view this is not an instinct; rather, social and group phenomena are explained as results of *identification*, the origin of which is to be found in the jealousy and hostility of childhood. It is said that the first child is jealous of his successors and desires to get rid of them. He realizes, however, that his animosity cannot be maintained without injury to himself. If the jealousy is maintained he will lose the admiration and love of his parents. He is eventually compelled to unite (to identify himself) with his brothers and sisters.

When identification takes place it is followed by reaction formation, that is, sympathy with the rival replaces hostility. The identification with the leader is of the same order as the earlier identification with the father. The leader is a new ego-ideal.

"It is possible and convenient to group instincts (or interests) under three great headings, ego-activities (self-preservation and aggrandizement), sexual proclivities (mating and parenthood) and herd or social functions." (MacCurdy, J.T. *The Psychology of Emotion*, 1925)

instinct, mastery According to Fenichel, mastery means the ability to handle outer demands and inner drives, to postpone gratification when necessary, to assure satisfaction even against hindrances. There exists, however, no instinct bent on mastering. Mastery "is a general aim of every organism, but not of a specific instinct." (*PTN*) See *mastery, oral.*

instinct need See *need.*

instinct, partial Part instinct. See *impulse, component.*

instinct, passive "Every instinct is a form of activity; if we speak loosely of passive instincts, we can only mean those whose aim is passive." (Freud, *CP*) For example, an instinct may be reversed into its opposite; an active instinct (e.g. sadism) may be reversed and appear as a passive one (e.g. masochism).

It appears that the *aim* of a passive instinct is the same as that of an active one. The difference rests in the object. When oneself is the object, the instinct is passive, while it is active when the instinct is directed away from oneself.

instinct, possessive The drive for power, the primitive urge to conquer and retain the love object. In the infant, the possessive instinct manifests itself in the acts of sucking and swallowing, and in the stubbornness with which the child holds on to the nipple of the mother. It is also shown in the capacity to control the anal sphincter and thus retain the feces. The possessive instinct is partly responsible for the child's excessive need of having exclusively for himself the parent's undivided love. Later the infant's crude possessive urge is transformed into a more socialized form; it becomes, one may say, "civilized," in order to be approved by the community and accepted by the person himself. In this more socialized form, the possessive instinct may express itself in stinginess, punctuality, the habit of collecting things, even the search for intellectual knowledge, and in many other character traits. In the adult, the crude possessive urge is sublimated under the constant exigencies of the superego (a code of moral behavior) and acquires a constructive quality, a proper intensity, and an acceptable direction toward admissible goals.

instinct presentation The mode by which an instinct is expressed.

instinct-ridden Beset or characterized by aggressive and/or libidinal impulses that are only inadequately modified or controlled by the superego; the instinct-ridden character typically keeps his superego "actively and consistently at a distance. Experience with the persons whose incorporation created the superego have made it possible for the ego to feel the conscience in one place or at certain periods (and for the most part in very distorted forms), but to be relatively free from the inhibiting influences of the superego, when tempted by the irresistible urge of strivings for instinctual gratification and for security.

"An isolation of this kind is fostered if the ego has previously experienced both intense erogenous pleasure and intense environmental frustrations, especially if experiences of this kind were encountered by a person already characterized by an oral regulation of self-esteem and an intolerance of tensions, developed under the influence of early traumata or orally fixating experiences." (Fenichel, *PTN*) See *disorders of impulse control; impulse disorders; impulsive.*

instinct, self-preservative See *instinct; instinct, death.*

instinct-training interlocking See *instinct.*

institution Typical social institutions in the broader sense are the family, the school, the church, the economic system, and the state. Each institution has its particular function to play in its service to its members and to society.

instrumentalism "An extreme form of *Self-Extension* in which one makes use of people for pleasure or profit; exploitation of others." (Hamilton, G. *A Medical Social Terminology,* 1930) See exploitative type under *assimilation.*

instrumentality theory The hypothesis that a subject's attitude about an occurrence (outcome) depends on his perception of how that outcome is related (instrumental) to the occurrence of other desirable or undesirable consequences.

insufficiency, apperceptive In his studies of the vitally important psychic process of symbolism (the indirect representation of objects or ideas by means of symbols), Silberer originated this term for the essential cause of symbolism—an incapacity of the apperceptive faculty of the mind. Because of this incapacity the mind cannot truly and correctly apperceive the nature of some hitherto unencountered object by appraising the attributes of this object *sui generis,* so to speak, but only by appraising similarities and/or dissimilarities of the new object in association with some old (known) object. The new object then becomes synonymous with the old object and is given the same name. One is the other: the other is the one. This is the origin of symbolism.

Silberer recognizes two types of apperceptive insufficiency: (1) of purely intellectual origin; (2) of affective origin. In the first type apperception is insufficient by reason of mental incapacity inherent in the organism (or by reason of a capacity *as yet undeveloped*), or by mental incapacity of functional nature, i.e. as induced by sleep, fatigue, drugs, etc. In the second type apperception is insufficient because of psychopathology existing in the interplay of affective (emotional) components attaching to the apperceiver or to that which is to be apperceived.

insufficiency, segmental In Adlerian psychology, inferiority of a body segment (using the term segment in its embryological, developmental sense); the inferiority of the internal organs is typically betrayed by some disorder of the skin of that segment—nevi, angiomata, telangiectasiae, neurofibromata, etc., all of which Adler termed the *external stigmata.*

insular sclerosis See *sclerosis, multiple.*

insularity, psychological The quality or state of being narrow-minded or circumscribed in outlook, mentality, and character. "The most important value to character formation of group experiences is the modification or elimination of egocentricity and psychological insularity." (Slavson, *IGT*)

insulin treatment See *treatment, insulin.*

insurance, narcissistic "It is the narcissistic satisfaction derived from the fulfilling of an ideal which benumbs the critical judgment of the ego, and secures gratification of the forbidden aggressive tendencies. This economic mechanism may be described as a kind of *narcissistic insurance.*" (Rado, S. *International Journal of Psychoanalysis IX,* 1928)

intake The initial interview of the patient (or, in the case of a child, a member of the patient's family) by the therapist (or any member of the psychiatric team); usually in reference to a patient who is admitted into a psychiatric clinic or a mental hospital.

intake, family group An initial interview technique, devised by the Riley Child Guidance Clinic (Indianapolis), that substitutes the family unit (usually the child and his parents) for the usual single informant and a psychiatric team (consisting of a psychiatrist, a psychologist, and a social worker) for the usual single interviewer. One member of the team acts as the principal interviewer and opens the way to a discussion by the family of the presenting problems as they see them. The other team members later enter into the discussion as active participants. Interaction between family members is interrupted only

if one member is too aggressively attacked (verbally or physically) by another.

The major objectives of such a technique are "(1) clarification of the presenting problems for all persons involved, including the child, (2) observation of the family interaction, and (3) information which will lead to tentative hypotheses about the relationship between the family dynamics and the child's symptoms." (Tyler, E.A., et al. *Archives of General Psychiatry* 6, 1962)

integration Act of bringing together the parts into an integral whole. In early infancy the components of the mind operate independently, as separate entities. One component does not influence another by any so-called combination of forces. The singleness of individual parts remains a characteristic of the mind during the greater part of the infantile period. From the psychoanalytic point of view, for example, oral, anal, and genital factors remain essentially discrete for a considerable period. Gradually, however, through various mechanisms the individual parts begin to act in cooperation with one another. It is the harmonizing of separate parts that is called integration.

During the infantile period, extending approximately through the fifth year of life, integration is relatively simple, being manifested chiefly in the form of knowledge on the part of the child that its body and mind are distinct from the environment. The integration at this stage of development is called *primary.* Subsequent integration that coordinates individual components into unified and socialized action is termed *secondary integration.*

When integration, having once been established, breaks down into its component parts, that is, when there is a reversal of the processes of integration, the condition is known as *disintegration.*

When disintegration is followed by a reorganization of the individual parts into a harmonious whole, the process is called *reintegration.* Hence it is said that a manic-depressive patient is disintegrated during the illness and reintegrated following it.

intellect From the standpoint of analytical psychology, intellect is "directed thinking." "The faculty of passive, or undirected, thinking, I [Jung] term *intellectual* *intuition.* Furthermore, I describe directed thinking or intellect as the *rational* function, since it arranges the representations under concepts in accordance with the presuppositions of my conscious rational norm. Undirected thinking, or intellectual intuition, on the contrary, is, in my view, an *irrational function,* since it criticizes and arranges the representations according to norms that are unconscious to me and consequently not appreciated as reasonable." (*PT*)

intellectual inadequacy See *retardation, mental.*

intellectualization See *brooding.*

intelligence According to Thorndike, there are three distinctive types of intelligence: *abstract, mechanical,* and *social.* The capacity to understand and manage abstract ideas and symbols constitutes abstract intelligence; the ability to understand, invent, and manage mechanisms constitutes mechanical intelligence; and the capacity to act reasonably and wisely as regards human relations and social affairs constitutes social intelligence. See *developmental psychology.*

Tolman's pragmatic viewpoint regards intelligence as the interrelated capacities of an organism (1) to perceive its environment through its various sensory modalities (discriminanda); (2) to integrate these sensations into total configurations (gestalt apperceptions); (3) to attribute meaning and personal reference (symbolization and value) to them in terms of retained past experiences (memory); and (4) to respond to such differentiated apperceptions by internal and external reactions of various degrees of finesse, versatility, and efficiency (manipulanda capacities).

Spearman's *g* is an overall index of general intelligence, made up of *p* (perseveration factor); *f* (fluency factor); *w* (will factor); and *s* (speed factor).

intelligence, artificial (AI) Use of a computer to manipulate symbols instead of following a rigid and precisely defined algorithm, so that the machine imitates the human intellect. The term was coined by Dartmouth mathematician John McCarthy, one of the "Dartmouth tetrad," whose members are considered to be the founding fathers of artificial intelligence. (The others were Marvin Minsky, then a fellow in mathematics and neurology at Harvard, and Allen Newell and Herbert Simon, who were then with the Rand Corporation in Santa Monica and later at the Carnegie Institute of Technology in Pittsburgh). The four met at Dartmouth in 1956 to consider the possibility of producing computer programs that could "behave" or "think" intelligently.

Artificial intelligence seeks to produce, on a computer, a pattern of output that would be considered intelligent if displayed by human beings. Computers can behave intelligently using two basic ingredients: (1) search, to find all the possibilities available, and (2) knowledge, which includes both factual data and heuristic knowledge (the rules of thumb built on previous experience that allows all the possibilities uncovered by the search to be reduced to manageable proportions). Such heuristic knowledge might be expressed in a number of logical propositions following the formula "*If* such conditions prevail, *then* proceed along path A." See *style, cognitive.*

Although a microchip is much speedier than a neuron, the brain can make millions or billions of neuronal calculations simultaneously and in parallel, whereas computers do their manipulations sequentially, in a one-step-at-a-time fashion. Artificial intelligence has demonstrated that the computer can be a useful tool for studying cognition and that it serves as a reasonable model for some human thought processes. But whether it is the best model for the most important processes is still very much an open question. No machine yet developed gives any indication of possessing common sense, which appears to depend on knowledge of a great number of facts that have yet to be codified into a form that can be manipulated by computers. Computers can imitate some aspects of human intelligence—in playing chess, for example—but they are no match for the human brain in others—such as recognizing a human face, understanding a nursery rhyme, or appreciating the humor of a play on words.

intelligence, crystallized The ability to use an accumulated body of general information to make judgments and solve problems, an area of intelligence that continues to rise over the entire life span in healthy, active people.

intelligence quotient See *quotient, intelligence.*

intemperance Lack of restraint or control of any desire; in particular, immoderate use of alcohol. See *alcoholism.*

intensive care syndrome See *syndrome, intensive care.*

intent, criminal "Criminal intent is a knowing disregard of criminal law (bearing in mind that ignorance of a law is no defense as knowledge of the law itself is presumed). Any person manifesting this disregard is an outlaw, that is to say, he is a criminal in the eyes of the law. Intent is often wrongly confused with motive; motive is merely that which impels." (Singer, H.D., & Krohn, W.O. *Insanity and Law,* 1924) Years ago Sir FitzJames Stephen wrote that "intention is the result of deliberation upon motives, and is the object aimed at by the action caused or accompanied by the act of volition. Though this appears to me to be the proper and accurate meaning of the word it is frequently used and understood as being synonymous with motives."

intention "An impulse for action which has already found approbation, but whose execution is postponed for a suitable occasion." Freud stresses the forgetting of intentions, saying that they can "invariably be traced to some interference of unknown and unadmitted motives—or, as may be said, they [are] due to a *counterwill.*" (*BW*)

intention tremor See *tremor.*

intentional See *volition.*

intentional unvoluntary behavior Those types of disorder in which the subject acts intentionally but not voluntarily, in that although he can perform an action he cannot refrain from performing despite good reason to do so. Included are compulsions, addiction (which is further complicated by drug-induced physiologic changes that alter behavior and capacity for control), the avoidance behavior seen in phobic disorders, factitious disorders such as Munchhausen's syndrome, alcoholism, binge eating, kleptomania, and some forms of ego-dystonic sexual behavior. See *volition.*

interaction See *transactional analysis.*

interaction, accelerated One of the results of the intensity of the *marathon session.*

interaction theory of personality See *chronograph, interaction.*

interactional contract See *contracting.*

interactions, drug The effects that one drug has on the actions of one or more other drugs given at the same time. Many drug-drug interactions are known, but relatively few of them appear to be of major clinical significance. Some of the most significant in psychiatry include the interactions between monoamine oxidase inhibitors and sympathomimetic amines or tyramine and those between tricyclic antidepressants, neuroleptics, and anti-Parkinson agents.

intercalated (in-ter'-ka-lāted) Internuncial. See *reflex.*

intercortical Burrow's term for the interrelationship among individuals by means of the sign, word, or symbol. In man's intercortical functioning only the restricted cortical segment of one person is brought into contact with the cortical segment of another. Contrasted with intraorganismic. Synonyms: interindividual, social, symbolic, semiotic, linguistic. (*The Biology of Human Conflict,* 1937)

intercourse, buccal Oral intercourse; fellatio or cunnilingus.

interego Stekel's proposed substitute for the Freudian term superego. According to Stekel, the Freudian *superego* (q.v.) should be considered not as a simple "watchman" (the vigilant moral part of the ego), but rather as an intermediary between our inner crude impulses and the final conscious aims of those impulses. For this reason Stekel prefers to call the superego an interego—a structure functioning as a compromiser between crude subconscious trends and the moral principles. (*ID*)

interest To interest is to attract and hold the attention, to occupy and engage a person's concern to the extent of employing his time. This is one of the basic principles upon which occupational therapy is applied.

interest, social Adler's term for the desire to belong, to be a part of a social group, a desire that he felt was basic to all human beings. See *psychology, individual.*

interface See *network.*

interfaceable minds See *minds, interfaceable.*

interference pattern of discharge See *attack, obsessive.*

intergroup exercises See *Conferences, A.K. Rice Group Relations.*

intermarriage In genetics, marriage between two blood relations, especially in the sense of a *cousin marriage*, or the union between two individuals belonging to different racial groups of a mixed population.

Cousin marriages are of particular genetic significance in the case of *recessive* Mendelian inheritance. See *recessiveness.*

intermediate In genetics, the type of Mendelian inheritance characterized by the fact that the expressivity of a dominant character is not always complete, but is to a certain extent modifiable by the recessive member of a given pair of contrasting characters. The term denotes both this blended kind of inheritance and the particular hybrids who resemble neither parent exactly, but are *intermediate* in several respects between the original characteristics of the two parent types. For instance, pink hybrids would be intermediate when they have one red and one white parent. See *dominance.*

Within the intermediate mode of heredity, many cases are known in which one and the same genetic factor has a dominant effect on one set of characters, but a recessive effect on others.

Another modification is constituted by those cases in which each member of a contrasting pair of factors produces its own effect independently, so that the heterozygote is neither a blend nor an intermediate, but a *mosaic.*

intermediate brain syndrome due to alcohol See *blackout.*

intermediate sex *Homosexuality* (q.v.).

intermetamorphosis See *syndrome, intermetamorphosis.*

intermission When a psychiatric syndrome ends in a disappearance of symptoms for a temporary period, only to reappear at a subsequent time, the interval between attacks is called an intermission. When after an attack it is not known that the symptoms will reappear, the term *remission* (q.v.) is used. A patient in a state of remission may never have another attack.

intermodal fluency See *fluency, intermodal.*

internal capsule See *basal ganglia.*

International Classification of Diseases (ICD) The official list of disease categories issued by the World Health Organization. DSM-III is based on the ninth revision of the ICD, prepared in 1977. See *DSM-III.*

internuncial Intercalated. See *reflex.*

interoception The Pavlovian concept that the cerebral hemispheres analyze and synthesize not only impulses entering from the external world but also impulses arising from changes taking place within the organism itself. Russian neurophysiologists have investigated extensively the presence of receptors in internal organs.

interpenetration A speech or writing defect in which the intensity of the patient's preoccupations reduces his ability to respond directly to questioning; instead every now and then he will interject a few fragments of the topic suggested by the question. Interpenetration is also used to refer to intrusion of the patient's complexes and preoccupations into any direct response he may give to a question. Interpenetration is seen frequently in the schizophrenias but occurs in other disorders as well; it is therefore considered an accessory schizophrenic symptom.

interpersonal Often used to refer to Sullivan's theory of personality, the dynamic-cultural view of development.

interpretation The description or formulation of the meaning or significance of a patient's productions and, particularly, the translation into a form meaningful for the patient of his resistances and symbols and character defenses. "Interpretation consists of seeing beyond the facade of manifest thinking, feeling and behavior, into less obvious meanings and motivations. Involved in interpretative activities are different degrees of directiveness. The lowest degree consists of waiting for the patient to interpret things for himself, giving him as few cues as possible. Next, the patient is enjoined to attempt the interpretation of representative experiences. Of greater degree, is a piecing together of items of information, and of seemingly unrelated bits, so that certain conclusions become apparent to the patient. Leading questions are asked to guide the patient to meaningful answers. More directive is the making of interpretations in a tentative way, so that the patient feels privileged to accept or reject them as he chooses. Finally, the therapist gives the patient strong authoritative interpretations, couched in challenging, positive terms." (Wolberg, L.R. *The Technique of Psychotherapy*, 1954)

Interpretation has multiple functions, including providing the patient with insight and understanding; increasing the patient's awareness of his mental life; making unconscious aspects of experience conscious; undoing repression; constructing or reconstructing memories of critical and possibly pathogenic early experiences; educating the patient about what treatment is and how it works; serving as reward or punishment and thus shaping the patient's behavior in the therapy.

In structural interviewing, Kernberg differentiates among (1) *clarification*—the patient and the therapist discuss and examine in greater detail what the patient has said so that both are more fully aware of its implications; (2) *confrontation*—the therapist notes contradictions or inconsistencies in the clarified information and suggests the need for an explanation of them; and (3) *interpretation*—the therapist suggests a hypothesis to explain the observed discrepancies when the patient is unable to make the causal connections.

interpretation, action "The non-verbal reaction of the therapist of the group to the statements or acts of the patient. Action interpretation is employed almost exclusively in activity group psychotherapy." (Slavson, *IGT*)

interpretation, allegoric "A view which interprets the symbolic expression as an intentional transcription or transformation of a known thing is *allegoric*." (Jung, *PT*) See *semiotic.*

interpretation, anagogic H. Silberer's term for a form of dream interpretation. He says that every dream is capable of two different interpretations. The first he calls the *psychoanalytic*, referring particularly to interpretations from the standpoint of infantile sexuality; the second, the *anagogic*, "reveals the more serious and often profound thoughts which the dream-work has used as its material. . . . The majority of dreams require no overinterpretation, and are especially insusceptible of an anagogic interpretation." (Freud, *ID*)

interpretation, deep An ambiguous term that usually refers to any interpretation concerned with early developmental levels (e.g. pregenital as opposed to genital levels) and/or with earliest repressed material. The terms "deep" and "depth" belong to an early phase of psychoanalytic theory, when description of the psyche was mainly in topographical terms—Cs (consciousness), below which is Pcs (preconsciousness), and below that the Ucs (unconscious).

interpretation, defense Ego and superego interpretation; in psychoanalytic therapy, an interpretation that brings to consciousness the kind and sources of defensive resistances used by the patient.

interpretation, delirium of Sérieux and Capgras suggest that there are but two forms of paranoia. One is the *delirium of interpretation*, characterized by delusions of persecution; the other is the *delirium of revindication*, which has to do with a delusional organization based upon the urgency to gain justice for alleged offenses perpetrated against the patient. *Delirium* in this sense signifies a delusional, not a delirious state.

interpretation delusion See *delusion, interpretation.*

interpretation, ego See *interpretation, defense.*

interpretation, id See *interpretation, impulse.*

interpretation, impulse Id interpretation; in psychoanalytic therapy, an interpretation that overcomes a defense and permits certain painful thoughts or feelings to come into consciousness.

interpretation, mutative Any interpretation producing change; specifically, an interpretation that produces a breach in the neurotic vicious circle. First, the analyst in the role of auxiliary superego allows a particular quantity of the patient's id-energy to become conscious (e.g. in the form of an aggressive impulse); second, such id impulses will be directed onto the analyst; third, the patient "will become aware of the contrast between the aggressive character of his feelings and the real nature of the analyst, who does not behave like the patient's 'good' or 'bad' archaic objects. This is the point at which the vicious circle of the neurosis is breached, and, with the patient's recognition of the distinction between the archaic phantasy object and the real external object, the way is opened to the recovery of further infantile material that is being reexperienced by the patient in his relationship to the analyst." (Strachey, J. *International Journal of Psychoanalysis 15,* 1934)

interpretation, serial The elucidation of a consecutive number of dreams taken as a group. This gives the analyst important psychic material which no study of a single, individual dream can bring forward. This is the only way to elucidate deeply repressed material that expresses itself only in part in sundry dreams. After such a serial study the analyst can reconstruct the jigsaw puzzle of the whole conflict with the aid of the various pieces. "Serial interpretation is of great advantage. Should a symbol whose meaning seems inexplicable turn up, we can tranquilly await its reappearance in later dreams. It will recur often, until its meaning grows plain." (Stekel, *ID*)

interpretation, superego See *interpretation, defense.*

interpsychology A term used by Tarde, Janet, and others for interpersonal relationships.

interruption, thought See *symptoms, first-rank.*

intersex A sexually intermediate individual that has developed biologically as a male (or female) up to a certain point in its life and thereafter has continued its development as a female (or male).

Owing to the supersession of one type of sex tendency by the other, intersexes usually show a mixture of male and female parts and are almost invariably sterile. They are *not* gynandromorphs, because their structures are not definitely and clearly male or female.

In cattle, an intersex that "is made so by action of hormone of the opposite sex" is called a *freemartin.* According to Shull, all freemartins are modified females.

intersexuality Incomplete sex reversal, which leads to the production of individuals intermediate between the sexes, as the final result of a competition between opposed male and female tendencies, in which supremacy is gained at the "turning point" by the formerly less developed tendency. The time at which this switch takes place determines the degree of intersexu-

ality. Intersexuality is thought to be of common occurrence, even if it may not yet be exactly recognizable.

A special form of intersexuality, occurring in humans as well as in domesticated mammals, is probably caused by delayed or deficient hormone production and results in modifications of both internal and external sex organs and secondary characteristics.

Intersexuality is sometimes used to refer to severe *transsexualism* or *transvestitism* (qq.v.).

interstimulation Modification of behavior in response to the presence of others. For instance, a child's general conduct is altered by the presence of one or more other children. Interest is stimulated or diminished, activity is intensified or decreased, and anxiety is heightened.

interval psychosis Postoperative delirium, the major psychiatric complication observed in surgical intensive care units. Depending on the type of surgery and the degree of preoperative psychosocial intervention, reported incidence varies from 15 to 70%.

intervening act See *act, intervening.*

intervention, crisis See *crisis intervention.*

interview, Amytal (am'i-tal) See *narcotherapy.*

Interview, Renard See *Renard Diagnostic Interview.*

interviewing, structural See *structural.*

intimacy A subjective state of closeness to another person that gratifies a wish for warmth and relatedness and provides an opportunity for expression of sexual and aggressive drives. Intimacy depends on an established sense of self, trust in the other person, and a conviction that one will not be injured in the relationship. One can then relinquish control, at least temporarily, and allow dependency on the other to form. Intimacy can exist without sex, and vice versa, but when the two act together they add to pleasure and fulfillment in an erotic relationship.

intimacy vs. isolation One of Erikson's eight stages of man. See *ontogeny, psychic.*

intimidate To frighten or cow; to make another fearful that one will attack him verbally or physically or that one will shame or embarrass him. Intimidation is sometimes used as a defense against anxiety proceeding from conflicts over passive homosexual impulses.

intoxication, alcoholic Alcohol poisoning; the state resulting from excessive ingestion of alcohol. Psychiatrically, alcoholic intoxication generally refers to an acute brain syndrome that develops as a result of overdose of alcohol. This syndrome may be of two varieties: (1) acute intoxication, or (2) pathologic intoxication (also known as mania à potu).

Acute intoxication: Alcohol is a physiological depressant, but the release of higher control as a result of this depression leads to an initial heightening of physical and mental activities and to a greater psychomotor speed; during this initial period, organic tremors may be decreased. With increasing depression, however, there soon appear generalized muscular weakness, impairment of intellectual functions, and, because the cerebellar system is attacked early, ataxia, reeling gait, and coarse incoordination of the upper extremities. The marked loss of inhibition typically gives rise to many medico-legal problems. Walking a chalk line, repeating certain paradigmata, and chemical analysis of the breath, urine, and blood have all been used to determine the degree of intoxication, but none of these is completely valid because of the adaptation of the central nervous system to alcohol. Tolerance to alcohol varies greatly; the epileptic, the hysteric, many schizophrenics, and some psychopaths have a low tolerance, as do patients following a head injury.

Pathologic (idiosyncratic) intoxication: This occurs predominantly in people with a low tolerance to alcohol. Usually the syndrome lasts several hours, although it may continue for a whole day. It is characterized by extreme excitement ("alcoholic fury") with aggressive, dangerous, and even homicidal reactions. Persecutory ideas are common. The condition terminates with the patient falling into a deep sleep; there is usually complete amnesia for the episode.

intoxication, hypnagogic *Obs.* A rare condition in which a rough or stormy waking generates a dream and induces motility before the dream disappears; "In rare cases something clumsy is then per-formed, indeed, under the influence of terrifying ideas, an attack of murder may be perpetrated." (Bleuler, *TP*) *Hypnopompic intoxication* would be the more correct term for this condition.

intoxication, pathological See *intoxication, alcoholic.*

intracranial tumor See *tumor, intracranial.*

intralaminar system See *system, intralaminar.*

intrapsychic, intrapsychical Situated, originating, or taking place within the psyche.

intrinsic factor See *sclerosis, posterolateral.*

introject To withdraw psychic energy (libido) from an object and direct it upon the mental image of the object; to incorporate.

introjection The act of introjecting or state of being introjected. When one incorporates into his ego system the picture of an object as he conceives the object to be, the process is known as introjection. Libidinal and aggressive cathexes are then transferred from the object in the environment to the mental picture of the object. For example, when a person becomes depressed due to the loss of a loved one, his feelings are directed to the mental image he possesses of the loved one. He acts toward the image as if it were the loved one in reality.

The term introjection is sometimes used as if it were identical with *secondary identification* and perhaps also with *secondary narcissism.* See *identification; incorporation.*

From the point of view of analytical psychology, introjection is "psychologically . . . a process of assimilation, while projection is a process of dissimilation. Introjection signifies an adjustment of the object to the subject, while projection involves a discrimination of the object by means of a subjective content transveyed into the object." (Jung, *PT*)

"A *passive* and an *active* introjection may be discriminated: to the former belong the transference-processes in the treatment of the neuroses and, in general, all cases in which the object exercises an unconditional attraction upon the subject; while 'feeling-into,' regarded as a process of adaptation, should belong to the latter form." (Ibid.)

intropunitive Having the quality of turning anger against the self, as in the self-pejorative, demeaning, and belittling trend of the depressed patient. This is in contrast to *extrapunitive*, which refers to externally directed anger.

introversion Turning of the instincts inwardly upon oneself. "The libido in introversion is directed toward the inner world, the world of representation, instead of the world of reality. With object-love there is a desire for motor discharge, a going out toward the object, but with introversion there is no desire for motor expression: satisfaction is found in imagined response, in dwelling on phantasied activities in connection with images and ideas of external objects." (Healy et al., *SMP*)

Introversion is often used synonymously with *phantasy-cathexis*. Both imply a loss of contact with reality and because of it, they differ from *narcissism*, which does not imply such loss.

Freud's definition of introversion differs from Jung's. Freud says that introversion does not mean that the erotic relation with reality has been severed but that the subject "has ceased to direct his motor activities to the attainment of his aims in connection with real objects." (*CP*) Jung says it means "a turning inwards of the libido, whereby a negative relation of subject to object is expressed. Interest does not move towards the object, but recedes towards the subject. Everyone whose attitude is introverted thinks, feels, and acts in a way that clearly demonstrates that the subject is the chief factor of motivation while the object at most receives only a secondary value." (*PT*)

introversion, active "Introversion is *active* when the subject *wills* a certain seclusion in face of the object; it is *passive* when the subject is unable to restore again to the object the libido which is streaming back from it." (Jung, *PT*)

introversion, passive See *introversion, active*.

introvert One whose psychic energy (libido) is turned inwardly upon himself.

intrusive treatment See *forced treatment*.

intuition A literary and psychological term with no exact scientific definition or connotation. It refers to a special method of perceiving and evaluating objective reality. Intuition differs from foresight, conscious perception, and judgment in that it relies heavily on unconscious memory traces of past and forgotten experiences and judgments. In this way, a storehouse of uncon-

scious wisdom that had been accumulated (in unconscious memory) in the past is used in the present.

Intuition is characterized by accurate "predictability" in the engineering and mathematical sense. It is also characterized by the fact that people will feel and say "I don't know just how I know that, but I know it's correct," and it often is. The wisdom of the sum total of all past experiences, which have registered in some way or another in the individual and which may be unremembered, is the generally accepted concept of what is meant by intuition.

E.F. Sharpe (*Collected Papers on Psychoanalysis*, 1950) states: "The scientist who understands without having to learn to understand is working with and not against intuitive powers in the same way as the artist. He projects intuition which, when it works in reality to the discovery of real facts, must be initially based upon his own real bodily and psychical experiences." See *analytic psychology*.

intuition, intellectual See *intellect*.

invalidism Condition of being a chronic invalid. From the standpoint of the social worker: the habit of preoccupation with one's health not justified by one's actual condition. See *hypochondriasis*.

invalidism, psychological The mental state of a patient who, though he has been cured of his physical illness, refuses to accept this fact. He repudiates the idea of getting well and gives a thousand reasons why he should continue to live as he was compelled to live during the height of his physical illness.

Such an attitude is observed particularly among children. "When the situation is studied, it is found that he [the child] has learned that there are many benefits from being an invalid—extra attention, marked concern by his parents, extra food and toys, and frequent excuse from duties." The mechanism is largely an unconscious one, however; most children who suffer from chronic invalidism are not aware that they are using their disability as a means of gaining benefits. (Pearson, G.H.J. *Emotional Disorders of Children*, 1940) See *habit, complaint*.

invariance, developmental Stability over time, or failure to change with maturation, most often applied to speech organization in children. Believers in developmental invariance hold that speech organization in children is similar to that in adults and does not change with age. The developmental maturation position holds that children are born with hemispheric equipotentiality for language and that lateralization occurs as the child matures. Experimental and clinical evidence generally supports the developmental invariance position.

invasive treatment See *forced treatment.*

inverse agonist See *agonist, inverse.*

inversion See *inversion, sexual.*

inversion, absolute Freud speaks of those who are "absolutely inverted; i.e., their sexual object must always be of the same sex, while the opposite sex can never be to them an object of sexual longing, but leaves them indifferent or . . . may even evoke sexual repugnance." *(BW)*

inversion, amphigenous Psychosexual hermaphroditism; i.e. the sexual object may belong indifferently to either the same or to the other sex. See *androgyneity; bisexuality.*

inversion, occasional Accidental homosexuality, or homosexuality faute de mieux. See *homosexuality, male.*

inversion, sexoesthetic Eonism; *transvestitism* (q.v.).

inversion, sexual Homosexuality. Freud distinguished three types of sexual inversion: *absolute, amphigenous,* and *occasional.*

inversion, sleep Somnolence by day and insomnia at night; seen most commonly in organic brain disorders and in the schizophrenias.

invert A homosexual.

investment The affective charge given to an idea or object. See *cathexis.*

inveterate drinking Delta *alcoholism* (q.v.).

invisible college See *college, invisible.*

involution See *hereditary.*

involutional period *Climacterium* (q.v.).

involutional psychotic reaction See *psychosis, involutional.*

ion pump A metabolic mechanism that moves ions through a cell membrane. The calcium pump, for example, moves calcium ions out of the muscle cell with a consequent cessation of contraction; the sodium pump moves sodium ions out of cells and potassium ions into them. One proposed mechanism of lithium action in

affective disorders is based on the sodium pump (or through blockage of the calcium channel) reducing retention of sodium within the nerve cell.

iophobia Fear of poison.

ipsation *Rare. Autoerotism* (q.v.).

IPSS See *Schizophrenia, International Pilot Study.*

IQ Intelligence quotient. See *quotient, intelligence.*

iridoplegia Paralysis of the iris muscle; failure of the pupil to react to light. The Argyll Robertson pupil is a special form of reflex iridoplegia. Reflex iridoplegia may be caused by optic nerve lesions, optic tract lesions, lesions in the upper part of the midbrain, and lesions in the motor path (oculomotor nerve). The condition is occasionally seen in alcoholic polyneuritis and in diabetes.

IRM Inherited releasing mechanism. See *instinct.*

irradiation 1. Illumination. 2. In medicine, exposure to rays (heat, light, X-rays, etc.) for diagnostic or therapeutic purposes. 3. In neurophysiology, a spreading of the neural impulse within the central nervous system and, by analogy in psychodynamics, the spread of energy or tension outside the system in which the tension was originally generated. 4. In conditional-stimulus experiments (see *conditioning*), elicitation of the conditional response by a stimulus other than the one to which conditioning has been established; ordinarily such irradiation occurs only when the other stimulus is of the same general class as the original conditional stimulus.

irradiation, ultrasonic Used, in the prefrontal areas of the brain, as an alternative to lobotomy; it is said to cause less variable and less severe cerebral damage than the surgical procedure, to entail minimal risk, and to give comparable results. Irradiation is applied through bilateral trephine openings, using a frequency of 1000 kcps and an average intensity of 7 watts/cm^2 for 4 to 14 minutes.

irrational Though commonly used to mean unreasonable, Jung says: "As I make use of this term it does not denote something contrary to *reason*, but something outside the province of reason, whose essence, therefore, is not established by reason.

"Elementary facts belong to this category, e.g., that the earth has a moon, that chlorine is an element, that the greatest density of water is found at 4° centigrade. . . . Both thinking and feeling as *directed functions* are rational," while sensation and intuition are irrational. (*PT*) See *rational.*

irrational action Harming oneself without an adequate reason; causing, or not avoiding, some evil such as death; physical or mental pain; physical, cognitive, or volitional disability; or loss of freedom, opportunity, or pleasure without adequate reason.

irrational desire Desire to carry out an irrational action; wanting to suffer some evil without an adequate reason for doing so.

irregular *Obs.* Social workers' expression covering unlegalized unions, unconventional love affairs, and adultery.

irreminiscence Amnesia; inability to remember; more specifically, a type of agnosia with inability to form a mental picture of objects.

irresistibility See *responsibility, criminal.*

irresponsibility See *responsibility, criminal.*

irritability, acoustic Auditory hypersensitivity. A generalized, diffuse irritability is one of the common characteristics of the traumatic neurosis. "From the point of view of distribution, irritability is present in every case of traumatic neurosis. It chiefly concerns auditory stimuli, but in some instances there may be abnormal sensitivity to temperature, pain, or sudden tactile stimuli. From the physiologic point of view there exists a lowering of the threshold of stimulation; from the psychologic point of view—a state of readiness for fright reactions. This is intimately connected with the general hypertensity of these cases. Auditory hypersensitivity is the most common symptom, being occasioned by the most widely distributed sudden stimulus, perceived by the oldest sense organ which establishes contact with its environment, and the most intimately connected with fright." (Kardiner, A., & Spiegel, L. *War Stress and Neurotic Illness,* 1947)

irrumation Fellatio.

irrumo- Combining form for various terms that refer to oral sexual activity performed on the penis, from L. *irrumare,* to offer the penis for sucking.

IS *Index of sexuality* (q.v.); Ischemic Scale.

Isakower, Otto (1899–1972) Austrian psychoanalyst; described the phenonmenon that bears his name in the *International Journal of Psychoanalysis,* 1938.

Isakower phenomenon See *hallucination, blank.*

ischemia, cerebral See *TIA.*

ischnophonia, ischophonia (isk-nō-fō'ne-à) Stammering; *stuttering* (q.v.).

isocortex Neocortex; the most commonly found type of cortex of the cerebral hemispheres, composed of six layers of cells that have their embryologic origin in the mass of gray matter surrounding the ventricles—the outermost molecular layer, external granular layer, external pyramidal layer, internal granular layer, ganglionic layer, and the innermost fusiform layer.

isogamous (ī-sog'-à-mus) *Genet.* Pertaining to or characterized by gametes that are equal in size and similar in structure in both sexes. See *syngamy.*

isolate In the therapy group, anyone who does not participate in group activities or make contact with other members of the group. See *instigator; neutralizer.*

In psychoanalysis, to separate experiences or memories from their affect.

isolate monkey See *monkey therapist.*

isolated delusion See *monosymptomatic hypochondriacal psychosis.*

isolation In psychoanalysis, the separation of an idea or memory from its affective cathexis or charge, "so that what remains in consciousness is nothing but an ideational content which is perfectly colorless and is judged to be unimportant." (Freud, S. *Inhibitions, Symptoms and Anxiety,* 1936) For example, a patient remembered the many occasions on which he made ineffectual attempts to murder his father. The recollections were entirely without affect.

Isolation may also be observed in the motor sphere. There is a pause "in which nothing is to happen, no perception is made, no action carried out." (Ibid.)

Freud distinguishes between *isolation* and *undoing.* Isolation implies a kind of foresight that tries to check the appearance of something unpleasant; it is a rational process, according to Freud, whereas *undoing* is "irrational or magical in nature."

As a therapeutic regimen *isolation* has been practiced for centuries. Janet writes: "The chief difficulties in life arise in connection with social relationships, and it has long been felt that social activities are more exhausting than any other kind. On this recognition has been based a method of treatment which is often associated with the rest cure of nervous diseases, namely, treatment by isolation." (*PH*)

In sociology isolation is the separation of the person or group from social contacts.

Erikson describes *intimacy vs. isolation* as one of the eight stages of man. See *ontogeny, psychic.*

isolation, perceptual See *deprivation, sensory.*

isolation, psychic Jung's term for the sense of estrangement from one's fellows that is felt immediately upon experiencing material communicated from one's collective unconscious. Under certain conditions material from this area of the psyche irrupts into consciousness. "Such irruptions are uncanny, because they are irrational and inexplicable to the individual concerned. They signify a momentous alteration of the personality in that they immediately constitute a painful, personal secret that estranges the human being from his environment and isolates him from it. It is something that 'you can tell to no one,' except under fear of being accused of mental abnormality, and with some justification, for something quite similar befalls the insane. It is still a long way from an intuitively sensed irruption to pathological overthrow; but a layman does not know this.

"The result of the *psychic isolation* through a secret is, as a rule, the vivifying of the psychic atmosphere as a surrogate for the lost contact with the individual's fellow beings. . . . The experiencing of the unconscious is a personal secret communicable only to the very few, and that with difficulty. *It isolates the individual to whom it happens.* But isolation effects a compensatory animation of the psychic atmosphere, and this is uncanny." (*The Integration of the Personality,* 1939)

isolation, psychological Disinclination, aversion to, or fear of making contact with another member of the group.

isolation, sensory See *deprivation, sensory.*

isophilic Sullivan's term for affection or liking for others of the same sex, such affection lacking the genital element characteristic of homosexuality; approximately synonymous with homoerotic.

isozyme A genetically determined variant of a normally occurring enzyme. Isozymes catalyze similar processes as their normal counterparts, but because they differ slightly in protein linkage they differ also in optimal conditions for function.

issue, central In Mann's terminology, the particular theme on which the work of brief psychotherapy will focus. It is different from the complaints voiced by the patient, since they are derived from the central issue. The central issue itself is typically an affective statement to the self of how a person feels now and has always felt about the self. It is formulated to include time, affects, and the image of the self. The last will be found to fall within one of the five categories of feeling about the self: glad, sad, mad, frightened, or guilty. See *psychotherapy, time-limited.*

it *Id* (q.v.).

itching See *craving, autonomic-affective.*

ITPA *Illinois Test of Psycholinguistic Abilities* (q.v.).

J

Jack the Clipper The designation given to any person with a morbid propensity to clip hair or braids of girls; the name was first used in reference to a man in Chicago who for several years carried on the practice.

Jack the Ripper A London physician, an epileptic, who over a period of years during the 1880s committed brutal murders, presumably while in a postictal fugue state.

Jackson, John Hughlings (1834–1911) British neurologist; epilepsy, aphasia, dissolution, and disinhibition processes in brain damage.

Jacksonian epilepsy See *epilepsy, Jacksonian*.

Jackson's syndrome A bulbar syndrome due to involvement of the vagus, spinal accessory, and hypoglossal nerves. Symptoms are homolateral paralysis of the soft palate, pharynx, and larynx; homolateral paralysis of the sternocleidomastoid and trapezius muscles; and homolateral paralysis and atrophy of the tongue.

jactatio capitis nocturna A disturbance of sleep sometimes observed in children: it consists in rhythmical rolling of the head from side to side—which hinders normal sleep. See *head-rolling*.

jactitation, jactation Extreme restlessness or tossing about.

Jakob, Alfons (1884–1931) German psychiatrist; *Creutzfeldt-Jakob's disease* (q.v.). See *virus infections*.

Jakob-Creutzfeldt's disease (CJD) Presenile dementia with dysarthria and a syndrome of amyotrophic lateral sclerosis. Also known as Heidenheim's or Kraepelin's disease. See *Creutzfeldt-Jakob's disease*.

jamais vu A paramnestic phenomenon consisting of the erroneous feeling or conviction that one has never seen anything like that before. Such a *denial* (q.v.) produces a fragmentation or break in continuity of memory.

James-Lange theory See *theory, James-Lange-Sutherland*.

James, William (1842–1910) American philosopher and psychologist.

Janet's disease (Pierre Janet, French psychiatrist, 1859–1947) *Psychasthenia* (q.v.).

Janet's psychology A forerunner of Freudian psychoanalysis that recognized unconscious mental forces as significant factors in the production of dissociative states, hysteria, etc.

Janusian thinking (Janus, the Roman god of doorways and communication, whose two faces enabled him to look in opposite directions simultaneously) Oppositional thinking; the capacity to conceive and utilize two or more opposite or contradictory ideas, concepts, or images simultaneously. A. Rothenberg (*Archives of General Psychiatry 24*, 1971) suggests that Janusian thinking is one of the thought processes employed in creative thinking.

jargon aphasia See *aphasia, jargon*.

jargon, organ Adler applies this term to the "somatic language" (symptoms) that the neurotic uses to express a masculine protest. According to Adler, the child's ego-consciousness is in conflict with the facts of his environment. Thus the child wishes to be big and powerful but actually is small and weak. The child therefore constructs all its aggressive attitudes into one of masculine protest against all symptoms of weakness (femininity) such as tenderness, subordinacy, and, most important, manifestations of organ inferiority. The neurotically predisposed child, however, endeavors further to gain an effective weapon by associating with its organ inferiority such character traits as originate in the ego-consciousness—i.e. obstinacy, need of affection, exaggerated cleanliness, pedantry, covetousness, ambition, etc. Thus in order to gain attention and affection a psychogenic epileptic managed so that most of his "attacks" were preceded by obstipation, thereby worrying his family—all this to offset his degradation. In this way the masculine protest makes use of a somatic language or organ-jargon to gain expression. As one of Adler's patients expressed it in a dream, "My disease has its origin in my feeling of inferiority." (Adler, A. *The Neurotic Constitution*, 1917)

Jarisch-Herxheimer reaction (Adolf Jarisch, Austrian dermatologist, 1850–1902, and Karl Herxheimer, German dermatologist, 1861–1921) An inflammatory reaction in syphilis, involving skin, mucosae, viscera, and/or nervous system, often precipitated by antisyphilitic treatment and possibly due to an allergic reaction to liberated toxic products. Such reactions are much less common with penicillin than with older antispirochetal agents and rarely consist of more than transient fever during the first 24 hours of treatment. Some workers advise a course of bismuth and iodide before instituting penicillin treatment in an attempt to minimize such reactions.

Jaspers, Karl (1883–1969) Philosopher and psychiatrist, a member of the Heidelberg (Germany) school (others were Gruhle, Mayer-Gross, and Schneider); one of the founders of existentialism; *General Psychopathology* (1913).

jaw-jerk A deep reflex. The patient opens his mouth so that the lower jaw hangs a little; the examiner places his finger on the side of the lower jaw, and strikes it with a percussion hammer; this results in contraction of the masseter muscle and raising of the jaw.

jealousy According to Freud, normal jealousy is compounded of (1) grief, which is the pain caused by the thought of losing the loved object; this being associated with (2) narcissistic injury, i.e. a loss of self-esteem; (3) feelings of enmity against the successful rival; and, finally (4), self-criticism in which the person blames himself for his loss. This reaction is not completely rational, for it is disproportionate to the real circumstances, not completely

under the control of the conscious ego, and not derived from the actual situation. Rather it is rooted in the Oedipus complex. Frequently jealousy is experienced also bisexually: for example, a man will feel both "the suffering in regard to the loved woman and the hatred against the male rival," and "grief in regard to the unconsciously loved man and hatred of the woman as a rival." (Freud, *CP*)

jealousy, morbid *Pathologic jealousy; Othello syndrome; amorous paranoia; conjugal paranoia;* the delusion that the marital or sexual partner is unfaithful, typically accompanied by intense searching for evidence of infidelity and repeated interrogations and direct accusations of the partner that may lead to violent quarrels. Pathologic jealousy appears to be fanned by alcohol intoxication, and both show a high degree of association with violence, including homicide. Morbid jealousy most often is isolated or encapsulated, and phenomenologically it has much in common with the *monosymptomatic hypochondriacal pyschosis* (q.v.). Although their number is small, some reports suggest that tricyclic antidepressant drugs or pimozide (but not other neuroleptics, such as haloperidol) may be effective in diminishing or eliminating the delusion.

jealousy, projected The type of jealousy that is derived from the person's own actual unfaithfulness or from repressed impulses toward it. In this type of jealousy, the person who is being tempted in the direction of infidelity alleviates his guilt by projecting his own impulses onto the partner to whom he owes fidelity. Now, social conventions permit a certain amount of latitude to the married woman's desire to attract, and the married man's desire to possess, members of the opposite sex. Through these social flirtations the person exercises his tendency to unfaithfulness and the desire now awakened is gratified by a turning back to the marital partner. The jealous person, however, does not recognize these conventions of tolerance: having projected onto his partner his own impulses toward infidelity, he will interpret as actual infidelity this behavior that covers such unconscious impulses in his partner. (Freud, *CP*) See *paranoia, conjugal.*

Jelliffe, Smith Ely (1866–1945) American psychoanalyst; founded *Nervous and Men-*

tal Disease Monograph Series and, with William Alanson White, *Psychoanalytic Review* and *Diseases of the Nervous System.*

Jellinek's formula (E.M. Jellinek, U.S. physician, 1890–1963) A means of estimating the number of alcoholics in a population, based on the assumption that the relationship between alcoholism and cirrhosis remains fairly constant. Jellinek proposed (1959) that the formula be abandoned, and it is not generally used nowadays.

Jendrassik reinforcement (Ernest Jendrassik, Slovakian physician, 1858–1922) A weak response of the knee jerk may often be reinforced, that is, strengthened, by having the patient grasp his own hands and pull vigorously on them.

jerk, elbow See *reflex, triceps.*

jerk, knee Patellar reflex; the leg is flexed at the knee joint and the quadriceps tendon is tapped just below the patella; this results in extension of the leg with visible and palpable contraction of the quadriceps muscle. The femoral nerve contains both the afferent and the efferent pathways of the patellar reflex, whose spinal center is at L_{2-4}.

jerk, patellar Knee jerk.

jerk, pendular knee When tapping the patellar tendon, several oscillations of the leg occur before it comes to a stop; observed in disease of the cerebellum.

jet lag See *circadian desynchronosis; clock, biological.*

jhin jhinia A culture-specific syndrome that is said to occur in epidemic form in India, consisting of bizarre and seemingly involuntary contractions and spasms.

joint, Charcot See *arthropathy.*

Joint Commission on Mental Illness and Health Authorized by the U.S. Congress' Mental Health Study Act of 1955; a multidisciplinary study group that included 36 national agencies in the mental health and welfare fields; its final report, *Action for Mental Health,* was instrumental in the legislation and federal funding that made possible the development of community mental health centers for the mentally ill and mentally retarded. See *psychiatry, community.*

joint custody See *custody.*

Jones, Ernest (1879–1958) British psychoanalyst; one of the original group who gathered around Freud in the early days of

psychoanalysis; first to introduce psychoanalysis into English-speaking world (England, 1906); one of the founders of American Psychoanalytic Association (1911) and British Psychoanalytic Society (1913); honorary life-president of International Psychoanalytic Association; three-volume biography of Freud.

judgment A conclusion, decision, or verdict about a particular action and specifically about whether the action was morally right or wrong. See *principle; rule; theory.*

Of the many definitions of judgment, the one most commonly used in psychiatry has to do with the ability to recognize the true relations of ideas. This involves what is called *critical judgment.* "But if we speak in psychiatry and jurisprudence of the capacity to judge, we mean the ability to form judgments, that is, the capacity to draw correct conclusions from the material acquired by experience." (Bleuler, *TP*)

Some authorities distinguish between *critical* and *automatic* judgment, meaning by the latter the performance of action as a reflex. When a patient with good vision walks directly into a wall, instead of stopping or turning, it is said that his automatic judgment is impaired.

jumpers See *lata.*

jumps See *epilepsy, myoclonic.*

junctim "Purposive connection of two thoughts and affect-complexes that have in reality little or nothing to do with one another, in order to strengthen the affect. For example, a patient with *agoraphobia* [q.v.], in order, by a complicated mechanism, to raise his prestige at home and force his environment into his service and to prevent himself likewise from losing, while on the street or in open places, the 'resonance' so fervently desired, unites unconsciously and emotionally into a 'junctim,' the thought of being alone, of strange people, of purchases, search for the theatre, society, etc., and the phantasy of an apoplectic stroke, a confinement on the street, disease infection through germs on the street." (Adler, A. *The Practice and Theory of Individual Psychology,* 1924)

Jung association test See *association.*

Jung, Carl Gustav (1875–1961) Swiss psychiatrist; originally associated with Freud, later founded own school of *analytic psychology* (q.v.).

Jungian psychology The theory of human personality development and behavior proposed by Jung, who regarded the mind not only as a result of past experiences but also as a preparation for the future, with aims and goals that it tries to realize within itself. Merging of the personal unconscious with the racial or collective unconscious provides the background for all thought and emotion. Jung described archetypes within the collective unconscious, psychologic typology with attitude and function types, and the compensatory function of dreams and symbolism. See *analytic psychology*.

juramentado A culture-specific syndrome described in the Malays and Moros consisting of marked agitation and assault or stabbing of anyone they encounter, followed by a stupor and, upon awakening, amnesia for the episode.

jus primae noctis The "right to the first night" or "right of the lord" (*droit du seigneur*) is described as "a lascivious tribute levied by feudal lords upon their vassals, in accordance with which the lord enjoyed the first embrace of the vassal's bride." (Paolo Mantegazza, *Gli amori degli uomini,* 1883?) It was also called *virginal tribute*. Among certain primitive tribes the "right to the first night" belonged to the father of the bride and was supposedly symbolic of his authority.

justification A genetic-nutritional mechanism consisting of the ability of the fetus to alter its amino acid environment to a pattern requisite for its protein-synthesizing apparatus. The fetus that is homozygous for an amino acid disorder is almost always injured because it cannot justify the maternal mixture. If the condition occurs in nutritionally deprived areas, the heterozygous fetus in the heterozygous mother is also at high risk since he cannot adequately justify the deficient mixture that the mother also fails to justify because of nutritional deprivation.

juvenile The juvenile period extends from the beginning of the phase of puberty to the end of the stage of adolescence. See *ontogeny, psychic*.

juvenile general paresis See *neurosyphilis, congenital*.

juvenile tabes See *tabes, juvenile*.

juvenilism Persistently youthful appearance of the body in a mature individual exhibiting all the signs of having passed the puberal crisis.

K

Kahlbaum, Karl Ludwig (1828–99) German psychiatrist; catatonia.

Kahlbaum-Wernicke syndrome *Presbyophrenia* (q.v.).

kaif, kif Pleasure or feeling of contentment and ease, as in a dream or state of ecstasy. The term is used in Morocco to refer to hashish or *marihuana* (q.v.).

kainotophobia, kainophobia Fear of change or novelty. See *neophobia*.

kakergasia See *merergasia*.

kakidrosis *Obs.* Perspiration with disagreeable odor.

kakorraphiophobia Fear of failure.

Kalinowsky, Lothar B. (b. 1899) German-born neuropsychiatrist; in U.S. since 1940; electroconvulsive and other somatic treatments.

Kallmann, Franz J. (1897–1965) German-born psychoanalyst and geneticist; genetics of human behavior, especially schizophrenia, manic-depressive psychosis.

Kandinsky-Clérambault complex See *complex, Clérambault-Kandinsky*.

Kanner, Leo (1894–1981) Austrian-born psychiatrist; to U.S. in 1924; founded Johns Hopkins Children's Psychiatric Clinic (1930); wrote first text in *Child Psychiatry* (1935); early infantile autism.

Kardiner, Abraham (1891–1981) American psychoanalyst; cofounder of first psychoanalytic training school in U.S. in 1930; *The Individual and His Society* (1939); *Psychological Frontiers of Society* (1945).

karyotype A photograph of the chromosomes of a cell; the original photograph is enlarged and the chromosomes are cut out, paired, and mounted in order of decreasing size. A karyotype is unique, similar to a fingerprint. A schematic representation of the karyotype is termed *idiogram*. See *chromosome*.

katalepsia *Obs.* Same as *catalepsy*.

katasexual Necrophiliac.

katatonia See *catatonia*.

kathisophobia Fear of sitting down.

Kaufman, Moses Ralph (1900–77) Russian-born, Canadian-educated American psychiatrist; psychoanalysis, psychosomatic medicine.

Kayser-Fleischer ring (Bernhard Kayser, German ophthalmologist, 1869–1954, and Richard Fleischer, Munich physician, 1848–1909) See *degeneration, hepatolenticular*.

Keeler polygraph See *detector, lie*.

Kempf, Edward J. (1885–1971) American psychiatrist, psychosomatic medicine; *Basic Biodynamics* and *Autonomic Functions and the Personality*.

Kempf's disease See *homosexual panic*.

kenophobia Also spelled *cenophobia;* fear of barren or empty space, of voids. See *agoraphobia*.

keraunoneurosis H. Oppenheim's term for traumatic neuroses associated with electric shocks.

keraunophobia Fear of lightning. It is related to the fear of strong and superior forces, and as such it appears to stem from the fear of the father, arising during the stage of phallic primacy. It is therefore closely allied with the fear of castration.

kernel complex Oedipus complex. See *complex, Oedipus*.

kernicterus, kernikterus See *icterus gravis neonatorum*.

ketamine A surgical anesthetic or analgesic, 2-(2-chlorphenyl)-2-(methylamino)cyclohexanone, sometimes used in less than anesthetic doses as a psychedelic; manifested in a feeling of being disconnected from one's surroundings and perceptions of floating in space or being disembodied.

key concept Arnold Gesell and his coworkers at the Yale Clinic of Child Development formulated the idea that in all psychological studies of the preschool child the interpretation of individual differences should be governed by one key concept: that a child's abilities are all relative to one inclusive ability, the ability to grow. "Growth, therefore, becomes a *key-concept* for the interpretation of individual differences. There are laws of sequence and of maturation, which account for the general similarities and basic trends of child development. But no two children grow up in exactly the same way." (Gesell, A., et al. *The First Five Years of Life*, 1940)

The tempo and style of growth are different in every child and are characteristic of the child's individuality. Gesell holds that "mental growth is a patterning process: a progressive morphogenesis of patterns of behavior," and that "envisagement of the mind as a growing system puts us in a better position to observe and comprehend the determinants of the child's behavior."

kibbutz A form of collective education and upbringing of children, in use in Israel, in which the rearing of the child by his parents is replaced by upbringing in communal houses under the direction of specially trained "metapelets," or mother substitutes.

kif *Kaif* (q.v.).

kimilue A culture-specific syndrome described in Native Americans of Southern California consisting of general apathy, lack of interest in life, loss of appetite, and vivid sexual dreams.

kindling Progressively increasing responsiveness to successive electrical stimuli. Depending on the part of the brain that is stimulated and on the nature of the stimulus, the end result may be a generalized convulsion or behavioral alteration. The limbic system appears to be particularly susceptible to kindling. Because behavioral change can occur as a result of kindling, the mechanism is viewed by at least some investigators as a model for learning and for psychological development, including both normal behavior and psychopathology.

kinephantom (kin'e-fan-tum) An illusory phenomenon: the movement of an object that actually occurs is perceived as being different from what the movement really is. An example is perceiving the wheels of an automobile as moving in a counterclockwise direction when they are, in fact, moving in a clockwise direction. See *illusion*.

kinesalgia Pain induced by movement, common with organic lesions. Pain of psychic origin (psychalgia) may also be experienced in the absence of organic pathology. See *somatoform disorders*.

kinesics The study of movement and action, particularly as a part of communication. See *method, linguistic-kinesic*.

kinesis Generic term for motion.

kinesitherapy See *therapy, physical*.

kinesophobia Fear of motion or of motion sickness.

kinesthesia Perception of one's own movement; proprioception. The receptors for kinesthesia are located in the muscles, tendons, and joints. The cell bodies of these peripheral sensory neurons are in the spinal root ganglia. The central processes pass via the dorsal roots into the spinal cord and brain stem and, uncrossed in the posterior columns of the spinal cord, ascend to the gracilis and cuneate nuclei. Here they make synaptic connections with their second-order neurons, which cross and enter the medial lemniscus of the opposite side, and thence pass to the thalamus. Synaptic connections are made here with third-order neurons that ascend to the sensory projection center in the postcentral gyrus of the cortex (areas 3, 1, 2 of Brodmann).

kinesthetic hallucination False sensation of body movement, as in phantom limb. See *limb, phantom*.

kinetic Relating to movement.

kinky hair syndrome See *syndrome, kinky hair*.

Kinsey, Alfred Charles (1894–1956) American biologist; director of Indiana University's Institute for Sex Research; *Sexual Behavior in the Human Male* (1948), *Sexual Behavior in the Human Female* (1953).

kinship *Genet.* The blood relationship among individuals belonging to the same stock by common descent. See *consanguinity*.

KIPS Acronym for *knowledge information processing systems*, applied to "fifth-generation" computers, which are expected to be capable of handling 10^8 to 10^9 LIPS (logical inferences per second), as compared with the fourth-generation computers of the early 1980s that handle 10^4 to 10^5 LIPS.

Kirchhoff, Theodor (1853–1922) German psychiatrist; history of psychiatry.

Kirkbride, Thomas Story (1809–83) American psychiatrist; one of the 13 founders of the Association of Medical Superintendents of America (the forerunner of the American Psychiatric Association); mental hospital construction.

klazomania Compulsory shouting; usually a motor discharge phenomenon based on mesencephalic or other central nervous system irritation.

Klebedenken Adhesive, sticky, perseverative thinking. Klebedenken is one of the associational disturbances seen in the schizophrenias.

Klebenbleiben (klā′ben-blī-ben) A type of language disturbance occurring in schizophrenic patients in which the speaker remains glued to the same topic; he restates the topic in different words, elaborates it, qualifies it, explains it, but cannot leave it. See *circumstantiality.*

Klein, Melanie (1882–1960) British psychoanalyst (British Psychoanalytic Society-Institute); child analyst; a controversial figure whose theories of early psychic development (e.g. the ubiquity of "internal objects," the "depressive" and "paranoid positions," and her direct clinical application of the death instinct) were at variance with orthodox psychoanalytic theory.

Kleine-Levin syndrome See *syndrome, Kleine-Levin.*

kleptolagnia A morbid desire to steal; *kleptomania* (q.v.). A psychiatric term devised by J.C. Kiernan to designate "theft associated with sexual excitement"—on the analogy of "algolagnia." In 1896 La Cassague (and others later) had stressed that sex and kleptomania were often associated, but the prevailing view that "cleptomania was a syndrome of irresistible and motiveless impulses to theft based on constitutional 'degeneration' persisted. In 1908, Stekel observed that irresistible and apparently motiveless thefts were substitutive forms of sexual gratification [consequent to sexual deprivation or repression]. Ellis's concept of kleptolagnia represented the theft as a means of generating fear and anxiety

to 'reinforce' the 'feeble sexual impulse' in its drive for gratification. . . . [Ellis did] not appreciate that the states of anxiety which to him appeared to 'overflow into the sexual sphere' are in actuality, as in the theft itself, a form of defense of the ego against sexual impulses which threaten to overwhelm it." (Freedman, B. *Psychoanalytic Quarterly 11,* 1942)

kleptomania Morbid impulse to steal; pathological stealing; "senseless" stealing in that the objects are not taken for immediate use or for their monetary value and are often returned surreptitiously, given to others, or hidden away. Kleptomania is one of the *disorders of impulse control* (q.v.). From the psychoanalytic standpoint it is believed that obsessive stealing stems from the period of infantile sexuality. The thief steals objects that possess libidinal value to him (or her, for stealing is regarded by Staub as essentially a female problem). It is held that stealing is rooted in penis envy. When one steals from those in superior position, it is said that the theft traces back to original penis envy and active castration of the superior (father).

Abraham and Alexander believe that the motive for stealing arises at the suckling stage, when the mother refuses to give the child the breast. Abraham further maintains that obsessive stealers are those who were emotionally starved during the infancy period; they become antisocial because they were not loved. The narcissistic injury gives rise to revenge.

Adler says: "Lies, thefts and other crimes committed by children are manifestly attempts to extend the limits of power in this way [i.e. toward superiority]." (*The Neurotic Constitution,* 1917)

kleptophobia Fear of stealing or becoming a thief.

Klinefelter's syndrome See *syndrome, Klinefelter's.*

Klippel-Feil syndrome See *syndrome, Klippel-Feil.*

klismaphilia Love of enemas and a dependence on their use for sexual arousal; one of the miscellaneous paraphilias within the *psychosexual disorders* (q.v.); popularly referred to as "water sports." See *anal eroticism.*

klon See *clone.*

klopemania *Obs.* Kleptomania.

Klumpke-Déjerine syndrome See *syndrome, Klumpke-Déjerine.*

Klüver, Heinrich (1898–1979) Pioneer in brain research at University of Chicago.

Klüver-Bucy syndrome See *syndrome, Klüver-Bucy.*

knee, wobbly Laxness of the knee joint, indicative of lowered muscular tonus. The wobbly knee sign, elicited by shaking the knee, is seen in the cerebellar and pseudo-cerebellar syndromes and is probably indicative of disturbed proprioception.

Knight's move See *derailment, thought.*

knowledge information processing systems See *KIPS.*

knowledge test See *responsibility, criminal.*

Köhler, Wolfgang (1887–1967) U.S. psychologist, born in Estonia; author of the classic work *Gestalt Psychology* (1929).

Kohnstamm maneuver See *test, Kohnstamm.*

Kohut, Heinz (1913–81) Viennese psychoanalyst; to U.S. in 1940; narcissistic character disorder; self psychology; *Analysis of the Self* (1971); *Restoration of the Self* (1977); *Search for the Self* (1978).

koinotropy (koi-not'rō-pē) The state of being identified with the common interests of others or the public (Meyer).

kolyphrenia Cortical inhibitability.

kolytic (kō-lit'ik) Inhibitory. J.R. Hunt used this term in a way that is approximately equivalent to *schizoid* (q.v.).

kopophobia Fear of fatigue.

koro An acute delusional syndrome seen in Malaya and Southern China in which the patient suddenly experiences depersonalization and comes to believe that his penis is shrinking into his abdomen. Elaborate measures are taken to prevent such an end result, such as tying a red string around the penis or clamping a wooden box around it.

Although generally classified among the culture-specific syndromes, koro may be no more than a variant of castration anxiety in a susceptible person. A case has been reported of amphetamine-induced koro syndrome in a 20-year-old Canadian youth. (Dow, T.W., & Silver, D. *Journal of the Florida Medical Association 60*, 1973)

Korsakoff psychosis Also spelled Korsakov. See *syndrome, Wernicke-Korsakoff.*

Krabbe's disease (Korud H. Krabbe, contemporary Copenhagen neurologist) See *leukodystrophies.*

Kraepelin, Emil (1856–1926) German psychiatrist; psychiatric nosology and systematization; attempted to sort out definite disease entities and differentiated between manic-depressive psychosis and dementia praecox (schizophrenia), and between endogenous and exogenous psychoses; prognostic approach, by correlating basic symptoms with course of illness.

Kraepelin's disease *Jakob-Creutzfeldt's disease* (q.v.).

Krafft-Ebing, Richard von (1840–1903) German sexologist.

Kretschmer, Ernst (1888–1964) German psychiatrist; somatotyping and relationship of physique to character, personality, and mental illness.

Kronfeld, Arthur (1886–1961) German psychiatrist; psychotherapy.

Kuf's disease See *Tay-Sachs disease.*

kuru The first chronic degenerative neurologic disease of humans shown to be due to unconventional slow virus infection, perhaps transmitted via ritual cannibalism, and limited to a number of adjacent valleys in the mountainous interior of New Guinea. It was first described in 1957 by D. Carleton Gajdusek and V. Zigas and has been disappearing gradually since then as ritual cannibalism has been abandoned. In the Fore language, kuru means shivering or trembling. The disease is characterized by cerebellar ataxia and a shivering tremor that progresses to complete motor incapacity and death in less than one year from time of onset. See *virus infections.*

L

L-dopa See *paralysis agitans*.

L-K Linguistic-kinesic See *method, linguistic-kinesic*.

la belle indifference See *hysteria*.

LAAM L-α-acetylmethadol, a longer acting congener of methadone (72 hours as compared with 24 hours). See *methadone; narcotic blockade*.

labeling theory The sociologic hypothesis that deviance is determined by the reactions of others, in that defining a person as deviant automatically consigns him to a path of mental illness or criminality. Deviance thus is in the eye of the beholder, whose labeling of another as abnormal or delinquent constitutes a self-fulfilling prophecy. Also known as *societal reaction theory*.

labile (lāb′il) Characterized by free and usually uncontrolled expression of the emotions. See *lability*.

lability Volatility; instability. Emotional lability refers to emotions that are inordinately mobile and hence not under adequate control; seen most commonly in the organic brain syndromes and in the early stages of the schizophrenias.

labyrinthine A type of schizophrenic speech that wanders aimlessly, from one topic to another, without obvious connection between the various topics. Certain topics may be elaborated tangentially, others appear to be an outgrowth of circumstantiality; the overall effect on the listener is to produce a massive, vague, hazy maze of words, made all the more remarkable by the fact that typically the patient is able to return to the initial topic of conversation and appears to think that his incomprehensible ramifications have been appropriately related to that topic.

Lacan, Jacques (1901–81) French psychoanalyst; *Ecrits* (1966). Lucan replaced Freud's model derived from 19th-century physics with a model of modern structural linguistics: "The unconscious is structured like a language."

According to Lacan, experience occurs in three "registers": the Symbolic, the Imaginary, and the Real. Experience encoded in language is the Symbolic; what is absent can be made present through signs. The Imaginary is the realm of all phantasy, the world of the ego in which there is no experience of an "I" as subject (since this requires the ability to symbolize). The Real is the raw experience of what is happening, before it is imaged or symbolized.

laceration, cerebral A cerebral contusion of sufficient severity to cause a visible breach in the continuity of the brain substance. This may occur either directly below the site of the blow to the head, or by contrecoup on the opposite side of the brain. See *contusion, brain*.

Lachschlaganfall (läK′shläK än′fål) a condition described by Herman Oppenheim (German neurologist, 1858–1919) in which the patient falls unconscious due to violent laughing. See *epilepsy, gelastic*.

lactate challenge A technique used to provoke panic attacks in susceptible subjects, consisting of infusion of 0.5 M sodium DL-lactate over a 20-minute period. Approximately two-thirds of patients with *panic disorder* or *agoraphobia* (qq.v.) develop a panic attack when injected with lactate; imipramine blocks the lactate panic in 65 to 75% of those who develop it.

lacuna Small focal infarct due to occlusion of a branch artery in the brain. An accumulation of such lesions can cause progressive mental deterioration, the *lacunar state,* by many equated with *multi-infarct dementia* (q.v.). When the infarcts are limited to the subcortical white matter the condition is termed *Binswanger's disease.*

lacunae, superego Defects in the superego of delinquents and psychopathic personalities that are believed to originate from similar defects in the parents. Viewed in this way, some antisocial behavior would appear to be an acting out of unconscious wishes and impulses of the parents. (Johnson, A.M., & Szurek, S.A. *Psychoanalytic Quarterly 21,* 1952)

Laehr, Henrich (lär') (1820–1905) German psychiatrist; bibliography.

Lafora's disease (Gonzalo Rodriguez Lafora, Spanish neurologist, b. 1887) A rare form of epilepsy that begins in adolescence, with severe muscular spasms and seizures, and usually ends in death within five to ten years.

lagneia furor *Obs.* Mason Good's expression for *erotomania* (q.v.).

lagnesis *Obs.* Erotomania (q.v.).

lagneuomania *Obs.* Sadism in the male.

-lagnia (-lag'nē-à) Combining form meaning act of coition, salaciousness, lust, from Gr. *lagneis.*

lagnosis See *satyriasis.*

lagophthalmos, lagophthalmus (làg-of-thal' mus) A condition in which the upper lid fails to move down when the patient attempts to close the eye. It is one of the signs of affection of the seventh, or facial nerve.

Laing, R.D. (1927–) Scottish psychiatrist; radical therapy, which views therapy as a social and political activity; *The Politics of Experience* (1967).

Laingian view See *Equus-Laingian view.*

Lake v. Cameron See *consumerism.*

-lalia, lalo Combining form meaning talk(ing), talkative, chat, loquacity, from Gr. *laliá, lálos.*

laliophobia Fear of talking (and possibly stuttering).

lallation, lalling Unintelligible speech, such as infantile babbling; often used more specifically to refer to substitution of *l* for more difficult consonants such as *r.*

laloneurosis Nervous speech-disorder.

laloneurosis, spasmodic *Stuttering* (q.v.).

lalopathy (là-lop'à-thē) Any form of *speech-disorder* (q.v.).

lalophobia Fear of speaking.

laloplegia Inability to speak because of paralysis of speech muscles other than the tongue muscles.

lalorrhea See *tachylogia.*

lambitus (lam'bi-tus) See *cunnilinction.*

Landry's paralysis (Jean Baptiste Octave Landry, French physician, 1826–65) Acute ascending paralysis; a disorder of unknown etiology (?infectious; ?toxic, ?autoimmunity) consisting of flaccid paralysis beginning in the lower limbs and spreading upward to the bulbar and respiratory muscles. Males account for 80% of cases, and most cases occur during the third decade of life. Between 50% and 80% die by the fifteenth day; in the remainder, recovery is usually complete within three months.

Lange, Carl Georg (läng'ē) (1834–1900) Danish pathologist. See *theory, James-Lange-Sutherland.*

Lange's colloidal gold reaction (Carl Lange, German physician, b. 1883). A diagnostic test no longer in common use. It depends on the fact that cerebrospinal fluid in certain diseases is able to precipitate in a preparation of colloidal gold.

language A system that combines sounds to form words which arbitrarily represent knowledge about persons, objects, events, ideas, etc. Language includes not only words themselves and their grammatical relationships, but also how they are used in human intercourse to communicate feelings and thoughts.

Phonology is the study of speech sounds and how they form words. *Semantics* is the science of meaning. *Syntax* is the study of sentence structure and grammar, the rules for combining the units of sound and meaning. *Pragmatics* is the study of how language is actually used in conversation. *Psycholinguistics* (q.v.) is the study of the psychological aspects of language, including how it is learned by the child as the mind develops and matures. See *method, linguistic-kinesic.*

language and speech disorders Included within this type of specific developmental disorder are articulation disorder, stuttering, cluttering, expressive language disorder (impaired verbal or sign language), and receptive language disorder (impaired comprehension). See *developmental disorders, specific.*

language, artificial Bleuler speaks of the artificial language of schizophrenic individuals, meaning neologistic language.

language disability Difficulty in getting information out of the brain through the use of words, as in speaking. Typically, such disabilities involve difficulty with *demand language*, i.e. the subject has no trouble initiating conversation but finds it difficult to organize thoughts well enough to find the right words when language is demanded, as in being asked a direct question.

language disorder See *developmental disorders, specific.*

language, gestural-postural A method or form of communication between persons by means of gestures and/or postures without resorting to the use of words. Communication of this kind is better known by the more inclusive expression "communication by means of nonverbal language," and gestural-postural language is but one form of this. See *language, nonverbal.*

language, hypochondriac See *speech, organ.*

language, irrelevant Words, phrases, utterances that have meaning only for the speaker and for *no other person.* In listening to schizophrenic patients, the psychiatrist commonly encounters instances of irrelevant language. In the course of an otherwise wholly intelligible utterance, the patient has said a word, phrase, or even a sentence that conveys or communicates nothing to the psychiatrist. The patient has a clear understanding of what his utterance means to *himself*, for it is his own creation—he has made it up. According to Kanner, instances of irrelevant language occur in "the language of schizophrenia and early infantile autism." He points out that irrelevant utterances, "though peculiar and out of place in ordinary conversation, were far from meaningless. Some words or phrases were metaphoric substitutions." Kanner cites the following example where an irrelevant utterance of an autistic child was traced to an earlier source: "Jay S., not quite four years old, referred to himself as 'Blum,' whenever his veracity was questioned by his parents. This was explained when Jay, who could read fluently, once pointed to an advertisement of a furniture firm which said in large letters: 'Blum tells the truth.' Since Jay had told the truth, he *was* Blum." (*Child Psychiatry*, 1948)

language, metaphoric Used in psychiatry in a sense rather different than in rhetoric and, for that matter, in ordinary speech. *Metaphor* means the use of a word (or phrase) literally denoting one kind of object (or idea), instead of another word (or phrase) through suggested likeness (e.g. a *stream* of words). In the case of a psychiatric patient's metaphoric language, that other object (or idea), by which the metaphor has suggested itself to the speaker through likeness or similarity, remains an unrevealed entity and *eo ipso* makes the metaphor incomprehensible to the listener, though perfectly logical and legitimate for the speaker. Hence the term *irrelevant* for the language of psychiatric patients—often framed in this kind of meaningless metaphoric configuration.

language, nonverbal Communication by gestures, sounds, facial expressions, posturing, and so forth. In psychiatry, especially in child psychiatry, communication between doctor and patient by way of nonverbal language often tells more than any words that may be spoken.

language, primitive psychosomatic A phrase used by L.E. Hinsie to characterize the expression of feelings or thoughts by means of bodily movements rather than by words.

This primitive psychosomatic language can be easily observed in schizophrenics and in latent schizophrenics. Children who later in life develop catatonia often exhibit rather early a "tendency to stubbornness manifested through postures, gestures, immobility or exaggerated movements of the body. These children speak more with their muscles than with their mouths." For example, when they do not want to see anything they shut their eyes tightly, or they close the lips tightly when they do not want to talk. In advanced schizophrenics body movements often express specific beliefs or delusions. A patient may sway to and fro in the belief that this movement is necessary to keep the universe going or may drop his outstretched hand repeatedly in the belief that he thus destroys the universe. (*UP*)

language retardation See *retardation, language.*

lapse Same as *petit mal.* See *epilepsy.*

lapsus calami (kă'lă-mē) A slip of the pen. "A lady once told me that an old friend in writing to her had closed a letter with the curious sentence, 'I hope you are well and *un*happy.' He had formerly entertained hopes of marrying her himself, and the slip of the pen was evidently determined by his dislike at the thought of her being happy with someone else. She had recently married." (Jones, E. *Papers on Psycho-Analysis,* 1938) See *act, symptomatic.*

lapsus linguae (lin'gwi) Slip of the tongue. See *act, symptomatic.*

lapsus memoriae (me-mô'rē-ī) Lapse or slip of memory. See *act, symptomatic.*

lascivia (làs-kē'vē-à) (L. "jollity, wantonness, lewdness") *Nymphomania* (q.v.).

lasciviency Lasciviousness; lewdness.

lascivus (làs-kē'voos) (L. "wanton frisky, lewd, lustful, lascivious") Paracelsus's term in describing chorea, to denote the unrestrained character of the motor symptoms.

Lasègue sign (la-sâg') (Ernest Charles Lasègue, French physician, 1816–83) The Lasègue sign indicates disease of the sciatic nerve. Pain and resistance are caused by extending the leg on the thigh and flexing the thigh at the hip joint.

Lashley, Karl Spencer (1890–1958) U.S. psychologist, bacteriologist, and geneticist; psychology of learning; *Brain Mechanisms and Intelligence* (1929), numerous monographs in psychology, neurology, and the biology of behavior; directory of Yerkes Laboratory of Primate Biology.

lata, latah, lattah (là-tà) A behavioral pattern seen among the Malays, usually precipitated by sudden fright or tickling, consisting of imitative behavior (echopraxia), automatic obedience, and coprolalia. It is seen more often in women and usually before late adolescence. Some authorities consider latah and related states, such as the miryachit or olonism of Siberian tribes, the inu of the Ainu, and the Jumpers of New England (a 19th-century Shaker sect), as acute forms of schizophrenia. Others classify latah as a hysterical reaction or a startle pattern, and among the Malays themselves it is considered as a behavioral quirk rather than a disease.

latchkey Used as an adjective to describe a condition or situation in which a door was closed but not locked; more specifically, the phrase "latchkey children" refers to the estimated two million children in the United States who come home from school each day to a house or apartment that is empty because both parents are working.

late luteal phase dysphoric disorder *Periluteal phase dysphoric disorder; premenstrual tension; permenstrual dysphoric disorder;* the emotional or psychologic symptoms that may occur during the week prior to mensis (the last week of the luteal phase) and disappear within a few days of the onset of flow (the follicular phase). The most frequently reported symptoms are affective lability, persistent and marked anger or irritability, feelings of inner tension (feeling "on edge" or "keyed up"), and marked dejection with pessimistic, self-deprecating thoughts. Also common are fatiguability, lack of energy, craving for sweets or other food, difficulty in concentration, insomnia, and loss of interest. Physical symptoms include migraine-like headaches, abdominal bloating, weight gain, nausea, and vomiting.

There is disagreement as to whether the syndrome as described should be recognized as a specific psychiatric disorder. Critics contend that such a diagnosis stigmatizes as psychiatrically disturbed a woman who is only reacting to such biological discomforts as painful bloating. Further, there is no clear psychiatric treatment for the problem. Finally, some fear that such a diagnosis invites abuse in that it might be used as a legal defense against criminal charges related to violent acts. Because of these concerns, the category has been listed in the appendix of DSM-III-R and may be included within the regular text of later editions should new evidence warrant such a change.

latency In psychoanalysis, the period of one's life extending from the end of the infantile to the beginning of the adolescent stage. In point of years it normally begins at about the age of 5 and terminates at about the age of puberty.

Freud employed the term latency at a time in the development of psychoanalytic psychology when attention was focused largely on the sexual drive and libido; later work in the area of ego psychology has made it abundantly clear that the drives are by no means inactive during this period. Instead, what has happened is that the dangers of the Oedipus relationship have necessitated a strong blockade against libidinal impuses. The ego achieves this by mobilizing aggressive energies against the id. In effect, then, libidinal energies are redirected into elaborating a more effective web of defenses including the superego, and into increasing mastery in the social sphere, in socially condoned and desirable competitiveness, conquest, and domination. Mental development, in other words, has occurred in spurts. In the infantile years, libidinal forces are more in evidence as they are deployed in various areas in accordance with physiologic growth. With the appearance of the Oedipus, these forces must be held in check, and the aggressive forces of the ego acquire greater prominence. They are used as frontline combatants to prepare the way for the reappearance of libidinal strivings during adolescence.

latency, sleep The period of time between going to bed and the onset of sleep.

latent Not visible or apparent; dormant, quiescent. Latent homosexuality, for example, refers to homosexual tendencies or conflicts that have never been manifested overtly and/or are unrecognized by the subject. Latent psychosis refers to an existing disorder that has not erupted into full-blown or florid psychotic symptoms; sometimes also termed prepsychotic, borderline, or incipient, and almost always referring to an underlying schizophrenic disorder. See *schizophrenia, latent.*

laterality Handedness; preferential use of one side of the body for such acts as writing, eating, sighting, and listening. See *dominance, cerebral.*

lateralization See *dominance, cerebral.*

lateropulsion Rapid running sidewise with short steps, in paralysis agitans.

laughter, compulsive Inappropriate laughter, as seen in the hebephrenic form of schizophrenia.

"Among the affective disturbances [in schizophrenia] compulsive laughter is especially frequent; it rarely has the character of the hysterical laughing fit, but that of a soulless mimic utterance behind which no feeling is noticeable. It may often be provoked by allusion to a complex. Sometimes the patients feel only the movements of the facial muscles (the 'drawn laughter')." (Bleuler, *TP*)

laughter, drawn See *laughter, compulsive.*

Laurence-Moon-Biedl syndrome See *syndrome, Laurence-Moon-Biedl.*

law, autonomic-affective According to Kempf, "All of the autonomic-affective cravings, whether they compel an acquisitive or an avertive course of behavior or attitude toward the environment, follow the same two laws:

"1. When an autonomic-affective craving is aroused, either to compensate for the deficiencies due to metabolism (as in hunger) or through the influence of exogenous stimuli (as in fear), it compels the projicient (striped muscle) apparatus to shift the exteroceptors about in the environment so they will acquire such stimuli as are necessary to counterstimulate and neutralize the autonomic derangement, so that the segment will assume comfortable tensions.

"2. The projicient apparatus that shifts the receptors about so as to expose them to appropriate stimuli is organized and coordinated so as to bring a *maximum of affective gratification with a minimum expenditure of energy.*" (*PP*)

law, biogenetic mental According to the biogenetic law of the mind, "The history of the development of the species repeats itself in the embryonic development of the individual. Thus to a certain degree in his embryonic life man passes through the anatomical forms of primordial times. The same law is valid for the mental development of mankind. Accordingly, the child develops out of an originally unconscious and animal-like condition to consciousness; first to a primitive, and then slowly to a civilized consciousness." (Jung, *CAP*) See *perverse, polymorphous.*

law, Briggs's A law of Massachusetts named after L. Vernon Briggs (1921); the law provides that a person indicted by the grand jury who has previously been convicted of a felony, or who is known to have been indicted for any other offense more than once, will be examined by a psychiatrist-expertappointed by the State Department of Mental Health. The examiner is not asked to determine whether the accused can distinguish between right and wrong or whether the accused acted because of an irresistible impulse; instead, the psychiatrist is asked whether the accused suffers from a mental illness severe enough to affect his responsibility and to require treatment in a mental hospital. See *responsibility, criminal.*

law, Dale's See Dale's law.

law, health See health law.

law, Jackson's According to Hughlings Jackson's concept of the hierarchic development of mental functions, when there is organic brain disease the higher (i.e. the more complex and more recently developed) centers will be paralyzed or affected first, and the lower centers will resist deterioration the longest.

law of avalanche Law of the distribution of energy in the nervous system as framed by Cajal. Sensory stimuli reaching the central nervous system normally gain release through a number of paths of discharge, which take the form of reflex arcs. When some of these reflex arcs are closed, so to speak, as avenues of release for nervous energy, the energy is forced to flow through the remaining arcs. It is possible, as, for instance, in epilepsy, that, when discharged, the dammed-up energy produces a condition likened by Cajal to an avalanche.

"Such a conception would apply equally well to the 'idiopathic' or 'genuine epilepsy' with Ammon's horn gliosis and the typical character traits, and to the epilepsies associated with marked developmental defects (idiocy) in which it may be conceived that the wider paths for avalanche discharge have not been laid down." (Jelliffe & White, *DNS*)

law of initial values The tendency of extremes of pathology, whether physiologic or psychologic, to regress toward the mean over time, thus rendering the findings of response to early intervention highly suspect. Alcoholics, for example, usually do not present themselves for treatment until their symptoms are at their height; on short-term evaluation, almost all such patients will appear to improve, no matter what the treatment approach.

law of retrogenesis See *retrogenesis.*

law, Pitres' (Pē-tres') This law states that the first language to return in polyglottic patients with aphasia is the one which is easiest for the patient, usually the mother tongue.

law, Ribot's The law that states the first language acquired is the first to be restored in cases of aphasia. See *law, Pitres'.*

laws, Mendelian The Mendelian laws relating to the mechanism of inheritance account for the results of Mendel's breeding experiments in terms of the segregation, independent assortment, and recombination of the individual gene factors, which he postulated as existing in the gametes as independent units for every inherited character. This system consists of at least two different principles.

First, segregation, or clear separation of genetic factors during the formation of the gametes: the various characters of hybridized organisms are transmitted separately and distributed to the reproductive cells independently of each other so that they may form any possible combination. Every known hereditary trait operates in accordance with segregation, and this principle is to be regarded as the basic aspect of the Mendelian system of heredity. Although it was evolved from examples with both dominant and recessive characters, dominance is not an essential feature of Mendelian inheritance, as is demonstrated by many intermediate hybrids. While dominance alone does not necessarily presuppose the existence of unit characters, this element is essential to the law of segregation.

Second, the *independent* assortment of the genetic factors and their recombination. It is demonstrated by the 9:3:3:1 ratio in the redistribution of the four gene factors involved in the crosses with two different pairs of allelomorphic characters (see *Mendelism*). According to the same principle, the ratio 27:9:9:9:3:3:3:1 results, on the average, in the F_2 generation of a *trihybrid* mating, that is, one involving three pairs of allelomorphs, one member of each pair being dominant.

The simple formulation of the entire Mendelian law is: When two organisms unlike with respect to any character are crossed, the parent whose trait appears in the offspring is the *dominant,* the other parent is the *recessive.* When, however, the hybrids of this first generation are in turn crossed with each other, they will produce a variety of offspring. One-fourth of them will be like the recessive one, and the remaining half like the parents who resembled the dominant grandparent, yet failed to breed true to it. See *dominance; recessiveness.*

lay analyst See *psychiatrist.*

layers, cortical See *isocortex.*

LD *Learning disabilities* (q.v.).

lead pipe rigidity See *rigidity, lead pipe.*

lead poisoning *Plumbism;* although more common in children, it occurs also in adults, as in painters and workers with lead pipes (e.g. plumbers), and it may result from the use of some cosmetics, abortifacients, and from too close contact with lead-containing petrol. It has also been reported in frequenters of "shooting galleries" and in persons who have used metal-decorated drinking glasses. Poisoning is more frequent in summer, because the greater amount of vitamin D_3 formed in the skin by the sun's radiation increases absorption of lead from the gut.

Lead produces a selective degeneration of ganglion cells, especially in the spinal cord, and to a lesser extent in the cortex. Among the various syndromes of lead poisoning are (1) acute encephalopathy—with convulsions, delirium, coma; (2) chronic encephalopathy—with mental changes, convulsions, and occasionally optic atrophy; (3) neuritis—which is really a myopathy, affecting chiefly the extensors of the wrist and fingers and thus producing wrist-drop; (4) progressive muscular atrophy, due to anterior horn cell degeneration.

Prognosis is worsened if convulsions appear, and chronic encephalopathy responds little to treatment. As many as 35% of affected children die, and girls have a higher mortality than boys. Severe residua are common: epilepsy, cerebral atrophy, paresis, blindness, speech defects, tremor.

Treatment includes high-calcium diet to promote storage of lead in bones, followed by a high-acid/low-calcium diet to promote gradual elimination; and BAL (British anti-Lewisite) or EDTA (ethylenediaminetetraacetic acid or versenate) to form a stable, nontoxic, excretable compound with the lead.

leadership, dual See *psychotherapy, multiple.*

leaping ague *Choreomania.*

learned helplessness See *helplessness, learned.*

learning, accretion See *accretion.*

learning disabilities A nonspecific term referring to a variety of difficulties evidenced in the learning process, many of them due to developmental lags rather than the brain damage or inimical environmental influences implied in some of the terms applied to the group or the subtypes within it. See *developmental disorders; dyslexia; impulse disorder, hyperkinetic; reading disabilities.*

learning disability, specific As used by R. J. Schain (*California Medicine 118,* 1973) a term that has no etiologic implications and is applied to children with learning disorders who have no demonstrable illness (such as mental retardation, cerebral palsy, or seizure, auditory, ocular, or, progressive neurologic disorders). *Developmental hyperactivity* is applied to children who are normal or even precocious in development but show high activity levels as part of their temperament.

learning, dissociated See *state-dependent learning.*

learning, visceral See *biofeedback.*

least restrictive alternative See *consumerism.*

Leber's disease See *disease, Leber's*

lecanomancy (lek′a-nō-man-sē) "A method of divination by means of a suitable person looking into a bowl half-filled with water, on the surface of which the indefinite images of candle flames are reflected." Herbert Silberer used free association to find the meanings of the visions reported. This showed "how the divination[s] are merely the results of the medium's own complexes" and emphasized the close relation between the visions and dreams. (*Psychoanalytic Review I,* 1913–15)

lécheur (lā-shēr′) One who applies the mouth to the genitals of others, that is, practices fellatio or cunnilingus.

left-handedness See *dextrality-sinistrality.*

legal custody See *custody.*

legal divorce See *divorce, stations of.*

legal psychiatry Forensic psychiatry; the application of psychiatry in the courts of law. See *advocacy; consumerism; forced treatment.*

legasthenia Dyslexia with dysorthographia, consisting of difficulty in visual and acoustic synthesis of individual letters into a total word structure or, conversely, difficulty in analyzing the word back into its component letters. The deficit exists in the presence of adequate intellectual and perceptual abilities, and it appears to be both congenital and hereditary. See *dysgraphia; dyslexia.*

legs, restless See *restless legs syndrome.*

leipolalia Elision; *ellipsis* (q.v.).

lengthening reaction See *rigidity, decerebrate.*

Lennox, William Gordon (1884–1960) U.S. neurologist; epilepsy.

-lepsia (-lēp′sē-à) Combining form meaning seizure, attack, from Gr. *-lepsia,* as in *epilepsia, epilepsis.*

leptomeninges See *meninges.*

leptomeningitis See *meningitis.*

leptoprosophia In anthropology and constitutional medicine, a condition characterized by a narrow face and an elongated cranium.

leptosomal, leptosomic *Asthenic;* Kretschmer's term for the main structural characteristics of the anthropological type in question rather than a secondary and not universal property of the type. See *type, asthenic.*

leptosome A person of the asthenic body type.

lerema, leresis *Obs.* Garrulity; childish speech observed in patients with *senile dementia* (q.v.).

lesbianism Erotic or sexual love of women for other women; *Sapphism.* See *homosexuality, female.*

leschenoma (les-kē-nō′mà) Garrulity. See *lerema.*

Lesch-Nyhan syndrome See *syndrome, Lesch-Nyhan.*

lesion See *disease.*

lethal Deadly, fatal. This describes a hereditary character that in its homozygous condition produces an extreme modification that is fatal to the organism affected.

Lethal factors occur quite frequently in all kinds of animals and plants and are always recognizable by their drastic effect only in the form of homozygosity. "In the heterozygous condition they may be carried with impunity by perfectly normal individuals, but that portion of the offspring of such individuals in which segregation has brought two lethals together is killed." (Sinnott, E.W., & Dunn, L.D. *Principles of Genetics,* 1939)

lethal catatonia See *Bell's mania.*

lethality scale A rating of the likelihood that a subject will attempt suicide, based on factors such as age, sex, medical status, degree of stress, previous history of suicidal behavior, and presence of alcoholism, depression, or sleep disturbances.

lethe (lē′thē) *Obs.* Total loss of memory.

letheomania Morbid longing for narcotic drugs; *addiction* (q.v.).

lethologica Momentary forgetting of a name.

leucomoria *Obs. Melancholia agitata* (q.v.).

leucotomy, leukotomy; leucotomy, frontal See *lobotomy, prefrontal.*

leukodystrophies A group of heritable, progressive demyelinating disorders. One of them, metachromatic leukodystrophy (*MLD*), is due to a deficiency of the enzyme arylsulfatase A as a result of which sulfatide accumulates in the myelin, leading to demyelination and axon loss in the cerebral hemispheres, brain stem, spinal cord, cerebellum, and basal ganglia. Symptoms include early clumsiness, tremor, and speech difficulty followed by progressive motor and intellectual impairment.

Other forms of leukodystrophy are adrenoleukodystrophy (*Schilder's disease, Schaumberg's disease*), with adrenal insufficiency, motor symptoms, and dementia; and *Krabbe's disease,* due to decreased galactosylceramidase. See *sclerosis, diffuse.*

leukoencephalopathia myeloclastica primitiva See *sclerosis, diffuse.*

leukoencephalopathy, progressive multifocal (PML) Viral infection of the brain that causes progressive dementia. PML has been reported frequently in AIDS patients. See *syndrome, acquired immune deficiency.*

level, confidence See *confidence, level of.*

level, hedonic See *psychodynamics, adaptational.*

level, maintenance The dosage of therapeutic agent that must be repeated at stated intervals in order to sustain the desired effect. In subacute combined degeneration of the spinal cord, for example, maintenance level of vitamin B_{12} is commonly 4 µg weekly for 6 months; in various psychiatric patients, maintenance level of chlorpromazine hydrochloride may be 600 mg per day for an indefinite period of time.

level of care See *ALC.*

level of confidence See *confidence, level of.*

level of development See *developmental levels; ontogeny, psychic.*

level of risk See *confidence, level of.*

leveling As used in family therapy, giving free expression to aggressive feelings, on the (so far unproved) assumption that verbal aggression can substitute for and thus reduce the likelihood of physical aggression.

levels, mental From the standpoint of analytic psychology (Jung) there are three mental levels: (1) consciousness; (2) the personal unconscious; (3) the collective unconscious. The personal unconscious consists of all those contents that have become unconscious, because their intensity has been lost, they were forgotten, or because consciousness has withdrawn from them, i.e. so-called repression. Finally, this layer contains those elements—partly sense perceptions—which on account of too little intensity have never reached consciousness, and yet in some way have gained access into the psyche. The collective unconscious, being an inheritance of the possibilities of ideas, is not individual but generally human, even generally animal, and represents the real foundations of the individual." (*CAP*) See *id; topography, mental.*

levirate Marriage to a deceased husband's brother. See *sororate.*

levophobia Fear of objects to the left; opposite of *dextrophobia.*

Levy, David M. (1892–1977) Psychoanalyst; activity play therapy, maternal overprotection, sibling rivalry; introduced Rorschach test into U.S.

Lewin, Kurt (1890–1946) German psychologist; to U.S. in 1933; field theory of behavior; sensitivity group training (at the National Training Laboratory).

Lewis, Nolan D.C. (1889–1979) American psychiatrist; research in schizophrenia, history of psychiatry; director, New York State Psychiatric Institute, 1936–53.

Lewis, Sir Aubrey (1900–75) Australian-born psychiatrist who joined the staff of the Maudsley Hospital (London) in 1928; professor of psychiatry at the associated Institute of Psychiatry, which under his leadership became an international center for training and research.

lex talionis (L. "law of retaliation, retribution") See *dread, talion.*

liaison psychiatry See *consultant.*

liar, pathological Often grouped under the category of *psychopathic personality* (q.v.): "Pathological liars and swindlers are imaginative and champion tellers of 'tall tales,' in which they invariably play the leading role. They build up their stories by proper accessories, such as accents, uniforms, forged documentary evidence, and other items. From time to time newspapers report the exposure of a bogus nobleman, officer, diplomatic agent, or some other impostor. Their activity sometimes takes the form of sexual conquests, and they may obtain money under false pretenses, either on the promise of marriage or after a bigamous marriage." (Lowery, L.G. *Psychiatry for Social Workers,* 1946) See *impostor; lying, pathological.*

libidinal (libidinous) 1. Relating to psychic energy. 2. Relating to the erotic instinct.

libidinal-cathexis See *cathexis.*

libidinization See *erotization.*

libidinize See *eroticize.*

libido In psychoanalysis, the energy of the sexual drive; but because Freud's consideration of the death or destructive drive came relatively late in the development of his psychology, the term libido is commonly used in a more general sense to refer also to the energy of the death or aggressive drive. See *instinct, death; theory, libido.*

McDougall suggests the term *hormé* for libido. He adds that it is the equivalent of Bergson's *élan vital.*

libido-binding See *activity, immobilizing.*

libido, displaceability of A psychoanalytic concept pertaining to one aspect of the "libido theory" of sexual development from infancy to childhood. In order of their appearance and development, the libidinal phases are usually considered as (1) the oral, (2) the anal, (3) the phallic, and (4) the genital. See *ontogeny, psychic.*

Sexual excitations and gratifications are specifically related to the erogenous zones, characteristic of each specific phase of libidinal development, and have been called *partial* impulses, since they tend to form or contribute partial components to the total final pattern of fully achieved adult sexuality. These partial impulses are usually discernible in adult sexual life, in what is called foreplay or forepleasure activities or perversion traits. See *impulse, component.*

These partial impulses can substitute for and replace one another in both excitation and gratification. Dissatisfaction at one zone may make for earlier or later increased activity at another zone. This gives the metaphorical impression that the total sexual instinct energy, or libido, is fluid in nature, subject to metaphorical hydrostatic and hydrodynamic forces. From this impression are derived such psychoanalytic terms as *block, recanalization, displacement,* implying the shunting of excitation and gratification from one area of outlet to another. (Sterba, R. *Introduction to the Psychoanalytic Theory of the Libido,* 1942)

libido fixation See *fixation, libido.*

libido, mobility The ease with which libidinal energy can be shifted from one object to another, in contrast to fixation of the libido, in which the libido attaches itself to particular objects.

In Freudian psychology, the love instinct (Eros) is one of the two sources of all human activity and it aims at the satisfaction of its need, which is "to establish ever greater unities and to preserve them thus—in short, bind together." The other instinct, which likewise aims at the satisfaction of its need, is the death instinct, whose final aim is to destroy, "to reduce living things to an inorganic state." Basically the two instincts (both of somatic origin) represent the physiological demands of the human organism. "The interaction of the two basic instincts with and against each other gives rise to the whole variegation of the phenomena of life." For example, the biological function of eating both destroys the object and unites with it by incorporation.

Initially, all libido is stored up in the ego "and serves to neutralize the destructive instincts which are simultaneously present." This is the state of *primary narcissim.* Later, as the infant begins to discern an outside world, he begins to invest the objects of the outside world with libido (object libido).

libido, object See *ego libido.*

libido, plasticity of That specific quality of libido that makes for the adaptability of the sexual instincts (or the partial impulses of the libido) to modified discharge of tensions through indirect rather than direct avenues of gratification.

The general fate of instinctual energy that cannot be overtly or directly discharged in instinct gratification has been described under the general term of "the vicissitudes of the instinct." The four major vicissitudes, or indirect avenues for partial gratification and discharge of instinct, are (1) repression with subsequent symptom and dream formation; (2) sublimation; (3) transformation of the instinct aim into its opposite; and (4) transformation of the direction of the instinctual aim from an external object onto the self. See *libido, displaceability of.*

libido, primal See *force, central.*

libido, viscosity of A psychoanalytic term carrying still further the metaphorical idea concerning the fluidity of the libido. The concept of the libido's viscosity is apt because of the following two characteristics of the libido: first, the slow pace of emotional growth from infancy to maturity; second, the tendency of the libido to remain fixed at or return, at slight provocation, to earlier phases of infantile sexual gratification.

The forward movement of libidinal development is apparently more oscillatory than direct, with many strong reactionary expressions of a kind of stubborn inertia, as well as a tendency toward the maintenance and reactivity of old or earlier phases of libidinal development. This makes for an instability and undependability of the newer or more recently acquired phases of developmental maturity. (Sterba, R. *Introduction to the Psycho-analytic Theory of the Libido,* 1942)

libido wish See *wish, id.*

lie detector See *detector, lie.*

lie, life Adler uses this term for the tendency of the neurotic to include in his life plan the idea that he will fail because of the fault of others or owing to events beyond his control.

Liebeault, Ambroise-August (1823–1904) (lē-bō′) French psychiatrist; hypnotism.

liebestod (lē′bes-tōt) J.C. Flugel's term for phantasies involving dying with a loved one. Such phantasies may signify a wish to become pregnant by the partner and/or attempt to deny the possibility of death by phantasying eternal union with the mother.

life course See *closure, law of and life course.*

life event See *event, life.*

life-event stress theory See *continuity theory of aging.*

life goal See *goal, life.*

life history model D.F. Ricks and J.C. Berry (in *Life History Research in Psychopathology,* ed. M. Roff & D.F. Ricks, 1970) proposed a life history model for schizophrenia: Because his biological and social equipment provides small margin for error in development, the child is vulnerable to disorder. Often he is aware of his limitations and tries various ways to defend himself. If successful, he may move into a low-stimulation pattern of living. If unsuccessful, he retreats into psychosis, usually through the typical stages of protest, despair, and finally apathy. The major determinants of regression or recovery are IQ, social and vocational success, and a reasonably receptive environment.

life, mental See *mentality.*

life, noon of The dividing line between the first and second halves of a person's life. Referring to Jung's "functional" and "attitudinal" types J. Jacobi writes: "This opposition of the functions and of the conscious and unconscious attitude intensifies itself into a conflict in the individual, as a rule, only toward the second half of life; indeed, it is just that problem which indicates an alteration of his psychological situation in that portion of life. Often it is precisely the capable persons, well adjusted to the environment, who, once past their forties, suddenly find that they are, in spite of their 'brilliant mind,' perhaps not equal to domestic difficulties or are, for example, insufficiently suited to their professional position. If this phenomenon is correctly understood, it must be taken as a sign and warning that the inferior function, too, now demands its rights and that a confrontation with it has become a necessity. The latter, therefore, plays in such cases the greatest role at the beginning of analysis." (*The Psychology of C.G. Jung,* 1942) In current parlance, the phenomenon described would be termed *burnout.*

"The constitutionally given habitus must take the lead in the first half of life, because the individual can in all likelihood best find his place in the world with the help of his naturally given attitude. The task of letting the opposite habitus come into its own only emerges during the sec-

ond half of life. That it will be easier for the born extravert than the born introvert to accomplish the external adjustment that • the first half of life above all requires, • needs no further explanation. Perhaps one may then venture the assertion: the born extravert gets along in the world more easily in the first, the born introvert in the second half of his life; with which justice is done at least approximately. The danger threatening both types is onesidedness.... The neglected functions and the unlived attitudes revolt—as it were, demand their place in the sun—to be seized by means of a neurosis if not otherwise. For the goal is always totally the ideal solution, in which all four psychological functions and both forms of attitudinal reactions are at the person's command in as nearly the same degree of consciousness and disposability as possible. And once, at least, must a certain approximation to this ideal be attempted. If it does not make itself felt earlier as a demand, then the *noon of life* signifies the last summons to attain it now or never and thereby to "round out" the psyche, so that it may not go toward life's evening unfinished and incomplete." (Ibid.)

life plan See *plan, life.*

life space In Kurt Lewin's holistic theory of personality, the person plus his psychological environment, the "totality of possible events" for any person. Lewin maintained that the person can be defined only in relation to his environment, and that the whole person always maintains primacy over any part systems. Included within the life space are *valences,* positive and negative pressures upon the person for movement toward or away from a goal. Externally presented valences are incorporated within the inner structure of the person in the form of ambitions, aspirations, values, and ideals.

lifestyle See *constancy; psychology, individual.*

ligand Bond; a molecule that is bound to a specific site, such as to a particular protein; in neuropharmacology, any compound (agonist or antagonist) that has the capacity to bind to a specific nerve cell receptor.

lights, snow See *snow lights.*

Lilliputian (From Lilliput, an imaginary kingdom of 6-inch pygmies in Swift's *Gul-*

liver's Travels) Microptic hallucinations, in which the objects seen appear much reduced in scale. See *metamorphosia; micropsia.*

Lilliputian hallucinations have been reported in intoxication from alcohol, chloral, ether, trichlorethylene, and present in cholera, typhoid, scarlet fever, cocainism, tumors of the temporal or temporosphenoidal lobe, and in some cases of petit mal epilepsy.

limb, phantom The feeling that an extremity that has been lost is really present. Fenichel points out that phantom extremity phenomena are closely associated with what is termed the *body image.* In its development the infant is first able to discern self from non-self because its own body can be distinguished from all other parts of the universe, or the rest of the world, by the fact that the body is perceived through two types of sensation simultaneously: external tactile sensations and internal sensations of depth sensibility. Thus the first idea of self consists of the sum total of the mental representations of the body and its organs, the so-called body image. The nucleus of the ego is the body image. "Freud stated that the ego is primarily a bodily thing, that is, the perception of one's own body." *(PTN)* See *ego, body; image, body.*

In phantom limb phenomena, the basic importance of the body image is underlined. For, indeed, the patient finds great difficulty in correlating with his body image the objective fact of the absence of the extremity. In the body image, which is the basic mental representation of the body, and the nucleus of the ego, the extremities are of the greatest importance. Thus a phantom extremity can be included in the body image. (Ibid.)

Appearance of the phantom is the expected physiologic reaction to amputation, if this takes place after early childhood, and admission of the phantom is a healthy psychological response. In time, the amputee slowly reorganizes his body image, accepts the defect, resumes his social and occupational role, and uses his prosthesis appropriately. Failure in any of these steps is indicative of coexistent personality disturbance. In all patients with phantom limb, there occur mild tingling sensations which probably depend upon the sensori-

motor cortex; but the term "painful phantom" refers to patients who in addition complain of twisting, burning, pulling, or itching sensations in the nonexistent limb. Such pain seems to represent an emotional response to the loss of an important part of the body that had significance to the patient in terms of his relationships with others. Amputation produces an upsurge of anxiety related to the resultant distortion of the concept of the body and the self. Hostile feelings typically emerge toward those with whom the amputee identifies as having been similarly mutilated and toward those on whom he is dependent and whose rejection he anticipates. Sometimes patients are further threatened by guilt feelings related to the upsurge in hostility. While typically the phantom tends to shrink and eventually disappear into the stump, such reorganization may not occur in those whose self-esteem is dependent on a high evaluation of the part lost. Some patients deny their loss, and this is especially common after amputation of the breast or penis. Still others project their loss and tend to see those around them as suffering in a similar way. (Kolb, L.C. *The Painful Phantom,* 1954)

Most amputees experience the phantom only sometimes or infrequently, rather than most or all of the time. Some retain an extended phantom (i.e. of the same length as the missing limb) for many years; others experience it as somewhat shortened (a retracted phantom); and others have a completely telescoped phantom, in which the digits may be felt as protruding from the stump. In a few, the phantom is experienced as longer than the missing limb. (Weiss, S.A., & Fishman, S. *Journal of Abnormal and Social Psychology 66,* 1963)

limbus See *memory; rhinencephalon.*

limitation, sex See *sex limitation.*

limited-symptom attacks In DSM-III-R, anxiety attacks with too few symptoms to qualify as panic attacks. Four or more of the following symptoms warrant the diagnosis of panic attack: shortness of breath, choking, palpitations, chest pain, sweating, dizziness or faintness, nausea or abdominal distress, depersonalization or derealization, numbness or tingling sensations, flushes or chills, trembling, fear of dying, fear of going crazy or of doing something uncontrolled. An episode with fewer than four symptoms is a limited symptom attack.

limophoitas (lī-mō-foi'tas) Psychosis induced by starvation. See *anorexia nervosa*.

limophthisis (lim-of'thi-sis) Emaciation from insufficient nourishment. See *anorexia nervosa*.

limosis Mason Good's term for mental disorders associated with abnormal appetites. See *eating disorders*.

Lindau's disease (Arvid Lindau, contemporary Swedish pathologist) Angioma of the brain occurring in connection with angiomatosis of the retina, occasionally familial and hereditary.

line, pure This biological term was introduced by the Danish botanist Johannsen, to characterize the identical *genotypical* equipment of an autogamous stock of organisms descended from a common ancestor by self-fertilization. According to the pure line theory, these organisms will continue to breed true regardless of environmental differences, forming lines genetically pure for all their characters. Whenever such genetic purity has been attained, all differences except newly occurring mutations must be caused by environmental influences and therefore cannot be hereditarily transmitted.

linguistics The study of words and language. See *method, linguistic-kinesic*.

lingula See *cerebellum*.

link, peptide See *peptide, brain*.

linkage Act of linking, or state of being linked. This is an important exception to the Mendelian principle of independent assortment and is the foundation of the modern chromosome theory of inheritance as formulated by Morgan, in 1910, from his famous Drosophila experiments. It is characterized by the tendency of genes located in the same chromosome to remain in their original combinations and to be inherited as a *block* rather than independently of one another.

Apart from the assumption that *linked* genes must be located in the same chromosome, in order to permit such a *coupling*—the mechanism of linkage has been partly explained by the discovery that "the gametes of a plant or animal which is heterozygous for two linked traits are not formed in equal numbers, but that the gametes with the parental combinations of genes are always more numerous than the gametes with the new combination of genes." (Sinnot, E.W., & Dunn, L.D. *Principles of Genetics,* 1939)

Because of the frequent occurrence of *crossing over* (q.v.), most of the known instances of linkage are *incomplete*. Although it is theoretically possible that two linked genes may never separate, because they are so close together in the chromosome that a break cannot occur between them, actual cases of *complete* linkage are exceedingly rare.

Linkage is assessed by determining the frequency of *recombination* of the traits in question, which is dependent upon the distance between loci of the alleles on the chromosome. The closer they are together, the less likely will they be split up and recombined or exchanged during meiosis; the farther they are apart, the more likely will recombination occur. When the phenotype indicates that recombination has occurred, the offspring is termed a *recombinant;* when it has not occurred, the offspring is a *nonrecombinant*.

linkage, sex See *sex linkage*.

linonophobia Fear of string.

lip-pursing See *Schnauzkrampf*.

lipochondrodystrophy *Gargoylism* (q.v.). See *mucopolysaccharidosis*.

lipofuscin See *aging, theories of*.

LIPS *Logical inferences per second;* see *KIPS*.

lisping A type of defective articulation in which the sounds "s" and "z" (sibilants) are not pronounced perfectly, by pressing the tip and next narrow part of the blade of the tongue to the alveoli (the sockets where the upper front teeth are rooted), but are pronounced by carelessly pushing the tip of the tongue forward and touching the edges of the upper front teeth as when uttering the sound of "th." Like all speech disorders, lisping is more common in boys than in girls. Lisping may be based on any or all of the following etiological factors: (1) local conditions, secondary to congenital or acquired organic defects; (2) mental retardation; (3) faulty training, especially as a result of parental ignorance or carelessness and the use of "baby talk." It is this last factor that is the most important and the most common and when it is operative lisping is often found to be a behavior reaction acquired in the interest of some personal or social goal. Treatment is directed to the removal or correction of organic defects and to reeducation of parents and child. Speech classes are normally helpful in removing the defect.

Lissauer's dementia paralytica (Heinrich Lissauer, German neurologist, 1861–91) An atypical syndrome of general paresis characterized by (1) unusually well-retained intellectual functions and (2) severe focal symptoms, such as apoplectiform attacks, hemiplegia, and aphasia.

lithiasis, hysterical Literally, production of (kidney) stones on a hysterical or neurotic basis; in fact, used to refer to *factitious disorders* (q.v.), where the foreign bodies are used to mimic kidney stones or other means are used to stimulate renal colic, often in order to obtain opiates.

lithic diathesis See *diathesis, lithic.*

lithium A naturally occurring element, number 3 on the periodic table (1 is hydrogen, 2 is helium), and the lightest metal known. It is an effective treatment for manic states and an effective prophylactic agent against recurrent manic or depressive episodes. Mechanism of action is unknown; lithium may interfere with sodium retention within brain cells. Usually lithium is administered as lithium carbonate; side effects with overdosage include nausea, diarrhea, tremor, muscular heaviness, hypersensitivity to sights and sound, and irritability.

litigious paranoia See *paranoia querulans.*

Litten's sign (Moritz Litten, German physician, 1845–1907) In paralysis of the diaphragm—nonprojection of shadow by the diaphragm X-rayed during respiration.

Little Hans See *Hans.*

Little's disease (William John Little, English surgeon, 1810–94) Congenital diplegia; cerebral palsy; atrophic lobar sclerosis; congenital spastic paralysis; spastic diplegia. A congenital disorder, probably due to in utero degeneration, consisting of bilateral symmetrical atrophy of the nerve cells and gliosis, mainly of the pyramidal tracts. As a result the limbs (particularly the lower) become weak and spastic. Other symptoms include involuntary movements, ataxia and usually some degree of mental deficiency. Predominant symptoms are spastic in 65% of cases, athetoid in 25%, and ataxic in 10%. Few cases survive beyond the early adult years.

LMT Lowenfeld Mosaic Test. See *test, mosaic.*

load, case In psychiatric social work, a term for the number of clients, as well as for intensity of service being given.

loading, genetic See *model, diathesis-stress.*

lobar sclerosis, atrophic *Little's disease* (q.v.).

lobe, flocculonodular (flo-kū-lō-nod'ūlēr) See *cerebellum.*

lobe, frontal Portion of the cerebral hemisphere that lies in front of the central sulcus and above the lateral fissure. The principal areas of the frontal lobe, as designated by Brodmann, are: area 4 (*precentral gyrus;* principal motor area); immediately in front of 4 is area 6 (*premotor area;* a part of the extrapyramidal tract circuit); in front of this, area 8 (which is concerned with the eye movements and pupillary changes); and in front of this, at the frontal poles and continuing along the inferior surface of the frontal lobe, areas 9, 10, 11, and 12 (which are frontal association areas).

Cells of the precentral gyrus (*Betz cells*) control voluntary movements of skeletal muscle on the opposite side of the body via the pyramidal tracts; irritative lesions in this area may give convulsive seizures (Jacksonian epilepsy). Destructive lesions in area 4 produce flaccid paralysis; spasticity will occur if area 6 and intermediate cortex is also involved. *Forced grasping* is often seen following destructive lesions of area 6. Destruction of the frontal association areas (9, 10, 11, and 12) may produce facetiousness (*Witzelsucht*), change in moral and social behavior, loss of interest, intellectual deterioration, and distractibility.

Frontal lobe dysfunction is manifested in several areas.

1. *Motor*—symptoms include motor impersistence, inertia, impaired rapid sequential movements, catatonic behavior, and stimulus-bound behavior such as gegenhalten and echopraxia, loss of learned complex behavior, a stooped and shuffling gait.

2. *Language*—loss of verbal fluency, Broca's aphasia, transcortical aphasia, impaired spontaneous prosody and gesturing (aprosodia), loss of the ability to repeat with prosodic affective variation, verbigeration.

3. *Memory*—impaired short-term memory storage.

4. *Other*—impaired concentration, glo-

bal disorientation, impaired judgment, impaired problem solving, impaired abstraction ability, right spatial neglect.

5. *Specific syndromes associated with frontal lobe dysfunction*—the convexity syndrome and the medial-orbital syndrome.

There is evidence that the frontal lobes are lateralized for approach and avoidance behavior in that activation of the right frontal region is often associated with positive affects, whereas activation of the left frontal region is associated with negative affects. The frontal lobe is concerned not with the intellectual functions of analysis, synthesis, and selectivity but with the adjustment of the personality as a whole to future contingencies in the light of past experience. The prefrontal regions in humans are therefore concerned with foresight, imagination, and the apperception of the self, and these psychological functions are invested with emotion by way of the association fibers which link the hippocampus and the cingulate gyrus with the prefrontal region on the one hand and with the thalamus and hypothalamus on the other.

lobe, limbic See *memory; rhinencephalon.*

lobe, occipital The posterior lobe of the cerebral hemisphere; it is pyramidal in shape and lies behind the parietooccipital fissure. Visual function is localized in the occipital lobe, primarily in the calcarine cortex (area striata, area 17 of Brodmann). Neurons from the retina project to the external geniculate body, from which second-order neurons project to the calcarine cortex. Fibers from the nasal half of each retina cross in the optic chiasm and so are projected onto the visual cortex of the opposite side; fibers from the temporal half of the retina remain uncrossed. The posterior occipital poles are mainly concerned with macular (central) vision; the more anterior parts of the calcarine area are concerned with peripheral vision. The human loses both object vision and light perception when the calcarine cortex is removed. See *field defect.*

The calcarine cortex (area 17) projects to area 18 (parastriate lobule), which in turn projects to area 19 (preoccipital area). Areas 18 and 19 are visual association areas; lesions here cause disturbances in spatial orientation and visual word-

blindness (alexia). Area 19 receives projections from all parts of the cortex and then coordinates visual with other reflexes.

Occipital lobe dysfunction is manifested in impairment in visual memory and in impaired recognition of visual patterns (*visual agnosia*).

lobe, parietal Portion of the cerebral hemisphere that extends from the central sulcus to the parietooccipital fissure and laterally to the level of the Sylvian fissure. The *postcentral gyrus* (areas 3-1-2, the *somesthetic area*), the *supramarginal gyrus,* and the angular gyrus are portions of the parietal lobe. The postcentral gyrus receives projections from the relay nuclei of the thalamus; the latter receive the great ascending somatosensory tracts of the spinal cord and the trigeminal lemniscus. Areas 5 and 7, which make up the posterior parietal lobule, are sensory association areas. Experimental studies indicate that the body surface is projected dermatome by dermatome on the postcentral gyrus. It appears that taste is also a function of the sensorimotor area and is localized at the inferior end of the lobe, possibly on the opercular surface of the Sylvian fissure.

The dominant parietal lobe is concerned with ideokinetic (ideomotor) praxis and symbolic categorization. The nondominant parietal lobe has to do with constructional praxis, dressing praxis, kinesthetic praxis (of the contralateral hand), and the ability to recognize or be familiar with people and objects. Abnormalities associated with nondominant parietal lobe dysfunction are anosognosia, spatial nonrecognition, and prosopagnosia. See *metamorphosia.*

Graphesthesia, stereognosis, and kinesthetic praxis all test the parietal lobe contralateral to the hand being tested, as well as the connections between the hemispheres. Abnormalities indicating dysfunction are graphanesthesia and asterognosis.

lobe, temporal Portion of the cerebral hemisphere that lies below the Sylvian fissure and extends back to the level of parietooccipital fissure. The temporal lobe receives auditory projections from the medial geniculate body, and ablation of the temporal lobe in man results in partial deafness and contralateral disturbance in memory for auditory impressions. The temporal lobe also receives vestibular projections, but the source of these is unknown.

Symptoms of temporal lobe tumors include visual *field defect* (q.v.), auditory and speech defects, and minor seizures known as dreamy states (see *states, dreamy*). If the uncus is implicated, there may be hallucinations of smell and taste (uncinate seizures). See *fit, uncinate.*

Bilateral temporal lobe disease usually produces dementia. If the disease is in the dominant lobe, manifestations include euphoria, auditory hallucinations (often "complex" voices), thinking disorder, primary delusional ideas, cognitive deficits such as decreased learning and retention of verbal material (read or heard) and poor speech and reading comprehension.

If the nondominant lobe is affected, symptoms include dysphoria, depression, irritability, inappropriate emotionsl expression (aprosodia), cognitive deficits such as decreased recognition and recall of visual and environmental sounds, amusia (loss of ability to repeat musical sounds), poor visual memory, decreased auditory discriminations and comprehension of tonal patterns, and decreased ability to learn and recognize nonsense figures and geometric shapes.

lobotomy, Grantham Lobotomy performed by means of electrocoagulation of the ventromedial quadrant of the prefrontal lobe of the brain.

lobotomy, prefrontal A psychosurgical procedure consisting of ablation of the prefrontal area of the frontal lobe. The prefrontal area is that portion of the frontal lobe anterior to Brodmann's area 6, the premotor area. As a psychosurgical procedure, the operation is ordinarily performed bilaterally. In contrast to frontal lobectomy, which is an open procedure in which tissue is excised and therefore more direct cortical damage is caused, the lobotomy procedure is "blind." A hole is drilled through the skull and a leukotome is inserted to cut white nerve fibers connecting the frontal lobe with the thalamus. Thus, in lobotomy, there is less cortical damage than in lobectomy. This procedure interrupts frontothalamic and thalamofrontal fibers and also the association systems of the frontal lobe.

Prefrontal lobotomy was among the first psychosurgical procedures used in the United States. It seems to reduce anxiety feelings and introspective activities; feelings of inadequacy and self-consciousness are thereby lessened. Lobotomy reduces the emotional tension associated with hallucinations and does away with the catatonic state. Because nearly all psychosurgical procedures have undesirable side effects, they are ordinarily resorted to only after all other methods have failed. The less disorganized the personality of the patient, the more obvious are postoperative side effects. For this reason, bilateral prefrontal lobotomy is employed more commonly in schizophrenia than in any other disorder. Prefrontal lobotomy is of value in the following disorders, listed in a descending scale of good results: affective disorders, obsessive-compulsive states, chronic anxiety states and other nonschizophrenic conditions, paranoid schizophrenia, catatonic schizophrenia, and hebephrenic and simple schizophrenia. Good results are obtained in about 40% of cases, fair results in some 35%, and poor results in 25% or thereabouts. The mortality rate probably does not exceed 3%. Greatest improvement is seen in patients whose premorbid personalities were "normal," cyclothymic, or obsessive-compulsive; in patients with superior intelligence and good education; in psychoses with sudden onset and a clinical picture of affective symptoms of depression or anxiety, and with behavioristic changes such as refusal of food, overactivity, and delusional ideas of a paranoid nature.

Convulsive seizures are reported as sequelae of prefrontal lobotomy in 5 to 10% of cases. Such seizures are ordinarily well controlled with the usual anticonvulsive drugs. Postoperative blunting of the personality, apathy, and irresponsibility are the rule rather than the exception. Other side effects include distractibility, childishness, facetiousness, lack of tact or discipline, and postoperative incontinence.

Prefrontal lobotomy has also been used successfully to control pain secondary to organic lesions. In this case, the tendency has been to employ unilateral lobotomy, because of the evidence that a lobotomy extensive enough to relieve psychotic symptoms is not required to control pain.

Since the introduction of prefrontal lobotomy and prefrontal lobectomy various other psychosurgical procedures have been initiated—transorbital lobotomy, thalamotomy, cortical undercutting, and topectomy. The present trend is toward selective operation, the particular procedure being chosen on the basis of the nature of the disease, its duration and extent, the patient's age, etc. Also called *frontal lobotomy; prefrontal leukotomy; frontal leukotomy.*

lobotomy, transorbital A psychosurgical procedure consisting of partial ablation of the prefrontal area. The approach is through the superior conjunctival sac, and the operation is usually performed bilaterally. The plane of section corresponds roughly to that of *topectomy* but, like prefrontal lobotomy, the procedure is a "blind" one and white matter rather than gray matter is destroyed. The incision interrupts the frontothalamic and thalamofrontal radiations and also the frontal lobe association fibers. Some surgeons prefer the transorbital approach to classical prefrontal lobotomy, because they feel that incontinence, apathy, and other undesirable side effects are less frequent. See *lobotomy, prefrontal.*

locked-in syndrome See *mutism, akinetic.*

locomotor ataxia See *tabes.*

locus minoris resistentiae Area or point of least resistance. See *compliance, somatic; specificity, individual-response.*

Loeffler's syndrome See *syndrome, Loeffler's.*

logagnosia Sensory aphasia.

logamnesia Forgetting words; nominal or amnestic aphasia.

-logia, -logy (-lō'jē-à, -'lō-jē) Combining form meaning (1) speaking, speech; (2) science, doctrine, theory; from Gr. *-logia,* from *lógos,* word, speech, discourse.

logical inferences See *KIPS.*

logoclonia Logospasm. Reiterative utterances of parts of words; reported frequently in Alzheimer's disease and senile dementia.

logodiarrhea See *tachylogia.*

logomania See *tachylogia.*

logomonomania *Obs.* An abnormal mental state characterized only by great loquacity. It is difficult today to name a psychiatric state of which volubility is the only symptom.

logoneurosis *Obs.* Any neurosis associated with a speech defect; by some, used synonymously with *stuttering* (q.v.).

logopathy (lō-gŏp'à-thē) A general term for any type of speech disorder.

logopedics The study of speech and its disorders.

logophasia A form of aphasia, characterized by loss of ability to use articulate language correctly.

logoplegia *Obs.* See *aphasia.*

logorrhea See *tachylogia.*

logospasm Explosive speech; stuttering. Sometimes used as an equivalent of *logoclonia* (q.v.).

logotherapy Existential analysis; see *existentialism.* Logotherapy is a type of psychotherapy based on a system of spiritual values rather than on a system of psychobiologic laws. Logotherapy emphasizes the search for the meaning of human existence; lack of assurance in any meaning is believed to be one of the main causes of frustration in the present era.

Developed by Victor Frankel in the 1950s and 1960s, logotherapy emphasizes the subject's creative, experiential, and attitudinal values and encourages the incorporation of social responsibility and constructive relationships into solutions.

Lombroso, Cesare (1836–1909) Italian criminologist and psychopathologist.

longevity Length of life. In its medical and statistical sense, this term refers to the phenomenon of a long duration, or great length, of life.

The existence of *genetic* factors operating in human longevity has been conclusively demonstrated by a number of family studies, although the details of the genetic mechanism involved have not yet been elucidated. Certain experiments of Pearl have shown *long-livedness* to be dominant over *short-livedness* in Drosophila. A number of cases of short life span may thus be accounted for by single-recessive mechanisms. There is also the possibility of *lethal* (q.v.) genes that merit consideration as a factor of influencing life span, although the present evidence is to the effect that the significant role of lethal genes is in the fairly early (prenatal) stages.

Concerning the constitutional aspect of longevity it has been shown by Pearl that the long-lived are more asthenic and the short-lived more pyknic, that women have a decided biological advantage over men, and that in youth all individuals below average height have a greater mortality while overweight means greater mortality in individuals over 40 years of age.

Studies on the factor of *marital status* in longevity have demonstrated an advantage for the married over the unmarried in general, but this is mainly due to selective factors rather than to environmental benefits conveyed by marriage. Longevity is also positively correlated with a favorable *social* and *economic* status, and with professional work as opposed to manual occupations, although the question of the relative influence of genetic factors determining simultaneously low grade occupation and a poor constitution on the one hand, and the environmental disadvantages of manual occupations on the other has not been carefully worked out.

longilineal One of the two constitutional types distinguished by Manouvrier. Persons of this type are built on lines that tend to be long rather than broad, and are to be contrasted with the *brevilineal* (q.v.) type. The longilineal type corresponds roughly to the *asthenic* type of Kretschmer and the *dolichomorphic* type of Pende.

longitypical Identical with *longilineal* and *dolichomorphic*.

look, amphetamine Many patients on long-continued administration of amphetamine or its derivatives are said to show a characteristic facial appearance—a pale, pinched, serious facial expression with dark circles or hollows under the eyes.

look, metallic See *gloss, metallic*.

look, paranoid The facial appearance of a paranoid schizophrenic when he thinks about certain of his complexes. The patient appears to be watching or talking to someone, even though he may deny doing so.

loosening As applied to thinking, the term includes various disturbances of associations that render speech (and thought) inexact, vague, diffuse, and unfocused. The associations may drift aimlessly and wander from the central theme, which itself may be difficult to identify with certainty; instead of centering on a concept, thoughts veer widely off target until they may seem wholly unrelated to what seemed to initiate them. The subject's conversation seems muddled or illogical, and attempts to clarify it through further questioning of the subject tend only to make it still less comprehensible. See *associations, disturbances of; circumstantiality; tangentiality; thinking, allusive*.

Lorr scale See *MSRPP*.

LOS Length of stay. See *quality assurance; review*.

loser See *transactional analysis*.

loss of control See *alcoholism*.

love In psychiatry the most commonly accepted definition of love is contained in the word *pleasure*, particularly as it applies to gratifying experiences between members of the opposite sex. The manifestations of love are almost legion, ranging from those of the infantile period up to those of sublimated maturity.

In general it may be said to correspond to *eros* and *libido*. Freud defines libido as "the energy . . . of those instincts which have to do with all that may be comprised under the word 'love.' "

According to Freud the choice of a love object may be based on (1) the *narcissistic type*, with four possibilities; one may love (a) a person like himself; (b) a person resembling him as he once was; (c) a person who meets the requirements of being what one would like to be; and (d) someone who was once part of himself. (*BW*)

The love object (2) patterned after the *anaclitic type* may be (a) the woman who tends or (b) the man who protects.

love, anal-sadistic That type of ambivalent object relationship characteristic of the anal-sadistic period. See *anal eroticism; sadism, anal*.

love, Dorian Male *homosexuality, pederasty* (qq.v.).

love, genital The type of object love characteristic of the genital or adult stage; adult, mature, nonambivalent object love.

love, homogenic *Homosexuality* (q.v.).

love, monkey A literal translation of the German term *Affenliebe*. It refers to inordinate maternal love in which the mother caters unqualifiedly to all the wishes and whims of the child. See *love, smother*.

love, mother The feeling of affection, devotion, possessiveness, and the need of protecting the child born to a woman. "Mother love is frequently called an instinct, a proclivity that appears in a woman, because she becomes a mother and for no other reason. There may be something to this idea, but . . . 'instinct' is not all that is involved. In general, people love those for whom they have to make sacrifices, and babies demand sacrifices. Not only 'instinct' but many other types of pressures—social mores, the expectancy of the family for her to act in a motherly way, her husband's pride in her motherhood, pity for the helpless infant—are also involved in setting up the pattern of feeling and action we recognize as mother love." (Lemkau, P.V. *Mental Hygiene in Public Health*, 1949)

love, passive object See *narcissism*.

love, phallic The type of object love characteristic of the phallic period.

love, pregenital Abraham thus terms the behavior of the child toward the mother in particular, during the pregenital phase. Although the infant is relatively, if not completely, indifferent to the welfare of the object in the early suckling phase, it shows the first signs of caring for the mother during the biting stage. "We may also regard such a care, incomplete as it is, as the first beginnings of object-love in a stricter sense since it implies that the individual has begun to conquer his narcissism." (*SP*)

love, smother A phrase sometimes applied to the mother who overprotects her child so that he has little opportunity to develop independence, overindulges him so that he becomes unable to tolerate frustrations, dominates and controls his every action, and ultimately engenders multiple fears in him and doubts about his own adequacy and ability. Smother love predisposes to passive dependent types of mastery and is seen often in obsessive or phobic mothers. See *love, monkey; reciprocal regulation*.

loving, delusional Erotomania (q.v.).

low utilizer See *selection, adverse*.

low-volume hospital See *volume sensitive*.

LP Lumbar puncture. See *puncture, lumbar*.

LPU Least publishable unit, referring to the earliest report of research in progress that will be accepted by a publisher. In an age when scientific or academic merit is measured by number of publications rather than by the quality of their content, a situation disparagingly referred to as the publish-or-perish syndrome, it has become unfortunate practice to publish every investigation seriatim, in a series of generally disjointed progress reports, in order to gain credit for multiple publications when one study has been performed.

LSD See *psychotomimetic*.

LTB Life-threatening behavior, generally expressed as suicidal equivalents, chronic invalidism, or other self-defeating behavior that undermines health, nullifies treatment, or disrupts valuable and necessary personal relationships.

LTM Long-term memory. See *STM*.

lucidity From the legal point of view a lucid interval is not a perfect restoration to reason, but a restoration so far as to be able, beyond doubt, to comprehend and do the act with such perception, memory, and judgment as to make it a legal act.

ludic Unreal, playlike, quasi, pseudo. See *activity, ludic*.

luding out A term of the drug subculture referring to methaqualone abuse, similar to addiction to the short-acting barbiturates. Chief dangers are (1) severe withdrawal syndrome or (2) with overdose, cardiovascular complications and convulsions.

lues (lū'ēz) Originally, plague or pestilence; in current usage, syphilis.

lues divina (L. "divine plague") *Obs*. Epilepsy.

luetic curve See *Lange's colloidal gold reaction*.

lumbar puncture See *puncture, lumbar*.

lunacy *Obs*. Mental abnormality of such degree as to render the patient incompetent and bring him under the guardianship of the state.

lunacy commission A committee, usually of qualified psychiatrists, appointed by judicial order to determine the mental state of an individual whose case the court has under consideration.

lunacy, moral *Obs*. An old psychiatric term emphasizing social and moralistic attitudes toward symptomatic behavior disorders, for which the present-day synonyms are (1) *psychopathic personality;* (2) constitutional psychopathic inferiority; (3) *perversion* and *disorders of impulse control* (qq.v.).

lunatic One possessing a mental disorder.

lunatismus (L. "somnambulism") An old expression given to those somnambulists who only walk about at the time the moon shines. (Tuke, *DPM*)

lune *Obs.* A fit of insanity.

lust dynamism Sullivan's term for clearly expressed feelings of sexual interest and ability, such as the wish of the adolescent boy to reach orgasm.

Luys, body of (Jules Bernard Luys, French physician, 1828–98) See *subthalamus.*

lycanthropy (lī-kan'thrō-pē) The belief that one can change himself or others into a wolf or some other animal.

"The *delirium of metamorphosis* or transformation into some form of animal (lycanthropy) . . . is met with much more rarely today than in past centuries, including even the first half of the nineteenth century." (Bianchi, L. *A Text-Book of Psychiatry,* 1906)

lycomania Lycanthropy.

lycorexia See *bulimia.*

lygophilia Longing for dark or gloomy places.

lying, pathological Mendacity; falsification entirely disproportionate to any discernible end in view; such lying rarely, if ever, centers about a single event; usually it manifests itself over a period of years, or even a lifetime. Pathological lying is also known as mythomania or pseudologia fantastica. See *impostor; liar, pathological.*

lypemania *Obs. Depression* (q.v.). Esquirol, a pupil of Pinel, divided mental disorders into five classes:

1. Lypemania or melancholia.

2. Monomania, in which "the disorder of the faculties is limited to one or a small number of objects, with excitement and predominance of a gay and expansive passion."

3. Mania, characterized by "delirium" extending "to all kinds of objects" and accompanied by excitement.

4. Dementia, "in which the insensate utter folly, because the organs of thought have lost their energy and the strength requisite for their functions."

5. Imbecility or idiocy, "in which the conformation of the organs has never been such that those who are thus afflicted can reason justly." (Esquirol, J. *Des Maladies Mentales,* 1837)

lypothymia *Obs.* Melancholy.

lysatotherapy A form of treatment for clinical depression reported by Timopheyev that uses a lysate of the anterior hypophysis. Lysatotherapy is based on the assumption that hypophyseal hypofunction is of etiologic significance in the pathogenesis of pure depression or cyclothymia.

lysergic acid diethylamide See *psychotomimetic; psychotropics.*

lyssa (lis'ä) *Obs.* Insanity.

lyssophobia Fear of becoming insane.

lytic cocktail See *cocktail, lytic.*

M

M In Rorschach scoring, a human movement response, i.e. a response in which human figures are seen in movement or in a position of tension, or one in which animals behave physically like humans. According to Piotrowski the *M* responses reveal the subject's prototypal role in life, such as activity or passivity, aggressiveness or submissiveness. *M* indicates an interest in people and is positively correlated with creative imagination and the level of intelligence. Absence of *M* is frequent in deterioration secondary to intracranial pathology. (*Perceptanalysis*, 1957) See *type, M*.

m In Piotrowski's perceptanalytic scoring system, a response of movement or prevention of movement in reference to inanimate, inorganic, or insensate matter. Such responses are believed to indicate roles in life that are desirable and pleasant, but unrealizable, and thus to some extent they are a measure of motor restraint. (*Perceptanalysis*, 1957)

MA Mental age. See *quotient, intelligence*.

MAC Maximum allowable cost, or revenue cap, an element of some prospective payment plans for hospital reimbursement by governmental programs and other third-party health insurance payers.

machine fever Overdependence on an executive information system so that for the user the computer terminal becomes the organization or company. One well-recognized and undesirable effect of executive information systems is that the executives who use them become so mesmerized by the charts they can produce on their own that they ignore less tangible matters such as training managers. Also, they encourage chief executives to ask many, often irrelevant, questions on the basis of what they have discovered through the use of the information system, thus consuming a disproportionate amount of the managers' time. What senior executives see as guiding or monitoring, managers tend to interpret as meddling or second-guessing. See *information system executive*.

machlaenomania *Obs*. Masochism in women.

machlosyne (mak-lōs'-i-nē) *Obs*. Nymphomania.

macro- (mak'rō-) Combining form meaning large, enlarged, extended, exaggerated, from Gr. *makrós*.

macrobiotic Long-lived; tending to prolong life.

macrocephaly Abnormally large head.

macrogenitosomia A syndrome occurring in children before the age of puberty, due to tumors of the pineal gland. The condition is also known as *pubertas praecox* (precocious puberty). The sexual development is precocious with early ejaculation or menstruation and the growth of prematurely large genitals. The secondary sex characters occur early with gruff voice, facial, pubic, and axillary hair, and mammary gland development.

macrogenitosomia, precocious Pellizzi introduced this term for a particular form of *gigantism* (q.v.) occurring in children and characterized by premature, rapid, and exaggerated development of the entire organism, including the sexual organs. In addition to the overgrowth of stature and body mass, which may reach the dimensions of the adult in a few years, there are frequently dissociations and partial hypo-evolutisms of the sexual characteristics, and also adiposity and a certain degree of mental deficiency.

This syndrome is caused by tumors of the adrenal cortex, the testicle, or the pineal gland, or in rare cases by dyspituitarism and, in female children, sometimes by constitutional hypothyroidism.

macroglobulinemia, Waldenström's Described by Waldenström in 1944; a disease of unknown origin characterized by a serum globulin of very large molecular size, lymphocytosis, thrombopenia, weight loss, weakness, and often splenomegaly and a hemorrhagic tendency. The illness is fatal within 2 to 10 years of onset, and approximately 25% of cases have central nervous system symptoms (termed *Bing-Neel syndrome*) such as progressive encephalopathy, polyneuritis, polyradiculitis, strokes, subarachnoid hemorrhage, delirium, coma, convulsions and other focal central symptoms, loss of hearing, and any number of mental disturbances such as depression.

macrology Long speech with little reasoning.

macromania *Obs.* "That form of insanity in which the insane person conceives things, especially parts of his own body, to be larger than they in reality are." (Tuke, *DPM*)

macropsia A form of *dysmegalopsia* (q.v.); visual sensation of objects being larger than they really are.

macroskelic In Manouvrier's system of constitutional types, that type characterized by excessive length of the legs; it corresponds roughly to Kretschmer's asthenic type. See *type, asthenic.*

macrosomatognosia See *somatognosia.*

Madame Butterfly phantasy See *phantasy, Madame Butterfly.*

made impulse See *symtoms, first-rank.*

madness, myxedema See *hypothyroidism.*

maenad (mē'nad) *Obs.* A mentally sick woman.

maenas (mē'nas) *Obs.* See *mania.*

Magersucht Desire to be thin or underweight; *anorexia nervosa* (q.v.).

magic See *thinking, magical.*

Magna Mater Cybele, later known to the Romans most commonly as the Great Mother of the Gods, the symbol of universal motherhood; one of Jung's archetypes. See *archetype; archetype, mother.*

Magnan's sign Formication (q.v.).

magnetic apraxia See *utilization behavior.*

magnetism The property of mutual attraction or repulsion possessed by magnets; such a force was once believed to be the principal factor in hypnosis, which was thus called animal magnetism.

magnus morbus *Obs. Epilepsy* (q.v.).

magrums *Obs. Chorea* (q.v.).

Mahler, Margaret (1897–1985) Hungarian-born psychiatrist and child analyst; *The Psychological Growth of the Human Infant* (1976). See *psychosis, symbiotic infantile.*

maieusiomania (mā-ū-sē-ō-) *Obs.* Puerperal psychosis.

maieusiophobia (mā-ū-sē-ō-) *Obs.* Fear of childbirth.

mainliner A slang expression for addicts who take narcotics by intravenous injection.

Main's syndrome See *syndrome, Main's.*

mainstreaming Return of discharged patients to an appropriate level of functioning within the community. See *deinstitutionalization.*

maintenance level See *level, maintenance.*

maintenance therapy See *preventive therapy, long-term.*

maître de plaisir (mâtr' dē plâ-zēr') One who derives satisfaction from arranging for the sexual satisfaction of others; pimp.

major role therapy See *therapy, major role.*

makeup, mental Character or personality structure. See *character; personality.*

makeup, personality The constitution of the personality. See *character; personality.*

mal de pelea Fighting sickness. See *syndrome, Puerto Rican.*

mal d'orient Homosexuality. It is said that the practice spread to Europe through the influence of the Crusaders. In some countries a homosexual is called a Turk or a Bulgar; hence the French term *bougre* and the English *bugger*, both denoting a homosexual.

mal puesto See *curanderismo.*

maladaptation, common See *psychodynamics, adaptational.*

maladie des tics (mȧ-lȧ-dē' dā tēk') See *syndrome, Gilles de la Tourette.*

maladie du pays (mȧ-lȧ-dē' dü pā-ē') Nostalgia; longing for one's native land.

maladjustment, simple adult Adult situational reaction. See *adjustment disorders; transient situational disturbances.*

malady See *disease.*

malady, English *Obs.* Hypochondriasis.

maleness See *masculine.*

malformation, congenital See *teratology.*

malignant alcoholism See *alcoholism.*

malignant identity diffusion See *crime and mental disorder.*

malignant syndrome See *syndrome, neuroleptic malignant.*

malinger To feign or protract one's illness; to simulate, with intent to deceive.

malingering Simulation of symptoms of illness or injury with intent to deceive. Malingering occurs, usually, in one of the following situations: (1) in criminal cases, when psychosis or mental deficiency is advanced as a defense; (2) in personal injury actions and compensation cases; and (3) in military service or similar special situations where nervous or mental disease might afford an escape from hazardous or arduous duty. The diseases most likely to be malingered are amnesiae, psychoses, psychoneuroses, and mental retardation. Detection in the latter case is relatively simple with available psychometric tests.

Malingering is not a mental malady, for it involves the intentional and voluntary production of false or grossly exaggerated physical or psychological symptoms. External incentives provide the motive for symptom production, in contrast to factitious disorder, conversion disorder, and other somatoform disorders where the incentives are internal and related to emotional or intrapsychic conflict. See *volition*.

malleation Convulsive movements of the hands, as if in the act of hammering.

malo ojo See *curanderismo*.

malum caducum *Obs.* Epilepsy.

malum minus Petit mal form of epilepsy.

malvaria See *mauve factor*.

mammalingus Suckling on the breast. "The fellatio conception of coitus, in fact, would seem to be only one-half of the story. One finds also the complementary idea that the father not only gives to the mother, but receives from her; that in short she suckles him. And it is here that the direct rivalry with the father is so strong, for the mother is giving him just what the girl wants (nipple and milk). . . . When this 'mammalingus' conception . . . gets sadistically cathected, then we have the familiar idea of the man who 'uses' the woman, exhausts her, drains her, exploits her, and so on." (Jones, E. *Papers on Psychoanalysis,* 1938) See *cathexis; sadism.*

man, effeminated Passive male, often implying that the male is homosexual.

management risk See *risk.*

manager disease A type of occupational neurosis occurring in overworked employers and leading officials who are overbur-

dened with responsibility. The symptoms most commonly complained of are those relating to the heart and cardiovascular system.

mandala Jung's term for the magic circle that symbolizes total unity of the self. See *Tantra.*

mania 1. *Obs.* Any mental disorder, madness, especially when characterized by violent, unrestrained behavior. 2. When used as a suffix, a morbid preference for or an irrepressible impulse to behave in a certain way, such as *kleptomania* (q.v.). 3. One of the two major forms of mood disorder. See *affective disorders; psychosis, manic-depressive.*

Mania is characterized by (1) an elated or euphoric, although unstable, mood; (2) increased psychomotor activity, restlessness, and agitation; and (3) increase in number of ideas and speed of thinking and speaking, which in more severe forms proceed to *flight of ideas* (q.v.), often with a grandiose trend.

In mania, the main disturbances in the ideational sphere are *overproductivity; flight of ideas* (i.e. a rapid shifting from one topic to another), of which *distractibility* is a part, the patient changing from topic to topic in accordance with the stimuli from without and from within; shifting may be occasioned by what is called *clang association*—stimulation of a new train of thought by some external sound; *leveling of ideas,* that is, essentially all topics have about the same value to the patient; *ideas of importance, grandiose ideas,* the patient expressing delusions of greatness perhaps in all fields; the feelings of well-being are expressed also in the sphere of *physical excellence.* Often the ideas are reproductions of those relating to *infantile sexuality.*

The principal modifications in the emotional field are inflated self-esteem with exaggerated feelings of gaiety, well-being, extreme happiness—in consonance with the ideas expressed.

The expression *psychomotor overactivity* refers to physical overactivity. In extreme states it is incessant throughout the waking hours; the patient attempts to motorize, that is, to put into physical execution all the ideas that occur to him; this tendency therefore leads to a shifting of physical activity paralleling that in the mental sphere. The person with mania has a decreased need for sleep. His days are likely to be spent in activities with a high potential for painful consequences, such as buying sprees, sexual indiscretions, reckless driving, and foolish business investments.

Depending upon the degree of mania, there are three types: *hypomania*, which is a less intense form; *mania*, which is presumably the common or usual type; *hypermania*, or a more intense expression of the manic reaction.

Some authors use the term *acute mania* synonymously with *mania*, and *hypermania* is often referred to as *delirious mania, Bell's mania, typhomania, delirium grave*, or *collapse delirium*, with partial or complete disorientation as the rule.

When a patient has a succession of manic attacks the condition is known as *recurrent* or *periodic mania*. When manic and depressive episodes alternate, the condition is called *alternating* or *circular psychosis* or *insanity*.

Periodic mania is to be distinguished from *chronic mania*, a form described by Schott in 1904 in which manic symptoms continue uninterruptedly for an indefinite number of years (in Schott's series, for 30, 25, 21, and 17 years). In all such cases reported, the particular episode that becomes chronic began after the age of 40.

A patient in a manic phase may not talk; his state is then known as *unproductive* or *stuporous mania;* he is said to be in a condition of *manic stupor.*

When a patient presents the symptoms of mania, but does not move, his condition is called *akinetic mania.* Follow-up studies suggest that akinetic mania and manic stupor and all of Kraepelin's "mixed" or "intermediate" states are really schizophrenic.

"The psychoanalytic point is one that several analytic investigators have already formulated in so many words, namely, that the content of mania is no different from that of melancholia, that both the disorders are wrestling with the same 'complex,' and that in melancholia the ego has succumbed to it, whereas in mania it has mastered the complex or thrust it aside." (Freud, *CP*) In mania, the ego for a time has thrown off the yoke of the superego

and protests, "I don't need control any more." The removal of inhibition allows all those impulses (mainly oral) which had been kept down to come to the fore. But the freedom from the superego is not a real one, and the ego must deny its fear of the superego by overcompensation. The cramped nature of the symptoms is due to the fact that they are of reaction-formation type and deny opposite attitudes. Mania is not a genuine freedom from depression but rather a cramped denial of dependencies.

TABLE OF MANIAS AND PHILIAS

Used as a suffix, -mania refers to an exaggerated interest in or preference for something, in many instances of sufficient intensity to lead to compulsive or impulsive actions. The traditional terms for several of the impulse disorders employ the -mania suffix: kleptomania, trichotillomania, pyromania.

In general, -mania stresses behavior and action, whereas the suffix -philia emphasizes the feeling, attitude, disposition, or preference. Another suffix, used much less frequently, is -lagnia, which emphasizes the erotic element in the craving or activity; most words with this suffix refer to what DSM-III and DSM-III-R term paraphilias. Thus pyrophilia means an excessive interest in fires, pyromania refers to fire-setting, and pyrolagnia refers to fire-watching or fire-setting as an essential or contributing factor to sexual excitement in the subject.

There are, however, many exceptions to the general rule. Some -mania words, in fact, do not refer to desire or need at all; instead, they describe an aversion or loathing (a function more typically performed by the -phobia suffix). Examples are demonomania (fear of devils) and nautomania (the sailor's fear of the sea).

Acrasia, acolasis, agriothymia, and *hyperepithymia* are general terms for exaggerated interest, inordinate desire, and intemperance. Terms for more specific preoccupations or cravings, and impulsive or compulsive actions, include:

alcohol: acoria (although Hippocrates used it to mean moderation in eating), alcoholophilia, alcoholomania, dipsomania, dipsos avens, oenomania, oinomania, polyposia, poisomania, potomania

animals: ophidiophilia (snakes), zooerasty, zoolagnia

bathing, washing: ablutomania

beauty: callomania (also = delusion that one is beautiful)

biting: agriothymia hydrophobica, vampirism

bloodletting: phlebotomomania, vampirism (love bites)

buying: oniomania

children: pedophilia, philoprogeneity (one's own)

collecting books: bibliomania

collecting, greed: hoarding, pleonexia, plutomania

counting, numbers: arithmomania

death: necromania, necrophilia, pseudonecrophilia (dead bodies), taphophilia (graves, cemeteries)

destruction of other nations: agriothymia ambitiosa

destruction of other religions: agriothymia religiosa

drugs: cocainomania (cocaine), etheromania (ether, inhalants), opiomania (opiates), toxicomania

eating, food: allotriophagy (unnatural food, such as thread), bulimia, opsomania (sweets), polyphagia

enemas: klismaphilia

family, upbringing: ecomania, oikiomania

filth, excreta: coprolagnia, coprophilia, mysophilia, urolagnia, urophilia

fire, firesetting: pyrolagnia, pyromania

gift giving: doromania

hairbiting: trichophagy

hair pulling: trichotillomania

health, body functioning: hypochondriasis, nosomania

images: iconomania (collecting or worshiping)

imitate, mimic: echomimia, echopraxia, philomimesia

injury, pain: castrophilia (castration), flagellomania (whipping or being whipped), machlaenomania (masochism in female), sexual masochism, sexual sadism, tomomania (desire to be operated upon), traumatophilia (self)

lies, myths: mythomania

litigation: processomania

marrying: gamonomania

masturbation: chiromania, psycholagny

murder, blood: hemothymia, homicidomania, phonomania

nostalgia, homesickness, need to go home: nostomania, philopatridomania

novelty: philoneism

odors: osphresiolagnia, renifleur

old persons: gerontophilia, gerophilia

pain: algolagnia (both sexual sadism and sexual masochism), algophilia (not necessarily sexual), lagneuomania (sexual sadism in the male)

the past: délire ecmnesique

plucking threads: allotriorhexia

power: cratomania

questioning: Fragesucht

repeating actions: mania of recommencement

sadness: tristemania

self: autophilia, autosynnoia, egomania, folie vaniteuse

sex, hypersexuality: aphrodisiomania, acrai, brachuna

in females: aedoeomania, andromania, clitoromania, estromania, folie uterine, hysteromania, metromania, oestromania, nymphomania, sexual erethism

in males: Don Juan complex, gynecoania, satyriasis, pornolagnia (need for prostitutes)

elimination: sexual vandalism (destroying any representation of genitals)

watching: scop(t)olognia, scop(t)ophilia, voyeurism

solitude: agromania,
claustrophilia,
eremophilia,
lygophilia (dark, gloom)

speaking: garrulosity,
lalorrhea, logorrhea,
logomonomania,
mania concionabunda (public
speaking)

spending, buying: asoticomania

stealing: kleptolagnia, kleptomania,
klopemania, monomanie du
nol

stealing books: bibliokleptomania

suicide: thanatomania

sunlight: photomania

thoughts (intrusive): onomatomania

thrill-seeker: philobat

touching: délire de toucher,
peotillomania (one's own
penis),
phaneromania (one's own
body)

trees: dendrophilia

urine,

urination: undinism, urolagnia, urophilia

wandering: drapetomania, dromomania,
ecdemomania,
ecdemomonomania,
eidemomania,
eretodromomania,
mania errabunda, oikofugia,
planomania, poriomania,
wanderlust

words: hellenomania (the display of erudi-
tion by excessive use of Greek
or Latin terms),
logophilia

work(ing): erasionomania

writing: erotographomania (love letters),
graphomania, graphorrhea,
metromania (verses),
pornographomania (obscene
letters)

mania à potu A state, produced by alcohol,
characterized by extreme excitement and
sometimes leading to homicidal attacks.
The attack is usually brought on, in a
susceptible person, by the ingestion of
comparatively small amounts of alcohol.
See *intoxication, alcoholic.*

mania, absorbed Manic stupor. See *mania.*

mania, acute See *mania.*

mania, akinetic See *mania.*

mania, ambitious *Obs.* Delirium grandiosum;
megalomania (q.v.); folie ambitieuse.

mania, Bell's (Luther V. Bell, American
physician, 1806–62) Acute mania. See
Bell's mania; mania.

mania, biting A form of epidemic or mass
hysteria reported in 15th-century Germany: a nun began to bite her associates
compulsively, and the impulse spread
throughout convents in Germany, Holland, and other parts of Europe.

mania, brooding Morbid impulse to meditate
long and anxiously; obsessive doubting.

"We have already mentioned the important part played by the sadistic instinctual
components in the genesis of obsessional
neuroses. Where the epistemophilic instinct is a preponderant feature in the
constitution of an obsessional patient,
brooding becomes the principal symptom
of the neurosis." (Freud, *CP*) See *folie du
doute.*

mania, Caesar *Obs.* "A feeling of being absolute master of life and death among savages." (Bleuler, *TP*)

mania, chattering *Obs.* Uncontrollable urge
to talk gibberish; pressured speech.

mania, chronic Term first used by Schott for
the manic type of reaction that is more or
less permanent. See *mania.*

mania, chronic intellectual *Obs.* "A general
disturbance of the intellect characterized
by the existence of varying unsystematized
delusions, accompanied by periods of mental excitement or depression, with more or
less incoherence and mental weakness."
(Foster, F.P. *Medical Dictionary,* 1892–94)

mania, classification of See *depression, classification of; mania.*

mania, collecting The morbid impulse to
collect. It is seen in one of its most vivid
forms in patients with schizophrenia, who
often collect all sorts of articles, most of
them useless; they stuff their clothing with
trash. The collecting mania is often clearly
representative of anal erotism. The symptom is also frequent in senile dementia.
See *coprophilia; hoarding; soteria.*

mania concionabunda *Obs.* Mania for ad-
dressing the public.

mania, doubting An obsessive doubting in
which the patient finds it necessary to say
"no" to everything. This patient will raise
objections to whatever comes into his mind

from within or without. For example, the names of people known intimately for years may become uncertain to the patient. He may realize intellectually that what he objects to is correct, but his emotions deny the fact. Usually, under analysis, it emerges that unconscious instinctual demands are being denied through the doubting-mania. (Hinsie, *UP*) See *folie du doute.*

mania, ephemeral See *mania transitoria.*

mania errabunda *Obs.* Impulsive wandering from home, apparently without aim; occurs frequently in senile states.

mania, grumbling "The patients, indeed, display exalted self-consciousness, are pretentious and high-flown, but by no means of cheerful mood; they rather appear dissatisfied, insufferable, perhaps even a little anxious. They have something to find fault with in everything, feel themselves on every occasion badly treated, get wretched food, cannot hold out in the dreadful surroundings, cannot sleep in the miserable beds, cannot have social intercourse with the other patients." (Kraepelin, E. *Manic-Depressive Insanity and Paranoia,* 1921)

mania, homicidal *Obs. Homicidomania.* Any kind of mental disease where there is an attempt or desire on the part of a patient to kill.

mania, incendiary *Pyromania* (q.v.).

mania, inhibited One of Kraepelin's "mixed states," characterized by flight of ideas, cheerful mood, and psychomotor inhibition. See *mania.* "The patients of this kind are of more exultant mood, occasionally somewhat irritable, distractible, inclined to jokes; when addressed they easily fall into chattering talk with flight of ideas and numerous clang associations, but remain in outward behavior conspicuously quiet, lie still in bed, only now and then throw out a remark or laugh to themselves. It appears, however, as if a great inward tension, as a rule, existed, as the patients may suddenly become very violent. Formerly I classified this 'inhibited mania' with manic stupor; I think, however, that it may be separated from that on the ground of the flight of ideas which here appears distinctly." (Kraepelin, E. *Manic-Depressive Insanity and Paranoia,* 1921)

mania, metaphysical *Obs. Folie du doute* (q.v.); insanity of doubt; doubting mania.

mania mitis *Obs. Hypomania.* "The slightest forms of manic excitement are usually called "hypomania," mania mitis, mitissima, also, but inappropriately, *mania sine delirio.*" (Kraepelin, E. *Manic-Depressive Insanity and Paranoia,* 1921)

mania phantastica infantilis A rare syndrome of childhood consisting of exaltation stages, fugues, confabulations or *pseudologia fantastica* (q.v.), immaturity, and retardation of mental development. The syndrome may occur as part of the delirious state following infectious diseases, and also as a psychogenic or autochthonous reaction.

mania, puerperal *Obs.* Postpartum psychosis with manic features. "Where mania really appears in the puerperal state, it is, like every other kind of mania, only a link in the chain of attacks of maniacal-depressive insanity." (Kraepelin, E. *Lectures on Clinical Psychiatry,* 1913) See *psychosis, puerperal.*

mania, reactive *Hypomania* induced by some external cause. See *reactive.*

mania, religious *Obs.* An acute psychotic episode, usually schizophrenic or organic in origin, characterized by generalized hyperactivity, agitation, restlessness, and many hallucinations with a religious coloring. See *ecstasy.*

mania senilis *Obs. Senile dementia* (q.v.).

mania sine delirio *Mania mitis* (q.v.).

mania, stuporous See *mania.*

mania transitoria *Obs.* "This term is used to describe a somewhat rare form of maniacal exaltation, which comes on suddenly, is usually sharp in its character, and is accompanied by incoherence, partial or complete unconsciousness of familiar surroundings, and sleeplessness. An attack may last from an hour up to a few days." (Clouston, T.S. *Clinical Lectures on Mental Diseases,* 1904) It was also called *ephemeral mania.*

mania, wandering See *wanderlust.*

mania(co)comium *Obs.* Psychiatric hospital.

maniaphobia Fear of insanity.

manic-depressive See *psychosis, manic-depressive.*

manic episode A distinct period of *mania* (q.v.) of not less than one week's duration and severe enough to cause marked impairment in functioning or to require hospitalization.

manic syndrome *Mania* (q.v.).

manie de perfection Compulsive perfectionism; *scrupulosity* (q.v.). For the person affected with such a symptom, everything must be 100% good, moral, clean, efficient, or otherwise perfect.

manie de rumination Janet's term for the morbid tendency to recall to mind and consider past events again and again; seen commonly in obsessive-compulsive neurosis and in some involutional psychoses.

manie sans délire Pinel's term for patients who had outbursts of rage but were not delusional (and therefore lacked what was considered the essential element of mental illness). The group thus identified included not only manic states but also psychopathic personality and other personality disorders.

maniodes *Obs.* Maniacal; ferine, brutal, beastly.

manipulanda See *intelligence.*

manipulative Exploitative; skillful in getting what one wants from others, and able to control or manage others in gaining one's own ends. Most commonly the term is used in a pejorative sense to refer to patients whose artful maneuvers in getting their own way border on the fraudulent; therapists are likely to use the term when they feel they have been made to feel foolish or outsmarted by their patients. Manipulative behavior may be seen in anyone, but it is particularly characteristic of some children, of personality types labeled hysterical, and of some schizophrenic patients—all of whom may use threats of throwing a tantrum, of suicide, or of other behavior that plays on the guilt of others in order to achieve their own goals of the moment. See *syndrome, Main's.*

mannerism A frequently repeated complex movement that appears to be goal directed and meaningful for the subject but is excessive, superfluous, inappropriate, or unexpected so that to the observer it appears to be odd or bizarre.

mantra See *Tantra.*

manustupration *Obs.* An older term for *masturbation* (q.v.).

MAO *Monoamine oxidase* (q.v.).

MAOI Monoamine oxidase inhibitor.

maple syrup urine disease A cerebral degenerative disorder due to a genetically induced defect in oxidative decarboxylation of the branched-chain keto acids leucine,

isoleucine, and valine. It is transmitted as an autosomal recessive. Clinical manifestations are poor feeding, developmental retardation, hypertonicity, convulsions, and a urine odor resembling that of maple syrup. The latter is due to increased plasma level of the above-named amino acids, whose keto-derivatives are excreted in increased amounts in the urine. Central nervous system pathology includes defective myelin formation within the white matter of the entire brain, areas of edema and spongy change, an associated astrocytosis, and a decrease in oligodendroglia. Although genetically induced, the disease does not manifest itself clinically until after birth; death usually occurs within two years after onset of symptoms, which may be partially controlled on a diet low in the amino acids involved.

mapping, genetic See *marker, genetic.*

marasmic state See *detachment, somnolent.*

marasmus nervosus *Obs.* Neurasthenia; *anorexia nervosa.* (q.v.).

marathon session A long group therapy meeting that may last from three hours to as long as an entire weekend; used particularly at the beginning of ongoing groups where unremitting group pressure on the participants tends to remove barriers to communication and stimulate group cohesion.

marche à petits pas (mȧrsh à pu-tē̆-pȧ′) A disturbance in gait in which the patient takes very short steps. The condition may be observed in cerebral arteriosclerosis and striatal rigidity. See *gait, propulsion.*

Marchiafava-Bignami disease A rare neuropsychiatric syndrome associated with alcoholism; the essential pathology is central necrosis of the corpus callosum and sometimes of the anterior commissure. This syndrome appears most typically in alcoholics who are addicted to crude red wine; when the central necrosis begins, the patient develops an acute psychotic picture consisting of excitement, ataxia or apraxia, disorientation, and confusion. With progression (and presumably due to spread of the process to the cingulate gyri), the clinical picture changes markedly: the patient becomes totally apathetic, aboulic, quiet, and completely inattentive; he appears devoid of all conation, shows akinetic mutism, and may develop hemiplegia or hemiparesis. Once this stage is reached, death is the usual end result. It is generally believed that alcohol per se is not the cause of this syndrome, but rather that it is due to metallic impurities found in wine as a result of processing and/or that it is a manifestation of vitamin deficiency.

Marcus Gunn sign (Marcus Gunn, contemporary British surgeon) The raising of a ptosed eyelid on opening the mouth and moving the jaw to the opposite side.

margin, conscious See *fringe.*

marginal psychosis See *cycloid psychosis.*

Marie's ataxia See *ataxia, Marie's hereditary cerebellar.*

Marie's disease (Pierre Marie, French physician, 1853–1940) See *acromegaly.*

marihuana, (marijuana) A variety of cannabis sativa obtained from the flowering tops of the Indian hemp plant, which grows freely in all parts of the United States and Mexico; other forms are kief, ma, ganja, dagga, charas, hashish, and bhang. Marihuana (known also as pot, tea, weed, hay, grass, charge) is most commonly rolled in cigarette papers (reefers or joints) and then smoked. Smoking two or three reefers gives the desired effect: a dreamy state of partial consciousness in which ideas are disconnected, uncontrollable, and plentiful; at times, euphoria and an excited joyousness, at other times a moody reverie or panic and fear of death; imagination runs riot, and perception is crowded and disturbed; a peculiar distortion of time, so that minutes seem to be hours, and of space, which is broadened so that near objects seem far away; vivid, pleasant hallucinations, often with a sexual coloring; loss of discriminatory ability so that a three-piece honky-tonk band may seem like a symphony orchestra. Under the influence of marihuana behavior is impulsive, mood is elevated, and random ideas are quickly translated into action. Prolonged use in those with a psychopathic personality may result in a certain degree of mental deterioration, but no positive relationship between violent crime and the use of the drug has ever been demonstrated.

Cannabis abuse refers to continuous or episodic use of the substance for at least one month, social complications of use, and either psychologic dependence or a pathologic pattern of use. Withdrawal symptoms have not been established so some workers would not apply the term dependence to cannabis use; most, however, point out that tolerance develops in many long-term users and would apply the label cannabis dependence to them.

Marin Amat syndrome See *syndrome, Marin Amat.*

marital infidelity See *paranoia, conjugal.*

marital schism A type of abnormal family pattern reported by Lidz, Fleck, and their colleagues, in the families of schizophrenics, in which the parents hold contrary views so that the child has divided loyalties. Another pattern is *marital skew* (q.v.).

marital skew A type of abnormal family pattern reported by Lidz, Fleck, and their colleagues, in the families of schizophrenics, in which one parent's eccentricities (usually the mother's) dominate the family and the other parent regularly gives in. Another pattern is *marital schism* (q.v.).

marker, genetic A detectable sign of the presence of or vulnerability to inherited disease, such as a measurable biochemical abnormality. The marker may also be an inherited trait that occurs in association with another disease often enough to support the assumption that the second disease is at least in part genetically determined and that its gene occupies a chromosomal location close to the gene for the inherited trait.

Genes are essentially segments of DNA (deoxyribonucleic acid), comprising four subunits: adenine (A), guanine (G), cytosine (C), and thymine (T). The subunits are repeated many times in various combinations, to make up the chemical language of heredity. The sequence of hundreds or several thousands of subunits in a gene gives the living cell orders for manufacture of a particular protein. It is estimated that the gene system or *genome* carried on the 23 pairs of chromosomes in the human is composed of between 50,000 and 100,000 genes, which contain about 3 billion subunits. In gene mapping, a special enzyme, a *restriction enzyme*, is applied to DNA. It cuts the DNA strands whenever it encounters a particular sequence of subunits. Genetic variation (i.e. an abnormal gene) alters the sequence, however, and since the restriction enzyme does not recognize the different unit, it will not cut the strand at that point.

There are at least 100 restriction enzymes, each of which targets a particular sequence of DNA subunits. Using a battery of enzymes, a sample of DNA is cut into many fragments, which are sorted by length. The unusually long fragment becomes a marker (*RFLP*, restriction-fragment-length polymorphism) for the disease gene. For example, study of a family in which cystic fibrosis is common will show that the disease is almost always inherited with one particular DNA variation, which thus becomes a chemical marker for the disease and can be used in diagnosis early in pregnancy for any fetus conceived in that family. The marker is (usually) not the disease gene itself, but rather an innocent bystander that occurs near the abnormal gene. It is analogous to the search for a restaurant in a strange city: knowing that it is near a certain hotel and a certain church will help locate it, but those markers have no relationship to the restaurant itself other than being nearby.

About 1,000 genetic markers were identified in the 1980s. The gene defect in cystic fibrosis has been traced to a small region of chromosome 7; that for Duchenne's muscular dystrophy to the X (female sex) chromosome; that for some Alzheimer's disease patients to 21; that for neurofibromatosis (Elephant Man's disease) to a place close to the center of chromosome 17. Complete RFLP maps have been made for 12, 13, 21, and several others.

A complete genetic map would identify all the genetic material in the 23 pairs of chromosomes. It would spell out, in their correct order, the sequence of the estimated 3 billion subunits that make up the genome.

market basket A measure of the cost of goods and services used to adjust hospital prices annually. Its components include labor, supplies, and technology.

marketing An exchange of some commodity (e.g. money, services, ideas) between buyer and seller. To the extent that more than one seller is able to provide the same or a similar commodity, marketing also includes the special efforts required to con-

vince the buyer to buy A, for example, rather than B or Z. Beyond that, marketing usually includes assessment of the target audience's perceived needs, preferences, and attitudes in order to determine appropriate strategy. In the competition model that has become a favorite of many health legislators, marketing of medical services has become increasingly important as a means of ensuring that potential patients will continue to have a broad range of needed services available to them.

marketing type See *assimilation*.

Maroteaux-Lamy's syndrome See *mucopolysaccharidosis*.

marriage counseling See *counseling, marriage*.

marriage, group A family structure in which three or more adults (including at least one male and one female) live together, share labor and money and the bearing and rearing of children, and have sexual access to each other.

marriage, psychiatric aspects of Nearly one-half of the United States in the past have had laws whose interest was to prevent persons with mental disorder from marrying. In some cases, issuance of a license was interdicted; in others, performance of the ceremony was forbidden. The constitutionality of such laws has been challenged, and the question of legality of marriage typically arises only when one of the parties concerned seeks annulment of the marriage contract. The validity of the marriage can be questioned by the "incompetent" spouse on the ground that he was incapable of understanding what he was doing.

marriage, sandbox A dysfunctional *symmetrical* marriage in which both partners vie for control or each demands to be the one who gets the most nurturance. See *complementary*.

marriage, therapeutic As an adjunct to their treatment certain probably well-intentioned, but misguided, physicians advised marriage for their patients, with various rationalizations.

marriage therapy See *counseling, marriage; therapy marriage*.

masculine Referring to a set of sex-specific social role behaviors, unrelated to procreative biological function, that identify the person as being a boy or a man. Contrast with *maleness*, which refers to anatomic and physiological features relating to the male's procreative functions. See *gender identity*.

masculine attitude in female neurotics Adler uses this term to indicate the masculine protest against feminine or apparently feminine stirrings and sensations occurring in the female neurotic. She manifests unconscious tendencies to play the masculine (domineering, active, cruel) role with the use of all available means.

masculine protest See *protest, masculine*.

masculinity While *maleness* primarily relates to the proper sex chromosome structure of XY individuals, *masculinity* is preferably understood as a male's possession of the typical and well-developed *secondary* sex characteristics of a man. See *sex determination*.

mask Stekel uses this term to mean characterological disguise: "Less known are other masks of homosexuality which I now mention. The love of old women (gerontophilia) and passion for children often covers a homosexual tendency." (*Bi-Sexual Love*, 1922) See *persona*.

Maslow, Abraham (1908–70) American psychologist, founder of humanistic psychology; developed theory of the hierarchy of needs; *Motivation and Personality* (1956), *Toward a Psychology of Science* (1966).

masochism (From Leopold von Sacher Masoch [1836–95], an Austrian novelist whose characters indulge in all kinds of sex perversions, deriving sexual pleasure from being cruelly treated) When sexual satisfaction depends upon the subject suffering pain, ill-treatment, and humiliation the condition is known as masochism.

Krafft-Ebing defined masochism as "a peculiar perversion of the psychical *vita sexualis* in which the individual affected, in sexual feeling and thought, is controlled by the idea of being completely and unconditionally subject to the will of a person of the opposite sex, of being treated by this person as by a master, humiliated and abused. This idea is colored by sexual feelings; the masochist lives in fancies in which he creates situations of this kind, and he often attempts to realize them." (*Psychopathia Sexualis*, 1908)

Havelock Ellis notes that Stefanowsky termed it *passivism*.

Freud originally believed that masochism was always secondary and represented a turning of sadism against the ego under the influence of guilt. Later, however, applying his theories of Thanatos or the Nirvana principle, he differentiated three types of masochism:

1. *Erotogenic* or *primary masochism*, when masochism is a requisite condition for sexual gratification. The self-destructive tendencies arising from the death instinct are to a large extent disposed of early in life by displacement onto objects in the outer world; this is the origin of mastery, the will to power, and true sadism. The part which is not so disposed of remains as the original erotogenic masochism, elements of which can be traced through all the developmental stages of the libido: oral (fear of being devoured), anal (desire to be beaten by the father), phallic (castration phantasies), and genital (in situations characteristic of womanhood, the passive part in coitus and the act of giving birth).

2. *Feminine masochism*, as an expression of what Freud considered to be the characteristic passivity and receptivity of feminine nature.

3. *Moral masochism* or *ideal masochism*, when there is a need for punishment arising from unconscious needs relating to resexualization of the parental introjects and reactivation of the Oedipus complex. The basic desire is to have intercourse with the father passively, and through regressive distortion this becomes a desire to be beaten by the father. The moral masochist must act against his own interests, even to the point of destroying himself, in order to provoke punishment from authority figures. Asceticism is related to moral masochism, for the mortification is sexualized and the act of mortifying becomes a distorted expression of the blocked sexuality.

Wilhelm Reich agreed that behind the masochist's behavior lay a desire to provoke authority figures, but he disagreed that this was in order to bribe the superego or to execute a dreaded punishment. Rather, he maintained, this grandiose provocation represented a defense against punishment and anxiety by substituting a milder punishment and by placing the provoked authority figure in such a light as to justify the masochist's reproach, "See how badly you treat me." Behind such a provocation is a deep disappointment in love, a disappointment of the masochist's excessive demand for love based on the fear of being left alone.

Berliner emphasized the role of the infantile love object in the genesis of masochism; he regarded the masochistic attitude as a bid for the affection of a hating love object. "Masochistic suffering represents in the unconscious the original personal love object that once gave suffering. Masochism is the sadism of the love object fused with the libido of the subject." (*Psychoanalytical Quarterly 27*, 1958)

masochism, actual See *instinct, death.*

masochism, erotogenic One of the three types of masochism described by Freud— "the lust of pain." It is the form commonly implied by the term *masochism* (q.v.).

masochism, ideal Freud's term for mental, psychic, or moral masochism; when the masochistic injury is mental or psychical, rather than physical. See *masochism.*

masochism, mass By this term T. Reik denotes "the mixture of (a) renunciation of one's own power and (b) enjoyment of its being used by proxy," such as may be seen in the enthusiasm and devotion shown by the masses to a dictator, who demands hardships and sacrifices of the masses, which they would be unable to bear if they did not consider him to be their own idealized image. (*Masochism in Modern Man,* 1941)

masochism, mental See *masochism, ideal.*

masochism, primal See *instinct, death.*

masochism, psychic See *masochism, ideal.*

masochism, secondary During growth the main part of sadism or the death instinct is directed outward; the portion that remains in the individual is called primary sadism or (now being directed inward upon the subject himself) masochism. Under given conditions, for example, in states of deep depression, the objectivated sadism is withdrawn from objects and redirected onto the subject; that is, it is introjected. This involves the process of regression to its earlier condition. "It then provides that secondary masochism which supplements the original one." (Freud, *CP*) See *masochism.*

masochism, social A characteristic subordinate attitude toward life, forcing the person into submissive and passive behavior, which enables him to stand defeats, priva-

tions, and misfortune. Such a situation can be described as a "giving up" attitude. (Reik, T. *Masochism in Modern Man,* 1941)

masochism, verbal The condition in which a person craves to hear insulting or humiliating words and derives sexual excitement by imagining himself abused or insulted verbally. A certain choice, succession, or emphasis of words and sentences seems important for the sexual excitement. Dialogues during the masochistic phantasy are quite frequent. These imagined situations "are frequently maintained for years with little or no change, and yet remain exciting. Alterations are usually restricted to trifling displacements and substitutions of persons, times and places, while the main theme, if it may be called so, is adhered to." (Reik, T. *Masochism in Modern Man,* 1941)

masochistic personality disorder *Self-defeating personality disorder* (q.v.).

massa intermedia See *thalamus.*

massotherapy Treatment by massage.

mastery, oral Domination by means of mouth. Mastery is a technique that the infant utilizes in adapting itself to its environment when seeking to control (master) it. See *instinct, mastery.*

mastigophobia Fear of flogging.

mastodynia A type of intercostal neuralgia in which there is pain and tenderness of the breast and often hyperesthesia of the nipples.

masturbation Direct self-manipulation of the genitals, most commonly by the hand, usually accompanied by phantasies that are of a recognizably sexual nature typically resulting in orgasm. *Psychic masturbation* (psycholagny) is also recognized, where phantasy alone is sufficient to cause orgasm without any direct physical manipulation. The masturbatory act, then, has two aspects—form (the physical manipulations) and content (the nature of the accompanying or provoking phantasy).

As thus defined, masturbation first occurs in the phallic period, although autoerotic activity that includes the genitalia and any other areas of the body can certainly be observed from the earliest days of life. But in the phallic period, the major portion of psychic energy is invested in the genital area, and autoerotic activity at that time comes to be associated with oedipal phantasies and so can be termed true masturbation.

It is recognized that all children masturbate during the infantile period, most do during adolescence, and some do during the latency period. Masturbation, then, can be considered psychologically normal during childhood, and is a major avenue for the discharge of instinctual tension. Under present cultural conditions, masturbation is considered psychologically normal during adolescence, and in adulthood when gratification of a physical and emotional relationship with another person is not possible.

Kinsey found that masturbation occurred in 92% of American males and 58% of U.S. females, and these figures were in line with other surveys and estimates both in this country and in Europe. More recent studies indicate that the percentage for males may be closer to 100%, and for females 85%.

Those adolescents who do not masturbate during puberty show regularly in analysis an especially deep repression of infantile masturbation, threats about which have overwhelmed them with guilt and fear; such patients, incidentally, have a poor prognosis in psychotherapy.

The conflicts of the adolescent over his masturbatory activity are often solved by reaction formations; if he is successful, these contribute to the formation of valuable character traits; if unsuccessful, he must find substitutes for masturbation, or the masturbation itself becomes a neurotic symptom. Thus the control and inhibition of instinctual impulses, at least within certain limits, may well be salutary for the development of character and personality.

Probably the most important consequence of masturbation is the guilt which typically accompanies it, and the struggle to defend oneself against it which may last for years and absorb onto itself all the energy of the psychic system. Freud tended to the view that neurasthenia could follow upon excessive masturbation; it is nowadays felt that it would be more correct to say that neurasthenia is an outcome of insufficient orgasm—that is, if anxieties and guilt disturb the satisfactory character of the masturbation.

Clinically it is recognized that many adolescents have a deep need to believe that masturbation is a terrible thing and strongly resist enlightenment about its harmlessness. This is because the conscious masturbatory phantasies are distorted derivations of unconscious Oedipus phantasies, and if the adolescent did indeed believe that masturbation is harmless he would have to resurrect these phantasies and would have to face the oedipal desires which are responsible for the guilt.

masturbation, compulsive An ill-defined term used with various meanings by different authors. Some use it synonymously with habitual masturbation or pathological masturbation, i.e. when masturbation is preferred to sexual intercourse or when masturbation is used, not occasionally to relieve sexual tension, but so frequently as to indicate a disturbed capacity for sexual satisfaction. Others apply the term to the constant impulse to masturbate that is seen in some children, who stimulate their genitals frequently, without regard to their environment, and usually without accompanying sexual erotic phantasies. More properly, the term is confined to repetitive masturbatory activity performed without adequate sexual feelings or without any accompanying sexual feelings. "Symptoms that were created for the purpose of warding off masturbation, through penetration by the warded-off forces, eventually may be replaced by masturbation. A masturbation of this kind does not bring pleasure. The lack of satisfaction increases the striving for satisfaction. The protection-forgiveness of the gods, which would make a relaxing satisfaction possible, may be sought with the same aggressive fury by masturbating, with which it is sought by the gambler in his gambling. And like gambling, masturbation also may be performed for the purpose of punishment, being thought of as an equivalent of castration. The ego demonstrates its self-destruction equivalent to its superego, asking for forgiveness by ingratiation and by stubbornness. And the superego behaves as the gods did who punished King Midas' greediness by ruining him through the fulfillment of his wishes. The sexuality the ego wanted is granted but in a painful and devastating manner. . . . Instinctual behavior of this kind may also represent a desperate and inadequate attempt to discharge, in a sexual way, tensions of any kind. The act is carried out not only to obtain pleasure or to achieve punishment but also to get rid of an unbearable painful tension and to be relieved of a state of depression. In the same way that the drug may become insufficient in addictions and an ever increasing amount of the drug is needed, so the orgastic impotence in such cases may require more and more of the pseudosexual acts. In severe cases of 'sexual addictions,' sexuality loses its specific function and becomes an unsuccessful nonspecific protection against stimuli." (Fenichel, *PTN*)

Used in a more general sense as synonymous with habitual, pathological, or overfrequent masturbation or masturbatory *pseudosexuality*, the term compulsive masturbation implies a disturbance in the capacity for satisfaction. Such cases are often based on (1) conflicts over hostility and aggressiveness, especially in those who are afraid to manifest overt defiance; or (2) conflicts over the expectation of punishment, for which masturbation may represent a substitute; or (3) conflicts over "perverse" sexual impulses, where masturbation is felt to afford a higher pleasure than can be achieved in reality; or (4) attempts to forestall threatened depression, which typically is related to unsatisfied yearnings for love and narcissistic supplies; or (5) use of masturbation to withdraw from reality in those who are neurotically inhibited, shy, and afraid of interpersonal relationships.

masturbation, habitual See *masturbation, compulsive.*

masturbation, larval Psychic *masturbation* (q.v.).

masturbation, passive *Obs.* Fellatio.

masturbation, pathological See *masturbation, compulsive.*

masturbation, psychic See *masturbation.*

masturbation, symbolic The displacement of thinly disguised masturbatory activity upon bodily parts and organs that function as symbolic objects substituting for the clitoris or penis, even if they give no direct orgastic gratification. Such symbolic masturbation can consist of nailbiting, playing with hangnails, pulling cuticle, twisting the coat sleeve or handkerchief corners, pull-

ing at buttons, twisting and plucking hairs or hair strands, fingering nose or earlobe, or inserting of finger into nose, mouth, or ear.

materialization, hysterical Somatization; Ferenczi's term for that type of conversion hysteria in which unconscious conflicts are expressed as alterations of physical functions. See *hysteria.*

The particular alterations occurring in physical functions symbolize certain specific memories and phantasies, determined by the patient's history and centering around the repressed instinctual demands and the anxieties they cause. Sometimes the conversions can be analyzed in the same way as dreams and the underlying phantasies uncovered, for often the same distortion mechanisms are used. (Fenichel, *PTN*)

maternity blues Brief episodes of crying, irritability, and lability of mood, experienced by more than half of women following delivery of a normal child. Symptoms reach a peak on the third or fourth day postpartum and disappear spontaneously within a few days. See *psychosis, puerperal.*

mathematical biology See *biology, mathematical.*

mating, assortative The mating of individuals who resemble one another in some particular, such as intelligence or hair color. Since for any such quality there is likely to be some genetic basis, assortative mating implies also the mating of genetically similar people; but the term *inbreeding* (q.v.) is used to refer to the mating of related people.

matrix, therapeutic In marital therapy, the specific patient-therapist combination used (e.g. therapist with one spouse in classic individual therapy, a different therapist for each spouse in collaborative therapy, one therapist seeing both spouses separately in concurrent therapy). The most common form of marital therapy is *conjoint*, where the spouses are seen together by the therapist (or by a cotherapy team).

matronism, precocious In constitutional medicine, this term refers to a dysgenital syndrome in young girls, which owes its name to the physical and sexual forms of a mature woman occurring in them at such a very early age. The particular characteristics of this condition apply to the size and form of the pendulous breasts, the breadth of the shoulders, pelvis, and thighs, and the adiposity of the legs and ankles. The face also has an adult expression, menstruation appears prematurely, and the temperament is vivacious and irritable.

The morphological basis of this anomaly probably consists of a pluriglandular imbalance, in which follicular hyperovarism and cortical hyperadrenalism predominate.

Matthew effect See *effect, Matthew.*

mattoid A person of erratic mind, a compound of genius and fool. Eugenio Tanzi used the term for that subgroup of paranoia characterized by abstract delusions, garrulousness, and feelings of persecution. These patients have no hallucinations, but are erotic and ambitious types. G. Lombroso used the term mattoid for cranks, eccentrics, etc., who are not overtly psychotic but are rather on the borderline of a psychosis.

maturation In genetics the cell process (in sexual reproduction) that leads to the formation of gametes in the gonads. See *hereditary.*

Following the multiplication of the reproductive cells by repeated cell division of the ordinary duplicating type, some of these cells cease to divide by ordinary division and become the *primary spermatocytes* and *primary oocytes* in the respective sexes. When these cells mature, they grow in size, and the homologous chromosomes pair in them.

Two cell divisions follow to complete maturation: (1) the *equation* division in which the chromosomes are duplicated as in ordinary cell division and (2) the *reduction* division, in which the chromosomes are merely separated so that the number of chromosomes per cell is reduced to half. See *meiosis.*

maturation, anticipatory, principle of Carmichael's generalization that almost all functions in a wide variety of organisms can be elicited by experimental means at some time prior to the spontaneous appearance of the function in the normal life cycle of the organism. This principle intimates that such functions are fully developed before they are needed by the organism.

mature *Genet.* Reproductive cells that have undergone the process of *maturation* or *meiosis.*

mauve factor A lavender or lilac-colored spot that was found on chromatographs of urine from many schizophrenics by Hoffer and Osmond. They termed *malvaria* the disorder that was presumed to be present in persons who were mauve positive. Subsequent studies noted that about 10% of "normals" were also malvarians, as were about 40% of all psychiatric patients and about 55% of schizophrenic patients. It is possible that the mauve factor represents phenothiazine or other drug metabolites rather than anything basic to schizophrenic illness.

MBD Minimal brain dysfunction. See *impulse-disorder, hyperkinetic.*

MCAT Medical College Admission Test. See *pathway, fifth.*

McDougall, William (1871–1938) American psychologist and psychiatrist; classification of emotions.

MCE Medical care evaluation. See *audit.*

McNaughton See *responsibility, criminal.*

MCR *Mother-child relationship* (q.v.).

MDD Major depressive disorder. See *affective disorders.*

MDI Manic-depressive illness; major depressive illness.

MDMA A synthetic drug, 3,4-methylenedioxymethamphetamine, related structurally to both the stimulant amphetamine and the hallucinogen mescaline. It is usually taken in doses of 75 to 175 mg, by mouth, to produce intensification of feelings, self-exploration, relaxation, heightened self-esteem, and better relations with others. Although it has some abuse potential, MDMA is rarely used more than once a week, and despite its general availability it has not been reported as a significant problem by drug clinics.

Mead, Margaret (1902–78) American anthropologist; *Coming of Age in Samoa* (1928).

mean Arithmetic average.

mechanism In psychiatry the mode of action performed by a psychic structure. For instance, repression is called a mental mechanism; it refers to functions of psychic structures and to the forces that give rise to them. One of the functions of the ego is to repress unconscious elements that are unwanted in consciousness. The various activities involved in the repression, from the time that the unwanted impulse makes itself felt or known in consciousness until the ego represses it, constitute a mechanism. See *defense.*

The term mechanism is also used in a less specialized sense to refer to the way in which any machine or system operates; it is also used to refer to the philosophical doctrine that human behavior is wholly explicable in terms of laws of physical mechanics.

mechanism, compensatory "These persons [psychoneurotics] who are intolerant of themselves often develop a compensatory attitude of intolerance of others. It is very common to find that persons who are overbearing, over-certain, almost offensive in manner, are underneath shy, sensitive, and fearful of their own inadequacies. Frequently they will criticize harshly in others the very faults which they themselves display." (Kraines, S.H. *The Therapy of the Neuroses and Psychoses,* 1948)

mechanism, flight The ego's (or psychic structure's) mode of procedure to escape from unbearable suffering. "I pointed out one or two other methods by which the ego attempts to escape from the sufferings connected with the depressive position, namely either the flight to internal good objects (which may lead to severe psychosis) or the flight to external good objects (with the possible outcome of neurosis)." (Klein, M. *Contributions to Psycho-analysis,* 1921–1945, 1948)

mechanism, homogenic A mechanism described by T. Burrow in which *part-impressions* of an object are substituted for the actual contact with the object itself, and *part-feelings* or *affects* are substituted for the total feelings with which the organism natively responds to the object as a whole. This mechanism has to do with the picture-forming processes associated with interindividual affects. Contrasted with central constant orthogenic mechanism. Synonyms: graphogenic system, graphonomic system, index system. (*The Biology of Human Conflict,* 1937)

mechanism, mote-beam Ichheiser's term for that distortion of social perception where the person is exaggeratedly aware of the presence of an undesirable trait in a minority group although oblivious to its presence in himself. See *objectivation.*

mechanism, orthogenic The organism's total coordinative function. It preserves the balance of the organism as a whole in its relation to the total environment. Contrasted with homogenic mechanism. (Burrow T. *The Biology of Human Conflict,* 1937)

mechanism, scapegoat A term used to denote the mental state of a patient who has strong antisocial feelings and looks for incidents on which he can displace, project, and rationalize his hostilities. (Burton, A., & Harris, R.E. eds., *Case Histories in Clinical and Abnormal Psychology,* 1947) See *scapegoat; scapegoating.*

mechanophobia Fear of machinery.

MEDEX See *extender, physician; physician's assistant.*

media The different means or vehicles by which anything is accomplished; in current usage, the term unless otherwise qualified usually refers to advertising media including *print media* (newspapers, books, newsletters, journals, posters, etc.) and *electronic media* (radio, television, etc.). Sometimes the term is used even more broadly to refer to all communication in all its forms: all devices, techniques, processes, and systems that may be used in acquiring, processing, and disseminating any type of information to or from large numbers of people.

median If all items constituting a series with respect to any measurable character are arrayed from smallest to largest, in order, the median is that value that will divide the total frequency in half, with just as many below as there will be above.

Example: five subjects are aged 15, 20, 22, 25, and 26 years, respectively. The median age is 22, since two are younger and two are older.

mediation, divorce See *divorce therapy.*

mediating mechanisms In research on the etiology of psychiatric disorders, *mediators* or mediating mechanisms are abnormalities of function, neither ultimate causes nor mere precipitating factors, that provide a link between causal factors and the phenomena of the disease. They are the psychological, autonomic, biochemical, or other second-order channels through which the etiologic factor(s) manifest themselves. In schizophrenia, for example, deficits in attention and perception, abnormalities in arousal or in some pathways of neurotransmission have all been considered as possible mediating mechanisms for some genetic abnormality.

medical care evaluation See *audit.*

medical model In medical care, an orientation that emphasizes treatment of the disease from which the identified patient suffers. It has been asserted that, at least at times, such an approach ignores the psychological and social components of illness and their role in determining not only the development of the "disease" but also the subject's response to it and the readiness to participate optimally in appropriate interventions. See *psychiatry, community.*

medicine, behavioral "An interdisciplinary field concerned with the development and integration of behavioral and biomedical science, knowledge and techniques relevant to health and illness and the application of this knowledge and these techniques to prevention, diagnosis, treatment and rehabilitation." (Schwartz, G.E., & Weiss, S.M. *Journal of Behavioral Medicine 1*, 1978) See *psychosomatic medicine.*

medicine, constitutional That branch of medical science which occupies itself with the study of the heredo-constitutional elements governing the biological equilibrium of human organisms and controlling their resistence or susceptibility to disease. See *constitution.*

Its aim is a most comprehensive and synthetic conception of the natural history of humans, while its research procedure consists mainly of devising methods for classifying human beings according to both their disease potentialities and capacities for adaptation, and of establishing correlations between types of human morphology and the success or failure of these types in the struggle for existence. "The evidence of the outcome of this reaction between individual and environment is expressed in terms of health, physical disease, insanity, criminality, and other less sharply defined inadequacies both physical and mental." (Draper, G. *Disease and the Man,* 1930)

Another definition of the main purpose of constitutional medicine is that of Pende, stressing the evaluation of *correlational principles,* "according to which the various combinations of organs and organic fluids and the special relationship or anatomical and functional correlations between the parts of the body, which determine the different physical and mental constitutions, *vary* according to the characteristics that are dominant in the interorganic equilibrium." (Pende, N. *Constitutional Inadequacies,* 1928)

The four basic categories, or panels, which are distinguished by Draper as the primary objects of constitutional investigation are the hereditary unit characters found in the domains of anatomy, physiology, psychology, and immunity. See *panels, personality.*

medicine, physical See *physical medicine.*

meditatio mortis A feeling of impending death; frequent in anxiety states.

meditation, transcendental See *transcendental meditation.*

medulla oblongata The pyramid-shaped portion of the brain stem lying between the spinal cord and the pons. The ventral portion contains the pyramidal decussation; the lateral portion contains the funiculus gracilis and the funiculus cuneatus. The medulla also contains the nucleus of the hypoglossal nerve, the nucleus ambiguus (somatic motor nucleus of glossopharyngeal, vagus, and spinal accessory nerves), the dorsal motor nucleus, and the sensory nucleus of the vagus nerve, and the dorsal and ventral cochlear nuclei. The medulla oblongata is sometimes called the bulb; syndromes resulting from lesions of the medulla are therefore known as *bulbar syndromes,* whose characteristic symptoms are due to involvement of the various tracts passing through the medulla and particularly to involvement of the nuclei of cranial nerves IX, X, XI, and XII.

Meduna, Ladislas J. von (1896–1964) Hungarian-born U.S. psychiatrist; developed Metrazol therapy, carbon dioxide therapy.

megadose Very high dose of any drug, often of the magnitude of 1,000 times the usual dose. Megadose therapy of schizophrenics with fluphenazine, for instance, has often used 800 to 1,200 mg per day, equivalent to 40,000 to 60,000 mg per day of chlorpromazine. Less commonly, megadose treatment refers to rapid neuroleptization. See *depot neuroleptic; neuroleptization, rapid.*

megalo- Combining form meaning big, great, from Gr. *mégas, -álon,* akin to L. *magnus.*

megalomania A type of delusion in which the subject considers himself possessed of greatness. He may believe himself to be Christ, God, Napoleon, etc. He may think that he is everybody and everything. He is lawyer, physician, clergyman, merchant, prince, generalissimo, ace athlete in all divisions of sports, etc.

"The question arises: What is the fate of the libido when withdrawn from external objects in schizophrenia? The megalomania characteristic of these conditions affords a clue here. It has doubtless come into being at the expense of the object libido. The libido withdrawn from the outer world has been directed on to the ego, giving rise to a state which we may call narcissism." (Freud, *CP*)

The ideas in megalomania are called *delusions of grandeur* or *grandiose delusions.*

megalophobia Fear of large objects.

megalopia hysterica See *macropsia.*

megalosplanchnic In Viola's classification of the constitutional forms of body build, the type which has the abdominal portion of the body relatively large in proportion to the thoracic, owing to the large size of the abdominal viscera. This type is further characterized by a predominance of the trunk over the extremities.

megavitamin See *orthomolecular.*

megrim *Obs. Migraine* (q.v.).

Meige syndrome See *syndrome, Meige.*

meiosis *Genet.* That particular kind of cell division in sexual reproduction which occurs in the sex glands immediately preceding gametic formation and results in a reduction of the chromosomes from the double or *diploid* number, characteristic of all somatic cells, to the halved or *haploid* number, characteristic of gametes. The "reduction division" leads to the separation of the two elements of each chromosome pair and provides the necessary basis for the segregation of genetic factors. Meiotic divisions are thus genetically *segregation divisions.* See *chromosome.*

According to A.F. Shull, the following features of meiosis are most essential to the process of heredity:

1. The pairing of the homologous maternal and paternal chromosomes.

2. The separation of these paired chromosomes and their passage to different cells in the reduction division.

3. The consequent separation of the genes of each pair to different germ cells.

4. The independence of the several pairs of chromosomes in this separation.

5. The resultant assembling of various combinations of maternal and paternal chromosomes in the different mature germ cells.

6. The variety of combinations of genes thus produced in the different germ cells.

7. The reduction of the number of chromosomes in the mature germ cells to half that found in the reproductive cells before maturation.

meiotic Relating to or manifesting from meiosis.

melancholia *Depression* (q.v.). Although in earlier usage depression and melancholia were approximately equivalent, the current tendency, following DSM-III, is to use melancholia in a more limited sense to refer to a major depressive episode of severe degree characterized by altered psychomotor activity (agitation or retardation), intense and pervasive lowering of mood tone that is independent of (i.e. not "reactive" to) environmental changes, depressive delusions with self-pejorative ideas, loss of interest in pleasurable activity, significant weight loss, and decreased ability to concentrate. Symptoms tend to be worse in the morning, and early morning waking is characteristic of major depressive episodes with melancholia. Some differentiate retarded anhedonic and agitated delusional subtypes of melancholia. For many, the term implies an organic etiology and it is similar to what other classifications label as *autonomous, endogenous, endogenomorphic,* or *nonreactive.* See *melancholia gravis; melancholia, hypochondriacal.*

According to Freud, normal mourning is to melancholia as normal fear is to morbid anxiety. Briefly stated, the loss of love object leads to withdrawal of libido from reality and the introjection of the libido upon the mental picture of the lost love object. Abraham has shown that in these states libido regresses to the oral stage. See *psychosis, manic-depressive.*

melancholia, abdominal A rarely used term for depressions (mainly the agitated, involutional type) characterized by a delusional fixation on the gastrointestinal tract, with vociferous complaints of dyspepsia, eructation, flatulence, constipation.

melancholia activa *Obs. Melancholia agitata* (q.v.).

melancholia agitata Agitated depression; usually the term refers to involutional psychosis, although in the 19th century it was used to refer to catatonic excitement. See *psychosis, involutional.*

melancholia, alcoholic "Not very rarely alcoholics suffer from depressive conditions which cannot be distinguished symptomatologically from a melancholia of manic-depressive insanity even though the delusions remain rudimentary. But they do not last long, only about two weeks." (Bleuler, *TP*)

melancholia anglica *Obs.* English melancholy; suicidal insanity.

melancholia attonita *Obs.* The morbid state common in the catatonic form of schizophrenia, characterized by immobility and muscular rigidity.

melancholia canina *Obs. Lycanthropy* (q.v.).

melancholia, climacteric Melancholia developing at the climacteric period of life. See *psychosis, involutional.*

melancholia, excited *Motor melancholia;* agitated depression. See *psychosis, involutional.*

melancholia, fantastic *Obs. Melancholia gravis* (q.v.).

melancholia flatuosa (L. "flatuous melancholy") *Obs.* See *hypochondriasis.*

melancholia gravis *Obs.* Kraepelin's term for the depressive syndrome in which "the patients see figures, spirits, the corpses of their relatives; something is falsely represented to them, 'all sorts of devil's work.' Green rags fall from the walls; a coloured spot on the wall is a snapping mouth which bites the heads off children; everything looks black. The patients hear abusive language ('lazy pig,' 'wicked creature,' 'deceiver,' 'you are guilty, you are guilty'), voices which invite them to suicide; they feel sand, sulphur vapour in their mouth, electric currents in the walls." (Kraepelin, E. *Manic-Depressive Insanity and Paranoia,* 1921)

melancholia, homicidal See *mania, homicidal.*

melancholia, hypochondriacal A symptom complex consisting of depressive affect, inhibition of thinking and acting, and hypochondriacal delusions. When not organic, this symptom complex is almost always schizophrenic in nature. Monoideism, in contrast to the simple melancholias, may here be almost absolute. For long periods there seem to be no thoughts other than the constantly repeated wishes, complaints, or maledictions. Even though the affect seems to dominate the entire personality, it is typically stiff, superficial, and exaggerated. In this condition, ideas of grandeur may coexist with appalling fears and terrors in spite of logical contradictions involved.

melancholia, involutional See *psychosis, involutional.*

melancholia, motor *Obs.* See *melancholia, excited.*

melancholia nervea *Obs.* See *hypochondriasis.*

melancholia, paranoid Depression with an admixture of paranoid elements, usually persecutory in nature; involutional melancholia. See *psychosis, involutional.*

melancholia vera See *anxietas praesenilis.*

melancholia zoanthropia *Lycanthropy* (q.v.).

melancholy In current psychiatry the term is synonymous with *melancholia* (q.v.). In literature of the 19th century melancholy was distinguished from melancholia "in that there are no morbid sense perversions, no irrationality of conduct, no morbid loss of self-control, no sudden or determined impulse towards suicide or homicide, and where surrounding events and occurrences still afford a certain amount of interest, though lessened in degree, and where the power of application to ordinary duties is still present." (Tuke, *DPM*)

melissophobia Fear of bees.

Melkersson-Rosenthal syndrome See *syndrome, Melkersson-Rosenthal.*

melomania *Obs.* Psychosis characterized by incessant singing.

mem-element See *system.*

meme The basic unit of cultural inheritance, analogous to the gene in biological inheritance. The meme is considered to be a unit of information contained in the brain; its outward manifestations are *meme products.*

memory The ability, process, or act of remembering or recalling, and especially the ability to reproduce what has been learned or experienced. Memory is more than mere registration, retention, and recall. It is a complex mental function that includes at least the following:

    1. *Primary response*—perception, apper-

ception, recognition, and often some degree of understanding of the significance of what is to be learned; the primary response is affected by many factors such as previously learned responses, set, fatigue.

2. *Short-term retention*—a transient holding of information that decays rapidly with time.

3. *Long-term retention*, subdivided into (a) secondary elaboration—in accord with other memories, needs, wishes, etc.; (b) consolidation—memory traces become increasingly well established with the passage of time; (c) inhibition—blocking out of unessential memories, even though these may be brought back on demand; (d) extinction—eradication of previously reinforced but no longer useful memories.

4. *Retrieval*—bringing stored material into consciousness at will (and in some early dysmnesias, the first symptom is having to wait excessively long before the information can be retrieved—"It will come back to me in a moment"). See *reminiscence*.

5. *Activation* or *readout*—decoding retrieved material, a process that is affected by the rest of the mental apparatus so that what is finally reproduced is different from what was actually laid down as a memory trace.

Such fine differentiation can rarely be made at the clinical level, however; instead, memory is usually subdivided into *immediate memory* (the ability to recall or reproduce material that has been presented within the past few seconds, and up to about 25 minutes, corresponding to what is termed short-term retention above), *recent memory* (the ability to remember what has been experienced within the past few hours or days or weeks), and *remote memory* (the ability to remember what was experienced in the distant past).

Defects in memory *(dysmnesia)* are characteristic of many organic brain disorders, where immediate and recent memory tend to be disturbed first, while remote memory may be relatively well retained for some time. See *syndrome, organic*.

Even small lesions in the inferomedial portions of the temporal lobes—and especially in the amygdala, hippocampus, fornix, mammillary bodies, and medial dorsal nucleus of the thalamus, the area

comprising the *limbic lobe*—can produce a permanent dysmnesic syndrome with little disturbance in other aspects of mental functioning. The importance of this area of the brain in memory is further attested to by the symptom of *panoramic memory,* a well-recognized temporal lobe aura. There is general agreement that bilateral hippocampal lesions produce deficits in learning ability and in remote memory (or habit retention). Short-term memory, on the other hand—a transient holding of information that decays rapidly with time and forms no permanent trace—seems not to be affected by such lesions.

It is probable that short-term memory is an intrinsic capacity of each cortical processing system and that temporary information storage may occur within each brain area in which long-term memory (LTM) is ultimately stored. Memory is believed to be stored as changes in the same neural systems that ordinarily participate in the perception, analysis, and processing of the information to be learned.

The capacity for LTM requires the integrity of the medial temporal and diencephalic regions, which operate in conjunction with the assemblies of neurons that represent stored information. The interaction between the medial temporal region and memory storage sites located elsewhere in the brain continues until the ensemble of those distant and distributed sites attains enough coherence so it no longer requires the participation of the medial temporal region.

Most current theories of memory and learning propose modification of existing synapses as the crucial mechanism. The theories of the 1950s and 1960s, that memories are coded molecularly and that each memory is coded by RNA, have for the most part been abandoned.

memory, affect A type of recall memory based on emotions experienced rather than on language. Infant research suggests that the infant is able to encode emotional experiences at least by the age of 7 months and long before the establishment of a language-based memory code. This is in accord with *infantile amnesia*, which refers to loss of memory for affect-laden experiences but does not involve amnesia for motor memories or semantic memories, since the subject does not forget how to walk or how to speak.

memory, automatic Reactivation of an affective state or emotional complex by means of an associate link to the original situation, even though the subject is not aware of the association. The term, used by Morton Prince, is rare, although the phenomenon is well-known; one type of automatic memory, at least according to Freud, is *déjà vu* (q.v.).

memory, biological Inherited knowledge of how to react; inherited engram. Instincts, for example, may be an expression of such biological memories or inherited engrams. The collective unconscious of Jung probably springs from biological memories in that the motives and images that he includes in the term collective unconscious are not dependent upon the acquisitions of personal existence, but originate in the inherited brain structures. See *memory, physiological.*

memory, cover See *memory, screen.*

memory, cued See *memory, evocative.*

memory declarative See *memory, long-term.*

memory disability Difficulty with storage, and later retrieval of information.

memory, dislocation of Holland's term for complete but temporary forgetfulness or amnesia.

memory, episodic Personal memory, in contrast to general knowledge (*semantic memory*). Rather than being separate, the two form a continuum and are often intermixed. See *memory, long-term.*

memory, evocative The capacity to remember something even though it is absent. *Recognition memory* refers to the ability to identify something as familiar when it reappears or is presented to the subject. The differences between recall and recognition memory are probably quantitative rather than qualitative, in that some kind of cue is needed to produce or evoke the remembrance. For that reason, recall memory and *cued memory* are the same. See *object constancy.*

memory hallucination Reappearance of repressed material as a visual image.

memory, hyperesthetic Oversensitive memory, especially one that is too easily aroused according to the laws of association. Breuer and Freud hypothesized that the provocation of hysterical attacks was in large part due to associative reactivation of hyperesthetic memories.

memory, liquidation by Assimilation or incorporation of experiences in the sphere of memory or intellect. "A situation has not been satisfactorily liquidated, has not been fully assimilated, until we have achieved, not merely an outward reaction through our movements, but also an inward reaction through the words we address to ourselves, through the organization of the recital of the event to others and to ourselves, and through the putting of this recital in its place as one of the chapters in our personal history." (Janet, *PH*)

memory, long-term (LTM) Long-lasting, consolidated memory, as contrasted with immediate or short-term memory. Amnesia typically involves loss of long-term memory but not of short-term memory.

Long-term memory is differentiated into *declarative* or *propositional memory* and *procedural* or *motoric memory.* Declarative memory is explicit and conscious, and it consists of information based on specific facts or data. It can be brought to mind verbally as a proposition or nonverbally as an image. It is sometimes further subdivided into *episodic memory,* which concerns specific time-and-place events, and *semantic* or *reference memory,* consisting of facts, general information, and knowledge of concepts and rules.

Procedural knowledge is implicit and concerns the processing of motor skills. It is accessible only through performance, by engaging in the skills or operations in which the knowledge is embedded. Procedural knowledge is generally retained in amnesic patients.

memory, motor A type of recall memory based on muscular movement rather than on language, such as the infant's ability to recall a particular act and reproduce it on cue even before he has acquired language. See *memory, affect; memory, long-term.*

memory, panoramic See *absent state; memory.*

memory, physiological M. Prince's term for the process of registration, retention, and reproduction of a somatic experience outside the field of conscious awareness; conditioning of autonomic system reactions would be an example of physiological memory.

Since 1950, when Katz and Halstead hypothesized that memory depends upon structural chemical changes in a nucleoprotein template, it has been learned that ribonucleic acid (RNA) is probably the substance involved in storing memory traces in the brain, and that deoxyribonucleic acid (DNA) comprises the genes and carries a code of chemical information that is the basis for the phylogenetic memory of the species. Both personal and phylogenetic memory, in other words, are mediated through the same chemical systems. As a result of such knowledge, the terms *biological memory* and *racial memory* are sometimes used to refer to the DNA and RNA chemical systems, rather than to the older senses of the terms.

memory, procedural See *memory, long-term.*

memory, propositional See *memory, long-term.*

memory, psychophysiological "Still another variety of memory is *psycho-physiological.* This type is characterized by a combination of psychological and physiological elements and is important . . . because of the conspicuous part which such memories play in pathological conditions. Certain bodily reactions which are purely physiological, such as vaso-motor, cardiac, respiratory, intestinal, digestive, etc., disturbances, become, as a result of certain experiences, linked with one or another psychical element (sensations, perception, thoughts), and, this linking becoming conserved as a 'disposition,' the physiological reaction is reproduced whenever the psychical element is introduced into consciousness." (Prince, M. *The Unconscious,* 1916) See *memory, physiological.*

memory, racial The part of mental life that a person brings with him at birth, the archaic heritage of fragments of phylogenetic origin. This archaic inheritance consists, first of all, of the ability and tendency of all human organisms "to follow a certain direction of development and to react in a particular way to certain excitations, impressions, and stimuli." The differences among organisms in this respect are the constitutional element in the individual.

A particular memory becomes part of the racial memory when the experience is important enough or repeated often enough or both. Such a memory will become conscious again (though in an al-

tered and distorted form) when an actual repetition of the remembered event has recently occurred. The obsessive character of religious phenomena in particular demonstrates the altered and distorted return (to consciousness) of memory traces of experiences that had occurred in the distant past and remained in the racial memory. (Freud, S. *Moses and Monotheism,* 1939)

memory, recognitory See *memory, evocative; object constancy.*

memory reference See *memory, long-term.*

memory, replacement The substitution of one memory for another. One type of replacement memory is the screen memory. See *memory, screen.*

memory romance See *romance, memory.*

memory, screen When a memory, a real thought, not a phantasied one, is used as a shield to conceal an allied memory, it is called a screen memory or cover memory. Thus when a patient recalls playing in the basement, but does not remember the nature of the play, he is said to be providing a screen memory.

memory, semantic See *memory, long-term.*

memory trace The material that remains in consciousness when a painful experience is not completely repressed.

memory, unconscious Retention of mental impressions of an event, even though, in ordinary circumstances, they are not subject to recall into consciousness. Freud first applied the concept to his studies of hysteria. He found that certain events, usually sexual, occurred to the patient, but were so unbearable that they were actively put out of consciousness by being repressed. In the process of *repression* (q.v.), the ideational content as well as its affective component is relegated to the unconscious and kept there as an unconscious memory or unconscious image. "At puberty, when the sexual drive is stronger, this unconscious mental impression, under certain conditions, is reactivated. Because of the increased capacity for sexual feeling, the repressed memory acquires new force. It now produces the same result as an actual event in the present, an effect which the original experience itself lacked. Such a memory is not conscious. When, at puberty, it is reawakened, there is a liberation of affect, although the ideas associated with it remain repressed." (Thompson, C.

Psychoanalysis, Evolution and Development, 1950) In such instances, the goal of therapy is to bring back into consciousness the unconscious ideational content as well as the associated affect.

mendacity As used in psychiatry, pathologic lying. See *liar, pathological.*

Mendel, Abbot Johann Gregor (1822–84) An Augustinian monk (and later abbot) at Brünn, published in 1865 his *Experiments on Peas and Honeybees in the Monastery Garden.* In 1910 his findings and theories were rediscovered simultaneously by Correns, von Tschermak, and De Vries, and thus *Mendelism* (q.v.) became the new science of *genetics* (q.v.).

Mendelian laws See *laws, Mendelian.*

Mendelism The biological phenomena underlying the distributive mechanism of organic inheritance as discovered by Mendel.

The problem of how true-breeding varieties within a species are related was attacked by him from its simplest side by concentrating his attention upon the genetic mode of inheritance on sharply contrasted pairs of characters: he crossed round peas with wrinkled ones or a yellow species with a green one, and was thus able to determine that all hybrids of the first filial generation (F_1) resembled each other, but exhibited only one of the two alternative characters distinguishing the parents. In the crosses of round and wrinkled peas all the offspring were round and this "prevailing" member of a pair of individual characters was called *dominant,* while the other member, which was "repressed," was called *recessive.*

If the round F_1 plants were allowed to become self-fertilized and the seeds were harvested separately and sown separately, producing the second filial generation (F_2), the wrinkled form reappeared in this generation in the proportion of one wrinkled to.three round. By inbreeding, in turn, the wrinkled F_2 individuals, it was found that they constantly produced wrinkled peas while the round form completely failed to reappear; genetically speaking, every individual exhibiting the the recessive character bred true. Of the self-fertilized round *(dominant)* individuals one-third likewise produced only round offspring. The remaining two-thirds propagated themselves in the same proportion as the uniform first

generation, one-quarter wrinkled to three-quarters round, and similarly in all the subsequent generations.

These phenomena are explained by Mendel's theory that the hybrid does not produce any hybrid gametes, but merely pure gametes of various kinds, some of which bear dominant and others recessive characters. The hybrids of the first filial generation with round seeds contain the factor for wrinkled as well as the factor for round but the former is hidden and suppressed by the latter. Since the recessive character reappears in the next generation, the dominant and the recessive characteristics must necessarily separate at the moment when the hybrid forms its gametes. See *laws, Mendelian.*

mendicancy, pathological A syndrome characterized by the necessity on the part of the patient to beg, regardless of any real financial need.

meninges (men-in'jez) The membranous coverings of the brain and spinal cord. The outermost meninx is the *dura mater;* the middle one is the *arachnoid;* the innermost is the *pia mater.* The dura mater is known as the *pachymeninx;* fibrous processes of the dura mater form the falx cerebri (which separates the two cerebral hemispheres), the tentorium cerebelli (which forms a partition between the posterior and middle fossae of the skull), the falx cerebelli (which separates the cerebellar hemispheres), and the diaphragma sellae (which forms a roof to the sella turcica and through which passes the infundibulum). The arachnoid and pia mater are known as the *leptomeninges;* the space between them is the subarachnoid space, which contains the cerebrospinal fluid.

meningismus Meningeal manifestations closely simulating those of meningitis, but in which no actual inflammation of the meninges is present.

meningitic curve See *Lange's colloidal gold reaction.*

meningitis Any inflammatory process involving the cerebrospinal leptomeninges, producing mental symptoms of the organic reaction type, in its acute form, with severe headache, delirium, somnolence, or stupor. Localized or generalized convulsions, generalized rigidity, twitching, and monoplegia or hemiplegia may also occur.

meningitis, aseptic Meningitis without identifiable organisms in the gram stain or bacterial culture of the spinal fluid; usually due to virus infection.

meningitis, serous See *pseudotumor cerebri.*

meningitis, tuberculous A condition in which the tubercle bacillus infects the meninges of the central nervous system and produces mental symptoms of the organic reaction type. The disease is always secondary to a tuberculous focus elsewhere in the body, and without treatment the course is usually slowly progressive toward a fatal termination. Headache, delirium, stupor, and convulsions occur. The neck is rigid; often the tubercle bacillus can be demonstrated in the spinal fluid.

meningitophobia A hysterical presentation of meningeal symptoms; morbid dread of brain disease.

meningocele (mē-ning'gō-sēl) A developmental anomaly in which there is a protrusion of the membranes of the brain or spinal cord through a defect in the skull or spinal column respectively.

Menninger, Karl Augustus (b. 1893) American psychoanalyst; criminology, classification, unitary concept of mental illness; *The Vital Balance* (1963), *Theory of Psychoanalytic Technique* (1948).

Menninger, William Claire (1900–66) American psychoanalyst; military psychiatry, mental hospitals.

menopause Climacterium; the period of natural cessation of menses; the involutional period; known popularly as "change of life." See *psychosis, involutional.*

mens rea (L. "criminal mind") Guilty intent and/or the mental ability to have such an intention, often an important legal consideration in determining an accused person's criminal responsibility.

mensuration Measurement of areas and distances on the surface of the body.

mental deficiency See *retardation, mental.*

mental disorders, classification of See *DSM-III; nomenclature, 1968 revision.*

mental handicap See *retardation, mental.*

mental health See *health, mental.*

Mental Health Center See *psychiatry, community.*

mental health worker See *worker, mental health.*

mental hygiene See *hygiene, mental.*

mental makeup See *character.*

mental retardation See *retardation, mental.*

mental set See *set.*

mental status The psychological and behavioral appearance of a person; in clinical psychiatry this term is commonly used to refer to the results of the mental examination of a patient. The written report of the mental status usually contains specific references to the following areas (Lewis, N.D. *Outlines for Psychiatric Examinations,* 1943):

I. Attitude and General Behavior
  A. General health and appearance (?weak ?prematurely aged ?immature)
  B. General habits of dress (?overmeticulous ?slovenly)
  C. Personal habits (toilet and eating habits)
  D. General mood (elation, excitement, calm, apathy, dejection)
  E. Use of leisure time
  F. Degree of sociability
  G. Speech (productivity; disorders of speech such as stuttering; topics of conversation)

II. Attitude and Behavior During Interview
  A. Cooperativeness
  B. Poise (?stilted ?poised ?boisterous ?uncontrolled)
  C. Facial expression (pain, grief, anxiety, distrust, bewilderment, anger, defiance, contempt, exaltation, preoccupation, apathy)
  D. Motor activity (gestures, coordination, retardation, or acceleration)
  E. Mental activity (flow of speech; flow of thought; loss of continuity or alterations of language and speech structure)
  F. Emotional reactions (appropriateness, harmony)
  G. Trend of thought (persecutory, hypochondriacal, unreality, nihilism, dejection, grandiosity, hallucinations, delusions, illusions, obsessions, compulsions, fears)

III. Sensorium, Mental Grasp, and Capacity
  A. Orientation
  B. Memory and retention
  C. School and general knowledge
  D. Estimate of intelligence
  E. Abstraction ability

F. Test of absurdity, interpretation of proverbs

G. Judgment

Mental Status Examination Report See *Multi-State Information System.*

mentales *Obs.* Linnaeus, in 1763, divided mental disorders *(mentales)* into three classes: *ideales, imaginarii,* and *pathetici.*

mentalia *Obs. Psychalia* (q.v.).

mentalism The primitive tendency to personify, in spirit form, the forces of nature and the motions of things on earth and in the heavens; the endowment of inert matter with the quality of "soul"—synonymous with *animism* (q.v.). This philosophical concept implies the existence of spiritual or mental forces completely different from the somatic structures, and denotes the subjective, mental, or mind approach to psychiatry in contrast to the behavioristic approach, which stresses objective physiological activities.

mentality Mental action or power; the psyche in action. In psychiatry mentality is considered from two points of view: (1) that of intellectuality and (2) that of the instincts. The former refers to the intellectual capacity, such as superior, average, or inferior intelligence. The latter forms the basis of personality structure and function. Since the introduction of the formulations of Freud the mind or psyche has been conceived in the light of an organ of the body, with its own structures and functions, and with its correlative action with other body organs and with the environment.

According to such conceptions, the psyche is the central organ that expresses mentality from the instinctual point of view, while the brain occupies an analogous position with regard to the intellectual aspects of mentality.

mente capti *Obs.* See *furiosi.*

menticide Mind control; *brainwashing;* any organized system of psychological intervention in which the perpetrator injects his own thoughts and words into the minds and mouths of the victims. See *deprivation, sensory; implant, dynamic.*

mentiferous *Obs.* Telepathic. See *perception, extrasensory.*

mentism *Rare.* Mental derangement.

mentula (L. "penis") Originally used in the socially taboo sense in which cock and

prick are used today; "membrum virile," frequently used in Victorian medical jargon to disguise the nature of its original meaning.

meralgia paresthetica A rare neuritis of the lateral femoral cutaneous nerve, characterized by numbness, pain, burning, tingling, and hypersensitivity localized on the anterior and lateral surface of the thigh usually due to pressure from obesity, abdominal binders, or corsets. Suffering can be relieved immediately by nerve block with local anesthetic.

Mercier, Charles Arthur (1852–1919) British psychiatrist; forensic psychiatry.

mere-, -mere Combining form meaning part, share, from Gr. *méros.*

merergasia Partial ability to work or function; *kakergasia.* Term used by Adolf Meyer to designate a clinical psychiatric syndrome that causes only a partial disorganization of the personality. In general it may be stated that the psychoneuroses and neuroses constitute the merergastic reactions.

mergent, partial Burrow thus denotes the interverbal conditioning that occurs reflexly among individuals and is socially systematized within groups or communities. By virtue of this reflex community reaction coincident with the employment of words or symbols, two phenomena that are completely disparate and unrelated outside the organism may become united or merged socially (intercortically) into a common motivation or "meaning" within the organism. Through this mechanism the organism's primary feelings have been socially replaced by mere reflex partial affects. The partial mergent represents a false mergent in contrast to the organism's total or true mergent. Contrasted with total mergent.

mergent, total Burrow's term for the organism's response as a whole to the total environmental situation. Contrasted with partial mergent.

merogony (me-rog'ō-nē) The process in which the egg cytoplasm comes from one parent and the nucleus, through the sperm, from the other, thus making possible a comparison of their effects. Boveri fertilized enucleated eggs of one species with sperm from a markedly different one. The merogonous embryos resembled the species from which the sperm was derived.

Thus development seems to be controlled by the nucleus, even if it is surrounded by cytoplasm from a very different source. See *nucleus*.

merycism "Merycism is a voluntary regurgitation, moderate in degree and slow, but rather pleasant, of food from the stomach to the mouth, in which it is masticated and tasted a second time, as in rumination. This remarkable habit is special to certain idiots and dements of a very low type." (Tanzi, E. *Text-Book of Mental Diseases,* 1909) See *rumination*.

Despite the foregoing, the symptom has also been reported, although rarely, in persons of normal intellect. In such cases, it is believed to represent the inhibited unconscious wish to vomit at the face of the stranger, attacker, and/or authority figure.

mescaline The active principal of the cactus from which peyote is obtained. See *peyotism*.

Mescaline has been used as one of the two chief agents to produce an experimental or model psychosis (the other agent is lysergic acid). The major effects are personality disturbances and an increase in sympathetic tension in the experimental subject; the former include visual (and sometimes auditory) hallucinations, illusions, distortions of the body image, altered time sense, thought-language changes, and an increase in self-observation sometimes to the point of complete withdrawal and feelings of unreality and detachment. Both mescaline and lysergic acid are also substances of abuse. See *substance abuse and dependence disorders*.

The mode of action of mescaline is not fully understood. It is a powerful synaptic inhibitor, and its sympathomimetic effects may be due to inhibition of the opposing parasympathetic system. It seems more likely, however, that its effects are due to stimulation of the sympathetic system by reason of imitation of norepinephrine at the latter's receptor sites, this leading to arousal, sympathetic outflow, increased psychomotor activity, and enhancement of sensitivity to external stimuli. It has also been suggested that the mescaline psychosis is due to formation of a protein-bound

mescaline compound in the liver, which then acts as a toxic agent to sensitive areas in the brain.

mesencephalon *Midbrain* (q.v.).

mesenchyme, mesenchyma Although this term was introduced in embryology by O. and R. Hertwig to denote the part of the *mesoderm* (q.v.) that separates from the original mesothelium as a loose mass of anastomosing cells to form the connective tissues, it has lost some of its precise meaning. It is now generally assumed that the mesenchymal tissue, occupying practically all the intervals between the epithelial layers, does not arise from the middle germ layer alone, but probably from certain parts of the *entoderm* and *ectoderm* also (qq.v.), and that it forms not only the various forms of connective tissue, but also the skeletal system, the smooth muscular tissue, the stroma of the iris and the ciliary body, the cartilages and ligaments of the larynx, and, especially, the blood and blood vessels.

In constitutional medicine, Viola's ontogenetic law contrasts *ponderal* evolution, or increase of mass due to the mesenchyme with *morphological* evolution, or change of proportion due to the *parenchyma* (q.v.), and holds that these two evolutionary types are in inverse proportion to one another. It is believed by Viola that when there is evolutionary disharmony, one system preponderates over the other, giving rise to the two great antithetic types of deviation from the average human constitution, namely the *megalosplanchnic* and the *microsplanchnic* (qq.v.).

Godin's *law of alternations* is a corollary to Viola's. It also identifies the mesenchyme with mass and the parenchyme with morphological differentiation, and it stresses the fact that, in normal growth, phases of growth in width alternate with phases of growth in length.

Mesmer, Franz (or **Friedrich**) **Anton** (1733–1815) An Austrian who first gave a demonstration of hypnotism (animal magnetism) in Vienna about 1775. At first, Mesmer used magnets for what he believed to be their latent curative power. The latter was due to a magnetic fluid that permeated space; he invented the *baquet,* consisting of a large tub containing rows of bottles filled with magnetic water. Patients sat around the tub holding steel rods coming up through the lid of the tub or applying them to ailing body parts and often joining hands in order to facilitate the passage of the magnetic fluid. By 1778 Mesmer had been discredited in Vienna and moved on to Paris where, in 1784, a royal commission (headed by Benjamin Franklin, the United States ambassador to France) also concluded that Mesmer's claims had no scientific basis. ("Imagination is everything; magnetism nothing."—Franklin)

mesmerism Hypnotism; animal magnetism. See *hypnosis*.

meso- Combining form meaning middle, from Gr. *mésos*.

mesocephaly See *index, cephalic*.

mesoderm The middle or third germ layer that is developed in the tridermic stage of the embryo called *notogenesis* (q.v.), or the fundamental tissues subsequently derived from this layer.

The *medial* portions of the original mesoderm, the paraxial or segmental mesoderm, become subdivided into blocks of tissue, the mesodermic segments, or *somites*, while the *lateral* plates develop a splitlike cavity, the *celom*. The connections between somites and lateral plates are collectively known as the *intermediate cell mass*, the primordium of the urogenital system.

The main tissue derivatives developed from the primitive middle germ layer include all muscular, connective, and vascular tissues, with blood and lymph vessels and all lymphoid organs; the cortex of the suprarenal gland and the sex cells; the epithelium of uriniferous tubules, renal pelves, and ureters, of the seminiferous tubules and the associated excretory ducts of the testis; of oviduct and uterus; and of pleurae, pericardium, and peritoneum.

mesomorphic In Sheldon's system of constitutional types, the type characterized by a predominance of its third component (bulk), that is, the structures of the body that are developed from the *mesoderm* of embryo (q.v.). The mesomorphic type is contrasted with the *ectomorphic* or *endomorphic* (qq.v.) types; it corresponds roughly to Kretschmer's *athletic* type. See *type, athletic*.

mesontomorph In Beau's system of constitutional medicine, characterized by broad, stocky body with long intestines similar to the mesomorph or pyknic of other sys-

tems. Contrasted with the hyperontomorph, ectomorph, or asthenic of other systems. See *type, pyknic*.

mesopallium Limbic lobe. See *rhinencephalon*.

mesoskelic Possessing legs of normal length.

In Manouvrier's system of constitutional types this describes a type that is intermediate between the *brachyskelic* and the *macroskelic* types (qq.v.). See *type, athletic*.

messenger, external chemical Pheromone (q.v.).

messenger, neural A general term for a chemical substance that conveys impulses or information from one cell to another; it includes neuroregulator, neuromodulator, *neurotransmitter,* and *neurohormone* (qq.v.).

messenger RNA See *chromosome*.

messenger, second See *adenyl cyclase*.

met-, meta- Combining form meaning change, transformation, after, next, trans-, beyond, over, from Gr. *metá*.

meta-analysis A secondary analysis of data from a large number of studies, which overcomes the drawbacks inherent in simple comparison of studies. Meta-analysis transforms the results of each study into a common metric and thus avoids both the bias in favor of studies with larger sample sizes and assignment of equal weight to differences of unequal magnitude.

metabolic anoxia See *anoxia, cerebral*.

metabolic-nutritional model See *psychiatry, community*.

metabolism The biophysiological processes by which the living cells and tissue systems of an organism undergo continuous chemical changes in order to build up new living matter and to supply the energy necessary for the life of an individual.

The morphological effect of *metabolism* can be *anabolic* or *catabolic* (qq.v.), according to whether it is of a constructive or destructive nature.

metabolism, destructive Catabolism. See *metabolism*.

metabolism, first-pass A pharmacokinetic phenomenon based on partial conversion of a drug into one or more active metabolites, whose effect is additive to or synergistic with the original compound administered.

metabolism, mental The rate or speed of mental processes, assumed to have an energy exchange with the environment similar to that of somatic physiological processes. Thus Abraham described the manic as having an increased mental metabolism, continuously hungry for new objects whose incorporation will provide discharge for the patient's intensified, uninhibited, oral impulses.

metaerotism Phenomenon described by S. Rado in which intoxicants, e.g. morphine, effect changes principally in the abode of the libido. The whole peripheral sexual apparatus is left on one side as in a "short circuit" and the exciting stimuli are enabled to operate directly on the central organ.

metaethics The study of what it is to make a moral judgment and of the decision-making process that ultimately leads to that judgment; study of the meaning and justification of ethical terms. See *ethics.*

metagnosis The changing of one's mind or attitude.

metalanguage The rules for use of a language (e.g. grammar, syntax); or any language system that can explain, relate, or unite two or more subsystems.

In communications theory, the specific instructions that accompany the spoken word to insure correct interpretation. Such instructions are typically expressed by voice tone, gestures, sentence construction, etc.

metallophobia Fear of metals.

metalloscopia An obsolete method of treatment in hysteria by the application of metals to anesthetic areas.

metamorphopsia Faulty perception of objects, which appear to be distorted; seen most often in parietal lobe lesions and as a type of illusion in intoxication with *mescaline* (q.v.). The most common distortions are *macropsia* and *micropsia,* which are sometimes referred to as the *Alice in Wonderland effect.* See *dysmegalopsia; Lilliputian.*

metamorphosis, delirium of See *lycanthropy.*

metamorphosis sexualis paranoica *Rare.* Delusion, often seen in paranoid patients, that one's sexuality has been changed into that of the opposite sex.

metapelet See *kibbutz.*

metaphase The second stage of the division of a cell by mitosis. See *division, cell.*

metaphor A type of comparison in which one object is equated with another and qualities of the first are then ascribed to the second—"He was a tiresome psychoanalytical turnkey with a belt full of rusty

complexes." Metaphorical language is a form of primary process thinking.

metaphoric paralogia *By-idea* (q.v.).

metapsychological profile A systematic psychoanalytic classification of clinical data, developed by Anna Freud (1963), that relates symptoms and signs to the inner, unconscious mental life of the patient, and is used especially in treatment of the psychotic patient where therapy is directed toward rendering him less vulnerable to inner dangers.

metapsychology In psychoanalysis, a theory of cognition and affect that is not derived directly from clinical data but is advanced to provide the developmental background that will allow one to deal with the clinical findings of psychoanalysis as aberrations of, and deviations from, the normal and expected evolution of the thinking process. Its cornerstone is Freud's belief that thought depends on the forging of links between sensory perception of objects and their appropriate verbal descriptions. Freud was dissatisfied with his own metapsychology, but using what has been learned about development in infancy and childhood through the work of Piaget, Vigotsky, and others, it is now possible to formulate a theory that does justice to the varied complex findings uncovered by the application of the psychoanalytic method. The significance of Freud's postulated second censorship between preconscious and conscious, as well as the importance of the defense of disavowal emphasized by Freud in his writings after 1927, can be accounted for by a theory of thought formation that was not available to Freud.

metatropism See *transvestitism.*

metempsychosis Migration of the soul or rational spirit at death into another body; the doctrine of metempsychosis is part of the Hindu religion, which further teaches that the soul carries with it the memories of former existences for a thousand years. It then induces forgetfulness by drinking of Lethe and begins all over again. See *collective unconscious.*

metencephalon See *hindbrain.*

meteorophobia Fear of meteors or of being an overnight success.

methadone A dependence-inducing, synthetic, narcotic-analgesic with morphinelike effects; at the present time its chief use is as maintenance therapy for heroin addicts according to the method advocated by V.P. Dole and M.E. Nyswander (hence called the *Dole-Nyswander program*). Methadone maintenance differs from other methods in that the successive peaks of elation obtained by repeated intravenous or subcutaneous injections of heroin are replaced by a sustained and uniform drug action without notable elation, abstinence symptoms, or demand for escalation of dose.

Cyclazocine is another synthetic narcotic antagonist that prevents the actions of large doses of narcotics. Since it prevents the development of physical tolerance, it controls the factors that ordinarily lead to compulsive build-up in heroin dosage. See *addiction; dependency, drug; narcotic blockade; opium.*

methilepsia Morbid craving for intoxicants. See *narcomania; substance abuse and dependence disorders.*

method, co-twin control A method of study developed by Gesell and Thompson for use in medical genetics. In this method, observational twin data are obtained from a few selected one-egg pairs, whose aptitudes or adjustment under different life conditions are then compared.

method, concentric A concept of stratification of the personality employed by Laignel-Lavastine. Five concentric zones of personality are recognized: psychic, nervous, endocrine, visceral, and morbific. Personality difficulties and psychiatric symptoms result from abnormalities in any zone, or in any combination of zones.

method, cross-cultural Comparison of different cultures or societies to determine the effect of a particular variable on behavior.

method, linguistic-kinesic An approach to the study of disordered behavior as it manifests itself in disturbances of communication. *Linguistics,* the study of words and language, and *kinesics,* the study of movement, are methods designed to isolate and study infracommunicational systems and thereby reduce the data of interactional behavior to objective, significant, measurable, and manipulative units. This approach is often referred to as the L-K method.

method, need-press A technique of analysis of the TAT used by Murray (one of the originators of the test); in this method, each sentence of the subject's story is analyzed as to the needs of the hero and the press (environmental forces) he is exposed to. Each need and press is given a weighted score and a rank-order system of the needs and press is then tabulated. The method is not widely used clinically because it is too time-consuming to be practical.

method of successive approximations *Shaping* (q.v.).

method, pedigree Study of the family history to determine the frequency with which a familial trait occurs in the members of an affected family. This method does not ordinarily afford conclusive proof of heredity and is largely restricted to rare pathological traits that are fairly constant in penetrance and expressivity.

method, projective As distinguished from the direct question-and-answer method in psychiatric examination, the projective method seeks to gain information indirectly, through the use of certain test techniques specifically designed to provide opportunity for self-expression without direct verbal accounting.

"Thus, an essential characteristic of projective techniques is that they are unstructured in that cues for appropriate action are not clearly specified and the individual must give meaning to (interpret) such stimuli in accordance with his own inner needs, drives, defenses, impulses—in short, according to the dictates of his own personality. Whether the stimuli are inkblots (the Rorschach tests) or ambiguous pictures (the TAT), the patient's task is to impose or project his own structure and meaning onto materials which have relatively little meaning or structure and which, in a purely objective sense, are only inkblots or ambiguous pictures." (Carr, A.C. *International Psychiatry Clinics 1,* 1964)

method, sibship A method devised by Weinberg for use in psychiatric genetics. In this method, the blood relatives of a statistically representative number of probands or index cases are studied to determine whether or not a particular trait occurs more frequently in them than it does in the general population (or in a group of persons not related to the carriers by blood).

method, Turkish-bath *Rare.* A type of treatment based on transference relationship in which the therapist applies threats and reassurances one after the other—one day hot, the next day cold.

method, twin-study One of the two principal methods used in psychiatric genetics for differentiation between genetic and environmental influences in relation to specific forms of adjustment or maladjustment. In this method, the dissimilarities of one-egg twins, genotypically identical organisms, are compared with the behavioral variations seen in ordinary sibs or two-egg twins.

methodology The study of the systems and procedures that are used in scientific investigation. Methodology attempts to devise a set of rules or guidelines that will govern or at least influence the choice of procedures to be used in a particular study. When the study in question has, in fact, used procedures in accord with such rules, it can be said that "the procedures of the study were selected and applied in accordance with sound principles of methodology." In current writings this cumbersome sentence is typically abbreviated to "the methodology was sound." As a result, methodology and method are often used interchangeably.

Epidemiologic research relies on two main approaches, the *case-control study* and the *cohort study.* In the case-control study, the illness is the dependent variable; it must already be present for the subject to be identified, and such studies must therefore be retrospective. The cohort study, on the other hand, may be either retrospective or prospective. In the *retrospective cohort study,* populations are examined to see what association exists between the illness under study and various antecedent variables, which can be controlled for in the statistical analysis of the comparison of the illness with the without-illness group. In the *prospective cohort study,* the antecedent variable is defined and the population is divided into subjects with the variable and those without; the two groups are then followed over time to see if there is a difference in incidence of the illness in the different groups.

methomania *Obs. Methilepsia* (q.v.).

methysergide A serotonin antagonist. See *migraine.*

metonymy A disturbance of language seen most commonly in the schizophrenias in which an approximate but related term is used in place of the more precise, definite, or idiomatic term which would ordinarily be used. A young schizophrenic patient, for example, spoke in a labyrinthine, circumstantial manner for many minutes during a psychotherapy session, but suddenly became blocked. He recovered spontaneously after 5 to 10 seconds and said: "Now let's see. What was I saying? I seem to have lost the piece of string of the conversation." The phrase "piece of string," would be considered a metonymic substitution for the idiom "to lose the thread of conversation."

Metrazol Cardiazol. See *treatment, Metrazol.*

metromania 1. Mania for incessant writing of verses. 2. *Obs. Nymphomania* (q.v.).

Meyer, Adolf (1866–1950) American psychiatrist; "the mind in action"; psychobiology.

Meynert, Theodore (mī′nērt) (1833–92) German neurologist and psychiatrist.

MF Multifactorial; one of the models of *inheritance* (q.v.).

MHPG A major metabolite of norepinephrine, 3-methoxy-4-hydroxy-phenylglycol; MHPG content of 24-hour urine samples is measured as an indication of the adequacy of norepinephrine from noradrenergic neurons. See *depression, unipolar.*

micro- (mī′krō-) Combining form meaning small, little, from Gr. *mikrós.*

microbiophobia *Microphobia* (q.v.); fear of infection, infestation, or small animals.

microcephaly Smallness of the head; a condition in which there is defective development of the whole brain and premature ossification of the skull.

microcosm See *words, microcosm of.*

microgeny (mī-krȧ′je-nē) The sequence of the necessary steps inherent in the occurrence of any psychological phenomenon; psychodynamic formulations, for example, are a statement of the microgeny of the patient's symptoms or behavior in that they trace the steps through which a mental process goes.

microglia (mī-krog′lē-ȧ) See *neuroglia.*

micromania *Obs.* Delusion of belittlement; the delusion or conviction that one's body, or some part of it, is or has become abnormally small. Such delusions are most often found in organic depressions, but the *small penis complex* is also an example. See *délire d'énormité.*

micromelia Small limbs, associated with achondroplasia; seen in various types of mental retardation. See *syndrome, de Lange.*

microorchidism See *syndrome, Klinefelter's.*

microphobia Fear of small objects and, in particular small animals.

microphonia Weakness of the voice.

micropsia, micropsy Perception of objects as smaller than they really are; a form of *dysmegalopsia* (q.v.). This may be occasioned by organic or psychic causes. When the latter prevail the condition may also be known as Lilliputian hallucination. See *Lilliputian.*

micropsychia *Obs.* Mental retardation.

micropsychosis See *schizophrenia, pseudoneurotic.*

microsomatognosia See *somatognosia.*

microsome, (microsoma) In biology, one of the minute granules found in vegetable protoplasm; this should not be confused with the concept of *microsomia* used in constitutional medicine.

microsomia See *dwarfism.*

microsplanchnic According to Viola's classification of the constitutional forms of body build, this term refers to the type that has the abdominal portion of the body relatively small in proportion to the thoracic portion, owing to the small size of the abdominal viscera. It is further characterized by the overdevelopment of the vertical diameters of the body in comparison with the horizontal diameters, so that the body presents an elongated appearance.

This *microsplanchnic* or *dolichomorphic* type corresponds to the *hypovegetative* biotype of Pende, the *asthenic* type of Kretschmer. See *type, asthenic.*

Midas punishment See *masturbation, compulsive.*

Midas syndrome *Rare.* Increased sexual desire in the female associated with diminished desire and capacity in her male partner.

midbrain Mesencephalon; the portion of the brain lying between the pons and the cerebral hemispheres, containing the *corpora quadrigemina* (q.v.), the cerebral peduncles, and the aqueduct of Sylvius. The base of each peduncle contains the homolateral corticospinal, corticobulbar, and corticopontile tracts. The substantia nigra is a broad layer of pigmented gray substance occupying the central portion of the peduncle. The roof or dorsal portion of the base is the tegmentum, which contains lateral and medial lemnisci, median longitudinal fasciculus, red nucleus, spinothalamic and spinotectal tracts, superior cerebellar peduncle, the nuclei of the trochlear and oculomotor nerves, and the nucleus of the mesencephalic root of the trigeminal nerve.

Lesions of the corpora quadrigemina cause paralysis of upward eye movements; of the cerebral peduncle, spastic contralateral paralysis; of the red nucleus, substantia nigra, or reticular substance, involuntary movements and rigidity. In cats, destruction of portions of the tegmentum produces cataleptic manifestations similar to cerea flexibilitas.

middle class See *class, social.*

middle game See *game, middle.*

Midtown study A classic study of *Mental Health in the Metropolis* (Srole, L., et al., 1962) based on interviews of 1,660 adults who were felt to be representative "to a high degree of confidence" of the midtown (Yorkville area of New York City) population of 100,000. Of particular relevance to social and community psychiatry are the findings that even though almost 3% of the population was incapacitated by mental illness, less than half of them had any psychiatric contact; and that of the 20% of the population impaired by mental illness, less than one-third of them had any psychiatric contact. It can be concluded that the persons who do come to the attention of existing psychiatric facilities may not constitute a majority of those who need help and may well be a biased and nonrepresentative sample of the mentally ill. The findings further suggest that the mere existence of psychiatric services does not ensure their optimal utilization, and they raise the question of whether the services that are available are desirable or appropriate to those they claim to serve. See *psychiatry, community.*

mignon delusion See *romance, family.*

migraine A syndrome of periodic, unilateral headache with photophobia, vomiting, nausea, and various prodromata such as scotomata, occasional paresthesiae, and speech difficulties. After the attack there is often a marked sensation of well-being.

The headaches usually appear at irregular intervals; several attacks a month are common. The headache has a crescendo type of intensity; it may be dull, boring, pressing, throbbing, viselike, lancinating, or hammering in character. It may begin at any point on the head and spread to involve the entire side. Because of the frequency of associated gastrointestinal symptoms, migraine is often called sick headache or bilious headache. The headache rarely lasts longer than 12 to 24 hours. The present-day conception is that migraine is a result of functional disturbances in the carotid cranial vascular tree; these occur in response to various etiologic agents that apparently vary greatly in different cases.

About one-quarter of migraine sufferers have "classic migraine," in which a visual aura precedes the headache. Patients may notice that they cannot see clearly in a small area to one side of the eye fixation point. Sometimes the area has an irregular, scintillating, or colored outline—known as *teichopsia* or *fortification spectra*. Other sensory changes induced by changes in cerebral blood flow include hallucinations and micropsia. Because of them many migraine sufferers develop intense fears of going insane.

In classic migraine, the headache begins as the visual manifestations begin to wane. "Common migraine" lacks a sharply defined aura. See *headache, cluster.*

Heredity is an important causal factor. Some patients with migraine also develop hemiplegia as part of their attacks, which are recurrent and prolonged; the hemiplegia is severe, generally affecting not only the face and arm but also the leg. Such patients have a clear-cut family history of migraine, and affected family members also have hemiplegia with their migraine attacks.

Migraine sufferers often have an obsessive personality. In the predisposed person an attack may be precipitated by psychologic stress and by the release of stress ("holiday headaches"), by eating a particular food, by alcohol, or by menstruation. Treatment is symptomatic; successful results have been reported with beta blockers and with calcium channel blockers.

It is estimated that migraine affects between 5 and 10% of the world's population. It was recognized in the Sumerian literature as early as 3000 B.C. Among its famous victims are Julius Caesar, Charles Darwin, Sigmund Freud, Thomas Jefferson, Leo Tolstoy, Lewis Carroll, Charles Dickens, Virginia Woolf, Frederic Chopin, Edgar Allan Poe, and Peter Ilich Tchaikovsky.

migraine, cervical *Cervical vertigo syndrome; Bärtschi-Rochaix syndrome;* headache, dizziness, stiffness of the neck, and paresthesiae due to cerebral artery compression.

migrainous neuralgia See *headache, cluster.*

migrateur (mē-gra-tēr') A wanderer; vagrant.

migration psychosis Paranoid states or other mental illnesses whose appearance is related to leaving one's homeland and settling in a foreign country. There is disagreement as to whether there is an association between rate of mental illness and migration; if there is, evidence is somewhat in favor of the hypothesis that it is not migration that breeds psychosis but that emigration is more likely to occur in those who are already predisposed to mental illness. See *breeder hypothesis.*

milieu Environment; surroundings. In psychiatry, the *social setting*, emphasis being placed upon the setting from the emotional point of view. To a psychiatrist the most important milieu is the home. Other environments—scholastic, recreational, industrial, religious, etc.—play a leading role in the growth of the personality. See *therapy, milieu.*

Millard-Gubler syndrome (August L.J. Millard, French physician, 1830–1917, and Adolphe Gubler, French physician, 1821–79) Paralysis of the external rectus on one side and supranuclear paralysis of the bulbar muscles and limbs on the opposite side.

Milligan annihilation method A type of regressive electroshock therapy (REST) in which three treatments are administered the first day, and two treatments are given daily thereafter until the desired regression is obtained.

-mimesis, -mimia Combining form meaning imitation, from Gr. *mímēsis, mimía,* from *mimeísthai,* to mimic, imitate.

Minamata disease An unusual form of toxic neuropathy and/or encephalopathy seen in fishermen in Minamata Bay (Japan); cause is presumed to be eating of fish contaminated by a chemical (probably organic mercury) in the effluent from a nearby fertilizer plant. Pathology consists of widespread neuron degeneration most marked in the granular layer of the cerebellum and in the cortex. Symptoms indicate involvement of the peripheral nervous system, cerebellum, hearing, and vision, and in some cases there are signs of progressive brain damage. Mental symptoms include impairment of intelligence, of which the patient is often aware, and changes in disposition and personality in that patients are often testy, irritable, bashful, unsociable, etc.

mind *Psyche* (q.v.).

mind/body perception, altered See *perception, altered mind/body.*

mind control Brainwashing. See *brain control; menticide; propaganda; psychopolitics.*

mind, miniature *Psychoinfantilism* (q.v.); a symmetrical retardation in all aspects of mental life, in contradistinction to mental retardation. The psychoinfantile person is regarded as one with a *miniature mind,* a mental midget.

mind-stuff See *psychology, atomistic.*

mindreading See *perception, extrasensory; telepathy.*

minds, interfaceable Any mental state shared by more than one person; the term is used most frequently in the context of the infant's "theory of interfaceable minds," referring to the recognition somewhere between the seventh and ninth month of life that the child can share a state of mind, such as an intention, with another person.

mineralocorticoid See *syndrome, general adaptation.*

minimal, brain dysfunction See *impulse-disorder, hyperkinetic.*

minimal risk See *risk, minimal.*

minor, emancipated See *emancipated.*

minus complementarity See *complementarity.*

miolecithal (mī-ō-les′i-thal) Referring to the human type of *cleavage* (q.v.) in the development of an embryo.

miopragia In constitutional medicine, diminished functional activity of an organ. For example, subjects of asthenic habitus may possess a small, immature, and functionally diminished cardiovascular apparatus. Thus Lewis (*Constitutional Factors in Dementia Praecox,* 1923) reported, among other things, a hypoplastic heart with lessened functional capacity.

miosis 1. The period of decline of a disease in which symptoms begins to abate. 2. Contraction of the pupil.

miriasha A person affected with *miryachit* (q.v.).

mirror imaging In genetics, reversed *asymmetry,* quite frequent in twins, with respect to handedness, hair whorl, dental irregularities, fingerprints, and other symmetrical characters including certain morbid traits based on heredity. The presence of mirror imaging is confirmatory evidence of *monozygotic* twins, though monozygosity is not excluded by its absence. See *twin.*

mirror sign See *sign, mirror.*

miryachit (mē-ryǎ′chēt) (Russ. "to fool or play the fool") *Olonism;* a culture-specific syndrome consisting of indiscriminate and seemingly irresistible imitation of the actions and speech of people in the subject's presence. See *echolalia; echopraxia; Faxenpsychosis; lata.*

MIS Medical improvement standard, used to gauge the degree of improvement in a condition before the SSDI benefits for that condition are terminated.

misanthropy Hatred of, or aversion to, mankind. A profound morbid distrust of human beings individually and collectively.

misapprehension See *apprehension.*

misidentification, amnesic The inability of a subject to identify the person confronting him, due to impairment of the memory or to clouding of consciousness.

misidentification, delusional A failure to recognize well-known objects as such, due to the delusion that the objects have been transformed; e.g. a patient may believe that a woman has been transformed into a man; or that a young person has been changed into an old one; or a new coat into a shabby one, etc.

misidentification, hyperbolic A condition sometimes found in manic states in which the patient flippantly calls a person by someone else's name. This misidentification tion is rarely clung to with conviction.

miso- (mis′ō) Combining form meaning hate, hatred, from Gr. *mīsos.*

misocainia (-kī′nē-à) Hatred or fear of anything new or strange, sometimes expressed as an obsessive desire for preservation of the status quo. See *autism, early infantile.*

misogamy Hatred of marriage, often based upon an unresolved Oedipus complex. To some patients, and especially schizophrenics, marriage is equated with incest and misogamy is their defense against it.

misogyny Hatred of women. When the hate of women is part of a morbid mental state, it may be associated with a wide variety of nosologic entities. The most common explanation for the condition has to do with the events of childhood, particularly those relating to the parents. See *complex, Oedipus.*

Abhorrence of women is expressed alike by women and men and is often a reflection of a homosexual conflict. A hysterical woman detested all women and all things effeminate; she had always wanted to be a male; indeed, throughout her childhood her father chided her because she was a female; since early childhood she detested effeminacy and did as much as possible to become masculine.

Passive homosexual males may hold women in severe contempt, as a reaction to disappointment with their own masculinity. A paranoid homosexual patient killed a woman in order to gain her femaleness. Thereafter he denied that he had any attributes, physical or mental, of masculinity.

misologia, misology Hatred of speaking or arguing. One patient with catatonic schizophrenia, for example, remained mute lest the world be destroyed through her speaking.

misomania *Obs.* The syndrome characterized by delusions of persecution.

misoneism (mis-ō′-nē′iz′m) Hatred of innovation, *misocainia* (q.v.).

misopedia Morbid hatred of children. A patient had an obsession to kill all children, because they were produced through the intervention of the male sex. He devoted his life to the Doctrine of Immaculate Conception.

Behind the hatred of children is often the idea of incest, the parent unconsciously viewing the child as the consequence of incestuous relations.

misopsychia *Obs.* Hatred or weariness of living; synonymous with the obsolete terms *misozoeticus* and *misozoia.*

Missouri Foster Community Program See *domicile.*

mistake, category To mix elements from different realms on the incorrect assumption that they are alike in kind. Ethics, for example, deals with values, biology with facts; if science be likened to a ship belonging to the material world, then ethics is a nonmaterial set of beliefs that should guide the ship's tiller.

mistakes, basic See *basic mistakes.*

mistrust See *ontogeny, psychic.*

Mitchell, Silas Weir (1829–1914) American neurologist and psychiatrist; *rest cure* (q.v.).

Mitgehen One of the signs of motor dysregulation seen frequently in catatonia, consisting of limb movement in response to light pressure, even though the subject has been instructed not to move the limb. A similar sign, often associated with Mitgehen, is *forced grasping,* repeated grasping at the examiner's outstretched fingers even though the subject has been told not to do so.

mitissima (mē-tēs′sē-mà) Mania mitis; paraphrosyne; hypomania. See *mania.*

mitosis Originally meaning the division of the *nucleus* of a cell, the term is now often used for the entire process of cell division, involving all radical changes in the structure of a cell that are of utmost significance in inheritance. See *division, cell.*

mitten pattern An abnormal electroencephalographic complex, so-called because it consists of a slow spike-and-wave resembling the thumb and hand portion of a mitten. The pattern is found almost solely in adults and occurs significantly more frequently in psychotic patients than nonpsychotic controls; e.g. near 40% of adult schizophrenics and epileptics with psychosis, but near 3% in nonpsychotic epileptics and other unselected controls. It also occurs in high frequency in criminals.

mix See *case mix.*

mixed phobic See *phobic, mixed.*

mixoscopia A form of paraphilia in which orgasm is reached by watching the act of coition between the desired one and another person.

mixoscopia bestialis A name suggested for a type of paraphilia involving the watching of sexual intercourse between an animal and another human being; ordinarily, the other person is forced or compelled by the subject to submit to the practice that the subject wishes to observe.

mixovariation This genetic term is synonymous with *combination* (q.v.), signifying hereditary variations between related individuals, due to the sorting out and recombining of separate factors in the generations following crosses of mates with unlike hereditary equipment.

mixture, Cloetta's (Max Cloetta, Swiss pharmacologist, 1868–1940) A combination of paraldehyde, amylene hydrate, chloral hydrate, alcohol, barbituric acid, digitalin, and ephedrine hydrochloride that is usually administered per rectum in continuous sleep treament. See *treatment, continuous sleep.*

MLD Metachromatic leukodystrophy. See *leukodystrophies.*

MMECT Multiple monitored electroconvulsive therapy. Treatment consists of the induction of more than one seizure (typically four or five) in a single session, with concomitant monitoring of the EEG and EKG. The goal is to shorten the time needed for a course of treatment. See *therapy, multiple monitored electroconvulsive.*

MMPI See *test, Minnesota Multiphasic Inventory.*

MMT Multimodal therapy. See *BASIC-ID.*

M'Naghten rule See *responsibility criminal.*

mneme (nē'mē) Memory trace or *engram* (q.v.).

mneme, phylogenetic The racial ancestral memory preset in the deep unconscious of the individual. See *memory, racial.*

mnemic (nē'mik) Pertaining to or characterized by memory.

mnemism (nē'miz'm) Mnemic hypothesis that cells possess memory. See *mneme.*

-mnesia, -mnesis Combining form meaning memory, from Gr. *mnēsis*, memory, from *mnāsthai*, to remember.

mobility, social. The free interactions among, and the changing roles and status of, members in a group. This term is used in contrast to social fixity. See *fixity, social.*

modality Any method or technique of treatment; a class or group within the therapeutic armamentarium. Also any class or subdivision of sensation, such as vision or smell.

modality profile In multimodal behavior therapy, a chart that lists the patient's problems in each of the seven areas of the *BASIC-ID* (q.v.), and the treatments proposed for each of them.

mode The value in a frequency curve at which the height of the curve is greatest; i.e. the most frequently recurring score in a distribution. The mode is a very unstable measure.

mode, diploid The normal number of chromosomes; in humans, 46.

model A device for ordering information.

model, diathesis-stress *Genetic loading;* vulnerability (usually implied to be on a constitutional or genetic basis) to react to environmental stressors with abnormal or pathologic manifestations such as psychosis, regression, or other indications of impaired or defective coping or adaptive mechanisms.

model, medical Any conceptualization of psychiatric illness that corresponds to those used in general medical descriptions of a disease. Included are (1) infectious disease model—a specific agent causes a specific disease; (2) cellular pathology disease—a defect of cells or organs of the body produces the disease in question; (3) diagnostic model—disease is a variable process that moves from recognition of symptoms and palliative treatment to a definition of etiology and pathogenesis that allows rational and specific treatment. See *psychiatry, community.*

modeling A form of behavior therapy, based on the principles of imitative learning; it obviates the need for the patient to discover effective responses through trial-and-error emulation of the therapist.

modeling, behavior A training technique for supervisors based on a sequence of modeling, role-playing, and reinforcement that changes behavior directly through the fundamentals of social learning (imitation and reinforcement) rather than indirectly through traditional training approaches (such as lectures, the case method, or T-groups). It consists of imitation of effective behaviors, use of retention aids, intensive and guided practice of new and unfamiliar behavior, reinforcement or recognition for application of the specific behaviors, and transfer of training principles. Modeling consists of a concise and distinct display of the desired behavior in a specific job situation—by actors, on videotape, film, etc.—typically by a person whom the observer is likely to regard as competent. Repetition of viewing and mental rehearsal are typical retention aids, followed by behavior rehearsal, i.e. supervised reenactment of the model performance. Videotaping of sessions is often used as a way to provide detailed feedback to trainees.

models of illness See *model, medical; psychiatry, community.*

models, treatment See *psychiatry, community.*

modification In genetics, the term is limited to variations in the phenotype that are caused by environmental influences and modify the individual appearance without affecting the idioplasm. Drastic effects of the environment of living beings may lead to profoundly modified developments, but it is generally assumed that they do not become inheritable.

Of the modifying factors that interact to produce a human phenotype, the physiological effects of nutrition, light, and climate seem just as important as social, cultural, and psychological influences. These variations in environmental modifications can be best observed in identical co-twins reared apart under different life conditions. See *variation.*

modifier In accordance with the genetic principle that of the several hereditary factors that interact to produce a greater share than others of the total effect, this term is used to denote those factors that appear merely to modify the effect of other factors, having little or no effect when the main factor is not present.

A modifier is called *specific* when its effects are produced only upon a specific genotype. See *variation.*

Moebius, Paul Julius (mē'bi-oos) (1853–1907) German neuropathologist and sexologist.

mogigraphia Writer's cramp. See *neurasthenia, professional.*

mogilalia Hesitancy or difficulty in speaking and particularly the kind that appears as a type of resistance in psychotherapy.

mojo See *rootwork.*

molar Massive or gross, as contrasted with molecular, nuclear, minute, or discrete.

Molar is often used to refer to large-scale units of analysis and molecular for small-scale units. Related is the contrast between *top-down* and *bottom-up* approaches to a situation. In a bottom-up approach, the details of the task or setting are the determinants of how the subject performs. In the top-down approach the subject's own intentions, goals, and strategies are imposed on the situation and directly affect performance and outcome.

molilalia *Mogilalia* (q.v.).

molimen (mō-lē'men) Distress, malaise; specifically, the labored or difficult performance of a normal function or of a task that could ordinarily be performed with ease. *Molimen virile* was formerly used to refer to fatigue symptoms associated with the male climacterium; *menstrual molimen* is still used to refer to premenstrual tensions.

molimina, premenstrual Premenstrual tension; the term includes both physical and psychic symptoms referable to the premenstrual period.

molysmophobia Fear of contamination.

mongol 1. One belonging to the Mongolian race. 2. One who presents the clinical syndrome of mental deficiency called *mongolism*, now called Down's syndrome. See *syndrome, Down's.*

mongolism *Obst.* Trisomy 21; Langdon-Down disease. See *syndrome, Down's.*

monitor To supervise, invigilate; especially, to watch carefully so as to give warning should anything go wrong.

Moniz, Egas (1874–1955) Pen name for Antonio Caetano deAbreu Freire, Portuguese neurologist; development of cerebral angiography and of frontal leukotomy (the first psychosurgical procedure), for which he received the Nobel Prize for medicine in 1949.

monkey therapist A socially appropriate monkey, used in experiments with monkeys raised in total isolation, as a means of modifying the isolate's behavior and bringing it more in accord with normal behavior. In many cases, pairing of the isolate monkey with the monkey therapist results in a gradual improvement in the isolate's behavior, with only occasional lapses into inappropriate behavior, such as self-clasping and huddling.

mono- (mon'ō-) Combining form meaning alone, only, single, unique, from Gr. *mónos.*

monoamine oxidase (MAO) An enzyme, discovered by Hare in 1928, which has since been shown to be able to oxidize (and thus inactivate) various amines, including serotonin and the catecholamines and their methoxy derivatives. Of interest clinically is the fact that many inhibitors of monoamine oxidase are psychic energizers (antidepressants).

monobulia *Obs.* A wish, desire, drive, thought, obsession, etc., that dominates the psychic life and inhibits or eliminates all other forms of mental activity.

monecism (mō-nē'siz'm) See *hermaphroditism.*

monohybrid Differing with respect to only *one* hereditary character (in a hybrid individual). See *hybrid.*

monohybridity (monohybridism) The state of a hybrid whose parents differ in a single character, or the character of belonging to a type of individual heterozygous for a single pair of genes.

monoideism (mon-ō-ī'dē-iz'm) "The theory according to which an idea detached from other ideas will exercise an unusually powerful force in the mind. This notion was formulated long ago both by Descartes and by Condillac. The magnetisers were well aware that suggestion was more powerful when the subjects were 'isolated,' that is to say when they were apparently unable to perceive any phenomena except the personality of the magnetiser and his utterances." (Janet, *PH*)

The term is also used to refer to the symptom of harping on one idea, seen frequently in the senile group and in the schizophrenias.

monomania *Rare.* Partial insanity, in which the morbid mental state is restricted to one subject, the patient being of sound judgment and appropriate affect on all other subjects; impulsive act without motive.

In older psychiatry there were such expressions as *intellectual monomania* (e.g.

paranoia); *affective monomania,* which corresponded with *manie raisonnante,* characterized by emotional deviation; *instinctive monomania,* which in general is the equivalent of the compulsive-obsessive syndrome of modern psychiatry.

When monomania or partial insanity was associated with depressive states, Esquirol suggested that the term *lypemania* be used, to distinguish the monomania with exaltation of mood.

monomania, affective *Obs.* Used by Esquirol, most likely the equivalent of the manic phase of manic-depressive psychosis.

monomanie boulimique *Obs.* Bulimia; insatiable hunger.

monomanie du nol *Obs. Kleptomania* (q.v.).

monomoria *Melancholia* (q.v.).

mononoea *Obs.* Concentration on a single subject, as in monomania.

monopagia Clavus hystericus. See *clavus.*

monopathophobia Fear of a single, specific organic disease.

monophobia Fear of being alone.

monoplegia Paralysis of one limb or single part of the body, such as one arm, one leg, or the face alone, or only the finger.

monopsychosis *Obs.* Term, coined by Clouston, synonymous with *monomania.*

monosymptomatic Manifested by a single symptom. When a disorder is presented in the form of a single symptom it is said to be monosymptomatic.

monosymptomatic hypochondriacal psychosis A term for *isolated delusion* that emphasizes the severity of the disorder even though the false belief remains relatively separate from the rest of the personality, and also the frequency with which such delusions focus on somatic symptoms and loss of body integrity. The most common forms are the *olfactory reference syndrome,* the *dysmorphic delusion,* and *parasitophobia.* Closely related phenomenologically is conjugal paranoia. See *jealousy, morbid.*

monozygosity (monzygocity) Used in genetics with reference to the origin from one egg of *monozygotic* or *identical* twins.

monozygote One of the *monozygotic* (identical) co-twins.

monozygotic Referring to twins developed from a single egg and exhibiting extreme resemblances because of their identical genotypes. These *monozygotic,* or *identical,* or *one-egg* twin pairs are to be distinguished from the *dizygotic, fraternal,* or *nonidentical* twin pairs produced by two eggs. See *twin.*

Montessori, Maria (1870–1952) Italian physician and educator, the first woman to receive the M.D. degree from an Italian university; devised an educational system that provides a carefully prepared environment for self-education of the child with emphasis on practical living, sensorial response, mathematics, biology, geography, and reading. The first Montessori School in the United States was established in 1913.

mood The sustained emotional states that color the whole personality and psychic life; the pervasive or prevailing emotion at any specific time. See *affect.*

Howard Owens and Jerrold Maxmen (*American Journal of Psychiatry 136,* 1979) note that both mood and affect refer to a disposition to react emotionally in certain ways, and thus there is considerable overlap between the two concepts. In their usage, inferences about mood are drawn from the subject's past history as well as present observations, while inferences about affect are confined to current observations.

mood-congruent Referring to symptoms and behavior consistent with the subject's expressed or prevailing mood, used particularly in the subclassification of mood (affective) disorders.

Manic episodes, for example, are subdivided into those with and those without psychotic features (delusions, hallucinations, grossly bizarre behavior, etc.). Those with psychotic features are further subtyped as mood-congruent or mood-incongruent psychotic features. *Mood-congruent features* are delusions or hallucinations consistent with manic grandiosity, expansiveness, and inflated self-esteem. *Mood-incongruent features* are symptoms that contradict or at least fail to match manic features; examples are persecutory delusions, ideas of thought insertion or of being controlled, and catatonic symptoms such as stupor, mutism, or posturing.

In major depressive episodes mood-congruent psychotic features are delusions or hallucinations consistent with depressive lowering of self-esteem, feelings of guilt, and ideas of punishment through disease or death. Mood-incongruent features include persecutory delusions, ideas of thought insertion or thought broadcasting, and delusions of being controlled.

mood, delusional *Wahnstimmung* (q.v.).

mood disorders *Affective disorders* (q.v.).

mood, manic See *disposition, constitutional manic.*

mood, melancholic See *disposition, constitutional depressive.*

mood swings The oscillation between periods of the feeling of well-being and those of depression or "blueness." All people have mood swings, blue hours, or blue days. Mood swings are somewhat more marked in the neurotic than in the normal. In the manic-depressive patient, the swings are of much greater intensity and much longer duration. See *cyclothymia.*

moodcyclic disorders See *psychodynamics, adaptational.*

Mooney Problem Check List A questionnaire, used often as part of a rapid screening battery for high school and college students, in which the subject is asked to indicate which ones of a list of symptoms are frequent or troublesome to him.

moral hazard See *hazard, moral.*

moral philosophy *Ethics* (q.v.).

moral right See *right.*

moral treatment In psychiatry, humane treatment of the mentally ill. It was the French who spearheaded the late 18th-century move toward humane treatment of the insane. Jean-Baptiste Pussin, a tanner by trade who became the governor of mental patients at the Hospice de Bicêtre in Paris, taught Philippe Pinel the psychological methods he had developed for the care of the incurable mental patients on his ward. Among other things, Pussin replaced chains with straitjackets in 1787, although it is Pinel who is usually credited with the reforms. The unleashing of the mentally ill did not occur without severe resistance from the medical profession, from the politicians of the day, and from the Paris populace, and Pinel was more than once accused of harboring traitors in his hospital. One day he was set upon by a menacing crowd who threatened to lynch him for his "crimes." He escaped death only because his bodyguard, Chevigne, was able to fight off the mob—the same Chevigne who had been among the first group of patients to be released from their fetters.

Pinel's next step was to train hospital personnel in adequate care of the mentally ill, and it was his organization of mental hospitals that first demonstrated the value of hospital research and prepared the way for moral treatment and psychotherapy.

In the United States, Dr. Benjamin Rush (1745–1813) was a part of the movement toward humanization of treatment methods, including the abolition of mechanical restraint and the betterment of physical care. The period of moral treatment and humane care is the historical antecedent of the modern therapeutic community. See *social therapy*.

Advocates of psychological treatment in caring for the mentally ill in other countries between 1750 and 1850 included Willis, Haslam, and the Tukes in England, Fowler in Scotland, Daquin at Chambery, Chiarugi at Florence, the Brothers of Charity, and the French military medical inspector Jean Colombier. (Weiner, D. *American Journal of Psychiatry 136*, 1979)

moral turpitude See *turpitude, moral*.

morality See *ethics*.

morality, sphincter Ferenczi's term for those forerunners of the superego that arise from introjection of parental (usually maternal) prohibitions and demands having to do with toilet training.

moramentia *Obs*. Absolute amorality.

morbus astralis *Obs*. Epilepsy.

morbus eruditorum *Obs*. Hypochondriasis.

morbus sacer (så'ker) *Obs*. Epilepsy.

morbus Sancti Joannis *Obs*. Epilepsy.

morbus Sancti Valentini *Obs*. Epilepsy.

Morel, Benedict A. (1809–73) French psychiatrist and physiologist; introduced the term *dementia praecox* (q.v.).

mores Culture; traditions, and particularly those so valued by the group or society that failure to observe them incurs condemnation, ostracism, or some other punishment. One example that survives in some subcultures is "marrying one's own kind."

mores, social Codes of manners and morals imposed by tacit authority (or "unwritten" law) upon the individual to guide his social behavior in a given society, culture, or ethnic group and varying with the shift from one group, society, or culture to another.

moria A morbid impulse to joke. Sometimes used synonymously with gallows humor or, more commonly, to refer to any dementia (usually of the exogenous-organic type) characterized by silliness. See *humor, gallows*.

Morita therapy See *psychotherapy, Morita*.

morning after See *hangover*.

moron A person with mild mental retardation (IQ 52–67); in England, called *dullard*.

morosis *Obs*. Fatuity; also idiotism.

-morph Combining form meaning one endowed with (specific) form or shape. From this are further formed *-morphic, -morphous, -morphy*.

morphinism Morphine addiction. See *addiction; opium*.

morphinomania, morphiomania *Obs*. Morbid craving for morphine. See *addiction; opium*.

morphology The study of form and structure; anatomy.

Morquio's syndrome See *mucopolysaccharidosis*.

morsicatio buccarum (môr-sē-kả'tē-o boo-kảr'oom) Habitual self-mutilation by biting the cheeks. *Morsicatio labiorum* refers to biting of the lips.

mort douce (mawr' doos') (F. "sweet death") Some authorities (e.g. Hirschfeld) use this expression to refer to the phenomena attendant upon the completion of the sexual act.

Others use the phrase synonymously with *euthanasia* (q.v.).

mortido Federn's term for the destructive instinct; *destrudo* (q.v.).

morula The embryological stage of human organism, comprising the segmenting process of *cleavage* of a fertilized egg up to the 32-cell stage and the formation of the *blastula*.

Morvan's disease (Augustin Marie de Lannitis Morvan, French physician, 1819–97) See *syringomyelia*.

mosaic See *intermediate; test, mosaic*.

mosaicism See *nondisjunction*.

mother-child relationship (MCR) The reciprocal emotional interactions between mother and child, used particularly in reference to the effects of the mother's attitude on the emotional development of the child. Punitive mothers, for example, often have disobedient, hostile children; inconsistent mothers may have children with temper problems; critical, depreciatory mothers may have children who lie and are destructive. See *reciprocal regulation; retardation, psychosocial; separation-individuation.*

mother, complete A term used by Federn to refer to the ideal type of mother that every schizophrenic seeks both in phantasy and in reality. The complete mother loves her child unselfishly, for himself alone, and does not use him as a means of gratifying her own psychological needs. She shows a conspicuous and admirable absence of certain characteristics of "typical" mothers of schizophrenics, viz., a sense of resentful obligation and reluctant duty in regard to the mother's responsibilities toward her child, or sensual gratification in her relationship with her offspring. See *mother, schizophrenogenic.*

mother fixation See *fixation, mother.*

mother, great See *Magna Mater.*

mother hypnosis See *hypnosis, father.*

mother image See *image.*

mother, phallic In psychoanalysis the phantasy, which occurs early in the male's psychic development, that the mother has a phallus. In the course of his development, the male child reaches a stage in which his interest is concentrated on his genitals. Because this organ is so valuable and important to him, he believes that it is also present in other persons. Having seen no other type of genital formation, he will perforce assume that women also possess genitals like his. As part of the erotic activity developing around his genitals, the child manifests an intense desire to see the genitals of other persons, probably in order to compare them with his own. This erotic desire is very strong with regard to his mother, on whom his most intense feelings are concentrated at this age. He wishes to see the penis that he believes his mother possesses, and thus is developed the phantasy of the phallic mother in the male child.

This phantasy or belief may leave ineradicable traces in the child's subsequent psychic life. When he finds later that women, indeed, have no penis, his longing to see his mother's penis "often becomes transformed into its opposite and gives place to disgust which in the years of puberty may become the cause of psychic impotence, of misogyny, and of lasting homosexuality." And in fetishism the object that the patient reveres is "a substitutive symbol for the once revered and since then missed member of the woman." In mythology, too, "this revered and very early fancied bodily formation of the mother" is retained. It is personified in those maternal deities appearing in many cultures in which the goddess is represented as having, in addition to breasts, a phallus. (Freud, S. *Leonardo da Vinci,* 1922)

mother, schizophrenogenic A term used by those who believe that the attitude of the mother toward her child is the basic determinant of schizophrenia. To those who would subscribe to this viewpoint, the term usually includes (1) the overtly rejecting mother, who is domineering, aggressive, critical, and overdemanding (especially in regard to cleanliness and the observances of social forms); and (2) the covertly rejecting mother, who smothers her child with overprotectiveness. See *love, smother.*

Adherents of the schizophrenogenic mother hypothesis for the most part ignore the fact that of all the mothers who could be classified as fulfilling the above criteria, only a small percentage have schizophrenic children. Also ignored are the many studies indicating that there is no uniform pattern of family dynamics in the families of schizophrenic patients.

mother substitute See *surrogate, mother.*

mother surrogate See *surrogate, mother.*

mothering, pathologic See *love, monkey; love, smother; mother-child relationship; reciprocal regulation.*

motility disorder Any abnormality of motion or movement; used by many in a more specific sense to refer to the abnormal postures, gestures, etc., seen in catatonic schizophrenics and/or in childhood schizophrenics.

motility psychosis See *cycloid psychosis.*

motility, unconscious Movements that are dissociated from consciousness, such as hysterical convulsions and spasms that are the unconscious and distorted physical expression of repressed instinctual demands.

motivation The force or energy that propels an organism to seek a goal and/or to satisfy a need; striving, incentive, purpose. Sullivan termed *conjunctive* those strivings directed to long-range satisfaction of real needs, and *disjunctive* those substitute strivings that afford only immediate gratification.

motivation, unconscious An aim or goal that is not recognized consciously by the subject, and especially any such aim that is the basis for a symptom, slip of the tongue or pen, or dream. Hysterical vomiting in a pregnant woman, for example, may be determined by her desire to rid herself of the fetus, a desire of which she is not consciously aware.

Freud's early work with hypnosis in hysterical patients led him to the conclusion that the symptoms afford a release of excitation in response to certain events, usually sexual, which are so unbearable that they are actively put out of consciousness and relegated into the unconscious portion of the psychic structure. But even though there is no longer any conscious awareness of these events, it does not mean that they cease to affect the individual: they nonetheless produce excitation that seeks discharge, yet cannot operate within the field of awareness, and therefore finds *abnormal* discharge in symptoms, slips of the tongue, and dreams.

motive Any explanation for the performance of an action by a person. Reason, in contrast, is a belief that is able to render an otherwise irrational action rational.

motive, lay See *tendency, final.*

motor aprosodia See *aprosodia.*

motor cortex The area of the cerebral hemisphere that controls movement; sometimes used synonymously with *precentral convolution,* although this is inaccurate, since movements can be excited from other areas as well.

motor disability Difficulty in getting information from the brain for expression via the musculature, as in writing and drawing.

motor inertia See *perseveration.*

motor neurosis See *neurosis, motor.*

motor persistence See *persistence, motor,*

motor skills disorder *Coordination disorder* (q.v.).

motorium 1. The motor cortex. 2. The faculty of the mind that has to do with volition (as the function of the sensorium is perception and of the intellect, thinking).

Mott, Frederick Walker, Sir (1853–1926) British neurologist; law of anticipation, that mental illness occurs earlier in succeeding generations.

mourning Normal grief, as contrasted with *melancholia* or *depression* (qq.v.), which are pathological.

mourning, anticipatory Acknowledgment of and reconciliation with the inevitability of death of a child with a fatal illness, experienced by the child's parents and other relatives.

movement, decomposition of See *disorganization.*

movement, involuntary Forced movement; an unwilled, adventitious contraction of one or more muscles or muscle groups that gives rise to movement in a limb or some other part of the body. The most frequently observed involuntary movements are *athetosis, chorea, myoclonus, tic,* and *tremor.*

movements, eye See *movements, pursuit.*

movements, hypermetamorphic Wernicke's term for *touching* (q.v.).

MPD Multiple personality disorder; see *personality, multiple.*

MPI Maudsley Personality Inventory.

MPPS Massive parallel processing system, a type of artificial intelligence investigation concerned with the process of visual perception and modeled on the primate nervous system; also known as *parallel visual computation, neo-associationism,* and *neoconnectionism.*

MPTP A synthetic heroin, known among drug users as *China White.* It is a fentanyl derivative that is highly toxic to the nervous system and has produced parkinsonism in a significant number of people who have used it. A *designer drug* (q.v.), it is made to look, feel, and cost like a high-quality heroin.

MRI Magnetic resonance imaging. See *NMR.*

MSER Mental Status Examination Report. See *Multi-State Information System.*

MSIS *Multi-State Information System* (q.v.).

MSLT Multiple sleep latency test.

MSRPP Multidimensional Scale for Rating Psychiatric Patients; often called the *Lorr scale.*

MSUD *Maple syrup urine disease* (q.v.).

Much-Holzmann reaction (Hans Much, German physician, 1880–1932, and Wilhelm

Holtzmann, German physician) The alleged property of the serum from a person with schizophrenia or manic-depressive psychosis to inhibit hemolysis caused by cobra venom.

mucopolysaccharidosis Any group of autosomal recessive disorders of glycosaminoglycans (GAG), characterized by severe mental retardation, skeletal deformities, and deposits of GAG in the tissues and excretion in the urine. The group includes:

1. *Hurler's disease*—also known as *gargoylism*, Pfaundler-Hurler syndrome, dysostosis multiplex, lipochondrodystrophy. It usually manifests itself in the early months of life, and death usually occurs by the age of 10 years. The child resembles an achondroplastic dwarf and shows multiple skeletal deformities (short neck, dorsal kyphosis, deformed thorax and long bones, flexion deformities of all joints, and maldevelopment of the skull vault and facial bones), hideous features (thickened skin and soft tissues, large head with widely spaced eyes and flattening of the bridge of the nose, coarse lips, protruding tongue, stridulent mouth breathing, and an apathetic, bovine expression), hepatosplenomegaly, corneal clouding, mental retardation. Several siblings are often affected, but the parents are phenotypically normal; parental consanguinity is frequent. The deficient enzyme is α-L-iduronidase; the urine contains excessive dermatan sulfate and heparan sulfate.

2. *Scheie's syndrome*—although the enzyme deficiency and urinary mucopolysaccharides are the same as in Hurler's, the syndrome is compatible with a normal life span and normal intelligence; clinical features include stiff joints, cloudy cornea, and aortic regurgitation.

3. *Hunter's syndrome*—a sex-linked (rather than autosomal) deficiency of sulfoiduronide sulfatase enzyme, with excessive dermatan sulfate and heparan sulfate in the urine. There is no clouding of the cornea, but in the more severe form death occurs usually by the age of 15 years; in the mild form, patients survive to the thirties or even fifties.

4. *Sanfilippo's syndrome*—also known as polydystrophic oligophrenia. It usually starts between 18 and 36 months of age with retardation or cessation of psychomotor development, progression to erethetic oligophrenia and, finally, severe dementia. Usually there are accompanying signs of gargoylism and hepatomegaly; less common are moderate contractures of the large joints and splenomegaly. Sanfilippo's syndrome is of two types, A and B, both with excessive heparan sulfate in the urine, but type A with a deficiency of the enzyme heparan sulfate sulfatase, type B with a deficiency of the enzyme *N*-acetyl-α-D-glucosaminidase.

5. *Morquio's syndrome*—probably a deficiency of chondroitin sulfate enzyme, with excessive keratan sulfate in the urine, severe bone changes, cloudy cornea, and aortic regurgitation.

6. *Maroteaux-Lamy's syndrome*—a deficiency of arylsulfatase B enzyme, with excessive dermatan sulfate in the urine, osseous and corneal defects, but normal intelligence.

7. *β-glucuronidase deficiency*—with excessive dermatan sulfate in the urine, hepatosplenomegaly, dysostosis multiplex, white cell inclusions, and mental retardation.

Diagnosis of all the mucopolysaccharidoses can be made prenatally by examination of fluid obtained through amniocentesis.

multi-infarct dementia Cerebral arteriosclerosis; a relatively small group of persons in whom a clear-cut succession of strokes has produced enough brain tissue damage to cause *dementia* (q.v.), with disturbances in memory, abstract thinking, judgment, impulse control, and personality. The course of deterioration is patchy and fluctuating, rather than steadily progressive. See *arteriosclerosis, cerebral.*

Multi-State Information System (MSIS) An automated, clinical record-keeping system, developed by the Information Sciences Division and New York State Department of Mental Hygiene in cooperation with five other states (Connecticut, Maine, Massachusetts, Rhode Island, and Vermont) and the District of Columbia, for use in mental hospitals and community mental health facilities, to provide comparative multistate summary statistics for evaluation of programs and treatment procedures. Included in the system are the Mental Status Examination Report (MSER)—a four-page optical scan form made up of structured multiple-choice items that cover the usual mental status categories—and the Periodic Evaluation Record (PER), a one-page subset of the MSER that is administered at frequent intervals so as to provide a narrative of the patient's progress.

multiaxial classification See *DSM-III.*

multidetermination *Overdetermination* (q.v.).

multidimensional pain management See *pain management, multidimensional.*

multifactorial model See *inheritance.*

multimodal therapy See *BASIC-ID.*

multiple monitored electroconvulsive theory See *therapy, multiple monitored electroconvulsive.*

multiple personality disorder (MPD) One of the *dissociative disorders* (q.v.); the presence of two or more relatively distinct and separate subpersonalities in a single person, as in Dr. Jekyl and Mr. Hyde, or in Morton Prince's case of Miss Beauchamp, or in Cleckley and Thigpen's case of Eve.

Although previously considered rare, MPD has been reported in increasing numbers since the late 1970s. Greater awareness of the disorder has also permitted identification of a relatively specific historical antecedent with which it appears to be associated: child abuse, most commonly physical and sexual child abuse. Each alternate personality appears to deal with a related set of affects, such as rage in response to abuse or sexual affects and conflicts stemming from sexual abuse.

There appears also to be a relationship between MPD and temporal lobe epilepsy. Perhaps as many as 33% of patients with temporal lobe epilepsy experience dissociative episodes, and some such patients develop multiple personality disorder. It has been hypothesized that the dissociation is a product of intensely dystonic affects characteristic of the interictal period in temporal lobe epilepsy.

Multiple personality is popularly known as split personality, and this has led to the logical but incorrect inference that schizophrenia (*split personality*) is identical with multiple personality. The latter is actually a dissociative reaction, and thus a form of hysteria. Splitting is seen in both hysteria and schizophrenia, but the splitting is quite different in each. In hysteria, the splitting is massive or molecular and consists of division into complicated and relatively complete subpersonalities. In the schizophrenias, on the other hand, individual psychic functions are split off from the personality as a whole and attain an autonomy of their own unrelated to and often contradictory to the major personality trends; thus the splitting in schizophrenia is often termed discrete, nuclear, or atomic.

In multiple personality, the original personality is termed the primary personality, and the dissociated or split-off personality is termed the secondary (tertiary, etc.) personality.

multiple sclerosis See *sclerosis, multiple.*

multiplication of personality See *personality, multiplication of.*

multiplicity, target A term suggested by Slavson to indicate the multiple possibilities existing in a group for projecting or displacing hostility on other patients, who replace the therapist as the target.

multipolarity A term introduced by Slavson to stress the fact that in group psychotherapy transference is directed toward more than the one person of the therapist. The interpatient (sibling and identification) transference produces a state of multipolarity in transference.

mumbling Muttering; indistinct speech; asapholalia; mussitation. Continuous mumbling without apparent signs of excitation may be an outstanding manifestation of the terminal state in schizophrenia. The mumbling consists of inarticulate, indistinct, and incoherent phrases, usually uttered in low tones so that the patient appears to be talking to himself.

Munchhausen syndrome See *syndrome, Munchhausen.*

Munich cooperation model A type of group therapy in which the group is structured to allow for reproduction of typical intrafamilial conflicts. The ward staff observe the group sessions and apply interpretations from them to the patient-personnel interactions on the ward, and patients support one another in autonomous groups that form after the treatment period.

Munsterberg, Hugo (1863–1916) Prussian-born American psychologist; founder of applied psychology, especially to law, business, industry, and sociology.

muscarinic See *acetylcholine.*

musicomania, musomania *Obs.* "A variety of insanity in which the passion for music has been fostered to such an extent as to derange the mental faculties." (Tuke, *DPM*)

musicotherapy Treatment of nervous and mental disorders by means of music, such as David's harp playing, which is said to have cured King Saul of his depression.

musophobia Fear of mice.

mussitation Movement of the tongue or lips as if in speech, without the production of articulate sounds. See *mumbling*.

mutant (mutational, mutated) Pertaining to new hereditary characters originated by mutation.

mutation An alteration of the nucleotide sequence. Genetic information consists of sequences of building blocks (nucleotides) that constitute a molecule of DNA. Whether these mutational variations are minor or more conspicuous, it is their clear distinction from the parental type and their ability to reproduce the new type that distinguish them from other forms of variation. See *chromosome*.

Mutant characters arise suddenly, breed true from the beginning, and give rise to a new and distinct race. They seem to occur in each species, usually with irregular frequency and more or less "spontaneously." This means that very little is known about the real cause, although it has been possible experimentally to produce various mutations by such external influences as high temperatures, radium, or chemicals.

In human beings *factor mutations* are brought about by a change in one of the chromomeres. These mutated genes produce more or less *pathological* types that often have a restricted viability (*lethal* factors). It may be assumed that the majority of hereditary malformations are caused by such factor mutations. Other kinds of mutation arise from changes in equipment or in the position of genes.

Although all present evidence indicates that mutations are relatively common in nature and probably the starting point for every form of evolutionary development, it is clear that more differences among individuals are derived from combination than from changes of genes. As soon as a multiplicity of unlike genes have originated by mutation, the genes are brought together in every new combination as rapidly as crosses are effected between individuals differing with respect to them. In the last analysis, however, mutations must underlie the origin of each new stock, race, or species.

mutation, point Mutation of a single gene.

mutative Relating to or productive of change, variation, alteration. See *interpretation, mutative*.

mutilation See *self-mutilation*.

mutinus, mutunus *Obs.* Priapus; penis.

mutism The state of being mute, dumb, silent; voicelessness without structural alterations; silence due to disinclination to talk as the "vows of silence" in anchorites or monastics of various religious creeds or people who will not tell the reason for their mutism: they can, but they will not speak.

By usage the term *stupor* is often a synonym for *mutism*. The condition is frequently observed in the catatonic form of schizophrenia, in the stupor of melancholia, and in states of hysterical stupor.

mutism, akinetic First used by H. Cairns in 1941 (and hence also known as *Cairn's stupor*) to describe a state of disturbed consciousness due to a tumor of the third ventricle. The patient lay inertly in bed, mute and almost totally unresponsive, although he followed the movements of people around him with his eyes. The syndrome is most likely a result of interference with the reticular activating system, so that response to environmental stimuli is defective. The term has also been used to describe subjects with bilateral frontal lobe lesions who lack all drive and impulse to action, despite intact motor and sensory tracts.

A related condition is *coma vigil* (also known as the *deafferented state,* "locked-in" *syndrome,* and *pseudocoma*). The subject is conscious and aware but is unable to respond. The lesion is in the ventral pons with preservation of the dorsal tegmental area; the activating system is intact but interruption of the corticobulbar and spinal pathways makes it impossible for the subject to move or speak.

mutism, elective As first used by Tramer in 1934, mutism limited to absence of verbal communication with certain persons, even though speech itself is intact. The condition is rare, appears usually at about 3 years of age, and lasts for several months or up to 2 years. Since the original description, the condition has been reported in older children, and in many it has been of longer duration. Improvement is typically related to a change of environment, such as a change of school. See *phobia, school.*

mutualism *Symbiosis* (q.v.).

mutuality See *divorce, emotional.*

MVP Mitral valve prolapse; a deformity of one or both cusps of the valve between the left atrium and the left ventricle, rendering the valve incompetent or insufficient. As a result, the ventricular contraction is inefficient: instead of all the blood within the ventricle being propelled into the aorta, some regurgitates back into the left atrium. Part of the cardiac energy is thereby wasted in pushing blood backward against the stream coming from the pulmonary bed into the left atrium. The most common cause of mitral valve prolapse is infection (especially rheumatic). Other frequent causes are deformity and injury. MVP is not always of sufficient degree to cause symptoms or to lead to heart failure; when it does, the process tends to be gradual and to extend over many years.

Some reports find MVP to occur significantly more often than expected in subjects with *panic disorder* and *agoraphobia* (qq.v.), but the majority of research does not indicate any relationship between the two.

my- myo- (mī′ō-) Combining form meaning muscle, mouse, from Gr. *mys.*

myasthenia Weakness of the muscles; fatigability; seen often in schizophrenia and depression.

myasthenia gravis A chronic disorder of conduction at the myoneural junction. Acetylcholine does not move from the synapse to its appropriate receptors on the adjoining cell. The major factor is an antibody-mediated autoimmune attack, which leads to a reduction in the number of acetylcholine receptors at neuromuscular junctions.

The disorder shows a marked tendency to remissions and exacerbations; females are more commonly affected than males; and onset is usually between the ages of 20 and 50 years. The characteristic symptom is muscular fatigability; this begins in the ocular muscles (producing ptosis and diplopia) and eventually leads to the other common disturbances: snarling smile, nasal speech, difficulty in swallowing and articulation, etc. The upper limbs are more affected than the lower. Sooner or later, permanent paralysis of the affected muscles develops.

Treatment includes drugs to prevent natural enzymes from destroying the acetylcholine and immunosuppressive treatment to prevent the patient's disordered immune defenses from abnormally blocking or destroying the receptors: corticosteroids, other anti-immune drugs, thymectomy, and *plasmapheresis* (q.v.).

mydriasis Dilation of the pupil. Mydriatics include *parasympatholytic* agents (such as atropine, scopolamine) and *sympathomimetic* drugs (such as cocaine, epinephrine). The former are *cycloplegic* (i.e. they relax ciliary muscles); the latter are not.

myelasthenia *Obs.* Neurasthenia of the spinal region. See *camptocormia.*

myelencephalon See *hindbrain.*

myelinoclasis, acute perivascular See *encephalomyelitis, acute disseminated.*

myelitis Inflammation of the spinal cord.

myelo- (mī′el-ō-) Combining form meaning marrow, spinal cord, from Gr. *myelos.*

myelocystocele (mī-el-ō-sis′tō-sēl) Spinal cord substance contained in a *spina bifida* (q.v.).

myelogram An X-ray of the spine following injection of a suitable contrast medium (usually Pantopaque) into the spinal subarachnoid space by means of spinal puncture. Myelography is most commonly used to demonstrate herniations of the intervertebral discs.

myelomeningocele (mī-el-ō-me-ning′gō-sēl) Spina bifida with protrusion of both the cord and its membranes.

myoclonia Any disorder characterized by spasmodic muscular contractions, as in infectious myoclonia or chorea.

myoclonic epilepsy A type of petit mal epilepsy. See *epilepsy.*

myoclonic sleep disorder Insomnia disorder with repetitive, stereotyped leg muscle jerks preceding periods of micro- or macroarousal.

myoclonus A sudden regular or irregular contraction of a muscle that does not usually produce movement of the part supplied by the muscle; it occurs most frequently in the limbs, but it may be seen in the body and face.

myoclonus epilepsy See *epilepsy, myoclonus.*

myoclonus, nocturnal Repetitive, stereotyped jerkings of the leg muscles of variable duration and frequency that occur during the night and continually disrupt sleep. In contrast to *restless legs syndrome* (q.v.), nocturnal myoclonus is not associated with disagreeable sensations in the legs. See *sleep disorders.*

myodynia, hysterical Muscular tenderness, usually over the ovarian region, observed occasionally in hysteria.

myoedema Swelling of muscle; on tapping a muscle with a percussion hammer, a localized swelling appears and persists for a few moments; a sign of hyperirritability of atrophic muscles.

myokymia A transient quiver of a muscle, occurring in weak anemic subjects.

myopathy, menopausal A pseudomyopathic polymyositis that appears in women during the menopausal years; proximal muscles are affected, and pathology consists of muscle necrosis without cellular infiltration.

myopia Shortsightedness or nearsightedness, caused by an elongation of the globe of the eye so that parallel rays are focused in front of the retina. Farsightedness is the reverse condition and is known as *hyperopia.* See *ametropia.*

myotonia atrophica *Dystrophia myotonica* (q.v.).

mysophilia Pathologic interest in, and desire for, filth or dirt; the desire to become unclean or polluted by contact with dirty or filthy objects—the opposite of *mysophobia* (q.v.). Mysophilia is commonly associated with *coprophilia* and *urophilia* and related to *paraphilia* (q.v.). Mysophilia is demonstrated in the following statement of a patient: "I get more sex thrill from the idea of a dirty woman than I do from a clean one." See *psychosexual.*

mysophobia Fear of contamination. It is commonly observed in the form of incessant handwashing. Some patients spend the greater part of their waking hours washing their hands. They may exhibit the dread of uncleanliness by many other actions. Some refuse to touch anything unless they wear gloves; others must constantly wash everything in their surroundings.

mythomania Pathologic lying; pseudologia phantastica; excessive interest in myths and propensity for incredible stories and fabrications. See *confabulation; liar, pathological.*

mythophobia Pathologic fear of stories or myths; disbelief in everything one is told.

myxedema madness See *hypothyroidism.*

myxoneurosis A neurosis affecting the mucous membranes, marked by a mucous discharge from the respiratory or intestinal mucous membrane, unaccompanied by signs of active inflammation.

MZ Monozygote, *monozygotic* (q.v.).

MZA Monozygotic twins reared apart.

MZT Monozygotic twins reared together.

N

N-allylnormorphine See *psychotomimetic*.
Nachmansohn, David (1899–1983) American neurophysiologist. See *process, elementary*.
nail biting Onychophagia (q.v.).
naming A disturbance in association, peculiar to schizophrenia, in which the only recognizable association to external stimuli consists in naming them. Thus in a word-association test, even though the patient understands its purpose, his only responses may be an enumeration of the furniture in the examining room. This naming does not appear only in response to visual impressions. When asked to do something, the patient may name the act: "Now he is sitting down." Such patients appear to be completely dependent upon, and at the mercy of, external impressions. This seems to be related to the lack of a goal-concept, to the lack of directives and aims. See *touching*.
nanism (nā'niz'm, nan'is'm) Paltauf's term for a special form of *dwarfism* (q.v.), which is of dysglandular origin and may best be classified as partial hypoevolutism affecting especially the skeletal growth. A conspicuous exception to this underdeveloped skeleton is a very large skull, with which a normal development of brain and intelligence may be associated, although the face (saddle-nose) usually takes on a cretinoid aspect. Since the genitals also may be sufficiently developed, these dwarfs can procreate others of the same type.
nanism, senile See *progeria*.
nanosomia Obs. See *dwarfism*.
nanosomia, primordial Hansemann's term for a rare form of *dwarfism* (q.v.) with regular physical proportions of the dwarfed body and normal mental development. It seems to be hereditary, is more common in

the male sex, and is transmitted from the father. Although small from birth, these dwarfs accomplish their puberal crisis regularly and are able to reproduce.

This is practically identical with the other special forms of *microsomia* called *pygmyism* by the French school and *heredofamilial essential microsomia* (q.v.) by E. Levi.
Napalkov phenomenon See *phenomenon, Napalkov*.
narce (när'sē) Hippocratic term for mental torpor.
narcema (när-sē'må) *Obs*. Narcosis.
narcism A shortened (and incorrect) form of *narcissism* (q.v.).
narcissism This term was first used by Nacke to indicate the form of autoerotism characterized by self-love, often without genitality as an object. Not infrequently, however, narcissism is associated with genital excitation: Krafft-Ebing cited the instance of a man who masturbated before a mirror.

In psychoanalytic psychology, narcissism is a stage in the development of object relationships in which the child's estimation of his capacities is heightened to the degree of omnipotence. At the narcissistic stage, which follows the autoerotic or somatogenic stage, the infant is still in the primary undifferentiated phase of consciousness: he is ignorant of any sources of pleasure other than himself and does not differentiate between the breast (or other objects) and the self. The breast is thought of as a part of his own body, and since his slightest gestures are followed by satisfaction of his instinctual nutritional needs, he develops the "autarchic fiction of false omnipotence." This is the stage of *primary narcissism*. The ego believes itself to be omnipotent, but this is disproved by experience and frustration; the infant then comes to believe that the parents are the omnipotent ones, and he partakes of their omnipotence by introjection (the "primary identification"). Even though reality has destroyed the feeling of omnipotence, the longing for this primary narcissism remains—the narcissistic needs—and self-esteem is the awareness of how close the individual is to the original omnipotence. The desire to partake of the parental omnipotence, even though it arose originally from the basic desire for the satisfaction of hunger, soon becomes differentiated from the hunger itself, and the child craves affection in a passive way ("passive object-love"); he is even willing to renounce other satisfactions if rewards of affection are promised. Thus the narcissistic needs are developed in relation to the ego and superego (and the term *secondary narcissism* refers to such love of the ego by the superego); the sexual needs, on the other hand, are developed in relation to the object.

When applied to the adult, the term narcissism implies a hypercathexis of the self and/or a hypocathexis of objects in the environment and/or a pathologically immature relationship to objects in the environment. Because the concept of narcissism was developed before Freud had formulated his last theory of the instincts (i.e. the dual-instinct theory of the sexual and aggressive instincts), it is not clear how Freud would have incorporated the aggressive instinct into his formulation of narcissism as described above; the formulation given refers only to the sexual drive. See *narcissism, primary.*

narcissism, disease Ferenczi's term for overevaluation (hypercathexis) of parts of the self that are not involved in a disease process. He described a soldier "whose lower jaw had been almost entirely blown away by a shell. His face was horribly deformed by the injury. The only striking thing about his behaviour, however, was his naive narcissism. He requested that the nursing sister should manicure him thoroughly every day; he would not eat the hospital food, since much finer fare was due to him, and he reiterated these and similar requests increasingly, after the fashion of querulants—a case, therefore,

of true 'disease-narcissism.' " (*FCT*) See *narcissism.*

narcissism, negative An exaggerated underestimation of oneself. It is particularly expressed in states of melancholia, characterized by ideas of inadequacy, unreality, and self-accusation.

narcissism, primary According to Freud, the whole available amount of libido is at first stored in the ego. "We call this state of things absolute, primary narcissism. It continues until the ego begins to connect the presentations of objects with libido—to change narcissistic libido into object libido." (*International Journal of Psychoanalysis XXI*, 1940) But in later writings (*The Ego and the Id*, 1949), Freud stated that in the beginning all libido is stored in the id and is drawn into the ego as narcissism only secondarily. "Part of this (original) libido is sent out by the id into erotic object cathexes, whereupon the ego, now growing stronger, attempts to obtain possession of this object libido and to force itself upon the id as a love object. The narcissism of the ego is thus seen to be secondary, acquired by the withdrawal of the libido from objects."

Thus it would seem that there is no such thing as primary narcissism, although Freud (and most of his followers) continued to refer to it despite the above quoted denial of it. And there are further contradictions in Freud's theory in that at various times he considered object love to be the primary and most primitive type of relationship to the environment, while at still other times (as discussed above) it was narcissism that was considered the most primitive type of relationship.

narcissism, secondary The narcissism once attached to external objects but now withdrawn from those objects and placed in the service of the ego (and not to objects in phantasy) is called secondary narcissism. This means that object libido is transformed into ego libido. For example, when a schizophrenic patient regresses, he withdraws libido from reality. The libido becomes attached, for instance, to ideas of grandeur and is called secondary narcissism. It is closely related, as Freud says, to infantile manifestations of megalomania. See *omnipotence.*

Secondary narcissism is not introversion, as Freud describes the latter. In introversion libido goes into the service of phantasies of real objects.

narcissistic Relating to self-love or narcissism.

narcissistic personality disorder See *personality disorders*.

narcoanalysis See *narcotherapy*.

narcocatharsis See *narcotherapy*.

narcolepsy *Friedmann's disease; Gelineau syndrome;* a *sleep disorder* (q.v.) of the DOES class consisting of a classic tetrad of cataplexy on emotion (sudden transient loss of muscle tone in the extremities or trunk), excessive sleepiness (recurrent paroxysms of uncontrollable sleep, usually lasting minutes but sometimes lasting for more than an hour), hypnagogic imagery, and sleep paralysis. There is at least a partial hereditary component, and the disorder usually persists through the subject's lifetime even though sleep paroxysms can be controlled with amphetamines or other cerebral stimulants.

narcomania A morbid desire to gain relief from painful stimuli usually through pharmacologic agents (morphine, opium, etc.), but also occasionally through psychic measures (e.g. hypnosis). See *substance abuse and dependence disorders*.

narcosis, continuous See *treatment, continuous sleep*.

narcosuggestion See *narcotherapy*.

narcosynthesis See *narcotherapy*.

narcotherapy A form of treatment used extensively in the war neuroses of World War II. As a general group term it includes narcosuggestion, narcocatharsis, narcoanalysis, narcosynthesis, Amytal interview, Pentothal interview, "truth serum." The treatment consists of injecting a barbiturate drug intravenously, either sodium Amytal or sodium Pentothal. When slowly injected intravenously in a 5 to 10% solution in doses of from 0.2 to 0.5 g, either of these two drugs induces a state of complete relaxation and a feeling of well-being and serenity, with a desire to communicate thoughts and a capacity to verbalize easily. Previously repressed memories, affects, and conflicts are expressed and the therapist then guides the patient along the lines of narcosuggestion, narcoanalysis, or narcosynthesis.

Narcosuggestion implies the active utilization of suggestion and reassurance while the patient is in a state of complete relaxation in the process of receiving sodium Amytal or sodium Pentothal intravenously. Narcocatharsis or narcoanalysis (the two words are used interchangeably) implies either free association or direct questions by the therapist to uncover repressed memories and affects while the patient is under the effects of sodium Amytal or sodium Pentothal given intravenously. At the end of the narcoanalysis, after the effects of the drug have worn off, the therapist explains to the patient the significance of what he recalled. Narcosynthesis uses free association, dreams, and transference material obtained during the Amytal or Pentothal interview, but a day or so later the material is discussed with the patient, who is guided by the therapist to conative and emotional reintegration, behavioral adjustments, and social rehabilitation. Although this method is also known as truth serum treatment, a patient who does not wish to tell the truth cannot be made to do so by the intravenous injection of Amytal or Pentothal. Consequently, this method is of limited value in medicolegal work.

narcotic Sleep-inducing. Drugs that can relieve severe pain are sleep-inducing and usually also highly addictive. In consequence, narcotic generally refers to an addicting analgesic, typically an opioid, while *hypnotic* refers to sleep-inducing.

narcotic blockade Total or partial inhibition of the euphoriogenic action of narcotic drugs through the use of other drugs, such as methadone, LAAM, or cyclazocine, which can then be used for maintenance treatment without producing the peaks of elation, abstinence symptoms, or demand for escalation of dose that characterize addiction to opiates. It is presumed that the narcotic antagonist or blocking agent achieves its effect by occupying the receptor site that the narcotic itself would ordinarily occupy.

narcotism The state of being under the influence of narcotic drugs. As commonly used, the term refers to the condition in which the drug is present in amounts great enough to be toxic, or, in any event, sufficient to alter behavior. See *addiction; dependency, drug*.

natural See *unnatural.*

natural study See *study, natural.*

naturalia *Obs.* The sexual organs.

nature, experiment of A term frequently used in the field of objective psychobiology emphasizing the study and treatment of stressful situations and the ways in which a person reacts to such stresses. Meyer refers to "experiment of nature," meaning the reaction to real environmental situations, and in particular to stressful ones.

nautomania Seaman's mania. Not infrequently sailors are affected by a morbid fear of a ship or water.

NE Norepinephrine.

-nea (-nē′à) Variant of *-noia* (q.v.).

necro- (nek′rō) Combining form meaning dead, from Gr. *nekrós.*

necromania Morbid desire for a dead body, the interest in the corpse usually being of a sexual character.

necromimesis The delusion in which the patient believes himself to be dead and acts as though he were.

necrophilia *Katasexuality;* a paraphilia, whose condition is that the love object, whether heterosexual or homosexual, must be dead before orgasm can be achieved. Although a rare perversion overall, it is claimed by some that morticians, undertakers, etc., contribute a relatively high proportion of subjects who have the perversion in either a grossly overt or an attenuated form. See *sexual disorders.* Although usually thought of as a condition limited to males, necrophilia was described in a female in 1976. (Foerster, K., Foerster, G., & Roth, R., *Schweizer Archiv für Neurologie, Neurochirurgie und Psychiatrie, 119*) See *taphophilia.*

necrophilism (ne-krof′i-liz′m) 1. A morbid desire to be in the presence of dead bodies. 2. *Necrophilia* (q.v.).

necrophobia Fear of a corpse or of death.

need Any stimulus of instinctual origin. Need implies a goal and, further, that the existing state is deficient in one of the elements that define or describe that goal. Needs are sometimes defined in terms of distance from postulated ideal norms, or lack of minimal standards, or the subject's sense of deprivation (*felt needs*).

need, aboriginal See *psychodynamics, adaptational.*

need, acculturated See *psychodynamics, adaptational.*

need, affiliative The desire to be associated with or allied with others in order to promote gratification of love, sexual desires, dependency, etc.

need-fear dilemma The schizophrenic's inordinate need for other people or an institutional structure to provide him with the regulation and organization that his own psychic structure cannot provide, combined with an equally inordinate fear of influence or control since these are potentially disorganizing if not in exactly the right dosage.

need for punishment See *criminal from sense of guilt.*

need, neurotic In Horney's terms, a demand or insistence that others behave toward the subject in a certain, specific way.

need-press See *method, need-press.*

needology The study of the needs of a person or population, often used pejoratively by economists in referring to what sociologists or other behavior scientists define as significantly lacking in the group with which they work.

needs, narcissistic See *narcissism.*

negation *Denial* (q.v.). Délire des négations is nihilistic delusion; see *syndrome, Cotard's.*

negation, delusion of Nihilistic delusion; denial of the existence of externality and/or of oneself; often associated with *depersonalization* (q.v.).

negation, insanity of An older term introduced by J. Cotard as *délire des négations* for the syndrome known as *depersonalization* (q.v.).

negative period, first *Negativism* (q.v.) that normally occurs in children between the ages of 2 and 4.

negative practice See *therapy, paradoxical.*

negative therapeutic reaction See *resistance, superego.*

negative utilitarianism See *utilitarianism, negative.*

negativism Negative attitude or behavior. In psychiatry, equivalent to *resistance*, as when a person, aware of stimuli from without, actively or passively opposes conformation with the stimuli. It is sometimes called *contrasuggestibility* or *contrariety*, though the latter terms are used more frequently in psychology than in psychiatry. It is also called *command negativism.*

Negativism is said to be *active* when the subject does the opposite of what he is asked to do. For example, when a catatonic patient closes his fists tightly upon being requested to open his hands, he presents active negativism.

He is said to exhibit *passive negativism* when, without prompting, he does not do things he is expected to do. He remains passive to his physiological urges; he does not get out of bed in the morning, dress, or eat. Bleuler calls this *inner* negativism.

Some authorities use the expression *intellectual negativism* when a patient always expresses an opposite to a thought. Thus a patient thought: "I must go; I must not go. I am a man; no, I am a woman; I will tell him; I will not tell him." This is more properly termed *ambivalence* (q.v.).

negativism, sexual Anerotism; Hirschfeld thus denotes absence of sexual interests, due, he believes, to deficiency in the sexual glands. See *sexual disorders; sexual response cycle.*

neglect, child Disregard, indifference, or inattentiveness to the needs of a child by the person(s) responsible for him; as a result, the child experiences avoidable suffering and/or is denied elements that are essential to the adequate development of his physical, intellectual, or emotional capacities. Child neglect is estimated to be three or four times as frequent as child abuse. See *syndrome, battered child.*

neglect, sensory Failure to respond to stimuli, used particularly to refer to a group of symptoms characteristic of patients with cerebral lesions, including *allesthesia* (contralateral stimuli are referred to the ipsilateral side); *anosognosia* (denial that the affected extremities belong to the subject); *hemiakinesia* (failure to turn toward stimuli presented on the side opposite the lesion); *hemispatial neglect* (subject draws only half the object he is asked to copy); and *paralexia* (only part of a word is read).

neo-Freudian Referring to modifications, extensions, or revisions of Freud's original psychoanalytic theory, most commonly to those that emphasize social, cultural, and interpersonal elements rather than innate biological instincts such as sexuality and aggression. Among the major theorists described as neo-Freudian are Alfred Adler (see *psychology, individ-*

ual), Erich Fromm, Karen Horney, and Harry Stack Sullivan.

neoassociationism *MPPS* (q.v.).

neoatavism (nē-ō-at′à-viz′m) The recurrence, in a descendant, of characters or traits of a near or immediate ancestor.

neobehaviorism Skinner's operant *behaviorism* (q.v.).

neoconnectionism *MPPS* (q.v.).

neocortex See *isocortex.*

neographism (nē-og′rà-fiz′m) The graphic equivalent of neologism, i.e. the writing of new words. See *neologism.*

neography Neologistic writing.

neolalia Neologistic speech; frequent use of neologisms in patient's speech.

neologism "Words of the patient's own making, often portmanteau condensations of several other words, and having originally had a special meaning for the patients." (Henderson, D.K., & Gillespie, R.D. *A Text-Book of Psychiatry,* 1936)

"A paranoid female 'is a Billy-goat,' i.e., she is united with her beloved minister: minister = Christ = lamb = billy-goat." (Bleuler, *TP*) See *contamination.*

neomimism A type of stereotypy, analogous to neologisms, consisting of a seemingly senseless gesture that has a particular meaning to the patient.

neomnesis (nē-om-nē′sis) Memory for the recent past.

neonate The newborn infant. See *developmental levels.*

neonaticide See *filicide.*

neophasia, polyglot A type of neologism formation in which one or more languages are devised by the patient, sometimes with full vocabulary, grammar, and syntax. Polyglot neophasia is rarely seen except in expansive paranoiacs and, to a lesser extent, in manic states. See *glossolalia.*

neophobia Fear of anything new or unfamiliar.

neophrenia *Obs.* In 1863 Kahlbaum classified psychiatric conditions (then called insanity) in accordance with the patient's age: neophrenia (the insanity of childhood), hebephrenia (the insanity of adolescence), and presbyophrenia (the insanity of old age).

neoplasm, cerebral See *tumor, intracranial.*

neopsychic Of recent psychic development.

neosleep See *dream.*

neostriatum See *basal ganglia.*

neoteny Temporal extension of the juvenile period in succeeding generations, or retention of juvenile characteristics of early generations as adult characteristics in their descendants. An example is the long period of childhood in humans in comparison with its length in early primates. In consequence, family ties are retained longer and the period of childhood learning is extended.

nephelopsychosis *Obs.* Intense interest in clouds.

nerve, abducens The sixth cranial nerve. The abducens nerve arises in the lower portion of the pons and supplies the external rectus muscle of the eye. For symptoms of abducens nerve lesions, see *nerve, oculomotor.*

nerve, acoustic The eighth cranial nerve. The acoustic nerve is a sensory nerve with two separate portions, the cochlear or auditory nerve (hearing) and the vestibular nerve (orientation in space). First-order neurons pass from the receptor cells in the spiral organ of Corti to the cochlear nuclei; from here, second-order neurons proceed through the trapezoid body and lateral lemnisci to the medial geniculate bodies. From here, auditory radiations are projected to the auditory cortex. First-order neurons of the vestibular nerve pass from the receptor cells in the vestibular ganglion (Scarpa's ganglion) to the vestibular nuclei, and thence to the cerebellum.

Symptoms of cochlear nerve involvement include tinnitus, deafness, and, in the case of supranuclear disorders, auditory aphasia or word-deafness. Symptoms of vestibular nerve involvement include vertigo and nystagmus.

nerve, cochlear See *nerve, acoustic.*

nerve conduction See *conduction, nerve.*

nerve, facial The seventh cranial nerve. The facial nerve is primarily a motor nerve that originates in the posterior pons and supplies the stapedius muscle of the middle ear and the superficial musculature of the face and scalp. Parasympathetic fibers supply the glands and mucous membranes of the pharynx, palate, and nasal cavity. The facial nerve also has some sensory fibers that carry taste from the anterior tongue. Lesions of the facial nerve may be peripheral (Bell's palsy or prosoplegia), nuclear, or supranuclear. In peripheral facial pa-

ralysis, the following signs will be seen on the affected side: drooping mouth, inability to whistle or wink or wrinkle forehead, tearing of eye, loss of deep facial sensation, food collecting between cheek and gum, paralysis of the flaccid (lower motor neuron) type. In the nuclear type of facial palsy, the above signs are also seen and, in addition, contralateral hemiplegia due to pyramidal involvement. In the supranuclear type of facial palsy, the paralysis is of the spastic (upper motor neuron) type, the frontalis muscle is spared because of its bilateral cortical innervation, and reflexes and emotional responses are retained. Supranuclear facial paralysis is often associated with homolateral hemiplegia or monoplegia.

nerve, glossopharyngeal The ninth cranial nerve. The glossopharyngeal nerve is motor to the stylopharyngeus muscle and sensory to the pharynx, soft palate, posterior tongue, and to the carotid body (for reflex control of respiration, blood pressure, and heart rate). The glossopharyngeal nerve also supplies taste buds in the posterior third of the tongue. Symptoms associated with lesions of this nerve include loss of gag reflex, loss of taste in posterior tongue, and deviation of uvula to the unaffected side.

nerve, hypoglossal The twelfth cranial nerve. The hypoglossal nerve is motor to the muscles of the tongue. Peripheral paralysis results in homolateral flaccidity, paralysis and atrophy, and the tongue deviates to the side of the lesion. Supranuclear paralysis results in contralateral hemiplegia, contralateral spastic paralysis of the tongue, and deviation of the tongue to the side opposite the lesion.

nerve, oculomotor The third cranial nerve. The oculomotor nerve arises at the level of the superior colliculus and is the motor nerve to the following eye muscles: internal rectus, superior rectus, inferior rectus, inferior oblique, and levator palpebrae. Parasympathetic fibers originate in the Edinger-Westphal nucleus and proceed via the nasociliary branch of the oculomotor nerve to the ciliary ganglion, whence the short ciliary nerves pass to the sphincter muscle of the iris.

The other muscles of the eye are supplied by the trochlear and abducens nerves, which functionally are considered together with the oculomotor nerve. Symptoms of involvement of these three cranial nerves include lid droop (ptosis), nystagmus, double vision (diplopia), squint (strabismus), and conjugate deviation, in which both eyes are turned to the same side. Strabismus may be internal, in which case the visual axes cross each other, or external, in which case the visual axes diverge from each other.

J.G. Chusid and J.J. McDonald (*Correlative Neuroanatomy and Functional Neurology*, 1956) suggest the following classification of disorders of these three cranial nerves:

A. Ophthalmoplegias (paralyses)
  1. Oculomotor paralysis
      a. external ophthalmoplegia—divergent strabismus, diplopia, ptosis
      b. internal ophthalmoplegia—dilated pupil, loss of light and accommodation reflexes (total ophthalmoplegia refers to a combination of external and internal ophthalmoplegia)
      c. Argyll Robertson pupil—miosis with loss of light and cilio-spinal reflexes, and preservation of accommodation reflex (pretectal lesion)
      d. Paralysis of convergence (central lesion)
  2. Trochlear paralysis (rare)—slight convergent strabismus and diplopia
  3. Abducens paralysis (most common)—convergent strabismus and diplopia
  4. Chronic progressive ophthalmoplegia (Graefe's disease)—usually involves all three nerves
B. Myasthenic States
C. Spasmodic Ocular Disorders (supranuclear lesions)
  1. conjugate deviation spasm
  2. lateral or ventral association spasm
  3. central nystagmus: rhythmic (vestibular origin) or undulating (cerebral or cerebellar origin)

nerve, olfactory The first cranial nerve. The olfactory nerve is structurally a fiber tract of the brain; it is a sensory nerve that transmits olfactory (smell) stimuli. Symptoms due to olfactory nerve lesions include anosmia (loss of sense of smell), hyperosmia, parosmia (perverted sense of smell), cacosmia (sensation of unpleasant odors), and olfactory hallucinations. The *Foster Kennedy syndrome,* caused by tumors at the base of the frontal lobe, includes anosmia with atrophy of the optic and olfactory nerves, blindness, and contralateral papilledema.

nerve, optic The second cranial nerve. The optic nerve is structurally a fiber tract of the brain; it is a sensory nerve that transmits visual stimuli. The rods and cones of the retina of the eye are the first-order neurons; they connect with the bipolar cells of the retina, which in turn connect with the ganglion cells. These form the optic nerve fibers, which proceed to the optic chiasma, form the optic tracts, and then pass to the lateral geniculate bodies, the superior colliculi, and the pretectal region. From the geniculate bodies, fibers pass (as the geniculocalcarine tract) to the occipital cortex. Fibers from the superior colliculi pass to various cranial and spinal nuclei (for involuntary oculoskeletal reflexes); fibers from the pretectal region pass to the Edinger-Westphal nuclei (for the simple and consensual light reflexes).

Visual defects include scotomata (abnormal blind spots in the visual fields), amblyopia (reduction of visual acuity), amaurosis (complete blindness), *field defect* (q.v.), hemeralopia (day blindness), nyctalopia (night blindness), color blindness, and optic agnosia or word blindness.

nerve, spinal accessory The eleventh cranial nerve. The spinal accessory nerve is motor to the trapezius and sternocleidomastoid muscles. Unilateral paralysis results in inability to rotate head to unaffected side, atrophy of sternocleidomastoid, inability to shrug affected shoulder, and drooping of affected shoulder. Bilateral paralysis results in difficulty in rotating head or lifting chin and in a dropping forward of the head.

nerve, trigeminal The fifth cranial nerve. The trigeminal nerve has both motor and sensory components. Motor fibers arise from the motor nucleus in the pons and supply the muscles of mastication (masseter, temporal, internal and external pterygoids). Sensory fibers are in three divisions: the ophthalmic division supplies the forehead, eyes, nose, temples, and meninges; the maxillary division supplies the upper jaw and hard palate; the mandibular division supplies the lower jaw and tongue. Symptoms of trigeminal nerve lesions include pain, loss of sensation, paralysis of muscles of mastication with deviation of the jaw to the affected side, loss of jaw jerk, sneeze, lid reflex, conjunctival reflex and corneal reflex, and various trophic changes in the nose, face, and jaw.

nerve, trochlear The fourth cranial nerve. The trochlear nerve arises at the level of the inferior colliculus and is the motor nerve to the superior oblique muscle of the eye. For symptoms of trochlear nerve lesions, see *nerve, oculomotor.*

nerve, vagus The tenth cranial nerve. The vagus nerve is motor to the muscles of the soft palate and pharynx, sends parasympathetic fibers to the thoracic and abdominal viscera, and is sensory to the pharynx, larynx, trachea, esophagus, and the thoracic and abdominal viscera. Symptoms of vagus nerve lesions include aphonia, dysphagia, paralysis of the soft palate with loss of the gag reflex, cough, bradycardia (with irritative lesions), or tachycardia (with vagus palsies).

nerve, vestibular See *nerve, acoustic.*

nervous 1. Relating to a nerve or the nerves. 2. Easily excited or agitated; suffering from instability or weakness of nerve action.

nervous system, autonomic See *autonomic nervous system.*

nervous system, conceptual Any model whose operation is in accordance with known mechanisms of central nervous system functioning and which is capable of producing responses comparable to or identical with the behavior of the living organism. The value of the conceptual nervous system is primarily heuristic in that it affords a simplified and manipulatable analogy of the nervous system itself and thus stimulates hypotheses about how the nervous system operates. Often, however, it is accepted uncritically as an exact reproduction of the nervous system and then used incorrectly as a way to verify theories about the nervous system.

nervous system, parasympathetic See *autonomic nervous system.*

nervous system, sympathetic See *autonomic nervous system.*

nervous system, third See *third nervous system.*

nervous system, vegetative See *autonomic nervous system.*

network A system or structure of interlacing lines, threads, fibers, channels, etc. In social psychiatry, a field or patterning of interrelationships envisioned as a matrix of connected points that are the various types of stimuli impinging on the person— *taxic* (inanimate, such as humidity, temperature, terrain), *biotaxic* (people or animals), and *sociotaxic* (social groups and any other type of social stimulation).

In the network model of social psychiatry, attention is also given to the spaces between the interconnected points—the interface. When one is removed from familiar stimuli, he is considered to be in the empty space between cultural networks and is said to be experiencing *interface shock* (of which culture shock is an example). The person who goes from one culture to another and almost at once becomes what he believes people from the other culture are like demonstrates what is termed *interface penetration* (what would popularly be termed "going native"). *Interface stationing* refers to the enjoyment of being at the interface, as the visitor to a foreign country who acts "touristy." An extension of such behavior into becoming more like the original culture than the person ever was while he was in fact within his system of origin is *interface accentuation,* exemplified by the Brooklyn Jew who never follows dietary laws until he settles in Wyoming. See *therapy, network.*

network, psychological A set of interrelated social elements (individuals, families, etc.) whose cohesiveness, even though relatively loose, provides a mechanism for shaping social tradition and public opinion and also an emotional support system for those who are a part of it.

network, social That group of people who have an ongoing significance in a specific person's or a nuclear family's life in terms of meeting human needs; the social network is a largely invisible system that is rarely together at any one time.

neuradynamia (nū-rad-i-nā′mē-à) *Neurasthenia* (q.v.).

neural plate (tube) See *cephalogenesis.*

neural tube defect (NTD) Failure of the neural tube to close properly during development. Neural tube defects are among the most common major congenital malformations, occurring in approximately 1 out of every 600 pregnancies. Amniocentesis permits prenatal detection in 95% of cases by revealing an increase in α-fetoprotein (AFP), which leaks from an open lesion such as spina bifida or anencephaly. Elevated AFP is not specific to neural tube defects, however; it has also been reported in Turner's syndrome, duodenal atresia, and many other congenital anomalies.

neuralgia, Fothergill's See *tic douloureux*.

neuralgia, trifacial See *tic douloureux*.

neuralgia, trigeminal See *tic douloureux*.

neurasthenia Neurasthenic neurosis; nervous debility. The concept neurasthenia was introduced in the U.S. in 1869 by G.M. Beard; it had been outlined by Bouchut as nervosisme in 1860.

The clinical syndrome is characterized by a wide variety of symptoms, including easy fatigability, feeling of physical and mental weakness, aches, pains, paresthesias, and a number of other pathological physical sensations; inadequate functioning of any organ or organic system of the body; insomnia. While some subjects run the gamut of symptoms, usually complaints center upon some particular organ or system. See *hypochondriasis*.

The fatigue state is a defense against some intrapsychic conflict, and is itself defended against by a search for some physical cause to explain the fatigue. The emotional basis is sometimes wholly and always at least partially outside conscious awareness. Fatigue may be a symbolic expression of or a defense against consciously disowned needs or wishes. Unresolved anger may lead to hidden resentment, which in turn provokes fear of punishment or disapproval, and the latter fear is expressed as being tired, and not feeling well. Such fatigue states are often found in conjunction with feelings of failure, frustration, and disappointment. See *hypoglycemia*. Neurasthenic patients are typically narcissistic, self-centered, and manifest strong dependency needs.

In DSM-I, neurasthenia was classified as a psychophysiologic nervous system reaction. According to Freud's early theory (1894), "Neurasthenia arises whenever a less adequate relief (activity) takes the place of the adequate one, thus, when

masturbation or spontaneous emission replaces normal coitus under the most favorable conditions." Four years later he said that neurasthenia was an *actual neurosis*. "Psychoneuroses appear under two kinds of conditions, either independently or in the wake of actual neuroses (neurasthenia and anxiety-neurosis)." (*CP*)

neurasthenia, arrived *Obs*. Well-established, chronic neurasthenia in which intellectual fatigue and depression are paralleled by physical emaciation and weakness. J.J. Déjérine and E. Gauckler noted that some such patients develop episodes of agitation, of the nature of a periodic psychosis, during which intellectual activity accelerates as motor activity increases. (*The Psychoneuroses and Their Treatment by Psychotherapy*, 1915)

neurasthenia, aviator's "A chronic functional nervous and psychic disorder occurring in aviators and characterized by gastric distress, nervous irritabilities, minor psychic disorders, fatigue of the higher voluntary mental centers, insomnia, and increased motor activity." This condition is also known as *aeroneurosis* (q.v.), *staleness*, and *flying sickness*. (Sladen, F.J. *Psychiatry and the War*, 1943)

neurasthenia, professional Nervous prostration manifested principally in the inability to use the organ(s) habitually employed in the course of one's profession or occupation. See *neurosis, occupational*.

neurasthenia, traumatic A neurasthenic reaction pattern that develops in response to physical trauma, such as those caused by automotive or industrial accidents. Trauma is here considered to have precipitated an acute exacerbation of an underlying neurotic potentiality. See *neurasthenia; post-traumatic stress disorder*.

neurasthenia, war A term for neurocirculatory asthenia or effort-syndrome as observed in soldiers in time of war; *soldier's heart*. As described, the condition corresponds to what currently would be termed hyperventilation syndrome. See *asthenia, neurocirculatory; syndrome, hyperventilation*.

neurasthenoid Resembling neurasthenia.

neuraxon See *neuron*.

neuremia Laycock's term for functional disorders of the nervous system.

neuriatry, neuriatria Treatment of nervous diseases.

neurilemma See *neuron.*

neurinomatosis A tendency toward new growth of primitive neuroepithelial cells. See *diathesis, glial.*

neuritis, optic An inflammatory process affecting the head of the optic nerve, or that part within the bulb of the eye. The condition is usually bilateral, and early loss of vision is characteristic. Ophthalmoscopically, there is blurring of the margins of the disk with congestion, dilatation of the veins, and narrowing of the arteries. The retina may show hemorrhages, pigment deposits, exudates, connective tissue changes, and atrophic spots. Optic neuritis may occur in severe renal disease, syphilis, leukemia, carbon monoxide poisoning, diabetes, anemia, and other constitutional diseases.

neuro- Combining form meaning nerve, from Gr. *neuron.*

neuroadaptation Changes in the nerve in response to continued or repeated stimulation; more specifically, drug-induced dependency state, typically manifested by a characteristic withdrawal state. See *addiction; dependency, drug; withdrawal.*

neuroanatomy, chemical That branch of anatomy that is concerned with the biochemistry of nerve tissues and, in particular, the function of chemical transmitters in nervous system activity. Within the nervous system, electrical impulses are transmitted along axons, but transmission from one nerve cell to another depends on the release of neurotransmitters at synapses. Knowledge about such transmitters has broadened considerably with the development of methods that could localize specific chemical transmitters in the brain.

Before 1960, only acetylcholine and norepinephrine were known with certainty to be neurotransmitters, and then only in parts of the peripheral nervous system. In the early 1960s, a histofluorescence method was introduced that revealed the existence of previously unknown neural systems. In the early 1970s, immunohistochemical methods were used to identify various antigens associated with neurotransmitters. As a result, not only are acetylcholine and the biogenic amines known to play an active role in central nervous system transmission, but numerous peptides and amino acids have been identified as neurotransmitters or neuromodulators.

Current research in chemical neuroanatomy is directed to the identification of biochemically specific pathways in the nervous system and defining their relationship to those that have already been identified by the histological, electrophysiological, and behavioral approaches. See *neurohormone; neuromodulator; neurotransmitter.*

neuroarthritism A condition with a predisposition to nervous and rheumatoid or gouty disorders. See *diathesis, arthritic.*

neurocentral See *constant, central.*

neurochemistry The study of the chemical composition of neural tissue. Lipids account for about half the weight of the dry brain, and certain lipids—galactocerebroside and gangliosides—are found only in brain. Proteins, nucleic acids, nucleotides, amino acids, and amines are other important constituents. Unlike other organs of the body, the brain has only limited reserves of carbohydrate. Consequently, it is particularly vulnerable to hypoglycemia. It is highly dependent on a constant supply of both glucose and oxygen, and it consumes approximately 20% of the total oxygen consumption of the body.

neurochemistry, behavioral Study of the relations between chemical substances in the brain and behavior, including such areas as synthesis of neuroregulatory substances, genetic control of transmitter agents, different roles of compounds in different areas of the brain, biochemical effects of receptor excitation, interactions between different agents within the brain, actions of drugs on enzymatic and metabolic processes within the brain, and the relation of all such biochemical events to psychological events and behavior.

neuroethology A synthesis of neurobiology and behavior that attempts to explain how the brain produces behavior and views the properties and connectivity of neurons in the context of what they are doing.

neurofibromatosis Neurofibroblastomatosis; *von Recklinghausen's disease.* A congenital, hereditary disorder, transmitted as a Mendelian dominant, consisting of café-au-lait pigmentation of the skin and the formation of tumors in various tissues (e.g. cutaneous fibromas or mollusca fibrosa and perineural fibroblastomas of the peripheral and cranial nerves). The tumors are often associated with overgrowth of the skin and subcutaneous tissues. Of the cranial nerves, the eighth nerve is the most commonly involved. The disorder is sometimes progressive, but it does not always shorten life. It may be associated with varying degrees of mental retardation.

Two forms of neurofibromatosis have been differentiated. Von Recklinghausen's disease, or *Elephant Man's disease* (because it was cited as the cause of the disfigurement of Joseph Herrick, a 19th-century Englishman who was exhibited at sideshows as the elephant man). This form occurs in approximately 1 in 4,000 births, and its gene has been identified as occurring on chromosome 17. The second form is bilateral acoustic neurofibromatosis, which occurs in approximately 1 in 50,000 births. It causes multiple tumors on the cranial and spinal nerves, producing deafness, ataxia, and paralyses. The gene for this form is located on chromosome 22.

neurogenic Caused or produced by, born of, or engendered by nerves or a nerve.

neuroglia (nū-rog′lē-à) A fine web of supporting tissue in the nervous system, composed of modified ectodermal elements in which are enclosed the neuroglia (or glia) cells: astrocytes, oligodendroglia, and microglia.

neurogram "Whatever may be the exact nature of the theoretical alterations left in the brain by life's experiences they have received various generic terms; more commonly 'brain residual,' and 'brain dispositions.' I have been in the habit of using the term *neurograms* to characterize these brain records. Just as telegram, Marconigram, and phonogram precisely characterize the form in which the physical phenomena which correspond to our (verbally or scripturally) thoughts, are recorded and conserved, so neurogram precisely characterizes my conception of the form in which a system of brain processes corresponding to thoughts and other mental experiences is recorded and conserved." (Prince, M. *The Unconscious,* 1916) See *memory, physiological.*

neurohormone Neurohumor; a chemical messenger produced by neuroendocrine transducers, most of which are located in the hypothalamus. The neurohormone is carried to the anterior pituitary by means of the hypophyseal portal system and moves along axons to the posterior pituitary. From there the neurohormone binds to specific receptor sites on the plasma membrane of the other cells, whose activity it modulates. Neurohormones are similar to *neurotransmitters* (q.v.), except that they generally interact with a variety of cells whereas neurotransmitters interact only with other neurons. See *epinephrine; neuroanatomy, chemical; peptidergic; process, elementary; serotonin.*

neurohypnology The study of *magnetic sleep* (Braid). See *hypnotism; Mesmer.*

neurohypnosis *Obs.* Braid's original term meaning literally sleep of the nervous system; later Braid dropped the first part of the word, and used hypnosis instead, "for the sake of brevity."

neuroinduction Suggestion.

neurokym *Psychokym* (q.v.).

neuroleptic Referring to a specific antipsychotic effect of a pharmacologic agent on nervous system; the terms ataraxic and tranquilizer, in contrast, are merely descriptive of a sedative effect. See *psycholeptica; psychotropics; tranquilizer.*

neuroleptic malignant syndrome See *syndrome, neuroleptic malignant.*

neuroleptization, rapid Administration of multiple doses of an antipsychotic drug over several hours in an attempt to interrupt an acute psychotic episode; sometimes called *megadose* (q.v.) treatment, although that also refers to long-term or maintenance therapy with very high doses of any drug. The technique of rapid neuroleptization was introduced in the 1960s and achieved its greatest popularity in the 1970s. Since then, however, most reports suggest that high parenteral doses of neuroleptic are no more effective than standard oral doses but are associated with a much higher incidence of extrapyramidal symptoms.

neurolinguistics The study of language—including its acquisition, production, processing, reception—at the neurologic level. See *psycholinguistics.*

Neurolinguistics is particularly concerned with *aphasia* (q.v.) and disturbances of any part of the language system, such as disturbances in syntax and grammar, lexicon (vocabulary), semantics (meaning), phonology (sound systems), and prosody (intonation, accent).

neurology The branch of medicine that devotes itself to the study of the organization and function of the nervous tissue. The diseases of the peripheral nerves of the spinal cord and the brain, as far as they are based on organic pathology, are in the realm of neurology.

neurology, behavioral That branch of neurology which links normal and abnormal behaviors to functioning of specific areas or regional systems of the brain, such as the finding that stopping and starting motor tasks is a frontal lobe function and that perseveration or motor inertia is therefore suggestive of frontal lobe disturbance. The basic science of behavioral neurology is *neuropsychology* (q.v.).

neurometadrasis *Obs.* Animal magnetism or the influence of one body upon another.

neurometrics Computer-assisted studies and measurement of brain function, including brain electrical activity mapping (*BEAM*), brain wave activity measurement (*BWAM*), visual and auditory evoked potentials (*VEP, AEP*). See *NMR.*

The development of such techniques is associated with the name of E. Roy John, of the Brain Research Laboratories of New York University Medical Center. Using computer techniques, John and his colleagues analyze electroencephalograms and evoked potentials in order to gain quantitative data about brain functioning, particularly as it is related to information processing. The neurometric data obtained from subjects with a variety of behavioral symptoms, neurologic dysfunctions, and maturational/developmental levels are then subjected to the mathematical analyses of numerical taxonomy to construct objective, operational categories of brain dysfunctions. Such analysis provides identification of different types of brain functioning in persons whose behavior manifestations are similar. (E. Roy John et al. *Science 196,* 1977)

Two classes of slow waves can be recorded from the human scalp: (1) spontaneous fluctuations of voltage, reflected in the *elctroencephalogram* (EEG); and (2) transient oscillations of voltage in response to environmental stimuli, called evoked potentials (EPs) or event-related potentials

(ERPs), which can be extracted from the EEG by computer averaging methods.

The ERP is a succession of waves corresponding to the sequential processing of information by the subject. Some elements of the ERP are determined by the physical stimulus and the state of the afferent pathways ("exogenous" processes); others reflect the prior experience, expectation, or semantic processes of the subject ("endogenous" processes). At least in some brain regions, these different processes appear to involve different neurons. Exogenous processes are mediated by *stable cells,* which respond to physical features of the stimuli independent of their meaning. Endogenous processes are mediated by *plastic cells,* whose firing patterns are correlated with subsequent behavioral responses and not with the physical features of the stimulus.

P_{300} is a late-appearing component of the ERP. Its amplitude increases with unpredictable, unlikely, or highly significant stimuli and thereby constitutes an index of mental activity.

The *brain-stem-evoked potential* (*BSEP*; sometimes referred to as the *far-field evoked potential*) is a special type of exogenous ERP. The auditory BSEP is a sensitive measure of lateral lemniscus functioning, and the somatosensory BSEP is equally sensitive to the functional status of the medial lemniscus.

neuromimesis *Obs.* Mimicry of disease or disorder of a mental or nervous character. See *factitious disorders; syndrome, Ganser.*

neuromodulator A substance that conveys information to nerve cells by means other than neurotransmission. Neuromodulators regulate nerve cell function by amplifying or dampening neuronal activity; *neurotransmitters* (q.v.), in contrast, regulate neuronal activity by conveying information between adjacent cells.

Three types of neuromodulators have been differentiated: (1) synaptic neuromodulators, which act on nerve cells in synaptic contact; (2) hormonal neuromodulators, which affect cells relatively distant from the site of neuromodulator release; and (3) autoinhibitors, which modulate their own release or synthesis by means of presynaptic mechanisms. See *neuroanatomy, chemical; peptidergic.*

neuromyelitis optica *Devic's disease* (q.v.).

neuron (neurone) The unit of the central nervous system; the nerve cell, consisting of cell body, dendrites, and neuraxon. Conventional descriptions of the neuron usually follow that of Ramón y Cajal (1911), even though his morphological description has long been inadequate in terms of neuron function. This inadequacy is related primarily to his inclusion of the cell body as the focal point of functional polarization of the neuron, a view no longer tenable if recent advances in neurophysiology and cytology are to be taken into consideration.

In the classical description, the dendrons or dendrites are described as receptor portions of a neuron that arise from the nucleated cell body or perikaryon; they conduct nerve impulses toward the cell body. The axon is a nerve-cell process that also arises from the cell body, but it conducts nerve impulses away from the cell body.

D. Bodian (*Science 137,* 1962) has proposed the following redefinition of structure in terms of function:

1. *Dendrites*—neuron processes with response generator function; the dendritic zone is "the receptor membrane of a neuron, either consisting of a set of tapering cytoplasmic extensions (dendrites) which receive synaptic endings of other neurons or differentiated to convert environmental stimuli into local-response-generating activity."

2. *Nuclear cell body* or *perikaryon*—consists of an internal portion (the chromidial neuroplasm) and an external membrane; it is located in a variety of positions in various nerve cells. The membrane alone is involved in synaptic transmission; the chromidial neuroplasm is a separate functional component of the cell and is a cytoplasmic zone related primarily to the trophic aspect of nerve cell function. Its position within the neuron "is related to the outgrowth and metabolic maintenance of processes rather than to the conducting polarization of the neuron." "It may be located in the dendritic zone or within the axon, or it may be attached to the axon."

3. *Axon*—"a single, often branched and usually elongated, cytoplasmic extension morphologically and perhaps uniquely differentiated to conduct nervous impulses away from the dendritic zone. It is characteristically uniform in caliber and ensheathed by neuroglial or neurilemma cells." Functionally, "the axon may be said to arise from any response generator structure, such as receptor terminal, dendrite, cell body, or axon hillock. . . . According to this view, axons do not arise from 'cell bodies' which are separated from the response generating region."

4. *Axon telodendria*—"the usually branched and variously differentiated terminals of axons which show membrane and cytoplasmic differentiation related to synaptic transmission or neurosecretory activity. Mitochondrial concentrations, 'synaptic vesicles,' or secretory granules are commonly present in bulblike terminals. . . . They transmit electrical or chemical signals capable of producing generator potentials in the dendritic zone of other neurons and in muscle, and stimulatory effects in innervated glandular cells or in distant cells via the humoral route (neurohormones)." See *synapse*.

The above revisions of classical descriptions "make it possible to relate basic functional aspects of neuron function to general aspects of neuron structure, as follows: response (spike) generation, to the 'dendritic zone' (transducer and synaptic surfaces); impulse origin, at or near the axon origin (the initial axon segment or axon 'neck'); impulse conduction, to the axon; and synaptic transmission or neurosecretory emission, to the axon telodendria." See *neurotransmitter*.

neuropathy (nū-rop′ă-thē) Any (organic) disease of the nervous system; any disorder involving neural tissue. Formerly the term included disorders that currently would be termed neurotic or psychoneurotic. See *traits, neuropathic*.

neuropathy, huffer's See *huffing*.

neuropeptide See *peptide, brain*.

neuroplasm, chromidial See *neuron*.

neuropsychiatry Sometimes used as a synonym for psychiatry; the term emphasizes the somatic substructure on which mental operations and emotions are based, and the functional or organic disturbances of the central nervous system that give rise to, contribute to, or are associated with mental and emotional disorders.

neuropsychology That branch of clinical psychology concerned with the evaluation of brain dysfunction and particularly with the development, standardization, and validation of techniques to assess behavioral expressions of such dysfunction. Neuropsychological assessment employs batteries of tests to evaluate major areas of functioning, both quantitatively and qualitatively, not only to provide assistance in differential diagnosis but also to assess levels of impairment as part of planning a treatment and rehabilitation program for the patient. See *neurology, behavioral*.

neuropsychosis *Obs.* This term used to mean what *psychosis* means today. It is not interchangeable with *psychoneurosis*.

neurosal *Obs.* Pertaining to neurosis.

neuroses, class differences in Neuroses are considered by many authorities as consequences of the specific social and economic circumstances of a particular class. For example, some have felt that poverty and social misery are the chief conditions for the development of neurosis. Others, on the contrary, have said that only the idle and privileged classes have had the time to develop neuroses and that the hard-working lower classes are protected from neuroses by their all-absorbing preoccupation with keeping fed and sheltered.

Fenichel denies both views, pointing out that neuroses are equally widespread in all socioeconomic groups. Further, he remarks on the negligible differences between types of neuroses prevalent in different classes. See *class, social*.

neurosis As used today, this term is interchangeable with the term *psychoneurosis*. The term implies that the condition is not the result of organic brain disorder, that reality testing is not impaired, and that the underlying personality is not grossly abnormal. At one time it was used to refer to any somatic disorder of the nerves (the present-day term for this is *neuropathy*) or to any disorder of nerve function. In psychoanalytic terminology, neurosis often is used more broadly to include all psychical disorders; thus Freud spoke of actual neuroses (neurasthenia, including hypochondriasis, and anxiety neurosis); transference or psychoneuroses (anxiety hysteria, conversion hysteria, obsessional and compulsive neurosis; and Fenichel adds to this group organ neuroses, pregenital conversions, perversions, and impulse neuroses); narcissistic neuroses (the schizophrenias and manic-depressive psychoses); and traumatic neuroses. See *disorder, neurotic*.

The distinctions between neurosis and psychosis are symptomatic, psychopathological, and therapeutic. In the neuroses, only a part of the personality is affected (Meyer's *part-reaction*), and reality is not changed qualitatively although its value may be altered quantitatively (i.e. diminished). The neurotic acts as if reality had the same kind of meaning for him as the rest of the community. Psychopathologically, the psychotic change in reality is partly expressed as projection, and of a type that does not occur in the neuroses. In the neuroses, language as such is never disturbed, while in the psychoses language is distorted, and the unconscious may come to direct verbal expression. In the neuroses, the unconscious never attains more than symbolic expression and regression to primitive levels (e.g. soiling and wetting) is not found in the presence of clear consciousness. Symptoms of neurosis include sensory, motor, or visceral disturbances and mental disturbances such as anxieties, specific fears and avoidances, memory disturbances, trance states, somnambulisms, troublesome thoughts.

Charcot was the first to make a systematic study of the neuroses; he formulated a group of clinical pictures that he called hysteria, which was considered to be an outcome of hereditarily determined degeneration. Janet was the first to attempt a grouping of neuroses on the basis of their dynamics. He theorized that there are two kinds of psychological operations—easy ones, requiring the cooperation of only a few elements; and difficult ones, requiring the systematization of an infinite number of elements, involving a very new and intricate synthesis in each operation. When the nervous tension or psychological force is lowered (by puberty, disease, fatigue, emotion, etc.) there is a general lowering of the mental level and only the simpler acts can be performed. Psychasthenia (including obsessions, compulsions, fears, and feelings of fatigue) results from a generalized lowering of the mental level; in hysteria, the lowering is localized in one particular function, which disappears (is dissociated) in consequence from the rest of the conscious personality.

Since Janet, there have been many other attempts at dynamic formulation of the neuroses, but Freud's concepts are probably the most widely accepted and the most complete explanations at the present time. They developed out of his clinical experience with hysteria, where Freud and Breuer found that hysterical symptoms disappear when the patient recalls, under hypnosis, previous experiences that have been forgotten. These experiences were found to be traumatic and sexual in nature, and this led Freud to pursue an investigation of sexuality. He described the various stages of development, from autoerotism to object love, and he noted that the various erotogenic zones, which originally are autonomous, are finally subordinated to the primacy of the genitals and reproduction. Not all of the instinctual energy associated with these various zones is useful for procreation, however, and normality as defined by our culture is achieved when these component instincts are repressed and diverted into sublimation. There are three stages in cultural development that correspond with this development of the sexual instinct: a stage in which the sexual impulse is allowed free rein regardless of its usefulness in procreation; a stage in which the whole of the sexual impulse is repressed except for that portion that subserves procreation; and a third stage in which procreation itself is limited by various factors. It is this latter that is our current civilized sexual morality. But constitutionally, Freud believed, not all people are capable even of the second stage and there thus arise two forms of deviation from normal sexuality—the perversions and the inversions (homosexuality). In the perversions, there has been fixation on an infantile aim; in the inversions, the sexual aim has been deflected from its normal object onto one of like sex. In both cases, those tendencies that conflict with the cultural norms may be completely repressed, but such repression requires all of the energy that would otherwise be used in cultural activities. If such repression is not achieved, the individual may remain in conflict with his culture (the overt perversions), or repression may be only partially successful. In the latter case, the inhibited sexual impulses (and the painful memory of infantile sex experiences) are not expressed as such but reappear in a disguised form (symptoms of neurosis). Thus the neuroses are seen to be the negative of the perversions. If this disguise takes the form of somatic symptoms, the clinical picture is that of conversion hysteria; if conversion is not achieved, the conflict between the repressed material and the ego leads to conscious fear that is bound to some specific and apparently indifferent content, and the clinical picture is that of anxiety hysteria; if the material is allowed to remain in consciousness but is deprived of its affective cathexis, the clinical picture is that of obsessive-compulsive neurosis.

The above represents Freud's earlier theory of neurosis. He later came to recognize that aggression as well as the sexual instinct is important in the etiology of the neuroses, and he elaborated his theory of the death instinct (Thanatos or Nirvana principle). At the present time in psychoanalysis, it is believed that the neurotic conflict is essentially between the id (sexual and/or aggressive instincts) and the ego, with the superego taking either side. The external world may represent temptation or punishment so that the conflict may appear to be between the world and the ego. The ego attempts to defend itself against the instinctual impulses and does so successfully in the case of sublimation; but if the defense is unsuccessful, the warding-off process must be maintained at a high level of countercathexis. To escape the defenses, the impulses attempt indirect discharge through substitute impulses—the *derivative*. The defensive system requires a damming up of tension and an inhibition of impulses; what then happens is that the original impulse manages to break through, in which case a symptom will be formed, or intensification of the defense will in itself constitute a symptom, or both of these may occur and the impulse will find a substitute outlet that helps to ward off the remainder of the impulse. Thus three main types of precipitating factors can be recognized in the neuroses: (1) an increase in the warded-off drive; (2)

a decrease in the warding-off forces; and (3) an increase in the warding-off forces. An increase in the instinctual energy may be absolute, as in puberty and the climacteric; or relative, as in the case of exposure to temptation, or devaluation of other drives whose energy is then displaced onto the warded-off drive, or blocking of instinctual satisfaction that has hitherto been obtainable, or blocking of any activity that has supplanted instinctual satisfaction. A decrease in the warding-off forces is seen in fatigue, intoxication, and when the ego is strengthened at one point and in its false confidence allows some of its censorial activities to lapse. An increase in warding-off forces is found in instances of increase in anxiety or guilt feelings, when any means of support or reassurance are lost, and, finally, a reactive increase is ordinarily seen after any temporary diminution.

The type of defense mechanism (i.e. the *choice of neurosis*) depends on the nature of the warded-off impulse, the age of the patient when the decisive conflict was experienced, the intensity and nature of the frustrating factors, the availability of substitute gratifications at the time of the frustration, and, particularly, the specific historical situation, which forces certain types of reaction.

General symptoms of the neurotic conflict include (1) specific avoidances; (2) inhibitions of partial instincts (such as smoking and eating), of aggressiveness, of sexualized functions, and of emotions; (3) sexual disturbances such as impotence, premature ejaculation, and frigidity; (4) lack of interest in the environment and general impoverishment of the personality due to the constant drain of energy necessary to maintain countercathexes, and awareness of this impoverishment gives rise to inferiority feelings; (5) use of emergency discharges for the relief of tension; and (6) sleep disturbances, because of the many dreams and because of the fear of the ego to relax its guard during sleep.

neurosis, actual In Freud's terminology, a true neurosis, i.e. symptoms that develop as a result of actual, true, or real disturbances of the sexual economy. Forced abstinence, frustrated sexual excitement, incomplete or interrupted coitus, sexual efforts that exceed the psychical capacity, sexual outlet rendered inadequate by guilt feelings or other conflicts, the need to revert to more primitive and/or less satisfactory means of sexual expression—these are the common "present-day" disturbances of sexuality that give rise to actual neurosis. Psychoneurosis, on the other hand, is determined by infantile and childhood experiences, and present-day occurrences are significant only in that they represent or repeat earlier events. Freud considered neurasthenia (a form of which is hypochondriasis) and anxiety neurosis as true or actual neuroses.

neurosis, alternation of *Obs.* This is an older expression "calling attention to the fact that nervous disorders are frequently relieved by acute bodily disease, so that persons suffering from insanity may be temporarily or even permanently cured by the occurrence of some acute bodily ailment." (Tuke, *DPM*) The more usual present-day term for this phenomenon is *pathocure* (q.v.).

neurosis, analytic A neurosis that develops subsequent to, and as a result of, interminable analysis. Stekel is of the opinion that after a too lengthy analysis, conducted over a period of many years, the patient, even if cured of his neurotic symptoms, "loses his natural attitude toward life, and what should have cured him becomes his illness." In this manner, after maintaining an emotional dependency for several years the patient develops toward analysis and analysts a special attitude that is called analytic neurosis. Similarly, the harmful effects upon psychic life produced by an analysis that is carried out without the necessary skill are also known as analytic, or postanalytic, neurosis. (Stekel, *CD*)

neurosis, anxiety See *anxiety neurosis*.

neurosis, artificial See *neurosis, experimental*.

neurosis, association See *association, psychosis of*.

neurosis, character Used by most authorities to refer to *personality disorders* (q.v.).

In psychoanalysis the expression has acquired a nosologic implication. A neurotic character, in terms of mental deviation, occupies a position between the healthy and the clear-cut neurotic personality. Apparently the difference is largely one of degree. Alexander says that the neurotic character is one who suffers "from no very definite symptoms of illness, but whose behavior in life is in the highest degree impulsive and frequently even compulsive." Jones claims that the neurotic character exhibits "manifestations intermediate between normal character traits and neurotic symptoms." (*Papers on Psycho-Analysis*, 1938)

The neurosis is, as Jones expresses it, "built into the character"; character traits acquire the significance of symptoms. For example, a person presenting no formal symptoms, but excessively pedantic, meticulous, and cruel in an intellectual way, is said to be a neurotic character and to exhibit a *character neurosis* (of the obsessive-compulsive type). See *defense, character*.

neurosis, choice of See *compliance, somatic; neurosis*.

neurosis, combat See *post-traumatic stress disorder; shellshock*.

neurosis, compensation 1. Kempf so classifies a neurosis in which there is "persistent striving to develop potent functions and win social esteem initiated by fear of impotence or loss of control of asocial cravings." (*PP*)

2. A form of traumatic neurosis induced by desire of monetary recompense. It is believed that some people after sustaining an injury may develop a neurosis in the hope of gaining financially (and otherwise) as a result of the injury. See *gain, epinosic*.

Compensation neurosis has been defined as "a state of mind, born out of fear, kept alive by avarice, stimulated by lawyers, and cured by verdict." The degree and duration of the neurosis are often inversely proportional to the extent of injury. See *hebephrenia, insurance; pathosis, attitudinal*.

neurosis, compulsion A mental disorder, characterized by an irrestible impulse to perform a morbid act or an act considered morbid by the subject. See *obsession; obsessive-compulsive psychoneurosis*.

In every compulsion-neurotic, Adler states, "there inheres the function of withdrawing from external compulsion, so that he may obey only his own compulsion. In other words, the compulsion-neurotic struggles so definitely against the will of another and against every foreign influ-

ence, that, in his fight against these, he comes to the point of positing his own will as sacred and irresistible." (*The Practice and Theory of Individual Psychology*, 1924)

neurosis, compulsive-obsessive See *neurosis, compulsion; obsessive-compulsive psychoneurosis*.

neurosis, contagiousness of The alleged but generally disputed capacity of a person's neurosis to affect another through contagion. It is theorized that in cases of hysteria and traumatic neurosis, there is a tendency for the patient to pick up additional symptoms from other patients who may be in the same ward.

neurosis, desire See *neurosis, compensation*.

neurosis, dissociation Dissociative disorder; hysterical neurosis, dissociative type. See *conversion; dissociation; dissociative disorders; hysteria*.

neurosis, ego Traumatic neurosis. This neurosis "differs in mental content from the non-traumatic psychoneuroses in that the conscious ego is more vividly disordered than are the unconscious parts of the mind." There may be, for example, disturbances of orientation and memory, even delirious states and extreme fatigue and weakness, throwing out of gear almost all of the ego. (Hinsie, *UP*) See *neurosis, traumatic*.

neurosis, esophageal Psychogenic disturbances of the swallowing functions of the esophagus, usually manifested by choking on food, inability to get it down, or the sensation of a foreign body in the upper region of the esophagus, the *globus hystericus*. The major unconscious emotional basis for the symptom is the rejection of, or defense against, the process of "incorporation," which represents a guilty oral aggressive (castrative) wish.

A patient prone to cunnilingus, associated with phantasies of oral castration (eating off the female phallus, i.e. clitoris), developed frequent severe choking spells while voraciously eating symbolic foods such as asparagus or melon at meals, following such sexual activity.

neurosis, existential Chronic meaninglessness, apathy, and aimlessness, which typically arise within a person who sees himself as nothing more than an embodiment of biologic needs and a player of social roles. See *existentialism*.

neurosis, expectation *Obs.* Anxiety that develops over the anticipated performance of an act; performance anxiety. Such anxiety is often a symptom of *agoraphobia* (q.v.).

neurosis, experimental *Artificial neurosis;* disorganized behavior that appears in the experimental subject in response to inability to master the experimental situation. Such behavior was noted by Pavlov in his dogs; when the animals were unable to discriminate between sounds of similar pitch or test objects of similar shape, they "went to pieces." Experimental neuroses have been induced in other animals as well—monkeys, chimpanzees, cats, goats, pigs, etc.

Neurotic symptoms are based on insufficiencies of the normal control apparatus and can be understood as involuntary emergency discharges that supplant the normal ones. The insufficiency may be brought about in two ways (which are not mutually exclusive)—too much excitation may be presented so that it cannot be mastered, as in traumatic neurosis; or a previous blocking or inadequacy of discharge may lead to an accumulation of tensions within the organism so that previously innocuous stimuli may release them and thus operate as though they were traumatic. The experimental neurosis is an example of this second type. "Some stimulus which had represented pleasant instinctual experiences or which had served as a signal that some action would now procure gratification is suddenly connected by the experimenter with frustrating or threatening experiences, or the experimenter decreases the difference between stimuli which the animal had been trained to associate with instinct gratification and threat respectively; the animal then gets into a state of irritation which is very similar to that of a traumatic neurosis. He feels contradictory impulses; the conflict makes it impossible for him to give in to the impulses in the accustomed way; the discharge is blocked, and this decrease in discharge works in the same way as an increase in influx; it brings the organism into a state of tension and calls for emergency discharges." (Fenichel, *PTN*)

neurosis, fate Failure in one's career as a result of unconscious need for punishment; a type of moral masochism. See *destiny, neurosis of; masochism.*

neurosis, holiday See *neurosis, Sunday.*

neurosis, housewife's Also called *housewife's psychosis;* a compulsion neurosis characterized by constant preoccupation with cleaning house. Though justified by the patient, who explains that these exaggerated domestic activities are necessary in view of the danger inherent in the lack of hygiene in the place where she lives, in reality they constitute an external disguise of obsessive ideas concealed by the patient. According to Stekel, the inner "compulsions are covered up for many years until the decrease of the patient's working capacity, or the danger of complete isolation force the patient to confess her illness to other people." (*CD*) This is often the personality type of the woman who later develops an involutional psychosis.

More recently, the term *housewife's disease* or *housewife's syndrome* has been applied to a state of acute or chronic dissatisfaction and frustration that appears in some women as a type of mental stagnation secondary to marriage, motherhood, and separation from the stimulation of employment and free movement among people. Typical symptoms are loss of libido and fatigability at age 24–30, backache at age 30–35, and general somatic overconcern at age 40–55.

neurosis, iatrogenic See *iatrogeny.*

neurosis, indemnity Levy-Bruhl's term for compensation neurosis.

neurosis, infantile The neurosis that is to become manifest in the adult and is already present in the infant even though the symptoms are so mild that they go unnoticed.

neurosis, infinity Neurotic preoccupation with the infinity of space and time, usually encountered in adolescents and/or as an expression of an autistic, dereistic approach to life; *apeirophobia.*

neurosis insana *Obs.* Psychoneurosis.

neurosis, malignant A neurosis characterized by a progressive increase in the extent and severity of symptoms, which may ultimately prevent the performance of any activity. The patient may become a prisoner in his room or in his bed, or he may be paralyzed by indecisiveness and doubting. Many such cases are in actuality schizophrenics. See *agoraphobia; neurosis, progredient; schizophrenia, pseudoneurotic.*

Malignant neurosis is to be contrasted with *stationary neurosis,* in which the defenses operate successfully without further increase in anxiety or other symptoms.

neurosis, military War neurosis; *shellshock* (q.v.). See *post-traumatic stress disorder.*

neurosis, mixed In Freud's earliest psychoanalytic communications this (now infrequent) term denoted a neurosis that contained phenomena of two or more subdivisions of the neuroses. It is now recognized that many of these more properly belong to the schizophrenic group, and particularly to the subtype described by Hoch and Polatin, the pseudoneurotic schizophrenias. See *personality disorders; schizophrenia, latent; schizophrenia, pseudoneurotic.*

neurosis, motor A neurosis characterized principally by disorders of movement, such as tics.

neurosis, obsessional See *obsessive-compulsive psychoneurosis.*

neurosis, occlusal Grinding, pounding, or setting of the teeth, when the mouth is empty; that is, entirely apart from the perfectly normal activity of mastication. *Bruxism* is an occlusal neurosis occurring during the night.

neurosis, occupational A psychogenic inhibition of actions that are essential to the performance of the patient's occupation, such as writer's cramp (a painful spasm of the muscles of the fingers used in writing), seamstress's cramp, or musician's cramp. Such inhibitions of working often represent oral conflicts over dependence and independence, or anal conflicts over rebellion and obedience. See *inhibition, occupational.*

neurosis, organ See *psychosomatic.*

neurosis, parent as carrier of "The most common types of such parental carriers of neurosis to the children are : (a) The 'cold' parents, who cannot give the warmth and love the children need; (b) the over-indulgent parents, who cannot expose their children to the disciplines and reality frustrations necessary to the child's development of adult survival traits; (c) the sexually frustrated parents, who displace their sexual needs onto the establishment

of an over-intense emotional bond to their children as a substitute love-object; (d) the unconsciously hating parent, who visits repressed and denied aggression and hostility on his child, expressing repressed and denied jealousy and rivalry." (Weiss, E., & English, O. *Psychosomatic Medicine,* 1949)

neurosis, pension See *gain, epinosic; neurosis, compensation.*

neurosis, performance A mental disturbance that may take place in the course of any performance whose normal execution requires any degree of spontaneity. An illustration is an attack of trembling overcoming a violinst while playing. See *neurosis, occupational.*

neurosis, perhaps A type of obsessive neurosis, as exemplified in the formula: "*If* I had done this instead of that, *perhaps* my sister would still be alive."

neurosis, population *Obs.* A collective or group neurosis prevailing in the populace of a locality; group hysteria. See *psychosis, collective.*

neurosis, post-traumatic Traumatic neurosis. See *post-traumatic and postencephalitic syndromes, classification of; post-traumatic stress disorder.*

neurosis, postconcussion A form of traumatic neurosis following cerebral concussion. Depending upon the history, physical findings, and symptom picture presented the condition may be considered primarily organic (*organic personality syndrome* or mixed organic brain syndrome) or primarily psychologic (*post-traumatic stress disorder*).

neurosis, prison See *chronophobia.*

neurosis, progredient A neurosis that takes a progressive course, with increasing severity of symptoms. See *neurosis, malignant.*

In progredient neurosis, the damming-up of instincts increases more and more. Because there is neither adequate discharge nor adequate defense, the neurosis becomes increasingly severe. For example, at first a phobic patient may not be able to walk across a particular square. Later on he cannot go out of doors, and finally, perhaps, not even out of his room. In the case of the compulsion-neurotic, ambivalences and doubts increase, until no decision whatsoever can be made.

Another type of progression may occur

when neuroses that have been stationary for a time suddenly become progredient again. A compulsive equilibrium may change into uncontrollable vegetative attacks, or a rigid character neurosis into a symptom neurosis with anxiety attacks, depressions, or other symptoms.

neurosis, promotion Inability to function when given added responsibility or authority; seen most often in obsessional neurotics. See *success, failure through.*

neurosis, pseudoschizophrenic Roth's term for the phobic anxiety-depersopalization neurosis. See *depersonalization.*

neurosis, regression According to Kempf's classification of neuroses, this subdivision is characterized by "failure to compensate but regression to a preceding, more comfortable, irresponsible level, permitting wish-fulfilling fancies, postures and indulgences." The symptoms are built around "distressing visceral tensions, rare, but persistent maintenance of characteristic affective attitudes of the prenatal, infantile or preadolescent stage." (*PP*)

neurosis, repression A neurosis in which there is "vague consciousness to total unconsciousness of the nature and influence of the ungratifiable affective cravings." The symptoms are the same as those in the suppression neurosis "plus functional distortions of the projicient apparatus and changes in reactivity to the sense organs." (Kempf, *PP*)

neurosis, social Burrow's term for the common condition of disorder and conflict that exists throughout the social structure, though generally unrecognized by society. It is expressed symptomatically in nervous and mental disorder and also in so-called normal human interrelations—in peaceful social institutions, in economic conflict, crime, and war.

neurosis, space See *neurosis, infinity.*

neurosis, substitution *Obs.* Obsessional neurosis.

neurosis, Sunday Any psychiatric symptom or syndrome that is triggered or exacerbated by particular days or dates; called Sunday neurosis because of the frequency with which that day appears to be the significant one. The most frequent symptoms are feelings of uneasiness, dissatisfaction, dejection, and fear of what the future may bring. In some affective disorders,

recurrence of a manic or depressive episode seems to be an *anniversary reaction* (q.v.) that occurs at the same time of year as the significant past event.

neurosis, suppression From the standpoint of Kempf's psychopathology, in a suppression-neurosis there is "clear to vague consciousness of the nature and effect of the ungratifiable affective cravings." The symptoms are said to be due to "distressing hypertensions or hypotensions of autonomic (visceral) segments (mild to severe)." (*PP*)

neurosis, transference A "new artificial neurosis," occurs only during psychoanalytic treatment. It is the reappearance of the early infantile Oedipus situation. The analyst represents one or both parents as a love object, as if he were really the original parent in the original infantile setting of the patient. The patient also lives out all his old ego attitudes and incest prohibitions. See *transference.*

Transference neurosis represents a stage where the history of the patient's development, leading up to the infantile neurosis, is reenacted in the analytic room—the patient plays the part of actor-manager, pressing into service (like the child in the nursery) all the stage property that the analytical room contains, first and foremost the analyst.

neurosis, traumatic A psychogenic or nonstructural nervous disorder, shortly following a physical injury. Current thinking emphasizes the importance of psychologic rather than physical trauma as necessary for the development of the disorder. See *post-traumatic stress disorder; stasis, libido.*

While a traumatic experience can precipitate any of the well-known types of neurotic or psychotic disorders, the most common conditions seen in combat are hysteria, anxiety states, and exhaustion conditions. The essential features of traumatic neurosis are (1) fixation on the trauma with amnesia for the traumatic situation that may be total or partial; (2) typical dream life (dreams of annihilation, aggression dreams where the patient is the aggressor but is defeated, frustration or Sisyphus dreams, and occupational dreams in which it is the means of livelihood rather than the body-ego that is annihilated); (3) contraction of the general level of functioning, with constant fear of the environment, disorganized behavior, lowered efficiency, lack of coordinated goal activities, and profoundly altered functioning in the autonomic, motor, and sensory nervous system; (4) general irritability; and (5) a proclivity to explosive aggressive reactions. A malignant type of traumatic neurosis, *psychorrhexis* (q.v.), is seen in 2 to 3% of war neuroses.

neurosis, vagabond See *dromomania.*

neurosis, vegetative The expression of emotion, or unconscious emotional conflict, by disturbed functioning of the internal visceral organs. The term is usually employed in contradistinction to conversion hysteria: whereas conversion hysteria takes place in the voluntary neuromuscular, or sensory perceptive system, the vegetative neurosis has its site in the internal visceral organs. See *psychosomatic.*

It is found that chronic repressed, suppressed, and denied resentment and anger are invariable factors in the personality reactions of people with essential hypertension (high blood pressure). Similarly, those developing duodenal ulcer seem to suffer from longstanding chronic conflict between independency-aggressive strivings and dependency-submissive trends. "A vegetative neurosis is not an attempt to express an emotion, but is the physiological response of the vegetative organs to constant, or to periodically returning, emotional states." (Alexander, F. *Psychosomatic Medicine,* 1950)

Sometimes used synonymously with *acrodynia* (q.v.).

neurosis, wish Bing thus denotes a traumatic neurosis in which the wish to be afflicted seems to constitute the essential etiology; *traumatic hysteria.*

neurosthenia *Obs.* Excessive quantity of so-called nervous energy.

neurosurgery, functional *Psychosurgery* (q.v.).

neurosyphilis A generic term for all forms of involvement of the nervous system by the spirochaeta pallida.

neurosyphilis, asymptomatic Neurosyphilis without clinical symptoms but with physical signs and laboratory findings of syphilitic involvement of the nervous system.

neurosyphilis, congenital Intrauterine infection of the nervous system by the spiro-

chete; sometimes mistakenly called *inherited syphilis.* Approximately 10% of congenitally syphilitic children develop neurosyphilis, which, as in adult neurosyphilis, may be of the meningovascular or the parenchymatous type. Meningovascular syphilis is the more common form and resembles the adult form in pathology and clinical manifestations; these include mental retardation, convulsions, pupillary abnormalities, optic atrophy, diplegia or hemiplegia, and slight hydrocephalus of the communicating type. Deafness, a common symptom of congenital syphilis, is more often due to a temporal bone lesion than to N. VIII involvement. See *syphilis, cerebral.*

Juvenile or *infantile general paresis* probably occurs in no more than 1% of congenital syphilitics. Symptoms typically develop in early adolescence and mimic those of adult paretics except that the delusions are more puerile, the dementia is more complete and severe, and the course is more prolonged.

Congenital tabes often does not appear until early adult life. Symptoms mimic those of adult tabetics.

neurosyphilis, ectodermogenic Cerebrospinal syphilis. See *syphilis, cerebral.*

neurosyphilis, interstitial See *syphilis, cerebral.*

neurosyphilis, meningeal Tertiary syphilis involving the leptomeninges (the pia mater and arachnoid membrane). See *syphilis, cerebral.*

neurosyphilis, parenchymatous (par-eng-kī'mà-tus) A general term that includes paresis, tabes, taboparesis, and juvenile general paresis. See *paresis, general.*

neurosyphilis, vascular See *syphilis, cerebral.*

neurotic disorder *Neurosis* (q.v.). See *disorder, neurotic.*

neurotic process See *disorder, neurotic; self, actual.*

neurotigenic Producing or favoring the induction of a neurosis.

neurotization Direct implantation of nerve into a paralyzed muscle.

neurotransmission Propagation of an impulse along a nerve fiber, which is mediated electrically, and from one neuron to another across the synapse. Synaptic transmission is mediated chemically, by *neurotransmitter* (q.v.).

neurotransmitter A chemical messenger that carries information from one neuron to another at the synapse, sometimes referred to as a *neurohumor*. The neurotransmitter is synthesized within the neuron, stored in vesicles in the *bouton* (q.v.), and is released into the synaptic cleft when the bouton is depolarized. It binds to receptor sites in the postsynaptic cell and thereby exerts its effect on the cell ligand. See *conduction, nerve; neuroanatomy, chemical; neurohormone; process, elementary; synapse.*

Three categories of neurotransmitter are recognized:

1. *Biogenic amines,* which provide diffuse innervation throughout the neuroaxis; included within this group are dopamine, norepinephrine, *epinephrine, serotonin, acetylcholine* (qq.v.), and histamine.

2. *Amino acids,* which exert discrete excitatory or inhibitory effects within the nervous system; included within this group are aspartic acid, gamma-aminobutyric acid (GABA), glutamic acid, glycine, homocysteine, taurine.

3. *Neuropeptides,* which often act as co-transmitters with modulatory function; included within this group are angiotension, β-endorphin, bombesin, bradykinin, choecystokinin, corticotropin-releasing factor, dynorphin, gastrin, leucine-enkephalin, methionine-enkephalin, somatostatin, substance P, thyrotropin-releasing factor, vasoactive intestinal peptide, vasopressin. See *peptide, brain.*

Snyder estimated (1980) that known peptide transmitters represent 10% or less of the total that will be identified.

neurotrophasthenia *Obs.* Defective nutrition of the nervous system.

neurypnology *Obs.* Braid's term for the science of hypnosis.

neutrality The role of the therapist in activity group psychotherapy: here he is not only passive and permissive, but neither has nor applies criteria of right and wrong, proper and improper behavior on the part of the patient. According to Slavson, neutrality of therapist means "that each patient can utilize him in accordance with his own particular needs. Each member of the group projects on the therapist his unconscious attitudes toward adults. Neutrality on the part of the therapist makes this possible." (*IGT*)

neutralization In psychoanalysis, neutralization includes both *desexualization* and *desaggressivization* (qq.v.). "The term neutralization implies that an activity of the individual which originally afforded drive satisfaction through discharge of cathexis ceases to do so and comes to be in the service of the ego, apparently nearly or quite independent of the need for gratification or discharge of cathexis in anything which even approaches its original instinctual form." (Brenner, C. *An Elementary Textbook of Psychoanalysis,* 1955)

neutralizer A member of a therapy group who neutralizes, i.e. counteracts and controls, the aggressivity, impulsiveness, and destructiveness of other members of the group. See *instigator; isolate.*

névrospasmie *Obs.* Neurasthenia.

new health practitioners Medical paraprofessionals, including nurse practitioners and physician's assistants.

newborn screening See *screening, genetic.*

nexus Linkage of thoughts.

NFD Neurofibrillary degeneration, whose degree is positively correlated with the severity of neuropsychological impairment in *senile dementia* and *Alzheimer's disease* (qq.v.). Some workers claim that NFD is the primary neuropathology in over 80% of senile dementia, which is viewed as progressive "alzheimerization" of brain tissue, a secondary result of which is reduction in cerebral blood flow. There is also some suggestive evidence that aluminum may play some etiologic role in the pathogenesis of NFD.

NFT Neurofibrillary tangle, first described by Alzheimer in 1907, characteristic of the brains of patients with senile dementia, Alzheimer type (SDAT), where their density in the hippocampus is 6 to 40 times greater than that of nondemented age-matched subjects. Also known as *paired helical filaments (PHF)*, the tangles consist of massive proliferation of intracytoplasmic material containing unusual, cementlike protein that the neuron apparently cannot break down. There is some evidence that aluminum may play some role in the pathogenesis of the tangles, but how significant a factor it may be is controversial.

NFTT Nonorganic failure to thrive. See *failure to thrive.*

NGI, NGRI Not guilty by reason of insanity; insanity defense, insanity plea.

nicotinic See *acetylcholine.*

nicotinic acid deficiency Pellagra; symptoms of this disorder, which occurs nowadays primarily in alcoholics, include appearance of sucking and grasping reflexes, cogwheel rigidity of the extremities, progressive clouding of consciousness, and memory defects (which may persist despite otherwise successful treatment). Manic or melancholic states may also be seen, and there are usually accompanying diarrhea and skin lesions.

Niemann-Pick disease See *disease, Niemann-Pick.*

night-eating See *syndrome, night-eating.*

night hospital See *day hospital.*

night phantasy See *phantasy, night.*

night terror See *terror, night or sleep.*

nightmare A fright reaction during sleep. "In the nightmare (*ephialtes, incubus*) the child awakens in terror from a dream usually characterized by a feeling of suffocation and helplessness. He can ordinarily relate his bad dream; he is well oriented, can recognize people about him, and can be calmed readily. Nightmares are often very vivid and the memory of them accompanied by a sense of dread, sometimes recurs the following day when the child is awake. They are not uncommon and generally take place within an hour or two after going to bed." (Bakwin, H., & Bakwin, R. *Clinical Management of Behavior Disorders in Children*, 1953) See *terror, night or sleep.*

When nightmares are recurrent, in children or adults, they are termed *dream anxiety disorder* in DSM-III-R. The dream content typically involves threats to survival, security, or self-esteem and the memory of it, or the interference with sleep caused by it, cause significant distress. The awakenings usually occur during the second half of the sleep period.

nightshade poisoning See *poisoning, deadly nightshade.*

nihilism The delusion of nonexistence. The delusion may be widespread in the sense that it includes everything—the patient himself and the entire world—or it may refer only to parts of the world or of himself.

nihilistic delusion See *syndrome, Cotard's.*

NIMH-DIS National Institute of Mental Health Diagnostic Interview Schedule; a highly structured interview developed for use by lay interviewers in large-scale epidemiologic surveys in the United States. It is a modification of the SADS and the *Research Diagnostic Criteria* (q.v.).

Nirvana Death, extinction; oblivion to care, pain, or external reality.

In psychoanalysis the expression *Nirvana principle* (suggested by Barbara Low) is explained by Freud as a manifestation of the action of the death instinct, "the aim of which is to lead our throbbing existence into the stability of an inorganic state." Freud maintains that "the *Nirvana*-principle expresses the tendency of the death-instinct, the *pleasure*-principle represents the claims of the libido, and that modification of it, the *reality*-principle, the influence of the outer world." (*CP*) See *instinct, death.*

NMR Nuclear magnetic resonance; used in imaging or scanner systems; also called *MRI* (magnetic resonance imaging).

Brain *imaging* is a computer-assisted graphic representation of brain structure and function. Computer graphics uses colors to represent a range of numbers in measuring the phenomenon under study; measurements are taken at different positions in space and the computer constructs a colored picture representing the structure or function being measured. The two major types of imaging are tomographic methods and surface imaging methods.

Tomographic methods of brain imaging include X-ray computed tomography (CT scan), NMR, and positron emission tomography (PET). They are able to measure at closely spaced intervals and yield pictures that resemble slices of a brain. In CT, a rotating X-ray beam slices through the body in the desired plane while detectors on the opposite side of the patient record the degree to which the radiation is absorbed or attenuated by the tissues. The computer uses these density recordings to construct an image.

Surface imaging methods include regional cerebral blood flow (rCBF) and computer electroencephalographic topography (CET). See *neurometrics.*

NMR uses magnetic fields instead of radiation to produce diagnostic images similar to CT scans. In NMR, the patient is placed in a magnet that first aligns some of his hydrogen nuclei (protons), then disrupts that alignment with an energizing radio signal that temporarily excites the protons. As the signal ends, the protons surrender their excess energy while wobbling back into alignment. The computer converts these excess energy signals into an image. NMR scans take several minutes to produce their images as compared with the several seconds required for CT scans. NMR differentiates better than CT does between white and gray matter in the brain, and it may replace CT scanning except where very high resolution or information about cortical bone is needed.

Another imaging modality is PET, which provides slice images of any chemical tagged with a radioisotope. Low atomic weight isotopes with short half-lives are used. As they decay, positrons are emitted and interact with electrons in the brain. With the resulting annihilation two photons are emitted and travel in opposite directions. Detector crystals, located in a ring around the head, respond to the arrival of the photons on opposite sides of the ring and provide a highly precise reconstruction of the density of the isotopes. Because of the short half-life of the isotopes used, the technique requires a cyclotron to produce positron emitters and a radiochemistry laboratory for rapid synthesis of radiopharmaceuticals.

Single photon emission computed tomography (SPECT) employs a radiopharmaceutical agent such as isopropyl-iodoamphetamine or radioactive gas such as xenon-133 in combination with a scanning machine.

Another imaging technique is digital subtraction angiography (DSA), in which fluoroscopic images are converted into digital information. Before contrast material is introduced, a radiographic image is taken of the area in which the blood vessels under investigation are located. Images made after contrast material is injected are compared with the before image, and anything common to both is "subtracted" from the image. What remains is an image of the vessel through which the contrast material flows.

Surface imaging methods are less precise than tomographic methods. Typically they use between 16 and 32 sensors or detectors, and values for the intervening positions are filled by interpolation to produce a picture. In CET, the EEG or evoked potential is recorded at the 16 or more locations, and the amount of activity of each EEG frequency (alpha, delta, theta, etc.) is measured at each position. The brain map contains as many as several thousand tiny squares, called *pixels* (picture elements). For the 16 or more squares which have values recorded by the sensors, the color represents the exact measurement; for the pixels between those 16 to 32 "absolute" values, the color is interpolated by calculating the distance of each pixel from three or four closest squares with a known value. CET is less costly than PET, can be repeated any number of times without risk, and is about 100 times more rapid than PET.

NMS See *syndrome, neuroleptic malignant.*

noasthenia *Obs.* Mental debility; *neurasthenia* (q.v.).

nocar (nō′kēr) *Obs.* Lethargy.

noctambulation Night-walking; sleepwalking; *somnambulism* (q.v.).

noctiphobia See *nyctophobia.*

nocturnal hemiplegia or paralysis See *paralysis, sleep.*

nocturnal myoclonus See *sleep disorders.*

nocturnal penile tumescence See *tumescence, penile.*

nodal behavior See *behavior, nodal.*

-noea (-nē′à) Variant of *-noia* (q.v.).

noematic Relating to the mental processes.

Noguchi, Hideyo (1876–1928) Japanese bacteriologist, worked in New York, demonstrated spirochetes in brain of paretics (1911). Until this discovery, syphilis was not recognized as the etiologic agent in general paresis but was thought merely to predispose to its development.

-noia (-noi′à) Combining form meaning mind, mental state, from Gr. (*para*)*noia*, from *nóos, noûs.*

nomadism A pathological tendency to roam from place to place, which is so strong that it gives rise to serious social maladjustment. "Occasional and episodic nomadism apparently arises on the basis of a mental mechanism similar to that underlying resorting to alcohol or drugs. It is often associated with mental deficiency, epilepsy, and psychotic disease. It is not infrequently seen in children as residuals of epidemic encephalitis and may be part of the clinical picture of the residuals of cerebral birth trauma." (Selling, L.S. *Synopsis of Neuropsychiatry*, 1947) See *dromomania; wanderlust.*

nomenclature See *nosology.*

nomenclature, 1968 revision (DSM-II) This classification is based on the Section on Mental Disorders of the World Health Organization's Eighth Revision of the *International Classification of Diseases (ICD-8)*, which was adopted in May 1966, to become effective in 1968. The major deviations from ICD-7 are: (1) mental retardation is placed first in the listing, to emphasize that it is to be diagnosed whenever present and whatever its cause; (2) nonpsychotic organic brain syndromes are also placed out of numerical order so as to keep all the organic brain syndromes together, as is customary in the United States; (3) multiple psychiatric diagnoses are encouraged when one will not suffice to account adequately for the clinical picture; and (4) a fifth coding digit was introduced to provide further specification of additional characteristics of mental disorders—in ICD-8, the first three digits designate the major disease category; the fourth digit (which follows the period) specifies additional detail (such as etiology); and in the U.S. nomenclature, an additional fifth digit allows still greater detailing. Thus .x1 indicates acute, .x2 indicates chronic; .x5 indicates in remission.

nomenclature, 1980 revision *DSM-III* (q.v.).

nomological *Nomothetic* (q.v.).

nomothetic Giving or generating laws; legislative; in psychiatry, used particularly to refer to the deriving of general laws through observation of many cases, as contrasted with the *ideographic* approach, which is concerned with the explanation and prediction of behavior in the single or unique case (usually on the basis of extensive knowledge of the history and biography of the person).

non compos mentis Not of sound mind, mentally incapable of managing one's affairs. See *incompetence.*

non-winner See *transactional analysis.*

nondirective therapy See *therapy, client-centered.*

nondisjunction Failure to separate normally; used to refer to a chromosomal abnormality in which the two members of a given pair of chromosomes fail to separate during cell division. As a result, two abnormal gametes are formed: one with both members of a chromosomal pair instead of only one, and the other with neither. When such abnormal gametes unite with a normal sperm or ovum during fertilization, the resulting zygote will contain either one too many chromosomes (in the human, 47 instead of 46), or one too few. Cells of both types may be formed in the same person, and each may perpetuate its line so that the person has cells of two (or more) types; such a condition is referred to as *mosaicism.*

nonmalfeasance See *beneficence.*

nonrecognition Loss of familiarity with objects or people, suggestive of dysfunction of the nondominant parietal lobe. It can occur in various forms, such as *anosognosia* (failure to recognize serious medical disability), *prosopagnosia* (failure to recognize familiar people and faces), and *spatial nonrecognition* (failure to recognize one side of one's body, or objects in one side of the visual field).

nonrecombinant See *linkage; recombination.*

nonregressive schizophrenia More frequently used by Nordic or Scandinavian workers than in the United States to refer to borderline schizophrenia. See *dishabituation.*

nonreporting See *psychodynamics, adaptational.*

nonreproductive As used by G.E. Hutchinson (*American Naturalist 93*, 1959), descriptive of any form of sexuality that would currently fall under the label *paraphilia* (q.v.). According to his usage, homosexuality was included within the more general term "nonreproductive sexuality." By some, nonreproductiveness is used as an indicator of the "unnaturalness" of certain types of sexual activity. See *unnatural.*

nonrestraint Management of the psychotic patient without the use of the strait jacket or other forms of restraint.

nonsense syndrome See *syndrome, Ganser.*

nonspecific research. See *research, specific.*

nonsystematic schizophrenia See *schizophrenia, systematic.*

nontranssexual cross-gender disorder See *transsexualism.*

nooklopia *Obs.* N. Lewis defines the term as *thought theft obsessions,* i.e. the delusion that "one's thoughts are being sucked out of his brain by some sinister personal magnetism." (*Psychoanalytic Review XV,* 1928) Also known as *castrophrenia.* See *symptoms, first-rank.*

noology The doctrine of the mind; the science of the understanding.

noopsyche *Rare.* Stransky coined this term with the idea that there are two separate psychic factors: (1) the *noopsyche,* comprising all purely intellectual processes, and (2) the *thymopsyche,* made up of affective processes. In his opinion, intrapsychic ataxia, which results in marked incongruity between ideas and emotions, is a consequence of the more or less independent activities of the two psychic factors.

noosphales *Obs.* Mentally deranged.

noosteresis *Obs.* Dementia.

nootropic Affecting the mind, especially the intellectual aspects (cognition, memory, understanding, etc.); used to describe drugs that improve cognitive functioning in the organically impaired.

noradrenalin Norepinephrine. See *epinephrine.*

norepinephrine See *epinephrine.*

norm, psychic A psychically normal person is one who is in harmony with himself and with his environment. He conforms with the cultural requirements or injunctions of his community. He may possess organic deviation or disease, but as long as this does not impair his reasoning, judgment, intellectual capacity, and ability to make harmonious personal and social adaptation he may be regarded as psychically sound or normal.

It appeared that normality developed as the result of repression of certain component-instincts and components of the infantile disposition, and of a subordination of the remainder under the primacy of the genital zone in the service of the reproductive function. (Freud, *CP*) This means harmonious relationship of the forces of the id, superego, and ego. "The original urges are not unhealthily inhibited, but rather are domesticated in the service of the individual and society." (Healy et al., *SMP*) See *health, mental.*

normative ethics See *ethics.*

normative-referenced See *test.*

normatology The study of normal behavior and development, with emphasis on data obtained from people who are not patients.

normosplanchnic In Viola's system of constitutional forms of body build, this term denotes the type that has a normal or average relationship between thoracic and abdominal size, owing to medium size of the abdominal and thoracic viscera. This type is further characterized by a proportionality between vertical and horizontal diameters, resulting in a harmonious physique. Persons of this type correspond roughly to Kretschmer's athletic type. See *type, athletic.*

normothymotic Mood normalizer; specifically a pharmacologic agent that acts against a disorder of mood but does not affect normal mood.

normotonic In Tandler's system of constitutional types, a type characterized by normal or average tone of the voluntary muscles, in contrast to the *hypotonic* and *hypertonic* types.

normotype In constitutional medicine a term for the structurally or morphologically average person. It is synonymous with *eumorphic.*

normotypical In constitutional medicine three types of body build are recognized: (1) dolichomorphic or longitypical; (2) brachymorphic or brachytypical; (3) eumorphic, normotypical, or normosplanchnic.

norms See *review.*

Norrie's disease See *disease, Norrie's.*

nos(o)- Combining form meaning sickness, disease, from Gr. *nósos.*

nosocomion, nosocomium Where illnesses are taken care of, hence a hospital or sanatorium. The adjective *nosocomial* means relating to a hospital but most commonly is used in a specific sense to refer to a hospital-induced condition that is unrelated to the patient's primary condition. See *iatrogeny.*

nosogenesis, nosogeny Synonymous with *pathogenesis* (q.v.).

nosography The description of diseases.

nosology The study of diseases and, in particular, their classification, grouping, ordering, and relationship to one another; it includes the formulation of principles for differentiating one disease from another.

Ideally, nosology would provide a differentiation of discrete diseases and for each describe a specific cause, the typical clinical picture, its natural history and outcome, objective tests for its confirmation, and specific treatments.

Nosology, classification, nomenclature, and diagnosis are related, and to some extent overlapping, terms that refer to various aspects of the conceptualization of disease. *Classification* is the grouping of diseases according to a logical scheme for organizing and classifying them and assigning them their proper places.

Diagnosis is the process of distinguishing or recognizing the presence of disease from its symptoms or part-manifestations. The term is also applied to the end result of that process, a summary statement of the conclusion to which the process leads. Some prefer the term *assessment* for the process of collecting information relevant to the diagnosis, management, and treatment of the patient's clinical condition, and diagnosis for the process of using pertinent information to assign the patient to a specific nosological class or disorder.

Nomenclature is the label or term that is used to communicate the results of the diagnostic process. It is a shorthand name for the disease that has been identified. The term implies, in addition, that there is reason for using one term rather than another (e.g. Down's syndrome rather than mongolism, schizophrenia rather than dementia praecox, multi-infarct dementia rather than cerebral arteriosclerosis).

nosomania *Obs.* Hypochondriasis (q.v.).

nosophobia Fear of disease; usually associated with no discoverable organic illness, or if the latter is present, the fear is grossly exaggerated and has been superimposed upon natural concern about the illness.

nostalgia Longing to return home or to one's native land; homesickness. This is explained by psychoanalysts as intense yearning for the members of one's family or for some particular member of the family. It is related to the dread of being alone, which is but another way of saying that the subject feels at ease when he is with someone to whom he is emotionally bound.

nostomania *Obs.* An intense form of nostalgia; an irresistible impulse to return home.

nostras(is)ia *Obs.* Nostalgia.

not-me In Sullivan's system, symbolic representation of previous (usually infantile) interpersonal events that were associated with such overwhelming anxiety that they were dissociated from conscious awareness and memory; when the symbolic representations of such experiences threaten to invade consciousness (as in dreams, nightmares, fatigue states, intoxications, and schizophrenic reactions), the subject feels that the experience is foreign, unreal, and "not-me," and typically also is flooded with one or another of what Sullivan termed the "uncanny emotions"—awe, dread, horror, loathing. The feeling of unfamiliarity or foreignness is the opposite of *déjà vu* (q.v.), although in both phenomena the accompanying feelings are typically of the uncanny variety.

Nothnagel, Carl Wilhelm Hermann (not'nägel) (1841–1905) Austrian neurologist; described angiospastic acroparesthesia and a cerebral peduncle syndrome that bears his name, consisting of unilateral oculomotor paralysis combined with cerebellar ataxia.

notogenesis The later stages of *gastrulation* (q.v.) , in which the *notochord*, or embryonic backbone, is formed. This period is associated with the appearance and development of the third germ layer, the *mesoderm* (q.v.).

Subsequently, at a stage overlapping the next salient step of development, *cephalogenesis* (q.v.), the plates of the mesoderm become differentiated into a more robust *medial* portion, and a thinner *lateral* portion, the two connected by a constricted plate of the original mesoderm.

noumenal Intellectually, not sensuously, intuitional; relating to the object of pure thought divorced from all concepts of time or space.

novelty In information theory, *incongruity* (q.v.).

noxa Any injurious agent, mental or physical.

NPH Normal-pressure hydrocephalus; also known as Hakim's disease. See *hydrocephalus, normal-pressure*.

NPT Nocturnal penile tumescence. See *tumescence, penile*.

NREM Nonrapid eye movement. NREM sleep includes the four quiet stages of sleep. See *REM*.

NTD *Neural tube defect* (q.v.).

nuclear Pertaining to, or having the character of, a nucleus.

nuclear family See *conjugal unit, isolated*.

nuclear imaging See *encephalography, radioisotopic*.

nucleus In the minute structure of a typical cell, the nucleus is a denser body in the midst of its protoplasm, usually rounded in form and representing the directive center of most cellular activities. As it governs the mitotic process of cell division, it plays a decisive role in the chromosomal mechanism of hereditary transmission. See *chromosome*.

The actual seat of the genetic elements in the nucleus is a fine reticulum of various protein substances that stain very readily and are collectively called the *chromatin*. In addition to this chromatin network, the nucleus contains not only a liquid in which the chromatin floats, but frequently also one or more dense, rounded bodies, the *nucleoli*.

In a resting cell, the nucleus is surrounded by a thin membrane, the tension of which tends to keep the nucleus round. All cytoplasmic substances entering the nucleus must pass through this membrane.

nucleus, caudate See *basal ganglia*.

nucleus, dentate See *cerebellum*.

nucleus, Edinger-Westphal See *accommodation*.

nucleus, emboliform See *cerebellum*.

nucleus fastigius See *cerebellum*.

nucleus globosus See *cerebellum*.

nucleus pulposus See *disk, herniated lumbar intervertebral*.

nucleus ruber Red nucleus. See *midbrain*.

null hypothesis In statistics, the hypothesis that the true difference between any two samples or populations is zero, and that any apparent difference between them is due to chance. When the null hypothesis can be rejected at a high level of confidence, the difference is said to be statistically significant.

numbness, sleep See *paralysis, sleep*.

Nunberg, Herman (1884–1970) German-born U.S. psychoanalyst; synthetic function of ego.

nurse practitioner A registered nurse who has had special training in an approved continuing or graduate education program to provide primary care or special services. The nurse practitioner, although considerably more independent than the graduate nurse, usually works under the supervision of a physician. See *extender, physician*.

nursing facilities See *domicile*.

nyctalopia Night-blindness; inability to see well at night or in dim light; sometimes due to vitamin A deficiency. See *hemeralopia*.

nyctiplanctus *Obs.* Somnambulistic agitation.

nyctobadia, nyctobatia *Obs.* Somnambulism.

nyctophobia Fear of night or darkness.

nyctophonia Night voice; ability to speak at night but not during daylight hours; sometimes appears as a variant of elective mutism. See *mutism, elective*.

nympholepsy 1. A form of pedophilia consisting of obsessive craving for "nymphets"; Lolita complex. 2. *Obs.* Demonic frenzy, especially frenzy arising from desire for an unattainable ideal.

nymphomania Hypersexuality in a woman; sexual erethism; (o)estromania. Compare with male pseudohypersexuality; see *Don Juan; hypersexuality*.

nymphomania, active See *nymphomania, grave*.

nymphomania, grave *Obs.* Severe, active nymphomania in contrast to *slight, platonic,* or *lesser nymphomania*.

nymphomania, platonic See *nymphomania, grave*.

nystagmus An involuntary to-and-fro movement of the eyeballs induced when the patient looks upward or laterally. It is usually a sign of pathology.

Nystagmus may be *horizontal*, the most common form, when the oscillations of the eyeballs are from side to side; or *vertical*, when the movements are up-and-down; or *rotatory*, when the oscillations are in a circular direction.

O

oaf *Obs.* Idiot; mental retardate.

obedience, automatic Many patients, particularly those with the catatonic form of schizophrenia, carry out the orders of others through blind obedience, that is, without critical or automatic judgment. "The patients carry out any commands whatsoever, even if it is against their will, as for example, putting out their tongue when they know a pin will be stuck into it." (Bleuler, *TP*) See *automatism; automatism, command; echopraxia.*

obedience, deferred According to Freud, a prohibition, command, or threat received early in life may be repressed and the effect deferred for many years until a neurotic illness occurs and the original prohibition or command is obeyed.

In spite of his father's opposition, a man became a painter. "His incapacity to paint after the father's death would then . . . be an expression of the familiar 'deferred obedience.' " (Freud, *CP*) See *success, failure through.*

obesity A condition characterized by excessive accumulation of fat in the body, usually defined in terms of the degree of excess over normal body weight, such as a body weight that exceeds by 20% the standard weight listed in the usual height-weight tables.

obesity, hyperplastic Obesity in which the number of fat cells is increased. The other major form of obesity is *hypertrophic obesity*, in which the size of the fat cells is increased. Many obese persons, and most of those who are severely obese, show both types of change, a condition sometimes called *hyperplastic-hypertrophic obesity.*

obesity, psychogenic Corpulence or the state of being overweight as a result of emotional factors that lead to overeating.

Overeating may be a nonspecific response to emotional tension, a substitute gratification in intolerable life situations, a specific symptom of emotional illness such as hysteria or depression, or a type of addiction. Bruch has claimed that there is a characteristic psychologic constellation in psychogenic obesity in children, consisting of maternal ambivalence, hostility, and compensatory overprotection. Most other investigators have failed to confirm these claims. See *eating disorders.*

object From the instinctual point of view, "The *object* of an instinct is that in or through which it can achieve its aim. It is the most variable thing about an instinct and is not originally connected with it, but becomes attached to it only in consequence of being fitted to provide satisfaction. The object is not necessarily an extraneous one; it may be part of the subject's own body." (Freud, *CP*)

Freud points out that the object of an instinct may, and usually does, change from time to time throughout life; moreover, "The same object may serve for the satisfaction of several instincts simultaneously."

object addiction See *addict, object.*

object, bad In psychoanalysis, part of the dichotomous formulation "*good object* versus *bad object*." "Good" and "bad" as used in this connotation refer essentially to moral, conscience (superego) evaluation: "good" stands for nonsexual (clean), while "bad" stands for sexual (dirty). In the unconscious the ultimate good object is equated with God, while the bad object means the Devil. See *position, paranoid-schizoid.*

object blindness Visual *agnosia* (q.v.).

object cathexis See *cathexis.*

object choice See *finding, object; object love.*

object constancy The capacity to maintain object relatedness despite frustration or satisfaction, an outcome of successful *separation-individuation* (q.v.) and perhaps dependent upon the capacity to evoke a stable, consistent mental representation of the mother even when physically separated from her. Object constancy is the ability to develop *evocative*, as contrasted with purely *recognitory*, memory, so that stable, reliable, intrapsychic representations of significant others can be developed. *Object inconstancy* is often a prominent feature of borderline *personality disorders* (q.v.), where one of its typical manifestations is a relative poverty of waking phantasy life, nocturnal dreaming, or both. See *autonomy, sense of.*

object finding See *finding, object.*

object, good See *position, paranoid-schizoid.*

object, homoerotic See *homosexuality, male.*

object identification See *identification.*

object-ill Stekel's term for the compulsive-neurotic who expresses his own mental conflict in the form of symbolization of objects pertaining to the outer world (i.e. outside his body) and also through symbolization of "the function of his everyday life such as washing, dressing, eating, defecating. . . . In compulsive diseases it is the patient's relationship to an object (usually a close member of the family) that is disturbed."

In opposition to the object-ill patient, Stekel calls "subject-ill" the person suffering from phobias, who uses his own body to symbolize his emotions. "The patient shows an ambivalent emotional attitude toward this object, that is, the polar tension between the extremes of love and hate with regard to this object is also extreme. . . .

"The 'object-ill' is conscious of his abilities; he fails, because of his bipolar family fixations which create defiance, aggression and self-punishment; while the 'subject-ill' feels that he has failed in his relations with the outer world and feels inferior to the demands of life. . . . The 'object-ill' is introverted and makes no attempts at extraversion; the 'subject-ill,' however, makes efforts to extravert himself in order to adjust himself to the world." (Stekel, *CD*) See *subject-ill.*

object libido See *ego libido.*

object love That portion of the libidinal energy of the psyche that is attached to some object outside the person himself (or to the intrapsychic representation of that object). At various times, Freud appears to have considered object love to be the earliest type of relationship to the environment and thus to precede autoerotism and narcissism; but at other times he considered autoerotism or narcissism to be primary. See *narcissism, primary.*

object love, passive See *narcissism.*

object relations theory Formulation of the ways in which the experience of the external world is internalized, how experience contributes to the development of subjectivity and of the ego, and how interpersonal transactions are schematized as mental models. Object relations theory is a description of the psychodynamic processes by which the child handles conflicts with the parents by introjecting the relationship and dealing with it on an intrapsychic level. *Ego psychology*, or *psychoanalytic development psychology*, is associated particularly with Heinz Hartmann, Edith Jacobson, Margaret Mahler, René Spitz, Otto Kernberg, and Heinz Kohut. See *deprivation, emotional; self psychology.*

Even sexuality, despite its clear biologic base, is shaped by experience, and both the experience of sexual desire and the expressions of sexuality are influenced by the culture and other internalized elements of the outside, interpersonal world. Object relations theory was originally described by Klein (1959) and Fairbairn (1967) and applied to marital relationships by Dicks (1967) and others.

object, transitional A blanket, cloth, sheet, diaper, etc., that assures a special value for the infant under stress, particularly when going to sleep. Elaborating on Winnicott's initial description in 1953, Fred Busch and his co-workers (*Journal of the American Academy of Child Psychiatry 12*, 1973) differentiated between the primary transitional object (adopted in the first year of life, usually at age 6 months) and the secondary transitional object (adopted at about age 2). Characteristic of the primary transitional object are (1) time of attachment within the first year; (2) duration of attachment being one year or more; (3) effect being to soothe and reduce anxiety; (4) object not meeting a direct oral or libidinal need; (5) attachment made actively by the infant rather than passively accepting something such as a pacifier that is forced upon him; (6) object being distinguished from parts of the body, such as the thumb, that also bring comfort.

objectivation A type of projection in which one's own unrecognized impulses or feelings are quickly detected and recognized in others. Objectivation may lead to overemphasis of the importance or significance of such impulses in others and, when present in the analyst, may produce troublesome *countertransference* (q.v.) manifestations.

oblativity Capacity for renunciation of the mother or mother substitute; the ability to tolerate frustration in the process of achieving independence. See *mechanism, mote-beam.*

obliviscence The state or process of passing into oblivion; the tendency for a memory to fade with the passage of time.

obnubilation Clouding of consciousness; stupor.

OBS 1. Organic brain syndrome; see *syndrome, organic.* 2. Obstetrics.

obscenity Speech, gestures, writings, drawings, or other actions that are offensive to taste or modesty, and/or that aim to incite the viewer to lewd and prurient thought or action. See *pornography.*

observation, delusion of Delusion of being watched.

observer, participant In psychoanalysis, the analyst as he is viewed by those who feel that he must be something more than an authoritarian sounding board or a mirror in which the patient's problems are reflected. Although the therapist must be objective, he also takes active part in the interpersonal process of therapy. The so-called cultural interpersonal school of psychoanalysis particularly emphasizes the participant role of the analyst. See *process, interpersonal.*

obsession An idea, emotion, or impulse that repetitively and insistently forces itself into consciousness even though it is unwelcome. An obsession may be regarded as essentially normal when it does not interfere substantially with thinking or other mental functions; such an obsession is short-lived and can usually be minimized or nullified by diverting attention onto other topics.

Morbid or pathological obsessions, in contrast, tend to be long-lived and may constitute a never-ending harrassment of mental functioning; they are but little subject to conscious control and force the sufferer into all sorts of maneuvers in his vain attempt to rid himself of the thoughts.

Most commonly, obsessions appear as *ideas,* or sensory images, which are strongly charged with emotions: (1) *intellectual obsessions,* often in the form of preoccupation with metaphysical questions concerning one's purpose in life, ultimate destiny, whereabouts after death, etc.; see *brooding;* (2) *inhibiting obsessions,* in the form of doubts or scruples about actions, or multiple phobias that may paralyze all activity; (3) *impulsive obsessions,* which are repetitively intruding ideas that lead to action (e.g. arithmomania, kleptomania, and other so-called *manias*).

Less commonly, obsessions appear as feelings, unaccompanied by clear-cut ideas, such as anxiety or panic, feelings of unreality or depersonalization. Some authorities, in addition, classify motor tics as impulsive obsessions. See *obsessive-compulsive psychoneurosis.*

obsession, masked An obsession that appears in the disguised (masked) form of other symptoms. One of the most interesting forms is the obsessive idea that disguises itself in the form of pain. "The patients complain of pain, state that it drives them to suicide, yet they remain attached to the pain which—on closer scrutiny—may prove to represent pleasurable though tabooed memories.... Such pain (for which usually no organic cause can be found) then appears as a mask of the obsessive idea. The real idea is hidden behind the pain, so that the patients, instead of complaining of obsessions, complain of pain. It is diagnostically important that the usual sedatives are always ineffective in these cases or, if forced upon the patient, may lead to narcotomania." (Stekel, CD) See *somatoform disorders.*

obsession, somatic Morbid preoccupation with one's body or an individual organ. "Usually these obsessions concerning the body or individual organs are connected with [the] patient's feeling of guilt and inferiority. The somatic obsessions are mostly monosymptomatic, though they are always part of a more complicated neurotic system. A person not only is forced to think constantly of his nose, but also operates with a 'nose-currency,' so to speak, that is, in looking at people he sees only their noses and compares them with his own. No other human problem appears to be worthy of his attention." (Stekel, *CD*)

obsessive attack See *attack, obsessive.*

obsessive-compulsive psychoneurosis Obsessive-compulsive reaction; a type of psychoneurosis characterized by disturbing, unwanted, anxiety-provoking, intruding thoughts or ideas, and repetitive impulses to perform acts (ceremonials, counting, hand washing) that may be considered abnormal, undesirable, or distasteful to the patient. Typical are ruminations that recur even though the subject regards them as alien or absurd, voluntary motor actions that are reluctantly performed even though regarded as alien or absurd, or a combination of both. According to R. Stern and J. Cobb (*British Journal of Psychiatry 132*, 1978), the four most commonly reported compulsive rituals are cleaning, avoiding, repeating, and checking.

The "psychasthenia" of earlier writers usually included obsessive-compulsive neurosis, which was also known as substitution neurosis.

Psychoanalytically, obsessive-compulsive psychoneurosis is interpreted as a defense against aggressive and/or sexual impulses, particularly in relation to the Oedipus complex. The initial defense is by regression to the anal-sadistic level, but the impulses at this level are also intolerable and must be warded off—by reaction formation, isolation, and undoing. Because the use of these defenses renders superfluous the use of repression proper, the offensive impulses can exist in consciousness although when they do they are divorced from their affective significance and so remain meaningless to the patient. See *compulsion; obsession.*

obsessive-ruminative tension state Adolf Meyer's term for *obsessive-compulsive psychoneurosis* (q.v.).

obstipatio paradoxa Soiling associated with constipation. "The child retains the stools, which become very hard and can be felt through the abdominal wall. Small pieces of firm stool are passed from time to time and are retained between the buttocks, macerating the perianal skin." (Bakwin H., & Bakwin, R. *Clinical Management of Behavior Disorders in Children,* 1953) See *obstipation.*

obstipation Extreme or intractable constipation; when of psychologic origin, it may appear either as a conversion symptom or as an organ neurosis. Like all conversions, obstipation may be the somatic expression of a specific, repressed, unconscious sexual phantasy. Usually obstipation expresses retentive tendencies connected with pregnancy wishes or incorporation phantasies. This is "in accordance with the equation child = penis = feces."

As an organ neurosis, obstipation is a physiological change in organic function, resulting from an unconscious attitude or affect. In the particular case of obstipation, the unconscious attitude is a chronically frustrated retentive pressure, which may exist for several reasons. It may represent an anal erotic fixation, a desire for anal retentive pleasure, or the feces may represent introjected objects as in the case of the conversion. Again, in some other instances, the retentive pressure, with its resulting obstipation, might be associated with a continuous and repressed aggressiveness. (Fenichel, *PTN*)

obstruction *Blocking* (q.v.); "Among the formal disturbances of the mental stream [of thought] the *obstructions* (deprivation of thought) are the most striking and when they occur too readily or too often or become too general and too persistent, they are positively pathognomonic of schizophrenia." (Bleuler, *TP*) See *symptoms, first-rank.*

Thought deprivation or sudden cessation of thought may last for variable periods of time.

obstupescentia *Obs.* Stupor.

obtunded An inexact term indicating depression of cerebral function, ranging from sedated to comatose. See *clouding* (of consciousness).

occult Hidden from understanding or not susceptible to logical rational verification; includes magic, foretelling, telepathy, clairvoyance. See *perception, extrasensory.*

occupation, sedative In occupational therapy, a form of activity characterized by repetitious, uniform movements that, because of their monotonous recurrence, have a soothing and quieting effect. It is usually prescribed for overactive patients. An example of sedative occupation is simple weaving.

occupation, stimulating In occupational therapy, activity so varied that the lack of monotony and repetition tends to arouse and awaken to activity the slow, retarded, and depressed patient. For instance, the various activities associated with photography constitute a type of stimulating occupation.

occupational neurosis See *neurosis, occupational*.

occupational psychiatry See *psychiatry, industrial*.

occupational therapy See *therapy, occupational*.

oceanic feeling See *omnipotence*.

ochlophobia Fear of crowds.

ocnophile Balint's term for the person with that type of primitive two-person relationship in which the subject is clingingly dependent on the overvalued object and is unable to make any move toward independence. See *philobat*.

O'Connor v. Donaldson See *consumerism*.

oculocardiac reflex See *phenomenon, Aschner ocular*.

oculogyral crisis See *spasm, oculogyric*.

OD (Drug) overdose; less frequently, organization(al) development; right eye; each day.

odaxesmus (ō-dak-sez′mus) *Obs.* Marshall Hall's (English physician, 1790–1857) term referring to the biting of tongue, cheek, or lip during an epileptic seizure.

odontophobia Fear of teeth.

-odynia (-ō-din′ē-à) Combining form meaning pain of body or mind, sorrow, from Gr. *odýnē*.

odynophobia Fear of pain.

Odysseus pact An attempt to provide for the future on the basis of knowing what pitfalls the past has presented. The term is used to refer to the process involved in making a living will, and in making provisions for one's commitment to a hospital should there be a recurrence of a psychotic episode similar to one that the person has recovered from.

oedipal Pertaining to Oedipus. This adjective is occasionally encountered, though as

a rule the noun *Oedipus* is used unchanged as an adjective, as in *Oedipus complex*.

oedipism *Rare.* Self-inflicted injury to the eyes.

Oedipus, complete The simultaneous presence of both a positive and a negative (or inverted) Oedipus situation; the child displays mother object love and father identification, and father object love and mother identification. The quantity of cathexis (or emotional charge) given to each of these four conditions is a reflection in part of the strength of innate bisexuality, and in part of experiential factors.

Oedipus complex See *complex, Oedipus*

Oedipus, inverted Same as *Oedipus, negative* (q.v.).

Oedipus, negative Also known as *inverted Oedipus* (complex), the negative Oedipus complex is a form of infantile psychosexual development in which the parental object is the opposite or reverse of the usual love object. The usual oedipal love object for the male child is the mother; but should love for the father and hatred for the mother prevail, the boy would be said to demonstrate a negative Oedipus complex. In like fashion, should the girl's attachment remain fixed on the mother (instead of being transferred to the father, as is the usual course of events), she would be described as manifesting a negative Oedipus. See *complex, Oedipus*

oenomania (ē-nō-mā′nē-à) *Oinomania* (q.v.).

oestromania, estromania Nymphomania.

OFD See *syndrome, OFD I*.

offender, status A term applied to juveniles whose offenses are not criminal; included are runaways, truants, and "ungovernable" youths. The status offender is thus differentiated from the juvenile delinquent, a youth under 18 whose offense, if committed by an adult, would constitute a crime.

offset In insurance, the phenomenon of reducing total expenditure when the granting of one benefit (e.g. psychiatric) makes a second one (e.g. general medical) unnecessary; the declining use of medical services after and, according to some, because of institution of psychiatric services. The offset effect is most evident in people who receive brief psychotherapy at a relatively high intensity. Chronic users of psychiatric services, in contrast, are consistently higher users of medical care than other psychiatric care users.

oikiomania See *ecomania*.

oikiophobia See *oikophobia*.

oikofugic Pertaining to or swayed by the impulse to wander or travel.

oikophobia Fear of one's house or home.

oikotropic Homesick. See *nostalgia*.

oinomania *Delirium tremens; dipsomania* (qq.v.); craving for alcohol.

OIT Organic integrity test. See *test, organic integrity*.

olfaction See *rhinencephalon*.

olfactophobia Fear of odors.

olfactory reference syndrome The fixed and incorrect belief in a self-generated foul odor, a form of *monosymptomatic hypochondriacal psychosis* (q.v.). Some cases appear to have benefited from treatment with tricyclic or monoamine oxidase inhibitor antidepressants.

oligergasia (ol-i-gēr-gās′ē-á) Adolf Meyer's term for intellectual deficiency or mental retardation.

olig(o)- (ol′i-gō-) Combining form meaning small, pl. few, from Gr. *oligos*,.

oligodactyly (á-li-gō-dak′ti-lē) See *syndrome, de Lange*.

oligodendroglia See *neuroglia*.

oligomania *Obs.* Insanity on a few subjects; *monomania* (q.v.).

oligophrenia Mental deficiency. See *retardation, mental*.

oligophrenia, moral See *insanity, moral*.

oligophrenia, phenylpyruvic *Folling's disease*. Mental retardation secondary to an inherited biochemical defect, *phenylketonuria* (q.v.).

oligoria In certain forms of melancholia, an abnormal indifference toward or dislike of persons or things.

oligosthenic Kretschmer's variety of *asthenic* type characterized by moderate strength and intermediate between the *phthinoid* and the *eusthenic*.

oligothymia Poverty of affectivity; Davidson's term for *psychopathic personality* (q.v.).

olonism *Miryachit* (q.v.).

-oma, -ome Combining form meaning affected or diseased state, from Gr. *-óma*.

ombrophobia Fear of rain(storm).

omega melancholium *Obs.* Schuele's sign; a wrinkle (between the eyebrows) in the shape of the last letter of the Greek alpha-bet, the omega (ω), assumed to indicate a state of melancholy.

ommatophobia Fear of eyes or of the "evil eye."

omnipotence Feelings of omnipotence and self-esteem undergo extensive development and change, concomitant with the development of the ego. There is a feeling of omnipotence from the very beginning, even before the conception of objects exists. The outside world is perceived by the organism as part of it (the organism), within itself, though there is as yet no non-ego. Similar phenomena are observed in mental patients when they lose contact with reality and relapse to a childlike level of emotional behavior: the person loses the distinction between his personality (ego) and the environment (reality). Such a person is in a state of primitive all-powerfulness, believes that he is omniscient and omnipotent, and has phantasies which know no bounds. In such a state of omnipotence the patient can express ideas that he is able to move the universe, create war and peace, and give birth to millions of children. In delusional adults the symptom is more commonly called *megalomania*. (Hinsie, *UP*)

This feeling of unlimited omnipotence, often termed the "oceanic feeling," becomes limited as the ego and sense of reality develop: this occurs when the infant experiences tensions he cannot master, which in turn lead to uncoordinated discharge movements. "Something outside" becomes necessary to quiet the infant's tension and, through recognizing this "something outside," the infant makes his first distinction between ego and object. Also he develops a new concept of omnipotence. When his movements are understood by the environment to be a signal calling for a quieting of his tension, the child experiences this train of events as an "omnipotence of movements." However, he still longs for his original "oceanic feeling." His earliest reaction to objects is to swallow them; he tries to "swallow" or incorporate all pleasurable sensations and, through introjection, to make parts of the external world flow, like tributaries, into his ego. Unpleasurable sensations are perceived as being non-ego and are "spat out." Thus, through introjection, anything pleasurable becomes part of the ego, and through projection, anything unpleasant becomes non-ego. See *orientation, oral.*

These efforts to reestablish the "oceanic feeling" of primary narcissism and also the "omnipotence of movements" are doomed to failure, however, since, through his experiences, the child realizes he is not omnipotent. The adult is now considered omnipotent and, by reuniting with this omnipotent force in the external world, the child tries to share this omnipotence: either he incorporates parts of this world or has the phantasy of being incorporated by it. The latter type of omnipotence is at work in religious ecstasy and patriotism. Mass political movements may also attest to the participation of the powerless followers in the omnipotence of their leaders. The feeling of having been reunited with the omnipotent force is known as *secondary narcissism.* The longing for the omnipotence of primary narcissism is the "narcissistic need which all people experience. 'Self-esteem' is the awareness of how close the individual is to the original omnipotence." Originally, the longing for omnipotence was a longing for the removal of instinctual tension to restore the objectless narcissistic state: self-esteem was restored by getting rid of an unpleasant stimulus. This was done through nourishment. Thus the first regulation of self-esteem and satisfaction of narcissistic need was through food. After the infant relinquishes its feeling of omnipotence, however, and tends to participate in the adult's omnipotence, his self-esteem is regulated by tokens of love from the adults. The child gains self-esteem when he gains affection and loses self-esteem when he loses affection: through the promise of these and the threats of withholding or withdrawing them, the child becomes ready to obey authority and forgo other satisfactions. "This is what makes children educable."

In later development, needs for self-esteem, the narcissistic needs, are all-important: they develop in the relationship between ego and superego. Guilt-feeling lowers self-esteem and fulfillment of ideals raises it. But even in the relationship to objects in which the sexual needs develop, part of the relationship remains governed by the needs of self-esteem. In persons fixated at this level the dominant need from objects is narcissistic. Such persons may attempt to maintain their self-esteem either through aggressive or submissive behavior toward their objects or through both methods simultaneously. (Fenichel, *PTN*)

omnipotence, magic See *identification, cosmic.*

on-off A phenomenon described in parkinsonian patients treated with dopaminergic agents consisting of alternating akinesia ("off") and choreoathetotic dyskinesias ("on"). Lithium decreases the amount of off activity, at least in some patients, perhaps because of a dopamine receptor-stabilizing property. See *up-regulation.*

onanism Strictly speaking, sexual intercourse interrupted before ejaculation. Havelock Ellis says: "Onan's device was not auto-erotic, but an early example of withdrawal before emission, or *coitus interruptus.*" Some writers use onanism interchangeably with *masturbation.*

onanism, buccal *Fellatio* (q.v.).

oneirism (on'ĭ-riz'm) Dream state while one is awake; a waking dream.

oneir(o) (ō-nī-r[ō]-) Combining form meaning dream, from Gr. *oneiros.*

oneirodelirium Literally, dream delirium. Some French psychiatrists apply the term to that group of psychoses marked by delirium. Delirium tremens is the prototype of this group and is considered to be essentially a prolonged dream. Fever deliria are also part of this group, because they are so closely related to dreams. Although it is true that hallucinations can be interpreted in the same way as dreams, this does not mean that deliria, schizophrenic hallucinations, and dreams are etiologically the same, as this term would imply.

oneirodynia One of the four great divisions of insanity recognized by Cullen. The four were amentia, melancholia, mania, and oneirodynia (somnambulism and nightmare).

oneirogonorrhea Nocturnal emission of semen; wet dream.

oneirogonos (ō-nī-rog'ō-nos) *Oneironosus* (q.v.).

oneirology The science of dreams.

oneironosus Morbid dreaming.

oneirophrenia Meduna and McCulloch's term for a schizophreniform psychosis that, like schizophrenia, shows disturbances in associations and in affectivity but, unlike schizophrenia, shows in addition clouding of the sensorium. Onset is ususally acute, during the episode the patient is in a dreamlike condition, and prognosis is usually good.

By others, oneirophrenia is considered to be an acute form of *schizophrenia* (q.v.).

oneiroscopy Dream analysis, diagnosis of the mental state by a study of the person's dreams.

oniomania Irresistible impulse to buy, extending inordinately beyond the needs of the person; buying binge; spending spree.

onirism Régis's term for a state of prolonged dreaming.

onology *Rare.* Asinine talk.

onomatomania A type of obsessive thinking in which certain words of sentences obtrude themselves into the patient's thoughts. A patient with an obsessive-compulsive psychoneurosis was beset with anxiety, because a man's name was incessantly forcing itself upon him. It was the surname of a man with whose wife the patient had had intercourse; the anxiety was occasioned by the fear of being attacked by the husband, though the patient knew that he need have no fear of attack in the usual sense.

onomatophobia Fear of hearing a certain name.

onomatopoiesis, onomatopoesis The formation of an echoic word, i.e. in imitation of the sound associated with the thing or action. The words *hiss, crash, hush, buzz, click, chickadee* closely resemble the sound. In psychiatry the phenomenon is often observed in morbid form in patients with schizophrenia, who create a number of neologisms on the basis of sound association.

ontoanalysis Existential analysis. See *existentialism.*

ontogenesis, ontogeny In biology, the development of the individual organism as compared with the evolutionary or *phylogenetic* development of the species. This fundamental distinction was clarified by Haeckel, when in 1867 he formulated his famous "biogenetic law" that "ontogeny recapitulates phylogeny" (*Naturliche Schopfungsgeschichte*). If the histories of the genealogical and of the individual development are dis

tinguished in accordance with this law, it follows that "the organism in its development is to a great extent an epitome of the form-modifications undergone by the successive ancestors of the species in the course of their historic evolution."

In other fields of science one finds ontogenesis or ontogeny applied in a more limited and specialized sense. With bacteriologists it means the evolution of the individual germ. According to certain psychologists, ontogeny refers to factors in the life of human beings after their birth, as the psyche is believed to have its special form of development, its own embryology, physiology, structural evolution, and pathology. See *phylogenesis.*

ontogeny, psychic Development of the mind, and particularly the ways in which the organism relates its inborn needs to environmental demands. In psychoanalysis, psychic ontogeny includes (1) development of object relationships; (2) the vicissitudes of the drives in relation to reality; and (3) the development of mechanisms to achieve the foregoing.

The development of object relationships is generally described according to the following schema:

1. Autoerotic (or somatogenic) stage, from birth until about 3 years of age; see *autoeroticism.*

2. Narcissistic stage, from 3 to 6 years of age; see *narcissism.*

3. Homoerotic (or suigenderistic) stage, from 6 years until puberty; see *homoeroticism.*

4. Heteroerotic (or altrigenderistic) stage, during adolescence; see *heteroeroticism.*

5. Alloerotic stage, the stage of maturity; see *alloerotism.*

The vicissitudes of the drives are typically described in terms of libidinal phases, as follows:

1. Pre-superego sexuality, from birth until about 6 years of age, including

   a. Oral phase, from birth until 2 years; see *orality.*

   b. Anal phase, from 2 until about 4 years; see *phase, anal.*

   c. Phallic phase, from 2 until about 6 years; see *phallic; phase, phallic.*

2. *Latency* (q.v.), from 6 years to puberty.

3. *Genitality* (q.v.).

The mechanisms developed to achieve the foregoing are those involved in the development of the ego and superego and of the ego defenses. See *defense; ego; superego.*

Some critics believe that classical psychoanalytic psychology overemphasizes childhood as the beginning and end of personality development and have described psychic ontogeny in different terms. Erikson, for example, maintained that side by side with the psychosexual stages described by Freud were psychosocial stages of ego development, that personality continued to develop throughout the whole life cycle, and that each stage has a positive as well as a negative component. (See *developmental levels.*) Erikson's *eight stages of man* were:

1. *Trust vs. Mistrust* extends through first year of life (and thus corresponds roughly to Freud's oral stage). During this stage, the degree to which the child learns to trust the world, other people, and himself depends upon the quality of care he receives; if that care is inadequate or inconsistent, *basic mistrust* develops, an attitude of fear and suspicion of the world.

2. *Autonomy vs. Doubt* extends through second and third years (Freud's anal stage). Adequate care in this stage consists of allowing the child to do what he is capable of, at his own pace, so that he can develop autonomy, i.e. ability to control his muscles, his impulses, himself, and ultimately his environment. Inconsistent, overcritical, or overprotective care, on the other hand, fills the child with doubt about his own abilities to control his world and himself.

3. *Initiative vs. Guilt* extends through fourth and fifth years (Freud's genital stage). Adequate care provides freedom and opportunity for the child to initiate motor play, phantasies, and intellectual questioning of those around him so that he is no longer only an imitator of others. But if the child is inhibited or derided for his play activity or his inquisitiveness, he will develop guilt about self-initiated activities.

4. *Industry vs. Inferiority* extends from 6 to 11 years (Freud's latency period). During this period, the child learns to reason deductively, and to obey the "rules of the game." This is a *Robinson Crusoe age,* in that the child is concerned with the details of how things are made, how they work, and what they do. Adequate care involves encouraging the child in his effort to make and do practical things, rewarding him for results, and thus enhancing his sense of industry. Because the child's world at this stage includes more than his parents, adults outside the immediate family also play an important part in enhancing industry, or on the negative side, instilling in the child a sense of inferiority.

5. *Identity vs. Role Confusion*—adolescence extending roughly from age 12 to 18. During this period, the person can wonder about what other people think of him, he can compare his own family and society with what he conceptualizes as an ideal family or society, and he develops a sense of who he is, where he has been, and where he is going. But both the family milieu and the social milieu may interfere with the development of a sense of ego identity; when rapid social and technological change breaks down traditional values, the adolescent may develop a sense of role confusion in that he finds no continuity between what he learned as a child and what he is experiencing as an adolescent. For such a person, an identity as a delinquent, to cite but one example, may be preferable to having no identity at all.

6. *Intimacy vs. Isolation* extends from adolescence to early middle age; roughly, the period of courtship and early family life. During this phase, the person must learn to share with and care about another, without the fear of losing himself in the process; if he does not, he develops a sense of isolation, a feeling of being alone without anyone to share with or care for.

7. *Generativity vs. Self-Absorption*—middle age. In this stage, the person becomes concerned with others beyond his immediate family, and with the nature of society and the world in which future generations will live. On the negative side, the person without a sense of generativity becomes self-absorbed with his personal needs and comforts.

8. *Integrity vs. Despair*—old age. The person at this stage who can look back on his life with satisfaction, who can pause to reflect on the past and take time to enjoy

his grandchildren, manifests a sense of integrity. At the other end of the scale is the person whose past life is a series of missed opportunities and mistakes that cannot be undone; he is filled with despair at the thought of what might have been.

ontology Study of the nature, essential properties, and relations of being; *existentialism* (q.v.).

onychophagia, onychophagy Nail-biting, cited by Kanner as one of the habitual manipulations of the body encountered in neurotic children and considered by him as one of the several forms of motor discharges of inner tension.

oo- (ō-'ō-) Combining form meaning eggs, from Gr. *ō (i), on.*

oocyte (ō'ō-sīt) In sexual reproduction, the female germ cells or *oogonia* divide into two unequal daughter cells, the larger of which is called the *primary* or *secondary oocyte,* according to whether it is produced by the first or second meiotic division.

oogonia In sexual reproduction, the first stage in the development of mature reproductive cells in the female.

oophorectomy See *ovariotomy.*

open In group therapy, a group to which members can be added; a *closed* group is limited to those who started with the group. In questioning or interviewing, an open question is one that allows the person questioned maximal freedom in choosing the manner or content of his response.

open-door policy Approximately equivalent to *community, therapeutic* (q.v.). The term open-door emphasizes the growing trend in psychiatric hospitals to minimize or even eliminate completely any form of restraint or enforced confinement ("locked doors").

operant behaviorism See *behaviorism.*

operant conditioning See *conditioning, operant.*

operational planning See *strategic planning.*

operations, concrete See *adolescence.*

operations research (OR) A group of techniques that developed pragmatically in an attempt to apply scientific methods and tools to solve the problems of decision making in complex organizations and systems, where any one decision typically proves advantageous for some parts of the system but disadvantageous for others. Operations research searches for optimal solutions in situations of conflicting goals

and relies heavily on mathematic modes from which solutions for the actual problem may be derived.

ophidiophilia (ō-fid'i-ō-) A morbid fascination with snakes.

ophidiophobia Fear of snakes.

ophthalmoplegia See *nerve, oculomotor.*

ophthalmoplegia externa See *sign, Ballet's.*

-opia, -opy, -opsia Combining form meaning defect of sight, from Gr. *ōps, ōpós,* eye.

opiate See *opium.*

opioid Opiumlike; see *opium.* The opioids include natural substances such as heroin and morphine, as well as synthetics with morphinelike actions, such as meperidine and methadone.

The opioids are associated with patterns of abuse and dependence. Opioid intoxication is suggested by the following symptoms: constricted pupils ("pinning"), drowsiness, slurred speech, impaired attention or memory, euphoria or dysphoria, apathy and psychomotor retardation, impaired judgment, and failure to meet social, occupational, or academic responsibilities.

The characteristic withdrawal syndrome includes lacrimation, rhinorrhea, dilated pupils, gooseflesh, sweating, diarrhea, yawning, tachycardia, elevated blood pressure, insomnia, and fever. See *addiction; dependency, drug.*

opiomania Addiction to the use of opium or any of its derivatives.

opisthotonos (op-is-tot'ō-nos) See *arc de cercle.*

opium A narcotic and analgesic obtained from the juice of unripe seeds of the poppy plant. The juice dries in the air to form a brown, gummy substance, which is further dried and powdered commercially to produce the opiates (i.e. morphine and its transformation products). All the opiates are potentially addicting drugs, as are the synthetic analgesics; morphine possesses perhaps the greatest potentiality in this direction, followed by heroin, Dilaudid, metopon, Demerol, methadone, and codeine, in that order. Because it is easier to traffic in illegally, heroin is the most commonly used of the group by opiate addicts, at least in the United States. All the opiates are characterized by the development of a high degree of tolerance in their users, and severe deprivation or abstinence syndromes are therefore the rule. See *addiction; dependency, drug.*

opotherapy *Organotherapy* (q.v.).

Oppenheim reflex See *reflex, Oppenheim.*

Oppenheimer treatment (Issac Oppenheimer, New York physician, 1871–1943) A secret method of treatment of alcoholism and drug addiction.

Oppenheim's dystonia musculorum deformans (Hermann Oppenheim, Berlin neurologist, 1858–1919) See *dystonia, torsion.*

opposite, reversal into the One of the major defensive processes of a psychological nature by which the ego handles, or defends itself from, the sexual instinct, which impinges upon it while seeking direct gratification. The specific nature of this process consists of the transformation of the aim of an instinct into its opposite, and the substitution of the instinct itself for the external object. This process is called into play when the aim of a sexual instinct has been blocked from direct object gratification by internal intrapsychic or external environmental prohibition and restriction. In the process of reversal into the opposite, the active aim usually becomes a passive one.

oppositional disorder Also *oppositional-defiant disorder,* classified within the disruptive behavior disorders; a childhood disorder consisting of pervasive disobedience, negativism, and provocative opposition to authority figures (e.g. repetitive infractions of minor rules, temper tantrums, argumentativeness, stubbornness). Unlike *conduct disorders* (q.v.), behavior is not primarily an invasion of the rights of others.

oppositional thinking *Janusian thinking* (q.v.).

opsomania *Obs.* Pathologic craving for sweets, such as may occur in binge-eating syndrome. See *syndrome, night-eating.*

optimism, oral Optimism appearing as an oral character trait. Oral eroticism is extremely important for the formation of character. At the time when oral eroticism occurs in infantile development, children "become acquainted with objects and learn to assume relationships with them." Consequently, the way in which this happens "remains basic in determining the whole subsequent relationship to reality." Thus all positive or negative attitudes to taking and receiving have an oral origin. In particular, whenever there is unusually pronounced oral satisfaction in infancy, the results are a self-assurance and optimism which may persist throughout life. Fenichel remarks, however, that if frustration has followed this satisfaction, there may be created a state of "vengefulness coupled with continuous demanding." (*PTN*)

optimism, technologic(al) The disposition to employ technologies in the belief that the benefits deriving therefrom will outweigh any undesirable effects, and that the latter can themselves be controlled or eliminated through technologic developments.

OR *Operations research* (q.v.); operating room.

oral-aggressive See *defense, character.*

orality A general term referring to the oral components of sexuality, to manifestations of instinctual conflict centering about the oral stage of sexual development, to manifestations that indicate fixation at the oral stage of development, to manifestations of oral erogeneity. Orality is prominent in manic-depressive psychosis and addictions. A driving ambition in the field of oratory or speech making is often based on oral conflicts. Excessive generosity in a person often has the following significance: "As I shower you with love, in the same way do I want to be showered with love"; this mechanism is typical of the oral-receptive person. The oral-sadistic person often shows extreme niggardliness: "You must make up for the love denied me." Volubility, restlessness, haste, and a tendency to obstinate silence are also indicative of extreme orality. E. Bergler (*Psychiatric Quarterly 19,* 1945) believes that the mechanism of orality is as follows: (1) through his behavior the person provokes disappointment, thus identifying the outer world with the refusing, pre-oedipal mother; (2) he becomes aggressive, seemingly in self-defense; (3) he indulges in self-pity, a manifestation of his psychic masochism. See *character, oral.*

Probably for biological reasons, the main energies of the infant are concentrated first in the mouth area—feeding is his most important function and reality demands little else of him. Orality is, in essence, one of the steps in learning, and at this stage in ontogenetic development stress and distress stem primarily from the complex physiological processes that produce hunger. Gratification follows stimulation of the mouth area, and oral stimulation is what the infant seeks because of the pleasure it provides.

orbitomedial syndrome See *syndrome, orbitomedial.*

orchestromania Chorea; St. Vitus' dance.

orderliness, organic A characteristic symptom of patients with organic brain disease, consisting of a stereotyped, meticulous, compulsive approach to the environment; the patient's possessions must always be arranged in the same order, any action must always be performed in the same sequence or in the same way, etc. See *syndrome, organic.*

-orexia Combining form meaning appetite, desire, longing, from Gr. *órexis.*

orexis That part of an act or response which is not the cognitive aspect; specifically, affect and conation are the orectic aspects of an action.

organ choice See *compliance, somatic; specificity, individual-response.*

organ-erotic Relating to or characterized by the attachment of the erotic instinctual component to an organ of the body.

"The child's first sexual feelings have reference to its own body, more particularly to parts, segments, of its body; it is organ erotic." (Jelliffe & White, *DNS*)

organ erotism Libido or erotism situated in an organ.

organ, executive The organ that is used for the execution of responses to stimuli. "In the infant the technique of mastery has two chief executive organs, the hand and the mouth, the eye being the leading auxiliary organ." (Kardiner, A., & Spiegel, H.X. *War Stress and Neurotic Illness,* 1947) Thus when hunger is the stimulus, response to it is executed by way of the mouth; when the stimulus is the desire to grasp at an object, response to it is executed by means of the hand.

organ jargon See *jargon, organ.*

organ libido See *organ erotism.*

organ neurosis See *psychosomatic.*

organ pleasure The excitement and satisfaction attained in the extragenital erogenous zones; used particularly to refer to the *partial instincts* in the pregenital period. Characteristic of infantile sexuality is the fact that the genitals themselves are but one of many erogenous zones, and that sexuality is undifferentiated and contains all the later part-instincts, which are not as yet subordinate to genital satisfaction. In the child, every kind of excitation can become a source of sexual excitement—oral, anal, urethral, mechanical and muscular stimuli, skin, temperature, and even pain. "In time, however, the genitals begin to function as a special discharge apparatus, which concentrates all excitation upon itself and discharges it no matter in which erogenous zone it originated. It is called genital primacy when this function of the genitals has become dominant over the extragenital erogenous zones, and all sexual excitations become finally genitally oriented and climactically discharged." (Fenichel, *PTN*)

organ speech See *speech, organ.*

organ, target See *syndrome, general adaptation.*

organic anxiety syndrome In DSM-III-R, an organic mental syndrome in which the predominant disturbance is recurrent panic episodes or generalized anxiety.

organic brain syndrome See *syndrome, organic.*

organic drivenness See *drivenness, organic.*

organic mental disorders Mental disturbances resulting from transient or permanent dysfunction of brain tissue that is attributable to specific organic factors, such as aging (senile and presenile dementias), drugs and toxins, infection, cardiovascular disease, trauma, neoplasm, or metabolic disorders. These disorders manifest themselves as one or more *organic brain syndromes* that reflect the localization, progression, and duration of the underlying pathology, and with associated or secondary features that reflect emotional, motivational, and behavioral reactions to recognition of the primary deficits and the anticipation of their consequences. See *syndrome, organic.*

In DSM-III-R, organic mental syndromes and (non-substance-induced) disorders include *delirium, dementia, amnestic syndrome,* organic *delusional disorders,* organic *hallucinosis, organic anxiety syndrome* (qq.v.), organic mood disorder (manic, depressed, or mixed), and organic personality disorder. Intoxication and withdrawal, previously included within this category, have been placed under *psychoactive substance-induced organic mental disorders.*

organic psychosis See *syndrome, organic.*

organic reaction See *syndrome, organic.*

organicism 1. The theory that refers all disease to material lesions of organs. Disordered physiology may give rise to symptoms, yet there may be no demonstrable lesions.

2. The theory that all symptoms are organically determined.

3. In constitutional medicine, "the theory that the various organs of the body have each their own special constitution." (Pende, N. *Constitutional Inadequacies,* 1928)

organicist As currently used in psychiatry, a pejorative designation for the psychiatrist who can admit of only material lesions in organs as etiologic agents in psychiatric disorders. The organicist is typically contrasted to the *psychodynamist* or *psychogeneticist,* but all three terms represent an unwelcome regression to the days of the nature-nurture conflict. They focus upon a dualism that exists only on a conceptual heuristic level, and ignore the reality of the functioning whole person whose mental and emotional processes are interwoven with and interdependent upon neurophysiologic substrata and sociocultural factors. See *ecology; psychosomatic.*

organization, libido See *zone, primacy.*

organization, pregenital The arrangement of the libido in the stages prior to that of infantile genitality. See *ontogeny, psychic.*

organization, social "Socially systematized schemes of behavior imposed as rules upon individuals." (Thomas, W.I., & Znaniecki, F. *The Polish Peasant in Europe and America,* 1927)

"Every human group is organized; its individual components do not behave independently of one another, but are linked by bonds, the nature of which determines the types of social unit. Kinship, sex, age, co-residence, matrimonial status, community of religious or social interests, are among the unifying agencies; and in stratified societies members of the same level form a definite class." (Lowie, R.H. *Social Organization; Encyclopaedia of the Social Sciences,* 1934)

organogenesis *Somatogenesis* (q.v.).

organogenic, organogenetic Somatogenic.

organotherapy Treatment with preparations or substances as they are found naturally in the body. In general it is called *replacement therapy,* because usually the object is to restore to the body in sufficient quantity to maintain health something that is lacking in the body. *Endocrinotherapy* is one form of organotherapy.

orgasm The peak of excitation in the genital zone; the sexual *climax.* Erotic arousal involves a series of physiologic and psychologic phenomena in response to tactile stimulation or phantasy or a combination of mechanical and psychologic stimuli. These changes include increased pulse rate and blood pressure, raised skin temperature, flow of blood into the erectile tissues of the eyes, lips, ear lobes, nipples, penis or clitoris, and the genital labia; usually also there is some degree of hyperextension of the trunk. All such changes build up to a maximum, at which point tension is suddenly released. The latter produces local spasms of the perineal musculature or more extensive convulsivelike contractions. Technically, the term orgasm refers to the moment of sudden release of tension.

orgasm, alimentary Rado's term for the feeling of bliss and rapid reduction in tension experienced by the infant at the height of breast feeding; he related the wish to reexperience alimentary orgasm to mania, melancholia, and drug dependency.

orgasm, pharmacogenic The drug addict's satisfaction (and accompanying reduction of sexual and aggressive drives) following drug administration.

orgasmus deficiens Lack of sexual pleasure. See *psychosexual.*

orgone (or'gōn) Reich's term for the life energy, which he believed to be specific and identifiable. See *bion.*

Oriental nightmare-death syndrome *Bangungut* (q.v.).

orientation 1. Awareness of one's physical relationship to reality as measured by the parameters of person, place, and time. A person with intact orientation knows his own identity and can correctly identify the people who are a part of his usual environment; he knows where he is; and he knows the year in which he lives, the month of the year, the day of the week, and whether it is morning, afternoon, or evening. A patient may be disoriented in any one or in any combination of these spheres; *disorientation,* or *confusion,* is usually indicative of organic brain disease, although some patients with functional disorders of reality testing may become confused secondary to withdrawal from and/or inattention to their environment.

2. One's direction or position in relation to a person, object, concept, or principle. Thus when a psychiatrist is asked, "What is your orientation?" the questioner is trying to determine the general theory of human behavior to which the psychiatrist subscribes, his theoretical frame of reference, the "school of thought" within psychology or psychiatry that guides his formulations and methods of treatment.

orientation, autopsychic Appreciation of oneself, of one's own personality, one's psychic self. When a person is aware that changes take place in his personality he is said to possess intact autopsychic orientation. For example, the patient with a manic-depressive disorder usually has full knowledge of the changes that have appeared in his personality. The patient with schizophrenia, however, ordinarily denies that he has changed in any way. He is autopsychically disoriented.

orientation, delusion of See *orientation, double.*

orientation, double Bleuler's term for the schizophrenic's ability to maintain some adequacy in day-to-day functioning and at the same time to believe sincerely in the most contradictory and phantastic delusions, such as the patient who works conscientiously as an elevator operator and at the same time feels that he is the president of the United States. Also known as *delusion of orientation.*

orientation, illusion of Misinterpretation or misidentification of something real in the environment because of an unclear sensorium, as in the toxic deliria. The patient hears the voice of his nurse, for example, and believes it to be that of his wife.

orientation, oral A method of approaching, evaluating, and relating oneself to the environment on the basis of the hunger drive, oral needs, etc. The infant, for example, is primarily orally oriented; the mouth is his most differentiated organ and he uses it as his chief perceptive

apparatus. The primitive ego is an oral ego, for the infant first becomes aware of objects, identifies them, and recognizes the outside world by putting objects in his mouth. When the infant began to long for something already familiar to him, absent at the moment, but with the ability to gratify his needs, he became aware of an object for the first time. When the object appeared, the longing for it disappeared and sleep followed. Thus hunger compelled the awareness of objects, i.e. the recognition of the outside world.

Next, the experience of satiation which first banished the hunger that had disturbed sleep became "the model for the mastery of external stimuli in general." That is, the taking of objects into his mouth was one of the first reactions to objects on the part of the infant. Thus the first recognition of reality on the part of the infant is for him to judge whether he should swallow an object or spit it out. In the way described above, the reaction to recognition of the outside world, that is, to the perception of objects on the part of the primitive ego, is taking-into-the-mouth: oral introjection. "The incorporation which is the first reaction to objects in general and the precursor of the later sexual and destructive attitudes in a psychological sense destroys the existence of the object. The attitude that the object exists only for the ego's satisfaction and may disappear once satisfaction is achieved can still be observed in some childish types of love." Fenichel emphasizes, however, that the aim to incorporate objects does not necessarily reflect subjective destructive tendencies toward those objects. The fact that in incorporation the object disappears, i.e. is destroyed, is an incidental consequence and shows merely that oral incorporation is an urge to get satisfaction without any further thought of the object. Rather, this primary oral attitude of incorporation is the attitude out of which love and destructive hate grow at a later stage of development. (*PTN*) See *character, oral; orality.*

orientation, reality See *reality orientation; remotivation.*

orientation, reversed A state in which a person when walking in one direction feels that he is walking in the opposite direction. The condition is purely subjective; the person orients himself correctly by reasoning.

orientation sessions See *gatekeeper*.

orientation, sexual See *sexual orientation; sexual orientation disturbance*.

original response See *popular response*.

ornithinemia Excessive ornithine in the plasma, due presumably to reduced activity of hepatic ornithine ketoacid transaminase; the condition has been described in siblings, who manifested mental retardation with marked disturbance in speech development. Whether this is an inborn error of amino acid metabolism or a secondary result of hepatic disease is uncertain.

ornithophobia Fear of birds.

orofacial dyskinesia See *dyskinesia, orofacial*.

orphan drug Any pharmacologic agent that is not economical to produce because the condition for which it is indicated affects relatively few persons. Many such drugs are further difficult to market because they are already in the public domain and consequently are not patentable. The intent of the 1983 orphan drug law is to speed the production of such drugs and to ensure their availability to the persons who need them. See *syndrome, Gilles de la Tourette*.

orthergasia See *euergasia*.

ortho- Combining form meaning straight, right, correct, sound, from Gr. *orthós*.

orthomolecular Judicious, normal, or optimal arrangement of molecules; as used in psychiatry, the term ordinarily refers to a treatment program based on Linus Pauling's theory (1967) that the schizophrenias and other functional mental disorders might be a result of vitamin deficiency. The treatment regimen consists of high doses of vitamins (hence also known as *megavitamin* treatment), especially niacin, vitamin C, and vitamin B_6, but also occasionally other vitamins and hormones as well. Neither the original theory nor the worth of the treatment regimen(s) has so far been substantiated.

orthopathic Burrow's term for feeling that is primary, direct, whole. Contrasted with *autopathic*.

orthophrenia Soundness of mind; also, the curing of a disordered mind.

orthopsychiatry A subdivision of psychiatry that deals with the study and treatment of mental deviations known in general as borderland states; it also includes the study of methods of preventing mental disorders. The term is approximately equivalent to mental hygiene. See *health, mental; hygeine, mental*.

orthostatic epileptoid See *epileptoid, orthostatic*.

orthovagotonia Exaggerated functioning of the vagotonic or parasympathetic nervous system, but only when this exaggerated functioning is in harmony with that of the sympathetic nervous system.

orthriogenesis Federn's term for the recapitulation by the ego of its whole development, which he felt occurs at the moment of awakening when the ego, which has been without cathexis in deep sleep, suddenly has its cathexis restored.

-osis Combining form meaning action, state, condition, process, from Gr. *-ōsis*.

osmo- Combining form meaning smell, odor, from Gr. *osme*.

osmophobia Pathologic fear of (bad) odors.

osphresia, osphresis The sense of smell.

osphresiolagnia Morbid or fetishistic interest in odors, often associated with infantile sexuality. Some patients believe that their body sends out an odor that is disagreeable and harmful to others, that makes others sick or insane.

The schizophrenic patient, particularly the one with delusions of persecution, often projects the idea of bad odors upon others, coming to the delusion then that others force evil body odors upon him, the patient.

One who possesses a morbid idea regarding body odors is called an osphresiolagniac or *renifleur*.

Freud says that a tendency to osphresiolagnia, which has become extinct since childhood, may play a part in the genesis of neurosis. (*CP*) See *rhinencephalon*.

osphresiophilia Morbid attraction to or interest in odors and smells.

osphresiophobia Pathologic fear of (bad) odors or of being contaminated by them.

ossification Lewin's term for the relative rigidity of behavior patterns that have become second nature or autonomous because of frequent repetitions.

osteitis deformans *Paget's disease* (q.v.).

ostensive Referring to what can be demonstrated, manifested, or exhibited. An ostensive definition of a table consists of teaching the meaning of the word "table" by pointing to many different tables.

osteoarthritis See *arthritis.*

OT Occupational therapy. See *therapy, occupational.*

Othello syndrome See *jealousy, morbid.*

otiumosis (ō-shē-um-ō'sis) E. Bergler's term for *alysosis* (q.v.).

otohemineurasthenia (ō-tō-hem-ē-nū-ras-thē'nē-à) Functional deafness affecting one ear.

otoneurasthenia Functional deafness.

outframing A type of paradoxical therapy. See *therapy, paradoxical.*

outlier Beyond the acceptable or usual range. In insurance reimbursement terminology, outliers are patients with atypical characteristics relative to other patients in a DRG (diagnosis-related group), such as an unusually low or high length of stay, death, departure against medical advice, admission and discharge on the same day. Such patients fall within a low-volume DRG (a group with five or fewer patients in a hospital's base year), presenting an unusual combination of diagnoses or surgical procedures or one or more very rare conditions.

outpatient Ambulatory patient who is not listed on the hospital inpatient census.

output The amount of work performed or completed within a specified period of time; in communications theory, any action or response that cues or signals another person or another communication system.

outputs See *functional budgeting.*

ovariotomy Surgical removal of one or both ovaries. Bilateral ovariotomy is required for the castration of a female and usually leads, if performed before puberty, to such marked disturbance in the sex balance as to produce a eunuchoid symptomatology with secondary male sex characteristics (see *castration*). Also called *oophorectomy.*

overactivity, psychomotor See *mania.*

overadequate-inadequate reciprocity See *psychotherapy, family.*

overanxious disorders See *anxiety disorders of childhood.*

overcompensation The term has been made popular by Alfred Adler. When the feeling of inferiority is so great that the person fears he will never be able to compensate

for his weakness, his striving for power and dominance is exaggerated and intensified to a pathological degree.

Such people endeavor to secure their position in life by extraordinary efforts, by greater haste and impatience, by more violent impulses, and without consideration for anyone else. Their attitudes are apt to have a certain grandiose quality. See *complex, Demosthenes.*

According to Adler, overcompensation is the counterpose of an overwhelming feeling of inferiority that is profusely neutralized by steps toward a towering goal of dominance.

overconsciousness Exaggerated development of self-consciousness as the result of "oversocialization with leveling of the object relations." The term applies to parents who first identify themselves too strongly with their children as love objects, and then perform acts ostensibly of "self-sacrificing love," which, in psychiatric terms, are mere expressions of an increased narcissism on the part of the parents. Overconsciousness is a narcissistic attitude developed as a result of object relations of a special intensity and character. (Schilder, P. *Mind, Perception and Thought,* 1942)

overdependence, social See *psychodynamics, adaptational.*

overdetermination "As a rule neuroses are *overdetermined;* that is to say, several factors in their etiology operate together." (Freud, *CP*) More properly, *multidetermination.*

overflow, motor *Synkinesia* (q.v.).

overinclusiveness One of the many association disturbances that may be observed in schizophrenic speech; it is the inability to preserve conceptual boundaries, so that irrelevant or distantly associated elements become incorporated into concepts, making thought less precise and more abstract. See *associations, disturbances of.*

overprotection, maternal Overprotection of the growing infant by the parent can result in difficulties for the person in later life. Overindulged and overprotected at an early age, the infant has not learned to bear frustrations. As a result, at a later period of development, little frustrations that a less spoiled person could tolerate have the effect of a severe frustration. The infant will refuse to go further in development and will demand the withheld gratification associated with the particular little frustrations. Thus there will be fixations at the level of development at which the frustrations occur. These fixations resulting from overprotection produce personality difficulties such as various neurotic defense symptoms, or character attitudes, and primitive types of love.

An overprotecting parent predisposes the child to passive, dependent types of mastery. As a result, he will be unable to adapt himself objectively, but his passive dependent needs will color all his activities and relationships, causing the inevitable illusions and disappointments.

overreactive disorders See *psychodynamics, adaptational.*

oxycephaly (ok-sē-sef′a-lē) Tower-head; turrecephaly. A congenital anomaly in which there is premature closure (craniosynostosis) of the coronal and lambdoid sutures, resulting in an upward elongation of the head, which thus appears dome-shaped. The anomaly does not affect mentality or length of life, but in order to preserve vision the King corrective operation must be performed early in life.

P

P Rorschach scoring symbol for a *popular response* (q.v.).

P-element See *system*.

P-system See *system*.

P$_{300}$ wave *P$_{300}$ brain wave, P$_{300}$ amplitude;* a positive brain wave that appears between 300 and 500 msec after a stimulus. It is one of the endogenous components of the sensory-evoked response that is related to information processing of task-relevant information. The P$_{300}$ wave is associated with the psychologic processes of attention, expectancy, stimulus recognition, stimulus evaluation, and cognitive decision-making activity.

Computer-averaged brain waves are measured by exposing subjects to a train of stimuli (such as flashes of light) and asking them to discriminate a randomly occurring unusual stimulus. When the anticipated unusual event occurs (such as a light of greater brightness or duration than the others), a positive brain wave appears between 300 and 500 msec following the stimulus. Its amplitude and latency are related to the importance of the task, how unpredictable or infrequent the event is, and the subject's motivation. See *neurometrics; NMR*.

pacemaker, cerebral A hypothesized central neurophysiologic mechanism that regulates and synchronizes the EEG rhythms of the two cerebral hemispheres. The cerebral pacemaker is believed to be located in the reticular substance of the upper brain stem or in the adjacent posterior hypothalamic region. (Aird, R., & Garoutte, B. *Neurology 8,* 1958)

pachymeningitis See *meninges; meningitis*.

pachymeninx See *meninges*.

pack In psychiatric nursing, the application of sheets to the patient's body. The pack may be wet or dry, hot or cold. In each case the patient is wrapped in several sheets. When a *cold pack* is used the sheets are imersed in water at a temperature of 60° F.; the temperature of the water in case of a *hot pack* is 130 to 145° F.

Dry packs are sometimes used to induce increase of body temperature by lessening heat elimination. Their chief use is with agitated patients who have failed to respond to neuroleptics alone.

pact, suicide See *suicide pact*.

PAD Primary *affective disorder* (q.v.).

paederastia *Obs.* Pederasty.

paedicatio *Obs.* Pederasty.

paedico Although it appears as the root of various terms referring to sexual activity with children—and often specifically as homosexual activity with young boys, as in paederasty—the term means to penetrate the anus and does not imply either specific gender or age of either participant in the activity. Pederasty in ancient writing often has no more relation to the age of objects of desire than does the term "girl chasing" according to J. Boswell (*Christianity, Social Tolerance, and Homosexuality,* 1980). See *pederasty*.

paed(o)-, ped(o)- Combining form meaning childlike, or having to do with children, from Gr. *paid-*.

Paget's disease (Sir James Paget, English surgeon, 1814–99) Osteitis deformans; bony overgrowth often produces neurological complications by exerting pressure on the cerebral nervous system or nerve roots.

pagophagia Ice-eating, a type of *pica* (q.v.) suggesting an underlying iron deficiency anemia; the affected subject typically ingests at least one ordinary tray of ice daily for a period of two months or more.

paidicatio *Obs.* Pederasty; sodomy.

pain agnosia See *dwarfism, psychosocial.*

pain clinic An outpatient facility providing a multidisciplinary approach to the management of pain, typically through a combination of medical, physical, and behavioral modalities that may involve any or all of the following: anesthesiologist, neurologist, psychiatrist, physiatrist, orthopedist, nurse, physical therapist, and psychologist.

pain conduction See *gating, spinal.*

pain, ecstatic "The *hunger for excitement* of some people comes about in this manner. There are people who must always be doing something; it matters little whether the situation is of a pleasurable or painful nature. Sometimes a decided preference is shown for the latter; they experience 'ecstatic pain,' martyrlike pleasure, and forever consider themselves unfairly treated." (Bleuler, *TP*)

pain management, multidimensional The use of operant conditioning techniques in the treatment of chronic pain syndromes. It is sometimes helpful in short-term management, but benefits are rarely maintained.

pain, psychic *Psychalgia;* psychogenic pain disorder. See *somatoform disorders.*

pain, referred Irradiation of pain sensation, with or without hyperalgesia, into an area of skin when a viscus or muscle is the site of the lesion. Although the basis for referral of pain must be excitation of common pathways, it is uncertain whether the brain, the spinal cord, or the peripheral nerves are involved.

painting, finger Direct manipulation of the paint with the fingers and hands to achieve a graphic effect. In psychology, finger painting is used as a projective technique, the assumption being that finger painting is a form of expressive behavior, the analysis of which reveals significant characteristics of the subject. Finger painting was developed by Ruth F. Shaw (1934) as an educational technique, and it has since been used as a diagnostic projective technique, as a means for stimulating free associations, as a part of psychotherapy and play therapy, and by occupational therapists in rehabilitation of spastic patients, the deaf, and the blind.

pairing assumption See *group, basic assumptions.*

pal(a)eo- (pā'lē-ō-, pal'ē-ō-) Combining form meaning old, ancient, from Gr. *palaiós.*

paleologic Archaic or ancient logic; with this term, Arieti refers to the same method of thinking that has been variously designated as pre-Aristotelian, prelogical (Levy-Bruhl) or paralogical (Von Domarus). Paleologic is seen most clearly in schizophrenic thinking disorders. See *prelogical.*

paleomnesis Memory for the remote past in the life of the subject.

paleophrenia This psychoanalytical term, meaning literally ancient or primitive mentality, was suggested by O. Osborne to be used instead of schizophrenia to emphasize the regression to a primitive type of thinking that is often seen in schizophrenics.

paleopsychic Pertaining to or possessing primitive mentality.

paleopsychology The study of paleopsychic phenomena; it is believed by Freud, Jung, and many others, that remote ancestral modes of mental activity reside in the unconscious of modern man.

paleosensation The term of the Dutch school of neurologists (Brouwer, Kappers) for *protopathic* sensations in contradistinction to the epicritic and deep, which they call *gnostic* or new sensations. See *gnostic; protopathic.*

paleosymbol A private symbol, which is highly individualistic, fleeting, flexible, and mutable and which is evolved and maintained without regard for socialization or interpersonal relationships. Paleo-symbols are seen as a form of *paleologic* (q.v.) and are characteristic of immediately prehuman races although they probably exist also in apes in rudimentary form.

pali- (pal'ē-) Combining form meaning morbid or obsessive repetition or reiteration, from Gr. *pálin,* backward, again.

paligraphia The morbid or obsessive repetition of something (letters, words, phrases, etc.) in writing.

palilalia A rare speech disorder in which a phrase is repeated with increasing rapidity. The most common causes of palilalia are encephalitis or other conditions producing parkinsonism, Alzheimer's disease, and pseudobulbar palsy due to vascular lesions.

palilexia The morbid rereading of words or phrases.

palilogia Morbid or obsessive repetition of something spoken.

palingraphia Mirror-writing.

palinlexia Backward reading.

palinopia, palinopsia A rare visual phenomenon consisting of visual perseveration in time, i.e. a prolonged afterimage. Palinopia is suggestive of an occipital lobe lesion. See *polyopia*.

paliopsy Visual perseverance; brief persistence in vision of objects no longer in the visual field, usually indicative of occipital lobe pathology.

paliphrasia The morbid repetition of phrases in speaking.

pallesthesia The vibratory sensation felt when the foot of a vibrating tuning fork is placed over subcutaneous bony surfaces. Also known as *palmesthesia*.

pallidum (pȧ′lē-doom) See *basal ganglia*.

palmesthesia *Pallesthesia* (q.v.).

palsy Paralysis.

palsy, cerebral *Little's disease* (q.v.).

palsy, progressive bulbar See *sclerosis, amyotrophic lateral*.

palsy, pseudobulbar See *sclerosis, amyotrophic lateral*.

palsy, shaking *Paralysis agitans* (q.v.); Parkinson's disease.

pamphobia *Obs.* *Panphobia;* fear of everything.

pamplegia, panplegia *Obs.* Generalized paralysis (not the clinical entity, general paralysis).

pan-, pam- Combining form meaning all, whole, from Gr. *pān.*

pananxiety See *schizophrenia, pseudoneurotic.*

panchreston The state or quality of being adaptable to any and all uses; applied sometimes to the terminology of psychiatry and psychology, where words are used to explain everything, and in such a variety of ways as finally to become a meaningless jargon.

Pándy's reaction See *test, Pándy.*

panels, personality The concept of a four-panel Japanese screen, across which is painted a complete picture, moved Draper to introduce into the vocabulary of constitutional medicine the term *panels of personality* representing the four main divisions of the human individuality.

These panels relate to the anatomical, physiological, psychological, and immunological elements of a person, each of which "may be considered to occupy one panel of the great screen across which Man's personality is drawn." (Draper, G. *Human Constitution,* 1924) See *constitution; medicine, constitutional.*

panencephalitis, subacute sclerosing (SSPE) A rare disease of children and young adults due to a measles virus variant. Symptoms, which typically develop five to seven years after the child has had measles, consist of progressive deterioration of mental and motor performance and associated myoclonic movements. In the early stage, signs are mainly cerebral (awkwardness, stumbling, mental deterioration, memory loss); at the second stage, convulsions and repetitive myoclonus are characteristic. In the final stage, stupor, coma, and increased spasticity appear, with death within one to three years after onset. Within the United States, incidence is about one in one million; 85% are from rural areas, and males are four times as frequently affected as females.

panglossia Garrulity, especially psychotic.

panic An attack of overwhelming *anxiety* (q.v.). Some writers restrict the term to psychotic episodes characterized by unrealistically based and autistically determined anxiety of overwhelming proportions, such as is seen in *homosexual panic* (q.v.) . and in acute aggression panic. The latter term refers to cases where homosexual content is lacking and, instead, a picture of undue malignant influence, physical violence, or impending death is seen.

panic disorder A type of anxiety disorder consisting of sudden onset of intense apprehensiveness or terror and, often, a sense of impending doom, feelings of depersonalization or derealization or both, and a fear of losing control or "going crazy." Accompanying the mental state are emergency physical symptoms and signs of automatic hyperactivity, such as sweating, pallor, dyspnea, choking sensations, palpitations, dizziness, or vertigo. Attacks usually last minutes; some continue for more than an hour. Like some other *anxiety disorders* (q.v.), panic disorder tends to run in families, and there is evidence that it is transmitted as an autosomal dominant trait. (Pauls, D., et al. *American Journal of Human Genetics 32,* 1980)

DSM-III-R differentiates panic disorder

with *agoraphobia* (q.v.) and panic disorder without agoraphobia.

panic, homosexual See *homosexual panic*.

panic, lactate See *lactate challenge*.

panic, prepsychotic Arieti's term for that stage in the development of schizophrenia in which the patient's grotesque and disordered self-image leads to feelings of being unlovable, different, humiliated, guilty, under suspicion, etc., but the cognitive distortions are not yet expressed in such full-fledged psychotic symptoms as delusions and hallucinations.

panic, primordial Reactions of fright and anger combined with unfocused, disorganized motor responses akin to the infantile startle reaction; such reactions are seen in many schizophrenic children. Primordial panic is also termed *elemental anxiety* and is believed to be based on primary defects in the ego that result in an impairment in personal identity, self-awareness, and differentiation of the self from the non-self.

panmixia In genetic population studies this term indicates equal and unrestricted mating conditions of organisms with different racial characteristics in a mixed population group. See *homogamy*.

panneurosis See *schizophrenia, pseudoneurotic*.

panoramic memory See *absent state*.

panphobia, panophobia, pantophobia Fear of everything.

pansexualism The doctrine that all human behavior stems from sex. There is no school of psychiatric medicine today whose leaders profess such a doctrine. Freud specifically disavowed any connection between pansexualism and psychoanalysis.

Papez's circle See *emotion, Papez's theory of*.

papilledema (pap-i-le-dē′mȧ) Papilledema or choked disk is a condition in which the optic nerve is literally choked at the optic foramen by increased intracranial, and especially intraventricular, pressure, leading to an increase in the intraocular tension. The condition is usually bilateral, although there may be differences in the degree of choking on the two sides. Ophthalmoscopically, the disk is raised, at times to five or six or more diopters; the margins of the disk are blurred; the veins are tortuous and full, the arteries thin; and hemorrhages may occur. Papilledema is most commonly caused by tumor of the

brain. Other conditions producing choked disk include fracture of the skull, hydrocephalus, abscess of the brain, subarachnoid hemorrhage, sinus thrombosis, meningitis, encephalitis, and possibly multiple sclerosis and anemia.

para-, par- (par′ȧ) Combining form meaning beside, past, aside, beyond, i.e. perverted, amiss, wrong, faulty, irregular, disordered, abnormal, mis-, from Gr. *pará*, from (the side), beside, near, beyond, against.

parabulia Perversion of volition or will as when an impulse is partly or completely checked and is then replaced by another impulse. A patient had the impulse to strike his physician; he advanced toward the physician for that purpose, but suddenly stopped "to regulate the universal voices." Parabulia usually occurs as a manifestation of ambivalence of the will in schizophrenic disorders. See *will, disturbances of the*.

paracenesthesia Any abnormality of the general sense of well-being.

parachromatopsia, parachromopsia Partial color blindness, such as red-green color blindness.

paracope (par-ak′ō-pē) *Obs.* Hippocrates's term for delirium accompanying fever; later synonymous with *insanity*.

paracousia, paracusia Any abnormality of hearing other than simple deafness; in psychiatric writings the term is often used to refer specifically to auditory illusions. *Paracousia loci* is impaired ability to determine the direction from which a sound proceeds. *Paracousia willisiana* is the ability, demonstrated by some partially deaf persons, to hear better in the presence of loud noise.

paradementia Brugias' term for schizophrenia.

paradigm A model; presentation of a word to demonstrate each of its forms (as in a conjugation or declension); a classificatory system in which each of the terms is so defined that no term overlaps or includes another, every component is discriminated by at least one term, and all terms can be displayed on the same graph or system.

paradox, neurotic This term indicates that neurotic behavior often persists indefinitely despite the fact that it is seriously self-defeating and even inimical to the individual. Freud attempted to explain this paradox by assuming that it was due to the retention of an oversevere superego, evolved from too zealous childhood training. This explanation, however, is contrary to all learning theory, which says that learning tends to undergo extinction unless periodically reinforced. It is more likely that the paradox results from infantile ego resistance to socializing forces, so that the basic values and attitudes of society are faultily assimilated into the personality. It may also be that the neurotic behavior represents a means to an end that is unconsciously determined, the desire for which overcomes the wish to conform.

paradoxical intention (PI) A treatment technique for phobic patients that directs the subject to try to increase anxiety and become as panicky as possible.

paradoxical therapy See *therapy, paradoxical.*

paraerotism Perversion. See *metaerotism.*

paraflocculi See *cerebellum.*

parageusia (par-à-gū'sē-à) Perverted sense of taste.

paragnomen (par-ag-nō'men) An unexpected action, not understandable for the subject's environment or by reason of his usual conduct or behavior, which at the moment it is performed is considered to be consciously performed and adequate to the situation but which later appears inexplicable even to the subject. Paragnomens are seen frequently in schizophrenic patients.

paragnosia Irrelevant or approximate answers and, in particular, the "wild" guesses made by subjects with nondominant parietal lobe dysfunction who cannot state spontaneously where they are (even though they might select the right answer if offered a number of choices).

paragrammatism Any speech disturbance characterized by faulty grammatical or syntactical relationships; the disturbance may be a part of the organic asphasias, or it may be found in schizophrenic speech. "At times grammar fails them (*paragrammatism*). Many words are used incorrectly, thus, e.g. frequently the word 'murder' that designates all the tortures that the patients suffer." (Bleuler, *TP*)

paragraphia Perverted writing. Ordinarily, however, it does not refer to alterations in the handwriting itself, such as are manifested by tremors, rigid writing, flourishes and abnormalities in the size of the script; rather, it has to do with such errors as the omission and transposition of letters or words, or the substitution of a wrong letter or word, or the writing of nonexistent words. Errors of this kind are usually due to cerebral injury, although they may also occur in schizophrenic disorders. See *neologism.*

parahypnosis Abnormal sleep as in hypnotism or somnambulism; used particularly to refer to the suggestibility of patients under general anesthesia, when remarks or suggestions made by others in the operating or delivery room may be responsible for later development of symptoms by the patient.

parakinesia Bizarre and clumsily executed movement.

paralalia Any speech defect, especially the habitual substitution of one letter for another.

paralalia literalis Perversion in uttering certain sounds; usually combined with stammering.

paralanguage See *psycholinguistics.*

paraleresis *Obs.* Mild delirium.

paralexia Misreading of printed or written words, other meaningless words being substituted for them. See *neglect, sensory; reading disabilities.*

paralipophobia Fear of neglecting duty.

parallel distributed processing See *connectionism.*

parallel visual computation *MPPS* (q.v.).

paralogia Perverted logic or reasoning in speaking. "Evasion or *paralogia* consists in this, that the idea which is next in the chain of thought is suppressed and replaced by another which is related to it." (Kraepelin, *DP*)

paralogia, derailment or displacement See *acataphasia.*

paralogia, metaphoric See *by-idea.*

paralogia, thematic Perverted reasoning in relation chiefly to one theme or subject, upon which the mind dwells insistently. See *monomania.*

paralysis Loss of power of voluntary movement in a muscle due to injury or disease of its nerve supply.

paralysis, acute ascending *Landry's paralysis* (q.v.).

paralysis agitans Parkinson's disease; a chronic, progressive disease of the central nervous system, occurring more frequently in males than in females, most often between the ages of 50 and 70 years. Onset is usually insidious, with gradual, slow progression; the characteristic symptoms are cogwheel rigidity and spontaneous tremor, with immobile and masklike facies, loss of associated movements of the arms, dysarthritic speech, propulsive gait, etc. Tremors are often of the pill-rolling type, involving the thumb, index finger, or wrist, and are often accompanied by a to-and-fro tremor of the head.

Idiopathic or true Parkinson's disease is to be differentiated from *parkinsonism* (parkinsonian syndrome), which may be a side effect of tranquilizers; carbon monoxide, manganese, nitrous oxide, or carbon disulfite poisoning; brain tumor; brain injury; neurosyphilis; and encephalitis. Idiopathic Parkinson's disease (including the arteriosclerotic cases) is characterized by degeneration of cells and tracts of the striate bodies and substantia nigra, perhaps secondary to disturbed metabolism of brain amines. In this disorder, both dopamine and serotonin (or their derivatives) are decreased in brain and in urine, and this decrease may be related to a relative deficiency in the enzyme dopa-decarboxylase.

Treatment is symptomatic, with belladonna derivatives, synthetic compounds with atropinelike action, and/or antihistamines; some patients benefit from stereotactic operations that destroy portions of the globus pallidus or the ventrolateral nucleus of the thalamus. Treatment with L-dopa, the biosynthetic precursor of dopamine, produces favorable results in approximately 70% of patients.

paralysis, catatonic cerebral A term applied to rare cases of catatonic excitement or delirium that terminate abruptly in death, often following the development of fever of unknown origin. The syndrome is also known as *Stauder's lethal catatonia* and is generally regarded as a schizophrenic disorder; probably less than 1% of schizophrenic patients follow such a course. See *Bell's mania*.

paralysis, congenital spastic *Little's disease* (q.v.).

paralysis, divers See *disease, caisson* (q.v.).

paralysis, familial periodic A hereditary disorder consisting of abrupt, periodic attacks of flaccid paralysis that may last anywhere from hours to three or four days. The illness, which appears to be based on an abnormal demand for potassium, usually begins during adolescence. Prodromata such as hunger, thirst, or sweating are common, and the attacks themselves tend to occur in the early morning. The paralysis is at its height an hour after onset; the proximal limb is affected more than the distal portion and during the attack deep reflexes are abolished, but there is no loss of consciousness. Attacks may occur every few days, or only once every few years. They tend to be precipitated by exposure to the cold, excess sugar intake, fasting, or overexertion. Potassium chloride is used in the treatment of individual attacks and prophylactically when attacks occur frequently.

paralysis, hysterical A paralysis of psychogenic etiology, in contradistinction to a paralysis of organic origin. The organic paralyses are never so complete as the hysterical paralyses. The hysterically paralyzed limb will be absolutely inert; the hysterical aphasic is completely mute. Thus hysterical paralysis shows both an exact delimitation and an excessive intensity. These two characteristics of hysterical paralysis indicate that the hysterical lesion is entirely independent of the anatomy of the nervous system. See *conversion; hysteria*.

paralysis, immobilization "In wound-cases where there had been immobilization of a limb in splints for some time, the immobilization sometimes persisted long after the splints were removed—the so-called immobilization-paralysis. The patient had 'failed to realize when he had become well.' The hysterical purpose was the same as in the unwounded cases of functional paralysis. The same phenomenon is encountered in the 'traumatic,' of peace time." (Henderson, D.K., & Gillespie, R.D. *A Text-Book of Psychiatry*, 1936)

paralysis, infantile *Poliomyelitis* (q.v.).

paralysis, Landry's See *Landry's paralysis*.

paralysis, periodic See *paralysis, familial periodic*.

paralysis, progressive *Obs.* General paralysis.

paralysis, saturnine pseudogeneral Chronic encephalopathy due to *lead poisoning* (q.v.).

paralysis, sleep A benign neurological phenomenon, most probably due to some temporary dysfunction of the reticular activating system, consisting of brief episodes of inability to move and/or speak when awakening or, less commonly, when falling asleep. There is no accompanying disturbance of consciousness, and the subject has complete recall for the episode. The incidence of the phenomenon is highest in younger age groups (children and young adults) and much higher in males (80%) than in females. The terms by which the phenomenon has been known are nocturnal hemiplegia, nocturnal paralysis, sleep numbness, delayed psychomotor awakening, cataplexy of awakening, and post-dormital chalastic fits.

parameter In mathematics, a variable or constant that determines the shape of the mathematical object or function being studied (e.g. length or depth); by extension (regrettable, because imprecision will ultimately render the term meaningless), any limit or boundary.

In psychoanalytic therapy, any deviation from the neutral interpretive stance of the analyst; any interventions other than interpretation that might be necessary to initiate or maintain the analytic process. The term *pseudoparameter* is used to refer to technical devices which, though not strictly interpretations, nonetheless have the same dynamic effect, such as telling the right joke at the right moment or repeating to the patient the words he has just said.

paramimia Disturbance of sense for gestures or mimetic movements leading to incongruities between feeling and means of expression.

paramimism A movement or gesture that has a meaning for the patient different from the ordinarily accepted meaning.

paramnesia Disturbance of memory in which real facts and phantasies are confused. Thus a patient was unable to tell whether he had dreamed or actually experienced that of which he was given an account. Paramnesia is a common phenomenon in dreams, and in the schizophrenias where it often appears as false recognition such as déjà fait or déjà vu.

Such paramnesiae may also occur in the normal person.

paramnesia, reduplicative *Doppelganger* (q.v.).

paramyotonia congenita A rare muscle disorder transmitted by a single autosomal dominant gene with nearly complete penetrance, characterized by two sets of symptoms: (1) myotonic cramps of the facial musculature and hands precipitated by cold and myotonia of the lingual muscles in response to percussion, and (2) attacks of weakness and flaccidity in the proximal muscles lasting for minutes or up to 24 hours.

paranee (par-à-ně') A term introduced by Richard M. Brickner to designate the "victim" of a paranoid patient.

paraneoplastic See *encephalitis, paraneoplastic limbic.*

paranoia, paranoea Although paranoia in the sense of mental derangement, delirium, occurs in Aeschylus (Theb. 756), Euripides (Orestes 822), Plato (Laws 928E), and elsewhere, i.e. the term is even pre-Hippocratic, credit is generally given to Vogel for having introduced or reintroduced the term in medicine in 1764.

Following this, the term was inconsistently applied to a great number of diverse conditions until 1883, when E.C. Spitzka, a New York psychiatrist, defined paranoia as it is known at the present time. Kahlbaum was among the first to use the term in the way in which it is generally used today, to refer to gradually developing, systematized delusional states, without hallucinations but with preservation of intelligence, and with emotional responses and behavior that remain congruous with and appropriate to the persecutory or grandiose delusions.

Paranoid disorders—termed *delusional disorders* in DSM-III-R—constitute a group of rare conditions in which the central feature is the development of one or more persistent delusions that are not bizarre but involve mechanisms that occur in real life, such as being followed, being loved from afar, or being deceived by a lover. In any one patient, the delusions typically revolve about a single theme or a series of connected themes. *Paranoia* is sometimes used to refer to a chronic condition with fixed and typically systematized delusions, in a subject who in other areas does not appear to be odd or bizarre and who does not show prominent auditory or visual hallucinations.

Shared paranoid disorder corresponds to what other systems term *folie à deux* (q.v.) or psychosis of association (see *association, psychosis of*). In DSM-III-R it is termed *induced psychotic disorder* and is classified among "other psychotic disorders" rather than within the group of delusional disorders.

Atypical paranoid disorder has been used to refer to suddenly appearing paranoid states in persons who recently changed their living or work situation, such as immigrants, refugees, and inductees into military service. Such conditions rarely become chronic. Paranoid developments occur also in association with other disorders, and particularly in organic mental disorders; they are then classified under those disorders or as "organic delusional syndrome."

Types of paranoid disorder are usually described in terms of the predominant delusional theme: persecutory (the subject or someone close to him is being treated malevolently), jealous or infidelity type (the subject's sexual partner is unfaithful), erotic or erotomaniacal (some other person, usually of higher social or economic status, is in love with the subject), somatic (delusional conviction that one has a physical disorder), grandiose (delusions of great importance, wealth, social standing, special relationships to the deity or the famous), litigious (constantly seeking legal redress for imagined wrongs), etc.

On the basis of his analysis of the Schreber case, Freud concluded that the core of the conflict in paranoia (at least in males) is a homosexual wish-phantasy of loving a man. The forms of paranoia represent the contradictions of the proposition: I, a man, love him, a man. This proposition is contradicted (a) in the subject, by delusions of jealousy: "It is not I who love the man, it is she"; (b) in the predicate, by delusions of persecution: "I do not love him, I hate him, and because of this he hates me and persecutes me"; (c) in the object, by erotomania: "I do not love him, I love her, because she loves me"; and (d) by complete denial in megalomania: "I do not love anyone else at all, but only myself."

paranoia, acquired Krafft-Ebing described two principal forms of paranoia: (1) *original paranoia,* developing before or at puberty—always hereditary; (2) *acquired paranoia,* developing late in life, particularly at the involutional period.

paranoia, affect-laden In Leonhard's classification, a subtype of nonsystematic schizophrenia characterized by paranoid delusions and strong affective reaction to their content. See *schizophrenia, systematic.*

paranoia, alcoholic An inexact term, used by some writers as equivalent to alcoholic hallucinosis (see *hallucinosis, alcoholic*), by others to refer to infidelity delusions that develop in alcoholics. Although alcoholics can develop any of the forms of *paranoia* (q.v.), they seem especially prone to jealousy delusions. See *alcoholic paranoid state.*

paranoia, amorous *Obs.* By some, used to refer to the jealous or infidelity form of paranoia; by others, used to refer to the erotomaniacal form. The patient with amorous paranoia develops delusions of marital infidelity in relation to his spouse. According to Freud's analysis of the Schreber case, such delusions are based on a denial of unconscious homosexuality: "It is not I who love the man, it is she." See *jealousy, morbid.*

paranoia completa *Obs.* A term coined by Magnan (*délire chronique à évolution systématique*) equivalent to present conceptions of the paranoid form of schizophrenia.

paranoia, conjugal Morbid jealousy of the marital partner that constitutes the sole or primary delusion of an underlying paranoia or paranoid schizophrenia. See *jealousy, morbid.*

paranoia dissociativa (dēs-sô-kē-à-tē′và) *Obs.* An expression coined by Ziehen to designate states of acute confusion (amentia) with paranoid elements.

paranoia, eccentric See *paranoia, amorous.*

paranoia, hypochondriacal Hypochondriac paranoid psychosis; somatic delusion that constitutes the sole or primary delusion of an underlying paranoia or paranoid schizophrenia. See *dysmorphophobia.*

paranoia, intermediate *Obs.* Paranoia in which there are no delusions, but a tendency to quibbling or quarreling. See *paranoia querulans.*

paranoia, involutional The paranoid form of involutional melancholia. See *psychosis, involutional.*

paranoia, litigious (li-ti'jus) *Paranoia querulans* (q.v.).

paranoia, mystic Pike's term for psychosis of association. See *association, psychosis of.*

paranoia, negative Paranoia in which the false beliefs of the person have to do with matters *favorable* to him rather than with those *unfavorable.* The delusionary material is characterized by praise, protection, and defense instead of persecution, accusation, destruction, and the like.

paranoia querulans (kwe'roo-làns) A form of paranoia characterized by more or less incessant quarrelsomeness due to alleged persecution. Often starting from a factual injustice, the patient weaves a delusional trend about it and then seeks redress at the hands of the law.

paranoia, reformatory Zealotry; a form of megalomania sometimes expressed in psychotic delusions but more often as character or personality traits. The subject is determined to convert the world to his ideas or to convince all of the wonder of some discovery he has made (*inventive paranoia*).

paranoia, rudimentary *Latent paranoia.* "What distinguished the delusions of these patients [with rudimentary paranoia] from those of pronounced paranoia was their *vagueness* and the *absence of systematic working up.* Their fears and hopes were of a more indefinite kind, were brought forward as indications and conjectures, or they consisted in a strong personal valuation of actual events, which was not too far removed from the one-sidedness of normal individuals. As far as could be known, no internal connection of the individual component parts of the delusion with a paranoiac view of life had taken place." (Kraepelin, E. *Manic-Depressive Insanity and Paranoia,* 1921) The expression was coined by Morselli.

paranoia senilis A paranoid syndrome appearing during old age; late *paraphrenia.* "The forms showing a clear sensorium with delusional formation and eventually hallucinations are designated as *senile paranoia* (i.e. paranoid forms of dementia senilis); they are not frequent. Such people think they are spied on by neighbors, teased, robbed especially by those living in the same house; everywhere they find reference to themselves, and confirmation of their ideas in voices, etc." (Bleuler, *TP*)

paranoid (paranoidal) Relating to or resembling paranoia. Psychiatrists today speak of *paranoid* states, usually referring to clinical states that occupy a position between paranoia and the paranoid form of schizophrenia. In the eighth edition of his textbook Kraepelin uses the term *paraphrenia* to designate this group. He divided the group into four parts: (1) *paraphrenia systematica,* the equivalent perhaps of what today is known as paranoia; (2) *paraphrenia expansiva,* seen only in women and characterized by ideas of grandeur with exaltation; (3) *paraphrenia confabulans,* characterized by delusions of persecution and grandeur based upon falsification of memory; (4) *paraphrenia phantastica,* with auditory hallucinations, unsystematized delusions, and phantastic accounts of adventures.

paranoid dementia gravis See *dementia paranoides gravis.*

paranoid disorders See *paranoia.*

paranoid personality In this type of personality disorder, the affected person is hypersensitive, rigid, and unwarrantedly suspicious, jealous, and envious. He often has an exaggerated sense of self-importance, must always be right and/or prove others to be in the wrong, and has a tendency to blame others and to ascribe evil motives to them.

Often, the opposite-sex parent of such patients is domineering, overprotective, and ambivalent, while the same-sex parent is submissive, passive, and relatively unavailable as a suitable model or object for identification. In other cases, the same-sex parent has instilled feelings of inadequacy by intimidation, hostility, and the imposition of rigid controls. As a result of such rearing, the child fails to develop a stable self-image, gender role, or clear ego boundaries. He then may find it necessary to surrender to the omnipotent parent in a passive, more or less homosexual way; or he may resist and rebel defensively, but the necessary hypervigilance in his defensive operations may progress to ideas of reference.

paranoid-schizoid position See *position, paranoid-schizoid.*

paranoid schizophrenia See *schizophrenia, paranoid.*

paranoid state Like *paranoia* (q.v.), the paranoid state is characterized by persistent persecutory or grandiose delusions, affect in harmony with the delusional ideas, and preservation of intellectual functions but, ordinarily, an absence of hallucinations. This condition is differentiated from paranoia by its lack of extreme systematization, and from schizophrenia by its lack of fragmentation of associations and the absence of bizarre incongruities.

paranomasia See *homonym.*

paranormal Alongside or beyond the normal, as in paranormal cognition (telepathy). See *perception, extrasensory.*

paranosic Relating to the primary advantage derived from an illness or paranosis. See *gain, epinosic.*

parapathic proviso See *proviso, parapathic.*

parapathy (pà-rap'à-thē) Stekel's term for neurosis; he objects to the word neurosis because connotatively it indicates a functional nervous disorder. Parapathy, on the other hand, indicates that psychiatrists deal with emotions, not with nerves.

paraphasia Perverted speech; jargon; most commonly used to refer to a form of expressive asphasia in which the patient, although he hears and comprehends words, is unable to speak correctly—one word is substituted for another, and sentences become so jumbled as to be unintelligible. Paraphasia occurs in many organic brain disorders, but most characteristically in bromide delirium, Pick's disease, and delirium tremens.

paraphemia *Rare.* Distorted speech such as neurotic lisping.

paraphia (par-af'ē-à) Perverted sense of touch. Impairment of tactile sensibility; paresthesia.

paraphilia Perversion. See *nonreproductive; sexual disorders.*

paraphilic coercive disorder Suggested, but ultimately rejected, as a new category in DSM-III-R to refer to a paraphilia characterized by intense urges and sexually arousing phantasies whose main theme is forcing a nonconsenting person to submit to sexual contact (such as oral, vaginal, or anal penetration or grabbing a woman's breast). Paraphilic rapism had also been suggested, and also rejected, as a term for this disorder. It was differentiated from sexual sadism in that the arousing element is coercion rather than signs of psychological or physical suffering in the victim.

paraphora (par-af'ō-rà) *Obs.* A mild state of mental disorder.

paraphrasia Perverted sense or faculty of constructing a phrase; a speech disorder of a less severe nature than aphrasia from which it differs in degree, but not in kind. The difficulties of *aphrasia* (q.v.) and, consequently, of paraphrasia may be of mental origin and are not always due to cerebral pathology. The phenomenon is especially common in the schizophrenias. Thus a patient wishing to refer to a certain person says "Saturday" instead; it was on a Saturday that a particularly intense emotional reaction took place between the patient and the person in question.

"We shall have to keep apart two chief forms of paraphrasic disorders; firstly, *derailments in finding words*, secondly, *disorders in connected speech.*" (Kraepelin, *DP*)

paraphrasia, thematic This expression was used by Arndt to denote incoherent speech "wandering" from the theme or subject.

paraphrasia vesana *Obs.* "If the formation of ideas and of thought is disturbed in its whole extent, so that it is only with difficulty that a single proper judgment can be expressed, and if new words are coined to express the imperfect and strange thoughts, such neologisms being but maimed fragments of regular words, veritably heaps of syllables, then we have *paraphrasia vesana*, an effect of profound psychic decadence." (Bianchi, L. *A Text-Book of Psychiatry*, 1906)

paraphrenesis *Obs.* Delirium.

paraphrenia Severe paranoid illness without deterioration of other cognitive or affective processes.

Kraepelin used the term in a special sense; see *paranoid.* Freud uses the expression to refer to dementia praecox or schizophrenia.

In the early part of the 19th century, Guislain used this term synonymously with that of the clinical syndrome then known as *folly* (q.v.).

The most common usage of the term today is to denote a disorder characterized by phantastic, absurd, paralogical delusions without deterioration, dementia, or loss of contact with reality except in the area of the delusional system. In paranoid schizophrenia, on the other hand, there is deterioration and splitting off of many of the psychic functions, while in paranoia the delusions are so logical, at least on the surface, as to appear to be little more than an extension of the premorbid personality.

Late paraphrenia is the term applied to that relatively distinct group of older (seventh and eighth decades) patients with predominantly paranoid symptoms of a highly systematized kind, typically revolving about the delusion that neighbors are trying to kill the patient to get his money, or about the erotic delusion that someone is in love with or is about to marry the patient. In such cases, dementia is rare, even after some years. Most late paraphrenics are of the female sex; premorbid personality is typically schizoid or paranoid, and many such patients have severe defects of hearing or, less commonly, of vision.

paraphrenia confabulans See *paranoid*.

paraphrenia expansiva See *paranoid*.

paraphrenia, involutional *Involutional paranoid state*. It is generally recognized that there are two principal psychiatric syndromes associated with the period of involution: one closely resembles manic-depressive psychosis; the other, schizophrenia. Lerko calls the latter *involutional paraphrenia*.

paraphrenia phantastica See *paranoid*.

paraphrenia, presenile Among the many psychiatric syndromes having their onset after the involutional and before the senile phase of life, there is a schizophrenic form that Albrecht calls presenile paraphrenia.

paraphrenia systematica See *paranoid*.

paraphrenitis *Obs*. Mental derangement in general.

paraphrosyne (pà-rà-fros'i-nē) *Obs*. "It is a transitory insanity without a fever. A *delirium*. A symptomatic madness." (Motherby, G. *A New Medical Dictionary*, 1801)

parapithymia (par-ep-i-thim'ē-à, -thī'mē-à) Perverted desire or craving.

paraplegia Paralysis of the musculature of the lower extremities and of the torso, the latter to a lesser extent; when the upper extremities are paralyzed, the condition is called *superior paraplegia*.

paraplegia, ataxic Unsteadiness of station and gait in association with paraplegia.

paraplegia, hereditary spastic A familial disorder, usually affecting several siblings and occurring more frequently in males, which begins between the ages of 3 and 15 years with progressive destruction of the pyramidal tracts of the spinal cord, beginning in the lower limbs. To a lesser degree, there is also destruction of the posterior columns and of the cells of the precentral cortex. The disease is slowly progressive with a fatal termination after many years. Mentality is usually normal.

parapraxis Misaction. Freud applies this term to symptomatic acts such as slips of the tongue, mislaying of objects.

parapsychology The branch of psychology that deals with paranormal behavior and events such as telepathy, precognition, and clairvoyance, which are not explicable by present-day "natural" laws. See *perception, extrasensory*.

parapsychosis See *apsychosis*.

parareaction Abnormal reaction; specifically, overreaction to a situation followed by elaboration of its importance to a delusional degree. A person trips and falls to the floor and seems unduly embarrassed when helped to his feet; he refers to the incident repeatedly throughout the evening, and when seen again a day or two later cites it as evidence that his host is plotting to discredit him and have him discharged from his job.

parasexuality Perverted sexuality, comprising such practices as pederasty, voyeurism, pedophilia, sodomy, sadism, masochism.

"The various kinds of parasexuality are usually connected with a *premature appearance of the sex impulse* and hence can become known very early, at the age of three or four." (Bleuler, *TP*) See *paraphilia; perversion*.

parasitism See *symbiosis*.

parasitophobia A delusional state consisting of sensations of infestation of the skin or hair by insects; attempts to dig the "bugs" out of the skin typically produce irregular, linear excoriations that often become infected secondarily. Sometimes the delusion appears to be a part of an obsessional, depressive, or schizophrenic disorder, but it is also seen in organic psychoses and sometimes in association with vitamin deficiencies or as a complication of therapy with phenelzine (e.g. in some cases of hysteroid dysphoria).

Also known as *delusions of parasitosis* and *delusions of infestation*, parasitophobia is a form of monosymptomatic hypochondriacal psychosis. Pimozide, a dopamine-blocking agent used in Gilles de la Tourette's syndrome, has been reported to be effective in reducing or eliminating parasitophobia. See *monosymptomatic hypochondriacal psychosis.*

parasomnia Perverted or disordered sleep; sleep disturbance associated with lesion(s) of the nervous system. The term is used by some as a synonym for unconsciousness due to trauma, by others to refer to coma vigil. See *mutism, akinetic.*

parastriate lobule See *lobe, occipital.*

parasuicide Attempted suicide; suicidal gesture. See *suicide, attempted; syndrome, deliberate self-harm.*

parasympathetic nervous system See *autonomic nervous system.*

parasympathicotonia (par-à-sim-path-i-kō-tō′nē-à) Originally, in constitutional medicine this term denoted a particular hyper-irritability of the whole parasympathetic system; now it has become identical with *vagotonia* since the latter's meaning is stretched to cover the entire parasympathetic system.

parasympatholytic See *mydriasis.*

parataxic See *distortion, parataxic.*

parateresiomania Morbid impulse to observe; peeping-mania; *scopophilia* (q.v.).

parathymia Perversion of mood, as when a condition or occasion that should produce a certain mood evokes the opposite of the expected reaction. A patient, having asked for a new suit so that he might enjoy a coming party, was enraged when he received it.

"Parathymias are often indissolubly connected with *alteration of the impulses.*" (Bleuler, *TP*) Parathymia is one of the affect disturbances seen in the schizophrenias.

parathyroidism Excessive functioning of the parathyroid gland.

paratonia Any abnormality of muscle tension or tone, often a manifestation of catatonia. *Gegenhalten* is a particular form of paratonia consisting of uneven re-

sistance of the limbs to passive movement; its presence suggests frontal lobe dysfunction.

paratonia progressiva Bernstein's term for schizophrenia.

paratype The sum of all external, or *peristatic*, factors acting upon the phenotypical development of an organism or bringing about the individual manifestation of a genetic character. See *biotype.*

paravariation In genetics, synonym of *modification* (q.v.).

pareidolia A type of intense imagery that persists even when the subject looks at a real object in the external environment; image and percept exist side by side, but the image is usually recognized as unreal.

parenchyma, parenchyme (pà-reng′ki-mà, pàr′en-kīm) The specific or characteristic tissue of an organ or gland, as distinct from the connecting tissue or mesenchymal elements that support that gland. Paresis, for example, is also known as parenchymal syphilis because in this form of syphilis the spirochete invades and destroys nerve cells directly; cerebral syphilis, in contrast, is known as mesenchymal syphilis because it consists primarily of invasion of the arteries and arterioles within the meninges covering the brain and only secondarily does the process attack the cerebral tissue itself.

Parent egostate See *transactional analysis.*

parent therapist program A family-based treatment setting that is an alternative to residential treatment for emotionally disturbed children who can neither remain at home nor be managed satisfactorily in the usual foster home. The child is taken into the healthy nuclear family of the parent therapist, who receives support not only from the psychiatrist but also from discussion of experiences with other parent therapists.

parental perplexity See *perplexity, parental.*

parentectomy Removal of a parent; more specifically, the separation of a child from his parents for therapeutic reasons, as may be advisable in cases of intractable asthma.

parents, problem Parents who, because of their own unresolved unconscious conflicts, manifest unhealthy attitudes toward their children, who, in turn, become problem children. The problems of children may in part be merely a reflection of the problems of the parent or parents. The morbid attitudes of parents, such as perfectionistic, overconscientious, overly critical, overindulgent, overambitious, overanxious, and rejecting attitudes, may play a major role in setting up sequences that later cause symptoms in their child.

parerethisis (par-ē-reth'i-sis) *Obs.* Perverted excitement.

parergasia Perverted functioning; mismatched action. Kraepelin uses the term to refer to a form of parabulia in which the impulse to carry out an act is interrupted before the patient takes the first step toward performing the act. The interruption is occasioned by what he calls cross impulses, that is, by impulses which cross the path of the first impulse and thus check its further course. The process is also known as *derailment of volition.* For example, a patient who has the impulse to reach for a cup at the table suddenly brushes his hair. "The patient who is to show his tongue, opens his eyes widely instead; he flings the cup away instead of putting it to his mouth." (*DP*)

This is a psychiatric reaction type characterized usually by deep regression, abandonment of reality, and reconstruction of the conception of the self, and by delusions and hallucinations; this term, coined by Adolf Meyer, refers to schizophrenia and to schizophrenoid syndromes.

parerosia (par-ē-rō'sē-á) *Rare.* Sexual perversion.

paresis (pá-rē'sis, par'ē-sis) Partial paralysis.

paresis, alcoholic See *pseudoparesis, alcoholic.*

paresis, general *General paralysis of the insane (GPI), dementia paralytica, Bayle's disease;* the most malignant form of (tertiary) neurosyphilis consisting of direct invasion of the parenchyma of the brain producing a combination of both mental and neurologic symptoms. General paresis was first described by Haslan in 1798, and again by Bayle in 1822, and by Esquirol in 1826. The term general paralysis of the insane was first used by Delaye in 1824, and the relationship of the disorder to syphilis was first suggested in 1857 by Esmarch and Jessen. The identification of the spirochete as the cause, rather than merely a predisposing factor, was made possible in 1911, when Noguchi demonstrated the presence of organisms in the brains of paretic subjects.

Pathology includes shrinking and atrophy of brain substance and a thickening of the dura mater. Lymphocytes, plasma cells, and giant cells infiltrate the meninges and the brain itself, where the ganglion cells show severe large areas of softening.

Mental symptoms may appear in various forms: as (1) simple dementia, the most common type, with deterioration of intellect, affect, and social behavior; (2) paranoid form, with persecutory delusions; (3) expansive or manic form, with delusions of grandiosity; or (4) depressive form, often with absurd nihilistic delusions. No matter what the form, intellectual functions show increasing impairment, with loss of more and more memory, confabulation, disorientation (especially in the area of time), carelessness in personal appearance and hygiene, irritability and restlessness, alcoholic excesses, and sexual aberrations.

Neurologic symptoms and signs that may appear are (1) epileptiform attacks, which occur in 50% of cases; (2) Argyll Robertson pupil; (3) tremor, most on voluntary movement, that tends to affect the perioral musculature and also the muscles of the hands and fingers so that writing becomes tremulous, and words and letters are often left out or transposed; (4) vacant, masklike facies, giving patient a wrinkle-free, youthful appearance; (5) impaired oculomotor activity; (6) optic atrophy; (7) impaired motor function, including ataxia, poor coordination, unsteady gait, weakness; (8) slurred speech (dysarthria); (9) hyperactive reflexes (but hyporeflexia if tabes dorsalis coexists); (10) loss of bladder and bowel control. There are few or no sensory changes, unless tabes coexists.

Cerebrospinal fluid pressure is elevated, as are cells (usually lymphocytes or monocytes) and globulin. The Lange colloidal gold curve is of the paretic type (first zone reaction), and the Wassermann is usually strongly positive in both blood and spinal fluid.

Penicillin is the cornerstone of treatment, whose degree of success is related to duration and severity of mental and neurological symptoms before treatment is initiated.

paresis, infantile See *neurosyphilis, congenital.*
paresis, juvenile See *neurosyphilis, congenital.*
paresis, Lissauer type (Heinrich Lissauer, German neurologist, 1861–91) An atypical form of general paresis characterized by (1) unusually well-retained intellectual functions and (2) severe focal symptoms, such as apoplectiform attacks, hemiplegia, aphasia.
paresthesia Perverted sense of touch; paraphia. Unpleasant sensation, such as tingling, tickling, burning, caused by a tactile stimulus.
paretic Relating to or suffering from paresis.
paretic curve See *Lange's colloidal gold reaction.*
Parham decision A 1979 decision of the U.S. Supreme Court relating to due process provisions for children who are placed in psychiatric hospitals by their parents. The decision reaffirmed the appropriateness of traditional family and medical prerogatives in the rearing and care of children, indicating that due process at the point of admission is satisfied by an independent medical evaluation that confirms the need for hospitalization, and that parents have the right to admit their children to a psychiatric hospital for treatment.
parkinsonism (James Parkinson, English physician, 1775–1824) See *paralysis agitans.*
parkinsonism-dementia of Guam A degenerative disease of unknown etiology, limited to the Chamorro-speaking people of Guam and the Mariana Islands, similar clinically, pathologically, and biochemically to Parkinson's disease. It usually responds favorably to treatment with L-dopa.
parole A system of supervision of a patient who is away from the hospital or any of its adjuncts—such as colonies—prior to his legal discharge. While on parole, a patient is considered as still on the books of the hospital, and may, if necessary, be returned to the hospital without the necessity for formal court action.
paroniria (par-ō-nī′rē-à) Morbid dreaming; sleep disturbance. See *ecphronia.*
parorexia Perverted appetite, dysorexia. See *eating disorders.*
parosmia (pa-oz′mē-à) Any disturbance of the sense of smell, whether organic or psychic in origin; the term includes osphresiolagnia, osphresiophilia, olfactory hallucinations.
parosphresis (par-os-frē′sis) *Parosmia* (q.v.).
paroxysmal cerebral dysrhythmia *Epilepsy* (q.v.).
paroxysmal drinking See *alcoholism.*
Parry-Romberg's syndrome See *hemiatrophy, facial.*
pars pro toto (L. "part for the whole") In psychiatry a special form of psychic displacement. When a part of an object or a person stands for the whole object or person, the process is known as *pars pro toto.* A voice, a gesture, some physical trait, a bit of wearing apparel—each may be substituted for the total person.
part-brain See *third nervous system.*
part-instinct Partial instinct. See *impulse, component.*
parthenogenesis Virgin reproduction. The uniparental mode of sexual reproduction, in which an egg develops into a new organism without having first been fertilized by a spermatozoon. Although organisms produced in this way have only one parent, they originate sexually, as they undergo a process similar to that of typical maturation. See *reproduction.*

The best known example of parthenogenetic origin is supplied by the honey bee, in which the haploid egg, if unfertilized, develops into a male bee (drone).
parthenophobia Fear of girls.
partial adjustments Sullivan's term for the schizophrenic person's defensive maneuvers that are aimed at reducing environmentally generated stress during the period immediately preceding an acute psychotic episode. These include *compensatory activities* (substitution of simpler activities for more complex ones), *sublimatory activities* (roundabout but socially acceptable ways of achieving some degree of satisfaction in an environment where direct pursuit of a goal generates intolerable anxiety), and defense reactions (complex activities and phantasies that no longer maintain conformity with social standards; e.g. evasions, rationalizations, projection, negativism, hypochondriasis).
partial hospitalization All forms of inpatient treatment other than full, 24-hour programs; includes day hospital, night hospital, weekend hospital. See *psychiatry, community.*

partialism A form of sexual perversion in which the subject seeks gratification of the sexual impulse from a certain part of the partner's body—the leg, thigh, buttock, and so on. Partialism must be differentiated from fetishism, in which the partner is eliminated and displaced by an object symbolic of the genitals.

partialism, persistent Failure to gain genital primacy; continuation of part-object relations because development has been arrested before whole-object relations have been attained (see *genitality*). One form of partialism is expressed sexually (see *fetish; partialism*). Another form is expressed as a type of personality disorder, characterized by fixation at the depressive position, inability to work through separations and losses, vacillating or short-lived relationships, and a feeling of being incomplete or flawed. See *fault, basic; genitality; personality, "as if."*

partiality, multilateral A part of the process of family evaluation and family therapy in which the therapist comes to know each member of the family by being on each one's side. Family members can then feel that the therapist cares about each of them and understands each one's position within the family.

partiality, sexual *Rare.* Fetishism; sexual idolatry.

partitive In Burrow's usage behavior processes whose interaction socially has become independent of and at variance with the primary motivation of man's organism as a whole; those feeling-reactions that have ceased to issue as a direct expression of the organism as a totality but which have been secondarily displaced into the symbolic segment and now issue in mere images of feeling, or in affects. In accordance with investigations in phylobiology the artificial supremacy of this partitive (affectosymbolic) mode of behavior over the primary motivation of the organism as a whole constitutes the basis of both individual and social neurosis. Contrasted with total, organismic. Synonyms: affective, intercortical, symbolic. (Burrow, T. *The Biology of Human Conflict,* 1937)

passio hypochondriaca *Obs.* Hypochondriasis.

passive-aggressive personality See *personality trait disturbance.*

passive-dependency One of the subtypes of passive-aggressive personality, characterized by helplessness, indecisiveness, and a tendency to cling to others in a parasitic way. See *character, oral; character, receptive; dependence, oral; dependency; personality trait disturbance.*

passive tremor See *tremor.*

passivism A form of sexual perversion in which the subject, usually male, is submissive to the will of the partner. See *active; masochism.*

passivity One of the several modalities of adaptation. For example, it is possible for the organism to adapt itself to its environment by going either forward to meet it or backward to escape it. The first procedure would be termed the modality of *activity* in adaptive maneuvers, while the latter would be termed the modality of passivity.

In transference neurosis the consequences of inhibition of the modality of activity may find the organism simply abandoning this modality and falling back upon the modality of passivity. In traumatic neurosis, however, the modality of passivity cannot be resorted to when activity is inhibited, since it is impossible for the organism to remain completely passive to the outer world. One can retreat from an inhibiting *person,* but complete retreat from the inhibiting *forces* of the outer world is impossible—short of death.

past-pointing See *pointing.*

pastoral counseling See *counseling, pastoral.*

patentable life See *Chakrabarty.*

paternalism A distortion of fatherly or parental behavior in which some moral rule relative to the actions of one person toward another is violated without the consent of that other person. Because a moral rule is violated, the action requires justification, but that is not to say that paternalism is never justified. Paternalistic behavior is based on the belief of the actor, A, that his behavior toward the subject, B, benefits B even though it violates a moral rule and is performed without B's past, present, or immediately forthcoming consent, even though B is competent to give consent. Causing physical or mental pain, lying, cheating, and breaking a promise are the typical violations of moral rules that paternalism involves.

Paternalism is a form of control of one

subject or group by another, ordinarily rationalized as an expression of care and concern for the welfare of the group being controlled. Paternalism is not acting like a father; rather, it is an attempt to excuse one's actions as being better for the subject than the choice the subject might make were he not under control or domination. What is done under the label of paternalism is usually a violation of some moral rule, such as giving pain or depriving someone of liberty. Paternalism may, of course be justified or even necessary, but adequate justification for its need depends on the recognition that the action runs counter to a moral rule.

pathema (pà-thē′mà) *Obs.* Disease; often mental disease.

pathematology *Obs.* A general term for pathology, although it is ordinarily used to denote mental pathology. It has been replaced by the term *psychopathology.*

pathergasia Adolf Meyer's term for personality maladjustment in association with organic, functional, or structural changes. It is approximately equivalent to Ferenczi's *pathoneurosis.*

pathetism *Obs.* Mesmerism; hypnotism.

pathic 1. Pertaining to or affected by disease or disorder. 2. *Obs.* A male passive partner who submits to unnatural sexual practices. See *catamite; passivism.*

patho-, path- Combining form meaning suffering, passion, disease, from Gr. *páthos.*

pathobiology The study of diseased or disordered conditions arising from a biological source.

pathoclisis Sensitivity to disease or injury; often used in a more limited sense to refer to sensitivity to certain toxins; sometimes used to refer to the end result of a series of subclinical pathologic insults that, when added together, finally produce clinical manifestations. Some authorities have implicated pathoclisis as the mechanism responsible for most forms of parkinsonism and the senile and presenile dementias. In such a view, a transient viral infection early in life, for example, may produce a clinically undetectable degree of central nervous system damage. In subsequent years, any number of additional subclinical insults—other viral infections, minor head traumata, alcohol and other drugs, arteriosclerosis—gradually drain the sys-

tem's reserves until a critical point is reached when the neurons remaining intact can no longer maintain normal function.

pathocratia, pathocratoria *Obs.* Self-restraint.

pathoctonus (pà-thok′tō-nus) *Obs.* Killing of passion; self-restraint.

pathocure The disappearance of a neurosis upon the outbreak of an organic disease. Pathocure is seen in moral masochists whose neurosis is first of all, unconsciously, a suffering that pacifies the superego: the neurosis becomes superfluous as soon as it is replaced by another kind of suffering. Pathocure is the opposite of pathoneurosis, which is a neurosis developing as a result of somatic disease.

A pathocure was observed in a masochist who developed pulmonary tuberculosis. The patient had been a chronic failure in everything he undertook. Under analysis, he began to gain some insight into the masochistic nature of his character defenses. Analysis was interrupted by the tuberculous process, and after the patient's release from the hospital he went back to work. He functioned well on his job and previous symptoms did not reappear. The disease in this instance was one especially suitable for the character type of the patient—it was chronic, it necessitated definite limitations of activity, and the likelihood of recurrence was ever present. Other pathocures of a more temporary nature had been observed when the organic disease was short-lived and required no permanent or long-term changes in the patient's way of living. In such cases, neurotic symptoms tend to reappear with the disappearance of the organic condition.

pathoformic Referring to the beginning of pathological states; to the symptoms occurring in the transitional stage between health and disease or disorder proper.

pathogenesis, pathogenesy, pathogeny The way in which a disease or disorder originated or developed; also called *nosogenesis.*

pathognomonic, pathognomic (pà-thog-nō-mon′ik, path-og-nom′ik) Typical or thoroughly characteristic of a disease; diagnostic.

pathognomy The science of recognizing or diagnosing a disease or pathological condition.

pathognostic *Pathognom(on)ic* (q.v.).

pathography 1. Description of a disease. 2. The study of the effects of any illness on the writer's (or other artist's) life or art, or the effects of an artist's life and personality development on his creative work.

pathography, psychoanalytic The use of biography (and especially the biography of a predominantly pathological subject) to expand psychoanalytic knowledge or to demonstrate already existing psychoanalytic knowledge. See *biography in depth*.

pathohysteria See *hysteria, fixation*.

pathokinesis The course, development, or dynamics of an illness.

patholesia *Rare.* Any impairment or abnormality of the will. See *will, disturbances of*.

pathologic gambling One of the *disorders of impulse control* (q.v.).

pathology The study of the nature of diseases.

pathomania *Obs.* Mania without delirium; *moral insanity* (q.v.).

pathomimesis, pathomimicry The mimicry of a disease or disorder; not uncommon in hysteria and hysteroid conditions; *malingering* (q.v.).

pathomorphism Abnormal morphology such as extremes of bodily build.

pathoneurosis See *hysteria, fixation*.

pathopatridalgia *Obs.* Homesickness or *nostalgia* (q.v.).

pathophobia *Obs.* Fear of disease; *hypochondriasis* (q.v.).

pathophrenesis A nonspecific term for disturbance in the intelligence, regardless of its basis.

pathoplasty Birnbaum thus refers to the *form* of a disease, in contradistinction to the term pathogenesis, which relates to the *cause*.

pathopoeesia, pathopoiesis (path-ō-pē-ē′-sē-à, -poi-ē′sis) *Obs. Pathogenesis* (q.v.).

pathopsychology Wilhelm Specht's term for the study of abnormal psychic data from the point of view of general psychology. He proposed to restrict the expression to the study of the same data from the standpoint of medical psychology.

pathopsychosis When an organic process, such as brain tumor or general paresis, gives rise to a psychotic condition, the syndrome is known as a pathopsychosis. See *hysteria, fixation; syndrome, organic*.

pathosis, attitudinal Thorne's term for a type of personality disorder, seen frequently in compensation and postaccident cases, in which the patient's attitude and self-righteous belief that because he was injured he cannot work or deserves special consideration forms a central core in all his thinking about the effects of his injury. Kamman distinguishes this reaction from traumatic neurosis (which term he would reserve for latent psychoneurosis precipitated by accident) and from compensation neurosis (where, although it is usually unconscious, the basic motive is the desire for cash compensation), mainly because of the conscious volitional element in attitudinal pathosis. This disorder is presumed to fall somewhere between psychopathic personality and traumatic neurosis. See *neurosis, compensation*.

pathway, fifth For U.S. citizens who complete premedical education in the United States then complete all but the internship and/or social service components of the medical education outside the United States. On returning to the United States, such students must pass screening examinations designated by a school offering them a year of supervised clinical training and personal interviews; they must also have acceptable MCAT (Medical College Admission Test) scores and premedical grade point averages. About one-fourth of U.S. medical schools currently (1982) accept such students.

pathway variables See *recidivism*.

patient care audit See *audit*.

patient-government Patient participation in the ward administration of a psychiatric hospital; one of the ways of implementing the concept of the psychiatric hospital as a therapeutic community.

patient-oriented consultation See *consultant*.

patient, person in the A term expressing the basic key concept of the psychosomatic medical approach to the patient and emphasizing the patient's personality or character as a factor in the production of physical symptoms and complaints. Whereas the organic, or physical, approach tends to exclude awareness and interest in emotional, personality, and character factors as causative agents to be investigated and treated, the psychosomatic approach, conversely, tends to include these factors and give them central importance. It must be borne in mind, however, that the psychosomatic approach does not in any way exclude the usual physical and organic avenues of investigation.

patient responsibility As used clinically, the therapist's assumption of responsibility for the patient—defined operationally in terms of decision-making and effective limit-setting of five main types of behavior: destructiveness, disorganization, deviancy, dysphoria, and dependency. (Sternbach, R.A., Abroms, G.M., & Ricc, D.G. *Psychiatry 32,* 1969)

Paton, Stewart (1865–1942) American psychiatrist and neurologist; wrote first modern textbook of psychiatry in the U.S. (1905); founded first university mental health clinic in the U.S. at Princeton University (1910).

patroiophobia (pat-roi-ō-) Fear of heredity, and especially of hereditary disease.

pattern, expressive See *psychodynamics, adaptational.*

pattern, specific dynamic Franz Alexander's term for the specific nuclear conflict or dynamic configuration that is unique to a particular psychosomatic disorder or organ neurosis. See *psychosomatic.*

Pavlovian conditioning See *conditioning.*

Pavlov's reflex psychology (Ivan Petrovich Pavlov, Russsian physiologist, 1849–1936) The theory of human personality development and behavior proposed by Pavlov based on his discovery of the conditioned reflex and conditioned or internal inhibition. Mental processes and higher nervous activity were viewed as being identical with the neurophysiologic mechanisms through which they manifested themselves.

Pavlov's theory of schizophrenia A theory propounded by Pavlov, who held that the symptoms of schizophrenia are the result of a state of inhibition of the cerebral cortex.

pavor diurnus Fear reactions that occur in the young child during the afternoon nap, similar to night terrors but not so frequent as the latter.

pavor nocturnus *Sleep terror disorder* (q.v.).

pavor sceleris Fear of "bad men"—burglars, kidnapers, etc.

PBC Pregnancy and birth complication(s), found by some investigators to be more frequent in schizophrenic persons than in nonschizophrenic comparison groups.

PCP *Phencyclidine* (q.v.); pneumocystic carinii pneumonia.

pcpt *Perception* (q.v.).

Pcs *Preconscious* (q.v.).

PDD Primary degenerative dementia; includes what was formerly known as senile dementia of the Alzheimer type (SDAT) and presenile *Alzheimer's disease* (q.v.).

PEAQ *Personal Experience and Attitude Questionnaire* (q.v.).

peccatiphobia Fear of sinning. See *scrupulosity.*

pedantry, stool Exaggerated promptitude and punctuality that are overcompensations for the infantile anal-erotic tendency to hold back the stool as long as possible.

pederasty The meaning of pederasty varies among different authors, though it is most commonly defined as *coitus per anum* practiced on boys. It is not considered synonymous with *sodomy* (q.v.), though at times confused with it. See *paedico.*

pederosis *Obs. Pedophilia.* Auguste Forel coined this term in 1905 and defined it as sexual passion for children.

pedication *Pederasty; sodomy* (qq.v.).

pedigree See *method, pedigree.*

pediophobia Fear of dolls.

pedologia Infantile or childish speech that omits all but the principal words and substitutes easily pronounced sounds for more difficult ones; baby talk.

pedomorphism Describing adult behavior in terms more appropriate to behavior of a child. See *adultomorphism; anthropomorph.*

pedophilia Love of children. This term implies the love of prepubertal children by an adult (who is at least 10 years older than the child), for sexual purposes.

    Forel called it *pederosis;* Krafft-Ebing termed it *paedophilia erotica.*

    A man who was impotent with women was capable of sexual excitation only with young boys, with whom he frequently engaged in acts of anal intercourse and fellatio.

pedotrophy Literally, nurturance of a child; hence child rearing or "parentcraft."

peduncle, cerebral See *midbrain.*

peeping See *voyeurism.*

peeping Tom (From the name of the Coventry tailor who peeped at naked Lady Godiva riding through the city's streets by order of her husband, lord of Coventry) Voyeur.

peer review See *review.*

Pelizaeus-Merzbacher's disease (Friedrich Pelizaeus, German neurologist, 1850–1917, and Ludwig Merzbacher, German-born in Argentina, b. 1875) See *sclerosis, diffuse.*

pellagra Nicotinic acid deficiency, characterized by gastrointestinal disturbances (especially diarrhea), erythema followed by desquamation of the affected area, and mental disturbances. Symptoms vary widely in incidence and intensity but tend to be worse in the spring. The most frequent early picture consists of fatigue and lassitude combined with depression. Mania, convulsions, dementia, stupor, and unconsciousness may also occur, and if untreated the condition advances into delirious or subacute delirious states. Sucking and grasping reflexes may appear along with cogwheel rigidity of the extremities and progressive clouding of consciousness. Treatment with high doses of nicotinic acid or nicotinamide (and usually moderately high doses of the other B vitamins) usually results in amelioration of all symptoms, except that in some cases memory defects persist. Pellagra continues to be endemic in the Far East, Africa, and Mexico, and it can be seen as a complication of alcoholism in any part of the world.

penetrance See *chromosome; dominance; variation.*

penetration, interface See *network.*

penetration response See *barrier.*

Penfield, Wilder Graves (1891–1976) United States-born neurosurgeon, founded Montreal (Canada) Neurological Institute; epilepsy, speech disorders, memory.

penial *Penile* (q.v.).

peniaphobia Fear of poverty.

penile Relating to the penis.

penile tumescence See *tumescence, penile.*

penilingus Fellatio.

penis The male organ of copulation. In psychoanalysis it refers to the organ after the boy has reached the stage of genital love. See *phallus.*

penis captivus *Vaginismus* (q.v.) occurring during sexual intercourse so that withdrawal of the erect penis is impossible. The condition is the subject of many anecdotes, but the paucity of clinical reports indicates that such anecdotes are based more on male castration fears and female active castration tendencies than on real occurrences.

penis envy See *envy, penis.*

penis, female See *penis, women with.*

penis, women with A childhood theory or idea (that every woman has a penis), stemming from a universal, albeit usually forgotten, experience in the psychosexual development of all boys and girls. It generally appears between the ages of 2 and 5 as a consequence of the child's discovering the crucial anatomical difference between males and females, i.e. the absence of the penis in females. On finding the supposed organic deficiency or inferiority, most little girls react to their discovery with varying degrees of shock. In boys the same discovery tends to make their dread of castration more real for them, since it confronts them with the actuality of the "missing organ."

The idea that a woman once possessed or possesses a penis functions as a protective defensive denial of the horrible psychic reality, by which the child has theoretically explained to itself the observed absence of the penis in females.

pentothal interview See *narcotherapy.*

peotillomania *Obs.* False masturbation, pseudomasturbation; a nervous tic consisting in constant pulling at the penis.

peptide, brain *Neuropeptide, peptide neurotransmitter;* an element of a brain protein consisting of linkage of two or more amino acids by bonding of the carboxyl group (CO) of one with the amino group (NH) of the other. The CONH union is termed the *peptide bond* or *peptide link.*

There are two major families of endogenous opioid peptides, *enkephalins* and *endorphins* (qq.v.). Both can interact with opiate-binding sites and may thus modulate the perception of pain; endorphins, in addition, appear to modulate mood and responses to stressful stimuli.

The first peptide neurotransmitter was *substance P*, discovered by von Euler and Gaddum in 1931. Enkephalins were discovered in 1975. Many bioactive peptides have been discovered in the nervous system and proposed as neurotransmitters or neuromodulators, among them ACTH, angiotensin, bombesin, carnosine, cholecystokinin, gastrin, growth hormone, glucagon, insulin, luteinizing hormone-releasing hormone (LHRH), neurotensin, oxytocin, prolactin, secretin, somatostatin (growth hormone release-inhibiting hormone), thyrotropin-releasing hormone (TRH), vasoactive intestinal peptide (VIP), vasopressin.

Some of these substances undoubtedly have multiple roles, as neuronal, paracrine, or endocrine biological messengers, depending on their cells of origin and release. This is similar to other compounds; the catecholamines, for example, act primarily as endocrine messengers if released from the adrenal medulla, or as neurotransmitters if released from neurons. See *neuroanatomy, chemical; neurohormone; neurotransmitter; peptidergic.*

peptidergic Referring to interneuronal communication by means of neuropeptides, which may function in several ways: as neurosecretory neurons, for example, which signal to nonneural effector organs over long distances; as neurohormones, which communicate between the nervous system and the adenohypophysis; as neuron-to-neuron transporters of chemical signals by way of the acellular interstitium; or as neuromodulators, which enhance or depress a conventionally transmitted synaptic signal between two other neurons. See *neurohormone; neuromodulator.*

PER Periodic Evaluation Record. See *Multi-State Information System.*

perceived pseudohallucination See *pseudohallucination.*

percentile See *rank, percentile.*

percept The subject's meaningful interpretation of a sensory stimulus; a percept is a combination of subjective and objective elements and affords a link between the subject and his environment.

percept, body See *image, body.*

percept image "These are certain concrete images of hallucinatory clearness which may appear as phantasy or memory images. . . . This class of experiences, namely, the percept-images, which in general have been lost to adults, represents, according to the researches of Jaensch, a primitive level of intellectual life." (Storch, A. *The Primitive Archaic Forms in Schizophrenia,* 1924) The phenomenon is common among schizophrenic patients.

perceptanalysis Piotrowski's term for inferring personality traits from a subject's responses to the Rorschach inkblots. "The broadest and main assumption on which the logical structure of perceptanalysis rests states that the individual's sensory, intellectual, and motor handling, active and/or passive, of the blot stimuli corresponds closely to the habitual manner in which he handles, actively and/or passively, his interhuman relationships." (*Perceptanalysis,* 1957)

perception The mental process by which the nature of an object is recognized through the association of a memory of its other qualities with the special sense, sight, taste, etc., bringing it at the time to consciousness. Perception is a complex act of transferring physical stimulation into psychological information and includes at least four aspects: reception, registration, processing (i.e. further reorganization in accord with memory, affects, needs, intentions, etc.), and feedback (proprioceptive and autonomic processes that allow the subject to determine if the object sensed is the object sought).

perception, altered mind/body Any of a group of altered states of consciousness that are presumed to exist on a continuum ranging from ecstatic experiences of heightened awareness and integration to disorganizing episodes of psychotic decompensation with loss of identity. Characteristic of the group is subjectively experienced distortion of the normal spatial relationship between body and mind. The term includes out-of-body experiences, near-death experiences, body boundary disturbances, *autoscopy,* and *depersonalization* (qq.v.).

perception, delusional Misinterpretation of a percept as an indication that something sinister is occurring or is about to occur, before the development of a full-blown delusional idea. A young man looked at his television set and felt it was slightly tilted or off-center. This was a sign to him that people might think he was gay (off-center = not straight = gay).

perception, extrasensory (ESP) Cognition that is paranormal, or a response to an external event that has not presented itself to any of the five known senses. *Telepathy* and *clairvoyance* are two modalities of this single surmised basic function—extrasensory perception—and they differ only in the targets, thoughts, or objects upon which they operate: clairvoyance is the extrasensory perception of objective events; telepathy is the extrasensory perception of the mental activities of another person.

perception-hallucination See *hallucination of perception.*

perception, subconscious Perceptions of the environment that never even entered the fringe of the personal consciousness.

perceptions, abstract See *hallucination, blank.*

perceptivity The power of perception; the character of being perceptive.

perceptorium *Obs. Sensorium* (q.v.).

perceptual disability Difficulty in putting information into the brain through the five senses.

perceptual style See *style, perceptual.*

perceptualization The act or process of representing reality as it appears to the senses rather than to the intellect, as is seen in dreams and hallucinations. The term is also used to refer to regressive loss of higher conceptualization processes such as is seen in many schizophrenics whose ideas become more and more related to specific instances and less and less related to classes, groups, or categories. This is one of the expressions of *paleologic* (q.v.) and leads, among other things, to *concretism* (q.v.).

percipient In parapsychology, the receiver of telepathically transmitted messages.

peregrinating problem patients A term for patients with Munchhausen's syndrome. See *syndrome, Munchhausen.*

periblepsis The wild stare of a delirious person, with elements of bewilderment, consternation, and terror.

perichareia (-kȧ-rī′ȧ) Delirious rejoicing.

perikaryon See *neuron.*

periluteal phase dysphoric disorder *Late luteal phase dysphoric disorder* (q.v.).

period, Oedipus The period beginning at about the age of 3 during the phallic stage of development and reaching its height at 4 to 5 years. Psychoanalysts believe that the *Oedipus complex* is characteristic of all individuals, the boy, normally, becoming sexually attached to his mother, the girl to her father. In the phallic period, sexual interest at first is autoerotic: (1) the boy

identifies himself with the penis but soon merges his sexual interest into the sexuality of the mother; (2) the girl's clitoris sexuality leads to penis envy and the belief that the mother has been the castrator, and the girl turns to the father as a sexual object. In the *male,* the Oedipus period *ends because of castration anxiety,* for the oedipal object can be achieved only at the risk of losing the penis. In the *female,* on the other hand, the Oedipus period *begins* because of castration anxiety. Thus the Oedipus period in the female tends to be prolonged, for the father will be relinquished as object only when time has convinced her that her wishes will not be fulfilled, and only as time provides her the opportunity to find more suitable objects. The fate of the Oedipus complex in the female is still unclear. See *complex, Oedipus; superego.*

period, refractory See *refractory.*

periodic catatonia See *catatonia, periodic.*

Periodic Evaluation Record See *Multi-State Information System.*

peristasis The external environment. Some geneticists prefer this term to environment, to indicate that the environment of any genetic factor includes all the biophysiological processes that take place in the organism itself and are essential to the phenotypical development of the given genotype. According to modern physiological genetics, every inherited character necessarily becomes subject to the organisms' *peristatic* conditions. See *ecology.*

permissive hypothesis of affective disorders The hypothesis states that a deficit in central indoleaminergic transmission permits affective disorder but is not enough to cause it; changes in central catecholaminergic transmission when occurring in the context of indoleaminergic deficit cause affect disorders and determine their quality (excess catecholamine produces mania, catecholamine deficiency produces depression).

permissiveness See *environment, permissive.*

pernoctation *Obs.* Insomnia.

peroneal muscular atrophy See *atrophy, peroneal muscular.*

perplexity, parental A type of relationship of parents to their children that has been found relatively frequently in schizophrenic families (although it is as yet unclear whether the parental behavior and attitudes are productive of the child's disabilities, or whether it is the primary deviancy of the child that has generated the parental reaction). "This parental atmosphere is characterized by extreme parental indecisiveness, a lack of parental spontaneity and empathy with the child, the parents' inability to sense what the child's needs are and thus an inability to satisfy them at the proper moment, and an unusual absence of control and authority. In this type of unpatterned climate, positive re-inforcement of desirable traits and negative re-inforcement of undesirable traits are not administered. Instead, the child is left with feelings of confusion and an inclination to respond in a randomized, impoverished, and unpredictable fashion, when more focused, directed behaviors are lacking." (Goldfarb, W. *International Psychiatry Clinics 1*, 1964)

perplexity, vague A symptom seen most commonly in the organic psychoses, especially in the acute brain syndromes associated with systemic infection as part of the beginning of a toxic delirium. The patient feels "mixed-up in the head," shows a deficient grasp of the total situation, drowsiness, torpor, and disturbances of the association, memory, attention, and will.

persécuteurs persécutés (pâr-sā-kü-tēr′ pār-sā-kü-tē′) Term for those paranoid persecuted patients who also become persecutors, in an effort, as they believe, to defend themselves against their persecutors.

persecution syndrome See *syndrome, persecution*.

Persecutor See *transactional analysis*.

perseveration Difficulty in stopping a task once started, or continuing to perform a task that had been requested earlier when asked to perform a different task. The combination of perseveration with difficulty in initiating tasks is *motor inertia*. Perseveration and motor inertia suggest frontal lobe dysfunction.

The perseveration is often verbal, in which case the response is more appropriate to a preceding stimulus than to the succeeding stimuli that provoke it.

Perseveration occurs most often in association with brain damage (after head injury, in presenile and arteriosclerotic brain syndromes, in hepatic encephalopathy, etc.), and it may also appear with forced grasping, groping, and associated lesions of the premotor area (6a) of the brain. Perseveration may also appear in the schizophrenias as an association disturbance. See *verbigeration*.

Perseveration is often defined in a more operational way, particularly by experimental psychologists, as the inability to shift from one task to another or to break through an established set in order to perform a new task.

persistence, motor Ability to sustain a motor action, such as keeping one's eyes closed for 20 seconds on command. Inability to sustain motor action is motor *impersistence*, which, in a subject whose muscle strength is normal, indicates frontal lobe dysfunction.

person, composite A figure in a dream who is not an actual person at all but a composition or *composite* of two or more actual persons. The dreamer is not able to identify the composite person as any person known to him but, upon psychoanalytic interpretation of his dream, he is able to see that two or more persons who *are* known to him have been fused into one.

The composite person is produced by the mechanism of *condensation* in dream-making. "The condensation is effected in several ways. A figure in a dream may be constituted by the fusion of traits belonging to more than one actual person, with some belonging to another, or by making prominent the traits common to the two and neglecting those not common to them. . . . The same process frequently occurs with names. . . . The neologism thus produced closely resembles those met with in the psychoses." (Jones, E.J. *Papers on Psycho-Analysis*, 1949)

person, disturbances in the One of the fundamental symptoms of the schizophrenias, according to Bleuler. Such disturbances arise by reason of the tendency to splitting of the psyche and domination of the personality by one or another of the patient's complexes. The ego is never fully intact, resulting in a lack of homogeneity, wholeness, and stability of the personality organization.

persona With this term Jung denotes the disguised or masked attitude assumed by a person, in contrast to the more deeply rooted personality components. "Through his more or less complete identification with the attitude of the moment, he at least deceives others, and also often himself, as to his real character. He puts on a *mask*, which he knows corresponds with his conscious intentions, while it also meets with the requirements and opinions of his environment, so that first one motive then the other is in the ascendant. This mask, viz. the *ad hoc* adopted attitude, I have called the *persona*, which was the designation given to the mask worn by the actors of antiquity. A man who is identified with this mask I would call 'personal' (as opposed to 'individual')." (Jung, *PT*) See *analytic psychology; personality; personality disorders; pseudoidentification*.

persona, organic Burrow's term for the constellation of reactions embodied in the organism's total principle of motivation. The subjective correlate of the organism's primarily integrated or total behavior pattern. Contrasted with "I"-persona, symbolic persona. Synonym: organic identity. (*The Biology of Human Conflict*, 1937)

personal See *persona*.

personal disorganization See *disorganization*.

Personal Experience and Attitude Questionnaire (PEAQ) A screening questionnaire said to be a highly significant discriminator of psychopathic behavior. The test contains 150 items covering criminalism, emotional instability, inadequate personality, sexual psychopathy, nomadism, and other psychopathic traits.

personality *Character* (q.v.); the characteristic, and to some extent predictable, behavior-response patterns that each person evolves, both consciously and unconsciously, as his style of life. The personality represents a compromise between inner drives and needs and the controls that limit or regulate their expression. Such controls are both internal (e.g. conscience and superego) and external (reality demands). The personality functions to maintain a stable, reciprocal relationship between the person and his environment; it is thus a composite of the ego defenses, the autoplastic and the alloplastic maneuvers, that are automatically and customarily employed to maintain intrapsychic stability. See *defense, character*.

The personality, in other words, is a set of habits that characterize the person in his way of managing day-to-day living; under ordinary conditions, it is relatively stable and predictable, and for the most part it is ego-syntonic. Because the various defensive operations (*ego mechanisms*) that make up the personality are the very ones that appear in exaggerated form in recognized clinical entities, their identification will sometimes allow for prediction of what specific form of clinical disturbance the person is most likely to have, should he develop any kind of illness at all. Their identification does not, however, predict that any such illness will ever develop.

Because the personality is ego-syntonic, it is rare that the person will recognize his own personality as being deviant or abnormal (even if, in fact, it is). Any such evaluation is ordinarily a social diagnosis and an outgrowth of the effects of that personality on the people about him—who may view his behavior as destructive, frightening, nonconforming, or otherwise unacceptable. The subject, in other words, is unlikely to seek out ways to alter his personality, which for him is the best way of avoiding tension and fulfilling his potential that he has been able to develop; rather, he may consent to counseling or psychotherapy if this is urged by others or if he suffers social repercussions because of his usual behavior.

It is difficult to draw a clear distinction between normal personality and the variations of personality and character that extend beyond the normal range. To some extent, the stability of even the normal personality is achieved at the expense of an ideal mobility—perhaps unattainable—to deal effectively with new or unusual interpersonal problems and conflicts. Yet there is no doubt that in many persons the stability of their ways of being and living is a rigidly fixed, immutable pattern that severely limits their potentialities for effective functioning and satisfying interpersonal relationships. Such conditions are variously termed *personality disorders, character disorders,* or *character neuroses*. These are deeply ingrained, chronic, and habitual patterns of reaction that are maladaptive in that they are relatively inflexible; they limit the optimal use of potentialities and often provoke the very counterreactions from the environment that the subject seeks to avoid. See *personality disorders.*

personality, alternating Many consider this expression as synonymous with *split personality* (see *multiple personality disorder*), for the splitting of consciousness implies that the individual lives alternatingly now as one person and then as another (as in the familiar case of Dr. Jekyl and Mr. Hyde), but never as two persons simultaneously. Also known as *dual consciousness.*

personality, anal See *character, anal.*

personality, antisocial See *psychopathic personality.*

personality, "as if" A prepsychotic condition indicative of loss of object cathexis in which the subject's whole relation to life has something about it that is lacking in genuineness. The phenomenon is closely related to *depersonalization*, but, unlike the latter, the "as if" personality is not perceived as a disturbance by the patient himself. The expressions of emotion in such patients are formal, and interpersonal relationships are devoid of any traces of warmth. The person gives the impression of a good adjustment to reality, but this is based on mimicry and identification with the environment and leads to a completely passive attitude toward the environment and a readiness to adopt whatever attitudes or reactions seem to be expected. Thus there is no single, integrated personality; instead, the person seems to shift with the tide of his surroundings. According to Deutsch the schizophrenic goes through an "as if" stage before there is any delusional formation. She believes that the "as if" personality represents a deep disturbance of the process of sublimation, which results in a failure to synthesize various infantile identifications into an integrated personality; this leads to an imperfect, one-sided, and purely intellectual sublimation of the instinctual strivings. (*Psychiatric Quarterly II,* 1942)

M. Katan (*International Journal of Psycho-Analysis 39*, 1958), on the other hand, noting that this personality occurs almost exclusively in women, has suggested that the "as-if" personality arises as follows: while still in a stage of strong oral dependence, the little girl is deprived of the mother figure and this, combined with another "loss" (the absence of a phallus), forces the ego to remain dependent and to "rely for its reactions completely upon the examples which it receives from the chance object to which it is attached at the moment. But this attachment never developed beyond a primary identification as it existed at the time the patient lost her mother." The nature of this primary identification is clearly revealed in the patient's reaction to dissolution of an object relationship; "A relinquished relationship is never followed up by an identification, but, contrary to such sequence, the identification disappears with the relationship." (Ibid.)

Katan differentiates between the "as-if" personality and "*pseudo as-if*" (q.v.).

personality, compulsive See *defense, character; personality trait disturbance.*

personality, crowbar *Obs.* An example of post-traumatic mental deterioration that occurred in a patient who had a segment of a crowbar embedded in his left forebrain as a result of a premature dynamite explosion. Before the accident he had been a stable person of good character and exemplary conduct. After his head injury, he became a vulgar, short-tempered, irritable, disagreeable person who drank to excess, abused his wife and children, and finally abandoned them.

personality, cyclothymic See *personality pattern disturbance.*

personality disorder, post-traumatic The changes occurring in the disposition or personality as a result of head or brain injury due to force directly or indirectly applied to the head. The manifest symptoms may include headache, explosive emotional reactions, low resistance to alcohol, fatigability, vasomotor instability, and occasionally convulsive seizures.

personality disorder, transient situational A misnomer, in that personality by definition is long-lasting rather than transient, for *adjustment disorders* or *transient situational disturbances* (qq.v.).

personality disorders *Personality* (q.v.) is a set of relatively stable, predictable, and ego-syntonic habits that characterize the person in his way of managing day-to-day living; when those habits are enough beyond the normal range to warrant the appellation of personality disorder is difficult to define, and often the label is more a social diagnosis of nonconformity than a designation of disease process in the usual sense. In general, however, what are termed personality disorders are patterns of relating to the environment that are so rigid, fixed, and immutable as to limit severely the likelihood of effective functioning or satisfying interpersonal relationships. They are deeply ingrained, chronic, and habitual patterns of reaction that are maladaptive in that they are relatively inflexible; they limit the optimal use of potentialities and often provoke the very counterreactions from the environment that the subject seeks to avoid.

In DSM-III the following personality disorders are recognized:

1. *Paranoid*—characterized by unwarranted suspiciousness and mistrust of people, guardedness, hypervigilance directed toward detecting the earliest signs of anticipated trickery or harm, overconcern with hidden motives, hypersensitivity to criticism, tendency to be easily offended, cold and unfeeling attitude toward others, harboring grudges, reluctance to confide in others, concern with fidelity of sexual partner.

2. *Schizoid*—shyness, aloofness, insensitivity to others' feelings, seclusiveness, only one or two close friends, preference for solitary activities, claim to experience anger only rarely.

3. *Schizotypal*—oddities of thinking, perception, communication, and behavior in addition to the introversion and seclusiveness of the schizoid personality disorder; frequent admixture of dysphoric moods; proneness to eccentric convictions, bigotry, and zealotry, odd beliefs and superstitions; unusual perceptual experiences such as sensing the presence of a dead loved one, telepathic or clairvoyant experiences, marked social anxiety when exposed to unfamiliar people.

4. *Histrionic*—*hysterical personality* (q.v.).

5. *Narcissistic*—exaggerated sense of self-importance, belief that one's problems are unique and comprehensible only by "special" people, exhibitionistic need for attention and admiration, phantasies of unlimited power or brilliance, feelings of *entitlement* to special favors with no recipro-

cal responsibilities, lack of empathy and inability to recognize how others feel, exploitation of others while disregarding their rights and feelings, preoccupation with feelings of envy.

6. *Antisocial*—onset before age 15 as evidenced by truancy, expulsion from school, delinquency, running away, persistent lying, casual or promiscuous sexual intercourse, substance abuse, vandalism, fighting, etc., and continuing social difficulties after age 18 (e.g. inconsistent or unsustained work or academic record, irresponsibility as a parent, conflict with law or multiple arrests, impulsivity, recklessness); see also *psychopathic personality*.

7. *Borderline*—instability in multiple areas of functioning (behavior, mood, self-image, interpersonal relationships); impulsive behavior that is potentially self-destructive; shifting, inappropriate, or uncontrolled emotions; feelings of emptiness and boredom, cannot tolerate being alone, suicidal threats, self-mutilation, identity disturbance with uncertainty about self-image, long-term goals, values; see *borderline personality; borderline psychosis.*

8. *Avoidant*—hypersensitivity to real or imagined rejection, requires uncritical acceptance before venturing into relationships, avoids close personal attachments, low self-esteem.

9. *Dependent*—foists responsibility for his own life onto others and subordinates own needs to theirs, low self-esteem, cannot tolerate being alone.

10. *Compulsive*—also known as anal personality, anankastic personality; order, parsimony, and obstinacy are key traits; overconcerned with conformity and adherence to standards; rigid, overinhibited, overconscientious, overdutiful, indecisive, perfectionistic; a veil of smiling submissiveness and compliance often drops to reveal stubbornness, avarice, possessiveness, arrogance, and pretentiousness; obstructionistic, petty, irascible, and inordinately scrupulous.

11. *Passive-aggressive*—resistance to demands for adequate occupational or social performance, expressed indirectly through procrastination, dawdling, stubbornness, inefficiency, forgetfulness.

In DSM-II (1968 revision), several personality disorders were recognized that are not readily interchangeable with the above labels, such as:

1. *Cyclothymic* (affective)—recurring variations of mood, ranging from elated "highs" (with ambition, energy, warmth, enthusiasm, optimism) to dejected "lows" (with pessimism, worrying, low energy, feelings of uselessness and futility); see *affective disorders; cycloid; cyclothymia.*

2. *Explosive* (epileptoid)—see *personality, epileptic.*

3. *Asthenic*—easy fatigability, low energy, lack of enthusiasm, diminished capacity for enjoyment, oversensitivity to physical and emotional stress.

4. *Inadequate*—although neither physically nor mentally retarded, the person is nonetheless inept, unadaptable, and ineffectual in response to social, intellectual, and physical demands with a lack of physical and emotional stamina.

In DSM-I (1952 nomenclature), personality disorders were grouped under three headings: *personality pattern disturbance, personality trait disturbance,* and *sociopathic personality disturbance* (qq.v.).

personality, emotionally unstable See *personality trait disturbance.*

personality, epileptic It is not clear whether what is called epileptic personality is a true epileptic character or merely a reaction to the chronic invalidism of epilepsy. As usually described, in any event, it probably does not occur in more than 20% of known epileptics. Since its characteristics may appear in the form of a personality disorder in persons without evidence of epilepsy, it is better termed *epileptoid* or *explosive personality.* The characteristics of this personality type include rigidity, egocentricity, selfishness, religiosity, seclusiveness, explosive outbursts of emotion, and extreme rage reactions when frustrated (children especially become frenzied when refused their wishes). Enuresis is also said to be common. Probably the most frequently observed abnormality is a tendency to a certain morose egotism; and only one psychodynamic feature occurs in epilepsy that would in any way support the belief in a specific epileptic psychic constitution—phantasies of death and rebirth, which are more common here than in any other illness. See *dementia, epileptic.*

personality, hysterical See *hysterical personality.*

personality, ideal Jung's term for *ego* (q.v.).

personality, inadequate See *personality pattern disturbance.*

personality, intraconscious A co-conscious personality that knows another personality's thoughts. In one type of multiple personality, one personality functions subconsciously, and when it is aware not only of the outer world but of the thoughts of the conscious personality in the same person, it is termed intraconscious personality.

personality, multiple See *multiple personality disorder.*

personality, multiplication of A loss of continuity of ego boundaries seen most often in schizophrenia, where individual psychic functions may split off from the personality as a whole, attain an autonomy of their own, and then be identified by the subject as being different people within him. The term includes such phenomena as *appersonification, decomposition,* and *dedifferentiation* (qq.v.).

personality, panels of See *panels, personality.*

personality, paranoid See *personality pattern disturbance.*

personality pattern disturbance In the 1952 revision of psychiatric nomenclature (DSM-I), this term was used to refer to personality types or character structures that are more or less fixed and only minimally liable to any basic alteration. "The depth of the psychopathology here allows these individuals little room to maneuver under conditions of stress, except into actual psychosis." Included in this group are:

1. *Inadequate personality*—inadaptability, ineptness, poor judgment, lack of physical and emotional stamina, social incompatibility, etc.

2. *Schizoid personality*—avoidance of close interpersonal relationships, inability to express hostility, autistic thinking, etc.

3. *Cyclothymic personality*—extraverted type of relationships with reality, competitive, frequently alternating moods, etc.

4. *Paranoid personality*—hypersensitivity in interpersonal relationships, suspiciousness, envy, jealousy, stubbornness, and similar projection mechanisms.

See *personality disorders.*

personality, permorbid The personality as manifested before the appearance of any definite mental disorder, or before the development of symptoms that were unmistakably abnormal.

personality, prepsychotic The patient's personality makeup or the character structure considered usual for him before the development of a psychotic disorder.

personality, pretraumatic In the case of a person who has developed an emotional or mental illness in consequence of an injury, the personality as it was before the injury and illness. Knowledge of the details of the patient's pretraumatic personality is essential for proper therapeutic understanding and management in any of the traumatic neuroses and psychoses, i.e. psychiatric disorders attributable to injury.

personality, primary See *personality, multiple.*

personality, psychopathic See *psychopathic personality.*

personality, schizoid See *personality disorders.*

personality, secondary See *personality, multiple.*

personality, split See *personality, multiple.*

personality, stormy Arieti's term for a personality type, found often in preschizophrenic patients, consisting of repeated changes in the person's attitude to life that may be slow or abrupt and commonly are sudden, violent, and drastic. Such people have no stable sense of self-identity and are forever searching for their role in life, without success. Life often seems to be little more than a series of crises for them.

personality, subconscious M. Prince's term for any of the personalities in multiple personality that are not dominant at the moment. In his famous Beauchamp case, for example, Miss Beauchamp became the subconscious personality when Sally (another personality) took over, and vice versa. See *personality, multiple.*

personality trait disturbance In the 1952 revision of psychiatric nomenclature (DSM-I), this term was used to refer to "individuals who are unable to maintain their emotional equilibrium and independence under minor or major stress because of disturbances in emotional development. Some individuals fall into this group because their personality pattern disturbance is related to fixation and exaggeration of certain character and behavior patterns; others, because their behavior is a regressive reaction due to environmental or endopsychic stress." Included in this group are:

1. *Emotionally unstable personality*—excitability, ineffectiveness and poor judgment when under even minor stress; poorly controlled hostility, guilt, and anxiety; formerly called *psychopathic personality with emotional instability.* Some workers consider *EUCD* (emotionally unstable character disorder) to be a mood dysregulation and have reported successful results with long-term lithium treatment. Arthur Rifkin et al. (*Archives of General Psychiatry 27, 1972*) define EUCD as a disorder with chronic maladaptive behavior patterns characterized by short mood swings, both depressive and hypomanic. In their experience, most patients are adolescent girls, with difficulties in accepting reasonable authority and in being appropriately self-reliant. They are often overactive, abuse drugs, avoid schoolwork, malinger, and may be sexually promiscuous.

2. *Passive-aggressive personality*—passive-dependent type, passive-aggressive type, and aggressive type.

3. *Compulsive personality*—overinhibited, overconscientious, rigid adherence to standards of conscience or conformity.

See *defense, character.*

personality types Jung recognizes two "general attitude" types, described from the standpoint of the direction of the flow of libido. When the general direction of the flow of libido is away from the subject, the expression *extraversion* is used and the person is called an *extravert.* When the libido is mainly turned inwardly upon the person, the condition is known as *introversion* and the person as an *introvert.* These two are known as *temperamental* types.

Jung describes four basic *functional* types known as thinking, feeling, sensation, and intuition. Any one of these four functions may be(come) preponderant over the other three and, in that case, it is called the *superior function.* On the other hand, an *inferior function* is one less powerful than the other three. The remaining two functions are then said to occupy an intermediate position.

For a psychoanalytic description of personality types, see *defense, character.*

personification Endowing another with pleasant or unpleasant attributes as a result of frustration of one's desires or wishes. For example, one schizophrenic patient whose letter was not answered accused his doctor of intercepting the mail. Personification is a form of projection wherein the desirable or undesirable properties of reality are attributed to some person, even though the latter is unrelated to the happening itself. Thus schizophrenic persecutory delusions develop only after an obstacle to gratification is felt by the patient; a persecutor is chosen to take on the qualities necessary to explain the frustration. Delusions of persecution convert obstacles into machinations of certain people, the persecutors.

personification, eidetic See *eidetic personification.*

personology The science or study of the personality as a whole, of how people function in society, their perceptions, their actions, and especially their thoughts and feelings and their reasons for being. The scope of personology includes the totality of mental life, the dynamics and economics of the entire personality; and its task is to trace the laws and phases of personality development in the individual life. In contrast, metapsychology is the pure-science aspect of the study of personality and yields information regarding the general laws of mental life. Personology supplies the understanding of how to use this knowledge in relation to the specific individual as an organic-psychic whole whose every action can be understood only in terms of the whole. See *holism.*

persuasion A type of supportive psychotherapy in which the patient is encouraged to adopt the therapist's point of view and exhorted to follow the latter's advice. Persuasion is directive and limited in its goals. Ordinarily, it aims neither to provide the patient with insight nor to widen his range of coping mechanisms. Instead, it concentrates on the here and now, deals with the current crisis, and implies that the patient can accept an attitude of "The doctor knows best." See *psychotherapy.*

pervasive developmental disorders See *developmental disorders, pervasive.*

perverse, polymorphous Pertaining to one whose sexual behavior includes many different forms, expressing both adult and infantile tendencies, both normal and abnormal trends. Though it often appears during mental disorders, polymorphous perversion is said to be normal in early childhood, embracing activities observed in the period of infancy and also adulthood in the form of perversions. See *Haeckel's biogenetic law.*

perversion Abnormality, aberration, distortion, dysfunction; any deviation from the correct, proper, expected, or normal range. In psychiatry, most commonly used to refer to *sexual deviation,* i.e. any sexual practice that deviates from the normal, or any abnormal means of reaching genital orgasm. According to R.J. Stoller (*Archives of General Psychiatry 22,* 1970), a perversion is an indefinitely repeating conscious preference for a genitally stimulating exciting act that is not genital heterosexual intercourse.

Among the perversions (in DSM-III, *paraphilias* and other *psychosexual disorders*) are homosexuality, fetishism, pedophilia, transvestitism, frotteurism, exhibitionism, voyeurism, sadism, masochism, necrophilia, coprophilia, and urolagnia. Normal sexual behavior often includes elements of the perversions, typically as a part of *forepleasure* (q.v.). For the sexual pervert, in contrast, the activity is not merely an elective prelude to intercourse, but rather it has become an end in itself, usually sought after with an insistent, compelling, demanding quality that is reminiscent of compulsions. But unlike compulsions, the perverse activity brings positive pleasure and orgasm and does not merely serve to relieve the subject of psychic pain. The pervert likes something, and even though this be undesired it nonetheless is ego-syntonic; the compulsive, in contrast, is forced to perform an ego-alien action.

Early in the development of psychoanalytic psychology, the neuroses were considered to be "the negative of the perversions," in that neurotic symptoms seemed often to be a disguised expression of the very tendencies that were expressed overtly in the perversions. It is now believed that such an interpretation is tenable in few cases, for perverts are not notably free of neurotic conflicts. Most demonstrate instead a hypertrophy of one component

of infantile sexuality with a secondary repression of all else; often the pervert is
found to have regressed to an infantile
fixation point in order to reassure himself
against castration fears.

pervert One who practices perversions or
forms of genital activity not in accordance
with the general culture or mores of his
community or state.

pervigilium (pēr-vi-jil'ē-um) *Obs.* Coma
vigil.

PET See *NMR.*

petit mal (p'tē' màl') See *epilepsy.*

petrification Fixity, rigidity; used to describe the attitude and behavior of
chronic schizophrenics whose symptoms
in time tend to become colorless, repetitive, and robotlike.

Also, the process of turning, or being
turned, into stonylike substance or stone;
often in myths, fairy tales, etc., it is a
punishment for scopophilic or voyeuristic
impulses.

pettifog A popular term denoting mental
confusion.

peyotism Intoxication with peyote, the dried
blossoms of the mescal cactus. Peyote was
used by the Southwest American Indians
to produce ecstasies as part of religious
ritual. Results included beautiful visual
and sometimes auditory hallucinations, a
sense of timelessness, and a complete withdrawal from reality. Mescaline, the active
principle of the cactus, has also been used
in experimental psychiatry to produce a
model psychosis. See *mescaline.*

Pfaundler-Hurler syndrome *Gargoylism.* See
mucopolysaccharidosis.

PGR Psychogalvanic reflex. See *reflex, psychogalvanic.*

phacomatosis Van der Hoeve's term for
ectodermal disorders, the most common
of which are von Recklinghausen's disease,
or *neurofibromatosis* (q.v.); Pringle-Bourne-
ville disease, or tuberous sclerosis; *Lindau's
disease* (q.v.); Sturge-Weber's disease (intracranial hemangioma); and naevus epi-
theliomatodes multiplex.

phaged(a)ena (faj-ē-dē'nà) *Obs.* Bulimia; insatiable hunger. See *eating disorders.*

-phagia, -phagy (fā'jē-à -fa-jē) Combining
form meaning eating, food, from Gr.
phageīn.

phagomania Uncontrollable or insatiable desire to eat; *bulimia* (q.v.).

phagophobia Fear of eating.

phallic In psychoanalysis the term relates to
the penis during the phase of infantile
sexuality.

phallic love See *love, phallic.*

phallic pride See *pride, penis.*

phallicism, phallism Phallic worship.

phallus In psychoanalysis, the penis during
the period of infantile sexuality when it is
intensely charged or cathected with narcissistic love. When the narcissistic qualities,
associated with one's own genital organ,
are directed outwardly upon a love object,
it is said that the stage of *genital love* has
been reached. Thus genital love in the
male may be called penile love, in contrast
to phallic love.

phallus girl See *girl, phallus.*

phaneromania An irresistible impulse to
touch some part of one's own body especially an exterior growth on it. It is a form
of repetition-compulsion, related to ticlike
movements. A patient had the compulsion
to rub his nose; to him the nose, a centrally
placed, unpaired organ, was equated with
the penis. A homosexual woman, infuri-
ated by all manifestations of effeminacy,
constantly stroked her breasts, as if trying
to rub something off them.

phantasia *Phantasy* (q.v.).

phantasm A sense perception, appearing in
the form of illusion or hallucination.

Phantasms are classed as pseudohallu-
cinations in that they are usually recognized as being illusory or imaginary; often
the illusion is of an absent person seen in
the form of a spirit or ghost.

phantasmagoria The raising or recalling of
spirits of the dead.

phantasmatomoria *Obs.* Dementia with delusions.

phantasmophrenosis *Obs.* Daydreaming
(coined by Schultz).

phantasmoscopia *Obs.* Hallucinations involving specters, ghosts, or spirits.

phantastica See *psychotomimetic.*

phantasy (fantasy) A product of *imagination*
(q.v.) consisting of a group of symbols
synthesized by the secondary process into
a unified story, in which the subject appears as one of the actors. The phantasy
may originate from conflicts secondary to
unsatisfied instinctual wishes or secondary
to frustration in external reality; it may be
a substitute for action, or it may prepare

the way for later action; it may afford gratification for id impulses, it may serve the ego as a defense, or it may subserve superego functions by providing the imagery on which moral concepts, for example, are based. "Fantasies may be conscious or unconscious. In either case they are manifestations of ego functions. It is, I believe, a theoretical error to speak of 'id fantasies' or the 'repression of fantasies into the id.' The more accurate formulation is that unconscious fantasies indicate an unconscious ego function. They are, of course, derivatives of id impulses, and the motivating power or the unconscious fantasy take its energy from the id drives." (Beres, D. *International Journal of Psycho-Analysis XLI*, 1960)

A distinction made, but rarely observed, is to use *fantasy* for conscious constructions, *phantasy* for the content of unconscious constructions. In object relations theory as developed by Melanie Klein, *phantasy* denotes the whole inner world of one's unconscious feeling and impulse and therefore the source of all behavior.

phantasy, anal rape The idea or fear of being raped per anum. Mouth, anus, and vagina are often equated unconsciously by both sexes, and such phantasies may occur in either male or female. See *anal erotism; anality; cloaca.*

phantasy, beating See *beating.*

phantasy-cathexis See *cathexis.*

phantasy, forced A technique devised by Ferenczi, based upon his finding that there is a type of person who "both in analysis and life is particularly poor in phantasies, if not actually without them, on whom the most impressive experiences leave no apparent trace." Such people may reproduce experiences, but these are devoid of adequate or significant affects. Ferenczi advocated forcing affect into the memories, as by asking the patient to fabricate or guess about the memories, or even by telling him what he should have felt and phantasied.

Ferenczi believed that phantasies should be forced only at the end of a psychoanalysis. Moreover, he believed that there are mainly three topics that lend themselves to forced phantasies. They are (1) positive and negative phantasies of transference, (2) phantasies relating to infancy, and (3)

onanistic phantasies. (*FCT*) See *guided affective imagery.*

phantasy formation See *phantasy life.*

phantasy, hetaeral (hē-tē′ral) Phantasy in women of being, and in men of possessing, a courtesan or female paramour.

phantasy, king-slave A phantasy, in which the subject phantasies himself perhaps as now king, now slave, bound to service even by invisible golden chains.

phantasy life Daydreaming, in contradistinction to thinking that is logical and realistic. Varendonck says that phantasy life "gives the illusion that wishes and aspirations have been fulfilled; it thinks obstacles away; it transforms impossibilities into possibilities and realities." He adds that it is "a search for pleasurable representations and an avoidance of everything likely to cause pain." (*The Psychology of Day Dreams*, 1921)

Freud holds that there are two principal groups of phantasies, egoistic and erotic. Varendonck likens phantasy to a safety valve for the abreaction of strong affects.

Often the real meaning of a phantasy is not clear. In this condition it is called screen phantasy (see *phantasy, screen*), for it is believed to cover up a deeply repressed urge.

Phantasies may be conscious or unconscious. Unconscious phantasies are said to express the impulses of the infantile period of life. See *daydream; phantasy, unconscious.*

phantasy, Madame Butterfly The daydream of the return of a departed loved one, seen most frequently in children of divorce in the age range of 5 to 8 years, who cannot believe that the separation of the parents will endure and phantasize that the absent father loves them and someday will return to them.

phantasy, magic The phantasy based upon the idea of limitless power and authority attributed to the analyst by the patient, who consequently expects the impossible from the analyst.

phantasy, night In distinguishing night phantasies from dreams, in the psychoanalytic sense, Freud held that night phantasies occur during the sleeping state, but unlike dreams, do not undergo additions or alterations of any kind and in all other ways are similar to daydreams.

phantasy, Pompadour (Marquise de Pompadour [1721–64], mistress of Louis XV [1710–74], king of France) A hetaeral (mistress) phantasy, in which the woman imagines herself to be the mistress of a king or emperor. "The exaltation of the partner to kingly rank makes thoughts and wishes possible which would otherwise be rejected as immoral." (Ferenczi, *FCT*)

phantasy, primal See *phantasy, unconscious.*

phantasy, rescue See *romance, family.*

phantasy, screen A memory or phantasy that conceals or stands for another phantasy. See *memory, screen; phantasy life.*

phantasy, secondary See *phantasy, unconscious.*

phantasy-thinking *Autism* (q.v.).

phantasy, unconscious Unconscious phantasies "have either always been unconscious and formed in the unconscious, or more often, they were once conscious phantasies, day-dreaming" that were repressed into the unconscious. (Freud, *CP*)

Such phantasies are revealed through mental analyses of adults and children, and dream analyses. The unconscious phantasies of young children, the "primal phantasies" of Freud, are derived from several sources, such as the Oedipus situation, ideas of procreation, the phenomena of birth, the castration complex.

Secondary unconscious phantasies are as a rule some modification of the foregoing primal phantasies. For instance, the revival of the Oedipus complex at puberty gives rise to a new set of phantasies with certain adult sexual issues added.

phantasy, womb The phantasy of remaining within or returning to the womb, a frequent phantasy in psychiatric patients although almost always symbolically expressed. When it appears in consciousness it is highly disguised. It is commonly depicted as living alone on an island void of all things or as living in a cave of mother earth, or as being alone in a room or church.

Freud draws a distinction between womb phantasy and rebirth. For instance, while speaking of the homosexual fixation of a boy on his father, Freud says: "This instance, I think, throws light upon the meaning and origin of the womb-phantasy as well as that of re-birth. The former, the womb phantasy, is frequently derived (as it was in the present case) from an attachment to the father. There is a wish to be inside the mother's womb in order to replace her during coitus—in order to take her place in regard to the father. The phantasy of re-birth, on the other hand, is in all probability regularly a softened substitute (a euphemism, one might say) for the phantasy of incestuous intercourse with the mother." (Freud, *CP*)

phantom limb See *limb, phantom.*

phantom lover syndrome *Erotomania* (q.v.).

pharmacogenetics The study of inherited differences in responses to drugs due to interactions between genetically determined metabolic patterns and pharmacologic agents. Pharmacogenetic variations from the normal do not ordinarily cause disease; rather they predispose the persons who possess the gene variant to abnormal reactions to drugs. Women with blood group A, for example, are three times more likely than other women to develop thrombophlebitis as a complication of birth control pills.

pharmacogeriatrics The study of the use and effects of pharmacologic agents in the elderly. Older patients constitute 11% of the population but consume 29% of prescription drugs, have the highest incidence of adverse drug reactions, and take a greater variety and quantity of medication than younger patients do. Many studies indicate that the proper selection and use of drugs in elderly patients require as much specificity and individualization as does use of drugs in the infant or child.

pharmacokinetics Pharmacodynamics; the study of the actions of a drug within the living organism, particularly in regard to systemic availability of a drug as affected by time after administration, biotransformation (typically, in the liver), and excretion (e.g., renal clearance, biliary or pulmonary excretion).

pharmacopsychoanalysis Narcoanalysis. See *narcotherapy.*

pharmacothymia *Obs.* A neurotic or temperamental avidity for drugs.

phase, anal A psychoanalytical term designating (chronologically) the second stage of libidinal or psychosexual development, immediately following the primary or oral stage. The anal phase (or stage) is subdivided into the early or *first anal phase,* commonly occurring in the third and fourth year of life, and the late or *second anal phase*, occurring between the ages of 4 and 6. See *ontogeny, psychic*.

The first anal phase is characterized by pleasure in the passage of the fecal mass (or "fecal stick") over the anal mucous membrane at the sensitive mucocutaneous junction area. At this period children will hold back their stools for the purpose of increasing the sensory stimulus through increased size of the mass with secondary increased expulsive pressure. In addition to direct anal sensory pleasure, there may occur "hostility intent" pleasure, as the expelled stool mass may represent to the child an object that is destroyed in the expulsion.

The second anal phase occurs usually in the period between 4 and 6 years of age, in the libidinal (emotional) development of a child. It is marked by a predominant interest and pleasure in the *retention*, or holding back, of stool. This is in direct contrast to the first anal phase, which is characterized by *expulsive* excretory *anal pleasure*. In this second anal phase, stool is treated as a possession with an inordinately high value.

Many adult traits of stinginess, hoarding, and interest in hobby collections find here their original prototype. All folklore is replete with observations equating the identity of excrement with money and gold. As examples of this unconscious identity, we have such phrases as "filthy rich," "filthy with money," "money stinks," "he likes to be around the smell of money."

Often a mother's or nurse's oversolicitude toward the child's stool regularity serves to intensify this tendency to overvalue the stool; thus, when withheld, it becomes a powerful tool for getting inordinate attention and solicitude focused upon the child. When the stool is finally passed, it is bestowed as a gift, reward, or largess on the anxious mother or nurse. (Sterba, R. *Introduction to the Psychoanalytic Theory of the Libido*, 1942)

phase, magic A phase in the evolution of thinking in which the mere imagining of an object seems to the thinker the equivalent of his having created it. In other words, this is the magic-phase stage of thinking in which the world is seemingly created by the thinker. Freud referred to it as *omnipotence of thought*. The various phases in the evolution of thinking can be studied in the development of thought in primitive man, in the child, in the schizophrenic, and in the normal adult. Thinking receives its direction toward reality, its respect for facts, only in the last phases of its evolution. Before this maturity takes place, there is the magic-phase stage in which the child operates directly (without any intervening medium) in his thoughts in such a way that every effect will seem to him to be the result of his wish, or, in other words, that there can be action by wish only. (Schilder, P. *Mind, Perception and Thought*, 1942)

phase, oral incorporative The period (in early infantile development) marked by the appearance of possessiveness and its derivatives: voracity, greed, and envy, in association with "cannibalistic" urges toward incorporation of bodily parts, such as mother's nipple, breast, finger. In this way the danger of loss or separation from the loved or security object is obviated. Oral incorporation thus represents the ultimate of closeness.

When thwarted, the urge to possess becomes the drive for aggression, i.e. taking by force that which has been withheld. Later, these possessive, aggressive drives become the source of primary guilt feelings, or early conscience.

phase, phallic The stage of libidinal development in which libidinal and aggressive energies are concentrated mainly in the genital area (penis and clitoris); the phallic phase follows the anal phase and is generally in evidence during the period of 4 to 6 years of age. Concentration of drive energies in the genital area is due in part to increasing physical maturation, and in part to the child's increasing awareness of and natural curiosity about the differences between the sexes. Manipulation of the genitalia can certainly be observed before this phase, but masturbation now is characteristically accompanied by phantasies that relate to the use of the penis as an executive of libido and/or aggression. Object love in the phallic period is very close to what it will be in adolescence and adulthood, but there are two factors that decisively limit sexuality to a still infantile level.

One is physiologic immaturity, and maturation here will have to wait until adolescence; the other is the danger attendant upon the choice of the love object. The child is restricted in his social contacts, and the mother, who has been more or less the only other actor on his stage, retains her leading role. She will be the object of his psychic energies here, just as she was in earlier days; this is the relationship termed *oedipal*. The dangers of this relationship—rejection by the mother, retaliation by the father, etc.—necessitate a strong blockade against libidinal impulses. The ego achieves this by mobilizing aggressive energies against the id. Libidinal energies are repressed, and the child passes into the period of *latency* (q.v.). See *ontogeny, psychic*.

phase, preambivalent The earlier phase of the oral stage, when no conception of objects as yet exists. As infantile sexuality develops, it passes through several stages associated with the various erogenous zones. The libido is organized successively around these zones. The earliest stage in infantile sexuality is the oral stage, in which the libido is organized around the mouth, for the earliest tensions and satisfactions that the infant experiences are those of hunger and its satiation.

The development of object love is interwoven with the development of sexuality. As infantile sexuality develops, the type of relationship to objects changes, for associated with each stage and related to the particular erogenous zone around which the libido is being organized is a different type of relationship to objects. The stages of object love before real love is reached are denoted as ambivalent: in these stages, the process of achieving satisfaction destroys the object. This is based chiefly on the physiological nature of oral and anal erogeneities that are the usual models for these object relationships. For example, in the oral stage, the libidinous aim is to incorporate the object, that is, to put it into the mouth, but the object is thereby destroyed.

Oral incorporation is the first object relationship, for the first awareness of an object was the longing for something already familiar to the infant that could gratify his needs but that was not present at the moment. And the gratification of hunger was the earliest need.

Before this concept of object arose, the infant was not yet aware of the outside world: he was aware only of his own tension and relaxation. Thus, since in the earlier phase of the oral stage oral eroticism had no object, there could not be an ambivalent attitude toward the object. As a result this early objectless period of the oral stage in the development of infantile sexuality is known as the preambivalent phase. It has been noted that in the preambivalent phase oral erotic pleasure is gained not only from the gratification of hunger but also from stimulation of the erogenous oral mucous membrane. This is easily seen in thumb-sucking. Accordingly, this preambivalent phase is also characterized as the early oral sucking stage of libidinal organization or as the autoerotic stage in the development of object love. (Fenichel, *PTN*)

phase, presuperego The early years of life before the superego has been formed. It is generally believed that the superego comes into being when it replaces the Oedipus complex. The presuperego stage lasts until the child is 5 or 6 years of age, and includes the oral, anal, and phallic phases, as well as the development of the Oedipus complex in the phallic stage. A clear distinction is made between the presuperego stage and the superego stage because of the different type of anxiety that is typical of each. In the presuperego stage, anxiety is objective and more closely related to reality situations than in the adult superego stage, where anxiety is typically determined by the precepts of the fully developed superego, of whose role the individual is not consciously aware.

phase shift See *sleep disorders*.

-phasia (-fā′zhē-à) Combining form meaning faculty or power of speech, from Gr. *phásis*, saying, word, from *phánai*, to speak.

phasmophobia *Obs.* Fear of ghosts.

phasophrenias A group of benign degenerative psychoses with atypical symptoms that usually begin with cyclical phases or episodes from which the patient recovers spontaneously; called by Kleist *degeneration psychoses*. See *psychosis, reactive*.

phencyclidine A highly volatile analgesic-anesthetic and hallucinogen of the piperidine family, known chemically as 1-1-phenylcyclohexyl-piperidine HCl; Sernyl. Phencyclidine is rarely used, except in veterinary medicine, because of its high potential for abuse and because of the high incidence of intoxication, delirium, and other organic brain syndromes associated with its use. It is offered, illicitly, under any number of names, including *PCP*, PeaCe Pill, Crystal, Crystal Joints, CJ, KJ, *Angel Dust*, Hog, Rocket Fuel, sheet, goon, busy bee, and superjoint.

Phencyclidine produces a centrally mediated sensory deprivation syndrome by means of a blocking action on the thalamus and midbrain. It can be inhaled ("snorted"), injected or taken by mouth, but most commonly it is sprayed over parsley, mint leaves, or marihuana and then smoked. In small doses, it may give a "high" similar to alcoholic intoxication, with euphoria or mood swings. Larger doses, however, are apt to give rise to unpredictable outbursts of irrational rage or violent action, including suicide, mutilation, assault, and homicide. Convulsions, coma, and death may also result, as well as schizophrenialike psychotic episodes.

DSM-III recognizes phencyclidine intoxication, phencyclidine delirium, and phencyclidine mixed organic brain syndrome.

phengophobia Fear of daylight (comfort being felt only at night).

phenocopy A disorder, not genetic in origin, which imitates another disease. Schizophrenialike psychoses associated with drug-induced organic brain disorders are phenocopies of schizophrenia.

phenomena, release Hughlings Jackson's term for the unhampered activity of a lower center when a higher inhibiting center acting as a control is removed or destroyed, so that the "released" structure can spontaneously discharge motor impulses.

phenomenal field See *field, phenomenal.*

phenomenological reality See *psychotherapy, Morita.*

phenomenology The study of events and happenings in their own right, rather than from the point of view of inferred causes; specifically, the theory that behavior is determined by the way in which the subject perceives reality at any moment and

not by reality as it can be described in physical, objective terms. See *existentialism.*

phenomenon, Aschner ocular (Bernhardt Aschner, Austrian gynecologist, 1883–1960) Pressure exerted over the eyeball produces a slowing of the pulse; also known as the *oculocardiac reflex.*

phenomenon, autokinetic Perception of varying degrees of apparent movement by a stationary light; when exposed to a pinpoint of light at a distance of 12 feet in a totally dark room for 10 minutes, some subjects experience no apparent movement while others report varying amounts of movement.

phenomenon, Napalkov (A.V. Napalkov, contemporary Russian neurophysiologist) An exception to the usual conditioned reflex experiment occurring in some phobic patients in which the conditioning stimulus (e.g. a traumatic event) does not immediately produce a fear reaction; instead, the fear increases in time, rather than being extinguished as it ordinarily would during exposure to the unreinforced conditioning stimulus.

phenomenon, on-off See *up-regulation.*

phenothiazine Class name for a group of psychotropic drugs. The phenothiazines are *major* tranquilizers and are sometimes subdivided on the basis of chemical structure into (1) *alipathic group*—including chlorpromazine, promazine, triflupromazine; (2) *piperazine group*—including perphenazine, prochlorperazine, trifluoperazine, fluphenazine; (3) *piperidine group*—including mepazine, thioridazine.

phenothiazine death See *Bell's mania.*

phenotype The changeable picture of an organism's appearance as produced and modified by its external life situation. In contrast to the *genotypical* structure, the *phenotype* of an organism is the sum of all its manifested attributes. It is the outward manifestation of the subject's biochemistry, determined by the interaction of what is directed by the genes, the genotype, and the environment. See *directive, genetic; genotype.*

phenylketonuria (fē-nil-kē-tō-nūr′ē-à) A hereditary disorder of phenylalanine metabolism, inherited as a Mendelian recessive through a single autosomal gene. Phenylketonuria is the commonest inborn error of metabolism. Because the enzyme phenylalanine hydroxylase is inactive, phenylalanine is not converted into tyrosine but instead accumulates in the body, where it is converted into phenylpyruvic acid and excreted in the urine as phenylketones. The excess phenylalanine, and probably some of its abnormal metabolites, inhibit various enzyme systems and interfere with myelination of nerve tissue, thus producing severe mental retardation (most untreated patients have intelligence quotients below 20).

Because of the phenylketones it contains, the urine of affected children turns olive green in response to 10% ferric chloride (a normal reaction is red-brown color). The reaction was described in 1934 by Dr. Asbjörn Fölling of the University of Oslo and hence is often termed the *Fölling test.* Until the mid-1950s, urine testing was the standard procedure for identifying phenylketonuria (*PKU*), but the method was not wholly satisfactory in that 25 to 50% of affected children do not excrete detectable amounts of phenylpyruvic acid until after irreversible brain damage has already occurred.

A more sensitive test is the *Guthrie test,* a blood test based on bacterial-inhibition assay devised in 1961 by the American pediatrician Robert Guthrie. A drawback of this test is that it gives false positives, and dietary restriction of phenylalanine in children who do not have PKU may be fatal. Most authorities recommend repeated urine examinations and blood testing at birth and again at two weeks of age, to confirm the diagnosis.

Treatment is dietary restriction of phenylalanine; if begun early enough the child can be expected to achieve normal or near-normal intelligence. The dietary regimen can be eased when the child is about 6 years of age, by which time brain differentiation is complete.

PKU affects approximately one person in every 10,000 to 20,000; in institutions for the retarded, it accounts for about one patient in every 100.

phenylpyruvic oligophrenia See *phenylketonuria.*

pheromone A substance released by an organism whose odor affects the behavior of others of the same species. A number of insects, for example, produce attractant pheromones by which one sex finds the other. Alarm pheromones are secreted by some ants and beetles when they are attacked, causing others in their group or cluster to disperse. Some theorists have suggested that pheromones or *external chemical messages (ECM)* exist in the human and that the schizophrenic is aware of and responds to such stimuli that "normal" people ignore. Most investigators remain doubtful, however, of the applicability of the pheromone concept to mammals, and some believe that even for insects it is an oversimplification of behavioral responses.

philo-, phil- Combining form meaning loving, from Gr. *phílos.*

philobat Balint's term for the person with that type of primitive relationship to the environment characterized by an indifference to objects, which are typically considered as untrustworthy hazards, and a preference for objectless expanses such as mountains, deserts, sea, and air. Philobats are thrill-seekers who like adventure and travel and dislike being tied down. They typically have a history of shallow commitments as manifested in a long line of brief love affairs or a pattern of frequent job changes. See *ocnophile.*

philoenia (fi-lē'nē-à) *Obs.* Love of wine.

philogenitive *Rare.* Erotic.

philomimesia *Obs.* Morbid impulse to imitate or mimic.

philoneism (fi-lon'ē-is'm) *Obs.* Intense passion for novelty.

philopatridomania *Obs.* Nostalgia.

philoprogeneity *Rare.* Love of offspring.

philoprogenitive *Obs.* Erotic; manifesting abnormal love for children.

philosophy, coercive The attempt to force others by argument to believe things.

phlebotomomania (flē-bot-ō-mō-) *Obs.* A mania for bloodletting as a curative measure.

phlegmatic See *type, phlegmatic.*

phobanthropy (fō-ban'thrō-pē) *Obs.* Fear of people; anthropophobia.

phobia *Avoidance reaction; phobic disorder; phobic neurosis; anxiety hysteria.* A phobia is a type of anxiety disorder consisting of a morbid and irrational fear of a specific object or situation associated with severe anxiety, and recognized by the subject to be unreasonable or unwarranted. It is more than fear, however, for it requires that the feared object be avoided in order to stave off the panic it would otherwise engender. See *anxiety disorders; anxiety hysteria;* see also listings under *fear of.*

Three major forms of phobia are recognized: (1) *simple phobia*—phobia of objects such as animals or any of the things that people fear to some extent; it is frequent in children but may occur at any age; see *ailurophobia; phobia, bug;* (2) *social phobia*—phobia of function, most often observed in adolescents; see *phobia, social;* (3) *agoraphobia,* with or without panic—the severest form of phobia and the one for which professional help is most often sought (although, overall, simple phobia is probably more common); see *agoraphobia.*

phobia, bathroom A fear of the toilet or bathroom, seen often in children and obsessive-compulsive neurotics. The phobia is frequently expressed as a fear of falling into the toilet, of being attacked by some monster coming from it, or as a fear of being infected. As a rule, such phobias represent a condensation of ideas of dirt (representing anal-erotic temptations) with ideas of castration.

phobia, bug Fear of small animals such as insects, spiders, flies. Although animal phobias are usually distorted representations of the passionate, sexual, aggressive, "animal-like" father, fears of small animals may be a direct projection of one's own drives. Creatures of this sort commonly represent genitals, feces, or little children (brothers and sisters).

phobia, cancer A fear of being eaten away or eaten up by neoplastic cells. The fear of being eaten up, whatever rationalized form it takes, is common in neurotics and is based upon fears of retaliation for having sadistically introjected an object. The dangerous introject may have different meanings on different psychic levels; thus it may represent a child, a penis, the breast, milk, etc. In like manner, the fear may be expressed in various ways—as a phantasy of impregnation, as a delusion or fear of being poisoned, as a fear of infection, as a fear of cancer, etc.

phobia, death A morbid fear of dying, most commonly an outgrowth of the idea of death as a punishment for death wishes against other persons, or of the idea of death as the ultimate in relaxation consequent upon orgastic relief of one's own

excitement, or of the idea of death as a reunion with a dead person.

phobia, doorknob A phobia in which the situation to be avoided (because it produces anxiety) is the touching of a doorknob. On first examination it would appear that this anxiety is related to touching an object believed to be dirty, as a doorknob must be. Thus the patient is protected against anal-erotic wishes to be dirty or to soil, for in magical thinking the characteristics of an object are communicated by touching it.

As Fenichel points out, however, occasionally what appears to be only a protection against anal-erotic wishes may in reality be a protection against other impulses altered by regression, so that they seem to be anal-erotic impulses. He explains that the goal of all impulses involves touching an object, whether it be another person or one's own body. In this way, for example, the patient can achieve security against a wish to masturbate. "Not infrequently a wish to masturbate that has been warded off has been altered by regression, so that the phobia appears to be a protection against anal-erotic wishes to be dirty or to soil." (*PTN*)

phobia, hypochondriacal Morbid fear of organic disease in the absence of known pathology.

phobia, impregnation See *phobia, cancer.*

phobia, infection See *phobia, cancer.*

phobia, insect See *phobia, bug.*

phobia, landscape Fear of a particular locale or type of geography, or a wish to avoid such a setting because of the dysphoria it would engender. Whether it be a seascape, a mountain setting, a desert, an open plain, or a closed space, the object or situation feared is a symbol of unconscious conflict, whose meaning can be discovered only from the phobic subject himself. See *agoraphobia; anxiety hysteria.*

phobia, light-and-shadow A phobia or a morbid fear concerning light-and-shadow effects that works in a way similar to the mechanisms described in the *landscape phobia;* see *phobia, landscape.* "Probably many phobias of darkness or twilight contain memories of primal scenes." (Fenichel, *PTN*)

phobia, live burial A fear of being buried alive is a special "mother's womb" type of claustrophobia that represents the mother's womb, one's own body sensations, and/or the interior of one's own body. The patient attempts to rid himself of his aggressive or sexual sensations by projection and, as with other claustrophobias, the need for sudden escape is a need for escape from one's own feared excitement as soon as it has reached a certain intensity. See *agoraphobia*.

phobia, poisoning See *phobia, cancer*.

phobia, school School refusal syndrome; inability to attend school on a regular, five-day basis because of pervasive anxiety and somatic complaints (e.g. nausea, abdominal pain, headache). Usually, the condition is not a true phobia, but rather anxiety about separation from mother and home, often with obsessional concern about the safety of the mother. The central focus in management is prompt return to school. See *mutism, elective*.

phobia, simple See *phobia*.

phobia, social Fear of situations in which the affected person may be scrutinized by others and/or might act in a shameful fashion; included are fears of speaking in public, of blushing, of eating in public, of writing in front of others, of using public lavatories. See *anxiety disorders; anxiety hysteria; phobia*.

phobia, street A common, morbid fear of being in a street; *agoraphobia* (q.v.).

As with all phobias, the feared street may represent a temptation (especially a situation that would ordinarily call forth an aggressive or a sexual response), or it may represent punishment for the forbidden impulse directly or indirectly through symbolism, or it may be a fear that the anxiety will return because the initial anxiety attack occurred in the street. Any phobia may represent castration and punishment directly, or it may represent a loss of love.

phobia, toilet See *phobia, bathroom*.

phobia, traumatic See *neurosis, traumatic*.

phobia, vehicle A fear of trains, boats, airplanes, automobiles, and/or other forms of transportation. Often these represent a struggle against sexual excitation as perceived in the pleasurable sensations of equilibrium, or a fear that one will be unable to escape from a confined area, this latter representing a need for escape from

one's feared excitement as soon as it has reached a certain intensity.

phobic anxiety-depersonalization neurosis See *depersonalization*.

phobic companion See *agoraphobia*.

phobic, mixed The person who has spontaneous panic attacks but instead of massive *agoraphobia* (q.v.) develops a few specific avoidances such as flying or crossing bridges or driving through a tunnel. Such subjects usually respond to antidepressant medication in much the same way as agoraphobics with panic attacks.

phobic neurosis *Anxiety hysteria* (q.v.).

phobo-, phob- Combining form meaning fearing, from Gr. *phóbos*, flight, (panic) fear.

phobodipsia, phobodipson *Obs.* Hydrophobia.

phobophobia Fear of fearing.

phocomelia A deformity of the limbs in which the hands are attached directly to the shoulders without interposed arms; seen with some tetratogenic drugs and in some types of mental retardation.

phoneme (fō′nēm) In linguistics, a speech sound that serves to distinguish words from one another, such as the vowels in t*a*n, t*e*n, t*i*n, t*o*n, t*u*n; the consonants in *p*an, *b*an, *t*en, *d*en, *s*eal, *z*eal, *s*ink, *z*inc. There is a rigid sequence in the process of acquisition of new phonemes by a child learning to speak, and, accordingly, this process is reversed in various species of aphasic speech disorders; the patient loses those phonemes first that he has acquired most recently. In other words, the successive stages of speech disintegration are exactly contrary to the chronological process of their having been learned or acquired.

phonism See *sensation, secondary*.

phonology 1. The study of speech sounds or of the history of changes in the speech sounds of a language. 2. The sound structure of a language.

phonomania Homicidal mania.

phonophobia Fear of sounds; fear of one's own voice.

phosphene Sensation of flashes or spots of light when the subject is in darkness which a normal person would perceive as grayish rather than total blackness. Such sensations are entoptic phenomena that may be induced by pressure on the retina or by mechanical or electrical stimulation of other parts of the optic pathway. They are also known as *Eigengrauer* and have been reported in cocaine and other drug intoxications.

photic driving See *electroencephalogram*.

photism See *sensation, secondary*.

photogrpahy, spectral See *BEAM*.

photomania Morbid craving for light; sun-worship.

photophobia Literally, fear of light, but rarely used to indicate a phobic avoidance reaction. More commonly the term is used to refer to an organically determined hypersensitivity to light (as in many acute infectious diseases with conjunctivitis) that results in severe pain and marked tearing when the patient is exposed to light.

-phrasia (-frā′zē-à) Combining form meaning speech, way of speaking, phraseology, from Gr. *phrásis*.

phren-, -phrenia (-frē′nē-à), **phreno-** (fren′ō) Combining form meaning mind, brain, diaphragm, from Gr. *phren, phrenōs*.

phrenalgia *Obs.* Guislain classified mental disorders as follows: phrenalgia, or melancholy; phrenoplexia, or ecstasy; hyperphrenia, or mania; paraphrenia, or folly; ideophrenia, or delirium; aphrenia, or dementia.

phrenasthenia *Obs.* Mental retardation; feeblemindedness.

phrenatrophia *Obs.* Atrophy of the brain.

phrenesia *Obs. Encephalitis* (q.v.).

phrenesis *Obs. Phrenitis* (q.v.).

phrenetiasis *Obs. Phrenitis* (q.v.).

phrenetic Relating to or affected by phrenesis, phrenitis.

phrenhypnotic *Obs.* Pertaining to phrenology and hypnosis.

phreniatry (fre-nī′à-trē) *Obs.* Cure of mental disorders.

phrenic Pertaining to the mind or the diaphragm.

phrenicula *Obs.* Brain fever.

phrenismus *Obs. Encephalitis* (q.v.).

phrenitic Phrenic. See *phrenitis*.

phrenitis This term was used by Hippocrates for inflammation of the brain.

phrenoblabia *Obs.* Dementia.

phrenology Study of the conformation of the skull, based on the belief that the different mental faculties could be localized in particular sites on the brain surface, whose resultant conformation would be mirrored in the conformation of the overlying skull; thus a bump here might indicate intelligence, a bump there, willpower, etc.

phrenomania *Obs.* Collapse delirium; delirious mania; *Bell's mania* (q.v.); typhomania. See *mania*.

phrenopathia, phrenopathy *Obs.* Disorder or disease of the mind.

phrenophagia *Rare.* A term suggested by Radzinski to refer to the suppression and/or liquidation of those whose personalities and convictions are incompatible with or nonconforming to existing authoritarian standards.

phrenoplegia, phrenoplegy A sudden attack of mental derangement.

phrenoplexia Guislain's term for the clinical syndrome then (early part of 19th century) known as *ecstasy* (q.v.).

phrenopraxic One of the many terms used to describe the drugs that have an action on the mind or psyche; viz. the tranquilizers, ataractics, psychotropics, etc.

phrenorthosis *Obs.* Sound-mindedness.

phrenotropic Having an action on the mind. The term is usually used to describe certain pharmacologic agents, such as psychotomimetics, tranquilizers, and energizers, which have an effect on mental processes. See *psychotropics*.

phrenzy *Phrenitis* (q.v.); inflammation of the brain.

phricasmus (fri-kaz′mus) *Obs.* Shivering of psychic origin.

phrictopathia Sensation of touch, as unpleasantly tingling.

phronemophobia Fear of thinking.

phthinoid ([f]tin′oid) In Kretschmer's system of constitutional types this term refers to the variety of the *asthenic* type that is so underdeveloped as to represent a morbid condition in itself. This category of the asthenic type is contrasted with the *oligosthenic* and *eusthenic* varieties of moderately or considerably greater vigor, respectively.

In a more general sense, the term refers particularly to the flat, narrow chest characteristic of the tuberculous patient. Sometimes it is applied to any characteristic of the asthenic physique.

phthisiophobia ([f]thiz′ē-ō-) Fear of tuberculosis.

phylo- (fī′lō-) Combining form meaning race, tribe, clan, people, nation, from Gr. *phýlon*.

phyloanalysis A method developed by Burrow that induces in the patient an awareness of his partitive or dissipative behavior, personally and socially, by contrasting the internal tensions concomitant to this type of behavior reaction with an internal pattern of reaction that is concomitant to the organism's total motivation individually and as a phylum. Phyloanalysis regards the symptoms of the individual and of society as but outer aspects of impaired tensional processes that affect the balance of the organism's internal reaction as a whole. (*The Biology of Human Conflict*, 1937)

phylobiology The science of behavior that studies the organism's reactions in their phyletic motivation as these reactions mediate man's basic rapport with the external environment. Phylobiology posits a biological unity as a central governing principle motivating the behavior of the organism as an individual and as a species. (Burrow, T. *The Biology of Human Conflict*, 1937)

phylogenesis, phylogeny Originally a biological term denoting the genealogical history and evolutionary development of a species or group as distinguished from the *ontogenetic* development of the individual. According to Haeckel's biogenetic law, phylogeny is always recapitulated by *ontogeny* (see *ontogenesis*).

Jung speaks of psychic elements called *archetypes*, which he considers to be "the fundamental elements of the unconscious mind, hidden in the depths of the psyche, or to use another comparison, they are the roots of the mind, sunk not only in the earth in the narrower sense, but in the world in general. Archetypes are symptoms of preparedness that are at the same time images and emotions. They are inherited with the structure of the brain of which they represent the psychic aspect." (*CAP*)

If applied in such a special metaphorical sense, the term phylogeny becomes synonymous with *archaic inheritance*, thus losing all connection with its original biological meaning.

phylogenetic symptoms See *schizophrenia, hebephrenic.*

phyloorganism Burrow's term to denote the species man regarded as an organismic

whole in which the element or individual is a phylically integrated unit.

phylopathology The scientific investigation of the underlying causal factors in behavior disorders as envisaged from the background of phylobiology.

physiatrist See *physical medicine.*

physical custody See *custody.*

physical medicine The diagnosis and treatment of disease by physical means; a form of applied medical biophysics. The term includes physical therapy and rehabilitation. In 1947, a specialty board was established for this branch of medicine in the United States; a physician certified by this board is known as a physiatrist.

physician's assistant See *extender, physician; new health practitioners; nurse practitioner.*

physiogenesis Origin in the functioning of an organ of the body. Thus intellectual deficiencies due to impairment of organic (cerebral) functioning are described as physiogenic manifestations.

physiognomy The physical appearance of the face; also, judging personality from facial appearance.

physioneurosis See *neurosis, actual.*

physiopathology The study of disturbances of physiology, whether functional or organic in nature. The capacity for growth and adjustment inheres in physical structure and function. "The general psychological factors of an individual's personality are inherent in, and depend upon: (1) the nature of his physical state, (2) the degree of its effect upon his personal goals, (3) the cumulative effect of a physical deficiency affected by any other dysgenic element in the personality, (4) the local effect of the physical condition, but more especially in terms of the total personality, (5) the secondary effects of the physical condition in the light of social response to it as it conditions his education, occupation, recreation, social responsiveness and adaptability." (Wile, I.S. in *Handbook of Child Guidance*, ed. E. Harms, 1947)

physioplastic See *stage, physioplastic.*

physiotherapy See *therapy, physical.*

physique The *physical* structure of a human organism, the general build of the body as it is to be classified according to the various systems of constitutional types. See *type, constitutional.*

PI *Paradoxical intention* (q.v.).

pia mater A delicate fibrous membrane closely enveloping the brain and spinal cord.

Piaget, Jean (1896–1980) Swiss child psychologist and genetic epistemologist; emphasized the partial constancy of cognitive structuring across long time periods; *The Psychology of Intelligence* (1950); *The Language and Thought of the Child* (1952).

piblokot A type of disturbance reported in Eskimos, similar to *Imu, lata,* and *miryachit* (qq.v.). See *hysterical psychosis.*

pica Compulsive eating of anything, such as ice (*pagophagia*), dirt (*geophagia*), paint, clay, laundry starch. Typically, the subject eats one kind of food; the degree of compulsivity varies, but the person tries to hide the impulse and his behavior from his family and only rarely brings it up as a complaint to his physician. Although often ascribed to neurosis, superstition, rearing, and the like, pica most often is due to iron deficiency (which may or may not manifest itself simultaneously as iron deficiency anemia). About half of patients with iron deficiency have pica—half of those have pagophagia and the other half have food pica. Iron therapy is highly effective, and within one or two weeks not only does the pica disappear, but the original craving often becomes a revulsion.

In DSM-III, pica is included within the *eating disorders* and refers to the regular eating of nonnutritive substances for at least one month.

picatio *Obs. Pica* (q.v.).

Pick's disease (Arnold Pick, Prague psychiatrist, 1851–1924) A presenile psychosis; also known as *circumscribed cortical atrophy, lobar sclerosis.* It consists of progressive dementia with severe emotional impairment and social and ethical aberrations. Like *Alzheimer's disease* (q.v.), Pick's disease occurs more in women than in men and average age of onset is 55 years. Pathologically, there is focal atrophy of the cortical cells in the temporal and frontal regions. There is more often a family history of heredodegenerative traits in Pick's disease than in Alzheimer's, and while the dementia is less pronounced the emotions are more severely impaired.

picture, concrete "Perhaps the most prominent feature of primitive thinking is the tendency to employ 'full concrete pictures' instead of abstract ideas. The thought of primitive man works with total percepts of phenomena without analytic discrimination of their essential constituent parts; he thinks in full concrete pictures just as they are encountered in real experience. . . . In this connection it should be remembered that our own ideas of number have grown out of concrete sensory perceptions. The word *five* is derived from the Sanskrit *pancha,* meaning hand; the Roman number V represents the hand." (Storch, A. *The Primitive Archaic Forms in Schizophrenia,* 1924) Many psychiatric patients, particularly those with schizophrenia, abandon the use of abstract ideas, concrete ideas taking their place. See *abstract attitude; concretism.*

picture, inward An internally apprehended image or picture, as commonly presented in dreams, phantasies, and visions: the pictorialized expression of material from the deeper levels of the unconscious part of the psyche. It is an *inward picture* not only because it *occurs* "inwardly" but also because (according to Jung, whose expression it is) it is a picture of our most inward, innermost self—the *true* SELF.

"They are the real energy-transformers in psychic events. They have at the same time expressive and impressive character, expressing on the one hand internal psychic happenings pictorially, and on the other hand influencing—after having been transformed into images—through their meaningful content these same happenings, thus furthering the flow of the psychological processes. One can continually observe in the course of an analysis how the various pictorial motives determine and lead into one another. In the beginning they still appear in the guise of personal experiences; they bear the characteristics of childhood or other remembrances. As the analysis penetrates to deeper levels, however, they exhibit the outlines of the archetypes ever more clearly, the field becomes dominated ever more definitely by the symbol alone." (Jacobi, J. *The Psychology of C.G. Jung,* 1942)

pigmentary retinal lipoid neuronal heredodegeneration Spielmeyer-Vogt's disease, a type of *amaurotic family idiocy.* See *Tay-Sachs disease.*

pillow, psychological A specific form of catatonic catalepsy in which the patient lies for a long period with his head raised slightly above the pillow.

pineal substance See *therapy, pineal.*

Pinel-Haslam syndrome Schizophrenia; the phrase (suggested by Mark D. Althschule) recognizes that Pinel (1745–1826) formulated the concept of an illness manifested by diminished expression of affect, by looseness of associations and difficulty in forming abstractions, by dissociation of mood and content in thinking, and by inattention or withdrawal. Shortly after Pinel's description, Haslam elaborated the concept further.

Pinel's system Named after Philippe Pinel, a Parisian psychiatrist, 1745–1826, through whose efforts forcible restraint in the management of the mentally ill was abolished. See *moral treatment.*

pingponging Needless and repetitive referral of patients from one specialist to another in order to generate fees, alleged by some economists to be a significant factor in the continuing rise in the cost of medical care and usually considered a form of fraud and abuse by third-party payers.

pink disease *Acrodynia* (q.v.).

pink spot *DMPEA;* 3,4-dimethoxyphenethylamine, which when dipped in ninhydrin-pyridine reagent and treated with a modified Ehrlich's reagent takes on a pink color. In 1962, Friedhoff and Van Winkle reported that DMPEA was found in urine samples from schizophrenics but not in those of normals. Attempts to confirm those findings have yielded contradictory results, and there is some evidence that the finding is an artifact, related more to dietary factors than to schizophrenia.

pinocytosis Entrapment of fluid by the folds of undulating cellular membranes, with the formation of vacuoles that migrate through the cytoplasm; this is perhaps the major method by which the glia contribute to metabolic transport within the central nervous system.

Piotrowski, Zygmunt A. (1904–85) Polish-born psychologist, to U.S. in 1928; in *Perceptanalysis* he presented a system of interpretation of the Rorschach inkblots.

Pisa syndrome *Pleurothotonus* (q.v.).

pithiatism A forced suggestion; a method of removing hysterical symptoms by way of persuasion. The word was coined by Babinski, who held that everything that is hysterical may be caused by suggestion.

pithiatric Curable by persuasion or suggestion, referring to the class of hysterical symptoms that can be made to disappear or be reproduced by means of suggestion.

Pitres' rule A statement of the usual course of recovery of language functions in polyglots: a polyglot who becomes aphasic as the result of vascular ictus or craniocerebral trauma usually begins to understand and then to speak the language most familiar to him and in which he was most fluent at the onset of aphasia; only later are other previously known languages reestablished, more slowly and less completely.

pituitarism Overactivity of the pituitary gland. See *gigantism.*

pituitary cachexia See *cachexia, hypophysial.*

pity Compassion or sympathy for another's misfortune or sufferings. The term generally implies that the object of pity is regarded as inferior to the subject. Pity may appear as a character trait in persons with conflicts about unconscious passive-feminine wishes in which case it may signify "I shower you with love as I wish I had been loved." It may also represent a passive-feminine masochistic identification with the sufferer.

pixel Picture element. See *NMR.*

PKU *Phenylketonuria* (q.v.).

placebo (L. "I am to placate") Any medication used to relieve symptoms, not by reason of specific pharmacologic action but solely by reinforcing the patient's favorable expectancies from treatment. Also known as *dummy,* particularly in Britain. Although a placebo may be an inert substance, as used in present-day research placebos more commonly contain active substances that at least in part mimic the side effects of the specific therapeutic agent with which the placebo is being compared. Placebo effects include all those psychologic and psychophysiologic benefits and undesirable reactions that reflect the patient's expectations; they depend upon the diminution or augmentation of apprehension produced by the symbolism of medication or by the symbolic implications of the physician's behavior and attitudes.

The term may be defined even more

broadly to include *any* therapeutic procedure that has an effect on a symptom or disease, although objectively it has no specific action on the condition being treated.

placebo, balanced See *balanced placebo design.*

plan, life With this term Adler indicates the entire system of behavior by means of which the person prevents his "superiority" from being subjected to the test of reality.

plane, subjective "By interpretation upon the subjective plane, I understand that conception of a dream or phantasy in which the persons or conditions appearing therein are related to subjective factors entirely belonging to the subject's own psyche. It is common knowledge that the image of an object existing in our psyche is never exactly like the object, but at most only similar.

"In the analytical treatment of unconscious products, therefore, it is essential that the image shall not immediately be assumed to be identical with the object; it is wiser to regard it as an image of the subjective relation to the object. That is what is meant by the consideration of a product upon the subjective plane." (Jung, *PT*)

planning, social See *social policy planning.*

planning, strategic See *strategic planning.*

planomania *Obs.* Morbid impulse to wander from home and throw off the restraints of society.

planophrasia *Obs.* Wandering speech; usually used to refer to flight of ideas in manic syndromes.

plaques, senile See *senile dementia.*

plasm, germ The theory developed by Weismann conceives the germ plasm (the reproductive tissue that produces the germ cells) as separate and distinct from the other body tissues representing the *somatoplasm.* It is the basis of the important genetic concept that attributes acquired by the organism during the lifetime of its phenotype are never inheritable.

According to this concept (true only in higher animals and therefore of limited value) the germ plasm is the sole seat of hereditary characters and thus represents the potentially immortal part of an organism, through the continuing succession of its reproductive cells. The environment may cause many variations in the somatoplasm, but it has been shown by Weismann and other geneticists that these changes are not transferred to the germ plasm and therefore cannot be hereditarily transmitted to the offspring.

plasmapheresis *TPE* (therapeutic plasma exchange); a procedure to remove toxic elements from blood consisting of removing the blood, separating the plasma from the formed elements, and reinfusing the formed elements together with a plasma replacement. One major use of TPE is in neurological conditions in which autoimmunity is believed to play a role. Because effects are short-lived (four to six weeks), it is of greatest value in monophasic diseases of short duration, such as Guillain-Barré syndrome, or when used as a temporary expedient in chronic disorders such as myasthenia gravis, systematic lupus erythmatosus, and multiple sclerosis.

plasmid A hereditary unit, physically distinct from the chromosome, that has been used in genetic engineering to transfer a human gene into bacteria, which then copy the information and produce, for example, the hormone that the gene produces normally in the human. R plasmids are plasmids that are resistant to a variety of antibiotics; much genetic engineering has used naturally occurring R plasmids. See *recombinant DNA.*

plasmon This biological term was introduced by von Wettstein to characterize the independent genelike elements in the cytoplasm, in contradistinction to the nuclear system of Mendelian gene units for which he proposed the term *genome.*

plastic cells See *neurometrics.*

plasticity In neurology, changes in the developing organism induced by environmental influences and mediated through organization of the nervous system; one manifestation is the ability of axons and dendrites to grow, regenerate, or reorganize after injury or other environmental change.

plate, neural See *cephalogenesis.*

platonic nymphomania See *nymphomania, grave.*

platonization (From *platonize*, idealize, as in platonic love, which in Plato's view passed from physical passion on to higher contemplation of the ideal, i.e. to love free from sexual desire) A mental mechanism consisting of considering the desired act without actually performing it. Platonization is thus a mechanism of defense against impulses and would be considered by some as evidence of prelogical, primitive thinking wherein thought has become an equivalent of action by reason of infantile belief in the magical omnipotence of thought. Platonization is typical of paranoia, where thought rather than action reigns supreme. But, like any other mechanism of defense, such as repression, sublimation, or projection, platonization need not imply gross psychiatric abnormality in the person who uses the mechanism.

platybasia Basilar impression; an abnormality of the base of the skull, often congenital, in which the angle between the basisphenoid and the basilar portion of the occipital bone is widened. The neck is abnormally short and the head is sometimes mushroom-shaped.

platycephaly Flattening of the crown of the head.

play See *activity, ludic.*

pleasure-ego See *ego, pleasure.*

pleasure, function Enjoyment of functioning or doing or exercising one's own capacities. Function pleasure is obtained when an act can be accomplished without anxiety; such pleasure is the basis for subsequent repetitions of situations that originally induced excitation and anxiety, as is seen frequently in children who enjoy endless repetitions of the same game or of the same story, which has to be retold in exactly the same words.

pleasure, muscle Pleasure connected with body movements.

pleasure-pain principle See *principle, pleasure.*

pleasure principle See *principle, pleasure.*

-plegia, -plegy (-plē′jē-à, -plē′jē) Combining form meaning (paralytic) stroke, attack, from Gr. *plēge.*

pleiotropy (plī-o′trō-pē) The phenomenon of a single gene acting on very different characters; in the mouse, for example, a single gene is responsible for a ventral white spot, a flexed tail, and microcytic anemia.

pleniloquence Excessive talking.

pleocytosis Excess of cells; pleocytosis of the cerebrospinal fluid indicates meningeal irritation.

pleonasm Redundancy or the use of more than enough words to express an idea, as is seen in *circumstantiality* (q.v.).

pleonexia Greediness; a psychosis characterized by an uncontrollable desire for accquisition or gain.

pleurothotonus A torsion spasm in which the trunk of the body is bent to one side; sometimes called *Pisa syndrome.* Pleurothotonus may be seen as a form of tardive dystonia, which is sometimes a side effect of treatment with neuroleptics.

plot, melody See *speech, plateau.*

plumbism *Lead poisoning* (q.v.).

pluralism The concept that behavior is causally determined by a multiplicity of complexly interrelated factors. "Freud and Meyer were among the first to appreciate the importance of the setting, the *theme*, the emergence of a behavior item or action tendency from a complexly-integrated set of experiences and their meaning to the experiencing individual. Freud could show how the early 'family drama' was a theme which had a profound significance throughout a person's life, influencing his ambitions, identifications, choice of a mate, and even the contents of his dreams. Meyer's pluralistic orientation could not be satisfied with the study of behavior as a self-contained phenomenon: he was too much aware of the multiplicity of factors at play in any situation. His relativistic mode of thinking caused him to look for the cohesion and interdependence of these factors. . . . Behavior of the moment thus appears as the temporarily last scene of an uninterrupted plot or theme, during which a person has developed a certain readiness to perform in the particular manner in which he does perform." (Kanner, L. *Child Psychiatry*, 1948)

pluralistic utilitarianism See *utilitarianism, pluralistic.*

plus complementarity See *complementarity.*

plutomania Greediness; inordinate striving for wealth, possessions money, etc.

PML See *leukoencephalopathy, progressive multifocal.*

pneumoencephalogram An X-ray of the skull following replacement of measured quantities of cerebrospinal fluid with air or some other gas by means of lumbar or cisternal puncture.

pneumotherapy, cerebral Insufflation of oxygen or air into the ventrical or arachnoid spaces, once used as treatment for intractable epilepsy, circumscribed meningitis, and psychosis.

pnigerophobia (nī-jĕ-rō-) Fear of smothering.

pnigophobia (nig-ō-) Fear of choking.

Po Rorschach scoring symbol for a position response, i.e. a response determined or suggested by the location of the particular stimulus area on the card.

poena talionis The law of ancient Rome according to which the culprit was subjected to the identical injury or material loss as he had caused to the plaintiff. See *dread, talion.*

poiesis The making or composing of a word, and particularly the coining of a neologistic word or phrase; the term has been used specifically to refer to a type of schizophrenic neologism, in which language is constructed so as to affirm the patient's wishes, which are then believed by him to have been fulfilled.

poikilothymia (poi-ki-lō-thī'mē-à, -thim'-ē-à) E. Kahn's term for a mental constitution closely akin to cyclothymia, differing from the latter in that in poikilothymia the mood variations are more intense.

poinephobia (poi-nē-fō'bē-à) Fear of punishment.

point, critical The event, occurrence, or situation in which the patient's problem comes to a head and he mobilizes his resources for dealing with the problem. Slavson, who suggested the term, believes that in nearly all therapy an ultimum point is reached in the specific intrapsychic or environmental situation that is the culminating point of therapy. See *problem, nuclear.*

point, flicker-fusion Critical flicker frequency. See *flicker.*

pointing A test for vestibular rather than pure cerebellar function; patient is requested to extend his arm and perform the movements at the shoulder; examiner stands in front of him, and patient touches with his extended index finger the examiner's two index fingers, which are held together in a fixed position; with eyes open, there is no deviation normally; on closing the eyes, and knowing the position of the examiner's fingers, the patient should be able to touch the same spot every time; if he deviates to the left or right there is said to be *past-pointing.*

pointing the bone See *bone-pointing.*

poisoning, deadly nightshade *Strychnomania.* Deadly nightshade is a plant of the genus Solanum. Poisoning may follow ingestion of the black berries of the plant. The mouth and tongue become dry and vision is impaired; any or all of the following symptoms may then appear: visual hallucinations, mutism, restlessness, unresponsiveness, widely dilated pupils, disorientation and confusion, with increasing agitation. The patient then falls into a deep sleep and awakes asymptomatic but with amnesia for the agitated period. During the disturbed period, a misdiagnosis of acute schizophrenic reaction is commonly made.

polar body See *body, polar.*

polarity Possession of opposite properties, as if at opposite poles.

From the psychoanalytic point of view, "Mental life as a whole is governed by *three polarities,* namely, the following antitheses: Subject (ego)-Object (external world); Pleasure-Pain; Active-Passive." (Freud, *CP*)

policy, open-door See *community, therapeutic; open-door policy.*

policy, public A stated, conscious, and deliberate action (or decision not to take action) on the part of government, usually involving rules and regulations that prohibit or allow certain activity, or the allocation and distribution of social benefits and burdens, such as deciding that specific goods or services will be provided to one segment of the population and that their cost will be borne through taxation of another segment.

polioclastic Destructive to gray matter of the central nervous system; ordinarily used to refer to neurotropic viruses.

poliodystrophy, progressive infantile cerebral Also known as *Alpers's disease;* a nonlipid neuronal destruction of cerebral tissue with preservation of myelinated structures, probably most commonly due to cerebral anoxia, less commonly to maternal toxemia or genetic factors. Seizures and mental retardation are the usual symptoms.

polioencephalitis hemorrhagica superior See *Wernicke's encephalopathy.*

poliomyelitis Infantile paralysis; Heine-Medin's disease. An acute infectious disease due to a virus that attacks the anterior horn cells of the spinal cord and brain stem, causing muscular paralysis and atrophy. The usual route of infection is through the alimentary tract, via personal contact with healthy carriers and abortive carriers or by ingestion of contaminated food. From the alimentary tract, the virus reaches the central nervous system by ascending the peripheral nerves and through the bloodstream.

Before the introduction of inoculation the disease occurred in epidemics; now, for the most part, it occurs sporadically. Initially, immunity was conferred by three injections of inactivated poliomyelitis vaccine. Now, a live, attenuated Sabin-type vaccine is given orally; in epidemics, which still occur, gamma globulin gives temporary protection.

poliomyelitis, chronic See *sclerosis, amyotrophic lateral.*

political genetics See *genetics, political.*

pollakiuria (pol-à-kē-ū'rē-à) Abnormally frequent urination.

pollution *Obs.* The discharge of semen and seminal fluid in the absence of sexual intercourse; the term is often used synonymously with *nocturnal emission.*

pollution, air See *syndrome, air pollution.*

Pollyanna An optimist; someone who finds good and/or fails to see the bad in any situation. Often used as an adjective, as in comparing the "Pollyanna tendency" of normals to recall more pleasant than unpleasant material with the "anhedonic tendency" of schizophrenics to recall unpleasant and pleasant with approximately equal frequency.

polyandry The practice of having more than one husband at one time.

polychromate, abnormal One who distinguishes most colors, but fails to perceive one or two, or confuses two colors.

polyclonia epileptoides continua *Obs.* See *epilepsy, continuous.*

polycratism (pō-lik'rà-tiz'm) (From Polycrates, tyrant of Samos [535–512 B.C.], who wished to allay the envy of the gods, because all his enterprises were invariably highly successful. In a galley fitted out with regal splendor Polycrates sailed out on a pleasure trip. As if inadvertently his favorite signet ring fell overboard and with ostentatious grief Polycrates returned home, inwardly happy that he had

appeased the gods. Two or three days later a fisherman brought to the palace a huge fish he thought fit only for the ruler's table. When Polycrates carved the fish at the repast, he found his ring, which the fish had swallowed. The gods were not to be appeased—Polycrates met death by crucifixion.) "By analogy with Schiller's poem 'The Ring of Polycrates' one could give this name to the superstition that dreads lest things should 'go too well' with one, because then a proportionately heavier punishment is to be expected from God. In an analysis it could be traced to a bad conscience due to personal phantasies that were reprehensible." (Ferenczi, *FCT*)

polydipsia Excessive thirst.

polygamy The practice of having more than one mate at one time. This term is thus more general than *polyandry* and *polygyny* (qq.v.), both of which it includes.

polyglot See *reaction, polyglot.*

polyglot neophasia See *neophasia, polyglot.*

polygraph Also *Keeler polygraph.* See *detector, lie.*

polygyny The practice of having more than one wife at one time.

polyhybrid In genetics this characterizes *hybrids* that differ in more than three hereditary characters. See *hybrid.*

polylogia See *tachylogia.*

polymorph, polymorphous perverse See *perverse, polymorphous.*

polymorphism See *marker, genetic.*

polyneuritis A disease in which there usually is simultaneous inflammation of a large number of peripheral nerves. The signs and symptoms are usually bilateral and frequently symmetrical, although not all the nerves are affected with equal severity. The condition is due either to an infectious agent or an endogenous or exogenous poison, probably operating through the circulatory system. Prominent symptoms include severe pain, wasting of the muscles, and paralysis. Clinical examples are alcoholic polyneuritis, arsenic polyneuritis, diabetic polyneuritis, polyneuritis of pregnancy.

polyneuritis, acute toxic *Guillain-Barré syndrome* (q.v.).

polyneuritis, erythroedema *Acrodynia* (q.v.).

polyneuritis, rheumatic *Guillain-Barré syndrome* (q.v.).

polyopia Duplication or multiplication of a visual image, such as seeing two lights when there is only one or seeing hundreds of holes on a circular telephone dial. Polyopia may be organic in origin (associated with pathology in the ocular apparatus, with nystagmus, or with occipital lobe dysfunction), and it may also appear as a conversion symptom in hysteria. See *palinopia.*

polyparesis General paralysis of the insane. See *paresis, general.*

polyphagia Excessive eating; gluttony; *bulimia* (q.v.).

polypharmacy Simultaneous administration of more than one drug for the same disorder; in psychiatry simultaneous administration of more than one psychotropic drug; also known as *combination drug therapy, maxipharmacy,* or *orthopsychic tranquilization.* Such combinations are often no more effective than a single drug, but few of the combinations have been as dangerous as originally predicted by some opponents of polypharmacy. According to G. Gardos, A. Perenyi, and J. Cole (*Mclean Hospital Journal V,* 1980), "The best way to avoid drug induced toxic reactions is not to adhere rigidly to the principle of one durg only, but to be familiar with the drugs prescribed and to evaluate patients for side effects at appropriate intervals."

polyphobia Fear of many things.

polypnoea (pol-ip′nē-à) Deep, labored, and rapid respiration. It may be physically or psychically determined.

polyposia Craving for intoxicating drinks.

polypsychism The concept (sometimes found in psychotic patients) that each person possesses several souls.

polyradiculoneuritis *Guillain-Barré syndrome* (q.v.).

polysomnogram (PSM) The system of recording all-night measurements of various electrophysiologic and somatic variables, used in the study and diagnosis of sleep disorders. The variables include the electroencephalogram, electro-oculogram, submental electromyogram, ventilatory air exchange, respiratory effort, electrical heart activity, leg movement, blood oxygen saturation, and often also simultaneous video recording of the sleep behavior of the subject. The PSM provides precise data concerning the time at which the subject falls asleep, the number of wake periods experienced, and the quality and duration of sleep. Measurements are made during sleep without disturbing the sleeper.

polysomnography (PSG) The use of the *polysomnogram* (q.v.).

polyuria Excessive excretion of urine; profuse micturition.

Pompadour phantasy See *phantasy, Pompadour.*

POMR Problem-oriented medical record. See *problem-oriented record.*

ponopathy Synonymous with *nervous exhaustion.* See *neurasthenia.*

ponophobia Fear of overwork.

pons That portion of the metencephalon that forms the floor of the fourth ventricle; the pons is continuous with the midbrain anteriorly, and with the medulla oblongata posteriorly. The pons contains the pontine nuclei which connect the cerebellum with the cerebrum, and the nuclei of cranial nerves IV, V (in part), VI, and VII. Transverse fibers of the pons form the brachium pontis, or middle cerebellar peduncle; the longitudinal fibers of the pons contain the pyramidal tracts and the corticopontile fibers.

pontocerebellar angle tumor See *syndrome, pontocerebellar angle.*

popular response In Rorschach scoring, any response that is among those responses given more frequently by healthy subjects than any other responses. Various writers, on the basis of statistical analysis of their case protocols, have constructed itemized lists of the responses to be classified as popular.

A response is classified as *original* if it occurs not more than once in 100 records, and as *individual* if it is given by only one subject.

population genetics See *genetics.*

POR *Problem-oriented record* (q.v.).

porencephaly A developmental anomaly in which there occur small or large unilateral or bilateral cavities in the brain substance.

poriomania An irresistible impulse to journey. The latter may be carried out with the full and complete knowledge of the person or there may be complete amnesia for all activities associated with the trip. States of poriomania may be associated with criminal acts.

pornerastic Fond of prostitutes.

pornographomania Morbid impulse to write obscene letters.

pornography Obscene, lewd, lascivious, prurient drawing or writing, and especially that which aims to arouse the viewer or reader sexually. As R.J. Stoller points out (*Archives of General Psychiatry 22,* 1970), no written or pictorial material is pornographic in itself; instead, the observer's phantasies are projected into that material and only then does it become sexually and genitally exciting.

pornolagnia A perverted lustful attraction for prostitutes.

porphyria, acute intermittent A familial metabolic disorder of the pyrroles, resulting in the production of abnormal types of porphyrins, which appear in the urine; first described by Gunther and Waldenstrom. Females are four times as frequently affected as males, usually between the ages of 20 and 35. The first symptom is usually abdominal pain, often with nausea, vomiting, low-grade fever, leukocytosis, and tachycardia. These symptoms continue and to them are added psychic changes (irritability, tension, and often progression to a schizophreniform psychosis) and, later, neurologic symptoms (muscular weakness and other signs of peripheral neuritis). There is no known treatment. The disease is fatal in about half of the cases; mortality is higher (60–90%) in those with cranial nerve involvement.

porphyrinuria (por-fir-ē-nūr′ē-à) See *porphyria, acute intermittent.*

porphyrismus The mental changes associated with porphyria. See *porphyria, acute intermittent.*

porropsia Inability to gauge the real distance of objects, which appear more distant than they really are, without any alteration in their size.

port-wine stain See *angiomatosis, trigeminal cerebral.*

posiomania Dipsomania (q.v.).

position, depressive One of the stages in mental development hypothesized by Melanie Klein. This position succeeds the paranoid-schizoid position (see *position, paranoid-schizoid*) and is believed to be at its peak at the sixth month of life. Following the development of the paranoid-schizoid position, the ego continues to gain strength and shows a growing capacity for integration and synthesis. In the depressive position, the child's fear is of destroying and then losing the beloved and indispensable object. In contrast to the earlier position, the injured object in the depressive position appears not so much a persecutor as a love object toward whom the child feels guilty and wants to make reparation.

position, paranoid-schizoid One of the stages in mental development hypothesized by Melanie Klein. This position is believed to be at its peak during the third or fourth month of life and is an outcome of the method used by the infant to protect himself from destruction by his death instinct. Aggression is deflected (projected) onto the external object; this makes the object into a persecutor. But some aggression is retained by the ego, and this leads to aggression being turned actively against the persecutory object. The infant is thus compelled to destroy the object to escape persecution. At the same time, the primal process of introjection is used to defend the ego against the death instinct, and the breast is internalized and split into a helpful, loved object on the one hand, and into a frightening, hated object on the other. The internalized *good object* supports the ego in its binding of the death instinct by libido. Part of the death instinct is projected into a part of the ego itself and contributes to the formation of the superego. But some internalized *bad objects* are so terrifying that they are not handled in this way; instead, they are split off and relegated to the deeper layers of the unconscious.

The paranoid-schizoid position is normally succeeded by the depressive position. See *position, depressive.*

positioning, paradoxical See *therapy, paradoxical.*

positron emission tomography See *NMR.*

POSM Patient-operated selected mechanisms, i.e. electromechanical devices that can be controlled by patients with high cord lesions or extreme disability from other causes.

possession/trance disorder Once suggested as one of the *dissociative disorders* (q.v.) consisting either of altered consciousness with diminished or constricted responsiveness to external stimuli or of the subject's belief that he has been taken over by some spirit or other agent, or by both.

possum Same as *POSM* (q.v.).

post coitum triste (L. "gloom after sexual intercourse") See *impotence, psychic.*

post-torture syndrome See *syndrome, post-torture.*

post-traumatic and postencephalitic syndromes, classification of Blau (*Research Publications, Association for Nervous and Mental Diseases 34,* 1954) has suggested the following classification:

   I. Etiologic Classification

     A. Cerebral birth injury

       1. Direct injury—prolonged pressure applied to the cranium, disturbed labor, breech extraction, instrumental delivery, etc.

       2. Anoxemia—prolonged labor, abnormalities of pregnancy, placenta previa, strangulated cord, etc.

     B. Cerebral trauma—accidental head injury with or without skull fracture, concussion, contusion, subdural hematoma, etc.

     C. Cerebral inflammatory and degenerative diseases

       1. Encephalitis—epidemic, variola, vaccinia, rubella, measles, mumps, meningitis, etc.

       2. Encephalopathy—pertussis, burns, lead, epilepsy, etc.

  II. Psychiatric Classification (see *syndrome, organic*)

     A. Intellectual defect conditions

       1. Focal defects—memory disturbances, paraphasias, attention defects, concentration, etc.

       2. Generalized intellectual defect—general mental retardation, secondary dementia, learning difficulties, etc.

     B. Personality disorders—conduct and behavior disorders, delinquency, psychoneurosis, psychosis, character disorders, etc. See *constitution, post-traumatic; contusion, brain.*

post-traumatic stress disorder Traumatic neurosis; a group of characteristic symptoms that develop following exposure to a stressful situation or series of events that are outside the normal range of human experience (such as rape, child sexual abuse, assault, military combat, mass disasters, concentration or death camps). Although the older literature emphasized the importance of physical injury in precipitating the condition, current thinking emphasizes that a psychologic component is the essential element. Characteristic symptoms include reexperiencing the traumatic event either in recurrent dreams or as recurrently intrusive memories; a blunting or numbing of general responsivity to the external world, manifested as reduced interest in one or more significant activities, feelings of detachment or estrangement, or constriction of affect; exaggerated startle response; many different forms of sleep disturbance; difficulties in concentration and sometimes with memory; and in many of those exposed to mass disasters feelings of guilt about having survived. See *pathosis, attitudinal; syndrome, survivor.*

   Post-traumatic stress disorders are termed acute if they last less than six months after the traumatic event, and chronic if they last longer than six months and begin following a latency period of at least six months after the traumatic event. See *neurosis, traumatic.*

postambivalence See *stage, postambivalent.*

postcentral gyrus See *lobe, parietal.*

postconcussion neurosis See *neurosis, postconcussion.*

postdormital chalastic fits See *paralysis, sleep.*

postencephalitic syndromes See *post-traumatic and postencephalitic syndromes, classification of.*

posterolateral sclerosis See *sclerosis, posterolateral.*

posthallucinogen perception disorder See *flashback.*

posthion Small penis. (Greek *posthe* = penis or prepuce, although the preferred term for the latter was acrobystia. In most medical terms, however, the root *posth-, postho-, posthio-* indicates foreskin, and *phallo-, phallus* is used for penis.)

postpartum psychosis See *psychosis, puerperal.*

potamophobia Fear of rivers.

potence, potency The ability (of the male) to consummate the act of sexual intercourse.

potential, action See *action current.*

potential, event-related *ERP* (q.v.).

potential, evoked A specific electroencephalographic response to sensory stimulation, such as a light flash, a musical tone, a click, or a photograph. Because attention disturbances are frequently seen as a prominent part of schizophrenic disorders, average evoked potential (AEP) techniques have been widely used to investigate perceptual dysfunction in such patients. See *neurometrics*.

potential, specific action See *instinct*.

potomania *Obs.* Morbid impulse for intoxicating drinks; *delirium tremens; dipsomania* (qq.v.).

pototromania *Obs.* Delirium tremens.

Potzl's syndrome See *syndrome, Potzl's*.

poverty, clinical See *syndrome, clinical poverty*.

POW See *syndrome, prisoner of war*.

PPA Preferred provider arrangement(s), a term proposed as a substitute for *PPO* (q.v.) in recognition of the fact that a separate organization is not needed to develop preferred provider status.

PPO *Preferred provider organization;* an organized health care delivery system operating under the currently favored competitive concept of restricting health benefits to, or providing incentives to choose, designated providers. It is a form of selective contracting consisting of an arrangement or agreement between payer and specified provider(s) that establishes prices lower than those existing in the absence of such an arrangement. The services of the specified group or panel of providers (hospitals, physicians, or both) are marketed on the basis of cost efficiency, quality, accessibility, and effective management. Enrolled members are given incentives to "prefer" (use) certain providers, but they are not restricted to using only those providers. Payment by the purchaser is usually on a fee-for-service basis. A major element in a PPO is its utilization of a review program (such as preadmission certification and length-of-stay review) with supporting cost control information, which permits identification of lower cost alternatives, promotes reductions in length of stay, and assesses the intensity of ancillary services.

practice, programmed See *exposure, self-directed*.

practice, reinforced *Successive approximations; shaping;* graduated exposure of the phobic subject to the feared object or situation.

praecox, heboid "Not infrequently the principal changes [in dementia praecox] are shown in an emotional dulling, indifference and stupidity without the occurrence of hallucinations or developed delusions. These cases in which the dementia seems to be the principal symptom, and in which the accessory symptoms play a small part, have also been spoken of as simple or heboid praecox." (Barnes, F.M. *An Introduction to the Study of Mental Disorders,* 1923)

praecox, predementia The personality constitution of the schizophrenic prior to the appearance of overt symptoms of the disorder.

"Dementia praecox is thus the culmination of a long-continued series of faulty mental habits. The predementia praecox character is one in which the individual habitually ceases to apply himself vigorously to the real facts of life. His thoughts are devoted to day-dreams and fantasies, and by constantly seeking refuge in evasions he loses the capacity for grappling with difficulties. Thus, in the presence of some added stress, which the ordinary individual would be prepared to meet, 'the sensitive and weakened individual will react with manifestations constituting the deterioration process' of dementia praecox." (Kraepelin, E. *Lectures on Clinical Psychiatry,* 1913) Kraepelin credits Adolf Meyer with having first delineated the character syndrome observed in predementia praecox.

Prägung (prä'gooNg) *Imprinting* (q.v.).

-praxia (prak'sē-à) Combining form meaning action, doing, from Gr. *prāxis,* a doing, acting, action, from *prássein,* to achieve, accomplish, practice, do.

praxiology Dunlap's term for the science of behavior that excludes the study of consciousness and similar nonobjective metaphysical concepts.

praxis, ideokinetic Ability to perform an action from memory when requested to do so, without the need of external cues. Also known as *ideomotor praxis,* it is a function of the dominant parietal lobe.

praxitherapeutics An old term for occupational treatment; ergo-therapy.

pre- Combining form meaning earlier, before, ahead, from L. *pre-*.

pre-AIDS Early AIDS; also referred to as AIDS-related complex (ARC). See *syndrome, acquired immune deficiency*.

preadaptive attitude See *attitude, preadaptive*.

preambivalence See *phase, preambivalent*.

precentral area, convolution, gyrus See *lobe, frontal; motor cortex.*

precocity In a child, the premature or exceptionally early development of certain mental or physical capacities and endowments normally and characteristically exhibited only by children of a more advanced age group.

precognition Prescience; knowledge of future events, presumably by means of extrasensory perception.

preconscious Foreconscious; in psychoanalysis, one of the three topographical divisions of the psyche, and often abbreviated Pcs. The preconscious division includes those thoughts, memories, and similar mental elements that, although not conscious at the moment, can readily be brought into consciousness (Cs) by an effort of attention. This is in contrast to the unconscious (Ucs) division, whose elements are barred from access to consciousness by some intrapsychic force such as repression.

Burrow uses this term to denote the primary phase or mode of consciousness described by him; it represents the infant's original identification with the mother organism. This mode relates to a nonlibidinal, preobjective phase in the organism's development. It finds symbolic expression in poetry and in literature, in dreams, in the phantasies both of the psychoneurotic and of the normal individual. Not to be confused with the psychoanalytic term *preconscious* or *foreconscious.* Synonyms: primary identification, the nest instinct. (*The Biology of Human Conflict*, 1937) See *coconscious.*

predementia praecox See *praecox, predementia.*

predisposition The inherited ability of an organism to develop a certain attribute or morbid trait when the necessary peristatic conditions for the given character are present. According to genetic principles, there is no inheritance of fully developed hereditary characters, but only a transmission of *predisposing* genetic factors depending for their phenotypical manifestation on various constitutional and dispositional influences. See *heredity.*

preferred provider organization *PPO* (q.v.).

prefrontal lobotomy See *lobotomy, prefrontal; psychosurgery.*

pregenital Antedating the phase of genital primacy. See *ontogeny, psychic; organization, pregenital.*

pregenital organization See *organization, pregenital.*

preindustrial Prevocational.

prejudice, race See *racism.*

prelogical The mode of thinking may regress, as it often does in schizophrenic subjects, from the logical to the prelogical. It has frequently been pointed out that thought and language in their development change from *feeling, concreteness,* and *perception* in the direction of *reasoning, differentiation,* and *abstraction.* See *paleologic.*

premenstrual dysphoric disorder See *late luteal phase dysphoric disorder.*

premenstrual tension state *Late luteal phase dysphoric disorder* (q.v.).

premium, incitement *Forepleasure* (q.v.).

premorbid Existing before the appearance of symptoms or signs of pathology. See *personality, premorbid.*

premotor area See *lobe, frontal.*

prenubile Referring to the period of life from birth to puberty.

preoccipital area See *lobe, occipital.*

preoccupation The state of being self-absorbed or engrossed in one's own thoughts, typically to a degree that hinders effective contact with or relationship to external reality. Preoccupation may sometimes be no more than absentmindedness; in other instances, it is part of an autistic schizophrenic's withdrawal from reality and turning inward upon the self; in other cases, it represents a mild degree of interference with consciousness and the level of attention and thus betokens an underlying disturbance in brain cell functioning. See *stupor.*

preoedipal Relating to the stages of infantile development antedating the Oedipus complex (psychoanalysis).

"The pre-oedipal phase . . . is for both sexes that earliest period of attachment to the first love object, the mother, before the advent of the father as a rival. It is the period during which an exclusive relation exists between mother and child." (Brunswick, R.M. *Psychoanalytic Quarterly IX*, 1940)

prephallic Referring to the period of psychosexual development preceding the phallic phase; i.e. the oral and anal phases or stages. While the term pregenital is often used interchangeably with the term prephallic, this is not technically correct since the phallic and genital phases are distinct and separate.

prepotent Ascendant; dominant. In neurophysiology, that reflex is prepotent which, when two stimuli that would evoke dissimilar reflexes are applied simultaneously, displaces the second reflex. "The outcome of the rivalry depends upon a number of circumstances: (i) the nature of the reflexes, (ii) the intensity of the several stimuli and (iii) the duration of action of the reflex." (Fulton, J.F. *Physiology of the Nervous System*, 1949) In general, nociceptive reflexes, such as the flexion reflex, are prepotent to all other types of reflex competing for the final common pathway; other things being equal, the more intense stimulus results in prepotency of its reflex; and the longer a reflex has been in operation, the easier will its prepotency be lost.

prepsychotic Pertaining to the period before psychosis became evident. Some authors (e.g. Katan) use this term in a more restricted sense to refer to that phase of psychosis in which the patient, although he deviates from normality, has not yet proceeded to develop such grossly psychotic symptoms as delusions and hallucinations.

prepubertal Relating to the phase of life antedating puberty.

presbycusis The most common type of hearing loss in the elderly, consisting of slowly progressive, bilaterally symmetrical, sensorineural hearing loss. It often involves poor speech discrimination.

presbyophrenia Kahlbaum-Wernicke syndrome; one form of *senile dementia* (q.v.) . Its principal characteristics are marked confusional disorientation, confabulation, mistakes in identity, and agitation without accomplishment of any objective. Presbyophrenic confabulations typically show a poverty, monotony, puerility, and naiveté of content. Because ethical conduct is preserved for a relatively long time, the patient is able to fit into limited social contacts, and particularly so since his affect tends toward the euphoric and the amiable.

presenile Relating to the period of life antedating senility or old age. See *Alzheimer's disease; Pick's disease.*

presentation Freud uses this term to mean the mode by which an instinct expresses itself. He says that it is not possible to identify an instinct existing as an entity by itself; it is recognizable only when it is conveyed or presented by some vehicle of expression. For example, a patient had a dread of sharp instruments; the instruments comprised the *presentation* by which the dread was expressed.

This is a term used in a special sense by Jung (analytical psychology). "To my mind, a simple stringing together of representations, such as is described by certain psychologists as *associative thinking*, is not thinking at all, but mere *presentation*. The term 'thinking' should, in my view, be confined to the linking up of representations by means of a concept, where, in other words, an act of judgment prevails, whether such act be the product of one's intention or not." (*PT*)

pressure of ideas See *thought pressure.*

pressures, social Socially created sanctions which emanate from less sanctioned or less responsible sources than the direct authoritarian controls, effected through officials or other accredited social agents and expressive of established codes.

prestige-suggestion See *suggestion; suggestion, prestige.*

presumption, tender years See *custody.*

prevalence In epidemiology, prevalence is the number of cases presently existing and active in a given population at any particular time:

$$\text{Prevalence rate (or ratio) of illness} = \frac{\begin{array}{c}\text{Number of cases}\\\text{of illness existing}\\\text{on a specific date}\end{array}}{\begin{array}{c}\text{Number of per-}\\\text{sons in population}\\\text{on same date}\end{array}} \times 100{,}000$$

See *epidemiology; incidence; PSA; rate.*

prevention See *psychiatry, community.*

preventive therapy, long-term Pharmacologic treatment extending over long periods of time aimed at preventing recurrences of illness or reducing their severity and duration. Although it is a type of *maintenance therapy*, it is to be differentiated from *continuation maintenance therapy*, referring to continued pharmacologic treatment following initial control of acute symptoms, which is aimed at maintaining control over the illness.

priapism (prī'ap-iz'm) A term used by many in its psychiatric meaning as the equivalent of *satyriasis* (q.v.). It is also used to denote persistent erection of the penis, particularly when the erection is due to organic disease and not to sexual desire. Erection is prolonged, dysfunctional, often extremely painful, and it characteristically leads to impaired sexual desire. Sometimes surgery may be required to achieve detumescence. Priapism has been reported as a unusual complication of therapy with some antidepressant drugs, among them trazodone.

Priapus (prī-ā′pus) Priapus, the son of Venus and Mercury (or Bacchus), is the god of procreation and hence of gardens and vineyards, as the embodiment of the generative force in nature. The Priapic cult was associated with the worship of the membrum virile, and Priapus became equivalent to a satyr and the phallus, and *priapism* became a synonym of lewdness. Priapus has become a common noun and means the penis, though rarely so in psychiatry.

pride, brute *Real pride,* i.e. pride based on self-assertive rage. See *pride, domesticated.*

pride, domesticated Rado's term for the type of pride and overevaluation of self seen in the obsessive patient, whose pride is based on guilty fear and its resultant humiliation, which have been repressed. Such a patient has no awareness of the guilty fear that is the foundation on which his pride rests; this is in contradistinction to the individual with *real pride* in his self-assertive rage. Domesticated pride is also known as *moral pride.*

pride, moral See *pride, domesticated.*

pride, penis Phallic pride, a term employed to designate the feeling of superiority and power attendant to the possession of the male genital organ. The concept was emphasized by Melanie Klein in her analysis of the child's instinctual life. "In describing the development of the boy, I have drawn attention to certain factors which tend, as I think, to increase yet more the central importance which the penis possesses for him. They may be summed up as follows: (1) The anxiety arising from his earliest danger situations, his fears of being attacked in all parts of his body and inside it, which include all his fears belonging to the feminine position, are displaced onto the penis or an external organ, where they can be more successfully mastered. The increased pride the boy takes in his penis and all that this involves may also be said to be a method of mastering those fears and disappointments which his feminine position lays him open to more particularly. (2) The fact that the penis is a vehicle first of the boy's destructive and then of his creative omnipotence, enhances its importance as a means of mastering anxiety. In this ministering to his sense of omnipotence, assisting him in the task of testing by reality and promoting his object-relationships . . . in fact, in subserving the all-important function of mastering anxiety—the penis is brought into specially close relation with the ego and is made into a representative of the ego and the conscious; while the interior of the body, the imagos and the faeces—what is invisible and unknown, that is—are compared to the unconscious." (*The Psycho-Analysis of Children,* 1932)

pride, real See *pride, domesticated.*

prima facie duty See *duty, prima facie.*

primacy, complete genital From the psychoanalytic point of view, genitality is divided into two principal substages. The first is the phallic phase. The second is reached only at puberty; it is the stage of late genital, or complete genital primacy. See *ontogeny, psychic.*

primacy, early genital See *primacy, phallic.*

primacy, oral The infant's contacting and first comprehending the world primarily in terms of the mouth. According to Freud, this is determined by the erotic satisfaction derived from mouth contact. Other analysts believe that Freud overemphasized the erotization of a situation that may be purely developmental, and that the infant first contacts the world by mouth because it is his most efficient and adequate organ. Thus oral primacy is a generally recognized organic fact, but to many psychoanalysts the important aspect of the oral phase is not so much the biological background as the differences in experience that occur during this biologically determined period. "Moreover, the kind of world contacted through the mouth is not universally the same, and the differences in experience make a more significant impression on personality development than does the organic fact of a period of oral primacy." (Thompson, C. *Psychoanalysis, Evolution and Development,* 1950)

primacy, phallic When libido becomes preponderantly concentrated on the penis, during the stage of infantile sexuality. See *ontogeny, psychic.*

primal scene See *scene, primal.*

primary behavior disorders See *behavior disorders.*

primary degenerative dementia (PPD) *Alzheimer's disease* (q.v.).

primary health care Accessible, comprehensive, coordinated, and continual care provided by accountable providers of health services; the first level of personal health services (as distinguished from public, environmental, and occupational health services), where initial professional attention is given to current or potential health problems. Often it is associated with care of the "whole person" rather than treatment of an illness.

primary ictal automatism A type of psychomotor epilepsy. See *epilepsy.*

primary mental image See *eidetic; imagery, eidetic.*

primary microorchidism See *syndrome, Klinefelter's.*

primary physician See *caregiver.*

primary psychic process See *process, primary psychic.*

primary task See *task, primary.*

primary thought disorder See *thought disorder, primary.*

primitivation Regression of the ego to the primitive stage in its development with consequent loss of higher ego functions. Thus objective thinking will have been replaced by magical thinking or wish-fulfilling hallucinations; object relationships and love will be of the helpless, passive dependent type, or there may even be a lack of objects; sexuality will be colored with oral eroticism; all perceptions, even those associated with incorporation, may be completely blocked; uncoordinated discharge movements will replace purposeful actions. According to Fenichel, primitivation occurs in both the traumatic neuroses and schizophrenia. In the former, the patients often exhibit an attitude of utter helplessness and passive dependence in which the behavior is that of an infant. But in traumatic neuroses the

regression of the ego comes out most dramatically when perceptions and actions are temporarily blocked. The patient may show constant weakness and fatigue, be unable to undertake any active tasks, encounter difficulty in concentration and memory, show various levels of disturbance of consciousness. Of course, fainting is the most primitive response to a trauma. Fenichel explains that this primitivation appears in the traumatic neuroses as an emergency phenomenon. All mental energies are required to master the intruding overwhelming excitation. Thus the ego functions are blocked and have to relinquish their energies in favor of the emergency task. Moreover, in this way further excitations are excluded.

In schizophrenia, too, many of the symptoms are "direct expressions of a regressive breakdown of the ego and an undoing of differentiations acquired through mental development." There is a "return to the time when the ego was not yet established or had just begun to be established." For example, world-destruction phantasies are caused by the inner perception of the loss of object relationships; feelings of grandeur express the increase in narcissism that occurs as the psychic energy withdrawn from objects is invested in the ego; schizophrenic thinking is the archaic magical thinking that precedes the development of reality-testing in the small child; hebephrenia is a vegetative existence expressing the old passive receptive or even intrauterine adaptations. (Fenichel, *PTN*)

primitivization *Primitivation* (q.v.).

Prince, Morton (1854–1929) American psychiatrist and neurologist; hysteria, multiple personality; *Dissociation of a Personality* (1908).

principle The general foundation for a rule or action guide. See *judgment; rule; theory.*

principle, echo Imitative patterning, such as is seen in children who exhibit certain behavior or behaviorisms similar to those seen in their parents but not necessarily indicative of inheritance. For example, a child learns to speak English or French not because of specific genetic predisposition, but because English or French is spoken in his home.

principle, encoding specificity See *encoding.*

principle, homeopathic See *principle, isopathic.*

principle, isopathic Also termed *homeopathic principle;* E. Jones's terms for cure or relief of a symptom by expression of the very emotion that is being repressed, an instance of the cause curing the effect.

"It is curious, and seemingly a paradox, that guilt can be relieved by an exhibition of the very thing—namely, hate—which was the generating occasion of the guilt itself." (*Papers on Psycho-Analysis,* 1938)

principle of anticipatory maturation See *maturation, anticipatory, principle of.*

principle of inertia A term introduced in psychoanalysis by Alexander, the same as the principle of *repetition-compulsion* (q.v.). Alexander lays stress upon the consideration that the tendency to automatic action is greater than that involving constantly changing and active mental efforts.

principle, pleasure A hypothesized regulatory mechanism of mental life whose function is to reduce psychic tension that has arisen as a result of drives pressing for discharge. The pleasure-pain principle tries to undo the effects of disturbing stimuli (pain) in a way that will most easily provide satisfaction (pleasure). It comes into operation later than the repetition-compulsion principle and is concerned mainly with the stimuli afforded by the action of the drives or instincts, while the earlier principle is concerned with damping external stimuli and merely tries to restore the organism to as near its original state as possible. The pleasure-pain principle operates earlier than the reality principle. See *repetition-compulsion.*

principle, reality The reality principle, while entering into the service of the pleasure principle, causes the latter to be appreciably modified to conform with the demands of the outside world. As Freud maintains, "the *Nirvana*-principle expresses the tendency of the death-instincts, the *pleasure*-principle represents the claims of the libido and that modification of it, the *reality*-principle, the influence of the outer world." (*CP*)

principle, treble safeguard The variable regulation of all growth functions by means of integration of endocrine and individual organ activities with the molecular dynamics of the nervous system.

principle, utilitarian In policy and ethical decisions, a choice that is determined by whatever promises the greatest advantage to the common good. See *principle, weighted harm.*

principle, weighted harm In policy and ethical decisions a choice that is determined by whatever promises the least harm, without regard to benefits that might be anticipated if that particular action or approach is chosen. See *principle, utilitarian.*

print media See *media.*

prison neurosis *Chronophobia* (q.v.).

prison psychosis See *psychosis, prison.*

privacy The right of the subject to control both the amount of information he divulges about himself and the disposition of the information he has divulged. *Confidentiality* refers to how information, once collected, is treated so as to ensure that no harm will befall the subject as a result of having disclosed information about himself. See *communication, privileged.*

privilege See *communication, privileged.*

proband In genetic studies of tainted families, the original cases constituting the starting point of a family study. These cases are called *probands,* or *probati,* because they must be proved representative of the type of trait carrier whose blood relations are to be investigated as to the recurrence of the trait under observation. Although the probands are not the main object of such a family study, their examination comes first and is of preeminent importance, since it must determine the hereditary trait so positively that a group of their blood relations must have likewise inherited that trait.

The practicable statistical method of probands in the study of selective population groups was devised by Weinberg and is called the *proband method.*

probatus (prô-bä′toos) See *proband.*

probe Investigation, search. DNA probes, techniques for analyzing human genetic material, are often used in chorionic villus sampling. Once a DNA disturbance is identified, the genetic abnormality is reproduced synthetically; when mixed with DNA extracted from fetal cells, the synthetic probe will seek out only those cells that contain similar genetic abnormalities and thus allow the abnormality to be identified in the fetus. See *biopsy, chorion; marker, genetic.*

probe, ultrasound See *NMR*.

problem, behavior See *behavior disorders*.

problem child See *developmental disorders*.

problem drinker See *alcoholism*.

problem, feeding See *feeding problem*.

problem, nuclear The patient's central conflict on which therapy should be focused. It is believed that the manifestations of a number of maladjustments and defenses in a patient usually emanate from one central conflict. Examples of these are inadequate resolution of the oedipal conflict, feelings of inadequacy, unwholesome sexual identifications, and sibling rivalry. The critical event has a dynamic relation to the nuclear problem. (Slavson, *IGT*) See *conflict, actual; conflict, root*.

problem-oriented record (POR) POMR (for medical record); a method of organizing a patient's clinical chart devised by L. L. Weed (*New England Journal of Medicine 278*, 1968). The system consists of five parts:

1. *Data base*—a standardized collection of pertinent information derived from the patient's history, physical examination, laboratory and X-ray studies, social history, mental status examination and psychologic evaluation, and observation of the patient's behavior.

2. *Problem list*—a recording of the clinically significant and active problems that emerge from the data base, each with a different number to provide easy identification for later cross-referencing and a table of contents for the entire medical record.

3. *Treatment plan*—a comprehensive plan for the treatment of each active problem identified.

4. *Progress notes*—numbered to correspond with the number of the problem to which they refer, and often written in the SOAP format (S = subjective, the patient's report or complaint; O = objective, observations without interpretation of what the patient manifests clinically; A = assessment, evaluation and interpretation of the problem and of the patient's progress and response to date; P = plan, a statement of what is to be done about the problem).

5. *Discharge summary*—indicating the treatment for each problem and the patient's response to the intervention.

process, cultural The process by which the folkways, mores, and social values are transmitted from generation to generation and are modified in adjustment to social change.

process, elementary D. Nachmansohn's theory of neural excitation and transmission: excitation of the neural membrane results in a dissociation of bound acetylcholine into an active form (the ester); free acetylcholine acts on a protein receptor and thereby increases the permeability of nerve membrane to ions. Thus bioelectric potential is generated and acts as a stimulus to adjoining nerve segments or to the synapse, resulting in propagation and transmission of the impulse. Meanwhile, the free ester of acetylcholine undergoes hydrolysis by the enzyme cholinesterase, and the protein receptor returns to its resting condition. The barrier to ionic movement is thus reestablished.

process, interpersonal In psychoanalysis, this term refers to the fact that in the therapeutic situation the analyst is more than a mirror reflecting the patient's problems. Just as there is transference on the patient's part, so is there countertransference on the analyst's part. Still, not every attitude toward the analyst is a transference attitude. The patient can like or dislike the analyst for what he really is, and the analyst cannot completely conceal what kind of person he is. The analyst sometimes transfers elements from his past or present problems to the analytic situation.

"I think it is clear that Freud's conception of countertransference is to be distinguished from the present-day conception of analysis as an interpersonal process. In the interpersonal situation, the analyst is seen as relating to his patient not only with his distorted affects but with his healthy personality also. That is, the analytic situation is essentially a human relationship in which, while one person is more immediately detached than the other and has less at stake, he is nevertheless an active participant." (Thompson, C. *Psychoanalysis, Evolution and Development*, 1950)

process, neurotic See *disorder, neurotic*.

process, primary psychic Freud's term for the laws that govern unconscious processes; used to refer to a type of thinking, characteristic of childhood (and dreams), and/or to the way in which libidinal or aggressive energy is mobilized and discharged. The basic characteristics of the primary process are a tendency to immediate discharge of drive energy (i.e. immediate gratification) and an extreme mobility of cathexis so that substitute methods of discharge can be achieved with relative ease. Primary process thinking is characterized by the absence of any negatives, conditionals, or other qualifying conjunctions; by the lack of any sense of time; and by the use of allusion, analogy, displacement, condensation, and symbolic representation. Drive energy characteristically remains unneutralized during the period of operation of the primary process.

In essence, the primary process is identical with Freud's formulation of the pleasure principle. The difference between them is that while the pleasure principle is described in subjective terms, the primary process is described in objective terms.

process psychosis See *psychosis, process.*

process, secondary psychic A name given by Freud to the laws that regulate events in the preconscious or ego. The *ego* (q.v.) is that part of the individual's mental apparatus that regulates the discharge of excitations arising either from external stimuli or from internal stimuli (instinctual demands). In executing this function, the ego is concerned with self-preservation, i.e. avoiding danger. In the case of external stimuli, the ego determines when they should be avoided, when it should adapt itself, and when the external world can be modified. In the case of internal stimuli (those arising from instinctual demands) the ego decides when the demands can be satisfied, when the satisfaction should be postponed, and when the demands or excitations should be completely suppressed. (The dangers of instinctual demands are, first, that their satisfaction might involve dangers in the external world, and, second, that an excessive strength of instinct can damage the organization of the ego.)

By means of its faculties of judgment and intelligence, by the application of logic and reality testing, the ego blocks the tendency of the instincts toward immediate discharge. Instead, the ego decides

under what conditions it would be safe to satisfy the instincts, if at all. The process by which the ego regulates the discharge of instinctual demands, that is, through the above-mentioned logical thinking, is the mode of operation of the conscious and preconscious mind and is called the secondary process. (Freud, S. *An Outline of Psychoanalysis,* 1949)

processes, unconscious The processes going on in the unconscious part of the psyche; methods of handling the environment and the instinctual needs on a level outside that of conscious awareness. These include *repression, regression, reaction-formation, isolation, undoing, introjection, reversal, sublimation,* and the development of character structure (qq.v.).

"Freud saw the newborn infant as chiefly Id, that is, masses of impulse without an organizing or directing consciousness. Contact with the world gradually modifies a portion of this Id, and the Ego, a small area of consciousness, emerges from it. However, only a small part even of the Ego is conscious at any one time. A great part of the Ego exists outside of awareness, but can readily be recalled when needed. This part was called the preconscious. Still another part of the Ego is *unconscious* and cannot readily be made conscious. This consists of the experiences and feelings that have been repressed.

"In the course of time, the Ego takes over certain standards from the culture, chiefly through the training by parents in early childhood. These standards become incorporated as parent images within the Ego as a part of itself and this part is called the Super-ego. It exercises a criticizing and censoring power. It includes the parental attitudes, especially as these attitudes were understood and interpreted by the child in his early years. It includes also the person's own ideals for himself, and Freud even indicates that certain phylogenetic experiences such as those described by Jung under the concept of the collective *unconscious* may also be part of the Super-ego. Much of the Super-ego is *unconscious,* because it was incorporated by the child very early and without his awareness." (Thompson, C. *Psychoanalysis, Evolution and Development,* 1950)

processing, knowledge See *KIPS.*

processomania Bianchi's term for mania for litigation. See *paranoia querulans.*

proctalgia fugax Fleeting rectal pain, more often than not of psychologic origin and seen typically in anxious, tense perfectionists.

prodigy See *child, bright.*

prodigy, idiotic *Idiot savant* (q.v.).

prodromata The aggregate of *prodromes.*

prodrome Precursor. An early or premonitory symptom of a disease or disorder.

productive symptoms See *symptoms, deficit; symptoms, productive.*

profession "A cluster of occupational roles . . . in which the incumbents perform certain functions valued in the society in general and by these activities typically earn a living at a full-time job." (Parsons, T. *Essays in Sociological Theory,* 1954) "Professions control entry into their occupational roles by certifying that candidates have developed the requisite body of skills and knowledge. Thus, they have some degree of independence and autonomy in performing the functions valued by the society." (Beauchamp, T.L., & Childress, J.F. *Principles of Biomedical Ethics,* 1979)

professional code See *code, professional.*

professional neurasthenia See *neurosis, occupational.*

profile, modality See *modality profile.*

profile, structural See *structural profile.*

progeria (prō-jē'rē-à) Gilford introduced this term for a special form of dwarfism characterized by a combination of infantilistic traits and premature senility. The dwarfs of this type show infantile proportions of the skeleton, complete absence of hair, a senile face with a long, aquiline nose, deficient secondary sexual characteristics in spite of a fairly normal development of the sex organs, thickened ends of the long bones, average intelligence, and a tendency to vascular sclerosis; they are practically identical with the subgroup of dwarfism called *senile nanism* by Variot and Pironneau.

prognosis Forecast or estimation of the course, outcome, and duration of an illness—the opinion being formed during the course of the illness.

In schizophrenic psychoses, for example, the following have been found to be of value as predictors of outcome by one or more sets of investigators:

1. *Family history*—(a) presence of depression; (b) absence of schizophrenia.

2. *Premorbid characteristics*—(a) personality not schizoid or isolated, but stable and integrated; (b) adequacy of social relations functioning; (c) adequacy of psychosexual adjustment; (d) marital status (ever married, rather than never married, widowed, separated, or divorced); (e) intelligence not low; (f) good premorbid work record.

3. *Features of illness*—(a) acute onset (insidious onset and/or duration more than six months suggests a poor prognosis); (b) precipitating factors; (c) confusion or perplexity; (d) concern with death, guilt; (e) no emotional blunting; (f) previous hospitalization and duration of previous hospitalization (suggest a poor prognosis); (g) hebephrenic clinical picture (suggests a poor prognosis); (h) massive, defiant persecutory delusions (suggest a poor prognosis).

prognosis, direction Bleuler's term for the type of reaction that a disorder may be expected to develop. Thus, "Within the realm of schizophrenia there are again different directions such as the paranoid, catatonic dementia, etc., that have to be considered in the prognosis." (*TP*)

Direction prognosis is distinguished from *extent prognosis,* which has to do with the prediction relating to the progress of the disorder in a given period of time.

prognosis, extent See *prognosis, direction.*

programmed practice See *exposure, self-directed.*

programming, biologic See *aging, theories of.*

progredient See *neurosis, progredient.*

progressive degenerative subcortical encephalopathy See *sclerosis, diffuse.*

progressive teleologic regression See *regression, progressive teleologic.*

projection The process of throwing out upon another the ideas or impulses that belong to oneself. It is the act of giving objective or seeming reality to what is subjective. The expression implies that what is cast upon another is considered undesirable to the one who projects. The person who blames another for his own mistakes or seeks a scapegoat is using the projection mechanism.

It is to be recognized that the person orients himself by means of both inner and outer perceptions. The latter can be managed by motor activity, which is another way of saying that if reality is uncomfortable, one may alter or avoid it. Inner perceptions, such as the instincts and their representations, cannot be handled with the same facility; one cannot flee from the "merciless claims of his instincts." Whatever is painful or dangerous from within may be projected onto another person or upon some part of reality. When the conflicting issue has been externalized, the person may handle it as if it had always been an external situation. For example, the paranoid schizophrenic, beset with unconscious homosexual urges, projects the urges upon some man or men in the environment and then struggles against the urges as they seem to arise from outside sources.

In its morbid manifestations, the projection mechanism is clearly an unconscious process, at least in the sense that the conscious ego is not at all aware of the process.

According to Ferenczi, projection is one of the first defensive or protective measures employed by the child in defense of his narcissism. When the child realizes that he is not omnipotent, he begins to ascribe omnipotence to those about him and comes to realize that others control him. He does not, however, abandon the feeling of his own importance and of his magical powers. See *externalization; reality testing; reference, ideas of.*

projection fibers See *commissure.*

projection, impersonal Projection alone means attributing one's own ideas or impulses to another. By implication, this is done because one finds his own ideas or impulses objectionable. Impersonal projection refers to the same mechanism applied not to objectionable material but to impersonal or neutral material. One example of impersonal projection is found in the echo of reading aloud, when the subject feels that someone else is saying the words that he is reading. Approximately 47% of patients who admit to auditory hallucinations also hear the echo of reading. These patients do not feel that the echo occurs more with one type of reading material than with another, and it is therefore difficult to think of apparently innocuous reading material selected at random as

having assumed some objectionable significance to such a large percentage of patients. Marjorie C. Meehan feels that impersonal projection may indicate the extreme feeling of passivity and domination by an external agent so characteristic of certain schizophrenics; the symptom may also suggest that there is some mechanism, possibly physiological, that transforms internal speech so that it seems to the patient to be heard from without. (*Psychiatric Quarterly 16, 1942*)

projective test See *test, projective.*

projicient apparatus In the terminology of E.J. Kempf (*Psychopathology*, 1921), the striped muscle system and the cerebrospinal nervous system proper, which provide the autonomic apparatus with the means to master the environment.

prolactin Lactogenic hormone. The plasma prolactin level is used as a measure of the degree of dopaminergic blockade by neuroleptic agents. Neuroleptics decrease dopaminergic activity, and such a decrease stimulates prolactin secretion, which thus reflects neuroleptic activity.

prolonged sleep therapy See *treatment, continuous sleep.*

promiscuity Indiscriminate, casual sexual encounters; high frequency of sexual relationships with a large number of partners, such as found in nymphomaniacs, satyriasists, Don Juans, and many homosexuals.

promotion neurosis Inability to function when given added responsibility or authority; seen most often in obsessional neurotics and described by others as failure through success. See *polycratism; success, failure through.*

proneness, accident Liability or tendency toward involvement in mishaps that cause some pain or injury to the subject. It has long been recognized in industrial psychiatry that the majority of accidents occur within a comparatively small percentage of the total work force, and that that same percentage tends to be involved in multiple accidents. It was also noted in wartime that some soldiers appeared to be wounded largely because of their emotional state, and that the stress of battle often affected judgment and muscular control adversely. In some instances, accident proneness can be traced to a specific emotional state existing prior to the injury. In many others, however, a tendency to repeated accidents appears to be an expression of deep-seated personality traits and unconscious conflicts.

The typical accident-prone person is a young male who is decisive or even impulsive; he concentrates upon immediate pleasures and satisfactions and acts on the spur of the moment. He likes excitement and adventure, eschewing planning and preparation. Often he will be found to have been reared strictly and harbors an unusual amount of resentment against authority; he is a rebel who cannot tolerate even self-discipline. At the same time he feels guilty about his rebellion, but in the unconsciously provoked accident he is able to express his resentment and to atone for his rebellion through the injury.

proof, forensic The standard that testimony must meet in order to be probative. Proof of guilt beyond a reasonable doubt, for instance, requires a mass of evidence, each element of which must exclude every plausible inference except guilt. Many physicians and biomedical scientists feel that the law demands more certainty and concreteness than any probabilistic science can provide. Almost all states, however, require a "reasonable" degree of medical certainty rather than absolute certainty and thus allow medical testimony that reflects the current degree of knowledge within the field.

propaganda Any organized effort to spread a belief, doctrine, value system, etc.; of particular interest to psychiatry because of the possibility of controlling behavior with nonphysical means (*mind control*) and the ethical questions attendant thereon. See *psychopolitics.*

propfschizophrenia A schizophrenic syndrome superimposed or engrafted on mental retardation. Schizophrenia may, in fact, be engrafted on any organic disease, which manumits the schizophrenic disorder in a predisposed subject.

prophase The initial stage of a cell division by mitosis. See *division, cell.*

prophylaxis The branch of medical science that has to do with protection against the onset of a disease or disorder. For example, the treatment of a person showing marked schizoidism in an effort to prevent the

development of schizophrenia is termed prophylaxis. See *hygiene, mental.*

propinquity (prō-pin'kwi-tē) Proximity; in genetics, nearness of blood relationship.

proprioception The ability to appreciate sensations of muscle, joint, tendon, and vibration.

proprium See *Allport, Gordon Willard.*

propulsion Rapid, forward running with short steps, in *paralysis agitans* (q.v.).

prosencephalon *Forebrain* (q.v.).

prosody The tone or accent of speech; the study of the metrical structure of a poem. In psychiatry, prosody refers to the emotional tone or affective components of speech, which are served by the nondominant cerebral hemisphere. See *aprosodia.*

prosopagnosia Failure to recognize visually the faces of familiar persons, with retention of the ability to recognize them through other sensory channels. The condition is due to bilateral cerebral lesions involving the visual system. See *nonrecognition; syndrome, Capgras's.*

prosopalgia See *tic douloureux.*

prosoplegia, prosopoplegia Bell's palsy or peripheral facial paralysis. See *nerve, facial.*

prospective See *EPSDT.*

protanopia A form of color-blindness, usually referred to as red-blindness, in which red and blue-green are confused.

protection factor See *risk factor.*

protection, medical removal Insurance that a worker who has been removed from his or her regular employment on the basis of an examining physician's decision that such employment is hazardous to the employee's health will receive compensation. The specific amount and type of compensation vary but ordinarily are determined on the basis of maintained earnings, seniority, or other benefits.

protest, body A term coined by Esther L. Richards to indicate that physical dysfunctions may serve as outlets for worries, disappointments, frustrations, etc.

protest, masculine This is a technical term applied by Adler to both men and women, to describe a desire to escape from the feminine role. This concept he regards as the main motive force in neurotic disease. It represents the distorted apprehension of sex differences caused by the striving for superiority. If it takes an active form in women, they attempt from an early age to usurp the male position. They become aggressive in manner, adopt definitely masculine habits or tricks of behavior, and endeavor to dominate everyone about them.

The masculine protest in a male indicates that he has never fully recovered from an infantile doubt as to whether he really is male. He strives for an ideal masculinity invariably conceived as the possession by himself of freedom, love, and power.

protest psychosis See *psychosis, protest.*

prothymia (prō-thī′mē-à, -thim′ēà) Mental alertness.

proto- Combining form meaning first, original, primitive, from Gr. *prōtos.*

protocol The individual case record; the raw material of a study or experiment before it has been incorporated into the conclusions or overall results of the study. In clinical psychiatry, the protocol commonly refers to the complete case history and workup, in contrast to the case summary or final conclusions about the individual case.

protomasochism The primary, ancestral tendency of the death instinct to lead all human beings into annihilation; a drive into nothingness. Reik uses the term to describe "a pleasure of destruction directed against the ego, a kind of sadism which has chosen the ego for its victim." In Freud's opinion, the death instinct that is not neutralized by the erotic urges or channeled into the outer world remains effective within the organism, directing its forces against the ego proper, as it did in primitive man. (Reik, T. *Masochism in Modern Man,* 1941)

protopathic Of primary sensitiveness, i.e. pertaining to sensory nerves in the skin with a primary, grosser, or more limited sensibility to stimuli. The ability to appreciate deep pain sensation and marked variations in temperature such as hot and cold; distinguished from *epicritic* sensibility.

protophallic Jones says that there are two stages to what Freud calls the phallic phase: "The first of the two—let us call it the *protophallic* phase—would be marked by innocence or ignorance—at least in consciousness—where there is no conflict over the matter in question, it being confidently assumed by the child that the rest of the world is built like itself and has a satisfac-

tory male organ—penis or clitoris, as the case may be. In the second, or *deuterophallic* phase, there is a dawning suspicion that the world is divided into two classes; not male and female in the proper sense, but penis-possessing and castrated (though actually the two classifications overlap pretty closely)." (*Papers on Psycho-Analysis,* 1938)

protoplasm The cellular substance with which the life of living beings is associated. All vital activities of an organism, such as growth, repair, and reproduction, are ultimately referred to the properties of this transparent and jellylike cell material that usually shows a fibrillar structure with a honeycombed reticulum and consists of a mixture of proteins, carbohydrates, fats, lipoids, salts, and water.

The protoplasmic matter of each cell is endowed with the structural and functional peculiarities characteristic of the species of animals or plants to which the cell belongs. It is subject to the complex biochemical processes that are the fundamental basis of all cell functions.

Of particular importance in the biological mechanism of inheritance are the proteins, which are built up of one or more of the amino acids. They are very specific in their chemical relations and do certain things with such precision that the enormous number of different kinds of organisms can be maintained with a high degree of persistence.

prototaxic Of, or relating to, the earliest period in time or development; Sullivan applied the term to the early period of infancy, when the child has no awareness of himself as distinct from others and no concept of time or space.

prototheory Partial, incomplete, or untested theory; an initial "working" hypothesis; sometimes used to refer to an ad hoc rationalization that appears to justify a clinical practice or maneuver.

proviso, parapathic Stekel's term for a compromise or bargain that the neurotic makes with his illness—e.g. the patient who thinks that as long as he remains ill, his father will not die: it is a "clause," or stipulation with the neurosis in order to justify its existence. In other words, "If the patient accepts his neurosis, some disaster which he dreads will not happen." (*ID*)

Adler referred to this mental mechanism as *junctim;* another name for it is *neurotic proviso.*

proxemics The study and analysis of space, and particularly the study of interpersonal behavior in relation to density of population, placement of people within an area, opportunity for privacy. It is interesting to note in this connection that while the life span of animals in captivity is markedly reduced if they have no space for withdrawal into privacy, the conscious intent of the architecture of most mental hospitals is to reduce or abolish opportunities for their human residents' privacy. See *communication.*

prudery Exaggerated concern about minor points of the moral or ethical code. This is almost always a reaction formation, the prude decrying in others the very impulses and behavior he must deny in himself.

pruritus, psychogenic An itching dermatitis of a functional nature. Patients with functional pruritus are usually of the obsessive compulsive character type, are rigid, defensive, and not readily susceptible to suggestion or reassurance. The disease is difficult to cure.

Sullivan and Bereston distinguish four psychosomatic dermatological syndromes: psychogenic pruritus, neurodermatitis, psychogenic urticaria, and hyperhidrosis. (*American Journal of Psychiatry 103,* 1946)

PSA Proportion of survivors affected, the same as lifetime *prevalence* (q.v.) of disorder (the proportion of persons in a representative sample of the population who have ever experienced the disorder in question).

psammoma-body (sam-ō′mȧ) A collection of fibroglia, collagen fibers, and small calcified concretions seen often in meningiomas.

PSE See *Examination, Present State.*

psellism Stammering; indistinct or faulty pronunciation.

psellismus haesitans *Obs.* Stammering; ischnophonia.

pseudacusis *Obs.* Auditory hallucinations and illusions.

pseudesthesia Sensation or perception without a corresponding stimulus. An imaginary or illusory sensation, such as phantom limb.

pseudo- Combining form meaning false, from Gr. *pseudos,* falsehood, lie.

"pseudo as-if" Katan's term for a type of reaction, seen often within the framework of a hysterical disturbance, that simulates the "as-if" personality but differs from the latter in that the disturbance arises not from early loss of the mother but rather as a result of the mother keeping the child too dependent orally. In consequence, the ego is weakened and in response to stress it falls back on dependence on the mother or her substitutes. "Pseudo as-if" reactions are seen also in adolescents and in prepsychotic patients as temporary attempts at mastering conflicts during a process of disintegration. See *personality, "as if."*

pseudoaggression In psychoanalysis a false aggressiveness developed in neurotics as a result of denial of their basic psychic masochism; the basic desire is to be mistreated. This desire gains only reproach from the superego, and a defense of pseudoaggression is constructed. "No, I do not want to be mistreated by this person. The situation is just the opposite—I want to kill this person or mistreat him." This pseudoaggression also receives reproach from the superego and is itself denied, but the neurotic is more willing to accept the guilt for his pseudoaggression than that for his underlying masochism. Bergler believes that neurotics have no true ego aggression, for almost all of their aggression is in the superego. He explains *stage fright* (q.v.) in actors in this way. Superficially, the symptom refers to a fear of one's aggressive exhibitionism. In reality, however, this aggressiveness is a false front with which the patient deludes himself and others to deny the basic fear, that his masochism will be uncovered. Under successful psychoanalytic treatment, a more equitable distribution of aggression between superego and ego can be achieved and the patient can become truly aggressive as the need for aggression arises in reality situations. (*Psychoanalytic Quarterly Supplement 23,* 1949)

pseudoamnesia 1. False or feigned amnesia, as in Ganser syndrome. 2. Amnesia that is part of a dissociative disorder. 3. *Obs.* A transitory amnesia associated with organic brain disease.

pseudoathetosis Athetoid movement that is not spontaneous, but elicited when the patient closes his eyes and extends his hands; it occurs in those whose sense of position is impaired such as in tabes or combined sclerosis.

pseudoblepsis *Obs.* Visual hallucinations or illusions.

pseudocatatonia, traumatic A catatonic state following an injury. See *psychosis, traumatic.*

pseudocholinesterase An enzyme; of importance in psychiatry because it is the enzyme that normally breaks down suxamethonium, a muscle relaxant that is frequently used as part of electroconvulsive therapy. About one white American in 2,500 has a genetically determined abnormality or deficiency of pseudocholinesterase, and such a person is liable to severe and prolonged apnea when administered suxamethonium. The defect is much rarer in Blacks and virtually nonexistent in Orientals. See *pharmacogenetics.*

pseudocoma See *mutism, akinetic.*

pseudocommunity Norman Cameron's term for the progressive desocialization seen in the schizophrenias in which social language habits are replaced with personal, highly individual habits. The pseudocommunity is a behavioral organization that the patient constructs from his distorted observations, inferences, and phantasies; most commonly, the patient sees himself as the victim of some concerted action.

pseudoconvulsion An attack that simulates a convulsion, with falling and muscular contractions, but with no loss of consciousness, no pupillary changes, amnesia, or postconvulsive confusion. Such an attack usually occurs in hysteria. It may be consciously or unconsciously exaggerated for the sake of gaining sympathy or attention.

pseudocyesis (sū-dō-sī-ē'sis) Spurious pregnancy.

pseudodebility *Pseudoimbecility* (q.v.).

pseudodementia A condition of exaggerated indifference to one's surroundings without actual mental impairment; also, reversible decline in mental functioning such as occurs in depression. See *pseudosenility.*

pseudodementia, hysterical Wernicke's term for a syndrome of hysteria in which the patient appears unable to answer the simplest questions or to give any information about himself. The patient gives the appearance of being retarded.

As a rule the patient exhibiting this syndrome regresses to the behavior of early childhood, showing the condition known as *hysterical puerilism.* See *feeblemindedness, affective; syndrome, Ganser.*

pseudofeeblemindedness *Rare.* Feeblemindedness sometimes indicated by a low IQ but actually nonexistent. Untoward psychological and emotional factors operative at the time of testing can result in a low score misrepresenting the actual mental endowment: this blunder is especially likely to come about when children are tested. The label feeblemindedness resulting from a score of this nature is a misnomer, and the proper term is pseudofeeblemindedness.

pseudoflexibilitas A condition in which a person whose movements are more or less normal maintains for a relatively long period a posture imposed upon him.

pseudogeusia (-gū'sē-à) False perception of taste.

pseudogiftedness Apparent unusual talents in a child, resulting not from specific or permanent trends but rather from the ability of the bright child to imitate, adopt, and assimilate the behavior patterns of others. Pseudogiftedness is usually inspired by momentary influence from without rather than by any inborn ability or urge from within.

pseudographia Neologistic writing, such as an idiosyncratic alphabet that abolishes communication rather than enhancing it; observed most frequently in catatonic and paranoid forms of schizophrenia.

pseudohallucination A hallucination which the patient knows to be such; the patient has the vivid sensory experience, but realizes that it has no external foundations.

Two types of pseudohallucination have been recognized: *imaged pseudohallucination,* a particularly vivid mental picture, experienced as occurring within the mind but distinguished from the usual image by the subject's inability to change the image at will; and *perceived pseudohallucination,* an image experienced as located in external space but recognized by the subject as unreal.

pseudohomosexual Used in adaptational psychodynamic formulations to refer to the nonsexual motivations in homosexual behavior: specifically, dependency motivations and power motivations. "It should be emphasized that even in the overt homosexual, when the ultimate goal is orgastic pleasure, the sexual component does not operate in isolation, but always in association with the dependency and power components." (Ovesey, L., et al. *Archives of General Psychiatry 9,* 1963)

pseudohydrophobia *Cynophobia* (q.v.).

pseudohypersexuality A term used by Fenichel interchangeably with the term *hypersexuality* (q.v.).

pseudohypnosis See *captivation.*

pseudoidentification A method of dealing with people in the environment by apparently identifying oneself with, or assimilating oneself to, the person with whom one chances to be in contact at any given moment. Pseudoidentification is illustrated by the case of the man who asserted that he had found the ideal way of adapting himself to reality: he assimilated himself to the person with whom he chanced to be talking and so had no external conflicts. But in reality, such a method of adaptation led to many conflicts; the man found that he had assimilated himself to A at one time, to B at another, and that A and B were in disagreement. Since pseudoidentification is not insincerity, but rather the conviction that the subject has in fact become one with the other person, such conflicting identifications lead to many reality probelms. Pseudoidentification appears somewhat akin to paranoid projection in that the patient's ideas are prevented from entering consciousness and are ascribed to the object, with whom the patient then identifies himself. Unlike the ideas of paranoia, however, those of pseudoidentification are apparently innocent. The dynamics of the process are still poorly understood.

pseudoimbecility Pathological limitation and restriction of intellectual functions of the ego. This intellectual restriction or inhibition may mean (1) that intellectual functions have been erotized and so are given up to escape conflicts; (2) that the restriction disguises aggression in order to escape retaliation; (3) that it is a display of castration to escape the fear of literal castration and the loss of a love object; or (4) that it

represents an attempt to restore or maintain a secret libidinous rapport within the family. A mask of stupidity enables the child or infantile adult to participate in the sexual life of the parents and other adults to an amazingly unlimited extent, which, if overtly expressed, would be strictly and definitely forbidden. Such utilization of stupidity is widespread, because it affords an opportunity for the mutual sexual desires of parent and child to be gratified on a preverbal affective level without becoming conscious through word pictures. Thus repression or other defense measures are unnecessary, and the child and his parents can maintain a distorted but gratifying affective communion that would otherwise be limited to mother and infant.

The analysis of an 18-year-old pseudo-imbecile, who had manifested his pathological behavior since early childhood, revealed that in the phallic stage of psychic development he had had to give up competition with his aggressive twin brother. He was unable to pass the phallic stage successfully and so regressed to the immediately preceding anal stage. Acting as a counterpart to anal exhibitionism was an intense sexual curiosity against which he had to maintain strong defenses, because of the threats of his father. With pseudoimbecility, however, he was able unconsciously to satisfy his curiosity, for his parents and siblings permitted his presence even during intercourse. He was regarded as a pet animal that does no harm by its presence and neither understands nor participates in what it sees.

pseudointoxication *Obs.* A trancelike state in which there is a tendency to staggering and stammering with excitement and irritability.

pseudolalia Suggested by Stoddart to denote meaningless sounds produced by patients.

pseudologia fantastica An extreme form of pathological lying consisting of telling stories without discernible or adequate motive and with such zeal that the subject may become convinced of their truth. It has been reported in organic mental disorders and in character disorders (e.g. psychopathy), and it is often described as one of the three cardinal symptoms of the *Munchhausen syndrome* (the others being peregrination and disease simulation).

pseudologue Pathological liar. Kraepelin used the term as a subgroup of psychopathic personality. His distinction between the criminal liar and the pseudologue was not very clear.

pseudomania A symptom in which the patient accuses himself of having committed crimes of which he is really innocent; shame psychosis.

pseudomelancholia *Obs.* Juliusburger's term for the clinical syndrome characterized by subjective inhibition and depersonalization.

pseudomnesia *Obs.* The patient's belief in having a clear recollection of events that had never taken place or things that had never existed.

pseudomotivations Bleuler uses this term to refer to those after-the-fact justifications of behavior that are common in schizophrenia. One hebephrenic patient stated that he got into debt only to show that he could obtain money without his wife's assistance. Another patient flew into a rage and stated that he did so because his doctor was wearing a gray suit. "According to my experience the patient really becomes furious for quite different reasons which have some relationship to his complexes. He then, purely at random, mentions the grey suit as the reason for his fury." (Bleuler, E. *Dementia Praecox or the Group of Schizophrenias,* 1950) Although the patient himself believes in his ex post facto pseudomotivations, he may subsequently become aware that he has made up the motivations. Ordinarily, however, the patient is unaware of, and indifferent to, even the grossest contradictions.

pseudonarcotism Stupor of hysterical nature, not induced by drugs.

pseudonecrophilia Masturbation with phantasies of corpses as the sexual object.

pseudoneurotic See *schizophrenia, pseudoneurotic.*

pseudonomania Morbid impulse to falsify, to lie.

pseudoparameter See *parameter.*

pseudoparanoia An uncommon term for unsystematized paranoid trends that are not strictly associated with schizophrenia. For example, paranoid delusions may occasionally be observed in deaf people, sometimes in the retarded; the delusions are generally scattered and transitory or at least they do not constitute the preponderant part of the disorder.

pseudoparesis, alcoholic *Obs.* A clinical syndrome resembling general paresis but due to alcoholic encephalopathy. It consists of *dementia* (q.v.) with ideas of grandeur, hallucinations, delusions of jealousy, sometimes Argyll Robertson pupils, speech defect, tremors, and polyneuritis. Epileptiform attacks are frequent.

pseudopersonality A constellation of habits and reaction patterns consciously recognized as false by the subject. The development of a pseudopersonality is characteristic of many prostitutes, who strive to maintain an incognito quality in their sexual contacts and fortify this with fictitious tales about themselves and their families. Their pseudopersonality usually includes a false toughness, meanness, and indifference. It is obvious that, with time, the recognition of the falseness of the pseudopersonality may gradually dwindle so that it finally becomes a true *character defense,* and in therapy must be handled as such. See *defense, character.*

pseudopsia *Obs.* Visual hallucination or illusion.

pseudopsychopathic schizophrenia See *schizophrenia.*

pseudoquerulant A form of paranoid personality disorder. Pseudoquerulants regard trifling differences as grave injustices. A combination of irritability and arrogance leads them not only into quarrels, but into actual lawsuits. They are to be distinguished from the litigious paranoid type by the fact that in the pseudoquerulants the tendency exists from youth.

pseudoreminiscence *Pseudologia fantastica* (q.v.).

pseudoschizophrenia See *psychosis, process; psychosis, reactive.*

pseudosclerosis of Westphal-Strümpell (Adolf von Strümpell, German physician, 1853–1925, and Alexander Karl Otto Westphal, German neurologist, 1863–1941) See *degeneration, hepatolenticular.*

pseudosclerosis, spastic See *Creutzfeldt-Jakob's disease.*

pseudoseizure Pseudoepilepsy; *hystero-epilespy* (q.v.); "A clinical event which superficially resembles an epileptic attack, but under closer scrutiny is found lacking in an essential epileptic component such as a concomitant electroencephalographic dysrhythmia or possessing a feature not compatible with epilepsy such as the characteristic of being precipitated, modified or stopped by a simple command, a hypnotic suggestion or withdrawal of the attention of observers." (Liske, E., & Forster, F.M. *Neurology 14,* 1964)

pseudosenility *Pseudodementia* (q.v.); acute, reversible mental disorders in the elderly, which typically appear as confusional states or as depression. Among the more common causes of pseudosenility are drug effects (especially due to errors in self-medication), malnutrition, diminished cardiac output and other cardiovascular disorders, febrile conditions, alcoholism, trauma secondary to an unreported fall, intracranial tumor, endocrine disorders and other metabolic disturbances (e.g. hypernatremia, azotemia).

pseudosexuality See *masturbation, compulsive.*

pseudosmia False sense of smell.

pseudosphresia *Pseudosmia* (q.v.).

pseudotransference A result of inexact interpretations in psychoanalytic treatment in which the patient, responding to the suggestions of the analyst, builds up a relationship that is expressive of the analyst's hunches rather than related to problems of the patient that are of dynamic significance.

pseudotumor cerebri *Benign intracranial hypertension,* with headache, papilledema, and increased intracranial pressure in the absense of an intracranial mass. Spontaneous recovery generally occurs. It is associated with several conditions, although the mechanism producing the increase in pressure is unknown. Among the most common associated conditions are venous thromboses of the sagittal, straight, or lateral sinuses; disorders of the adrenal, ovarian, parathyroid, or thyroid glands; hypervitaminosis A in children and adolescents; antibiotic administration (particularly tetracycline or penicillin) to infants; high CSF protein, as in patients with polyneuritis or tumors of the cauda equina; intoxicants such as insecticides (termed *toxic pseudotumor cerebri*); and sometimes as a side effect of drug treatment (e.g. lithium). Also known as serous meningitis; arachnoiditis; toxic hydrocephalus.

PSG Polysomnography. See *polysomnogram.*

psi (sī) In parapsychology, this term refers to whatever it is that enables a person to perceive extrasensorially. See *perception, extrasensory.*

psi- (or ψ) **system** See *system.*

psittacism (sit′à-siz′m) A type of neologism which is totally devoid of any content. See *glossolalia.*

PSM *Polysomnogram* (q.v.).

psopholalia (sō-fō-lā′lē-à) Lallation; babbling, infantile, slovenly, incomprehensible speech.

PSR Physicians for Social Responsibility, an organization founded in 1961 to inform the public about medical consequences of nuclear testing and nuclear war.

PSRO *Professional standards review organization;* established by federal law (PL 92–603, Social Security Amendments of 1972) as a mechanism to ensure that the hospital care rendered under Medicare and Medicaid is medically necessary and of good quality. Initial review of care rendered is often performed by allied health professionals using standards set by the medical profession or medical specialty societies; final review, however, is performed by physicians (*peer review*). See *review.*

PST Prefrontal sonic treatment. See *irradiation, ultrasonic.*

psychagogy (sī′kà-gō-jē) Educational and reeducational psychotherapeutic procedures, with special emphasis upon the relationship of the patient to his environment. The general principles behind psychagogy are essentially in agreement with those behind objective psychobiology; both stress socialization.

psychal *Rare.* Psychical.

psychalgia, psychalgalia Discomfort or pain, usually in the head, which accompanies mental activity (obsessions, hallucinations, etc.), and is recognized by the patient as being emotional in origin. Depressed patients complain of peculiar head pains due to their horrible ideas. The schizophrenic patient complains, often with laughter, of the unbearable pains in his head, induced by electric currents that come from a distant machine operated by a persecutor.

Psychalgia is also used to refer to any psychogenic pain disorder. See *somatoform disorders.*

psychalia *Rare.* A mental syndrome characterized by auditory and visual hallucinations; also known as *mentalia*.

psychanopsia Hysterical blindness.

psychasthenia *Obs.* The nosologic syndrome characterized by fears or phobias. E. Strecker and F. Ebaugh say that "in the anxiety states belongs much of the material that was formerly described as psychasthenia, with a prominent display of the so-called phobias or fears." (*Practical Clinical Psychiatry*, 1935)

Pierre Janet recognized two subgroups of psychoneuroses, namely, hysteria and psychasthenia. In general he included under psychasthenia all psychoneurotic syndromes not classified under *hysteria* (q.v.).

"Psychasthenia resembles hysteria in that both of these psychoneurotic disorders may be traced to a conflict over a forbidden pleasure. The essential difference lies in the fact that the conscience of the hysterical person is intolerant of even the thought of such pleasure while the psychasthenic has an ambivalent attitude." (Henry, G.W. *Essentials of Psychiatry,* 1938)

psychataxia Mental confusion, inability to fix the attention or to make any continued mental effort.

psychauditory Relating to the mental perception and interpretation of sounds.

psyche The mind. In modern psychiatry the psyche is regarded in its own way as an "organ" of the person. The psyche, like other organs, possesses its own form and function, its embryology, gross and microscopic anatomy, physiology, and pathology.

The most comprehensive schematization of the psyche is that drawn by Freud, consisting in general of the conscious and unconscious divisions, each of which is made up of a great number of components. The mind, like all other organs of the body, has its own local functions and those functions that are intimately associated with adjacent and distant organs. It is like the cardiovascular system in that it reaches all parts of the body; it also serves to adjust the total organism to the needs or demands of the environment.

psyche, contrasexual component of Jacobi's term for the repressed side in Jung's theory of analytical psychology. Jung maintains that there is a male and a female side

to everyone, the side that is not dominant being repressed; i.e. in the male the female side is repressed and vice versa. "The second stage of the individuation process (self-realization through Jungian analysis) is characterized by the meeting with the figure of the 'soul-image,' named by Jung the ANIMA in the man, the ANIMUS in the woman. The archetypal figure of the soul-image stands for the respective contrasexual portion of the psyche, showing partly how our personal relation thereto is constituted, partly the precipitate of all human experience pertaining to the opposite sex. In other words, it is the image of the other sex that we carry in us, both as individuals and as representatives of a species. 'Jeder Mann trägt seine Eva in sich' (Every man carries his Eve in himself) affirms a popular saying. According to psychic law . . . everything latent, unexperienced, undifferentiated in the psyche, everything that lies in the unconscious and therefore the man's 'Eve' and the woman's 'Adam' as well, is always projected. In consequence one experiences the elements of the opposite sex that are present in one's psyche no otherwise than, for example, one experiences his shadow—in the other person. One chooses another, one binds one's self to another, who represents the qualities of one's own soul.

"The soul-image is a 'more or less firmly constituted functional complex, and the inability to distinguish one's self from it leads to such phenomena as those of the moody man, dominated by feminine drives, ruled by his emotions, or of the rationalizing, animus-obsessed women who always knows better and reacts in a masculine way, not instinctively.' (Wolff, T.)" (Jacobi, J. *The Psychology of C.G. Jung,* 1942)

psycheclampsia *Obs.* T.S. Clouston's synonym for *mania*.

psychedelic Mind-manifesting; sometimes used to describe certain pharmacologic agents (and particularly hallucinogens) that have an effect on mental processes. See *psychotropics*.

psychehormic Mind-rousing; sometimes used to describe certain pharmacologic agents that have an effect on mental processes. See *psychedelic; psychotropics*.

psycheism Mesmerism; animal magnetism.

psychelytic Mind-releasing; sometimes used to describe certain pharmacologic agents that have an effect on mental processes. See *psychedelic; psychotropics.*

psychentonia Mental (usually high) tension.

psychephoric Mind-moving; sometimes used to describe certain pharmacologic agents that have an effect on mental processes. See *psychedelic; psychotropics.*

psycheplastic Mind-molding; sometimes used to describe certain pharmacologic agents that have an effect on mental processes. See *psychedelic; psychotropics.*

psycherhexic (sī-ker-ek′sik) Mind-bursting forth; sometimes used to describe certain pharmacologic agents that have an effect on mental processes. See *psychedelic; psychotropics.*

psychezymic (sī-ke-zī′mik) Mind-fermenting; sometimes used to describe certain pharmacologic agents that have an effect on mental processes. See *psychedelic; psychotropics.*

psychiasis (sī-kī′à-sis) *Obs.* Spiritual healing.

psychiater (sī-kī′à-tēr) *Obs.* Psychiatrist.

psychiatria (sī-kē-at′rē-à) *Obs.* Psychiatry.

psychiatric social work See *social work, psychiatric.*

psychiatrics The theory or practice of psychiatry.

psychiatrism (sī-kī′àtriz′m) The injudicious and fallacious application of psychiatric principles in an unwarrantedly mechanistic way, without careful investigation of the dynamics of the individual case to which the principle is applied. Psychiatrism is perhaps best illustrated by the novice student of psychology who reads Freud's work on dream interpretation and begins blandly to interpret all his friends' dreams on the basis of the symbols mentioned by Freud. Thus psychiatrism tends to standardize and oversimplify complex problems of relationship and causality, and ignores the enormous importance of individual variation. It is based on the fallacy of hypothetical concepts of unconscious personality forces being accepted in an unscientific, matter-of-fact fashion.

psychiatrist One versed in the branch of medicine that deals with the prevention, diagnosis, and treatment of mental and emotional disorders. Although with the development of behavioral neurology there is increasing overlap between the medical specialties of psychiatry and neurology, it may generally be said that psychiatry is concerned with disturbances in emotion, thinking, perceiving, and behavior, whereas neurology is concerned with disorders of identifiable parts of the nervous system. (It has been suggested that a psychiatrist is a noninvasive neurologist.) A psychiatrist is a physician who has had advanced training in the diagnosis and treatment of mental disorders. This advanced training ordinarily includes the study of *psychotherapy* (q.v.) , and since the methods of psychotherapy are often based on a particular theory or system of psychology, the individual psychiatrist will often characterize his orientation as "psychoanalytic," "Freudian," "Jungian," "Adlerian," etc. Such appellations are to be considered as indicative of the philosophy or psychological system to which the psychiatrist adheres; they are, as it were, subgroupings within the more general field of psychiatry. A certain amount of confusion has arisen in regard to differentiation between the terms psychiatrist and psychoanalyst. In the United States, the term psychoanalyst generally refers to a physician who has had advanced training in the specialty of psychiatry and whose theoretical background is psychoanalytic. There are, however, certain people (particularly in Europe) who are psychoanalysts but not psychiatrists; these "lay analysts" are not physicians but have had intensive training in the psychoanalytic method of psychotherapy and their theoretical orientation is psychoanalytic.

psychiatrize To exert psychiatric influence.

psychiatry The medical specialty concerned with the study, diagnosis, treatment, and prevention of behavior disorders.

psychiatry, asylum Ernest Jones's term for the field of psychiatry that deals with major mental disorders under treatment in institutions.

psychiatry, C-L Consultation-liaison psychiatry. See *consultant; consultation-liaison.*

psychiatry, child The science of healing or curing disorders of the psyche in children.

psychiatry, community The branch of psychiatry concerned with the provision and delivery of a coordinated program of mental health care to a specified population. While following the medical model in general, with the methods and techniques of clinical psychiatry as its cornerstone, community psychiatry in addition uses public health methods to assess the psychiatric needs of any specified population, to identify the various environmental factors that contribute to or otherwise modify psychosocial disorder, and to evaluate the effects of therapeutic intervention on the identified patient and the social units of which he is a part.

The techniques of community psychiatry are not new, but their fusion into a coordinated, comprehensive program designed to ensure equal care of high quality and ready accessibility for all is a departure from the usual clinical emphasis on the individual patient or patient-therapist dyad. It carries with it the acceptance of continuing responsiblity for the mental health needs of a community. Although the importance of intrapsychic conflict in the production of some kinds of emotional disorder is not ignored, the emphasis in community psychiatry is on extrapsychic, interpersonal, environmental, and cultural forces that engender, precipitate, intensify, prolong, or otherwise complicate maladaptive patterns and their response to treatment.

The core concept of the *Community Mental Health Center* is that it will function as the nucleus for mental health services of the community it serves—usually defined geographically and termed the *catchment area.* An essential element in the delivery of such services is *continuity of care*—often misinterpreted to mean that the patient has the same therapist throughout every phase of his treatment and rehabilitation program, although more properly it refers to the provision of an organizational structure that will guarantee that the patient receive whatever kind of care he needs at the time he needs it and will ensure a relatedness between past and present care in conformity with the therapeutic needs of the patient. The therapy program is thus flexible, and tailored to the shifting needs of the patient, his pathology, and his community, rather than limited to the one or two techniques that may constitute the total armamentarium of a particular therapist.

Quite clearly, the mere existence of men-

tal health services does not ensure their optimal utilization, for those who do come to the attention of established psychiatric agencies may not even constitute a majority of those who need psychiatric help. Providing health services, particularly for that nonparticipant, voiceless segment of the population currently labeled *the disadvantaged,* is not enough. Truly comprehensive health centers must in addition function as agents in effecting social change that will promote mental health. They will be equally committed to *prevention,* in all its forms: *tertiary prevention* (rehabilitation)—the return of the identified patient to his peak potential of functioning, by concentrating on his assets and recoverable functions rather than on the liabilities of his psychopathology, by focusing on complications of disuse (such as the social breakdown syndrome) that have often been mistaken as part of the basic disease process; *secondary prevention*—early case-finding; and *primary prevention*—promotion of mental health, and prevention of psychosocial disorder.

But how this is to be done, and where, and when, and by whom, remain unsettled issues in *social psychiatry* (the body of knowledge and theory on which the methods and techniques of community psychiatry are based). Is community psychiatry a medical science or a social movement? Does it address itself to the mentally ill, or to the whole population, or to the entire social system within which it exists? Many in the field believe that evaluation of psychosocial disorder should include not only analysis, but ultimately also manipulation of existing social structures and systems. Others term such direct social or community action *social engineering* and include it as a part of social psychiatry. Still others view this as an unwarranted and potentially dangerous assumption of political power that is beyond the realm of medicine.

In view of the continuing controversy over the orientation, ideology, and philosophy basic to community psychiatry, it is little wonder that currently operating Community Mental Health Centers are organized along very different lines, or with different models. In the *medical model,* the focus is on treatment of the identified patient. In the *crisis-intervention model,* the focus is on transitional-developmental and accidental-situational demands for novel adaptational responses. Because minimal intervention at such times tends to achieve maximal and optimal effects, such a model is more readily applicable to population groups than the medical model. In the *metabolic-nutritional model,* the focus is on long-term studies to assess the presence of deprivations, toxins, etc., in population groups, and on attempts to modify, reduce, or abolish those threats to health. A subtype of this model is the *social integration-disintegration model,* whose basic premise is that, other things being equal, a better organized society promotes better adaptation. The *educational-socialization model* views a population as a social system containing people who have certain roles. This is a sociologic approach that asks how well are people fulfilling their roles, and whose focus is often on newcomers to the group (children, immigrants, etc.) and on refitting to appropriate roles those who have deviated (rehabilitation and tertiary prevention of residual defects). In the *public health model,* the focus is on epidemiology and the population at risk, not only to assess the incidence and prevalence of disease but also to discover the conditions that produce it. Finally, there is the *ecological systems model,* which views disorder not only as a deviance of the person himself but as a reflection of deviance or disequilibrium in that series of systems with which he articulates.

Ecology is the study of the mutual relationships of living things and their environments. The ecologist (or social psychiatrist) is particularly interested in why one person falls ill while his neighbor (or sibling, or parent) maintains good health. The ecological model provides a network approach to psychosocial disorder that may try to manipulate the expectations that impose specific roles on subsystems, and this is the model that involves itself most directly in social engineering and community action. In such a model, the primary role of the psychiatrist is as a *change agent* in social action and community organization, who uses his knowledge of group process to mediate and reconcile opposing forces that produce social dis-

equilibrium and to stimulate new approaches through interpersonal transactions. See *social policy planning.*

psychiatry, comparative Cultural psychiatry; that branch of psychiatry concerned with the influence of the culture on the mental health of members of that culture. Comparative psychiatry has also been termed social psychiatry, ethnopsychology, and clinical sociology. When the focus is on different cultures, rather than differences within a single culture, the term *transcultural psychiatry* is used. See *ecology; psychiatry, community.*

psychiatry, consultation See *consultant.*

psychiatry, cultural See *psychiatry, comparative.*

psychiatry, descriptive See *descriptive.*

psychiatry, dynamic See *descriptive.*

psychiatry, experimental As used today, this term generally refers to the use of chemical agents in the development of a science of human behavior, and particularly to research on the properties and pathways of action of the *psychotomimetics* (q.v.). In experimental psychiatry, drugs that alter behavior (including drugs that affect symptoms of psychiatric disorder) are used as devices for the detection and manipulation of significant variables in naturally occurring mental disorders.

psychiatry, forensic Legal psychiatry; psychiatry in its legal aspects, including criminology, penology, commitment of the mentally ill, the psychiatric role in compensation cases, the problems of releasing information to the court, of expert testimony.

psychiatry, geriatric The branch of psychiatry that deals with disorders of old age; it aims to maintain old persons independently in the community as long as possible and to provide long-term care when needed. Its future hinges on research into senile dementia (primary degenerative dementia) and cerebrovascular disease (including multi-infarct dementia) which, if prevented, would allow 90% of the people over 75 years of age to be free of physical and mental disability instead of the 50 to 75% who now are free of such disorder.

psychiatry, industrial The branch of psychiatry that deals with the worker's adjustment to his job and with the effects of the business organization on its members; specifically, it includes such areas and functions as (1) personality factors in the worker that affect his work fitness; (2) early detection of psychiatric illness within the unit; (3) rehabilitation of the worker who has had a major mental illness; (4) placement, promotions, transfers, etc.; (5) assessment of psychiatric factors in compensation cases, accidents, and absenteeism; (6) training of management for appropriate handling of their subordinates' behavior.

psychiatry, infant That branch of psychiatry concerned with mental and personality development in the first years of life, with emphasis on direct observation of the infant and the mother-infant relationship from the moment of birth. The aim is to identify subtle signs of infant psychopathology, differences from the normal that can interfere with or distort ego development. See *infancy research.*

psychiatry, liaison See *consultant.*

psychiatry, orthomolecular See *orthomolecular.*

psychiatry, pastoral The branch of psychiatry related to religion, and particularly to the integration of psychiatry and religion for the purpose of alleviating emotional ailments—the psychotherapeutic role that the clergyman must often play in his relationship to his parishioners. The term includes such things as vocational and marriage counseling.

Organized religion as a whole represents centuries of interpersonal experiences that have given pragmatic validation to certain tenets and doctrines. Therefore, when based on these doctrines, advice and other therapeutic measures are often psychologically valid, even though the dynamics as such may not be recognized or understood. And, at least with certain types of patients, the results may be excellent. The many cures at the shrine of Lourdes, France, afford an example of this.

Pastoral psychiatry at the present time is confined largely to reassurance and relief of guilt feelings, affording opportunity for catharsis, and alleviation of anxiety in general by directive and noninterpretive methods. In addition, religion offers the possibility of identification with the omnipotent Father, and engenders reaction

formations and sublimation. In certain aspects, organized religion may be likened to group psychotherapy of an educative type. Unlike the latter, however, religion is generally devoid of an understanding of the psychodynamics involved.

psychiatry, political See *psychopolitics.*

psychiatry, psychoanalytic See *psychoanalysis.*

psychiatry, social In psychiatry, the stress laid on the environmental influences and the impact of the social group on the individual. This emphasis is made not only with regard to etiology, but also for purposes of treatment and, more important, in preventive work. See *ecology; psychiatry, community; psychiatry, comparative.*

psychic 1. Of or pertaining to the mind or psyche. 2. Psychologic or psychogenic, rather than physical or somatic. 3. Sensitive to psychic pheonomena, as of a medium or spiritual healer.

psychic divorce See *divorce, stations of.*

psychic equivalent Psychomotor epilepsy. See *epilepsy.*

psychic suicide See *suicide, psychic.*

psychical Psychic.

psychical reality See *reality testing.*

psychicism Psychical research.

psychics Psychology.

psychiety A form of individualism which maintains that society resides within the individual rather than in the group. A person's emotions, ethics, and social experiences are emphasized, with the implication that more nearly perfect states of private experience and personal demeanor can be reached, perhaps through solitary meditation, self-help groups, or some form of more structured therapy.

psychinosis *Rare.* Psychosis.

psychlampsia *Obs.* Mania.

psychnosia *Rare.* A term used by Moshcowitz for syndromes of physical symptoms on the basis of emotional conflicts (e.g. essential hypertension, Grave's syndrome, cardiospasm, irritable colon, mucous colitis).

psychnosis *Rare.* Psychopathy.

psychoactive When used in reference to psychopharmacologic agents, the term usually means psychic energizer (antidepressant), although it is sometimes used less specifically to refer to any drug (stimulant, depressant, or tranquilizer) with an effect on mental processes.

psychoactive substance dependence Behavioral evidence of dependence on alcohol, sedatives or hypnotics, opioids, cocaine, amphetamine, phencyclidine, hallucinogens, cannabis, tobacco, or inhalants—either singly or in combination—manifested in one or more of the following: preoccupation with using the substance, taking it in larger amounts or for a longer period than intended, tolerance to the drug, development of typical withdrawal symptoms on discontinuance of the drug or use of the drug to relieve withdrawal symptoms, repeated efforts to reduce or control intake, interference with social or occupational obligations or opportunities by drug use, and continuing use of the drug in the face of clear-cut social, legal, or medical contrainidications.

Psychoactive substance abuse refers to a maladaptive pattern of substance use that is not severe enough to meet the criteria for dependence.

psychoactive substance-induced organic mental disorders In DSM-III-R intoxication, withdrawal, and posthallucinogenic perception disorder are recognized as organic mental disorders that may complicate psychoactive substance use, in addition to those organic mental syndromes that occur also in conditions other than psychoactive substance use (delirium, dementia, amnestic disorder, organic delusional disorder, organic hallucinosis, organic mood disorder, organic anxiety disorder, and organic personality disorder). See *flashback.*

psychoactive substance use disorders In DSM-III-R this category includes *psychoactive substance dependence* (q.v.) and *psychoactive substance abuse.*

psychoanaleptic See *analeptic.*

psychoanaleptica See *psycholeptica.*

psychoanalysis The separation or resolution of the psyche into its constituent elements. The term has three separate meanings: (1) a procedure, devised by Sigmund Freud, for investigating mental processes by means of free association, dream interpretation, and interpretation of resistance and transference manifestations; (2) a theory of psychology developed by Freud out of his clinical experience with hysterical patients; and (3) a form of psychiatric treatment developed by Freud that utilizes the psychoanalytic procedure (1 above)

and is based on psychoanalytic psychology (2 above). In the third sense, psychoanalysis is " an attempt to decode, i.e., interpret, a patient's communications according to a loosely drawn set of transformational rules concerning underlying meanings, motivations, and unities of thought." (A. Cooper, *American Journal of Psychiatry 142,* 1985)

Freud considered the cornerstones of psychoanalytic theory to be the assumption of unconscious mental processes, recognition of resistance and repression, appreciation of the importance of sexuality (and aggressivity), and the Oedipus complex. Ernest Jones delineated seven major principles of Freud's psychology: (1) determinism—psychical processes are not a chance occurrence; (2) affective processes have a certain autonomy and can be detached and displaced; (3) mental processes are dynamic and tend constantly to discharge the energy associated with them; (4) repression; (5) intrapsychic conflict; (6) infantile mental processes—the wishes of later life are important only as they ally themselves with those of childhood; (7) psychosexual trends are present in childhood. For a short summary of Freud's instinct theories, see *neurosis.*

Other schools of thought within psychology and psychiatry are sometimes referred to (loosely and not wholly correctly) as psychoanalytic. Chief among these are:

1. Jung's analytical psychology, which emphasizes the *collective unconscious,* a concept bearing on ethnological psychology. Jung considers that libido arises not from the sexual instinct but from a universal force or life urge; mind is not only a Has Been but also a Becoming, that is, it has aims and strives to realize certain goals within itself. Reminiscences of experience are relegated to the personal unconscious and then link up with and are used to express fundamental ideas and trends, the *archetypes,* which represent not only the past stages but also the future potentials of race development.

2. Adler's individual psychology, which is based on the egoistic side of man's nature, on the striving for power as a compensation for inferiority (psychic and organic). Neurosis is an attempt to free oneself from the feeling of inferiority.

3. Sullivan's dynamic-cultural school (see *Sullivan, Harry Stack*).

4. Horney's dynamic-cultural school (see *Horney, Karen*).

5. Rado's adaptational school (see *psychodynamics, adaptational*).

psychoanalysis, applied The use of established psychoanalytic knowledge to contribute to the understanding of psychic phenomena that occur outside the realm of psychoanalytic therapy, as in *biography in depth* (q.v.), art, history, anthropology, education, sociology, etc.

psychoanalysis, wild Psychotherapeutic techniques that use a limited amount of interpretation or that attack the patient directly with deep interpretations.

psychoanalyst One who adheres to the doctrine and/or uses the methods of psychoanalysis. See *psychiatrist; psychoanalysis*.

psychoataxia *Rare.* Intrapsychic ataxia. See *ataxia*.

psychobacillosis *Obs.* Treatment of schizophrenia by bacterial preparations.

psychobioanalysis See *bioanalysis*.

psychobiogram E. Kretschmer devised the psychobiogram for purposes of practical investigation of the personality. It is made up of several parts. The first two parts consist of the data concerning the patient's heredity and past history. The other parts consist of a detailed description of the person's temperament, his sociological attitude, intelligence, physical findings, etc., and the classification from the point of view of the somatotype. (*Textbook of Medical Psychology*, 1934)

psychobiology Biopsychology; the study of the biology of the psyche. It includes such subdivisions as the organization (anatomy), physiology, and pathology of the mind.

The term was used with a variety of meanings in the early part of the 20th century. Adolf Meyer first used the term in 1915, and in the United States, it is generally associated with his name. Meyer generally calls his point of view *objective psychobiology*, with particular stress upon the relationship of the individual to his environment.

Meyer's school of objective psychobiology concerns itself with the overt and implicit behavior of the individual, which is a function of the total organism. The mind is the integration of the whole-functions of the total personality. Ideal mental health is the maximal ability of, plus the best opportunity for, getting along with people, without the interference of inner conflicts or external frictions, in a manner that would make for full mutual satisfaction on a constant give-and-take basis. Psychobiology is a genetic-dynamic science that studies personality development in the light of environmental setting and longitudinal growth. Meyer's central theme is "the mind in action" and he stresses the relationship between the conscious drives and the environment. The aim of objective psychobiology as it is applied to patients (*distributive analysis and synthesis*) is to adapt the patient to his surroundings, both directly by working with him and indirectly via environmental manipulation and work with other social agencies. The therapist attempts to correct the patient's faulty mental habits. Psychobiology is particularly useful in the psychoses, where the conflict to a large extent is between the ego and the environment; but in the neuroses, the conflict is between the ego and the id.

psychobiology, developmental The study of the relationship between emotional experiences in childhood and later pathology, of the biological determinants of behavior and its psychological components. Developmental psychology is a broad field that includes (1) ethology and comparative psychology, with emphasis on how behavioral traits enable the organism to meet environmental demands and how they are maintained in the face of natural selection; (2) toxicology and teratology, with emphasis on the particular susceptibility of immature organisms to environmental events; and (3) the neurosciences, with emphasis on how the nervous system develops and its relationship to reproduction, communication, learning, memory, sleep, etc.

Animal studies, for example, have shown that early separation from the mother disrupts neurochemical and neuroendocrine growth processes, sleep-wake organization, emotional behavior, and immune reactivity. Psychosocial dwarfism appears to be a similar phenomenon in humans, and when such children are removed from the stressful situation their growth retardation, bizarre eating behavior, and deficiencies of adrenocorticotrophic and growth hormones disappear. See *dwarfism, psychosocial; failure to thrive.*

psychobiology, objective See *psychobiology.*

psychocatharsis Catharsis (q.v.).

psychochemistry Freeman's term for biochemistry as applied to psychiatric problems.

psychochromesthesia Sensation of color produced by any nonvisual stimulus.

psychocinesia See *psychokinesia.*

psychocoma *Obs.* Clouston's term for *stupor.*

psychocortical Relating to the cortex of the brain as the seat of the mind.

psychodiagnostics A term used by German writers to designate the Rorschach test.

psychodietetics The application of the principles of nutrition to the treatment of psychiatric disorders, and especially the replacement of assumed dietary deficiencies with supplemental vitamins, minerals, etc. See *orthomolecular.*

psychodometer An instrument for measuring the rapidity of psychic processes.

psychodometry The measurement of psychic processes.

psychodrama "The psychodrama deals with the private personality of the patient and his catharsis, with the persons within his milieu and with the roles in which he and they have interacted in the past, in the present, and in which they may interact in the future. Techniques have been devised to bring the underlying spontaneous processes to expression. Psychodramatic work is usually best organized in a therapeutic theatre, but it may be carried out wherever the patient lives, if his problem requires it.

"One of the techniques is that of self-presentation. The psychiatrist asks the patient to live through and portray or duplicate situations which are a part of his daily life, especially crucial conflicts in which he is involved.

"Another technique of the psychodrama is that of soliloquy. It is used by the patient to duplicate hidden feelings and thoughts which he actually has or had in a situation with a partner in real life, but which he did not or does not express.

"In the technique of spontaneous improvisation the patient acts in fictitious or symbolic roles which are carefully selected by the psychiatrist on the basis of the patient's problem.

"In the case of patients with whom any sort of communication is reduced to a minimum, the psychodrama attempts to create an auxiliary world, or a world within which the patient functions. This may require the use of a staff of auxiliary egos who are to embody the psychotic world of the patient. In this manner, the psychiatrist (through the auxiliary egos making up the auxiliary world) is able to 'act with' the patient on the patient's spontaneous level.

"*Psychodramatic catharsis* is a process which takes place between the actual partners in a problem or mental disturbance. Analysis before or after psychodramatic action may prepare a cathartic development, but the genuine phase of catharsis takes place in the course of the psychodrama itself." (Moreno, J.L. *Das Stegreif Theater,* 1936)

psychodrama, forms of

1. *Psychodrama*—focuses on the individual, being a synthesis of psychological analysis with drama (action). Psychodrama aims at the *active* building up of private worlds and individual ideologies.

2. *Sociodrama*—focuses on the group, being a synthesis of the *socius* with psychodrama. It aims at the active structuring of *social* worlds and collective ideologies.

3. *Physiodrama*—focuses on the soma, being a synthesis of physical culture (sports) and psychodrama. The physical condition of the participants before, during, and after the production is *measured.* It gives diagnostic (possibly also prognostic) clues for training requirements, provides the setup for retraining.

4. *Axiodrama* (Gr. *axios,* worth, worthy of value, goodly)—focuses on ethics and general values, and aims to dramatize eternal verities (truth, justice, beauty, grace, piety, eternity, peace, etc.).

5. *Hypnodrama*—the synthesis of *hypnosis* (q.v.) and psychodrama.

6. *Psychomusic*—a synthesis of *spontaneous* music with psychodrama.

7. *Psychodance*—a synthesis of *spontaneous* dancing with psychodrama.

8. *Therapeutic motion picture*—a synthesis of motion picture with psychodrama. (Moreno, J.L. *Sociometry 1,* 1937)

psychodynamic Relating to the forces of the mind. Ideas and impulses are charged with emotions, to which the general expression *psychic energy* is given. For example, delusions of persecution or obsessions or compulsions are described as psychodynamic phenomena, in that they are said to represent the results of activity of psychic forces. See *psychodynamics.*

psychodynamic cerebral system See *psychodynamics, adaptational.*

psychodynamics The science of mental forces in action. Essentially, psychodynamics are a formulation or description of how the mind develops, and of how the hypothesized energies of the mind are distributed in the course of its various adaptational maneuvers. See *ego; id; ontogeny, psychic; superego.*

psychodynamics, adaptational Rado's system of psychoanalytic psychiatry. "This science is based on the psychoanalytic method of investigation. As we have just seen, it studies the part played by motivation and control in the organism's interaction with its cultural environment. It deals with pleasure and pain, emotion and thought, desire and executive action, interpreting them in terms of organismic utility, that is, in an adaptational framework. In the theory of evolution, the pivotal concept is adaptation; since the organism's life cycle is but a phase of evolution, it is consistent to make the same concept basic to the study of behavior.

"We define ontogenetic adaptations as improvements in the organism's pattern of interaction with its environment that increase its chances for survival, cultural self-realization, and perpetuation of its type. Autoplastic adaptations result from changes undergone by the organism itself; alloplastic adaptations from changes wrought by the organism on its environment. In ontogenetic adaptations, the master mechanisms are learning, creative imagination, and goal-directed activity." (*Psychoanalysis of Behavior*, 1956)

"The organism's systemic requirements are known as its needs. Like its other traits, they are an outcome of the interaction between inherited predisposition (genotype) and environment. We speak of aboriginal needs that show predominantly the forming influence of the culture in which the organism lives." (Ibid.)

In Rado's terminology, the psychody-namic central system refers to mind and unconscious mind and includes (1) that range of the brain's neurophysiologic activity that comes to the awareness of the organism, the self-reporting range, and (2) that range of nonreporting activity accessible to extrapolative investigation by psychodynamic methods and/or to investigation by physiologic methods. The aim of adaptational psychodynamics is to discover the mechanisms by which the psychodynamic cerebral system accomplishes its integrative task. The integrative apparatus of the system is composed of four units, which are hierarchically ordered levels reflecting the course of evolutionary history—hedonic, brute emotions, emotional thought, and unemotional thought. At the hedonic level, the organism moves toward pleasure and away from pain. In the next two levels, the emotions are the controlling means of integration (divided into the emotions based on present pain or the expectation of pain, such as fear, rage, retroflexed rage, guilty fear, and guilty rage; and the welfare emotions based on present pleasure or the expectation of pleasure, such as pleasurable desire, affection, love, joy, self-respect, and pride). At the level of unemotional thought, reason, common sense, and science prepare the ground for intelligent action and self-restraint.

Behavior disorders are disturbances of psychodynamic integration that interfere with the organism's adaptive life performance, its attainment of utility and pleasure. The simplest forms of behavior disorder occur when the organism responds to danger with an overproduction of the emergency emotions; such emergency dyscontrol is in itself a threat to the organism from within and leads to processes of miscarried prevention and miscarried repair.

More complex behavior disorders arise when emergency dyscontrol acts in combination with additional pathogenic agents. With emergency dyscontrol as a point of departure, Rado classifies behavior disorders according to the increasing complexity of their patterns and mechanisms as follows:

"Class I. Overreactive Disorders.

"(1) Emergency Dyscontrol: The emotional outflow, the riddance through dreams, the phobic, the inhibitory, the repressive, and the hypochondriac patterns; the gainful exploitation of illness. (2) Descending Dyscontrol. (3) Sexual Disorders: The impairments and failures of standard performance. Dependence on reparative patterns: Organ replacement and organ avoidance; the criminal, dramatic and hidden forms of sexual pain-dependence; the formation of homogeneous pairs. Firesetting and shoplifting as sexual equivalents. (4) Social Overdependence: The continuous search for an ersatzparent; the mechanisms of forced competition, avoidance of competition, and of self-harming defiance. (5) Common Maladaptation: A combination of sexual disorder with social overdependence. (6) The Expressive Pattern (expressive elaboration of common maladaptation): Ostentatious self-presentation; dreamlike interludes; rudimentary pantomimes; disease-copies and the expressive complication of incidental disease. (7) The Obsessive Pattern (obsessive elaboration of common maladaptations): Broodings, rituals, and overt temptations. Tic and stammering as obsessive equivalents; bed wetting, nailbiting, grinding of teeth in sleep, as precursors of the obsessive pattern. (8) The Paranoid Pattern (nondisintegrative elaboration of common maladaptation): The hypochondriac, self-referential, persecutory and grandiose stages of the Magnan sequence.

"Class II. Moodcyclic Disorders.

"Cycles of depression; cycles of reparative elation; the pattern of alternate cycles, cycles of minor elation; cycles of depression marked by elation; cycles of preventive elation.

"Class III. Schizotypal Disorders.

"(1) Compensated schizo-adaptation. (2) Decompensated schizo-adaptation. (3) Schizotypal disintegration marked by adaptive incompetence.

"Class IV. Extractive Disorders.

"The ingratiating ('smile and suck') and extortive ('hit and grab') patterns of transgressive conduct.

"Class V. Lesional Disorders.

"Class VI. Narcotic Disorders.

"Class VII. Disorders of War Adaptation." (Ibid.)

Rado divides the methods of psychotherapy into two classes—reconstructive (adaptational technique of psychoanalytic therapy) and reparative (less ambitious treatment methods with limited goals but in general also of shorter duration).

psychodynamy *Obs.* Animal magnetism. See *magnetism.*

psychodysleptica See *psychotropics.*

psychoeducation Training in psychologic principles and their application to specified problems, conditions, or situations, often used to refer to *psychoeducational family therapy,* developed by Anderson, Hogarty, and Reiss (1980) for families of schizophrenics. The procedure includes a *survival skills workshop,* during which information about the technical and subjective aspects of schizophrenic disorders is presented to a group of families, along with guidelines for interactions between patients and family members. Sessions during the next months or years focus on how the guidelines can be applied within specific families, and continuing multiple family meetings at fortnightly intervals widen the supportive networks for all the families participating.

psychoembryological schedule of ego See *dedifferentiation.*

psychoendocrinology The study of the hormonal system in relation to psychiatric disorders and, particularly, the study of the endocrine system as a likely site for the manifestation of biochemical abnormalities that are significant factors in the production of mental disorders.

Psychoendocrinologic research has concentrated particularly on cortisol, estrogen, growth hormone, progesterone, prolactin, testosterone, and thyroxine because they are hormones that are controlled by the central nervous system through the regulatory neurochemical agents of the hypothalamic-anterior pituitary complex.

psychoepilepsy By some, this term is used synonymously with idiopathic or genuine epilepsy; an unfortunate term in that it implies a psychogenic basis for epilepsy, evidence for which is minimal. See *epilepsy.*

psychoexploration A generic term used to refer to the various procedures known as abreaction, psychocatharsis, narcoanalysis, narcosynthesis, etc.

psychogender The psychological or emotional sex of a person; the term is ordinarily confined to intersexed patients to differentiate psychological sexual identification from somatic sex.

psychogenesis Origination within the mind or psyche.

psychogenia *Rare.* Mental disorder due to impaired mentality.

psychogenic, psychogenetic Relating to or characterized by psychogenesis; due to psychic, mental, or emotional factors and not to detectable organic or somatic factors.

psychogenic amnesia One of the *dissociative disorders* (q.v.).

psychogenic fugue One of the *dissociative disorders* (q.v.).

psychogenic pain disorder Psychalgia; kinesalgia. See *somatoform disorders.*

psychogeny *Psychogenesis* (q.v.).

psychogerontology Geriatric psychiatry; the study of the psychosocial aspects of old age.

psychogeusic Pertaining to taste perception.

psychognosia 1. Awareness of one's own mental state, insight. 2. Study of another's mental state as a step in the diagnosis of psychiatric disorder. A rarely used term.

psychogogic Mentally stimulating.

psychogonical Psychogenic.

psychogony The doctrine of the development of the mind. See *ontogeny, psychic.*

psychogram *Psychograph* (q.v.).

psychograph A chart or profile that describes the personality traits of the subject; *psychogram.*

psychographic disturbances *Obs.* Bombastic speech or pretentious, prolix writing as the major manifestion of personality disorder.

psychography The history of the psychologic and emotional development of the subject as it relates to the development of the symptoms of which he now complains.

psychohistory Application of psychologic theory, and particularly psychoanalytic psychology, to history so as to understand the human forces at work in the production of past events. Its most common application is to the history of a particular person; this is termed psychobiography.

psychohygiene *Obs.* Mental hygiene. See *hygiene, mental.*

psychoimmunology *Behavioral immunology;* study of the relationship between the immune system and behavior, and in particu-

lar the effect of the brain and psychological phenomena on immune responses. The immune system is responsive to emotional stress, and it seems likely that the central nervous system, neurotransmitters, and neuroendocrine processes mediate hypothalamic influences on the immune system.

psychoinfantilism "Persistence, in the adult, of mental qualities characteristic of the child. Psycho-infantile behavior is referable to the hopelessness, uncertainty, and desire for guidance and authority distinctive of childhood. It is manifested in tractability and dependence, which often takes the form of a strong emotional fixation frequently to the mother or the father, but sometimes to other persons, even chance acquaintances. The psycho-infantile person gives the normal adult the same feeling of detachment and the same urge to protect as the child. It is the latter attribute which lies back of the terms 'naive,' 'childish' and 'artless' so often used to describe his personality." (Lindberg, B.J. *Psycho-Infantilism,* 1950)

"*Psycho-infantilism* is not a disease, nor is it the common denominator for psychoneurotic or psychosomatic disorders. It is a form of mental weakness, inasmuch as the psycho-infantile person is particularly vulnerable to mental insufficiency when confronted with decisive events in his life. He is specially apt to break down when he himself has to make an important decision, the more so if circumstances have deprived him of the person he has been used to leaning upon." (Ibid.)

psychokinesia, psychokinesis T.S. Clouston's term for defective inhibition; formerly it also referred to the clinical syndrome known as *impulse insanity.* See *impulse disorders.*

psychokym(e) "Psychic processes conceived physiologically, namely, that which is conceived analogous to a form of energy, that something which flows through the central nervous system and which is at the basis of psychic processes. 'Neurokym' is used to designate the nervous processes in general." (Bleuler, *TP*)

psycholagny Sexual excitation that begins, continues, and ends with mental imagery; mental or psychic masturbation, that is, the occurrence of masturbatory phenomena stimulated by mental forces alone. See *masturbation*.

psycholepsy, psycholepsis Sudden, intense lowering of psychic tension, associated with morbid ideas and actions.

"Individuals in whom psychological tension is unstable, suffer from sudden relaxations of this tension, succumb to psycholeptic crises which have been brought on by their relationships with certain persons in their immediate circle." When psychic tension mounts to great heights, "in which feelings of ecstasy and indescribable happiness" appear, there may be a sudden fall in tension "culminating in a psycholeptic crisis and even in an epileptic fit." (Janet, *PH*) Some people who have triumphed in a given work may terminate the triumph with a morbid clinical syndrome. See *crisis, psycholeptic*.

psycholeptica Delay's term for phrenotropic drugs, whose principal effect is on the psyche, in contrast to neuroleptica, whose principal effect is on psychomotor activity. The psycholeptica include (1) the minor tranquilizers or ataractics, i.e. diphenylmethane derivatives and substituted propanediols (see *tranquilizer*); (2) psychoanaleptica (psychic tonics, euphoriants, and antidepressives); and (3) psychodysleptica, which produce disintegration of psychic functions (lysergic acid, mescaline, etc.). See *psychotropics*.

psycholinguistic abilities See *Illinois Test of Psycholinguistic Abilities*.

psycholinguistics The "study of the relation between messages on the speech channel and the cognitive or emotional states of human encoders and decoders who send and receive the messages." (Markel, N.N. *Psycholinguistics: An Introduction to the Study of Speech and Personality*, 1969) Linguistics, or philology, is the scientific study of human language or speech. Two subfields of psycholinguistics are recognized: (1) verbal learning and verbal behavior, concerned with the relation between messages on the speech channel and the cognitive states of the encoders and decoders; and (2) speech and personality, concerned with the relation between message on the speech channel and the emotional, attitudinal, or motivational states of the encoders and decoders. Included in this part are: *stylistics*, the study of individual differences

in the selection of words in various contexts; and *paralanguage*, nonlanguage sounds; language sounds are those that are essential for the production of words of a language (e.g. to say "tin" the sound of a "t" must be produced) and the speaker has little option in producing those sounds or their distribution; but he has many options in producing nonlanguage sounds, e.g. voice set, voice qualities, vocalizations (discrete sounds that are not used to produce morphs in a particular language, such as the *tsk-tsk* sound used to indicate "too bad").

psychologic(al) Relating to psychology; mental functioning; functional, rather than organic; of emotional origin.

psychologist A person trained as a professional in the science of psychology; a person with a degree in psychology granted by an accredited training program or educational institution. The individual psychologist often specializes in one of the branches or fields of psychology, and is then identified as that type of psychologist (e.g. a comparative or animal psychologist, research psychologist, educational psychologist, industrial psychologist).

A *clinical psychologist* usually holds a doctoral degree from an accredited training program, has had at least two years of supervised experience in a clinical setting, and often is licensed under applicable state laws. Whether working individually or as part of the clinical (treatment) team, the clinical psychologist applies psychologic principles to the therapeutic management of the mental, emotional, and behavioral disorders and developmental disabilities of individuals and groups. In addition, the clinical psychologist is skilled in research methodology and has assumed increasing importance in evaluating the effectiveness of mental health services and in planning clinical programs.

As with other mental health professionals, the clinical psychologist's functioning will vary with the setting within which he or she works and with his or her theoretical orientation. He may be involved mainly in individual therapy, group therapy, marriage or family therapy; his techniques may be largely psychoanalytic, behavioral, transpersonal, or Gestalt. Among the areas in which most clinical psychologists have had special training are development of attitudes and opinions, motivation, norms and scales of measurement, experimental design, perception and thinking, memory and learning, language and communication, psychological development, and group processes.

psychology The science that deals with the mind and mental processes—consciousness, sensation, ideation, memory, etc.

psychology, applied Utilization of all knowledge available in the areas of psychology, sociology, etc., in order to achieve optimal effectiveness in any operation. Applied psychology is ordinarily subdivided according to the field in which the operation occurs; e.g. business psychology, educational psychology, industrial psychology.

psychology, atomistic Any psychology based on the doctrine that perceptions, thoughts, and all mental processes are built up through the combination of simple elements or atoms. According to the doctrine of atomism, the physical universe (or, as is sometimes taught, the whole universe both physical and mental) is composed of simple, indivisible, and minute particles or atoms. Many thinkers have endeavored to interpret atomism from a psychical point of view, treating the atoms either as *mind stuff* or as composed of sense elements. Mind stuff, a term first used by W.K. Clifford, is the elemental material held to be the basis of reality and to consist internally of the constituent substance of mind and to appear externally in the form of matter.

"The distinguishing feature of Freud's instinct theory is that it is based on a conative-appetitive-striving, rather than a structural principle like sensation or reflex. But, as with the classical psychologies and behaviorism, psychoanalysis is an *atomistic psychology* which attempts to derive complex entities from the action of a synthetic principle (association, conditioning, integration) on or about a basic unit. A conative principle is used as an atomic unit to reconstruct the molecules of experience." (Kardiner, A., & Spiegel, H. *War Stress and Neurotic Illness*, 1947)

psychology, "blame" The tendency of persons with serious inhibitions in social competitive relationships to find expression for these inhibitions in hatred and perse-

cution of some blameless scapegoat. It also permits the individual to harbor a secret grandiose conception of himself. See *projection.*

psychology, centralist The subdivision of psychology that emphasizes the role of higher brain centers in determining behavior. In contrast to this is *peripheralist psychology* (including *behaviorism*), which attributes the major role in behavior to the receptor and effector organs.

psychology, cognitive See *style, cognitive; therapy, cognitive.*

psychology, educational The branch of psychology concerned with the derivation of psychological principles and methods that can be applied directly to problems of education.

psychology, ego See *object relations theory.*

psychology, gestalt A school of psychology that is concerned primarily with perceptual processes. Its development is associated particularly with Max Wertheimer, Wolfgang Koehler, and Kurt Koffka, and it represents an outgrowth of opposition to the traditional association psychology.

"Gestalt psychology holds that the whole or total quality of the image is perceived. This is in contrast to association psychology, which states that stimuli are perceived as parts and built into images. According to gestalt psychology, the organization of the stimuli into the image is based upon laws of perception which include proximity, similarity, direction, and inclusiveness of parts of the stimuli. The perceptual experience is a gestalt or configuration or pattern in which the whole is more than the sum of its parts. Organized units or structuralized configurations are the primary form of biological reactions. In the sensory field, these gestalten correspond to the configuration of the stimulating world.

"The organism has a 'gestalt function' which is defined as that function of the integrative organism whereby it responds to a given constellation of stimuli as a whole, the response being a constellation or pattern or gestalt which differs from the original stimulus pattern by the process of the integrative mechanism of the individual who experiences the perception. The whole setting of the stimulus and the whole integrative state of the organism determine the pattern or response.

"There is a tendency not only to perceive gestalten but to complete gestalten and to reorganize them according to principles biologically determined by the sensory motor pattern of action which may be expected to vary in different maturation or growth levels and in pathological states organically or functionally determined." (Bender, L. *Child Psychiatric Techniques,* 1952) See *therapy, Gestalt.*

psychology, individual Adlerian psychology, a discipline elaborated by the Viennese psychiatrist Alfred Adler. The complete name of his system is comparative individual-psychology. "By starting with the assumption of the *unity of the individual,* an attempt is made to obtain a picture of this unified personality regarded as a variant of individual life-manifestations and forms of expression. The individual traits are then compared with one another, brought into a common plane, and finally fused together to form a composite portrait that is, in turn, individualized." (Adler, A. *The Practice and Theory of Individual Psychology,* 1924)

Among the key concepts of individual psychology are (1) *fictional finalism,* the idea that expectations about the future rather than experiences in the past are the significant determinants of motivation; (2) *striving for superiority,* an innate tendency to develop one's capacities to the fullest; (3) *inferiority feelings,* springing from the recognition that one has failed to achieve perfection or to develop capacities to the fullest; (4) *social interest,* an innate tendency to involvement with others; (5) *lifestyle,* each person's unique way of striving for perfection; and (6) *creative self,* the center of personality, which interprets experience and guides the responses to it.

psychology, mob The psychology of mob behavior is considered by Fenichel to have much in common with a certain type of character defense against guilt feelings. In this type of defense, the guilt-laden character feels admiration and relief when someone else does something that he has been striving to do, but has been inhibited from doing through guilt feelings. The meaning of the admiration and relief is "Since others do it, it cannot be so bad after all."

The attainment of relief from guilt feelings in this way is a powerful force for group formation. Others have dared to do what the individual has felt guilt about doing. And "If my whole group acts this way, I may, too." In this way, the relief from guilt feelings is described as "one of the cornerstones of 'mob psychology.'" Indeed Fenichel points out that "individuals acting as a group are capable of instinctual outbreaks that would be entirely impossible for them as individuals." (*PTN*)

psychology, peripheralist See *psychology, centralist.*

psychology, rational Any system of psychology in which a priori assumptions (usually of a philosophical or theological nature) form the background into which any observed facts must be fit.

psychology, social See *sociology.*

psychology, topographical See *topography, mental.*

psychology, uprooted The changed mentality exhibited by one who has been uprooted by force of circumstance, i.e. has had to leave his native place with its physical, social, and cultural background that had surrounded him all his life.

When removed from their customary environment and dislocated from their protective moral background, uprooted people deviate markedly from their inculcated reverence for original values and show symptoms parallel to those found in migrating hordes: recklessness, unregulated and indiscriminate sexuality, a marked lowered responsibility toward human life and property. (Baynes, H.G. *Mythology of the Soul,* 1940) See *network; syndrome, survivor.*

psychometrics Mental testing. See *examinations, psychometric.*

psychometry Measurement of the duration and force of mental processes.

psychomimic See *syndrome, psychomimic.*

psychomotility Any motor action, attitude, or habit pattern that is influenced by mental processes and thus reflects the individual's personality makeup. Certain psychomotor phenomena such as tics, sterotypies, catatonia, dysarthria, stammering, and tremor have long been used in diagnosis as signs of psychomotor disturbance. Recently, postural attitudes and gait have been under investigation by clinicians as objective signs of psychomotor disturbance. Handwriting, also, has long been known as a valuable aid in investigating psychomotility, for it gives some indication of the individual's motivation. Certain features of handwriting have been regarded as suggestive of certain personality traits. Preliminary investigations of a nature more scientific than mere palmistry indicate that correlations do exist between handwritings of different types and symptoms, syndromes, and character traits noted in the patient's records.

psychomotor Relating to movement that is psychically determined in contradistinction to that which is definitely recognized as extrapsychic or organic in cause.

psychoneuroid Resembling or like psychoneurosis or psychoneurotic.

psychoneurosis See *neurosis.*

psychoneurosis, battle War neurosis. See *neurosis, traumatic.*

psychoneurosis, defense Freud's term for hysteria and various neuroses and psychoses caused by some idea or sensation so painful that the sufferer endeavors to dismiss it from the mind; at times, instead of being absolutely forgotten, the thought sinks down into the unconscious and acts as the hidden cause of the psychoneurotic disturbances.

psychoneurosis maidica (mȧ-id′i-kȧ) *Pellagra* (q.v.).

psychonoetism (-nō′e-tiz′m) A term introduced by L.E. Hinsie to designate the transference of personal conflicts to the intellect. Often patients are seen "who shift their doubts, fears, obsessions and delusions from their original source in the unconscious to the sphere of the intellect. Thus a patient who was a great objector and had to contradict everything and everyone was really denying a strong Oedipus complex and unconscious instinctual demands directed toward his mother. However, he had transferred his denial of his unconscious instincts to the intellectual sphere, where it became an obsessive doubting of all ideas and statements. This is the process termed psychonoetism." (*UP*)

psychonomics The science of the laws of mind: psychology.

psychonomy The branch of psychology concerned with the laws of mental action.

psychonosema *Obs.* Mental disease.

psychonosology The classification of mental disorders. See *nosology.*

psychoparesis *Rare.* Mental enfeeblement.

psychopath, sexual See *psychopathia sexualis.*

psychopathia Psychopathy.

psychopathia martialis *Obs.* Shell shock.

psychopathia sexualis Referring to sexual perversions; introduced by the German sexologist Richard von Krafft-Ebing (1840–1903), whose classical book on sexology bears that title.

psychopathic personality Antisocial personality. Although the 1980 revision of psychiatric nomenclature does not recognize psychopathic personality as a discrete entity, the attempts to define more clearly the nature of the various behavior patterns that make up this poorly understood group have not been wholly successful, and the term continues to appear in the psychiatric literature.

It was J.C. Prichard who first offered a systematic description of the so-called *moral disorders;* in 1835 he described a series of cases (which he termed moral insanity and moral imbecility) that were the prototypes of the psychopathic state as it is generally understood today. In 1888 Koch introduced the term *psychopathic inferiority,* and Kraepelin later included in this group a variety of syndromes described in terms of the most obvious presenting symptom, e.g. excitability, impulsivity, lying, criminality. The term *constitutional psychopathic inferior* was used by Adolf Meyer in 1905; it should be noted, however, that Meyer did not use the term constitutional in the sense of congenital, but rather to indicate that the traits in question were acquired early and were thoroughly ingrained in the personality. In general, at least according to current usage, psychopathic personality (or psychopathic disorder) is any behavioral dysfunction that is primary (idiopathic or nonorganic) and manifests itself in abnormally aggressive or seriously irresponsible conduct.

Cleckley (1941), who considers psychopathic personality a psychosis, because of the lack of integration of the affective components into the personality, lists the following characteristics: "(1) Superficial charm and good 'intelligence.' (2) Absence of delusions and other signs of irrational 'thinking.' (3) Absence of 'nervousness' or psychoneurotic manifestations. (4) Unreliability. (5) Untruthfulness and insincerity. (6) Lack of remorse or shame. (7) Inadequately motivated antisocial behavior. (8) Poor judgment and failure to learn by experience. (9) Pathologic egocentricity and incapacity for love. (10) General poverty in major affective reactions. (11) Specific loss of insight. (12) Unresponsiveness in general interpersonal relations. (13) Fantastic and uninviting behavior with drink and sometimes without. (14) Suicide rarely carried out. (15) Sex life impersonal, trivial and poorly integrated. (16) Failure to follow any life plan." (*The Mask of Sanity*, 1941) The maladjustment is a chronic one, and the psychopath tends to project the blame for his actions onto others. He tends to act out his conflicts so that the environment suffers, rather than the patient. He is a rebellious individualist and a nonconformist.

E. Glover classifies psychopathy into three main subgroups: (1) sexual psychopathy, with predominantly sexual symptoms combined with some degree of ego disorder; (2) "benign" psychopathy, manifested in the main as social incapacity, but usually with accompanying psychosexual disorder; and (3) antisocial psychopathy characterized by an unstable ego, delinquent outbursts, and some degree of sexual maladjustment. (*The Technique of Psychoanalysis*, 1955)

The etiology is unknown; some claim an exclusively organic etiology, others maintain that it is due to psychogenic factors. Many writers have emphasized difficulties in identification leading to a formless or confused ego-ideal. An unstable, inconsistent maternal figure or rejection and emotional deprivation early in life are believed to produce such difficulties in identification. According to M.S. Guttmacher (in *Current Problems in Psychiatric Diagnosis*, ed. P.H. Hoch & J. Zubin, 1953), psychopathic behavior is generally the result of affect starvation during the first years of life. The most malignant antisocial psychopaths are probably the products of affect starvation plus sadistic treatment in early childhood. See *syndrome, battered child.*

Karpman suggests that those cases of psychogenic etiology be termed secondary or symptomatic psychopathy; the others he calls primary psychopathy or *anethopathy* (q.v.). See also *psychopathy, passive parasitic.*

Various workers have noted a high incidence of cerebral dysrhythmia in patients diagnosed psychopathic personality; a high alpha index and theta activity are among the most commonly observed abnormalities.

Many European workers (among them Kurt Schneider) used psychopathic personality as a generic term for the entire range of personality disorders and did not restrict its application to the antisocial group.

psychopathist (sī-kop'ă-thist) *Obs.* Psychiatrist; alienist.

psychopathology The branch of science that deals with the essential nature of mental disease—its causes, the structural and functional changes associated with it, and the ways in which it manifests itself.

psychopathosis Southard's term for what is more commonly termed *psychopathic personality* (q.v.).

psychopathy General term for mental disease or disorders.

psychopathy, autistic *Asperger's syndrome,* described in 1944 as a hypertrophy of intellect at the expense of feeling and manifested as one or more of the following: lack of sensitivity, empathy, intuition, and normal human understanding; inappropriate one-sided social interaction; pedantic speech, which is more a proclamation than a conversation; inability to make friends; clumsiness and poor motor coordination. Some authorities consider that early childhood autism and autistic psychopathy may be parts of the same pathologic spectrum.

psychopathy, benign See *psychopathic personality.*

psychopathy, passive parasitic A clinical subdivision of anethopathy (*psychopathic personality*). Karpman suggests the term *anethopathy* (q.v.) to replace idiopathic, constitutional, or primary psychopathy. Anethopathy is subdivided into two distinct clinical types: the aggressive predatory type and the passive parasitic type. In regard to the latter, Karpman says: "Instead of being actively aggressive, this type of an individual has much less of energy output and feeds himself by 'sponging' on his environment for all his needs in a passive and entirely parasitic way. Such aggression as there may be is very minimal and no more than is absolutely necessary to satisfy immediate needs." (*Psychoanalytic Review 34*, 1947) Typical of such patients is the lack of any positive or generous human emotions, of sympathetic or tender affect, of gratitude or appreciation. These patients show no guilt, remorse, or regret. Their total picture is one of self-gratification. There are almost no unconscious mechanisms, because there is no repression of instinctual demands and no deferment of pleasure. Further, the patients are completely lacking in insight into the nature of their disturbances.

psychopedagogy A combination of conventional pedagogy and Adlerian psychology that aims to stimulate, cultivate, and amplify the natural qualities of the child and do away with unnecessary authority.

psychopetal (sī-kop'e-tal) Literally refers to objects that seek the psyche. Ordinarily, however, psychiatrists prefer the term *centripetal*. "I do not speak of 'psychopetal' functions, because although there is a given 'direction' yet both incoming and outgoing functions, as far as psychology is concerned, take place within the psyche." (Bleuler, *TP*)

psychopharmacology The study of drugs that affect mental and behavioral activity, and in particular those drugs classified as *psychotropics* (q.v.).

psychophysical *Psychosomatic* (q.v.).

psychophysics The science of the relation between mental action and physical phenomena.

psychophysiologic disorders *Psychosomatic disorders, somatization reactions, organ neuroses,* etc. These disorders are disturbances of visceral function secondary to chronic attitudes or long-continued insufficiency of affective discharge and may present themselves as dysfunction involving any of the organ systems: skin, musculoskeletal, respiratory, cardiovascular, hemic and lymphatic, gastrointestinal, genitourinary, endocrine, nervous system, or organs of special sense. In this system of classification, ulcerative colitis, for example, would be labeled "psychophysiologic gastrointestinal reaction." See *psychosomatic*.

psychophysiology Physiology in relation to the mind and its processes.

psychoplegia *Rare.* A rapidly developing form of *dementia* (q.v.).

psychopneumatology Study of the interactions of mind and body; psychosomatology.

psychopolitics Application of psychiatric knowledge or theory to the process of government; any effort to gain acceptance of psychiatric principles as a significant factor in the shaping of public policy.

In a century marked by a tendency to designate socially undesirable conduct as illness, rather than as the crime or sin of earlier generations, psychiatry has often found itself the arbiter of right and wrong. Technologic advances, in the form of mind-altering drugs, operant conditioning, electrode implantations, and the like, have raised the specter of their use as ways to coerce, oppress, or control behavior, or to supplant independent thinking and freedom of choice. In consequence, the ethics of medical and psychiatric practice has become an important aspect of psychopolitics. Of no less importance are those political actions designed to improve the lot of the mentally ill and to ensure the availability of a broad range of appropriate services for anyone who might need them. Such actions may be directed at any, or every, level of government—legislative (Are the right laws being written?), judicial (Have the courts given due consideration to the mental health implications of their decisions?), and executive (Are the laws being implemented appropriately, and are the decisions of the courts being honored?).

psychoreaction Much and Holzmann's term for psychophysical interrelationship. They asserted that when they injected cobra poison into patients with schizophrenia, they observed lysis of the red blood corpuscles in a way that was characteristic of schizophrenia. Their claims were short-lived.

psychorhythm T.S. Clouston's term for *alternating insanity. See psychosis, manic-depressive*.

psychorhythmia Involuntary repetition, by the mind, of its formerly volitional action.

psychorrhagia, psychorraghy *Obs.* The death-struggle.

psychorrhea A form of hebephrenic schizophrenia characterized by vague and often bizarre theories of philosophy; usually the stream of thought is incoherent.

psychorrhexis A malignant type of anxiety reaction seen in 2–3% of war neuroses, according to Emilio Mira. Anguish and perplexity, rather than fear or excitement, are the cardinal features. Pulse remains above 120, respiration about 40. Temperature rises rapidly after seven days, the tongue becomes ulcerated, and jaundice and tympanitic abdomen may appear. Patients become restless, develop automatic movements and facial spasms. In fatal cases, death ensues after three or four days. Psychorrhexis occurs in patients with preexisting lability of the sympathetic system, with sudden severe mental trauma in conditions of physical exhaustion, and when there is long delay before sedative treatment is instituted. See *neurosis, traumatic.*

psychosensory Pertaining to (1) the mental perception and interpretation of sensory stimuli, or (2) a hallucination that, by an effort, the mind is able to distinguish from an actuality (pseudohallucination).

psychoses, alcoholic See *alcoholism.*

psychosexual In DSM-III-R, the categories included under this label are now termed *sexual disorders* (q.v.).

psychosexuality Psychosexual condition or state; distinguished from sexuality expressed somatically (somatosexual). For example, ideas of a sexual character are manifestations of psychosexuality. See *ontogeny, psychic.*

psychosis Loosely, any mental disorder (including whatever is meant by the obsolete terms *insanity, lunacy,* and *madness*); more specifically, the term is used to refer to a particular class or group of mental disorders, and particularly to differentiate this group from neurosis, sociopathy (or psychopathy), character disorder, psychosomatic disorder, and mental retardation. Traditionally, the psychoses or *psychotic disorders* are subdivided into:

A. Organic Brain Syndromes
B. Functional Psychoses
  1. Schizophrenias
  2. Affective psychoses (involutional melancholia; manic-depressive psychosis)
  3. Paranoid states
  4. Psychotic depressive reaction

While there might be general agreement that the term psychosis should be used as indicated above in a qualifying sense to refer to a particular group of psychiatric disorders, use of the term in fact has not been so precise or definite. Instead, "psychosis" (and its adjectival form, "psychotic") has often been used in a quantifying sense to indicate severity of disorder; thus a person with the psychosis schizophrenia may be labeled psychotic only at certain times when the symptoms of his disorder reach a certain intensity and/or adversely affect his mental competence.

In the 1968 DSM-II, psychosis was defined in terms of impairment of mental functioning of such degree as to interfere grossly with the capacity to meet the ordinary demands of life. D.F. Klein and J.M. Davis (*Diagnosis and Drug Treatment of Psychiatric Disorders,* 1969) define psychosis as "persistent misevaluation of perception not attributable to sensory defect or afferent abnormality and not accounted for on the basis of special social indoctrination or unusual life experience." See *psychotic.*

As a result of conflicting usage, there is no single acceptable definition of what psychosis is. In general, however, the disorders labeled psychoses differ from the other groups of psychiatric disorders in one or more of the following:

1. *Severity*—the psychoses are "major" disorders that are more severe, intense, and disruptive; they tend to affect all areas of the patient's life (in Adolph Meyer's terms, a psychosis is a *whole-reaction* rather than a *part-reaction*).

2. *Degree of withdrawal*—the psychotic patient is less able to maintain effective object relationships; external, objective reality has less meaning for the patient or is perceived in a distorted way.

3. *Affectivity*—the emotions are often qualitatively different from the normal, at other times are so exaggerated quantitatively that they constitute the whole existence of the patient.

4. *Intellect*—intellectual functions may be directly involved by the psychotic process so that language and thinking are

disturbed; judgment often fails; hallucinations and delusions may appear.

5. *Regression*—there may be generalized failure of functioning and a falling back to very early behavioral levels; such regression is more than a temporary lapse in maturity and may include a return to early and even primitive patterns.

psychosis, accidental *Rare.* Organic psychosis.

psychosis, acute shock An acute psychiatric disturbance occurring during war. Its most prominent symptoms are a completely unconscious state (with flaccid limbs and closed eyes), lasting from minutes to hours; insensitivity to pain with no reaction to external stimuli; the eyelids flutter, the eyeballs are mobile and are rolled outward and upward. The condition occurs most commonly during active warfare, especially on forced marches and in active campaigns. See *psychorrhexis.*

psychosis, affective A general term used to refer to any of those psychoses whose prominent feature is a disturbance in mood or emotion, viz. manic-depressive psychosis and involutional melancholia. See *affective disorders.*

psychosis, akinetic Wernicke's term for that extreme of catatonia that is marked by stupor, attonita, and cerea flexibilitas. Flexor action of the musculature predominates, and movement may be reduced almost to zero. At the other extreme of catatonia is the hyperkinetic motor psychosis, which corresponds to what is currently termed catatonic excitement.

psychosis, alcoholic Korsakoff When associated with alcoholism, the *Korsakoff psychosis* is also known as *chronic alcoholic delirium.* Some authors also refer to it as *chronic delirium tremens,* because the syndrome frequently follows (acute) delirium tremens. Bleuler says that "the Korsakov psychosis in the majority of cases begins with a delirium tremens that recedes somewhat slowly and leaves behind the organic syndrome." The basic symptom picture includes memory defects, confabulations, impairment of apperception and attention, disorientation, ideational and affective disorders, in addition to such physical symptoms as are associated with general neuritis (pains, paralyses, atrophies, etc.). (*TP*) See *syndrome, Wernicke-Korsakoff.*

psychosis, alternating The circular form of manic-depressive psychosis in which manic episodes alternate with depressive episodes in the same patient. This form was originally described by Falret, Jr. as *folie circulaire.* It is not as common as either the recurrent depressive or the recurrent manic type of manic-depressive psychosis. See *psychosis, manic-depressive.*

psychosis, arteriosclerotic Organic brain syndrome associated with cerebral arteriosclerosis; *multi-infarct dementia.* See *arteriosclerosis, cerebral.* The term cerebral arteriosclerosis refers to degenerative changes in the arteries of the brain, the most important causes of which are (1) primary degeneration of the intima; (2) degeneration secondary to high blood pressure; (3) endarteritis (usually syphilis); (4) thromboangiitis obliterans; (5) polyarteritis nodosa or periarteritis nodosa, and (6) temporal arteritis. The effect of progressive occlusion of the cerebral blood vessels is an impairment of circulation in the regions they supply. As a result of this, impairment of cerebral function occurs before any vessel is completely blocked.

Pathologically, the primary and most important changes are in the elastic tissues, especially in the internal elastic membrane of the cerebral arterioles. Two main types of elastic alterations are seen, hyperplastic and hypoplastic degeneration. Focal parenchymatous changes in the brain tend to be associated with hyperplastic degeneration, while gross hemorrhagic softenings are more prevalent in the hypoplastic type. The hyperplastic type tends to be associated with focal neurologic symptoms; the hypoplastic type shows predominantly mental symptoms.

The onset of the disease is often insidious, and its course is slowly progressive. Mental symptoms consist of a general reduction in intellectual capacity with memory impairment and emotional instability. The patient becomes self-centered and hostile to change in all forms. In more severe cases, loosely constructed delusions occur, often with a paranoid coloring. Depression is not uncommon and there may be attacks of confusion. Still greater deterioration leads to a profound dementia.

Neurologic symptoms include epileptiform attacks, various forms of aphasia, agnosia, and apraxia, signs of pyramidal tract lesions, senile tremor, athetosis, parkinsonism, and often some degree of visual impairment.

psychosis, autistic See *psychosis, symbiotic infantile.*

psychosis, barbed wire A psychosis reported in prisoners of war, characterized by irritability and loss of memory for prewar occurrences.

psychosis, borderline See *borderline psychosis.*

psychosis, buffoonery A form of hyperkinetic catatonia (catatonic excitement) in which the patient constantly makes disconnected caricatured grimaces and gestures. This psychosis probably represents a flight into disease as an escape from reality. "One has the impression that these patients want to play the buffoon, though they do this in a most awkward and inept fashion. They contrive any number of stupidities and sillinesses, such as beating their own knees, interchanging pillows for blankets when they go to bed, pouring water out on the floor instead of into a cup, lifting doors off their hinges. The patients will do all this while they are seemingly well oriented. As a rule they speak very little or not at all and what they have to say is, in the main, completely illogical cursing or other nonsense. Undoubtedly the 'faxen-psychosis' has an origin similar to that of the Ganserian twilight state. It usually involves individuals who for some unconscious reason pretend to be mentally deranged." (Bleuler, E. *Dementia Praecox or the Group of Schizophrenias,* 1950) See *factitious disorders; syndrome, Ganser.*

psychosis, circular See *mania; psychosis, manic-depressive.*

psychosis, circulatory Confused mental state associated with cardiovascular failure.

psychosis, climacteric Any psychotic reaction associated with the climacterium or "change of life." See *psychosis, involutional.*

psychosis, collective Psychic defensive mechanisms utilized by an entire group in adapting to other cultures and societies. Freud's instinctual theories recognized two basic drives, sex and aggression. Freud felt that people's aggressive trends lead them and their culture to fatal conflicts. Human aggressiveness within a cul-

ture is diverted to people outside that culture's psychic mass. This diversion of hostile trends implies a process of projection of the superego's aggressive component, so that an individual's hostility can be ascribed to other groups. Flescher thinks that this paranoid projection is inherent in the formation of the mass and constitutes the collective psychosis.

Perhaps the best demonstration of collective psychosis is given by countries at war. The citizens of each country unite in a concerted effort to destroy the opponent, their previous differences of opinion fade as all espouse a common conviction of right against might, and there is a tendency to view the opposing country as being wrong in every way and to perceive its citizens to be the embodiment of every undesirable human trait.

psychosis, defect *Obs.* Mental retardation; feeblemindedness.

psychosis, defense *Obs.* A general term used by Freud to emphasize the defensive value of a psychosis. He later employed the phrase *defense-neurosis* to express a similar concept in the neuroses.

psychosis, degeneration A group of atypical affective psychoses that show, in addition to the more typical manic-depressive symptoms, periodic hallucinosis, stupor, excitement, and paranoid phases. The term *degeneration* refers to the genetic loading found in families in which such variants occur. See *phasophrenias; psychosis, reactive.*

psychosis, degenerative *Obs.* Any psychosis with regressive tendencies or manifestations; by some, used in a more specific way to refer to organic psychoses with irreversible dementia.

psychosis, exhaustive *Collapse delirium.* Binswanger subdivides exhaustive psychosis as follows: *exhaustion stupor; exhaustive amentia; delirium acutum exhaustivum.* See *delirium, collapse.*

psychosis, febrile *Obs.* Infective-exhaustive psychosis.

psychosis, functional See *functional.*

psychosis, "furlough" An episode of the acute schizophrenic type secondary to the sudden emotional readjustments required by a military furlough or leave. Dynamically, the outbreak of the psychotic behavior seems to be related to the sudden release of the soldier from military authority, on which he has become dependent. Symptoms appear suddenly a few days after the apparently well-adjusted person has returned home. Affect becomes inappropriate, delusional trends and ideas of reference are prominent, and suicidal tendencies are frequent. In the ensuing week or two, severe confusion with blocking of thought processes becomes marked. Gradual improvement occurs within two months, irrespective of any particular form of therapy. The patient cannot return to duty, because flattening of affect and unpredictable behavior usually remain. (*American Journal of Psychiatry 102*, 1945–46)

psychosis, gestational *Obs.* Psychosis developing during pregnancy.

psychosis, governess "For decades, the idea has been preserved that governesses were especially prone to develop schizophrenia. Some authors even spoke of a 'governess-psychosis'; and it has even been maintained that' governesses suffer a particularly severe (and unpleasant) form of the disease." (Bleuler, E. *Dementia Praecox or the Group of Schizophrenias*, 1950) Statistics do not, in fact, indicate that the incidence of schizophrenia is higher in governesses than in other vocations.

psychosis, housewife's See *neurosis, housewife's.*

psychosis, hysterical See *hysteria; hysterical psychosis.*

psychosis, iatrogenic See *iatrogeny.*

psychosis, idiophrenic *Obs.* Organic psychosis.

psychosis, infective-exhaustive *Obs.* An older term for acute brain syndrome associated with systemic infection; also known as acute toxic encephalopathy, acute toxic encephalitis, or acute serous encephalitis.

psychosis, influenced Gordon's term for psychosis of association. See *association, psychosis of.*

psychosis, invocational A rare psychotic reaction to incantations, prayers, etc., such as is sometimes seen in revival meetings.

psychosis, involutional Climacteric psychosis; *involutional melancholia;* involutional psychotic reaction; *agitated depression* of middle life—all these terms are used more or less interchangeably to refer to depressive psychoses appearing during the involutional period (40 to 55 years for women,

50 to 65 years for men) in people who have no history of previous mental illness. See *anxietas praesenilis.* Characteristically, such depressions manifest a triad of symptoms, consisting of delusions of sin and guilt and/or of poverty, an obsession with death, and a delusional fixation on the gastrointestinal tract, all in a setting of agitation and dejection. In some (involutional paranoid state), a fourth major symptom is present in self-referential or persecutory delusions, and this second group with a vivid admixture of paranoid symptoms has a poorer prognosis than the more purely depressive variety. Concern over finances, physical illness, bereavement, enforced retirement, and "loss" of children to marriage or other forms of independence are frequent precipitants. Involutional psychoses account for 5–10% of first admissions to mental hospitals; their actual incidence is difficult to estimate because many respond favorably to antidepressant drugs or to electroconvulsive therapy administered on an outpatient basis.

psychosis, juvenile A psychosis occurring between the ages of 15 and 25, approximately; sometimes used, incorrectly, as synonymous with schizophrenia. All psychoses occur in this age group, and because schizophrenia is the most common of the psychoses, it is also the most common in this age group. But there is no characteristic juvenile psychosis or psychosis typical for the age of puberty.

psychosis, Korsakoff (Sergei Sergeevich Korsakoff, Russian neurologist, 1854–1900) A chronic brain disorder that may arise as a toxic complication of any chronic brain disease, but probably associated more often with brain damage due to alcoholism than with any other single entity. In approximately half of those affected there is an associated polyneuritis, but the characteristic mental symptom is *confabulation* (q.v.). The patient develops a marked memory retention defect and is unable to integrate new material into his memory; he fills the memory gaps with his confabulations. Often, in addition, grandiose delusions and emotional incontinence appear, and although the former may subside some degree of emotional lability generally persists. See *syndrome, Wernicke-Korsakoff.*

psychosis, malignant Fenichel's term for that type of schizophrenia which is progressive (slowly or rapidly) and terminates in permanent dementia. He contrasts these malignant psychoses with schizophrenic episodes that are temporary attacks in persons who are apparently well both before and after their psychotic episode.

The question arises whether these two general types of schizophrenia can have anything in common. Fenichel believes that both the malignant *schizophrenia process* and the shorter term *schizophrenic episode* have certain common features. These are "the bizarrity of the symptoms, the absurdity and unpredictability of the affects and intellectual ideas and the obviously inadequate connection between these two." Moreover, the symptoms in both types can be explained by the concept of regression of the ego to a much deeper level than in the neurosis, i.e. to the time of "primary narcissim" when "the ego was not yet established or had just begun to be established." Apparently no factors, of either an organic or a psychogenic nature, have yet been discerned that might explain the different courses taken by these different types of schizophrenic illness. (*PTN*) See *schizophreniform*.

The term *malignant psychosis* is approximately equivalent to the terms *process psychosis* and *nuclear schizophrenia,* and to *dementia praecox* as used by contemporary European psychiatrists.

psychosis, manic-depressive A term introduced by Kraepelin in 1896 to differentiate between those psychoses that typically progress to profound dementia (dementia praecox, or the group of schizophrenias) and those that do not lead to a true deterioration (manic-depressive psychosis). The term thus came to include periodic and circular insanity, simple mania, melancholia, and many types of confusion or delirium. Although involutional melancholia was later included in the manic-depressive group, until recently (in DSM-III) the tendency in both the United States and Great Britain has been to keep the involutional group separate; and in many classificatory schemes, involutional melancholia and manic-depressive psychosis are considered the two major subdivisions of the broader category of affective psychoses. See *affective disorders.*

Manic-depressive psychosis accounts for 5–15% of the total first admissions to mental hospitals in the United States; it occurs more frequently in women, who account for approximately 70% of cases, and is more common among Jews than is any other mental illness. Kallmann estimates that the general average frequency of manic-depressive psychosis does not exceed 0.4%; but the expectancy in half-siblings is approximately 17%, in siblings and in parents approximately 23%, in dizygotic co-twins approximately 26%, and in one-egg twin partners approximately 100%. These numbers are based upon fairly strict diagnostic criteria; Kallmann used as manic-depressive subjects only those whose illness is cyclic, with periodicity of acute, self-limited mood swings, onset before the fifth decade, and with no progressive or residual personality disintegration before or after psychotic episodes of elation or depression. Reactive and situational depressions, hallucinatory episodes, and agitated anxiety states associated with hypertension are excluded. Primary menopausal and presenile depressions and other nonperiodic forms of depressive behavior in the involutional period are placed in the category of involutional psychosis. Kallmann concludes: "The recurring ability to exceed the normal range of emotional responses with extreme but self-limited mood alterations seems to be associated with a specific neurohormonal disturbance, which depends on the mutative effect of a single dominant gene with incomplete penetrance. The dynamics identified with this specific ability cannot be considered to be part of a person's normal biological equipment nor are they out of line with current concepts of psychodynamic phenomena as observed in potentially vulnerable persons." (Kallmann, F. J., in *Depression,* ed. P.H.Hoch & J. Zubin, 1954)

Clinically, manic-depressive psychosis may appear in any of several forms: as a depressive episode in varying degrees of severity (simple depression or simple retardation, acute depression, and, according to some, depressive stupor, although many feel that this latter form is always a manifestation of catatonic schizophrenia);

or as an elated or manic episode in varying degrees of severity (simple mania or hypomania, acute mania, and delirious mania, the latter being also known as Bell's mania, typhomania, delirium grave, and collapse delirium). A fourth type of mania, chronic mania, has also been described; the symptoms here are of the same degree as acute mania, but they continue uninterruptedly for an indefinite number of years.

Some manic-depressive patients have only manic attacks throughout their lives (recurrent mania); others have only depressive episodes (recurrent depressions), and in a few the circular or alternating form is seen: a continuous alteration for years between states of depression and states of elation. In addition to these types, Kraepelin described a number of mixed states (e.g. maniacal stupor, unproductive mania), but closer scrutiny usually reveals these to be types of schizophrenic episodes. See *depression, unipolar; melancholia; suicide.*

psychosis, model Experimental psychosis and, particularly, such as is produced by mescaline or lysergic acid or similar psychotomimetic drugs.

psychosis, monosymptomatic See *dysmorphophobia.*

psychosis, motility A type of manic-depressive psychosis described by Ewald; symptoms are mainly hyperkinetic in character, and the episode often occurs only once in a lifetime, with complete remission.

psychosis, motor See *psychosis, sensory.*

psychosis of association See *association, psychosis of.*

psychosis of degeneracy *Obs.* That class of psychoses intimately associated with the environment, in contradistinction to the so-called real psychoses in which the environment plays no essential role.

psychosis, organic See *syndrome, organic.*

psychosis, perplexity A subdivision of manic-depressive psychosis, characterized by marked distress that goes with subjective perplexity. Hoch and Kirby first described this type in 1919.

psychosis, polyneuritic Korsakoff's psychosis. See *syndrome, Wernicke-Korsakoff.*

psychosis, postinfectious Mental disturbances may follow such acute diseases as influenza, pneumonia, typhoid fever, and acute rheumatic fever in their postfebrile period or may occur during the period of convalescence. These mental disturbances may be observed as mild forms of confusion, or suspicious, irritable, depressive reactions. Occasionally states of mental enfeeblement occur following such acute infectious diseases.

psychosis, prison *Stir-fever;* a mental disorder precipitated by anticipated or actual incarceration; the form of psychiatric syndrome depends on the type of person affected; thus a prison psychosis may resemble or be a schizophrenic, manic-depressive, or psychoneurotic disorder. See *syndrome, Ganser.*

psychosis, private Used by Ferenczi as a synonym of *neurotic character,* because as he says, it is tolerated by the ego.

psychosis, process The malignant type of schizophrenic psychosis that terminates in permanent dementia. It has always been recognized that schizophrenic phenomena have many diverse manifestations: there are the passing schizophrenic episodes in persons who apparently are well both before and after these periods; then, there are the severe psychoses that sooner or later end in permanent dementia. All the schizophrenic manifestations, however, have the common features of queer and bizarre symptoms, absurd and unpredictable affects and intellectual ideas, and the obviously inadequate connection between these two.

The question arises whether there is any etiological basis for differentiating schizophrenic episodes and schizophrenic processes. Some authors have felt that schizophrenic episodes result from traumata and impediments in early infantile life, whereas the process psychosis is due to unknown organic factors. Fenichel feels, however, that there is no basis for such a differentiation and that both psychogenic influences and organic disposition are contributory causes in the majority of cases. Certainly the prognosis in the "process" type of cases (in which there has been slow chronic development of the disease) is very poor. The prognosis is better in the acute cases, because some of them recover quickly and entirely. This is especially true of the cases in which the episode is the reaction to an acute and severe frustration or narcissistic hurt. (*PTN*) See *psychosis, malignant; schizophreniform.*

"The European tendency is to use the term nuclear or process schizophrenia, or dementia praecox, to refer to unquestionable cases with a high tendency to deterioration and little tendency to remission or recovery. The others are called by Ruemke the pseudoschizophrenias, by Lunn (Denmark) the schizophreniform psychoses. The nuclear types may or may not show the accessory symptoms of Bleuler (delusions, hallucinations, etc.), but the fundamental symptoms are prominent. In the other types, the accessory symptoms are in the foreground and the fundamental symptoms may not be readily apparent. As Bleuler pointed out, the accessory symptoms are not diagnostic of schizophrenia for they occur also in many other disorders, especially in the organic group." (Campbell, R.J. *Psychiatric Quarterly 32,* 1958) See *psychosis, reactive.*

psychosis, progressive Same as *psychosis, process.*

psychosis, protest A short-lived reactive schizophreniclike psychosis described among black prisoners charged with aggressive crimes. Onset is abrupt, following arraignment or indictment. Symptoms include mutism, destructiveness, incoherence, bizarre utterances and mannerisms, and auditory or visual hallucinations. W. Bromberg, F. Simon, and T.A. Pasto labeled the reaction *protest psychosis* because it contained elements of African and Muslim ideology and anti-Caucasian hostility related to white domination of nonwhites (*Israel Annals of Psychiatry and Related Disciplines 10,* 1972).

psychosis, puberty *Obs.* Adolescent psychosis; the term implied a condition unique to puberty, but it is now recognized that such a condition does not exist.

psychosis, puerperal Postpartum psychosis; any psychosis associated with the puerperium (the period from the termination of labor to the complete involution of the uterus). There is no single psychiatric condition that occurs during this period, and except for those states that are definitely connected with organic disorders, there is nothing in the puerperium as such that gives rise to a psychosis. The expression puerperal psychosis has about the same

weight as that given to *pregnancy psychosis, lactation psychosis,* etc.

psychosis, purpose While all psychiatric states serve a purpose, usually an unconscious one, there are some (such as the Ganser syndrome) whose motives are quite clear-cut. "The maximum of wish fulfillment is achieved by the ecstasies. These syndromes are also called *purpose psychoses.*" (Bleuler, *TP*)

psychosis, reactive When a psychosis is believed to be instigated principally by an environmental condition, it is designated as a *reactive* or *situational* psychosis.

"One class of the psychoses shows itself as a morbid reaction to an affect experience, as a prison psychosis to a confinement, and an hysterical twilight state to a jilting on the part of the beloved (*reactive psychoses, situation psychoses*)." (Bleuler, *TP*)

Currently, the term is often used to refer to functional psychoses that are neither schizophrenic nor primarily affective and/or to schizophrenic "episodes" with a good prognosis (in contrast to process or nuclear schizophrenia). Such psychoses with favorable outcome and little genetic evidence of any major relationship to schizophrenia are described under various labels: *schizophreniform states* (G. Langfeldt; Lunn), the *pseudo-schizophrenias* (Ruemke), *acute delusional psychoses* or *bouffées délirantes* (by the French), *cycloid psychoses* (K. Leonhard), *atypical psychoses* (Mitsuda), and the *acute schizophrenia reactions* within the schizophrenia spectrum described by S. Kety. See *psychosis, process.*

psychosis, schizoaffective A subtype of schizophrenia in which manic or melancholic symptoms are prominent. The affective symptoms are often so pronounced in the early stages as to mask the underlying schizophrenic process, and such cases account for the majority of diagnoses of manic-depressive psychosis in children and adolescents. Later in the course of the disease, however, the affective symptoms tend to abate as the schizophrenic elements become more obvious. Such cases usually end in hebephrenic or simple deterioration.

In DSM-III, *schizoaffective disorder* is included in the group "Psychotic Disorders Not Elsewhere Classified" along with schizophreniform disorder, brief reactive psychosis, and atypical psychosis. Schizoaffective disorders are those conditions in which the clinician cannot decide with certainty whether they are *affective disorders*, on the one hand, or *schizophreniform disorders* or *schizophrenia*, on the other.

psychosis, schizophreniform See *psychosis, process; psychosis, reactive.*

psychosis, senile See *senile dementia.*

psychosis, sensory Bucknill and Tuke suggested that mental disorders be divided into two large classes, called sensory psychoses and motor psychoses. The former were to include all forms of psychiatric syndromes in which feeling, emotion, sensory perception, and ideation predominated. The latter would comprise those reactions characterized by disorders in the intellectual and motor spheres. The classification (suggested in the latter half of the 19th century) was not adopted.

psychosis, septicemia An acute organic psychosis due to severe infection and characterized mainly by a delirium. Nosologically, this condition belongs to the toxic psychoses (deliria) associated with toxic-infectious diseases, and would today be classified as organic brain syndrome associated with systemic infection, with psychosis.

psychosis, shock A particular type of mental reaction observed in soldiers overcome by shock or fright in combat. Many of the soldiers who were picked up immediately after the shock and sent to a hospital had initial anxious deliriums, during which they regarded everything in the environment as hostile, and anybody who approached them excited violent fear reactions. Wild motor activity with mutism, depression, and disturbances of sleep sometimes followed.

"The most common form of this psychosis was perhaps the acute, passive, negativistic stupor, with mutism, complete immobility, total anesthesia, inability to take food, incontinence, total unconsciousness at first and cloudy states later, and inability to stand or walk. These patients had gradually to relearn sphincter control and the enunciation of words; at first they said only 'yes' and 'no' and then answered to their names. Very gradually they were taught how to grasp objects and how to feed themselves. Familiarity with the environ-

ment was also regained slowly; some time elapsed before these patients began to take an interest in their destiny. Of interest is the fact that most of them were able to recall the traumatic event; they remembered some details of their behavior such as making certain efforts to save themselves just before they lost consciousness. Gaupp reported a patient with no recollection of the accompaniments of the exploding shell which caused him to lose consciousness. This observation is important, because the psychic experience—the feelings and ideas excited by the explosion—called forth the powerful action of the entire organism, that is, unconsciousness and other symptoms of fright, as a defense against it. Gaupp believes that, between the moment of the explosion and the following psychic disturbance, an interval exists during which the perception of the effects of the explosion, the sight of mutilated comrades, and the excitation of fright aggravate the reaction to the trauma.

"Patients in fright stupor were not always passive and without feeling. Very frequently they shouted in their stupor: 'The enemy is coming!' 'They are coming!' 'Get em!' 'Fight em!' " (Kardiner, A., & Spiegel, H. *War Stress and Neurotic Illness,* 1947)

psychosis, situational See *psychosis, reactive.*

psychosis, somatic Dunbar's term for the somatic expression of tension, aggression, and resentment in diabetic patients. "Much of the aggression and resentment in these patients seems to have been driven inward in a manner which suggests patients with rheumatic heart disease, but they have not given in so much to the passive masochistic role. In addition to being expressed in tension of striated and smooth musculature, it gnaws at their vitals, and, probably because of their infantile regression and extreme ambivalence, brings about what might be called a *somatic psychosis.*" (*Psychosomatic Diagnosis,* 1943)

psychosis, symbiotic infantile Mahler's term for a disturbance seen in certain children at the time when separation from the mother would ordinarily be effected. Under the threat of separation, the symbiotic child's rage and panic are projected into the world, which is perceived as hostile and destructive. The child defends himself by maintaining or restoring the infantile delusion of omnipotence and oneness with the mother, by means of omnipotence phantasies, introjection, projection, delusions, and hallucinations.

Mahler differentiates between the symbiotic psychosis and the autistic psychosis. The latter arises in a child with a constitutionally defective ego anlage and thus the symbiotic mother-infant relationship is interfered with from the beginning. Autism is used as a major defense against external stimuli and inner excitations. See *anxiety, separation; depression, anaclitic.*

psychosis, symptomatic Brain dysfunction as a result of some general physical disease, the most common feature of which is a delirious state. This may occur in the course of an acute infectious disease such as pneumonia, influenza, typhoid fever, meningitis, or in the course of acute chorea, pellagra, or pelvic infections following childbirth.

psychosis, tardive See *dysmentia, tardive.*

psychosis, toxic Organic brain syndromes due to intoxication.

psychosis, toxic-infectious Mental condition accompanying or following an infective illness or poisoning by some exogenous toxin. The symptoms include delirium, dazed and stuporous conditions, epileptiform attacks, hallucinoses, incoherence, and confusion. Examples of diseases that may produce this reaction type include influenza, malaria, acute rheumatic fever, pneumonia, typhoid and typhus fever, smallpox, and scarlet fever.

psychosis, transitory A syndrome "characterized by emotional turmoil, various kinetic phenomena, and dissociation with confusion and hallucinations, followed by complete recovery and amnesia" for the episode. (Kasanin, J. *American Journal of Psychiatry 93,* 1936–37)

psychosis, traumatic Mental disorder caused by or associated with brain injury, often manifested as an organic personality syndrome. See *constitution, traumatic; contusion, brain; neurosis, traumatic; organic mental disorders; post-traumatic and postencephalitic syndromes, classification of; post-traumatic stress disorder.*

psychosis, zoophil *Obs.* A psychosis marked by morbid affection for or interest in animals.

psychosocial Referring to psychological attributes of subjects or their social environment that play a contributory role in the onset, course, or treatment of their disorder(s).

psychosocial dwarfism See *dwarfism, deprivational.*

psychosocial retardation See *retardation, psychosocial.*

psychosoma The union of physical and psychical components. For example, conversion hysteria comprises psychosomatic phenomena, in that a mental conflict gains outlet through somatic agencies.

Infrequently the term *psychosoma* is condensed into *psysoma.*

psychosomatiatria *Obs.* Medical treatment of mind and body.

psychosomatic This term may be used in a methodological sense only, to refer to a type of approach in the study and treatment of certain disturbances of body function. More commonly, however, the term is used in a nosological or classificatory sense to refer to a group of disorders whose etiology at least in part is believed to be related to emotional factors; in the 1968 revision of psychiatric nomenclature such *psychosomatic disorders* were called *psychophysiologic disorders.*

As used in the second sense, the term psychosomatic is unfortunate, for it implies a dualism that does not exist. No somatic disease is entirely free from psychic influence, just as even in the purest psychic disturbances there are organic-constitutional factors, somatic compliance, etc. While it is generally recognized that many symptoms and diseases occur in the setting of difficult life situations, there is no accepted answer as to why some people get one disease, some get another. Various hypotheses have been put forward: some have tried to show that there is a personality pattern common to all patients with the same disease; others have tried to demonstrate a single personality trait associated with a particular disease; others have maintained that a specific nuclear conflict or dynamic configuration is unique to a particular disease; others have emphasized what has happened to the patient previously, especially in childhood, as in a search for toilet-training problems in patients with intestinal disorders; and, finally, some have tried to correlate the occurrence of particular symptoms with particular life situations. None of the attempts has been wholly satisfactory. Not all patients fit into the pattern they should; many patients show more than one of the illnesses in question, and this is difficult to reconcile with the idea of fixed personality patterns; many patients show the specific dynamic configuration without developing the expected disease; and often there is little similarity between the various situations that provoke recurrences in the same patient.

Physical/organic disorders or symptoms are related to emotions in various ways: acute emotions, such as fright, may induce physiologic changes, such as cardiac arrhythmias, that may be fatal; chronically maintained emotions may induce physiologic changes that over time produce tissue damage ("psychosomatic disorders"); emotions may provoke self-destructive behaviors such as substance abuse, dietary inadequacies, and careless vehicular operation; diseases or their treatments, or both, can arouse intense emotions that secondarily affect the original disease and the patient's cooperation with treatment measures (see *pathocure; pathoneurosis*); emotions that are not permitted release may find symbolic expression in conversion symptoms or somaticization.

Many psychoanalysts (e.g. Fenichel, *PTN*) prefer the term *organ neurosis* to *psychosomatic disorder*. An organ neurosis is defined as a type of functional disorder that is physical in nature and that consists of physiologic changes caused by the inappropriate use of the function in question. Thus organ neuroses and conversion neuroses are quite different—in conversion neuroses, the symptom has a specific unconscious meaning and is an expression of a phantasy in body language; in organ neuroses, the change in function per se has no unconscious meaning, but instead the chronic, unconscious attitudes of the patient have secondarily produced a change in function. In other words, in the organ neuroses a persistent emotional disturbance has secondarily altered the physiology of an organ system; but in the conversion neuroses, a persistent emotional disturbance is directly symbolized by a disturbance in bodily function, and the physiology of the organ system in question need not be altered.

F. Alexander (*Psychosomatic Medicine, Its Principles and Applications,* 1950) maintains the theory of specificity in organ neuroses: physiological responses to emotional stimuli, both normal and morbid, vary according to the nature of the precipitating emotional states. He differentiates two types of organ neuroses, the sympathetic and the parasympathetic. "Whenever the expression of competitive, aggressive, and hostile attitudes is inhibited in voluntary behavior, the sympathetic adrenal system is in sustained excitation. The vegetative symptoms result from the sustained sympathetic excitation, which persists because no consummation of the fight or flight reaction takes place in the field of co-ordinated voluntary behavior, as exemplified by the patient suffering from essential hypertension who in his overt behavior appears inhibited and under excessive control." Besides essential hypertension, the sympathetic group includes migraine and hyperthyroidism. "In those cases in which the gratification of help-seeking, regressive tendencies is absent from overt behavior either because of internal denial of these tendencies or because of external circumstances, the vegetative responses are apt to manifest themselves in dysfunctions which are the results of an increased parasympathetic activity. Examples are the overtly hyperactive, energetic peptic ulcer patient who does not allow gratification of his dependent needs, and the patient who develops chronic incapacitating fatigue whenever he tries to engage in some activity requiring concentrated effort." Bronchial asthma and ulcerative colitis are also in this parasympathetic group.

psychosomatic disorders See *psychophysiologic disorders; psychosomatic.*

psychosomatic medicine An interdisciplinary approach to illness that emphasizes the interaction of medical, psychological, and social factors in the predisposition to, and the development and severity of, organic illnesses and their response to treatment.

At the time of its introduction in the 1930s, psychosomatic medicine was narrowly defined within the traditional medical or psychodynamic model. Alexander's seven "classical" disorders (bronchial asthma, rheumatiod arthritis, ulcerative colitis, hypertension, thyrotoxicosis, peptic ulcer, and migraine) were believed to have psychological determinants. Later, as technology became more sophisticated and experimental designs more rigorous, disease was recognized as being considerably more complex than had been envisioned by earlier writers. Psychosomatic medicine came to include consultation-liaison (C-L) psychiatry and it concerned itself with the diagnosis and treatment of psychiatric and psychosocial problems of the person who entered into the medical care system. Currently, its greatest application is within the areas of primary care and family medicine, where its focus on instrumental ways of influencing symptoms has come to be known as *behavioral medicine*. Its range has broadened from the classical specific diseases to such conditions as pain, cancer, organ transplantation, and eating disorders. Its major functions are psychiatric consultation to patients in medical settings, education of nonpsychiatrist physicians and other health care professionals, and research in both the subject matter of psychosomatic medicine and the processes of consultation and liaison.

psychosomimetic *Psychotomimetic* (q.v.).

psychostimulant See *psychotropics*.

psychosurgery *Functional neurosurgery;* any neurosurgical operation or intervention whose primary aim is to modify emotions or behavior in the absence of known physical disease. The term does not apply to surgical treatment of conditions that are known to cause emotional or behavior disturbances, such as epilepsy or parkinsonism.

psychosynthesis A system of psychology and a group of therapeutic techniques devised by the Italian psychoanalyst Robert Assagioli. He founded the Institute of Psychosynthesis in Rome in 1926; the major expositions of his system are to be found in *Psychosynthesis* (1965) and *The Act of Will* (1973).

Assagioli divided the psyche into the lower unconscious (the personal psychological past), the middle unconscious (where skills, states of mind, and everything that can be brought into the level of consciousness reside), and the supercon-

scious (the source of higher feelings, creativity, ecstasy, inspiration, and our urges to future heroic action). The goal of therapy is to bring together the diverse inner elements of the psyche so they will merge into successively greater wholes rather than compete or clash with one another. Therapeutic techniques include analysis, to assess blocks within the psyche; mastery training, to cultivate coordination of different aspects of the personality; transformation, to encourage reorganization of the personality around a different set of values; meditation, to facilitate exploration of the superconscious; and relational techniques, to foster more openness and better communication with others.

Jung used "constructive" and "synthetic" to differentiate his approach from the "reductive"(psychoanalytic) method.

psychotaxis T.V. Moore's term "to signify the mental adjustments of individuals to pleasant and unpleasant situations. . . . The tendency to enjoy pleasant states of mind or to make use of pleasant emotions and feelings . . . by analogy with the tropism or taxis could be termed a positive psychotaxis. The opposite tendency to avoid unpleasant situations is a negative psychotaxis." (*Psychoanalytic Review* 8, 1921)

psychotechnics The practical application of psychological methods in the study of economics, sociology, and other problems.

psychotherapeusis, -therapeutics *Psychotherapy* (q.v.).

psychotherapy Any form of treatment for mental illnesses, behavioral maladaptations, and/or other problems that are assumed to be of an emotional nature, in which a trained person deliberately establishes a professional relationship with a patient for the purpose of removing, modifying, or retarding existing symptoms, of attenuating or reversing disturbed patterns of behavior, and of promoting positive personality growth and development. See listings under *therapy*.

There are numerous forms of psychotherapy—ranging from guidance, counseling, persuasion, and hypnosis to reeducation and psychoanalytic reconstructive therapy—and many possible applications of each form—including disabling psychosomatic symptoms, interpersonal conflicts and pathologic attitudes secondary to recognizable (organic) disturbance of central nervous system functions, the so-called functional psychoses, character and behavior disorders, psychoneuroses, and marital conflict, to name a few; but in general it may be said that all forms of psychotherapy in all their applications employ the relationship established between patient and therapist to influence the patient to unlearn old and/or maladaptive response patterns and to learn better ones.

Psychotherapy has also been characterized as "an undefined technique applied to unspecified problems with unpredictable outcome; for this technique we recommend rigorous training." (Conference on Graduate Education in Clinical Psychology, 1949) While such a definition may seem so pessimistic as to approach nihilism, it emphasizes what would seem to be an irrefragable fact: despite centuries of its use, and despite decades of study of its various forms, psychotherapy and the means by which it achieves its results are but poorly understood.

"The patient's experience in the therapeutic relationship is assumed to be a sample in microcosm of the significant factors that brought on or related to his problems. Observing the patient's behavior (both verbal and non-verbal), and using his empathic understanding of the patient's behavior in relation to himself, the therapist comments on what he observes. The patient, witnessing the same behavior, and viewing it in the light of the therapist's comments as well as in the light of his own reactions, is now in a position to re-evaluate his own past behavior and to prepare for or begin to change. While all the factors involved in the change are not clear, it is assumed to involve the general principles of learning." (Stein, M.I. *Contemporary Psychotherapies*, 1961)

Because the term psychotherapy has been applied to a variety of dissimilar operations, the phrase *definitive forms of psychotherapy* has been suggested to exclude such procedures as environmental manipulation, general medical treatment as psychotherapy, physical examination as psychotherapy, and all procedures in which more than two people participate. In this sense, psychotherapy is a proce-

dure undertaken in order to foster the acquisition of self-knowledge. "The patient seeks self-knowledge for the purpose of changing his feelings and/or his behavior. The therapist, as participant-observer, fosters learning by decoding and interpreting the patient's unconscious messages. As in all sustained and important relationships, some learning or change also occurs as the result of imitation, identification, and various subtle influences. The situation is not (and cannot be) value-free, but the highest premium is placed on the patient's self-determination." (Hollender, M.H. *Archives of General Psychiatry 10*, 1964)

L.R. Wolberg (*The Technique of Psychotherapy*, 1954) distinguishes three types of psychotherapy: supportive, reeducative, and reconstructive.

1. *Supportive therapy* consists of encouraging or promoting the development of maximal, optimal use of the patient's assets; its objectives are to strengthen existing defenses, elaborate better mechanisms to maintain control, and restore to an adaptive equilibrium. Included in supportive therapy are guidance, environmental manipulation, externalization of interests, reassurance, pressure and coercion, persuasion, catharsis, desensitization, and inspirational group therapy. (It might be noted that in psychoanalysis the term *reassurance* has a slightly different meaning: any method of reducing or removing anxiety other than interpretation.)

2. *Reeducative therapy*, which aims at giving the patient insight into the more conscious conflicts, with deliberate efforts at goal modification and maximal utilization of existing potentialities. Included in reeducative therapy are relationship therapy, attitude therapy, psychobiology, counseling, reconditioning, and reeducative group therapy.

3. *Reconstructive therapy*, which aims at giving the patient insight into his unconscious conflicts and extensive alteration of his character structure. Included in reconstructive therapy are psychoanalysis (Freudian), Adlerian and Jungian therapy, the treatment techniques of the cultural-interpersonal school (Sullivan, Horney), and psychoanalytically oriented psychotherapy.

Another way of classifying the many different forms of psychotherapy is according to the recipient or target of treatment, as in individual psychotherapy, group psychotherapy, family therapy, marital therapy, divorce therapy, etc.

Psychotherapy may also be classified in terms of the theory espoused by the therapist: Freudian, Jungian, Adlerian, Kleinian, Rogerian client-centered therapy, behavior, body-centered, cognitive, existential, Gestalt, multimodal, paradoxical, transactional, transpersonal, Yoga, etc.

psychotherapy, active analytical See *analysis, active.*

psychotherapy, analytic group See *psychotherapy, group.*

psychotherapy, brief Any form of *psychotherapy* (q.v.) designed to produce therapeutic change within a minimal amount of time (generally not more than 20 sessions). The term sometimes refers to treatment lasting up to a year, with a frequency of one or two sessions per week. Brief psychotherapy is usually active and directive; it is most clearly indicated with well-defined symptoms and/or with specific, limited goals.

Also known as *short-term therapy,* brief psychotherapy is typically circumscribed, focused, action-oriented, concerned with immediate crises and with ways of dealing with the social unit or matrix of which the patient is a part. "Basic principles which are generally adhered to include early formulation of the problem, focusing, bypassing areas of resistance, and accepting, indeed sometimes strengthening defenses rather than challenging them." (Barten, H. H. *Brief Therapies,* 1971) The success of short-term therapy appears to be related to the following variables: easy accessibility to permit speedy restoration of equilibrium; modifying therapy techniques in accordance with the shifting needs of the patient and trials of different modalities when patient fails to improve; and maximal utilization of ancillary persons and agencies (*community supportive network*).

J. Burke, H. White, and L. Havens divide the principal types of short-term dynamic psychotherapy into (1) *interpretive*—which stresses insight produced by the therapist's interpretations; (2) *corrective*—where the therapist is more active, directive, and manipulative; and (3) *existential*—where pressure is exerted by limiting time and through an increase in the therapist's empathy.

psychotherapy, brief and emergency (BEP) A form of short-term, intensive psychotherapy developed by L. Bellak as an extension of his experience with the emergency psychotherapy of depression and with crisis intervention in a walk-in clinic. Based on dynamic psychotherapy and particularly on ego psychology, intensive brief and emergency psychotherapy is systematic, focused, and highly conceptualized. It is usually limited to five sessions.

psychotherapy by reciprocal inhibition See *behavior theory.*

psychotherapy, cooperative See *psychotherapy, multiple.*

psychotherapy, didactic group A strictly tutorial practice in which definite outlines, texts, and visual aids are used for teaching patients in special subjects.

psychotherapy, family A form of treatment (for the most part confined to therapy of schizophrenics) in which all members of the family attend all psychotherapy sessions together. Family psychotherapy is based on the hypothesis that the patient's psychosis is a symptom manifestation of a problem involving all members of the family. (Bowen, M., in *Schizophrenia—An Integrated Approach,* ed. A. Auerback, 1959) Bowen and his coworkers find that the father, the mother, and the patient (the *interdependent triad*) are the primary members involved. These investigators have further noted that in all their schizophrenic families there is a striking emotional distance between the parents (*emotional divorce*) that is maintained by a combination of controlled positiveness and physical distance. In such families, both parents are immature and true family teamwork is never possible. Instead, one parent will seize authority and make decisions for himself and his spouse, forcing the latter into a submissive, helpless role. This pattern has been termed *overadequate-inadequate reciprocity.*

psychotherapy, group A method of treating emotional disturbances, social maladjustments, and psychotic states in which two or more patients participate simultaneously in the presence of one psychotherapist or more.

The techniques in group psychotherapy vary to a great extent in accordance with the different schools of psychiatric thought and the preferences of individual psychiatrists and other psychotherapists. Slavson (*IGT*) separates group psychotherapy under three major categories: activity, analytic, and directive.

1. *Activity group therapy,* which he originated, is suitable for children in latency. Children selected by criteria he had described are given the opportunity to act out their aggressions or withdrawal in the presence of a neutral, permissive, and understanding adult. The patients draw upon one another for support. The accessibility of the patients to each other and to the environment, and their interaction, generate certain inhibitive controls that improve the superego formation and strengthen the ego of each participant. Slavson believes that this type of therapy is predominantly ego therapy and is an experience in which character changes occur. He therefore recommends selecting patients on the basis of these two factors. No interpretation is given to the children and a minimal restraint of their behavior is exercised by the therapist and, at that, only when the group cannot bring itself under control.

2. *Analytic group psychotherapy* is a technique in which interpretation is given to the patients, activity and verbalization are encouraged and interpreted, and insight is evoked. In this technique the therapist is more active than he is in activity group psychotherapy, where he is predominantly a passive agent. Slavson divides analytic group psychotherapy into three subdivisions: play group psychotherapy; activity-interview group psychotherapy; and interview psychotherapy. *Play group psychotherapy* is suitable for young children in the prelatency period, where the catharsis occurs through play with specially selected materials through which the children in the group can act out their preoccupations, phantasies, and anxieties. *Activity-interview group psychotherapy* has been designed by him for children in latency who suffer from severe psychoneuroses, who are given the opportunity to act out against each other and against their environment as in activity group psychother-

apy, but interpretation of the latent meaning of the behavior is given by the children to each other and by the therapist. Spontaneous and planned discussions are held with individual children or with a number of the children in the group or the group as a whole. These are intended to stimulate understanding by the children of the meaning of their behavior and to evoke insight into the unconscious motivations and phantasies. *Interview group psychotherapy* is intended for adolescents and adults who are selected by definite criteria and are grouped together so that the patients would have a therapeutic effect upon one another. The basic criterion suggested by Slavson is syndrome (not symptom or diagnosis) homogeneity. Other group psychotherapists do not use this criterion but group the patients without any special considerations, provided the patients can accept and gain from a group experience. In analytic group psychotherapy the procedure is the same as in individual psychotherapy. Since the patients are adolescents and adults, the catharsis occurs through verbalization and free association. The psychotherapist here, as in individual treatment, interprets, explores, and helps patients to uncover their repressed, guilt-producing, and anxiety-evoking feelings, attitudes, values, and behavior.

3. *Directive group treatment,* under which Slavson includes such activities as didactic or therapeutically educational group work, particularly with psychotics, group guidance, group counseling, therapeutic recreation, and many other group efforts to help patients, particularly psychotic patients, adjust to their environment.

Group psychotherapy is also synonymous with *group therapy.*

H.G. Whittington (*Clinical Practice in Community Mental Health Centers,* 1972) divides group therapies in relation to *control* and *expectation.* Control refers to the demands made of the patient, the limits imposed on him, and the structuring of the therapy situation. Expectation refers to the assumption that because of the group experience the patient can improve insofar as his feelings, thoughts, or behavior is concerned.

1. Group therapies with a relatively high level of control and expectation in-

clude the following. *In-hospital community meeting,* which is both psychotherapy and sociotherapy; it promotes a sense of shared plight among the participants. *In-hospital small group,* with a lower level of control and higher expectation; often focuses on insight derived from interaction with other patients and staff, on plans for posthospital adjustment. *Child activity group,* with high control and high expectation; helps the child to learn to trust an adult, to resolve conflict by discussion and compromise and to learn culturally valued skills. *Psychodrama,* with moderately high control and very high expectation; expects the patient to reexperience feelings and events and thereby to learn about himself and develop better ways of dealing with himself and others. *Adolescent group therapy,* with high expectation and high control. *Prevocational group,* prepares the patient to look for a job, effectively handle the interview situation, and then function adequately at work.

2. In the high control/low expectation group are the following. *Anaclitic group therapy,* to dampen the intensity of dependency strivings. *Addict and alcoholic groups. Social hour,* a large group after-care session that combines patient government, resocialization, remotivation, and recreation therapy as a way to encourage interpersonal relationships and minimize regression. *Boarding home group counseling.*

3. In the low control/high expectation group are the following. *Postemployment group,* for the patient moving from the prevocational group into active employment. *Marital group therapy. Expressive group therapy. T-group, sensitivity, and encounter groups,* typically to increase the quality of "humanness" in essentially normal people. *Family therapy.*

4. The *drop-in lounge* is a type of low expectation/low control situation; the patient consults with the staff member on duty if he experiences some adaptational failure, mixes with others who happen to be in the lounge at the time, etc.

psychotherapy, Morita Introduced by Professor Shoma Morita of Jikei University (Japan) during 1910–20 and said to be particularly effective in neurotic patients with prominent hypochondriacal tendencies. Morita therapy begins with absolute bed rest for four to seven days, during which time the patient may not smoke, read, talk, etc. He may only sleep or suffer and is instructed to accept any experience that might occur. After the first phase, the patient takes on increasingly difficult and tiring work, usually in a communal setting, so that he may learn to work well and behave normally no matter what his symptoms. The patient is thereby trained, with advice and encouragement from his therapist, to accept *phenomenological reality*—a process called *arugamama,* the acceptance of life as it is for him at the moment. (Iwai, H., & Reynolds, D.K. *American Journal of Psychiatry 126,* 1970). See *psychotherapy, Naikan.*

psychotherapy multimodal See *BASIC-ID.*

psychotherapy, multiple Role-divided, three-cornered therapy; cotherapy; cooperative psychotherapy; dual leadership all refer to the use of more than one therapist at one time in individual or group psychotherapy.

psychotherapy, Naikan A form of treatment developed in Japan which uses the subject's guilt to prod him into purposeful action, self-sacrifice, and service to repay his debt to those who have nurtured him and been kind to him. Naikan is said to be particularly effective for alcoholics and criminals. It is sometimes used in combination with Morita therapy. See *psychotherapy, Morita.*

psychotherapy, rational Also known as *rational-emotive therapy (RET);* a type of cognitive behavior therapy in which the patient learns to identify the irrational, self-defeating beliefs, emotions, and attitudes that block the development of potential abilities and provoke conflict with the environment. It is said to have been first used by Albert Ellis in 1955. RET is an action-oriented, problem-solving approach that employs a variety of experiential techniques—including direct confrontation and emotional focusing—to emphasize the person's responsibility for creating his own problems and disturbances in living.

psychotherapy, reconstructive See *psychodynamics, adaptational; psychotherapy.*

psychotherapy, short-contact Treatment of mental disorders, similar to brief psychotherapy, but used in child-guidance clinics when the therapy is of short duration.

psychotherapy, short-term anxiety-provoking (STAPP) A form of brief psychotherapy developed by P. Sifneos in the 1950s for patients with circumscribed problems. STAPP emphasizes systematic selection criteria and outcome studies as a way to assess the validity of its techniques in specific kinds of patients.

psychotherapy, time-limited (TLP) A form of brief psychotherapy developed by J. Mann. It has a strict limit of 12 sessions, and the date of termination is set at the start of treatment. In contrast to the short-term anxiety-provoking therapy of Sifneos, selection criteria are broad and the dynamic focus is on separation and reunion rather than on oedipal issues.

psychotic Showing signs of or having the characteristics of severe mental disorder; afflicted with *psychosis* (q.v.). This term has various meanings, and the reader will ordinarily have to depend on context to determine the specific meaning intended by the author. Sometimes the term is used in a quasilegal sense, in which case it is approximately equivalent to the term insane; or it may refer to a patient in an acute episode of psychosis, without reference to competence or other legal issues; or, less commonly, it may refer to a patient with chronic mental disorder, such as schizophrenia, even though he may not be in an acute phase of psychosis and even though he may not be insane in the legal sense.

In DSM-III, the term denotes the existence of one or more of the following: delusions, hallucinations, incoherence, repeated derailment or loosening of associations, marked poverty of thought, marked illogicality, and grossly disorganized or catatonic behavior.

psychotic disorder See *psychosis*.

psychotica See *psychotomimetic*.

psychotogenic *Psychotomimetic* (q.v.).

psychotoid According to Selling, psychotoid personalities are "individuals who might be classed as very mild cases of some psychosis, by virtue of their symptoms. However, they are not psychotic persons and their symptoms are of long standing without change and do not respond to the same treatment as the true psychoses which have similar but more exaggerated symptoms. They have more insight than psychotics." (*Synopsis of Neuropsychiatry*, 1947)

psychotomimetic Resembling or mimicking naturally occurring psychosis, especially schizophrenia; also known as psychosomimetic, schizomimetic, hallucinogenic. While any number of drugs can produce a psychosis, the term psychotomimetic agent is confined to those substances that produce psychological changes in a high proportion of subjects exposed to the drug without producing the gross impairment of memory and orientation characteristic of the organic reaction type. Among the known psychotomimetics are lysergic acid diethylamide (LSD), mescaline, adrenochrome, harmine, tetrahydrocannabinol, diisopropyl fluorophosphates (DFP), tetraethylpyrophosphate (TEPP), *N*-allylnormorphine, and bufotenin. Such drugs are also known as *phantastica*. See *ergotropic*; *psychotropics*.

psychotoxicomania Toxicomania; drug dependency or addiction.

psychotropics Drugs with an effect on psychic function, behavior, or experience; also known as *phrenotropics*. The term can include a wide variety of pharmacologic agents, but in psychiatry six groups of phrenotropic or psychotropic agents can be differentiated on the basis of clinical efficacy:

1. *Neuroleptics*—also known as *antipsychotics, ataractics, major tranquilizers;* they have antipsychotic and sedative effects; many of them also have neurologic effects, particularly on the extrapyramidal system; included in the group are phenothiazines, butyrophenones, thioxanthenes, reserpine derivatives, benzoquinolizines, and dihydroindolones.

2. *Anxiolytic sedatives*—also known as *minor tranquilizers, psycholeptics, antianxiety agents;* they reduce pathologic anxiety, tension, and agitation without therapeutic effects on disturbed cognitive or perceptual processes; they usually do not produce autonomic or extrapyramidal effects, but they may lower the convulsive threshold and have a high potential for drug dependency; included in the group are meprobamate and derivatives, benzodiazepines, and barbiturates.

3. *Antimanic agents*—lithium.

4. *Antidepressants*—also known as *psychic energizers, thymoleptics;* they reduce pathologic depression; included in the group are

monoamine oxidase inhibitors and imipramine and other tricyclic compounds.

5. *Psychostimulants*—these increase the level of alertness and/or motivation; included are amphetamine, methylphenidate, pipradol, and caffeine.

6. *Psychodysleptics*—also known as *hallucinogens, psychedelics, psychotomimetics;* they produce abnormal mental phenomena, particularly in the cognitive and perceptual spheres; included in the group are D-lysergic acid diethylamide, mescaline, psilocybin, dimethyltryptophan, and cannabis. See *dependency, drug; ergotropic.*

psychralgie (psē-kral′zhē) *Obs.* A morbid state characterized by painful subjective sensations of cold.

psychropophobia Fear of the cold or of anything cold.

psychrotherapy *Obs.* Treatment by the application of cold in any form. It was at one time extensively employed in the form of hydrotherapy as a stimulating agent for inactive or retarded patients, e.g. those with the depressive type of manic-depressive psychosis.

psyoma (sī-sō′mà) *Rare.* Contracted form of *psychosoma.*

PTA 1. Parent-teachers' association. 2. Post-traumatic amnesia, generally considered to be one of the most sensitive and reliable indices of severity of head trauma.

pteronophobia Fear of feathers.

ptosis (tō′sis) Lid-drop See *nerve, oculomotor.*

ptosis, waking A functional paralysis of the upper eyelid, occurring temporarily in the anemic or neurotic person on awaking.

puberal (pubertal) Relating to the age of puberty, extending from the termination of the period of puerilism to the beginning of the adolescent period.

puberism, persistent Condition characterized by hypogenesis and prolongation, or even lifelong persistence, of puberal characteristics. The individual seems an eternal adolescent with incompletely developed secondary sexual characteristics in contrast with the types distinguished by *infantilism* or *juvenilism.*

pubertas praecox Premature puberty. See *macrogenitosomia.*

puberty (puberism) The stage of growth extending from the termination of the puerile to the beginning of the adolescent period. It begins with the acquisition of

secondary sexual characteristics and continues for approximately two or three years thereafter.

puberty, precocious *Macrogenitosomia* (q.v.).

pubescence (pubescency) Puberty.

public health model See *psychiatry, community.*

publishable unit See *LPU.*

pudendum (pudenda, pudibilia) *pl.* Genitals; the private parts.

puella publica *Obs.* (L. "public girl") Hirschfeld's term for a prostitute.

puer aeternus Jung's term for the specific archetype of the eternal youth. See *archetype* (in Jung's psychology), *archetype, mother.*

puerilism Childishness; the stage following infantilism or infantility and followed by the stage of puberism or puberty.

puerilism, hysterical See *pseudodementia, hysterical.*

puerperium The period of time and/or the state of the mother following childbirth. See *psychosis, puerperal.*

pulling, ear Pulling of the ears is believed by Kanner to be a substitute for thumb-sucking; in psychoanalysis it is believed to be a masturbatory equivalent.

pulvinar See *thalamus.*

pump, sodium See *conduction, nerve.*

punch-drunk Martland's term to denote a concussion syndrome observed among pugilists; the symptoms are a reflection of an encephalopathy following repeated concussions. See *dementia, boxer's.*

"The early symptoms of punch-drunk usually appear in the extremities. There may be only an occasional and very slight flopping of one foot or leg in walking, noticeable only at intervals; or a slight unsteadiness in gait or uncertainty in equilibrium. . . . In some cases periods of slight mental confusion may occur as well as distinct slowing of muscular action. . . . Many cases remain mild. . . . In others a very distinct dragging of the leg may develop and with this there is a general slowing down in muscular movements, a peculiar mental attitude characterized by hesitancy in speech, tremors of the hand and nodding movements of the head." (*Journal of the American Medical Association 91,* 1928)

punch-drunkenness A chronic traumatic encephalopathy, occurring frequently in boxers, characterized by deterioration of the personality, impairment of memory, dysarthria, tremor, and ataxia.

puncture, cistern A technique for gaining access to the subarachnoid space by means of introduction of a needle into the cisterna magna. Cistern puncture is performed when lumbar puncture is for some reason impossible; it is also used for the injection of air or opaque media for diagnostic purposes and for the introduction of therapeutic substances. It is contraindicated in cases of tumor or abscess in the posterior fossa, in cases of increased intracranial pressure, and when the cisterna magna is likely to be obliterated by inflammatory adhesions. See *puncture, suboccipital.*

puncture, lumbar A technique for gaining access to the subarachnoid space by means of introduction of a needle into the lumbar cul-de-sac of the subarachnoid space below the termination of the spinal cord at the first lumbar vertebra. Lumbar puncture (LP) is used to obtain cerebrospinal fluid for diagnostic purposes, to relieve increased intracranial pressure, to introduce therapeutic substances or local anesthetics, to introduce air preparatory to encephalography and myelography, and to introduce opaque media for radiography.

puncture, suboccipital Suboccipital or *cisternal puncture* is a procedure introduced by Ayer and his coworkers for determining spinal subarachnoid block and for therapeutic purposes.

"The method consists in withdrawing fluid from the cisterna magna at the base of the brain behind the medulla. With the patient on the side, the head bent forward, the needle is introduced in the midline at a point midway between the external occipital protuberance and the spine of the axis or second cervical vertebra. The needle is directed forward and upward in the direction of the eyes or glabella." (Wechsler, I.S. *Textbook of Clinical Neurology*, 1939) See *puncture, cistern.*

puncture, ventricle A surgical technique for gaining access to the intraventricular space of the lateral ventricles. The principal indications for ventricle puncture are (1) to relieve increased intracranial pressure before operation for intracranial tumor; (2) to inject air for ventriculography; (3) to inject therapeutic substances such as penicillin or streptomycin; (4) to obtain cerebrospinal fluid for diagnostic examination when lumbar or cisternal puncture cannot be performed.

pundning The stereotyped, purposeless searching and grooming behavior of amphetamine abusers; stereotyped and/or compulsive behavior patterns are found in many species when adminstered high doses of amphetamines.

punishment, Midas See *masturbation, compulsive.*

punishment, unconscious need for See *criminal from sense of guilt.*

pupil, Adie's See *pupil, tonic (of Adie).*

pupil, Argyll Robertson (Douglas Argyll Robertson, Scottish physician, 1837–1909) "A usually but not invariably myotic pupil with sound vision that does not respond to light, even in a darkroom, but does to accommodation, and reacts slowly to mydriatics is known as an Argyll Robertson pupil." (Jelliffe & White, *DNS*)

It is usually found in patients with neurosyphilis, although it may appear in other conditions (traumatic brain injury, brain tumor, infectious disorders of the brain, multiple sclerosis, etc.).

pupil, fixed A pupil that does not react to light, to accommodation, or to convergence.

pupil, tonic (of Adie) (William John Adie, British neurologist, 1885–1935) A unilateral condition in which the pupil responds poorly to light and very slowly to convergence.

pupillary reflex The alterations in size of the pupil in response to light, convergence, and accommodation. Certain abnormalities of reaction are associated with lesions affecting portions of the pupillary reflex arc.

pupillotonia Adie's syndrome. See *pupil, tonic.*

puppy-love A state of love in the late adolescent or young adult period, highly romantic in nature, with little stability in the relationship formed, so that the courtship swiftly disintegrates. This is in the nature of a developmental activity, occurring in the course of emotional maturation; another designation for this emotional phenomenon is *calf-love.*

pure line See *line, pure.*

Purkinje cell See *cell, Purkinje; cerebellum*.

pursuit eye movements See *eye movements, pursuit*.

Pussin, Jean-Baptiste (1746–1820?) Superintendent of Hospice de Bicêtre and the originator of the psychological methods that were the basis of *moral treatment* (q.v.). Although Philippe Pinel is ordinarily given credit for the reforms, Pinel himself repeatedly attributed them to Pussin, who left the Bicêtre in 1802 to help Pinel reorganize the Salpêtrière.

putamen (poo-tà′men) See *basal ganglia*.

Putnam, James Jackson (1846–1918) American psychiatrist; Putnam-Dana syndrome (subacute combined degeneration of the spinal cord).

pycnic (pik′nik) See *type, pyknic*.

pycnoepilepsy Repeated slight epileptic seizures.

pycnolepsy *Pyknolepsy* (q.v.).

Pygmalion effect Self-fulfilling prophecy, most commonly used in reference to an assumed effect on students of their teachers' expectations of their abilities or potentialities.

pygmalionism (Pygmalion, the legendary king of Cyprus who fell in love with an ivory statue he had carved and asked Venus to give it life; subsequently, the live statue bore him a daughter) The condition of falling in love with one's own handiwork, sometimes manifested as the author's resentment of the editor who would dare to shorten or modify his work. A paranoid patient demonstrated a more severe form in devising a "perpetual-motion" machine to which he ascribed all masculine attributes. The machine was called "Albert" and was treated as a human being to whom the patient vowed his unqualified love.

The term is sometimes applied to the psychotherapist who assumes that his patient knows little or nothing and must be treated as a child, whose parent (the therapist) always knows best.

The term has also been applied to a fetishist whose sex object was a dressmaker's dummy.

pygmyism The constitutional anomaly characterized by a *dwarfed*, but well-proportioned stature as compared with the average type of the given racial group. It corresponds to the other special forms of microsomia, called *nanosomia primordialis* by Hansemann and *heredofamilial essential microsomia* by E. Levi and occurs in certain peoples as a more or less physiological condition (African bushmen, etc.).

pyknic (pik′nik) Compact, thick-set, round-bodied. See *type, pyknic*.

pyknoepilepsy See *pyknolepsy*.

pyknolepsy (pycnolepsy) A disorder characterized by frequent, brief interruptions in consciousness, and usually discussed in conjunction with epilepsy, although Furstner, Heilbronner, and others, classified it as a hysterical disorder. In children who are otherwise healthy, it occurs as a rule before the age of 7, as frequent, short, and incomplete cloudings of consciousness. The onset is usually abrupt, the disease runs a monotonous course without intellectual deterioration and shows little response to therapy, but the prognosis is generally favorable. During attacks, which may be as frequent as 150 times a day, the eyes turn upward, arms and trunk become somewhat tonic; but pulse and respiration are unaffected, there are no convulsive movements, and spontaneous recovery is common. J.W. Owen and L. Berlinrood (*American Journal of Psychiatry* 98, 1941–42) believe that "pyknolepsy is a form of petit mal epilepsy because of: (1) the similarity in the clinical picture; (2) the electroencephalographic pattern in the active phase showing a wave and spike formation found in petit mal epilespy; (3) the lack of evidence of definite psychogenic factors; (4) the high incidence of epilepsy in families of patients with pyknolepsy as revealed by a study of the literature." Lennox used *pyknoepilepsy* (which is by many considered synonymous with pyknolepsy, or dart and dome dysrhythmia) for the ordinary *petit mal* form of epilepsy (q.v.).

pyknophrasia Thickness of utterance.

pyramid The prominence on the anterior surface of the medulla oblongata where the pyramidal tract decussates. See *tract, pyramidal*.

pyramis See *cerebellum*.

pyrexiophobia Fear of fever.

pyrolagnia Sexual excitement aroused by the sight of conflagrations; erotic pyromania.

pyromania Morbid impulse to set fire to things; the term, however, generally means the actual setting on fire. See *disorders of impulse control*.

"The analysis of many neurotics and the observation of the doings of children show us that 'setting on fire,' the delight in conflagrations, indeed, too, the tendency to incendiarism, is an urethra-erotic character trait. Many incendiarists were excessive bed-wetters. . . . In a collec-tion of criminal cases of incendiarism there were quite a number in which incendiaries set fire to the *beds,* as though to indicate the still active enuristic primitive source of the pyromanic character trait." (Ferenczi, *FCT*)

pyromania, erotic *Pyrolagnia* (q.v.).
pyrophobia Fear of fire. See *pyromania*.
pyrosis Heartburn.

Q

Q-sort A personality rating technique, developed by William Stephenson (1953), in which statements or phrases about those aspects of personality or performance that are relevant to the needs of the person or organization requesting the rating are written on separate cards. The rater (who may be the subject himself) sorts the cards into 11 piles, with those most descriptive of the subject in the first pile, those least descriptive in the last pile. Q-sorts are of particular value for obtaining complex, comprehensive descriptions of a single subject, especially since they permit evaluations by multiple raters whose results can be compared.

QB See *Battery, Quantitative Electrophysiological*.

quadrantanopia, quadrantanopsia See *field defect*.

quadrantic, hemianopia See *field defect*.

quadriplegia Tetraplegia; paralysis affecting the four extremities.

quadruplet One of four children born at the same birth. See *birth, multiple*.

quality assurance Quality assessment; measurement and evaluation of services provided, with particular regard for their effectiveness, efficiency, appropriateness, and acceptability; it is generally understood that such evaluation will trigger corrective or remedial action for services that do not meet the desired standards. Quality assessment comprises such parameters as need for care, appropriateness of length of stay (*LOS*) and of site of treatment, adequacy and timeliness of diagnostic evaluation, appropriateness of treatment, and measures of outcome (*medical audit, medical care evaluation* or *MCE*). See *audit; review*.

quality, determining A term used by Freud in connection with the etiology of hysteria.

He states: "Tracing an hysterical symptom back to a traumatic scene in question fulfills two conditions—if it possesses the required *determining quality* and if we can credit it with the necessary *traumatic power*." (*CP*)

By this he means that a traumatic scene must be sufficient, alone, or more usually through another association, to explain the hysterical symptom. For example, a hysterical symptom of vomiting was attributed to the shock of a railway accident. This derivation of the symptom lacks *determining quality*, although it may be said to possess traumatic power. However, on further analysis this accident woke the memory of another event that had happened previously, during which the patient saw a decomposing corpse, a sight that aroused in her horror and disgust. This connection now supplies the *determining quality* for the hysterical symptom of vomiting. The antecedent experience justifiably gave rise to a high degree of disgust.

quasiaction See *activity, ludic*.

quaternity Any unit composed by the union of four factors; a group of four. In psychiatry, the term quaternity refers to the fact that Jung's system of psychology "is based on an archetype that finds its special expression as 'tetrasomy,' four-foldness—cf. the theory of the four functions, the pictorial arrangement of the four, the orientation according to the four points of the compass, etc. The number four can often be observed in the arrangement of dream contents as well. Probably the universal distribution and magical significance of the cross or the circle divided into four can be explained through the archetypal quality of the quaternity." (Jung, C.G. *The Integration of the Personality*, 1939) "It is a peculiar *lusu naturae* [play of nature] that the principal chemical constituent of the bodily organism is carbon, characterized by four valences; the 'diamond' too is, as is well known, a carbon crystal. Carbon is black; the diamond is 'brightest water.' . . . Such an analogy would be a regrettable lack of intellectual taste if the phenomenon of the four were a mere creation of consciousness and not a spontaneous product of the objective-psychic, of the unconscious." (Ibid.) "It might even be considered more than a mere coincidence that in an epoch which, particularly in consequence of revolutionary discoveries in the domain of the exact natural sciences, stands on the verge of transition from 'three-dimensional' to 'four-dimensional' thinking, the most modern system of depth psychology, the complex-psychology of Jung, taking its start from an altogether different point, has elevated the archetype of the four to the central structural concept of its doctrine." (Jacobi, J. *The Psychology of C.G. Jung,* 1942)

querulent Ever suspicious, always opposing any suggestion, complaining of ill-treatment and of being slighted or misunderstood, easily enraged, and dissatisfied with conditions as they exist.

question, key In the Adlerian approach, a question designed to uncover the purpose of the patient's psychiatric symptoms (e.g. What would you do if you were well?). The answer should indicate the patient's purpose in being sick and the personal things to which his symptoms are directed.

question, Pigem's A projective question asked of the patient such as, "What three things would you like most to change (or to do, or to be) in your life?" or, "If you could be changed into something else by a fairy, what would it be?" Such questions are often used as part of the mental status examination.

Quételet, Lambert Adolphe Jacques (1796–1874) Belgian statistician and astronomer; showed that the distribution of human characters such as height could be described by the normal curve. The law was first described in mathematical language by Abraham DeMoivre (1664–1754), a French Huguenot who went into exile in London in 1688. The law was later rediscovered independently by Pierre Simon, Marquis de Laplace (1749–1827), a French mathematician and astronomer (*Théorie analytique des probabilités,* 1812) and Johann Karl Friedrich Gauss (1777–1855), a German mathematician (*Theory of Numbers,* 1801).

Quincke disease (Heinrich Irenaeus Quincke, physician in Kiel, 1842–1922) See *edema, angioneurotic.*

quintuplet One of five children born at the same birth. See *birth, multiple.*

quotient, intelligence (IQ) The ratio of a subject's intelligence (determined by mental measures) to so-called average or normal intelligence for his age. The most common method for determining the intelligence quotient is to divide the assigned mental age by the chronological age.

R

R In Rorschach test scoring, the total number of responses to the cards.

rabbit syndrome See *syndrome, rabbit.*

rabies *Hydrophobia* (q.v.); a virus infection of the central nervous system, transmitted by the bite of a rabid animal (dog, jackal, cat, wolf; rarely, horse or cow).

race "Applied to human beings, the term race implies a blood related group with characteristic and common hereditary traits. . . . Primary races or sub-species—the Caucasian, the Mongoloid, and the Negroid—are generalized racial types, hypothetical stocks, rather than living races." (Reuter, E.B. *The American Race Problem,* 1938) See *racism.*

race, disease Group of individuals susceptible to the same disease. G. Draper uses the term *race* in a special way. In his efforts to establish correlations between constitutional characteristics of an individual and disease entities, he uses the expressions gastric ulcer race, gall-bladder race, etc. Thus he says, "By the same token, any other series of constant similarities, whether physiologic, psychologic, or immunologic, might as justifiably be used as proper criteria of racial entity. One might conceive, therefore, as well of a gastric ulcer race, a manic-depressive race, a meningococcus susceptible race, or gall-bladder race, as of the present customarily accepted black, yellow, or white divisions of mankind." (*Disease and the Man,* 1930)

rachischisis (rā-kis'ki-sis) See *spina bifida.*

racism The system that divides life roles and status according to race, assigning to one race the status of inferior, submissive, uneducable laborer, etc., and to another the status of superior, industrious, intelligent, patronizing manager/ruler. In similar fashion, *sexism* views status and role in terms of sex alone, *ageism* in terms of age alone.

Race hatred or racial prejudice is considered by many to be a group-related paranoia. Group members are more securely bonded to one another if they can project denigrating, destructive, and disruptive impulses onto targets outside the group instead of onto one another.

rackets See *transactional analysis.*

radiation In neurophysiology, the spreading of excitation to adjacent neurons.

radiation somnolence syndrome See syndrome, radiation somnolence.

radical, free See *aging, theories of.*

radical therapy An imprecise term for a group of interventions whose basic theme is that much of what is termed psychiatric illness is in fact a reflection of the subject's relationships to society, and that social problems need social rather than medical solutions. Most such "therapies" rely heavily on peer counseling and self-help networks.

radiculitis (rä-dik-ū-lī'tis) Inflammation of the intradural portion of a spinal nerve root prior to its entrance into the intervertebral foramen or of the portion between that foramen and the nerve plexus.

radioisotope See *encephalography, radioisotopic.*

radix Nerve root.

Rado, Sandor (1890–1972) Hungarian-born psychoanalyst; established the first graduate school of psychoanalysis at a United States University (Columbia University's College of Physicians and Surgeons) in 1944; adaptational psychodynamics.

rage Fury; violent, intense anger; often used in psychoanalytic writings to emphasize the overpowering and unbridled aspect of infantile anger. See *aggression*.

rage, defiant In Rado's terminology, the angry resistance or opposition to demands and orders, as in the child whose temper tantrum more or less obviously expresses the idea "I won't." Defiant rage is a typical reaction, at least in the American culture, to bowel training; opposed to this reaction is guilty fear and fearful obedience, which arise in response to the mother's punishments, threats, and demands for expiation. The resulting conflict between the opposing tensions of defiant rage and guilty fear is of particular significance in the genesis of obsessive behavior. See *attack, obsessive*.

rage, retroflexed See *psychodynamics, adaptational*.

rage, sham The term first used to denote the spontaneous outbursts of motor activity resembling fear and rage that occur in decorticate or diencephalic animals. (Cannon, W.B., & Britton, S.W. *American Journal of Physiology 72*, 1925) Such outbursts are accompanied by changes in the internal organs and in the composition of the blood similar to those characteristic of human emotional behavior. It has been shown that sham rage depends on the functional integrity of the caudal hypothalamus. The question naturally is: "How real or sham is such behavior? Does uninhibited action of the hypothalamus give rise to the experience of fear and rage, or does it affect merely the sympathetic and motor concomitants of the emotions?" Sham rage differs from normal rage in animals as follows: (1) the animal rarely attempts to avoid the stimulus that called forth the reaction; and (2) the response of sham rage rarely outlasts the duration of the stimulus, i.e. after-discharge is minimal. These differences are also seen in cases of sham rage in humans, which is never purposeful. In humans sham rage has been observed as a result of extensive cortical damage secondary to prolonged hypoglycemia and carbon monoxide poisoning: the response pattern was uniform to all strong stimuli, it lasted from 30 seconds to 1 minute, and the strength of stimulus had no apparent effect on the duration of the sham rage. In these cases, loud noises and painful stimuli produce

dilation of the pupil, widening of the palpebral fissures, exophthalmos, and marked increase in pulse rate and systolic pressure. A patient with carbon monoxide poisoning clenched and ground her teeth and emitted hissing sounds.

All in all, both animal and human data would seem to imply that the hypothalamus is not the emotional center. "It would, therefore, seem that while subcortical centers (the hypothalamus) may integrate and possibly reinforce the effector neural responses controlling some of the sympathetic and motor manifestations of fear and rage, there is little or no basis for the thesis that the hypothalamus governs or even mediates the emotional experiences themselves." (Wortis, H., & Mauer, U.S. *American Journal of Psychiatry 98*, 1941–42) See *Cannon hypothalamic theory of emotion; emotion, Papez's theory of; ergotropic*.

rami communicantes Branches of the spinal nerves that pass to the sympathetic trunk. The white ramus is present only in thoracic and upper lumbar nerves; the gray ramus is present in all spinal nerves.

random Uncontrolled, spontaneous, unplanned, occurring by chance. The term is used most commonly in statistics to refer to the choosing of experimental subjects on the basis of chance rather than on the basis of particular selective factors.

randomized clinical trial (RCT) *Controlled clinical trial;* an experimental design in which subjects are randomly assigned either to an experimental group (which receives the treatment under investigation) or to a control group (which receives no treatment or a placebo).

rank Position in a series when the components of the series are arranged in order of magnitude; thus a rank of 20 indicates that the component part is 20th from the top (or bottom) when all components have been arranged in order of size. Because the meaningfulness of any given rank will depend upon the number of component parts in the series, rank is more meaningful if expressed in relative terms as a percentile rank. See *rank, percentile*.

Rank, Otto (1884–1939) Viennese psychoanalyst; birth trauma, will therapy.

rank, percentile Position in a series expressed as a number that represents the percentage of cases in the total group lying below the given score value. Example: If a subject makes a score of 82 in an examination, and it is found that this score is higher than that made by 93% of the total number of those taking that examination, we would say that he is at the 93rd percentile on this particular examination. Percentile ranks are used to facilitate the interpretation of a single measure in a distribution of such measures, as a means of describing the variability and form of a frequency distribution, and as a means of comparing measures that were originally expressed in different units. Thus a student may make a score of 82 on one test and a score of 127 on a second; as raw scores these would be relatively meaningless, but when it is known that the score of 82 represents the 93rd percentile on the first test, and that the score of 127 represents the 92nd percentile on the second, the subject's performance on the two tests is seen in more meaningful perspective.

rap sessions See *consciousness raising*.

Rapaport, David (1911–60) Hungarian-born U.S. psychologist; systematizer of psychoanalytic theory; *Emotions and Memory* (1942); *Diagnostic Psychological Testing* (1945–46, with Roy Schafer and Merton Gill); *Organization and Pathology of Thought* (1951).

rape phantasy, anal See *phantasy, anal rape*.

rapism See *paraphilic coercive disorder*.

rapport A conscious feeling of accord, sympathy, trust, and mutual responsiveness between one person and another; to be differentiated from *transference* (q.v.), an unconscious process.

rapport, psychological In Jung's terminology, *transference* (q.v.).

rapprochement See *separation-individuation*.

raptus A type of action seen in some catatonic schizophrenics consisting of uncoordinated discharge movements that tend to relieve extreme tension. Cataleptic general muscular rigidity is a common form of raptus action.

raptus impulsive *Rare.* A sudden, unprovoked attack of extreme agitation that occurs sometimes in cases of catatonic schizophrenia.

raptus melancholicus An attack of extreme agitation or frenzy occurring in the course of *melancholia* (q.v.).

RAS Reticular activating system. See *formation, reticular*.

Rat-Man The patient reported on by Freud in a 1909 paper, "Notes upon a Case of Obsessional Neurosis," so called because of the experience that was the direct occasion of his consulting a psychiatrist: on military maneuvers he had heard a story of a type of punishment used in the Far East, the punishment consisting of overturning a pot of rats onto the buttocks of the prisoner so that the rats would bore their way into his anus.

rate In epidemiology, the rate is the level of occurrence of a disease or reaction in relation to a given population, such as 10 cases per 1,000 population, or per 10,000, or per 100,000. See *incidence; prevalence*.

rate, death The ratio of the number of persons dying within a specified period, usually a year, to the number who were in the original group. In institutional statistics the true death rate is usually approximated by finding the ratio of deaths to the average number under treatment during the period. The number of admissions and the total number under care have been used incorrectly as the base for the death rate.

rate, discharge The ratio of the number discharged within a given period (usually a year) to the total number in the original group. In institutional statistics this rate is usually approximated by relating the number discharged in a given period to the number who were admitted during the same period. See *readmission*.

Example: If there are 620 admissions to a mental hospital during the calendar year, and if there are 527 discharges from that hospital during the same period, the discharge rate is 85%.

rate, improvement The improvement rate is the ratio of the number discharged as improved within a given period (usually a year) to the total number in the original group. In institutional statistics this rate is usually approximated by relating the number discharged as improved in a given period to the number who were admitted during the same period.

Example: In one psychiatric hospital in New York City, 616 patients were admitted during the year. During the same period, 542 patients were discharged as improved. The improvement rate is 88%. See *rate, discharge*.

rate of first admissions The rate of first admissions (i.e. to hospitals for mental disease) is the ratio of all first admissions within a year to the average general population during that year.

Between 1922 and 1950, there was a definite increase in mental disease in the United States as a whole, and in New York State. But as shown in the following table (adapted from Malzberg, B. in *American Handbook of Psychiatry*, ed. S. Arieti, 1959), that increase was due not to any great increase in the incidence of functional psychoses, but rather to a great increase in the number of first admissions diagnosed cerebral arteriosclerosis or senile brain disorders. (Current rates are not comparable because of the effects of deinstitutionalization policies, the availability of psychopharmacologic agents, and preadmission diversion of potential inpatients—all of which have been introduced since 1950.)

New York State First Admissions per 100,000 Population

Total	Male	Female	Total	%of Total
1922	69.3	61.0	65.1	100
1950	109.9	102.4	106.0	100
Cerebral arteriosclerosis				
1922	6.6	4.3	5.4	8.3
1950	24.6	20.4	22.4	21.1
Senile brain disorders				
1922	4.9	8.0	6.4	9.8
1950	12.9	19.4	16.3	15.2
Paresis				
1922	12.6	2.9	7.7	11.8
1950	3.8	1.4	2.6	2.0
Alcoholic psychoses				
1922	3.6	0.7	2.2	3.4
1950	11.0	3.2	7.0	6.7
Manic-depressive psychosis				
1922	6.8	12.1	9.4	14.4
1950	1.9	3.1	2.5	2.3
Schizophrenias				
1922	19.2	16.3	17.8	27.4
1950	31.5	31.0	31.2	29.1

In general, both in the United States and Europe, males exceed females in the incidence of schizophrenia, organic brain disorders (except for the senile and presenile psychoses), and alcoholism, while females lead in manic-depressive disorders, neuroses, psychopathy, and senile and presenile psychoses.

rate, recovery The ratio of the number discharged as recovered within a given period (usually a year) to the total number in the original group. In institutional statistics this rate is usually approximated by relating the number discharged as recovered in a given period to the number who were admitted during the same period.

rate, residence In institutional statistics, the residence rate is based upon the population actually in institutions of a given type on any specified date. For example, it is the ratio of the resident population to the total population of the state. See *readmission*.

rate, specific A rate is specific when it is based upon a population and a class of that population both of which are homogeneous, or nearly so, with respect to a specific character: e.g. the number of male patients dying at ages 20–24 per 1,000 male patients aged 20–24.

rate, standardized A hypothetical rate that would prevail if a given population had the same relative distribution (i.e. with respect to age) as another population called the standard.

ratification theory See *theory, thank you*.

ratio, affective The ratio of the total number of responses to the colored Rorschach cards (cards VIII, IX, and X) to the total number of responses to the achromatic cards (I through VII). This ratio is an expression of the degree to which color increases responsiveness and is interpreted as an index of affectivity.

ratio, critical See *CR*.

ratio, sex The proportional distribution of males and females at birth. The usual sex ratio 106:100 has been cited as evidence that boys are stronger and better able to survive the ordeal of being born.

Recent genetic studies have shown, however, that more boys are born because more boys are *conceived*, and that the excess of males over females conceived is still greater than the ratio at birth. Investigation of embryos aborted when about three months old has shown that males outnumber females almost four to one. It must be assumed, therefore, that male embryos are not stronger, but just the contrary, *weaker* than female ones, and therefore more likely to perish under adverse intrauterine conditions.

ratio, type token An index of the balance between repetition and variety of words, used as a quantitative measurement of certain aspects of verbal communication during psychiatric sessions. Repetition gives a low index, variety of words gives a high index.

ratio, ventricle-to-brain *VBR* (q.v.).

rational Reasoning, sensible. From the standpoint of Jung, "The rational is the reasonable, that which accords with reason. I conceive reason as an attitude whose principle is to shape thought, feeling, and action in accordance with objective values." (*PT*)

"Thinking and feeling are rational functions in so far as they are decisively influenced by the motive of reflection. They attain their fullest significance when in fullest possible accord with the laws of reason. The irrational functions, on the contrary, are such as aim at pure perception, e.g., intuition and sensation; because, as far as possible, they are forced to dispense with the rational (which presupposes the exclusion of everything that is outside reason) in order to be able to reach the most complete perception of the whole course of events." (Ibid.)

rational psychotherapy See *psychotherapy, rational.*

rational type See *type, rational.*

rationality According to Culver and Gert (1982), there are two classes of rationality: (1) *required*—that which it would be irrational not to do, or believe, or desire; (2) *allowed*—that which it would not be irrational not to do, or believe, or desire. Whatever is not irrational is rational, either rationally allowed or rationally required.

rationalization This term was introduced into psychoanalysis by Ernest Jones. It means justification, or making a thing appear reasonable, when otherwise its irrationality would be evident. It is said that a person covers up, justifies, rationalizes an act or an idea that is unreasonable and illogical. For example, when a dehypnotized subject obeys a command received while under hypnosis and of which he is not consciously aware, and then proceeds to give a specious explanation for his act, he resorts to rationalization. Let us assume that he had been commanded to remove his shoes, when there was no reason for the removal. When the hypnotic stage is ended and he begins to take off his shoes, he explains that the shoes are too tight, or there are pebbles in them, or he gives some explanation that has the appearance of rationality. In other words, "Rationalization is a *screening process*, intended to cover a flaw in repression, e.g. to cover ideas or actions which are intended to gratify an unconscious need." (Glover, E. *The Technique of Psycho-Analysis*, 1955)

rationalize To invent a reason for an attitude or action, the motive of which is not recognized.

Ray, Isaac (1807–81) American psychiatrist; mental hygiene; forensic psychiatry; one of the founders of the American Psychiatric Association.

RBD *REM behavior disorder* (q.v.).

rCBF Regional cerebral blood flow. See *NMR.*

RCT *Randomized clinical trial* (q.v.).

RDC *Research Diagnostic Criteria* (q.v.). See *SADS.*

reaction Counteraction; response to a stimulus.

reaction, alarm The first stage of the general adaptation syndrome. The alarm reaction is a response to stress and as observed in experimental animals consists of adrenocortical enlargement with histologic signs of hyperactivity, thymicolymphatic involution, gastrointestinal ulcers, and often other manifestations of damage or shock. See *syndrome, general adaptation.*

reaction, alcohol-Antabuse See *Antabuse.*

reaction, all-or-none In psychiatry this expression means that instinctive processes, when stimulated, respond with full force or not at all.

In neurophysiology, the all-or-none (or all-or-nothing) principle refers to the fact that individual neurons either transmit their messages maximally or not at all. Differences in intensity are conveyed by means of spatial and temporal summation of impulses.

reaction, antisocial See *psychopathic personality.*

reaction, anxiety According to the 1952 revision of psychiatric nomenclature, this is the acceptable term for conditions formerly diagnosed anxiety state, or anxiety neurosis. See *anxiety neurosis.* In DSM-III, such conditions fall within *anxiety disorders.*

reaction, arousal See *arousal.*

reaction, aversion A response of avoidance or turning away from disturbing or frightening stimuli.

reaction, behavioral See *personality disorders*.

reaction, defensive *Defense* (q.v.).

reaction, delirious See *syndrome, organic*.

reaction, dissociate-dysmnesic substitution Adolf Meyer's term for conversion hysteria, which emphasizes the fundamental role of memory dissociation in the development of symptoms. See *hysteria*.

reaction, duplicative A perceptual disturbance described most commonly in schizophrenic children; because he does not conceptualize objects as continuing and unitary when they are out of direct sensory contact, the schizophrenic child "seeing the same person in different settings or at different times thinks he is seeing more than one person." (Goldfarb, W. *International Psychiatry Clinics 1*, 1964)

reaction formation Reversal formation; "The development in the ego of conscious, socialized attitudes and interests which are the antithesis of certain infantile unsocialized trends which continue to persist in the unconscious." (Healy et al., *SMP*) When, for instance, oversolicitude is the conscious response to unconscious hate, the condition (oversolicitude) is known as a reaction formation.

Reaction formation is a form of defense against urges that are unacceptable to the ego. It is one of the earliest of the defense mechanisms and one of the most fragile. As Freud says, it is "insecure and constantly threatened by the impulse which lurks in the unconscious." There is always the danger in reaction formation of a return of the repressed impulse to consciousness.

"Repression, as it invariably does, has brought about a withdrawal of libido, but for this purpose it has made use of a *reaction-formation*, by intensifying an antithesis. So here the substitute-formation has the same mechanism as the repression and at bottom coincides with it, while yet chronologically, as well as in its content, it is distinct from symptom-formation." (Freud, *CP*)

Reaction formation, then, is a type of repression, but it is distinguished from the latter by two features: (1) in reaction formation, the countercathexis is manifest in the form of the denying attitude, and thus the necessity for often repeated secondary repressions is avoided; and (2) the countercathexis is constantly manifested as a definitive change of personality rather than a momentary arousal of defensive maneuvers in response to an immediate danger.

"In a sense the superego can be considered a reaction formation of the ego, a complicated reaction to the oedipus complex. The fully developed superego in turn stimulates the ego to further reaction formations. The ego has to change its structure according to internal and external needs. It has the difficult task of maintaining itself in the face of three kinds of influences—the superego, the external world, and the id. Although its core is stable, the structure of the ego as a whole changes according to the influences to which it is subjected. Instead of reacting to these influences, that is, perceiving and discharging or abreacting them, the ego assimilates them and creates something new." (Nunberg, H. *Principles of Psychoanalysis*, 1955) Such reaction formations contribute extensively to the final structure of the character. Two commonly observed reaction formations are disgust (a reaction formation of the ego to an oral sexual impulse) and shame (a reaction formation to exhibitionistic impulses).

It is to be emphasized that reaction formation is an unconscious defense mechanism of the ego; conscious dissimulation or hypocrisy is not reaction formation. Further, reaction formation is not to be confused with sublimation; in the former, the unconscious impulse is repressed, and the constant countercathexis required to maintain such constant repression drains off energy that would otherwise be available to the ego. In the case of sublimation, on the other hand, the original impulse is superseded and its energy remains available to the ego for the fulfillment of its various tasks.

"To clarify the relation between reaction-formation and sublimation let us compare (a) a child who learns to write well and enjoys it very much, (b) a child who has an inhibition for writing, (c) a child who writes very constrainedly and meticulously, and (d) a child who smears. All of them have displaced anal-erotic instinctual quantities to the function of writing. In the first child a sublimation has taken place; he no longer wishes to smear but to write. The other children have not succeeded in channelizing this impulse. They are forced to inhibit it through a countercathexis, or to 'robot' through reaction-formations, or even to retain the original impulse in an unchanged way." (Fenichel, *PTN*)

While reaction formation can be seen as an element of any neurosis or psychosis, it is a typical mechanism of the obsessive compulsive psychoneurosis.

reaction, hand-to-mouth Observed in young infants, bringing to the mouth, for the purpose of sucking, all objects within reach of the infant's hand. These may be parts of the infant's body (hand, foot) or any outside object. According to Gesell this reaction disappears at about 12 months of age.

reaction, Herxheimer See *Jarisch-Herxheimer reaction.*

reaction, manic-depressive See *affective disorders; depression, unipolar; psychosis, manic-depressive.*

reaction, Much-Holzmann (Hans Much, German physician, 1880–1932, and V. Holzmann, German physician) The alleged property of the serum from a person affected with schizophrenia or manic depressive psychosis, to inhibit hemolysis by cobra venom.

reaction, polyglot In aphasia, any exception to the general rule that in persons who are multilingual, the mother tongue is the first to return.

reaction, psychotic See *psychosis; psychotic disorder.*

reaction, spoiled child Behavior reaction of children due to parental oversolicitude, overindulgence, and overprotection. Such children do not learn the value or even the meaning of regularity, self-care, responsibility, or independence.

reaction, thymonoic "Thymonoic reactions are closely related to catathymic reactions. They are distinguished by the presence of strong affective factors and equally strong tendency to systematization of thought (in the direction of depressive delusion), each factor springing from the same experiential and personality sources, and each feeding on and becoming more strongly fixed because of the other. These are the strongly 'intellectualized' and 'rationalized'

depressions, with marked systematized content, at times entirely autopsychic, but also at times with allopsychic manifestations." (Muncie, W. *Psychobiology and Psychiatry,* 1939)

reaction time Length of delay between application of stimulus and appearance of response. In word association tests, a long reaction time signalizes a complex.

reaction type A syndrome described in terms of the preponderating or essential symptoms. Adolf Meyer, for example, described six reaction types: organic, delirious, affective, paranoiac, substitutive, and deteriorated.

reaction type, affective A syndrome whose preponderant symptoms are of an affective or emotional nature, such as manic depressive disorder.

reaction type, delirious Adolf Meyer's expression for a type of psychiatric response due to toxic, infective, or exhaustive influences. The syndrome is characterized by dreamlike imaginations, hallucinations, and impairment of the sensorium. See *syndrome, organic.*

reaction type, deterioration When regression, accompanied as a rule by delusional and hallucinatory phenomena, is a principal characteristic of a psychiatric syndrome, as it is in schizophrenia, Adolph Meyer classifies the syndrome as a deterioration or deteriorated reaction type.

reaction type, organic See *syndrome, organic.*

reaction type, substitutive When mental conflicts are repressed into the unconscious and appear in the field of consciousness in disguised or substituted form, Adolf Meyer classifies the syndrome as *substitutive.* The psychoneuroses in general are substitutive reaction types.

reactive Secondary to, resulting from, or precipitated by an identifiable happening; thus a depressive episode following the death of a loved one could be termed reactive depression. In general, reactive episodes—be they depressive, manic, or schizophrenic in nature—carry a more favorable prognosis than those which arise endogenously and without apparent relationship to adversity or trauma in the patient's life. This fact has favored a regrettable equating of "reactive" with "non-psychotic" or "neurotic," even though it is well known that the same patient can have both reactive and endogenous episodes in the course of a recurrent or relapsing psychosis.

reactive psychosis See *cycloid psychosis.*

readiness, complex The tendency of unconscious feelings or impulses to find substitute expression in the behavior or routine of everyday life, as in lapses in speaking, reading, and writing.

readiness, explosion Readiness to explode, or burst forth violently. See *diathesis, explosive.*

reading disabilities The term includes a variety of clinical entities of apparently different etiology and treatment need; see *developmental disorders, specific.*

"In our total caseload, which now numbers some 250 children and adolescents, we have been impressed with the emergence of three major groups:

"1. Those in whom the reading retardation is due to frank brain damage manifested by gross neurologic deficits. In these cases there are clearly demonstrable major aphasic difficulties, and they are similar to adult dyslexic syndromes. An example is that of a 9-year-old boy who sustained a severe head injury with prolonged coma, followed by a right hemiparesis and expressive aphasia.

"2. Those with no history or gross clinical findings to suggest neurologic disease but in whom the reading retardation is viewed as primary. The defect appears to be in basic capacity to integrate written symbols. On the basis of findings to be presented later in this paper a neurologic deficit is suspected and, because the defect is basic or biologic in its origin, we have called these cases *primary reading retardation.*

"3. Those cases demonstrating reading retardation on standard tests but in whom there appears to be no defect in basic reading learning capacity. These children have a normal potential for learning to read but this has not been utilized because of *exogenous* factors, common among which are anxiety, negativism, emotional blocking and limited schooling opportunities. We diagnose these cases as *secondary reading retardation.*" (Rabinovitch, R., et al. *Research Publications, Association for Nervous and Mental Diseases 34*, 1954)

Failure to distinguish between these major types of reading disability has led to confusion among workers in the field, and innumerable terms have been coined to describe various types of reading defects, many terms frequently referring to the same concept. Among such terms currently in use are word-blindness, congenital symbolamblyopia, congenital typholexia, congenital alexia, amnesia visualis verbalis, congenital dyslexia, developmental alexia, analfabetia partialis, bradylexia, strephosymbolia, constitutional dyslexia, specific dyslexia.

In the primary group described above, "the defect appears to be part of a larger disturbance in integration. Our findings suggest that we are dealing with a developmental discrepancy rather than an acquired brain injury. The specific areas of difficulty manifested in the clinical examinations are those commonly associated with parietal and parietal-occipital dysfunction." (Ibid.)

readmission A person admitted or entered on the rolls more than once to any institution of a given class (e.g. mental hospitals). Until recently, the number of hospitalized mental patients increased each year in most states. In New York State, for example, the resident population of state hospitals doubled between 1929 and 1955, at which time a peak of 93,300 patients was reached. That upward trend was abruptly halted and inverted into a decline coincident with the use of tranquilizing drugs, which more than any other single factor made possible an increasing discharge rate. To some extent this has been balanced by an increasing readmission rate, since patients enabled to be discharged earlier than previously may require more frequent periods of rehospitalization. For some groups of patients, a pattern of early admission/speedy discharge/readmission(s) seems to have been established; such a pattern is often referred to as the *revolving door* phenomenon.

readout See *memory.*

reality The whole of the objective world, embracing all that may be perceived by the five senses.

reality confrontation See *therapy, social.*

reality-ego See *ego, reality.*

reality orientation A type of *remotivation* (q.v.), particularly useful for patients who are confused or disoriented from any cause. The patient is helped to regain his sense of identity by repeated reminders of who he is, where he is, the day of the week, the month of the year, what meal comes next, and similar basic information. The patient is thus oriented to his own identity and is taught to interact appropriately with others. "A successful reality orientation program requires a number of conditions: a calm environment, a set routine, clear but not necessarily loud responses to patients' questions with the same type of questions asked of the patients, clear directions and assistance in directing or guiding patients to and from their destinations if they need it, constant reminders of the date and time, interruption of the patients who start to ramble in their speech or actions, firmness when necessary, sincerity, requests of patients in a calm manner, and consistency." (Phillips, D.F. *Hospitals 47*, 1973)

reality principle See *principle, reality.*

reality system See *ego, stability of.*

reality testing A fundamental ego function that consists of the objective evaluation and judgment of the world outside the ego or self. Reality testing depends upon the simpler ego functions of perception and memory and upon differentiation between ego and non-ego. Reality testing provides the ego with a mechanism for handling both the external world and its own excitation, for it makes it possible for the ego to anticipate the future in the imagination. External objects represent a threat to the ego and/or potential gratification, and the ego can best protect itself against threats and can secure maximal gratification by using reality testing to judge reality objectively and direct its actions accordingly.

A stage of primary hallucinatory wish fulfillment precedes the development of reality testing, and a counterpart of the former is the ability to deny unpleasant parts of reality. As reality testing develops along with the acquisition of speech and thinking proper, such wholesale falsification of reality becomes impossible. Serious and important denials, then, are seen only in very early childhood and in pathological conditions such as psychosis, where the ego has been weakened by narcissistic re-

gression. Projection, too, can be used extensively only when reality testing is seriously impaired, as in psychosis, or when adequate demarcation between ego and non-ego has not yet been achieved, as in childhood. Only when the boundaries between ego and non-ego are blurred can the ego ward off the unpleasant by "spitting it out" and feeling it as being outside the ego.

Neurotics do, however, show some impairment of reality testing at least to the extent that warded-off impulses and their derivatives interfere with differentiated thinking and block the ego's capacity to organize its experiences, and insofar as present-day objects become mere transference representations of past objects and are reacted to with inappropriate and anachronistic feelings.

reason See *motive.*

reasoning mania Folie du doute, doubting mania.

reassociation A process of renewed or refreshed association occurring in hypnoanalysis of the war neurosis, during which the patient relives the traumatic event with emotional vividness. Such forgotten experiences will then become a part of his normal personality and consciousness.

reassurance A type of supportive psychotherapy.

rebound insomnia See *insomnia, rebound.*

rebound phenomenon of Gordon Holmes (British physician, 1876–1965) A test for ataxia, specifically illustrating the loss of cerebellar "check" on coordinated movement; if an attempt is made to extend the flexed forearm against resistance and suddenly let go, the hand or fist flies unchecked against the mouth or shoulder.

recall See *memory.*

recall memory Evocative memory. See *memory; object constancy.*

recapitulation, pubertal sexual The concept that the successive stages in the development of adult sexuality recapitulate those of infantile sexuality. The development of adult sexuality begins with puberty and is normally completed somewhere between the ages of 16 and 21. The developmental stages of adult sexuality "repeat" those of infantile sexuality, and rarely are conflicts found that have not had their forerunners in the earlier development. "At puberty a regression takes place in the direction of infancy, of the first period of all, and the person lives over again, though on another plain, the development he passed through in the first five years of life. This correlation between adolescence and infancy is of considerable importance as affording the key to many of the problems of adolescence." (Jones, E.J. *Papers on Psycho-Analysis*, 1949)

While it is true that conflicts in adolescent sexual development that have not had their forerunners in infantile sexual development are rarely encountered, nevertheless "experiences in puberty may solve conflicts or shift conflicts into a final direction; moreover, they may give older and oscillating constellations a final and definitive form. Many neurotics give an impression of adolescence. They have not succeeded in getting on good terms with their sexuality. Therefore, they continue the behavior patterns of adolescent children, that is, of an age at which it is usually considered normal not to have achieved these good terms and to feel life as a provisional state, with 'full reality' still waiting in an indefinite future." (Fenichel, *PTN*)

receiving type See *assimilation*.

receptive Passive, accepting, dependent. See *character, receptive*.

receptive dysphasia See *developmental dysphasia*.

receptor complex, supramolecular The association of two or more receptor groups in a functional unit, the net result of which is typically to enhance the effects of activation of one or both receptor groups. One well-known example is the benzodiazepine-GABA receptor complex, consisting of functional and structural coupling of the benzodiazepine receptor to the GABA receptor. By itself, GABA receptor activation inhibits neuronal excitability by increasing the permeability of the neuronal membrane to chloride ions. Benzodiazepines markedly potentiate that effect by increasing the frequency of GABA-mediated openings of chloride channels. It has been postulated that the benzodiazepine-GABA receptor complex is the common site of all minor tranquilizer action.

receptors, distance The visual and auditory apparatus, as contrasted with *proximal receptors* (touch, taste, smell). Schizophrenic children typically avoid distance receptors and prefer the use of proximal receptors, the reverse of the normal situation. As a result of avoidance of distance receptors, such children often have a glassy, nonseeing stare; they seem to look through others rather than at them, and often cannot meet the direct gaze of the examiner.

receptors, proximal See *receptors, distance*.

recessiveness The meaning of this genetic term is best understood as the mirror image of *dominance* (q.v.); a recessive factor remains *hidden* as an independent genetic entity, as long, and as far, as it is covered by the dominant member of a given allelic pair of hereditary factors.

A recessive character can be phenotypically manifested only in a *homozygous* condition when it is inherited by a hybrid from both parents. In the case of a single-recessive cross, this is true in 25% of the entire hybrid generation.

In the recessive or *indirect* mode of inheritance, as a rule, the heterozygotes are germinally affected, but phenotypically healthy. Since a recessive trait can appear only in the phenotype of a homozygote, all trait carriers must be homozygous. The occurrence of such a trait among the offspring is not possible, unless both parents are at least heterozygotes.

The probability of a union between two recessive trait carriers (heterozygotes) is clearly the greater the more frequent this recessive trait is in the general population. The probability is the greatest in the cases of *intermarriage* between blood relations, unless the trait in question is very common in the normal average population. Apart from this particular instance of *cousin marriages*, the direct transmission of a recessive trait is the exception and the indirect inheritance through the collateral lines is the rule.

recidivism Repetition of delinquent or criminal acts by the same offender who is called, accordingly, a recidivist or repeater.

Less commonly, recidivism is used to refer to relapse or recurrence of a psychiatric disorder. See *schizophrenia, recidives in*.

Victim recidivism refers to involvement of the same subject more than once as a victim in the same type of crime; surveys of victims of violent crime and of rape indicate that approximately one-quarter were prior victims of violent crime or rape. See *diathesis, traumatophilic.*

Differences in recidivism rate for psychiatric patients appear to depend on a combination of *gatekeeper variables* (number and length of previous admissions, severity of disorder) and *pathway variables* (age, sex, social class, number of dependents). Some types of patients, such as the elderly, women, and those with few or no dependents, tend to have a high risk of readmission regardless of the severity of their problems. Patients tend to have long stays because of the severity of their problems.

reciprocal inhibition psychotherapy See *behavior theory.*

reciprocal regulation A style of pathologic mothering described by J. MacMurray (*Psychiatric Annals 6,* 1976) in which the mother's oversolicitude controls the child's ability to think, test reality, and incorporate new ideas, but the child's behavior in turn controls the mother's self-esteem. See *love, smother; mother-child relationship.*

reciprocity, overadequate-inadequate See *psychotherapy, family.*

recognition memory See *memory; object constancy.*

recognition site See *synapse.*

recollections, early See *memory.*

recombinant DNA Genetic material (deoxyribonucleic acid) that has been transferred from one organism (human or animal) to another (the host cell, typically a bacterium such as *E. coli*). The foreign DNA is sectioned from the donor organism by *restriction enzymes* (*endonucleases*) and combines with the DNA fragments from a vector, usually a bacterial virus (*bacteriphage*) or *plasmid* (circular bacterial DNA). In multiplying, the host bacterium faithfully copies the genetic message of the insert DNA and thus is able to produce antigens, antibodies, interferon, hormones, etc., or can provide a normal gene when one is deficient or lacking. See *splicing, gene.*

recombination The genetic process by which linked factors break up their original combinations, so that originally separate genes become united in one gamete, or originally united genes become separated. These recombining phenomena are also known as *crossovers.*

"Under independent assortment the parental combinations and the recombinations are approximately equal in number. Under linkage the parental combinations are always more numerous than the recombinations. Linkage may vary greatly with different genes, producing all the way from very few to nearly 50% of recombinations." (Sinnott, E.W., & Dunn, L.C. *Principles of Genetics,* 1939)

When crossovers occur and lead to a separation of linked genes, the genes that have crossed over are bound to enter different gametes and to appear in different individuals among the progeny. See *linkage.*

recommencement, mania of Janet's term for the behavior of some obsessive-compulsive patients who must do things many times before they can feel some assurance that they have been done correctly—opening and shutting doors, locking and unlocking doors, dressing and undressing, constant repetition of prayers and penances, etc.

reconditioning A type of psychotherapy based on the belief that neurosis is a result of faulty conditioning. In Salter's method, the patient is authoritatively directed to abandon destructive patterns of behavior and to practice new habits that will be of value to him. The patient is considered to be in a state of pathologic inhibition which is itself a conditioned response that blocks free emotional expression (*excitation*). Treatment is directed to unlearning conditioned inhibitory reflexes and replacing them with conditioned excitatory reflexes by means of deliberate practicing of excitatory emotional reactions until they are established as conditioned reflexes.

reconstruction See *psychotherapy.*

recreation Leisure activity engaged in for its own sake. The term is also used to refer to a type of ancillary treatment and is then called recreation(al) therapy (RT). John E. Davis (*Clinical Applications of Recreational Therapy,* 1952) defines recreation therapy as "any free, voluntary and expressive activity; motor, sensory or mental, vitalized by the expansive play spirit, sustained by deep-rooted pleasurable attitudes and evoked by wholesome emotional release; prescribed by medical authority as an adjuvant in treatment."

Recreation therapy includes such activities as dressmaking, drama, puppetry, lectures, films, music appreciation, dancing, discussion groups, clubs, painting, singing, excursions, bowling, and athletic games of all sorts.

recreation, active In occupational therapy any form of diversional endeavor or pastime in which the patient actually engages and in the participation of which it is necessary for him to make some physical exertion. For example, dancing is a form of active recreation.

recreation, passive Entertainment or amusement planned and presented by others for the patient and in which he does not participate, but plays the passive part of onlooker. For example, moving pictures or a concert are forms of passive recreation.

recruiting system See *system, intralaminar.*

recruitment In neurophysiology, spread of response if stimulation is prolonged.

red nucleus See *midbrain.*

redintegration Hollingworth's term for the process in which part of a complex antecedent provokes the complete consequent that was previously made to the antecedent as a whole. The conditioned response is an example of redintegration. Redintegration is the basis of the value of souvenirs and keepsakes, which tend to arouse the same attitudes as were originally connected with the experiences to which they pertain.

Redintegration is also sometimes used synonymously with reintegration. See *integration.*

reductionism The philosophy, theory, or belief that everything is to be, and can be, explained in terms of simple, elemental components. Many theories of human behavior are based on the *drive-reduction theory:* the aim or function of every instinct, defense, action, habit, or phantasy is to reduce or eliminate either stimulation or excitation within the nervous system. That theory implies that in the absence of such motivation, the organism will become quiescent; in fact, however, the organism does not, and in their attempts to overcome such a basic contradiction between hypothesis and observed data many theorists have taken refuge in naming instincts, postulating drives in terms of their telic significance, and/or

speculating on the existence of spontaneous activity.

reductive "I employ this expression to denote that method of psychological interpretation which regards the unconscious product not from the symbolic point of view, but merely as a *semiotic* expression, a sort of sign or symptom of an underlying process. Accordingly the reductive method treats the unconscious product in the sense of a leading-back to the elements and basic processes, irrespective of whether such products are reminiscences of actual events, or whether they arise from elementary processes affecting the psyche. Hence, the reductive method is orientated backwards (in contrast to the constructive method), whether in the historical sense or in the merely figurative sense of a tracing back of complex and differentiated factors to the general and elementary." (Jung, *PT*)

redundancy, genetic See *aging, theories of.*

reduplicative paramnesia *Doppelganger* (q.v.).

reeducation See *psychotherapy.*

reefers Slang expression for marihuana cigarettes. Possibly the weed was first carried by sailors from the reefs of Mariguana Island in the Bahamas.

reenactment, emotional See *abreaction.*

reference, delusion of See *reference, ideas of.*

reference, ideas of When a person projects his own, usually unconscious, ideas upon another or other persons and then proceeds to act toward those ideas as if they originated from an outside source, he is said to show ideas of reference. For instance, a patient with an unconscious impulse to steal, was preoccupied with the idea, delusional, that others asserted he intended to steal. The psychic process involves criticism of the projected urges, so that the patient may not know that he is really criticizing some undesirable impulse within himself.

The term also includes the tendency to read a personal meaning into everything that goes on about one, to feel that every action or happening in the outside world is specifically and purposely related to the patient.

The paranoid patient almost always exhibits ideas of reference. He misinterprets the activities of others, believing that they have personal reference of a derogatory character to him. See *projection.*

referred pain See *pain, referred.*

reflection In psychiatry and psychology, this may refer (1) to a type of thinking characterized by introspection, deliberation, or contemplation, or (2) to a psychotherapeutic technique in which a patient's statements are restated or rephrased to the patient so as to emphasize their emotional significance.

reflex A sensorimotor reaction, the simplest form of involuntary response to a stimulus. Stimulation of the receptor organ or cell excites the afferent neuron, from which the impulse travels to one or more intercalated neurons in the central nervous system and then, via the efferent neuron, to the effector organ or cell. For specific reflexes, see listings below and under *sign.*

reflex, abdominal The upper (or epigastric) and lower abdominal reflexes are superficial skin reflexes tested by stroking the skin of the abdomen. This results in contraction of the abdominal muscles beneath the skin area stroked and usually also movement of the umbilicus in the direction of the area stroked. The upper abdominals depend on thoracic nerves 7 to 10; the lower abdominals depend on thoracic nerves 10 to 12.

reflex, accommodation See *accommodation.*

reflex, acute affective Kretschmer's term for the earliest indications of emotional discharge (usually, tremors) in response to great stress.

reflex, bar A pathologic postural reaction consisting of involuntary following by one leg when the other leg of the recumbent patient is moved laterally or vertically. The bar phenomenon is seen mainly in cases with lesions of the prefrontal areas (especially in cases of brain tumor).

reflex, biceps A deep reflex; patient's forearm is placed halfway between flexion and extension and slightly pronated; examiner's finger is on the tendon, and a blow on this digit results in flexion of the forearm. This reflex depends upon the musculocutaneous nerve for its afferents and efferents; its center is C_{5-6}.

reflex, Chaddock (Charles Gilbert Chaddock, American neurologist, 1861–1936) Dorsal extension of the great toe, induced by stroking the skin over the external

malleolus. This is one of several pathologic reflexes that may be seen when the lower motor neuron is released from the normal suppressor effect of higher centers, as in pyramidal tract lesions.

reflex, consensual When light enters the pupil of one eye only, the iris of the other eye contracts; the phenomenon is known as the consensual light reflex.

reflex, corneal Bilateral blinking induced by touching the cornea with a wisp of cotton. The afferent nerve of the corneal reflex is N V, its efferent is N VII, and its center is in the pons.

reflex, cornealpyterygoideal Touching the cornea is followed by contraction of the external pterygoid, which produces deviation of the lower jaw of the opposite side.

reflex, cremasteric A superficial reflex; stroking the inner and upper side of the thigh causes contraction of the cremaster and elevation of the testicle on the same side. The afferents of this reflex depend upon the femoral nerve, the efferents on the genitofemoral nerve; the center is L_1.

reflex, cuboidodigital See *Bechtereff-Mendel reflex.*

reflex, deep Any one of the tendon and periosteal reflexes, which include the jaw jerk, pectoral, triceps, biceps, radial, ulnar, knee jerk, suprapatellar, tibioadductor, flexion of the leg, ankle jerk, and Bechtereff-Mendel reflexes.

reflex, dorsocuboidal See *Bechtereff-Mendel reflex.*

reflex, emptying See *reflex, gastrocolic.*

reflex, epigastric See *reflex, abdominal.*

reflex, flexion, of the leg A deep reflex; patient's leg is semiflexed at the knee; the examiner's finger grasps the tendons of the semimembranosus and semitendinosus muscles; this finger is tapped, which results in contraction of these muscles and flexion of the leg.

reflex, gastrocolic Contraction of the colon following stretching of the muscle wall of the stomach (as by filling of the stomach); also known as emptying reflex.

reflex, gluteal A superficial reflex; stroking the buttocks causes contraction of the glutei.

reflex, Gordon (Alfred Gordon, American neurologist, 1874–1953) Dorsal extension of the great toe, induced by compression of the calf muscle.

reflex, grasp Same as forced grasping, forced groping, or instinctive grasp reaction. See *lobe, frontal.*

reflex, Landau A reaction normally present from the age of 3 months to about 1 year of age, consisting of raising the head and arching the back with the concavity upward when the infant is supported horizontally in the prone position. Absence of the reflex is seen with motor weakness, such as occurs in cerebral palsy, motor neuron disease, and mental retardation.

reflex, mass In very severe injury to or complete interruption of the spinal cord, stimulation below the level of the lesion produces the following reflexes: (1) flexion reflex; (2) contraction of the abdominal wall; (3) automatic evacuation of the bladder; (4) sweating of the skin below the level of the lesion. This *mass reflex* was described by Riddoch.

reflex, menace Blinking in response to a feint with the (examiner's) hand or other object toward the subject's eye.

reflex, Moro A type of mass reflex seen in the neonate in response to the examiner's slapping the surface on which the infant is lying; it consists of immediate flexion of the limbs and contraction of the abdominal wall with later interruptions of the spasm that produce cloniclike jerkings.

reflex, myxedema (miks-e-dē′mà) Also known as *Woltman's sign;* the myxedema reflex is the symptom of pathologically slow relaxation of reflexes in myxedema.

reflex, oculocardiac Slowing of the pulse in response to pressure exerted on the eyeball; also known as the Aschner ocular phenomenon.

reflex, Oppenheim (H. Oppenheim, German neurologist, 1858–1919) Dorsal extension of the great toe, induced by stroking distally along the median side of the tibia. This is one of several pathologic reflexes that may be seen when the lower motor neuron is released from the normal suppressor effect of higher centers, as in pyramidal tract lesions.

reflex, palmar A superficial reflex; scratching or irritation of the palm results in flexion of the fingers.

reflex, palmomental Contraction of the mentalis muscle following mechanical stimulation of the thenar and hypothenar eminences. This reflex is rare in normal

persons and is considered to be indicative of diffuse toxic brain damage. Also known as the *palm-chin* or *pollico-mental* reflex.

reflex, patellar See *reflex, suprapatellar.*

reflex, periosteal The response to tapping certain bones that lie just beneath the skin; for example, the radial and ulnar periosteal, and the tibial adductor reflexes.

reflex, plantar A superficial reflex; stroking the sole of the foot causes flexion of the toes. This reflex depends upon the tibial nerve for its afferents and efferents; its center is at S_{2-1}.

reflex, pollicomental See *reflex, palmomental.*

reflex, psychogalvanic (PGR) Changes in skin resistance to the passage of a weak electric current that occur as part of the physicochemical response to emotional stimuli. Also known as galvanic skin response (GSR), electrodermal response (EDR), Féré phenomenon.

reflex psychology See *Pavlov's reflex psychology.*

reflex, quadrupedal extensor Russell Brain described this reflex in organic hemiplegia. It consists in the extension of the hemiplegic flexed arm on the assumption of the quadrupedal position. An additional feature may be the further flexion of the arm if the head is bent forward and extension of the arm if the head is bent back.

reflex, radial A deep reflex; also known as the extension reflex of the wrist. When the styloid process of the radius is tapped, the wrist extends. This reflex depends upon the radial nerve for its afferents and efferents; its center is C_{7-8}.

reflex, Rossolimo's (Grigoriy Ivanovich Rossolimo, Russian neurologist, 1860–1928) Plantar flexion of the toes, induced by tapping the balls of the toes; one of several pathologic reflexes that may be seen when the lower motor neuron is released from the normal suppressor effect of higher centers, as in pyramidal tract lesions.

reflex, Schaeffer (Max Schaeffer, German neurologist, 1852–1923) Dorsal flexion of the great toe, induced by pinching the Achilles tendon; one of several pathologic reflexes that may be seen when the lower motor neuron is released from the normal suppressor effect of higher centers, as in pyramidal tract lesions.

reflex, scrotal By stroking the perineum or applying a cold object to it, a slow, vermicular contraction of the dartos muscle occurs. This is a purely automatic reflex with the cremasteric reflex.

reflex, superficial The response to stroking or pressing upon certain portions of the skin; for example, the plantar, cremasteric, and abdominal reflexes.

reflex, suprapatellar A deep reflex; patient's leg is extended with patella movable; examiner places index finger above patella, pushing down slightly, then striking this finger; the result is a kickback of the patella.

This reflex is also known as the patellar reflex. It depends upon the femoral nerve for its afferents and efferents; its center is L_{2-4}.

reflex, tendon The contraction of a muscle in response to tapping its tendon; for example, the triceps, quadriceps femoris (patellar), and gastrocnemius (Achilles or ankle) reflexes.

reflex, thumb-chin See *reflex, palmomental.*

reflex time, central See *facilitation.*

reflex, triceps A deep reflex; the patient's forearm, partly flexed at the elbow, is held by the examiner; the striking of the tendon just above the olecranon process results in extension of the forearm. This reflex depends upon the radial nerve for its afferents and efferents; its center is C_{6-7}.

reflex, ulnar A deep reflex; also known as the flexion reflex of the wrist; when the styloid process of the ulna is tapped, the wrist flexes (pronation and adduction of the hand). This reflex depends on the median nerve for its afferents and efferents; its center is C_{6-8}.

reflex, wrist See *reflex, radial; reflex, ulnar.*

reflexes, grasping and groping These reflexes are elicited when the palms and the fingers are stroked, causing a closure of the hand on the stimulating object. Normally this occurs in infants below 1 year of age. Otherwise it is indicative of frontal lobe lesions.

reformist delusion See *delusion, reformist.*

refractory Resistant, unresponsive, unmanageable, obstinate, stubborn. In neurophysiology, the refractory period is the time following stimulation during which a nerve or muscle remains unresponsive to a second stimulus. The absolute refractory period is that during which there is no response to any stimulus; the relative refractory period is that during which response can be elicited only if the stimulus is very strong.

reframing Viewing from a different perspective; reconceptualizing; redefining. The term is used most frequently in family therapy, where many approaches emphasize the positive aspects of symptoms or dysfunction as they support and protect the integrity and continuity of family life. Treatment entails a cognitive restructuring of behavior to indicate its positive qualities. Thus in *relabeling,* a particular form of reframing, excessive dependence on the mother may be viewed as a means of contributing to the mother's self-esteem by making her feel needed and wanted.

refrigerator parents Kanner's original description of parents of psychotic (autistic) children—cold, intellectual, stimulate their children less than parents of normal children. Most recent workers have failed to confirm such differences.

refusal, school See *phobia, school.*

regimen The specific details of a treatment plan, including the scheduling and regulation of diet, medication, and other therapeutic measures designed to operate over a period of time. The term regime is often used incorrectly in this sense.

registration In learning psychology, registration refers to impressibility or notation ability and implies the ability to notice, the ability to make a record, or both. Impaired registration of recent impressions is the most striking symptom of Korsakoff's psychosis. See *memory; syndrome, Wernicke-Korsakoff.*

regression The act of returning to some earlier level of adaptation. The mentally healthy individual progresses through many so-called levels. Following the designations of Freud, they are (1) intrauterine; (2) infancy (early and late; extending from birth to approximately the fifth year; this period includes, among other things, the phases of oral, anal, and genital organization); (3) latency (extending from about the age of 5 to puberty; one of its chief characteristics is sublimation); (4) puberty (beginning at the onset of manhood or womanhood and continuing for two or three years; one of its main attributes is adult sexuality); (5) adolescence (beginning in the early or middle twenties; its principal characteristics revolve around the reality principle, heterosexuality, and sublimated interest); (6) adulthood (extending from the termination of the adolescent period to senescence; the characteristics of adolescence are amplified during this stage); (7) climacterium; (8) senescence (the phase of decadence). See *ontogeny, psychic*.

When a person, say, at the age of 40, begins to show symptoms of schizophrenia and subsequently undergoes deep regression, he sometimes passes through the various levels of adaptation formerly lived through by him. Thus, with the abandonment of the qualities of adulthood, he regressively becomes, so to speak, adolescent, puberal, puerile, and finally infantile; he may also regress to a stage resembling that of the intrauterine period of existence. As a rule, regression in schizophrenia or in any of the psychogenic psychiatric disorders is accomplished by means of symbolic manifestations.

From the psychoanalytic standpoint, regression and *fixation* (q.v.) are commonly associated with each other. When fixation is intense, frustrations on the part of reality may easily lead to regression. But internal frustrations are even more important, according to Freud.

"According to the concept of finality, causes are understood as means to an end. A simple example is the process of regression. Regarded causally, regression is determined, for example, by 'mother fixation.' But from the final standpoint, the libido returns to the mother-imago in order to find there the memory associations by means of which further development can take place, as, for instance, from an emotional system into an intellectual system." (Jung, *CAP*)

regression, progressive teleologic Arieti's term for the tendency of the schizophrenic to return to the level of the primary process or primary cognition in an attempt to deal with a world and self-image that are grotesque, threatening, and terrifying. The regressing is teleologic in that it is purposeful, as when an inner threat is changed into a threat from the outside world that can be defended

against. But unlike other types of regression, schizophrenic regression is progressive because it usually fails in its purpose and still further regression is necessary until, finally, the process may lead to complete dilapidation.

regressive alcoholism See *alcoholism*.

regressive EST See *therapy, regressive electroshock*.

regulation, reciprocal See *reciprocal regulation*.

rehabilitation The use of all forms of physical medicine in conjunction with psychosocial adjustment and vocational retraining in an attempt to achieve maximal function and adjustment, and to prepare the patient physically, mentally, socially, and vocationally for the fullest possible life compatible with his abilities and disabilities. Rehabilitation is a dynamic, purposeful program in which, ideally, activities are scheduled for each patient for the entire day; such schedules are built around activities prescribed by the physician, with guidance, psychological services, adult education, prevocational shop training, and directed socialization supplementing the prescribed therapy and retraining. See *remotivation*.

Rehabilitation is sometimes called the fourth leg of medical practice, the others being prevention, diagnosis, and treatment.

Rehabilitation aims to restore a handicapped person to a situation in which he can make best use of his residual capacities within as normal as possible a social context. The handicaps themselves are of two varieties: *primary*—the chronic symptoms that are an inherent part of illness plus the accumulated losses of skills through illness; and *secondary*—unhealthy personal reactions to illness plus unfavorable, inappropriate attitudes toward the handicapped person that develop in his relatives, employers, hospital staff, etc. (see *syndrome, social breakdown*). In general, rehabilitation techniques are more applicable to decreasing or preventing secondary handicaps, and to increasing social acceptability of patients, than they are to modifying or removing chronic symptoms of psychosis.

In psychiatry, rehabilitation generally is concerned with the patient with chronic mental illness (specifically, organic dementia or schizophrenia), where the goals are (1) to prevent relapse and rehospitalization by achieving successful community tenure; (2) to improve the quality of life by assisting the patient in assuming responsibility over his or her life; and (3) to achieve an adequate social role with appropriate instrumental performance in the community. Included within the latter are vocational, homemaking, social, and interpersonal adjustment competencies, all of which aim to help the patient function as actively and independently in society as possible. Rehabilitation programs focus not only on strengthening the patient's skills but also on developing the environmental supports necessary to sustain him or her within the community. It has generally been observed that fewer than 20% of chronically mentally ill patients are able to adapt acceptably to average community life. Successful rehabilitation depends on a network of community care services such as halfway houses, adult homes, sheltered workshops, special schools, supervised residences for the handicapped and developmentally disabled, home care, satellite clinics, etc. See *care, long-term; domicile.*

rehearsal, behavioral See *therapy, behavior.*

rehearsal, obsessional A preliminary "try-out" often used by obsessional patients, who must carry out their compulsions but at the same time try to make their behavior conform to the requirements of the social milieu. In the obsessional rehearsal the patient performs his compulsion, but surveys the scene to determine how he can best work his compulsive activity into the pattern of behavior expected of him at some later date. Reik cites the case of the man whose compulsion was a stamping of the foot to ward off danger as he crossed the border of a country. The patient had arranged to go driving with a woman friend, and their tour was to include crossing a border. On the day before their meeting, the patient drove out to the border and surveyed the scene.

On the following day, when he was in his car with the woman friend, he was able to introduce a discussion of waltz music at just the right moment, so that when the car did cross the border, he could beat time with his foot. In this way his compulsion could be performed without alerting anyone to its pathological features. The obsessional rehearsal was necessary so that the patient would know when he was approaching the border, and so know when to introduce his discussion of waltz music. (Reik, T. *American Imago* 2, 1941)

The obsessional neurotic also often shows peculiar deliberations and anticipations in thought. These are test phantasies, which Reik calls *thought-rehearsals.*

Reich, Annie (1902–71) Austrian-born psychoanalyst; countertransference; lived in New York City after 1938.

Reich, Wilhelm (1897–1957) Austrian-born psychoanalyst; character analysis and ego psychology, orgone energy; practiced in the U.S. In 1957 he was arrested by the Federal Food and Drug Commission, which charged that his orgone boxes were a fraud. Reich died awaiting trial in the federal penitentiary at Lewisburg, Pennsylvania.

reification Treating the abstract as though it were concrete; a type of thinking seen often in schizophrenia but observable also in essentially normal subjects. See *concretization.*

reinforcement In neurophysiology, facilitation; i.e. the enhancement of response to a stimulus by simultaneous excitation of response(s) in other neural circuits, as when the knee jerk is facilitated by having the subject clasp his hands tightly at the same time that his patellar tendon is tapped. In conditioning theory, reinforcement refers to reintroduction of the original, unconditioned stimulus along with the conditioned stimulus, thus strengthening the conditioned response; reinforcement in this sense is sometimes loosely referred to as a reward. See *behaviorism; conditioning, operant.*

reinforcement, Jendrassik (Ernst Jendrassik, Slovakian physician, 1858–1922) A weak response of the knee jerk may often be reinforced, that is, strengthened, by having the patient grasp his own hands and pull vigorously on them.

reinforcement, reactive "Repression is often achieved by means of an excessive reinforcement of the thought contrary to the one which is to be repressed. This process I call *reactive reinforcement*, and the thought which asserts itself exaggeratedly in consciousness and (in the same way as a prejudice) cannot be removed I call a *reactive thought*." (Freud, *CP*)

reinstinctualization Deneutralization of drive energy that would normally be available to the ego for the execution of its various functions. As a result, the functions may be affected adversely by the wishes or conflicts arising from the drives. Reinstinctualization is one aspect of the phenomenon of regression.

In hysterical blindness, for example, the neutralized drive energy that made seeing possible regardless of inner conflict has been lost to the ego; the energy is deneutralized or reinstinctualized so that the function of seeing must be suspended just as the drive itself (aggression or sexuality) must be denied.

reintegration See *integration*.

rejuvenation A special *vasectomy* operation introduced by Steinach to mitigate in men certain pathological symptoms of old age, sexual impotence, hypertrophy of the prostate, or eunuchoidism.

While the ordinary vasectomy technique resulting in sterilization is bilateral and leaves the proximal end of the seminal ducts open, the rejuvenating operation is performed unilaterally and provides for ligatures at both ends of the given vas deferens. The effect of rejuvenation is said to be achieved by a renewed activity of the proliferating and regenerating interstitial secretory tissue of the testicles, which is considered to be the hormone-bearing apparatus mainly responsible in men for sexual libido and potency, as well as by an equally favorable response of the other endocrine glands.

No similar surgical technique has as yet been developed for the rejuvenation of women.

relabeling See *reframing*.

relapse A patient who has recovered or improved and who subsequently suffers a recurrence of symptoms is said to have experienced a relapse.

relatedness The interrelation between two or more people who reciprocally influence each other: patient-therapist, mother-child, etc. Normal relatedness is based on security in interpersonal relations and in large part is a result of early childhood experiences. S. Arieti (*Archives of General Psychiatry* 6, 1962) emphasizes that *basic trust* is essential for the development of normal or satisfactory relatedness. "Basic trust is an 'atmospheric feeling' which predisposes one to expect 'good things' and is a prerequisite to a normal development of self-esteem. . . . The mother expects the child to become a healthy and mature person. The child later perceives this faith of the mother and accepts it. . . . He finally introjects this trust of the significant adults, and he trusts himself."

relatedness, functional The arrangement of objects that are organically and dynamically related to each other: for example, placing woodworking tools near the woodworking bench and nails and other objects involved in woodworking nearby; placing drawing paper near crayons and paints in the proximity of an easel.

relation, fiduciary See *fiduciary relation*.

relationship, calamitous See *group tension, common*.

relationship, inversion of A transposition of natural roles, as a young girl taking the mother's responsibilities or place in the home.

relationship, mother-child See *mother-child relationship*.

relative risk See *risk factor*.

relaxation response A hypothesized coordinated physiologic reaction due to stimulation of hypothalamic regions, which results in generalized decreased sympathetic nervous system activity.

release In neurology, the removal of the inhibitory effect of higher centers on the activity of lower nervous centers. In psychiatry, a form of psychotherapy in which the patient is allowed to express wishes, thoughts, and impulses which he is unable to discharge adequately under usual environmental conditions; in this sense, release is approximately equivalent to catharsis. In child psychiatry, release therapy refers to the use of play methods as an avenue for the expression of the child's anxieties.

release phenomena See *phenomena, release*.

releaser, social Any object or situation that serves as an adequate stimulus to instinctive behavior; e.g. the shadow of a toy airplane moving overhead under certain conditions will make newborn chicks run for cover, as if they had sighted a flying hawk. Permanent modification of behavior by a social releaser is termed *imprinting* (q.v.).

releasing mechanism, inherited See *instinct.*

reliability The degree to which a test measures consistently; the dependability of a measure; the standard deviation is used as a measure of variability and when so used is known as a standard error. See *deviation, mean.* Reliability is inversely proportional to the standard error.

reliance In psychopharmacology, continuing need or desire for recommended doses of a drug, but without the induction of a withdrawal syndrome when the drug is discontinued.

REM Rapid eye movement. REM sleep is active sleep, characterized by increased metabolic rates, elevated temperature, and arousal-type EEG patterns. See *dream; NREM.*

REM behavior disorder (RBD) A parasomnia characterized by altered dreams and violent behaviors during REM sleep (electromyographic atonia and a flaccid paralysis are the usual accompaniments of normal REM sleep). The disorder affects older adults (over 60 years of age) and is associated with various neurologic disorders, including dementia. Successful treatment with clonazepam, a benzodiazepine with serotonergic properties, has been reported. (Schenck, C.H., et al. *Journal of the American Medical Association 257,* 1987)

REM latency The number of minutes from the onset of the first Stage I sleep to the first REM period, reported as being often shorter than normal in some types of depressed patients who are responsive to antidepressant medication. Normal REM latency is 80 to 100 minutes, but it may fall to half that length in depressed patients.

REM sleep efficiency See *sleep efficiency.*

reminiscence Recalling or recollection of past experiences, particularly when the recall has a "now you see it, now you don't" quality. In contrast to memory, reminiscence consists of a peculiarly irregular alternation between remembering and forgetting so that a memory apparently lost suddenly appears, while one that was just there disappears. See *memory.*

remission Abatement of the symptoms and signs of a disorder or disease. The abatement may be partial or complete.

remorse Feelings of regret or guilt about something that has been done; Freud differentiated between remorse and guilt, in that the latter refers to aggressive wishes that have not yet been satisfied.

remotivation Any planned group activity that aims to tap dormant areas of functioning and help the patient to find parts of himself that he has lost and/or that are unaffected by the pathologic process. Originally remotivation referred to a single technique, evolved to deal with severely regressed senile or schizophrenic patients. Remotivation is currently used to refer to a family of rehabilitation techniques that meet a variety of therapeutic needs. Included within the group are:

1. *Reality orientation* (q.v.)—to decrease the confusion of the organic patient, who needs help in relating himself to time, place, and person.

2. *Remotivation activities*—recreational and occupational therapy, rhythm and movement exercises, and the like, used to initiate communication with restless, agitated patients or with those who are silent and withdrawn; remotivation activities often crystallize group feeling and prepare for more meaningful group involvement and verbal communication.

3. *Primary remotivation*—stimulation of the various sensory modalities as a way to encourage group participation and communication.

4. *Advanced remotivation*—which involves some problem solving within the remotivation group setting, such as discussion of concepts or ideas, discussions about social issues and tour groups into the community. (Ward, E., Jackson, C., & Camp, T. *Hospital and Community Psychiatry 24,* 1973)

removal protection See *protection, medical removal.*

Renard Diagnostic Interview A structured interview developed in 1977 at the Washington University (St. Louis) Department of Psychiatry (by L.N. Robins, J. Helzer, and J. Croughan) to elicit enough information so that the criteria established for the diagnosis of 15 major psychiatric disorders could be applied. See *Research Diagnostic Criteria.*

renifleur (rē-nē-flĕr′) See *osphresiolagnia.*

renunciation, instinctual Disavowal of and refusal, on the part of the ego, to satisfy an instinctual (id) demand, for any number of reasons. In the first place, instinctual renunciation takes place in obedience to the reality principle when the satisfying action would bring serious danger to the ego from the outside world. In this case, the unsatisfied instincts would engender a lasting painful tension unless the strength of the instinctual urge were diminished through a displacement of its energies. Second, instinctual renunciation takes place in obedience to the demands of the superego. That is, the ego will not satisfy the instincts if such a satisfying would run counter to the individual's conscience, the prohibitions of his superego. In this case, too, painful tension will spring from the unsatisfied instinct. When, however, the instinctual renunciation takes place because of the superego's objections, it brings about, besides the pain, "a gain in pleasure to the ego—as it were, or substituted satisfaction." This gain in pleasure through obedience to the superego is a direct outgrowth of the child's relationship to its parents' love. He achieves this by renouncing his instincts and, instead, obeying his parents' precepts and thus avoiding a threatened loss of love. This gives him security and satisfaction. In later life, "The super-ego is the successor and representative of the parents (and educators)" and "perpetuates their functions almost without a change." Thus the ego is concerned with retaining the love and appreciation of the superego, which is experienced as relief and satisfaction, a pleasurable feeling. This will occur when an instinctual renunciation, a sacrifice to the superego, has taken place. (Freud, S. *Moses and Monotheism,* 1939)

repersonalization Morton Prince suggested this term in place of *hypnotism.*

repetition compulsion "The blind impulse to repeat earlier experiences and situations quite irrespective of any advantage that doing so might bring from a pleasure-pain point of view." (Jones, E. *Papers on Psycho-Analysis,* 1938)

The impulse to redramatize or to reenact some earlier emotional experience. The principle is more fundamental, according to Freud, than the pleasure principle and generally differs widely from it, in that the experience repeated is usually a painful one, which contains "no potentiality of pleasure and which could at no time have been satisfactory.

"It must be explained that we are able to postulate the principle of a *repetition-compulsion* in the unconscious mind, based upon instinctual activity and probably inherent in the very nature of the instincts—a principle powerful enough to overrule the pleasure principle, lending to certain aspects of the mind their daemonic character, and still very clearly expressed in the tendencies of small children." (Freud, *CP*)

repetition reaction See *repetition compulsion.*

replacement In psychiatric occupational therapy the substitution of normal and healthy thoughts and actions for unhealthy, abnormal ones. The means used to achieve this result include the employment of various activities such as the handicrafts, recreation, and other interests of a constructive nature.

replacement formation See *formation, replacement.*

replacement memory See *memory, replacement.*

representation See *sensorimotor stage.*

representation, coitus The representation of sexual intercourse in terms of symptom formations or by other symbolizations. "In this analysis the girl's stammering proved to be determined by the libidinal cathexis of speaking as well as of singing. The rise and fall of the voice and the movements of the tongue represented coitus." (Klein, M. *Contributions to Psycho-analysis, 1921–1945,* 1948)

representations, collective The concepts that embody the objectives of group activity.

representative intelligence See *developmental psychology.*

representatives, instinct The psychic manifestations, such as strivings and emotions, that ally themselves with ideas and give rise to wishes, of an instinct or drive. The instincts are not observable directly but are expressed by means of such representatives.

repress To force material from the realm of consciousness into the unconscious; to prevent material that was never conscious from gaining the level of consciousness.

repressed, return of the The return to consciousness of an idea or set of ideas that had been repressed into the sphere of the unconscious.

"So far as we know at present, it seems probable that the two [substitute-formation and symptom-formation] are widely divergent, that it is not the repression itself which produces substitute-formations and symptoms but that these later constitute indications of a *return of the repressed* and owe their existence to quite other processes." (Freud, *CP*)

repression The active process of keeping out and ejecting, banishing from consciousness, ideas or impulses that are unacceptable to it.

When an instinct presentation (i.e. an idea or group of ideas charged with affect) is painful to the contents of consciousness, an effort is made to thrust it into the sphere of the unconscious. It is possible to reduce to a minimum the influence of such an instinct presentation by first breaking it up into its two basic components: the idea and the affective charge. This means that there are three things that are subject to repression: (1) the instinct presentation; (2) the idea; (3) the affect. In many instances, when the entire instinct cannot be successfully repressed, either the ideational or the affective part may be. If the idea is repressed, the affect with which it was associated may be transferred to another idea (in consciousness) that has no apparent connection with the original idea. Or, if the affect is repressed, the idea, remaining, so to speak, alone in consciousness, may be linked with a pleasant affect. Finally, if the whole instinct presentation is repressed, it may at some later time return to consciousness in the form of a symbol.

For example, a son may consciously hate his father. The idea and the affect are repellent to him. He may repress both, but if the idea is strongly charged with affect, it strives to reenter consciousness. It may return to consciousness in disguised form, for example, as hatred for some superior, unconnected with the father. If the idea alone of the father is repressed, the hate may be transferred to someone else, who is not recognized as standing for the father. If the hate alone is repressed, the idea (father) may be cathected with love; in this last instance the hate may return to consciousness to be connected with someone not known to be a father substitute.

All the foregoing observations refer to *repression proper*, which Freud at times calls *after-expulsion*, because the material repressed is that which was once in the conscious realm.

There is another subdivision called *primal repression*. The ego has the task of keeping repressed in the unconscious material that has never been in consciousness. "Now we have a reason for assuming a *primal repression*, a first phase of repression, which consists in a denial of entry into consciousness to the mental (ideational) presentation of the instinct. This is accompanied by a *fixation;* the ideational presentation in question persists unaltered from then onwards and the instinct remains attached to it." (Freud, *CP*)

Primal repression is maintained by means of anticathexis, which Freud says "is the sole mechanism of primal repression."

Anna Freud pointed out that "repression occupies a unique place among the defences. It accomplishes more than others, acting once only through the anticathexis. It is also the most ego-limiting, because whole tracts of mental life are withdrawn from the ego in repression. In distinguishing repression from the other mechanisms of defence, she says 'it may be that these other methods (other defences) have only to complete what repression has left undone, or to deal with such prohibited ideas as return to consciousness when repression fails.' " (Leveton, A.F. *International Journal of Psycho-analysis XLII*, 1961)

According to Jung, when the *superior function* is *thinking* (e.g. the extraverted thinking type), the *feeling* function is subordinated. When the individual tries to meet all the requirements of living by the *thinking function*, "sooner or later—in accordance with outer circumstances and inner gifts—the forms of life repressed [i.e. feeling, intuition, and sensation] by the intellectual attitude become indirectly perceptible, through a gradual disturbance of the conscious conduct of life. Whenever disturbances of this kind reach a definite intensity, one speaks of a neurosis." (Jung, *PT*)

repression, organic A special type of amnesia that occurs in cases of head injuries independently of any personal problems that the patient wishes to forget. It is a retroactive amnesia: as in (the so-called) psychogenic amnesia, the subject turns away from a part of his experiences. In organic repression, however, no specific personal motives are discernible. The person forgets, more or less extensively, the events of his life prior to the accident, as if he were trying to get rid of knowledge of his experiences, although such a desire is not present even in the subconscious. See *amnesia.*

repression, primal See *repression.*

repression proper See *repression.*

repression resistance See *resistance, ego.*

repression, secondary Synonymous with *repression;* the word *secondary* is seldom used.

repressive personality *Hysterical personality* (q.v.).

repressors See *anxiety typology.*

reproduction The creative process by which organic life is transmitted from one organism to a succession of new ones. Although the origin of new organisms takes place in very different ways, the ultimate aim and sense of the reproductive process is always to maintain the preservation of a species and to guarantee the continuity between successive generations.

Plants and the simplest types of animals originate by *asexual* or *vegetative* reproduction, which simply divides the parental body into two or more parts, each of which grows into a new organism. The division into two *equal* new cells usually occurs in unicellular organisms like amoebae and is called *fission.* However, even in the case of *unequal* division, or *budding,* it holds true that the offspring can be expected to be practically identical with the parent. If differences between offspring and parents arise in asexual reproduction, they may primarily be attributed to *mutations* that do not depend on the type of reproduction and constitute the basis of most evolutionary developments. See *mutation.*

The typical form of *sexual* reproduction is biparental and presupposes the differentiation of a species into two sexes capable of producing individual germ cells. Among higher animals, the two types of specialized *sexual cells* or *gametes* are known as *spermatozoa* and *ova,* according to whether they are produced in the testis of a male or in the ovary of a female. At fertilization a male and a female gamete unite, the nucleus of one fusing completely with that of the other, and they form one *single* cell, the fertilized egg or *zygote,* from which a new organism develops by cell division.

Wherever sexual reproduction occurs, it is bound to lead to variations among the offspring as well as to differences between offspring and parents. Mature germ cells have only half of the chromosomes of the individual producing the germ cells, and homologous chromosomes are similar, but not usually identical. The nature of a germ cell depends on which of the two chromosomes it has received from each pair. See *meiosis.*

In certain groups of animals, for instance in the honey-bee, an egg may develop into a new organism without having been fertilized by a spermatozoon. Such uniparental mode of reproduction is called *parthenogenesis* and is regarded as sexual, although offspring produced parthenogenetically have only one parent.

reproductive failure Lack of success in bearing a child as in infertility or miscarriage, and usually also extended to include neonatal death.

reproductive mortality Deaths associated with fertility control, including deaths due to adverse effects of temporary contraceptive methods and sterilization and deaths due to complications of pregnancy.

repulsion A modifying process in the recombination of genetic factors, which was discovered by Bateson and Punnett both as an exception to the Mendelian principle of independent assortment and as the antithesis of the phenomenon of *coupling* (q.v.). Its mechanism consists of an "aversion" of the genes introduced by different parents to entering the same gametes, and its effect is similar to that of coupling, leading to the formation of an excess of the parental combinations of genes and a deficiency of the new type of combinations.

According to Morgan's chromosome theory repulsion and coupling are manifestations of a single important phenomenon now usually called *linkage* (q.v.).

required relationship See *group tension, common.*

rescue phantasy See *romance, family.*

Rescuer See *transactional analysis.*

research, action Scientific study of ongoing process, such research being aimed toward achieving some improvement in the methods of the operating program.

Research Diagnostic Criteria (RDC) A modification of the criteria developed by Washington University (St. Louis) for diagnosis of psychiatric disorders. The RDC was developed by R. Spitzer and coworkers at Columbia University (New York) and expanded the number of disorders from the original 15 to 25. (New York State Psychiatric Institute, *Biometrics Research*, 1978) It focuses on present or past episodes of illness and gives inclusion and exclusion criteria for diagnosis of the different disorders. It is supplemented by the *Schedule for Affective Disorders and Schizophrenia (SADS)*, designed to elicit information on signs and symptoms and their duration. See *Renard Diagnostic Interview*.

research, infancy See *infancy research*.

research, operations See *operations research*.

research, specific Any investigation or study that is designed primarily to gain knowledge about a disease or condition of the specific person being used as a subject of an experiment. Nonspecific research, in contrast, uses subjects to gain knowledge about a disease or functioning even though the results may be of no value or relevance to the experimental subjects. Some believe that it is never ethical to conduct nonspecific research, whereas others believe that if fully informed and mentally competent, subjects have the right to volunteer for such investigations.

research, strategic Studies whose focus is treatment and care, as opposed to *tactical research*, which emphasizes the action taken to implement the findings of strategic research. Development of a vaccine, for example, is based on strategic research; the public health programs devised to administer it and evaluation of its effect on the populations to whom it has been administered depend on tactical research.

residential centers See *domicile*.

residua, brain See *neurogram*.

residual Remaining, left behind, with the implication that some effect continues to be exerted. Some authorities recognize a psychoactive substance-induced organic mental disorder, the *organic residual syndrome*, which may develop after prolonged heavy use of a psychoactive substance. Also called the *amotivational syndrome*, it consists of reduction in goal-directed behavior such as attending school or going to work, and it may be accompanied by depression, irritability, difficulties in attention and concentration, and other mild cognitive deficits. See *syndrome, amotivational*.

residual schizophrenia See *schizophrenia*.

residue, archaic Remnants of primitive mentality. See *function engram; memory, biological; memory, racial*.

residue, night Persistence of any psychic material from sleeping and dreaming during the waking day; the manifest dream (i.e. the dream as remembered by the subject) is the most common example of night residue. The night residue persists because of failure of repression at the time the sleeper wakes, at least according to some theories of dream function. See *dream*.

resignation, neurotic In Horney's terminology, avoidance of any part of reality that brings inner conflicts into awareness, whether by means of withdrawal into inactivity, pressured hyperactivity in all other parts of reality, or neurotic rebelliousness against all rules and regulations.

resistance The instinctive opposition displayed toward any attempt to lay bare the unconscious; a manifestation of the repressing forces.

resistance, character See *defense, character*.

resistance, conscious Freud's term for the intentional withholding of information by the patient because of distrust of the analyst, shame, fear of rejection, or the like. In his early work, Freud discovered that patients cannot maintain free association uninterruptedly, and sooner or later fail to mention something that occurs to them. They show other signs of difficulty with the treatment process—tardiness or failure to keep appointments, loss of interest in their own problems, and turning all their attention to trying to win the analyst's love or to engaging in a battle of wits with him, etc. Exhortation can usually induce the patient to overcome these conscious difficulties.

Unconscious resistance, on the other hand, is more significant and more difficult to overcome, arising as it does from the ego as a defense against uncovering the repressed material, which the ego constantly strives to avoid, since it produces anxiety. Unconscious resistance is more than a phenomenon appearing early in treatment and later overcome once and for all. It is a conservative force seeking to maintain the status quo and appearing throughout the analysis whenever significant data are under discussion. See *silence, selective.*

resistance, ego Much of the resistance to be overcome in analysis is produced by the ego, "which clings tenaciously to its anti-cathexes." In other words, the ego "finds it difficult to turn its attention to perceptions and ideas the avoidance of which it had until then made a rule, or to acknowledge as belonging to it impulses which constitute the most complete antithesis to those familiar to it as its own." This resistance of the ego is known more specifically as repression resistance. It is often unconscious.

Freud describes two more categories of ego resistance. One, which is of the same character as repression resistance but exists specifically with reference to the analytical situation, is transference resistance: the repression constantly exerted by the ego is in this case related specifically to the person of the analyst and thus appears in the analysis in different and more definite ways than simple repression resistance. The other (third) category of ego resistance is related to the gain of the illness. Symptoms in warding off dangerous instinctual impulses both relieve anxiety and serve as a means of gratifying these instinctual impulses. The ego opposes the renunciation of both the gratification and relief that are "based upon the inclusion of the symptom in the ego."

It should be added that in analysis there are also resistances that derive from sources other than ego. These are (1) the "'resistance of the unconscious' or of the id, which derives from the "'repetition-compulsion,'" and (2) the "resistance of the super-ego," which derives from "the sense of guilt or need of punishment." (Freud, S. *The Problem of Anxiety,* 1936)

resistance, id A type of resistance, seen most clearly in patients in psychoanalytic treatment, that derives from the repetition compulsion and is manifested typi-

cally as situations of mistrust, grievance, depreciation, and the like, which dominate the analytic situation during periods of seeming stalemate. No matter how many interpretations are given by the analyst, and no matter how valid each interpretation seems to be, the same material continues to recur. "In short, having exhausted the possibilities of resistance arising from the ego or the super-ego, we are faced with the bare fact that a set of presentations is being repeated before us again and again. That is, at the same time, a clue to the understanding of the situation, because the nearer we get to seemingly blind repetition, the nearer we are to a characteristic of instinctual excitation." What has happened is that "the id has made use of weakened ego defenses to exercise an increased attraction on preconscious presentations.... For this reason Freud described the manifestation as being the *resistance of mind.*" (Glover, E. *The Technique of Psycho-Analysis,* 1955) The only method with which to counter id resistance is *working-through* (q.v.).

resistance, state of See *syndrome, general adaptation.*

resistance, superego *Negative therapeutic reaction;* a type of resistance encountered in patients in psychoanalytic treatment in which the need for punishment, as manifested in guilt feelings and masochistic behavior, continues to produce symptoms and is the only barrier to their resolution. Superego resistance is most frequently manifested by obsessionals whose anxiety is a fear of the loss of the superego's love.

Negative therapeutic reaction is sometimes used loosely to refer to any therapy that does not go well, although most authors use it more specifically to refer to patients whose conditions worsen during therapy. The patient with severe borderline personality disorder of the narcissistic, sadomasochistic, or paranoid subtypes is particularly likely to show a negative therapeutic reaction.

resistance, transference See *transference resistance.*

respiratory impairment sleep disorder Sleep apnea. See *sleep disorders.*

respondent conditioning See *conditioning.*

response, barrier See *barrier.*

response, conditioned See *conditioning.*

response, galvanic skin See *reflex, psychogalvanic*.

response (in marriage) Understanding, cooperative, sympathetic, or affectionate interreaction between two persons married to each other. Mowrer says: "The desire for response is universal among human beings. In the marriage relation it involves the demonstration of affection, the sharing of interests, aspirations, and ideals by husband and wife." (Lemkau, P.V. *Mental Hygiene in Public Health*, 1949)

response, negativistic A tendency to do the exact opposite of what is requested or ordered. When asked to open his eyes, the patient shuts them tightly; when asked to come forward, he backs away. This condition is most common in the catatonic type of schizophrenia. See *negativism*.

response, penetration See *barrier*.

response prevention See *therapy, delay*.

responsibility, criminal The culpability of a person, as determined by due process of law, for any of his actions that are defined as criminal. Determination of such responsibility is a legal function, not a psychiatric one, although a psychiatrist may be called upon to present evidence to the court in order to aid the judge or jury in reaching a decision as to responsibility. Determination of responsibility varies with the laws of the state in which the accused is being tried, but in general all states base their laws on three famous judicial decisions concerning criminal responsibility:

1. *The M'Naghten* (or McNaughton) *rule,* also known as the *right and wrong test* or the *knowledge test*—In 1843, Daniel M'Naghten shot and killed Drummond, private secretary to Sir Robert Peel. He had mistaken Drummond for the latter. For some years, M'Naghten had suffered from delusions of persecution and had finally woven Sir Robert Peel into his delusional system. He was determined to right his imaginary wrongs by killing Peel. When he was brought to trial the court recognized that the killing was an outcome of his delusions of persecution; he was declared of unsound mind and committed to an institution for the criminally insane. Following this trial, the Judges of England enunciated two rules to determine the responsibility of an accused who pleads insanity as a

defense: (a) to establish such a defense the accused, at the time the act was committed, must be shown to have been laboring under such defect of reason as not to know the nature and quality of the act he was doing, or (b) if he did know it, he did not know that what he was doing was wrong.

2. *The irresistible impulse test,* recommended as an addition to the M'Naghten rule in 1922—"A person charged criminally with an offense is irresponsible for his act when the act is committed under an impulse which the prisoner was by mental disease in substance deprived of any power to resist."

3. *The Durham decision*—A 1954 ruling by the United States Court of Appeals that "an accused is not criminally responsible if his unlawful act was the product of mental disease or mental defect." Prior to this decision, psychiatric testimony relating to the mental status of the accused was confined to a determination of whether the accused could distinguish right and wrong, or acted under an irresistible impulse at the time of the offense. Under the Durham test, however, the psychiatrist may give any relevant testimony concerning the mental illness issue.

Traditionally, the defense of nonculpability has been limited to very young children and the mentally disturbed. Controversy revolves about the question of defining "mentally disturbed." So long as the accused was clearly psychotic and obviously unable to understand what he was doing, it seemed only logical to absolve him of responsibility for his actions. But studies of persons found not guilty by reason of insanity (NGRI) reveals that between 10 and 30% of such acquittees are diagnosed as personality disorders, not as psychotic. In consequence, there is concern that the defense may be abused, particularly in the case of persons charged with violent crime. That concern has been reflected in recent tightening of the standards and procedures used to determine an accused person's culpability, both to prevent the misuse of the NGRI defense in the first place and also to protect the public against premature release of potentially dangerous people.

responsibility, limited See *insanity, partial*.

REST Regressive electroshock therapy. See *therapy, regressive electroshock*.

rest cure The term is usually associated with the American psychiatrist Silas Weir Mitchell (1829–1914), who stressed the value of rest, environmental change, fattening diet, massage, and mild exercise. It has not achieved much distinction as an isolated method of treatment, though the individual procedures (rest, environmental change, etc.) are known to be highly valuable.

rest tremor See *tremor.*

restitution See *schizophrenia, restitutional symptoms.*

restless legs syndrome *Ekbom's syndrome; restless legs sleep disorder; tachyathetosis;* a form of *insomnia* (q.v.) caused by sensations of quivering or fluttering inside the calves when lying or sitting down, a sense of tightness as if the muscles of the leg could no longer be contained within the skin. When symptoms occur at bedtime, they interfere with sleep onset. The syndrome may represent an extrapyramidal hyperkinesis, and it sometimes occurs as a side effect of neuroleptics. See *sleep disorders.*

restraining therapy See *therapy, paradoxical.*

restraint A generic term for measures taken to prevent a patient from injuring himself or others. Most frequently the term refers to physical interventions designed to control or reduce the patient's ability to commit dangerous or violent actions, but the term also includes limitation or restriction of movement in patients unable to function independently when they are at risk of falling (out of chair or bed), wandering, etc.

Four-point leather cufflets, cold wet packs, and camisoles have been used to achieve total or almost complete physical restraint. Such methods require constant, skilled nursing care, and if the restrained patient is also being treated with phenothiazines, the likelihood of temperature dysregulation and potentially dangerous hyperthermia increases. Further, the psychological effects of being tied down and totally dependent on others for feeding and toileting are generally negative.

For these reasons, most clinicians prefer to use *seclusion* of violent or potentially violent patients. The seclusion room is free of all objects the patient might use to harm himself or staff—including not only furniture, mirrors, and other room ap-

pointments but also any of the patient's belongings that might be used in self-mutilation or in an outwardly directed attack (belt, shoes, rings, etc.). The seclusion room is also called the *quiet room,* not as a way to deny what it is, but in recognition of the fact that many patients request seclusion when they feel themselves to be on the verge of an agitated or destructive outburst that they doubt they can control.

restraint, situational Employed especially in activity group psychotherapy, this type of restraint is differentiated from direct or authoritative restraint in that it is practiced by creating a situation that by its very nature will prevent the individual from committing dangerous or destructive acts. In activity group psychotherapy, windows are screened so that they will not be broken and furniture is placed in such a way that the children will not need to or cannot move it about. Placing materials according to their *functional relatedness* is also a form of situational restraint.

restricters Persons with anorexia nervosa who achieve and maintain their low weight by restricting their food intake. Restricters are contrasted with bulimics, who alternate between starvation and engorgement (a condition also known as *bulimia nervosa, bulimarexia,* and *dietary chaos syndrome*).

restriction enzyme See *marker, genetic; recombinant DNA.*

restructuring, cognitive See *therapy, behavior; therapy, cognitive.*

resymbolization A new symbolization adopted in the life of a patient on regaining a healthy mentality. "A recovered patient, as he makes a new adaptation to life, must redefine all his conceptions, particularly those related to his own conflict. This is essentially a resymbolization of his life concepts and in itself denotes a healthy attitude and a good prognosis. ... Resymbolization is a universal phenomenon in our daily life and of which the resymbolization as used by psychotics is only one of the pathological forms." (Karpman, B. *Psychoanalytic Review 9,* 1922)

retardation 1. Slowness or backwardness of intellectual development; *mental retardation.* 2. Slowness of response, a slowing down of thinking and/or a decrease in psychomotor activity; *psychomotor retardation*. Psychomotor retardation is characteristic of clinical depressions.

retardation, Amsterdam type See *syndrome, de Lange.*

retardation, developmental See *acceleration, developmental.*

retardation, language Delay in the development of language skills, not due to mental retardation, hearing impairment, or structural abnormalities of the organs of speech, but assumed instead to be based on lag in cerebral maturation. Included are numerous manifestations, variously called baby talk, lalling, lisping, congenital auditory agnosia, word deafness. Some authorities subdivide the group into *developmental dysphasia* and *developmental articulation disorder* (qq.v.).

retardation, mental *Mental deficiency; intellectual inadequacy; feeblemindedness; hypophrenia; oligophrenia; oligergasia;* subnormal general intellectual functioning that originates during the developmental period (before 18 years of age), and is associated with impaired learning and social adjustment or maturation. It is subdivided on the basis of degree of intellectual impairment into four subtypes: (1) *mild*—Wechsler IQ 69–55; in educational terms, the *educable* retardates, who account for about 75% of the total group; (2) *moderate*—IQ 55–40; the *trainable* retardates; (3) *severe*—IQ 39–25; together, the moderate and severe retardates account for about 20% of the total group; (4) *profound*—IQ below 25.

Intellectual deficit, or mental subnormality, denotes a lack of equipment, motivation, or opportunity to acquire knowledge at the usual pace. By some, mental deficiency is used specifically to refer to cases with demonstrable cerebral impairment. Others, however, do not make such a distinction or even use the terms in exactly the opposite way. Thus W.F. Windle (*Science 140,* 1963) defines mental retardation as "An organic condition of arrested or limited neural development that blocks successful evolution of the capacity of the brain to function; as a result of this block, behavior and (at least in man) intellectual ability are impaired. Forms of behavioral and intellectual impairment that are related solely to socio-environmental factors are excluded, since in these cases there is no detectable pathology." See *amentia; dementia.*

Fashions in labeling this group change almost from year to year; in the 1960s, mental retardation was the favorite appellation, and justifiably so in that it does not imply that inheritance or constitutional defects are always the cause of mental retardation. In 1941, Gregg demonstrated the association of rubella in the first trimester of pregnancy with mental retardation and thereby showed that the condition could result not from an inferior constitution but from birth conditions. Since then, there has been increasing recognition of the importance of psychosocial factors in exaggerating or even, in some cases, producing mental retardation, and two major approaches to such factors have developed.

The *stimulation theory* supposes that mental retardation may be a consequence of lack of stimulation, lack of opportunities, or deprivation. The *disorder theory* regards mental retardation as a disorder of mental processes due to failure of the family to give sufficient protection from stress or overstimulation during critical periods of learning in early childhood. As with some habits in animals (see *imprinting; releaser, social*), there are believed to be optimal periods in the human during which learning proceeds rapidly, although at other times those habits will be learned only slowly or not at all. Thus a child may not learn because family conditions or other elements in his environment are not favorable to acquiring the habit when he is in a critical or sensitive period; or if he is exposed to adverse circumstances soon after acquiring a habit, it may regress and his skill may disintegrate; and even if later moved into more favorable circumstances he may fail to learn because the sensitive period has passed.

retardation, mental, psychosis with Occasionally, mental retardates may show psychotic reactions that are usually of an acute transitory nature. These psychotic manifestations include episodes of excitement with depression, hallucinatory attacks, or paranoid trends.

retardation, psychopathology of Primary psychopathology of the mental retardation syndrome includes the intellectual impairment plus the characteristics of emotional development that are more closely related to the degree of retardation than to any other factors such as deprivation. The primary psychopathology consists of the intellectual impairment or specific learning difficulty, the slow rate of development, and disturbances in the quality of emotional development such as impairment in differentiation of ego functions producing infantile or immature character structure, nonpsychotic autism, repetitiousness, inflexibility, passivity.

retardation, psychosocial Mental retardation associated with, accentuated by, or caused by such interactional or environmental factors as defective mother-child relationships, disturbed attachment, inadequate enrichment at home (in the social, emotional, or intellectual sphere), impaired learning because of severe emotional disorder, and insufficient emotional interaction in institutional settings. See *attachment disorder of infancy; mother-child relationship.*

retardation, reading A term suggested by Rabinovitch et al. (1954) to describe all subjects in whom the level of reading achievement is two years or more below the mental age obtained in performance tests. See *reading disabilities.*

retardation, simple See *melancholia; psychosis, manic-depressive.*

retention Nonevacuation of the bladder or bowels. In psychological testing, retention refers to the ability to learn, remember, or recall (see *memory*). In psychoanalytic psychology, retention refers to any number of traits or symptoms believed to develop on the basis of the need or desire to withhold the feces during the anal stage of development; collecting mania, stubbornness, secretiveness, niggardliness are generally considered to be instances of anal retention or retentiveness.

retention, anal In psychoanalysis, the holding back of the fecal mass as part of toilet training and the characterologic or symptomatic carryovers of this in later life. Frugality, for example is considered to be a continuation of the anal habit of retention; stubbornness and obstinacy are more complicated developments of this same habit that are related to the child's ability to spite parental efforts by tightening his sphincters. Psychodynamically,

anal retention is seen to contain two components, fear of loss of body contents or of control over instinctual impulses, and enjoyment of erogenous pleasure; and later anal character traits represent an outgrowth of one or the other or both of these components. See *anal erotism; character, anal.*

reticular activating system See *formation, reticular.*

reticular formation See *formation, reticular.*

reticulum *Biol.* A finely meshed network in a cell or in some delicate tissue system.

rétifism (Rétif de la Bretonne, 1734–1806, a famous French educator, known for this paraphilia) Ivan Bloch coined this term for fetishism of the foot and shoe; in this form of sexual perversion the foot or shoe or both possess the value of the genital organs for the rétifist. A patient "loved," as he put it, the female shoe to the same degree that "others are attracted to the female genitals." He looked upon the shoe as if it were a real person—gaining full and complete sexual satisfaction, including "intercourse," with the object; he used it as an agency of masturbation.

retinodiencephalic degeneration See *syndrome, Laurence-Moon-Biedl.*

retreat, vegetative The tendency of some neurotic persons to meet an inimical or dangerous reality situation not by appropriate self-assertive behavior and actions, but by recourse to infantile or childish function of the visceral apparatus, which, to them, anachronistically stands for praise or succor from strong or omnipotent parents. It thus represents a return to the pseudopower of the "helpless" and dependent child and warrants the descriptive term *regressive,* because it is a resort to the old infantile ways of handling frustration and stress. See *hypoglycemia.*

A common example of this phenomenon is the man who develops diarrhea when in danger instead of carrying out an appropriate action directed against the dangerous enemy or situation. As a harbinger of protection and approval, this vegetative reaction, or achievement, is inappropriate for adult life, but logical for infancy, where it brought mother's care. There is on record the case of a married woman who found herself sucking her thumbs whenever thwarted or rejected by her husband. (Alexander, F. *Psychosomatic Medicine*, 1950)

retrieval See *memory*.

retroflexion A turning backwards, especially upon the self. In psychoanalysis, the term is used particularly by Rado, who speaks of retroflexed rage, i.e. one's own rage turned back upon the self. See *psychodynamics, adaptational*.

retrogenesis The regression to earlier or lower stages that is often essential before further development can be achieved; Staercek termed it the *Law of Retrogenesis*. "It is remarkable to know in the matter of conscience the universal rule once more applies: that that which is newly formed does not develop from the highest (in the sense of the most recent) existing formation but out of a lower part which has remained hitherto undeveloped. Every line of development is a blind-alley: the new sprouts from a bud which is further, sometimes much further, down. The path of development is not that of *evolution* but of *revolution*. Only out of temporary chaos does renewal proceed." (*International Journal of Psychoanalysis X*, 1929)

retrograde See *amnesia, retrograde*.

retrogression A return to earlier behavior or techniques when more recently developed techniques prove unsatisfactory. The term is synonymous with *regression* but avoids the psychoanalytic connotations of the latter.

retropulsion Rapid running backward with short steps, in paralysis agitans; as if drawn by an uncontrollable force.

return of the repressed See *repressed, return of the*.

revenge Retaliation; vindication; the wish of the injured person to retaliate against the aggressor, which often leads in the neurotic to a fear of retaliation and a consequent need to repress or deny his own aggression.

reverie (revery) A type of phantasy in which the subject is lost in thought or abstract musing that is not purposely directed.

reverie, hypnagogic The phantasies occurring between sleep and waking. Kubie has shown that the institution of a state of hypnagogic reverie can bring about easier access to unconscious material. When employing hypnosis, the analyst can take advantage of it by "permitting his patients to associate freely in the waking state, until a resistance is manifested. Hypnosis is then induced and the last few statements uttered by the patient before the onset of resistance are repeated to him. Usually free association will continue during hypnosis from this point on." (Wolberg, L.R. *Hypnoanalysis*, 1945)

reversal In psychoanalysis the reversal of an instinct into its opposite means a change of it from an active to a passive instinct or vice versa. The *aim* of the instinct does not change; its object does. For example, the destructive instinct may be directed outwardly, as sadism, or it may be turned against oneself, as masochism. "The passive aim (to be tortured . . .) has been substituted for the active (to torture . . .)." (Freud, *CP*)

Freud says also that there may be *reversal* of content. "Reversal of content is found in the single instance of the change of love into hate." (Ibid.) See *opposite, reversal into the*.

reversal formation See *reaction formation*.

reversal of affect See *affect, inversion of*.

reversal, role See *role reversal*.

reversal, sex The phenomenon in which chromosomal sex, as determined by any of the various sex chromatin tests, differs from anatomical sex. Etiology is unknown; chromosomal abnormalities, early deficiency of primordial germ cells, and/or hormonal imbalance have been suggested as playing an important role.

It has been produced in many animals "to the extent of changing the histological character of the gonads and to some extent the ducts, but the change has seldom gone far enough in an adult animal, to permit the individual to function as of the new sex." (Shull, A.F. *Heredity*, 1938)

The most remarkable instance of complete sex reversal was observed by Crew, in an adult hen that had laid normal eggs producing normal chicks, before she changed into a cock that became the father of two normal chicks. An autopsy showed that the original ovary had been destroyed by a tumor, and a testis had been produced in its place by regeneration.

reversion A genetic phenomenon that occurs in crosses between true-breeding varieties and produces offspring resembling a remote ancestor more than either parent.

These "throwbacks" had been observed for many years by plant and animal breeders, but for lack of satisfactory explanation had been regarded as due to some mysterious force that caused the retention and subsequent reappearance of a remote ancestral trait.

According to E.W. Sinnott and L.C. Dunn (*Principles of Genetics*, 1939) every kind of reversion is now readily explained in terms of ordinary Mendelian inheritance. "The reappearance of an old trait is usually due to the reunion of the two or more factors, necessary for its production, which had become separated in the history of the plant or animal."

Reversion is also used synonymously with regression or retrogression; less commonly, it is used synonymously with reversal formation or reaction formation.

review Critical examination or evaluation; assessment of medical care or services is no longer a matter solely of evaluating the quality of care, for it must also be judged in terms of cost effectiveness.

Third-party payers (insurers) have had criteria for reimbursement of medical claims for many years. In 1965, Medicare legislation established more uniform control over reimbursement for health care to the aged. The Social Security Amendment of 1972 established *PSROs (professional standards review organizations)*, with utilization control over inpatient (and ultimately outpatient) treatment of Medicaid and Medicare patients and of those covered by maternal and child health programs. Since those developments, there has been increasing emphasis on formalized *peer review*, evaluation of the treatment process by one or more colleagues. The review process includes utilization review, quality review, continuing education, advocacy with intermediaries for improved care, and cost control.

Peer review is a system of professional judgment of individual or group medical performance. Most systems depend upon professionally developed *screening* criteria for measuring quality of care, and the cases that do not meet those criteria are selected out for review in greater depth by professionals who make the final decision about adequacy of care. Peer review emphasizes continuing education as a way to improve methods of practice and quality of care. Like the more traditional forms of evaluation of treatment process—such as case conferences, grand rounds, and continuing case supervision—its objectives are professional growth and development and not reduction of psychiatric practice to a mechanical or pedestrian ritual.

Peer review for medical purposes attempts to systematize and document the treatment process with the ultimate goal of improving the quality of care. Peer review for insurance purposes, on the other hand, is focused on cost containment and medical necessity; such a process is termed *claims review*. See *audit*.

Utilization review is analysis of admissions to service from the point of view of determination of the medical necessity for the level of particular services provided and for the duration of stay within the institution. Utilization review is *concurrent* rather than retrospective in that it occurs while care is being provided: *admission certification* of the necessity for admission and *continued stay review (CSR)* for assessment of the need for care to be continued. CSR in large part consists of comparison of the case under review with regional *norms*, which usually are expressed as average *length of stay (LOS)* for each diagnosis.

revindication, delirium of, insanity of See *interpretation, delirium of*.

revolution A sudden and far-reaching change, a major break in the continuity of development; that mass movement that seeks to change the mores by destroying the existing social order.

Three major types of revolution are *cultural*, where profound changes take place in the mores; *industrial*, where sudden changes result from technological discoveries and inventions; and *political*, where violent change takes place in the political order.

revolution, sexual See *sexual revolution*.

revolving door See *readmission*.

RFLP Restriction fragment length polymorphism. See *marker, genetic*.

rhabdophobia Fear of the rod, instrument of punishment.

rhathymia Outgoing, carefree, happy-go-lucky behavior such as is seen in so-called oral optimists.

rhembasmus *Obs.* Indecision, mental uncertainty.

rheobase The lowest amount of current that will produce contraction (or other reaction) of a muscle.

rheumatism A variety of disorders characterized by pain and stiffness referable to the musculoskeletal system; rheumatism involving the joints themselves is termed *arthritis* (q.v.).

rheumatoid arthritis See *arthritis*.

rhinencephalon A phylogenetically old portion of the cerebral hemispheres that includes olfactory bulb and tract, anterior perforated substance, subcallosal gyrus, hippocampus, uncus, amygdala, fornix, and anterior commissure. Rhinencephalon is sometimes used synonymously with olfactory brain. In man, the olfactory brain is overshadowed by the neocortex (isocortex), but olfaction appears to be important in the psychic apparatus of the human. The physiology of the rhinencephalon is poorly understood and is largely based on inferences drawn from its anatomical relations. Animal experiments indicate that the olfactory tract terminates in the prepyriform area, the amygdala, the periamygdaloid cortex, and the opposite olfactory bulb. Although the hippocampus is generally regarded as part of the olfactory system, it is to be noted that no anatomical connections of the hippocampus with the olfactory tract have been demonstrated. Instead, the hippocampus appears to be primarily an efferent system projecting to the medial and lateral mammillary nuclei of the hypothalamus, and as such it is probably concerned with control of autonomic functions. Rhinencephalic structures may exert an inhibitory effect on brain-stem mechanisms concerned with emotional expression. Lesions of these structures result in restlessness and hyperactivity.

The *limbic system* (sometimes called the *visceral brain*) includes the olfactory areas, the hippocampus and amygdaloid complex, the cingulate cortex, and the septal area. It regulates the hypothalamic area and so is critical for emotional and affective display. It overlaps with both the sensory and the motor systems and so is also critical in learning and *memory* (q.v.). Positioned between brain areas concerned with sensory perception and motor action, the limbic system analyzes the significance of sensory input and then chooses behavior patterns that will maintain homeostasis, promote self-perpetuation, and ensure perpetuation of the species.

rhinolalia Nasality of speech. Rhinolalia is of two types: rhinolalia aperta, in which the passages at the back of the nose and mouth fail to close during speech; and rhinolalia clausa, in which obstructions in the nasopharynx interfere with nasal resonance.

rhombencephalon *Hindbrain* (q.v.).

rhypophagy *Obs.* The eating of filth or excrement; scatophagy.

rhypophobia *Obs.* Fear of dirt or filth.

rhythms, biologic *Clock-driven behavior;* time-specific cyclical variations in biochemical and physiologic functions and levels of activity (including variations in emotional state and psychomotor reactivity). *Circadian* rhythms have a cycle of about 24 hours, *ultradian* are shorter than one day and *infradian* are longer (weeks or months); *circalunar* have a duration of about one month; and *circannual* are about a year.

Although biologic rhythms are endogenous, a *Zeitgeber* (exogenous timegiver) often is instrumental in maintaining synchrony between the endogenous rhythm and environmental cycles, a process sometimes referred to as *entrainment*. When the Zeitgeber is removed, as under constant laboratory conditions, the internal clock is said to be *free-running,* and the rhythm may drift slightly from the norm. See *clock, biological*.

ribonucleic acid See *chromosome*.

ribosomal RNA See *chromosome*.

Ribot's law See *law, Ribot's*.

Rice Conferences See *Conferences, A.K. Rice Group Relations*.

riddance This term, coined by S. Rado, refers to "many reflexes designed to eliminate pain-causing agents from the surface or inside of the body. The scratch reflex, the shedding of tears, sneezing, coughing, spitting, vomiting, colic bowel movement are but a few well-known instances of this principle of pain control in our bodily organization. This principle I have called the *riddance principle,* and its physiological embodiments the *riddance reflexes*." (*Psychoanalytic Quarterly VIII,* 1939)

riddling See *alpha sleep*.

right A claim that a person or group can justifiably make upon others or upon society. A *moral right* is a claim that is justified by moral principles or rules.

right and left According to W. Stekel, when the concepts *right* and *left* appear in dreams they are understood in an ethical sense. "The right-hand path always signifies the way to righteousness, the left-hand path the path to crime. Thus the left may signify homosexuality, incest, and perversion, while the right signifies marriage, relations with a prostitute, etc. The meaning is always determined by the particular moral standpoint of the dreamer." (*Bi-Sexual Love*, 1922)

right and wrong test See *responsibility, criminal.*

right-handedness See *dextrality-sinistrality.*

right-left disorientation See *syndrome, Gerstmann.*

right to refuse treatment See *consumerism; forced treatment.*

right to treatment See *consumerism.*

rigid families See *family types.*

rigidity, affective When the emotions or affects remain constant in the face of topics that normally call for changes in affect, the condition is known as affective rigidity. Many patients with schizophrenia show no mood changes in spite of discussions covering a wide variety of experiences.

Rigidity of the affect, or affect-block, is common also in obsessive-compulsive neurosis. See *block, affect.*

rigidity, decerebrate A syndrome of exaggerated posture in continuous spasm of muscles produced by transection of the brain at a prepontine level. The extensor muscles are particularly affected and exhibit lengthening and shortening (clasp-knife) reactions.

rigidity, lead pipe *Rare.* Used ironically to indicate waxy flexibility. See *catalepsy.*

ring, Kayser-Fleischer (Bernhard Kayser, German ophthalmologist, 1869–1954, and Richard Fleischer, German physician, 1848–1909) See *degeneration, hepatolenticular.*

risk Hazard, peril, or exposure to loss or injury; the sum of the probability of harmful effect and the magnitude of such effect(s) resulting from any procedure or situation. See *risk factor.*

Children at risk are those who the clinician predicts will have some kind of emotional difficulty or psychiatric disorder in the future. For the researcher, however, the phrase is more likely to mean children of mentally ill parents, and most commonly the illness is schizophrenia and the ill parent is the mother.

The *high risk approach*, first employed by Doctors Sarnoff Mednick and Fini Schulsinger in Denmark, is a research method that studies vulnerable persons from their early years through the period of risk, in an attempt to identify those biochemical, physiological, or psychologic factors that differentiate between those who ultimately develop the disorder and those who do not.

Risk management consists of the identification, analysis, evaluation, and elimination of the factors that predispose to loss or injury and is most frequently applied to a hospital's program to control factors affecting the safety and security of its patients, visitors, and employees.

risk factor Any specific characteristic or condition whose presence is associated with an increased likelihood that a disorder is present or will develop at a later time. *Relative risk* is the ratio of the occurrence of a disorder in those exposed to the risk factor to the rate of disorder of those not exposed. *Attributable risk* is the absolute difference between the rate of the disorder in those exposed and the rate of the disorder in those not exposed to the risk factor.

In contrast with *vulnerability,* which is an actual, existing variation in structure or function that predisposes to disease, risk refers to a statistical probability. It includes any element whose occurrence has been demonstrated statistically to be associated with later development of the disease. See *vulnerability, genetic.*

Although many epidemiologic studies have been devoted to identifying putative risk factors for various diseases, not even the scientific community has appeared to appreciate fully the tentativeness of their implications. The demonstration of risk factors, for example, neither quantifies the risk for any individual nor measures the importance of the specific factor relative to that of many other risk factors that ordinarily operate. Further, it can rarely be determined that identified risk factors constitute the total number of risk factors predisposing to the disease in question. Finally, few studies of risk factors give more than fleeting recognition to possible antirisk or *protection factors,* whose potential for offsetting risk factors might alter profoundly the likelihood of any person or subpopulation developing the disease.

risk level *Confidence level* (q.v.).

risk management See *risk.*

risk, minimal The amount of hazard encountered by normal persons in their daily lives or in routine medical or psychologic examination of such persons.

risk, morbid The probability of having a first episode of illness during one's lifetime. Within a specified population, the morbid risk is the proportion of subjects who would be affected if all lived through the age of risk. See *epidemiology.*

risk-rescue rating A method of assessing the lethality or deadliness of suicide attempts devised by Avery Weisman and J. William Worden (*Archives of General Psychiatry 26,* 1972), expressed by the formula

$$\frac{A}{A + B} \times 100$$

where *A* is the risk score (the agent, the impairment of consciousness, lesions, toxicity, reversibility, treatment required) and *B* is the rescue score (location of attempt, person initiating rescue, probability of discovery by a rescuer, accessibility to rescue, delay until discovery).

rites, puberty In many primitive cultures it is customary for children at puberty to undergo certain initiatory rites as a part of the religious pattern of that culture. One of the commonest rituals is a pretense of killing the child and bringing him to life again. In another primitive group, part of the proceedings consists of knocking out a tooth and giving a new name to the child being initiated, indicating thereby the change from youth to adulthood. In still another tribe, the puberty rites comprise operations of circumcision and subincision. All of these ceremonies are conducted in absolute secrecy, and only those already initiated may attend them.

ritual Formal behavior for occasions not given over to technological routine that occur both as spontaneous invention of the individual, especially of the compulsion neurotic, and as a cultural trait.

ritual-making One of Rado's subdivisions of obsessive attacks is called *bouts of ritual-making:* repetitive sequences that must be continued until the patient is exhausted. Typically, these rituals are ceremonial, distortive, and stereotyped elaborations of some routine of daily life, such as bathing, dressing, and sexual activity.

rivalry A sublimated form of conflict where the struggle of individuals is subordinated to the welfare of the group.

rivalry, sibling The usual family situation wherein brothers and sisters engage in an intense and highly emotional competition, one against the other, for the love, attention, affection, and approval of one or the other or both of the parents. This intense competition between rival sibs (brothers or sisters) can be an important determinant of later specific character or personality traits.

Sibling rivalry, however, is usually evaluated in relation to other important experiences in the child's early life, such as the oedipal relationship to the parents; the discovery of and reaction to sexual differences; that specific reaction that is called the *castration complex;* self-comforting trends, such as thumbsucking and masturbation, and conflicts concerning their prohibition and gratification.

RLS person A person who finds difficulty in pronouncing the sounds of *r, l, s;* by hardly justified extension—a *stammerer.* See *stuttering.*

RNA Ribonucleic acid. See *chromosome.*

Robinson Crusoe age In Erikson's description of the eight stages of man, the stage of *industry vs. inferiority.* See *ontogeny, psychic.*

rocking See *stereotyped movement disorders.*

rocks See *crack.*

role The pattern or type of behavior which the child—and the adult—builds up in terms of what others expect or demand of him.

An automatic, learned, goal-directed pattern or sequence of acts developed under the influence of the significant people in the growing child's environment; such patterns provide the child with a repertoire of expected or appropriate responses to the behavior of those with whom he interacts. When the person's behavior does in fact conform with what is expected in a given situation or relationship, his role is termed *complementary* to the roles of the other people in the situation; such complementarity is desirable and comfortable. Noncomplementarity or disequilibrium of roles, as occurs when people's expectations of others are disappointed, leads to disruption of interpersonal relationships and breakdowns in group living. See *complementarity; complementary*. Roles are labeled *explicit* when they are consciously motivated and exposed to observation and awareness of the interacting participants; roles are *implicit* when they are more remote from consciousness and awareness and often are not recognized as such by actor or participant. Typically, implicit roles express personality attributes originating in early internalizations or identifications; they are an outgrowth of early transactions between mother and child, child and teacher, etc.

role confusion See *identity crisis; ontogeny, psychic.*

role, gender See *gender identity.*

role reversal Adopting or assuming the pattern of behavior that is expected of the other in a relationship. Probably the most common form is that in which the child is given parental authority because the parent is absent from the home or unable to shoulder the burdens of parenthood. Such role reversal can become a significant problem for the child, and the family as well, if the demands exceed the child's abilities.

role, sex See *sex role.*

rolfing After Ida Rolf, Ph.D., a biochemist who developed *Structural integration* while working with consciousness expansion at the Esalen Institute: deep massage to release the connective tissue that binds together the muscle groups in which both psychic and physical pains are stored. Typically, rolfing is given in ten hour-long sessions spread over several weeks.

romance, family A type of phantasy in which the subject maintains that he is not the child of his real parents, but is instead the offspring of other parents (usually of higher station). The *rescue phantasy*, of saving the life of the father (or king, or emperor, etc.) or of the mother, is a common variant of the family romance. Another variant, the *Mignon delusion*, is the

fixed belief that one is the child of a distinguished family. Usually, the family romance arises on the basis of disillusionment with the real parents (who have failed to demonstrate the omnipotence with which the child has endowed them) and/or as a defense against the aggressive sexual elements of the oedipal period.

romance, memory In psychoanalysis, the phantasy standing between infantile impressions and later symptoms. Thus in speaking of hysteria Freud says that the symptoms now no longer appeared as direct derivations of repressed memories of sexual experiences in childhood; "on the contrary, it appeared that between the symptoms and the infantile impressions were interpolated the patient's phantasies (memory-romances), created mostly during the years of adolescence and relating on the one side to the infantile memories on which they were founded, and on the other side to the symptoms into which they were directly transformed." (*CP*)

Romberg sign See *sign, Romberg.*

rooming-in The modern concept in pediatrics that recognizes the essential unity of mother and child after the birth of the child in a hospital. The mother and child are housed in the same room, the infant's crib standing alongside or near the mother's bed. It is essentially a rooming-in of the baby with the mother. The usual hospital nursery plays no role in this practice. The rooming-in process permits the mother to touch, fondle, and caress her child, to feed it when it is hungry, and to diaper it when it soils. This is said to make her immediately familiar with her baby and to allay considerable anxiety in the mother as well as in the child.

root-pain Pain in the segmental area innervated by the affected nerve root, usually excited or intensified by coughing, sneezing, or changes of posture.

rootwork A form of *folk healing* (q.v.) found among both Blacks and Whites in the southeastern United States, based on a belief in malign magic or evil spell. The rejected person in a love triangle or an envious coworker is most often the one suspected of "working roots" (also called *hexing or mojo*). The rootworker, or spirit doctor, has innate healing powers including the ability to counteract the effects of rootwork and return the spell to the one who instigated it. Herbal medicines are often prescribed for the victim, who may consult a physician concurrently.

Rorschach test See *test, Rorschach.*

Rosenbach's sign See *sign, Rosenbach's.*

Ross-Jones test See *test, Ross-Jones.*

Rossolimo's reflex See *reflex, Rossolimo's.*

rotation See *system, rotation.*

Rouse v. Cameron See *consumerism.*

RSBT Rhythmic sensory bombardment therapy. See *therapy, rhythmic sensory bombardment.*

RT Reaction time, also, recreation(al) therapy. See *recreation.*

rubber bands See *transactional analysis.*

rubella, congenital See *retardation, mental.*

rubidium An alkali metal, Rb, used in the 1880s in the treatment of syphilis and epilepsy, and more recently considered to have some antidepressant potential. Its primary effect appears to be on intracellular metabolism of potassium (lithium's major effect, in contrast, is on sodium metabolism). Most studies have failed to find evidence of significant antidepressant activity.

Rüdin, Ernst (1874–1951) German psychiatrist and geneticist; genetics of mental disorders.

rule A statement that because an action is right, or wrong, it should, or should not, be done. See *judgment; principle; theory.*

rule, basic The fundamental precept governing the activity of the patient in psychoanalytic therapy: to think aloud, and by means of free association to overcome censorship and resistance to unconscious content. See *association, free.*

rule, M'Naghten (or McNaughton) See *responsibility, criminal.*

rule utilitarianism See *utilitarianism, act.*

ruler, negative, of the soul See *ego, negation of the.*

rum fits *Obs.* See *delirium tremens.*

ruminate To regurgitate, remasticate, and reswallow; to ponder; to meditate. See *merycism.*

rumination A rare *eating disorder* of infancy consisting of the returning of food from the stomach without nausea or retching; often, indeed, the child seems to derive pleasure or satisfaction from the process. Rumination begins after a period of normal gastrointestinal functioning, usually within the first year of life, and is not associated with any known gastrointestinal illness. It leads to loss of weight, failure to thrive, and interference with growth and development; in some (perhaps as many as a quarter), the disorder pursues an unremitting course until death. In the older literature, *merycism* implied an association between rumination and mental retardation; in current usage, the terms are interchangeable in recognition of the probability that the retardation is a manifestation of developmental delays produced by the disorder.

Rumination is also used to refer to the persistence of some content of mind that has ceased to serve any adaptive purpose, the inability to turn one's attention from dominating, unpleasant ideas, and/or an obsessive preoccupation with ideas, recollections, or plans (and thus Meyer's term, *obsessive-ruminative tension state*). Although rumination more often than not falls within the range of normal mentation, it is also reported frequently in obsessional states, hypochondriasis, and personality changes following brain injury. See *manie de rumination.*

ruminative tension state *Obsessive-ruminative tension state* (q.v.).

Rumpf's sign See *sign, Rumpf.*

runche A crying syndrome described in Nepalese children between 1 and 4 years of age. The condition typically followed episodes of diarrhea and fever or measles and consisted of whining, crying, refusal to eat, and secondary weight loss. Until the condition was recognized as a manifestation of malnourishment, it was interpreted as the a spell placed upon the affected child by the touch of a pregnant woman.

rupophobia *Rhypophobia* (q.v.).

rush See *cocaine.*

Rush, Benjamin (1745–1813) Father of American psychiatry; first American to propose an original systematization of psychiatry.

rypophobia *Rhypophobia* (q.v.).

S

S An abbreviation for experimental subject or for stimulus; also used as a Rorschach scoring symbol to indicate a response to the white space on the card. Rorschach believed the *S* indicated habitual oppositional tendencies.

sabotage, masochistic The self-defeating attitude or behavior of some patients that aims unconsciously to provoke insult, punishment, scorn, etc., from the environment. It appears in many forms during analytic treatment, ranging from obstinate silence to insolent remarks and behavior directed against the analyst or the analytic setting. (Reik, T. *Masochism in Modern Man,* 1941)

saccade A rapid eye movement that puts the eye on a target that has moved. The saccadic system corrects position errors and the pursuit system corrects velocity errors in focusing on a moving object. Both schizophrenic patients and their asymptomatic family members have a high prevalence of abnormal pursuit eye movements, such as saccadic tracking in which smooth pursuit is replaced by small saccadic jumps, and saccadic intrusions in which extraneous eye movements that have no corrective function interrupt eye pursuit movements. The abnormality is believed to be a disinhibitory cortical dysfunction in which the saccadic system is not turned off during pursuit, as it should be.

sadism (After Marquis de Sade [1740–1814], a French writer who described persons whose sexual pleasure depended upon inflicting cruelty upon others) A *sexual disorder* (q.v.) in which orgasm is dependent upon torturing others or inflicting pain, ill-treatment, and humiliation on others. Krafft-Ebing defined sadism as sexual emotions associated with the wish to inflict pain and use violence. Moll defined it as a state in which the sexual impulse is manifested as a tendency to strike, misuse, or humiliate the love object.

Viewed as a paraphilia, sadism is a defense against castration fears and fears of one's own sexual excitement. What might happen to the subject passively is done actively to others—"identification with the aggressor." Further, the castration performed in the sadistic act is a symbolic one, not a real one, and such pseudo-castration assures the sadist that his fears are ungrounded. The sadist tries to force his victim to love him; this love is conceived of as a forgiveness, which removes the guilt feelings that interfere with sexual satisfaction.

While sadism is sometimes considered to be a deflection outside the self of the destructive or death instinct, it will be seen that the paraphilia of sadism depends upon fusion of destructive energy with libidinal energy. The discharge of aggression in itself may be pleasurable, but sadism further implies pleasure in the destruction of others. But at the same time, the manifestations of the aggressive drive progress through the same developmental stages as the sexual (oral, anal, phallic), and in this context such manifestations are generally called sadistic—thus oral-sadistic, anal-sadistic, and phallic-sadistic.

sadism, anal The aggression, destructiveness, negativism, and externally directed rage that are typical components of the anal stage of development; manifestations of the death instinct during the anal phase; the second portion of the anal stage of development, and its holdovers in later life. See *anal erotism; instinct, death; phase, anal; sadism, oral.*

sadism, id The primary primitive instinctual destructive urges, which are seen in their unmodified form in the early years of infancy. They are closely allied with drives toward omnipotent gratification and security, and seem to be brought out by frustration in early infancy. Much of this primary sadism suffers repression under the aegis of the striving for goodness and approval, and the fear of the reality consequences to the subject of external retaliation and its internal equivalent, conscience pangs.

sadism, larval (L. *larva*, "ghost, specter, mask") Hirschfeld's term for masked or concealed sadism.

sadism, manual A type of sadism in which the torture of the object is achieved through muscular eroticism. Any sadistic activity in which the sexual pleasure achieved by the sadist is intimately associated with the use of his musculature (as, for example, in beating or kicking his partner).

sadism, omnipotent infantile See *sadism, id.*

sadism, oral The expression of infantile, primordial, aggressive, instinctive urges toward omnipotent mastery, through phantasy function of the mouth, lips, and teeth. These phantasy functions represent distortions of the reality functions of the mouth, lips, teeth, tongue, cheeks, and pharynx.

Oral sadistic wishes, strivings, and phantasies appear normally in the earliest stages of infantile development, immediately after birth. As the child matures and develops, these wishes and strivings undergo various vicissitudes, to appear and persist later in adult life in modified and disguised form as components of neurotic symptoms; as paraphilias and foreplay desires and gratifications; as character traits; and as socially approvable and desirable sublimation activities. See *orality; phase, oral incorporative; sadism.*

sadism, phallic Aggression associated with the phallic stage of development. The child ordinarily comprehends sexual intercourse as an aggressive and sadistic act on the part of the male, and specifically on the part of the penis. Evidence that the penis is phantasied as a weapon of violence and destruction comes from unconscious productions of normal adults. Limericks, for instance, often refer to the penis as square, or too large, so that intercourse is dangerous and painful for the partner. This may well be a projection of the male's own fear of coitus.

Scop(t)ophilia may result at the phallic stage, secondary to such sadism. The looking gives reassurance that the sadistically perceived object is not yet dead. See *scopophilia.*

sadism, primal A certain portion of the death instinct that always remains with the person; according to Freud it is identical with masochism. "After the chief part of it [i.e. the death instinct] has been directed outwards toward objects, there remains as a residuum within the organism the true erotogenic masochism, which on the one hand becomes a component of the libido and on the other still has the subject itself for an object." (*CP*)

sadism, superego The intense cruelty, rigidity, and pain-giving punitive aspects of conscience (superego). In the developing child, the infantile sadism (primordial aggressivity) is eventually mastered by the development within the child of equally powerful controlling and countervailing forces. These forces of character, warning the child of the reality consequences of its unbridled aggressive trends, become organized into what is called *the conscience*, "that still small voice" that silently warns us when we are about to succumb to our urges and do something wrong. The warnings emanate from the internalized (introjected) pictures or images that the child has, not necessarily of his real parents, but rather of what he conceives the parents would be if they discovered the attempt to carry out his own violently aggressive wishes against them.

The internal image of the violently angry, discovering parent is formed in the old talionic formula of an "eye for an eye." The child feels that the discovering parent must become the punishing parent, seeking vengeance in proportion to the strength and enormity of the child's own phantasies and aggressives wishes. Thus, in the last analysis, the intensity of the sadism of the superego, or conscience, stems from the enormity and violence of the child's own infantile, primordial, sadistic phantasies and strivings, which have succumbed to the control of an equal and opposite repressive power.

(Sharpe, E.F. *Collected Papers on Psycho-analysis, 1950*)

sadistic personality disorder A pattern of cruelty and harshness toward others, ranging from intimidation or humiliation of others to enjoyment of inflicting physical pain or torturing other people or animals. Such a person is often fascinated with violence of any sort and interested in weapons, the martial arts, etc.

sadomasochism A condition of combined sadism and masochism: coexistence of submissive and aggressive attitudes in social and sexual relations to other persons, with a considerable degree of destructiveness present; a condition assumed to be charged with libidinal energy. The subject is affected by an interplay between the two instinctual components of love and hate, in which the destructive impulses momentarily have the upper hand. In a general way, in human relations a person may have three different kinds of attitude toward other persons: first, he is interested in having the other exist as his equal; second, he considers himself either superior or inferior to the other person, though still remaining interested in the other person's existence; and third, he is swayed by aggression and submission simultaneously in such a way that he wishes the other person's destruction and preservation at the same time. In normal social relations the existence of the other person not only is necessary but fulfills the inner psychic demands, although a certain amount of destructive impulse is always present. Only when a high degree of destructiveness is present in the relationship between two persons may one speak of sadomasochism.

SADS Schedule for Affective Disorders and Schizophrenia; a structured instrument designed to record the information necessary to establish diagnosis on the basis of the *RDC* (Research Diagnostic Criteria). The latter defines *inclusion criteria* for the clinical features that warrant or support the diagnosis, and *exclusion criteria* for features that are incompatable with the diagnosis. The SADS, Part I, includes information pertaining both to the history of the present illness and to the mental status examination. The PSE (*Present State Examination*), another structured interview schedule, restricts itself to data obtained from the mental state examination. See *Examination, Present State; Research Diagnostic Criteria.*

safeguard, treble See *principle, treble safeguard.*

SAHS-UAO Sleep apnea hypersomnolence syndrome associated with upper airway obstruction. See *sleep disorders.*

Saint Dymphna's disease See *disease, Saint Dymphna's.*

Saint John's evil *Obs.* Epilepsy.

Saint Martin's evil *Obs.* Dipsomania(q.v.).

Saint Vitus' dance (St. Vitus, a Christian child, martyred under Diocletian, 245–313 A.D., whose chapels, especially the one at Ulm, were filled with sufferers from epilepsy, invoking the saint for cure) Chorea. See *chorea, Sydenham's.*

Sakel, Manfred (1900–57) Polish psychiatrist trained in Vienna; in 1933 reported his discovery of the hypoglycemic insulin treatment of schizophrenia and soon after came to the U.S., where he remained until his death.

salaam spasm See *spasm, salaam.*

salad, word See *word salad.*

Salk vaccine See *poliomyelitis.*

Salmon, Thomas W. (1876–1927) American psychiatrist; mental hygiene, military psychiatry.

salpingectomy A general medical term for the *sterilization* of the woman by cutting and tying off the Fallopian tubes; also called *tubectomy, fallectomy,* or *tubal ligation. Vasectomy* is the corresponding operation on the male. Removal of the ovaries, resulting in the *castration* of the woman, is usually called *ovariectomy* or *oophorectomy.* See *sterilization; castration.*

saltatory Pertaining to leaping or dancing; proceeding by leaps and bounds rather than in measured, even progression. See *spasm, saltatory.*

sanable Curable.

sanatorium An institution for the treatment of chronic diseases, such as tuberculosis, nervous and mental disorders, chronic rheumatism, and a place for recuperation under medical supervision; often improperly called sanitarium.

sanction The defensive measure that the obsessional neurotic is obliged to adopt in order to prevent a phantasy from being fulfilled. Often it takes the form of repeating a word or other action as a way of diverting attention from the phantasy itself.

sandbox marriage See *marriage, sandbox.*

Sandler's triad A symptom group consisting of low self-esteem with confusion of identity, sadomasochistic behavior toward military authorities, and impotence, seen frequently as an essential part of *camptocormia* (q.v.).

sane Sound of mind.

Sanfilippo's syndrome Type III *mucopolysaccharidosis* (q.v.).

Sanger, Margaret Higgins (1884–1966) American nurse; pioneered in family planning and coined the phrase *birth control* (q.v.).

sanguine See *type, sanguine.*

sanity Soundness of mind. See *responsibility, criminal.*

sa(p)phism (After Greek poetess Sappho, born 600 B.C. on the island Lesbos, who was a homosexual) The sensual and sexual desire of a woman for members of her own sex; lesbianism; female homosexuality. See *homosexuality, female.*

satanophobia Fear of the devil.

satellite housing A type of long-term care facility, consisting of one or more residences for patients who require minimal supervision; the residences are related organizationally to a treatment center, such as a hospital, and thus provide ready access to more intensive levels of monitoring and care should a need for them arise. Sometimes a satellite house is located on or near the grounds of the hospital, but more often it is situated in a residential area close to a school or workplace. See *care, long-term; domicile.*

satisfaction "A better term for a stimulus of instinctual origin is a 'need'; that which does away with this need is 'satisfaction.' This can be attained only by a suitable (adequate) alteration of the inner sources of stimulations." (Freud, *CP*)

In occupational therapy this term means a feeling of gratification, of accomplishment; often used in relation to the progress of an activity or interest.

satyriasis 1. *Hypersexuality* (q.v.) in the male; sexual erethism. See *Don Juan.* 2. *Obs.* Leprosy.

Saunders-Sutton syndrome *Delirium tremens* (q.v.).

savant, idiot "Amentia is often characterized by an irregular as well as a defective mental development, and in a small number of patients this is so marked as to result in special aptitudes which are quite phenomenal, not merely in comparison with aments, but often with the acquirements of ordinary persons. These persons are conveniently described as 'idiot savants.' Usually such 'idiots' are not of the lowest grade of mental deficiency." (Tredgold, *TMD*) See *syndrome, savant.*

scabiophobia Fear of scabies.

scale, Columbia Mental Maturity See *CMMS.*

Scale, Global Deterioration See *GDS.*

scale, Lorr See *MSRPP.*

scan, brain See *encephalography, radioisotopic; NMR; tomography.*

scan, CAT See *NMR; tomography.*

scanning Skimming; a method of rapid reading in which the reader searches for specific content or tries quickly to grasp the general sense of the passage but does not attempt to read the complete text. *Scanning speech* is a slurred, ataxic, drawling monotone or singsong; it occurs, for example, in some cases of multiple sclerosis.

Scanning is also used to denote a method of diagnosis employing radioisotopes; see *encephalography, radioisotopic.*

scapegoat The person or object who is blamed for actions of others; the object of *projection* (q.v.). See *mechanism, scapegoat.*

scapegoating A form of intrafamilial behavior, largely unconsciously determined, in which one member (the child, the patient, etc.) becomes a repository or hiding place for the emotions that the rest of the family will not see in themselves.

Characteristic of scapegoating is *conflict detouring*, when the parents define the child as sick or defective and unite to protect him, or they see him as the cause of the family's problems and unite in attacking him. A form of scapegoating is *triangulation*, in which a dyad within the family preserves its stability by directing its hostility to a third person. See *mechanism, scapegoat.*

scar, psychic "*Cure with a defect* is also spoken of by formulating the conception, suitable only to a few cases, that the acute disease has left a defect just as a healed wound leaves a scar. A 'psychic scar' may be formed by definite 'residual symptoms,' as in the case of a delusion which in spite of returned clearness following a delirium is no longer corrected." (Bleuler, *TP*)

Scarpa's ganglion (Antonio Scarpa, Italian anatomist and surgeon, 1749–1832) See *nerve, acoustic.*

scatology The study of excrement and/or preoccupation with excrement and filth; lewdness (as in telephone scatologia). "The whole significance of the anal zone is mirrored in the fact that there are but few neurotics who have not had their special scatologic customs, ceremonies, etc., which they retain with cautious secrecy." (Freud, *BW*) See *anal erotism* and the several words beginning with *copro-.*

scatophagy Eating of excrement. See *rhyphophagy.*

scatophobia A morbid dread of contamination by excrement.

scattering One of the schizophrenic thinking disorders in which associations are sometimes irrelevant or tangential, with the result that speech productions are occasionally incomprehensible. The term is also used in clinical psychology to refer to widely divergent test scores, as when a schizophrenic patient passes all the year X items in an intelligence test but shows many failures at the year VI level, or as when there is marked inconsistency on subtest scores. See *age, basal.*

scelerophobia *Pavor sceleris* (q.v.).

scene, primal A child's first observation of sexual intercourse between the parents. In his description of the "wolf-man" case, Freud claims that the primal scene was influential in determining later morbid personality reactions.

scene, traumatic Any psychic experience that the subject wishes to forget or repress because it is disagreeable, painful, threatening, or unbearable. Freud speaks of traumatic situations and emphasizes that neurotic symptoms are "complete reproductions of such situations." It is as if the patient cannot get rid of the original painful experience and remains attached to it, an attachment that Freud called "fixation to traumas." Such is the case of the girl who had developed an abnormal erotic attachment to her father (traumatic situation, or scene) and was constantly ill after his death, so that she would be in no condition to marry and

could thus remain with her father, her original love object.

In the opinion of Breuer and Freud, the psychic energies that cannot be lived out in the normal way, when the patient tries to forget or repress the traumatic scene, are diverted into other pathways and there provoke symptoms in the somatic sphere. Later, Freud referred to it as a *psychosexual trauma.*

Schaeffer reflex See *reflex, Schaeffer.*

Schaumberg's disease See *leukodystrophies.*

schedule A form on which may be given many summarized items of information concerning a patient; it is arranged so that each item may be easily abstracted and made available for tabulation.

Schedule for Affective Disorders and Schizophrenia *SADS* (q.v.).

schedule, self-demand See *feeding, self-demand.*

Scheid cyanotic syndrome Scheid attempted to explain sudden death in excited manic patients and in catatonic states as a somatic condition somehow related to a somatic febrile or toxic etiology of the psychosis itself. This view is not widely held at the present time, it being more generally believed that such deaths are due to physiologic exhaustion secondary to pathologic overactivity; but some authors continue to speak of a catatonic cerebral paralysis as a primary somatic change that explains the occasional (probably not more than 1%) occurrence of unexpected death in this group. See *Bell's mania.*

Scheie's syndrome See *mucopolysaccharidosis.*

schema, body Same as body percept, which is one part of the body image. See *image, body.*

scheme, schemata See *cognitions.*

Schicksal analysis See *analysis, Schicksal.*

Schilder's disease (Paul Ferdinand Schilder, Vienna and New York neurologist and psychiatrist, 1886–1940) Encephalitis periaxialis diffusa. See *leukodystrophies.*

schism, marital See *marital schism.*

schizo- Combining form meaning to split, cleave, rive, from Gr. *schizein.*

schizoaffective disorder Combination of a manic or major depressive syndrome with symptoms of schizophrenia; in DSM-III-R, such a diagnosis also requires that delusions or hallucinations of at least two weeks' duration be present during an episode of illness in which there are no prominent affective symptoms. This requirement brings the definition closer to earlier uses of the term, which referred to affective episodes in subjects with an underlying schizophrenic illness. DSM-III and DSM-III-R classify this disorder with "Other Psychotic Disorders" rather than as a subtype of schizophrenic disorders.

schizobipolar *Schizomanic* (q.v.).

schizocaria *Obs.* An acute and highly malignant form of schizophrenia that leads to rapid deterioration of the personality. Mauz uses the term *catastrophic schizophrenia* synonymously with schizocaria.

schizogen See *psychotomimetic.*

schizoid Resembling the division, separation, or split of the personality that is characteristic of schizophrenia.

The term is an inexact one and used in different ways by different authors. By some, it is used to refer to a personality type characterized by shyness, sensitivity, aloofness, introversion, etc. (see schizoid personality under *personality* and *personality pattern disturbance*). It has been used by others to refer to any kind of psychiatric disorder that is not schizophrenia that occurs in family members of schizophrenics; or to refer to psychiatric disorders that occur more commonly in family members of schizophrenics than in other families, even though the particular case under consideration may not be from a schizophrenic family; or to refer to a trait or disorder that is believed to indicate an underlying genetic predisposition to schizophrenia. See *schizoidia; schizoidism.*

schizoid disorder of childhood Reduced capacity to form social relationships, preference for aloneness, bland or constricted affect, self-absorption, excessive daydreaming; the diagnosis should not be made before the age of 5 years, when socialization can ordinarily be expected to develop.

schizoid personality See *personality disorders.*

schizoid position See *position, paranoid-schizoid.*

schizoidia Schizoidism; also used synonymously with *schizophrenic spectrum disorders* to refer to a variety of abnormalities that are found among nonschizophrenic relatives of schizophrenic patients. Although the concordance rate for schizophrenia in monozygotic twins may be no higher than 45%, probably an equal percentage of the twins have some other significant abnormality. The latter are subsumed under the name *schizoidia*. In males these include impulse crimes such as arson, assault and poorly planned theft; extreme social isolation; heavy alcohol intake; and sexual deviance. In both males and females they include eccentric reclusiveness; incapacitating panic in ordinary social situations (especially in females); paranoid types with suspiciousness, sensitivity, moroseness, jealousy, litigiousness; giggly, opinionated, pedantic, or narrow-minded eccentrics; cruel, calculating, cold, unsympathetic persons who seem to lack feeling; reserved, haughty, snobbish, unsociable types; and anergic personalities with dependency, unreliability, or subservence.

It has been suggested that the whole group of schizophrenic disorders and schizoidia may be alternative expressions of a single genotype, perhaps due to a single autosomal gene that is modified by any number of other genes.

schizoidism The aggregate of personality traits known as introversion, namely, quietness, seclusiveness, "shut-in-ness." The schizoid person splits or separates from his surroundings to a greater or lesser degree, confining his psychic interests more or less to himself.

The intensely schizoid person may become schizophrenic; it is estimated that no fewer than 60% of schizophrenic patients show exaggerated schizoid tendencies prior to the development of schizophrenia.

Many contemporary European writers use the term schizoidism to refer to the hereditary or *nuclear* factor in schizophrenia. These same authors tend to use the term *dementia praecox* to refer to a type of schizophrenia showing a high tendency to deterioration and little tendency to remission or recovery.

schizomanic *Schizobipolar;* referring to a schizoaffective patient with manic features.

schizomimetic *Psychotomimetic* (q.v.).

schizophasia "Word salad"; in Leonhard's classification, a subtype of nonsystematic schizophrenia characterized by grossly disorganized speech. See *schizophrenia, systematic.*

schizophrene One affected by schizophrenia.

schizophrenese The associational defects of the schizophrenic patient as manifested in his speech; it is to be recognized that there is no specific schizophrenic language and schizophrenics' thinking disorders vary from patient to patient. "What is uniform is merely an absence of normal expectancy. It is also noteworthy that in the absence of such culturally standard cues for meta-communicative expression, the listener feels disengaged and the schizophrenic child is further isolated from human rapport." (Goldfarb, W. *International Psychiatry Clinics 1,* 1964)

schizophrenia Bleuler's suggested replacement for the now obsolete term *dementia praecox* (q.v.). Bleuler meant to designate what he considered to be one of the fundamental characteristics of patients so diagnosed, namely, the splitting off of portions of the psyche, which portions may then dominate the psychic life of the subject for a time and lead an independent existence even though these may be contrary and contradictory to the personality as a whole. Bleuler rejected the term dementia praecox because in his experience profound deterioration (dementia) was not the inevitable end result of the disease process, and because it did not always appear by the time of adolescence.

"In 1911, Eugen Bleuler described the schizophrenias as a slowly progressive deterioration of the entire personality, which involves mainly the affective life, and expresses itself in disorders of feeling, thought and conduct, and a tendency to withdraw from reality. Bleuler noted that the schizophrenias were at times progressive, at times intermittent, and could stop or retrogress at any stage; but that they showed a tendency toward deterioration and, having once appeared, did not permit of a full *restitutio ad integrum.* Bleuler established the multidimensional nature of the schizophrenias and believed them to be organic; but at the same time, he stressed the interaction of psychogenic and physiogenic features in their psychopathology and development." (Campbell, R.J. *Psychiatric Quarterly 32,* 1958)

The diagnostic criteria for this group of disorders vary considerably. In DSM-III, operational criteria are suggested for each diagnostic category so as to minimize false positive diagnoses and increase the reliability of diagnoses among different workers in different settings. The criteria suggested for the schizophrenic disorders are thus more narrow that the Bleulerian criteria, and schizophrenia is defined as a large group of disorders, involving disorganization of a previous level of functioning, the presence of some psychotic features (such as delusions or hallucinations) during the active phase of the illness, evidence of chronicity and disturbances of multiple psychologic processes (language and communication, content of thought, perception, affect, sense of self, relationship to the external world, volition and/or motor behavior). The following subtypes are recognized: disorganized (hebephrenic), catatonic, paranoid, undifferentiated, and residual (i.e. in partial remission). Illnesses with similar manifestations but of briefer duration are labeled *schizophreniform disorders;* illnesses that have not shown psychotic features (such as the latent, borderline, or pseudoneurotic form of other classificatory systems) are classified as *personality disorder.*

Bleuler subdivided the symptoms of the schizophrenias into two groups: (1) the fundamental, primary, or basic symptoms, which are characteristic and pathognomonic of the disease process; and (2) the accessory or secondary symptoms, which are often seen in the schizophrenias and which may even occupy the forefront of the symptom picture, but which are seen in other nosologic groups as well, particularly in the organic reaction types (acute and chronic brain syndromes). In this second group are included such symptoms as hallucinations, delusions, ideas of reference, memory disturbances (e.g. déjà fait, déjà vu). The fundamental symptoms of the schizophrenias include (1) disturbances in associations, (2) disturbances of affect, (3) ambivalence of the affect, intellect, and/or will, (4) autism, (5) attention defects, (6) disturbances of the will, (7) changes in "the person," (8) schizophrenic dementia, and (9) disturbances of activity and behavior. See *symptoms, first-rank.*

While the specific etiology remains unknown, mounting evidence favors the conception of the schizophrenias as a heredogenetic disease involving particularly certain enzyme systems of the body. The average expectance of schizophrenia in the general population probably does not exceed 1%; it is not, therefore, a universal potentiality and not everyone could become a schizophrenic under certain conditions. It occurs in every segment of the population, without regard for race, culture, or social class. It occurs, too, in all the forms generally recognized, although the content of the symptoms appears to be determined in large part by the culture. To state this in a different way: the fundamental symptoms are the same, no matter where schizophrenia appears.

Forms of the disease. Bleuler subdivided the schizophrenias into acute and chronic forms, depending upon the predominant symptoms of any particular episode. As already indicated, the predominant symptoms are often the accessory symptoms, and before subtyping of an episode is made the diagnosis of schizophrenia is first established by reason of the presence of the fundamental symptoms.

The acute syndromes are:

1. *Melancholia*—in contrast to non-schizophrenic depressions, the affect here tends to be superficial, inappropriate, and/or unconvincing, and hypochondriacal delusions are frequent.

2. *Mania*—the prevailing mood is capriciousness rather than euphoria or triumph, and withdrawal can usually be seen.

3. *Catatonia*—stupor, cerea flexibilitas, *Faxenpsychosis* (q.v.), or other hyperkinetic syndromes.

4. *Delusional states with hallucinations*—often visual and less stereotyped than the hallucinations seen in the chronic syndromes.

5. *Twilight states*—including religious ecstasies and other dreamlike conditions in which desires, impulses, or fears are represented in a direct or symbolic way as being already fulfilled.

6. *Benommenheit* (psychic "benumbing")—in which there is a slowing up of all psychic processes, usually in conjunction with an incapacity for dealing with any relatively complicated or unusual situation.

7. *Confusion, incoherence*—as a result of fragmentation of associations, speech is disconnected, sentences are broken,

and activity is excessive, purposeless, and random.

8. *Anger states*—with cursing, vilification, uncontrolled rage outbursts, often in relation to seemingly insignificant external events.

9. *Anniversary excitements*—episodes of agitation appearing only on definite calendar days, usually related to a specific event in the patient's past.

10. *Stupor.*

11. *Deliria*—acute hallucinatory episodes often resembling the fever deliria. These states are sometimes termed oneirophrenia and include those patients who become dazed and bewildered with narrowing of consciousness, often following specific traumata such as childbirth, postoperative exhaustion, and battlefield experiences. While such cases are often said to be benign, there is a percentage of cases that recur with decreasing recovery after each episode.

12. *Fugue states*—running away in intercurrent episodes of agitation and excitement, sometimes in response to a hallucinatory command.

13. *Dipsomania*—tense, anxious moods drive some patients to drink heavily until they become exhausted.

The chronic forms are:

1. *Paranoid*—see *schizophrenia, paranoid.*

2. *Catatonic*—see *schizophrenia, catatonic.*

3. *Hebephrenic*—see *schizophrenia, hebephrenic.*

4. *Simple*—see *schizophrenia, simple.*

Various other forms have been described since Bleuler's subdivision, among which are:

1. *Schizophrenia, childhood* (q.v.).

2. *Schizophrenia, pseudoneurotic* (q.v.).

3. *Schizophrenia, ambulatory* (q.v.).

4. *Acute episode schizophrenia*—those acute forms in which clear-cut crystallization into one of the generally recognized chronic forms has not yet occurred.

5. *Chronic undifferentiated schizophrenia*—mixed forms and also those termed latent, incipient, borderline, prepsychotic, etc.

6. *Schizoaffective schizophrenia*—including the acute melancholic and manic forms of Bleuler; this type often has its onset during adolescence and with recurrences the affective picture tends to abate and to be re-

placed by hebephrenic or simple or paranoid symptoms.

7. *Pseudopsychopathic schizophrenia*—with predominant asocial, dyssocial, or antisocial trends.

8. *Residual schizophrenia*—cases in a state of relative remission or improvement between acute psychotic episodes.

schizophrenia, acute The predominant clinical features are delusions, hallucinations, and thinking disturbances—sometimes referred to as *positive symptoms.* According to the World Health Organization (1973) the most frequent symptoms of acute schizophrenia are lack of insight (found in 97% of cases), auditory hallucinations (74%), ideas of reference (70%), suspiciousness (66%), flatness of affect (66%), voices speaking to the patient (65%), delusional mood (64%), delusions of persecution (64%), thought alienation (52%), and thoughts spoken aloud (50%). See *symptoms, positive.*

schizophrenia, ambulatory The term ambulatory schizophrenia (nonhospitalized) has been applied to the disease of the group of schizophrenics who, on the surface, appear normal, but can suddenly commit acts that reveal their abnormality. (Zilboorg, G. *Psychiatry 4,* 1941) The puzzling aggressive, asocial acts committed by apparently sane persons have very often turned out to be acts of ambulatory schizophrenics. (Abrahamsen, D. *Crime and the Human Mind,* 1944)

schizophrenia, arrest of The subsidence of acute schizophrenic symptoms. This may occur at any time in the process of the disease, and if the disease itself is not too far advanced, there may be little of a pathological nature to appear. In other words, schizophrenia does not necessarily imply progressive deterioration.

schizophrenia, catastrophic See *schizocaria.*

schizophrenia, catatonic One of the subgroups of schizophrenia (in the older literature, dementia praecox) that may appear as a chronic form or as an acute episode in the course of a schizophrenic pattern. As with any type of schizophrenia, the fundamental symptoms afford the basis for the diagnosis, although the subgrouping into the catatonic type is largely dependent upon certain secondary or accessory symptoms—catalepsy, stupor, hy-

perkinesiae, stereotypies, mannerisms, negativism, automatisms, and impulsivity.

Onset is acute in 41% of cases; in 31% of cases chronic paranoid symptoms precede the development of catatonic symptoms, and in the remaining cases the onset is subacute. In general, symptoms may be seen to fall into one of two categories: (1) catatonic stupor, including catalepsy, stupor, and negativism; and (2) catatonic excitement, including hyperkinesiae, stereotypies, mannerisms, automatisms, and impulsivity.

Catalepsy may appear as immobile or masklike facies, as posturing, resistance to movements, decreased spontaneity in movement, or less commonly, as cerea flexibilitas (waxy flexibility). The hyperkinesiae include arbitrary, automatic, pseudospontaneous movements while the stereotypies include movements, actions, posturings, speech, writings, or drawings that are monotonously repetitive and that bear little obvious relationship to external reality. *Schnauzkrampf* (q.v.) is a particular type of stereotypy. Mannerisms are not necessarily stereotyped but they are nonetheless inappropriate, inadequately modifiable, and caricaturelike. Negativism may appear in several forms: (1) external negativism, or negation of commands; (2) inner negativism, or oppositional thoughts (actually a type of intellectual ambivalence, but often misinterpreted as "obsessive thinking"); (3) active negativism, the active opposition of commands; (4) passive negativism, which often appears as stubbornness or uncooperativeness; (5) command-negativism, or doing exactly the opposite of what is ordered. Automatisms may also be expressed in various ways, such as echopraxia or echolalia (forms of command-automatism), or as fugues, self-injuries, or coprolalia. Impulsivity is commonly seen in catatonic schizophrenia and on occasion can lead to suicidal attempts or homicidal outbursts.

schizophrenia, childhood A clinical entity occurring in childhood, usually after the age of 1 and before the age of 11, characterized chiefly by disturbance in the ability to make affective contact with the environment and by autistic thinking. It has long been believed by many clinicians that such pictures represented early appearing schizophrenia rather than any different or unique syndrome, and Kallmann's genetic studies support this view. The criteria for establishing such a diagnosis, however, are not as well defined as in adult schizophrenia, so that various definitions of the disorder (or group of disorders) are given by various authors. Thus Bender says: "We now define childhood schizophrenia as a maturational lag at the embryonic level in all the areas which integrate biological and psychological behavior; an embryonic primitivity or plasticity characterizes the pattern of the behavior disturbance in all areas of personality functioning. It is determined before birth and hereditary factors appear to be important. It may be precipitated by a physiological crisis, which may be birth itself, especially a traumatic birth." (Caplan, G. *Emotional Problems of Early Childhood*, 1955) Mahler distinguishes between symbiotic infantile psychosis, which she described in 1952, and early infantile autism (Kanner's term), and considers both of them types of childhood schizophrenia. Others would limit the term childhood schizophrenia more narrowly and consider it as a separate entity from early infantile autism and from psychoses associated with mental deficiency. See *developmental disorders, pervasive; psychosis, symbiotic infantile.*

Bender describes the following symptoms:

1. vasovegetative—undifferentiated homeostatic functions; unpredictable temperature responses in illness; flushing, sweating, color changes, cold extremities; disturbed rhythm of sleeping and fluctuation in and out of torporous states of consciousness; disturbances in eating, elimination, and respiration; growth discrepancies; soft visceral tone leading to many "psychosomatic disturbances";

2. motility—undifferentiated reactions and hypersensitivity to external stimuli; lack of suppression of early reflex patterns (e.g. startle response); soft muscular tone, plasticity, awkwardness, infantile posture; insecurity with new motor patterns; residual primitive reflex patterned activities; oral mannerisms; head-turning and *whirling* (whose persistence after the age of 6 years she considers almost pathognomonic);

3. dependence on contact with others—

motor compliance; wooden, mechanical voice;

4. disturbances in the perceptual, thought, and language spheres, with incongruous early and late patterns; and

5. deep concern with problems of identity, body image, body functions, and orientation in time and space.

schizophrenia, coenaesthetic G. Huber's term (1957) for a chronic form of schizophrenia characterized by abnormal phenomena in the sphere of bodily sensation and by associated vegetative, motor, and sensory symptoms. According to Huber, this form is steadily progressive, and is organically determined by disturbances in the diencephalic and thalamic areas.

schizophrenia, compensation N.D.C. Lewis's term for a type of schizophrenia characterized by overcompensation for feelings of inferiority. Delusions of grandeur form the core of this psychosis.

schizophrenia deliriosa Menninger's term for a form of schizophrenia that starts as a delirium and is frequently associated with or directly follows a physical illness such as influenza.

schizophrenia, engrafted See *Propfschizophrenia.*

schizophrenia, hebephrenic A chronic form of schizophrenia characterized by marked disorders in thinking, incoherence, severe emotional disturbance, wild excitement alternating with tearfulness and depression, vivid hallucinations, and absurd, bizarre delusions which are prolific, fleeting, and frequently concerned with ideas of omnipotence, sex change, cosmic identity, and rebirth (the so-called phylogenetic symptoms). The hebephrenic forms tend to have an early onset, usually before the age of 20. Bleuler classified as hebephrenic all those schizophrenias with an acute onset that were not characterized by catatonic symptoms (e.g. the manic, melancholic, amented, and twilight states) and also all those chronic forms where the accessory symptoms are not dominant. Others have depended upon the presence of the silly, inappropriate "teenager" symptoms to establish the diagnosis.

Hebephrenic schizophrenia in almost all reported series has been associated with a poor prognosis; i.e. with a relatively rapid deterioration and schizophrenic dementia.

It is this form which contributes most heavily to the group termed nuclear or process schizophrenia by other workers.

schizophrenia, iatrogenic See *dysmentia, tardive.*

schizophrenia, induced Delusions or other schizophrenic symptoms imposed by one member of the family on other members. (See *association, psychosis of.*) In one such case, a schizophrenic mother transmitted her ideas of grandeur to her two daughters, one of whom was clearly schizophrenic, while the other could be convinced of the falsity of her beliefs and then showed no further evidence of the disease. This case, incidentally, is an example of *folie à trois* (q.v.). "Therefore, we must assume that an energetic patient can suggest his delusions to other members of the family if and when they articulate with the complexes (wishes and desires) of these same members. However, schizophrenia will only develop if the disease is already latent in those individuals. In induced insanity, not the disease as such is determined by induction but only its delusional content, and perhaps also the manifest outbreak." (Bleuler, D. *Dementia Praecox or the Group of Schizophrenias,* 1950) See *folie à deux.*

Schizophrenia, International Pilot Study (IPSS) A 1973 transcultural investigation of 1,202 schizophrenic patients in nine countries—Colombia, Czechoslovakia, Denmark, India, Nigeria, People's Republic of China, Union of Soviet Socialist Republics, United Kingdom, and United States. The major objective of the study is to define an operational base from which future international epidemiologic studies of schizophrenia and other psychiatric disorders can be developed. One part of the study is to define symptoms in such a way that psychiatrists all over the world can agree they are present, and then to determine what individual symptoms or groupings of symptoms are associated with clinical diagnoses.

schizophrenia, latent That form of schizophrenia in which, despite the existence of fundamental symptoms, no clear-cut psychotic episode or gross break with reality has occurred. Pseudoneurotic, pseudopsychopathic, borderline, ambulatory, and similar forms are included here so long as there has been no acute psychotic episode (a requirement that differentiates latent schizophrenia from the *residual* type).

The latent type of schizophrenia includes what some authors variously term incipient, prepsychotic, pseudoneurotic, pseudopsychopathic, or borderline schizophrenia, and these latter are more appropriately included under the latent group than with the chronic undifferentiated forms.

The group named *schizophrenia, residual type,* includes only those patients who, having had a psychotic episode, improve to the degree that they are not considered psychotic, even though signs of the schizophrenic disorder remain.

schizophrenia, mixed An instance of schizophrenia that shows symptoms of more than one of the disease's four generally accepted and clearly distinguished categories; simple, paranoid, catatonic, hebephrenic. Such cases are often called chronic undifferentiated schizophrenia.

schizophrenia, paranoid One of the chronic forms of schizophrenia. In addition to the fundamental schizophrenic symptoms, the paranoid type shows the following features: a feeling that external reality has changed and somehow become different; suspiciousness and ideas of dedication; ideas of reference; hallucinations, especially of body sensations; delusions of persecution or of grandiosity. Some paranoid schizophrenics may act in accord with their delusions and turn on their tormentors, while others may become suicidal in an attempt to escape their persecutors.

Several types of paranoid schizophrenia are recognized: litigious, depressed, persecutory, grandiose, erotomaniacal, etc. In general, paranoid forms of schizophrenia develop later than do the other forms, the highest incidence being between the ages of 30 and 35. In contrast to *paranoia* (q.v.), in paranoid schizophrenia the delusions are multiple, less highly systematized, changeable, illogical, and bizarre.

schizophrenia, postemotive In a person constitutionally predisposed, schizophrenia may be precipitated by an emotional trauma, especially in the face of situations that threaten self-preservation, the social self, or the sexual life. See *psychosis, reactive.*

A 21-year-old schizoid man, who had made a happy work adjustment for the preceding six years in a candy factory, developed postemotive schizophrenia. His right arm was caught in a machine pulley belt and he suffered severe muscular contusions. He was hospitalized for two weeks, but was unable to return to work after discharge from the hospital, because of his "nervous state caused by the accident." After two months, he finally went back to work, but did poorly and seemed terrified by machine work. He worked for several days but had to leave his job, because he began to tremble all over, could not sleep, developed numerous hypochondriacal complaints and crying spells, became generally apprehensive, with acute fear reactions. Shortly thereafter he began to neglect his personal appearance, and a widespread retraction of interest was noted. He became absorbed in himself, talked and laughed senselessly in a childish voice, and at times demonstrated verbigeration. He was institutionalized, and a diagnosis of schizophrenia, hebephrenic type, was made. After seven years, there was no improvement in his condition.

Most postemotive reactions eventually and spontaneously disappear and are self-limited syndromes. But when emotional stress precipitates a psychosis in a predisposed person, prognosis is made on the basis of the psychosis itself rather than on the nature of the precipitating factor. Many authorities feel that schizophrenia is nearly always postemotive, that detailed anamnestic investigation would reveal specific emotional traumata as precipitating factors in the majority of cases.

schizophrenia, pseudoneurotic P.H. Hoch and P. Polatin (*Psychiatric Quarterly 23,* 1949) apply this term to those patients whose defense mechanisms are, at least superficially, neurotic in type, but who, on close investigation, show the basic schizophrenic mechanisms. The most important diagnostic features are *pan-anxiety* and *pan-neurosis*. The all-pervading anxiety structure leaves no life approach of the person free from tension. Usually not only one or two different neurotic mechanisms are seen, but all symptoms known in neurotic illness tend to be present at the same time—anxiety, conversion symptoms, gross hysterical or vegetative manifestations, phobias, and obsessive-compulsive mechanisms. These neurotic mechanisms dominate the patient; they constantly shift but are never completely absent.

The life approach of these patients is always autistic and dereistic, although this may be very subtly expressed. Withdrawal from reality is more general than is the case even in the neurotic with schizoid features. Some inappropriate emotional connections are usually manifest, and there is a lack of modulation and flexibility in emotional display. Often, these patients appear cold and controlled in responding to major frustrations, but overreact to trivial ones. Hate reactions, particularly toward the family, are more open and less discriminating than in the neurotic. Commonly there is depression or an *anhedonic* state wherein the patient derives pleasure from nothing. Thinking disorders may also be too subtle to be on the surface; condensations and concept displacements, catathymic thinking, expression of omnipotence emanating from the patient, or the feeling of an omnipotential attitude of the environment toward the patient. Unlike neurotics, such patients do not try to rationalize their symptoms in a logical and coherent fashion. Instead, the component elements of their story always remain vaguely conflicting; they are unable to give details of the development of the symptoms, and repeat and reiterate their complaints in a stereotyped and sterile way. There is usually an inability to associate freely in spite of their ordinarily good intelligence and signal ability to verbalize. Psychosexually, such patients show a chaotic organization and a mixture of all levels of libidinal development. Marked sadistic or sadomasochistic behavior is often linked with this sexual material. The Rorschach test in such patients often shows thinking disorders such as concrete thinking, an unpredictable attitude toward various situations, lack of constructive planning, passive opportunism, and marked anxiety. In the Rorschach results there is often noticed that marked variability of performance which is so characteristic of schizophrenia. Amytal interviews frequently release some of the more overtly psychotic material.

Many of these patients develop psychotic episodes that are often of short duration with complete reintegration. These short-lived attacks are called "micropsychoses" and are characterized by the simultaneous development of three very significant features: hypochondriacal ideas, ideas of reference, and feelings of depersonalization. The patients zigzag, repeatedly trespassing beyond the reality line.

The following case illustrates pseudoneurotic schizophrenia. The patient was a single white female, 38 years old. Though an unwanted child, she had a normal early development, was very affectionate and obedient, and mixed well with her contemporaries. With advancing age the patient appeared to grow progressively more schizoid in personality, but never enough to interfere with her functioning. After completing high school, she obtained a position with a dentist, and several years later was discharged, because her employer felt that she had lost interest in her work, had become listless. Her arms hung down at her sides and she slouched as she walked. After that, the patient found employment in a hospital and began to complain of abdominal pain. Appendectomy was performed, but her complaints continued, including new ones about marked weakness and lack of strength, but there was no real depression. Later, constipation and a "foggy feeling" began to trouble her. She was much irritated by her mother and sister because they did not understand her and regarded her complaints as caused by laziness. She also complained that her heart hurt her. On admission to the hospital, the patient appeared cooperative but somewhat self-absorbed. Whenever she had to talk with people in the course of social contacts, she showed fear and shame, and marked feelings of inferiority. Later the patient complained that her subconscious mind played tricks on her, that she had a feeling as if a voice were telling her to go to sleep. Finally, this last complaint crystallized into frank ideas of reference and persecution and auditory hallucinations.

schizophrenia, recidives in (res'i-divz) Recurring, intermittent, acute episodes of schizophrenia, or other evidences of deterioration that begin after prolonged remission. The recurring attacks often duplicate the previous ones, but new features may appear. There is no definite correlation between initial disease symptoms and recidives.

schizophrenia, regressive symptoms Those schizophrenic symptoms that represent an undoing or primitivization of differentiations acquired through mental development; included here are such symptoms as phantasies of world destruction, physical sensations and delusions, depersonalization, delusions of grandeur, archaic speech and thought, most hebephrenic symptoms, and certain catatonic symptoms (negativism, echolalia, echopraxia, automatic obedience, posturing, stereotypy). See *schizophrenia, restitutional symptoms.*

schizophrenia, residual Interepisodic schizophrenia; the condition of being without gross psychotic symptoms following a psychotic schizophrenic episode. To be contrasted with *schizophrenia, latent* (q.v.).

schizophrenia, restitutional symptoms Those schizophrenic symptoms that represent an attempt at regaining reality, which has been lost by regression; included are such symptoms as hallucinations, delusions, most of the social and speech peculiarities of schizophrenia, and certain catatonic symptoms (stereotypy, mannerisms, automatic obedience, rigidity).

schizophrenia, reversible Menninger's term for a schizophrenic state with a potentiality for recovery. See *psychosis, process.*

schizophrenia, simple One of the chronic forms of schizophrenia; historically, called dementia praecox, simple type; dementia simplex; schizophrenia simplex; primary dementia.

In the simple form of schizophrenia, there is an insidious psychic impoverishment that affects the emotions, the intellect, and the will. Chronic dissatisfaction or complete indifference to reality are characteristic, and the simple schizophrenic is isolated, estranged, and asocial. Affect is markedly blunted and dulled, there is little phantasy life, and there may be few or no accessory symptoms. Dementia, in Bleuler's sense, is marked—patients make many foolish mistakes, are highly suggestible and gullible, and speech is filled with senseless generalizations. Thought is vacuous and banal, ideas are insipid and unintegrated. Such patients tend to sink to low and relatively simple social levels that make few or no demands on them and may come to lead almost a vegetative existence. They often become day laborers, peddlers, or vagabonds, and they contribute heavily to the group of eccentric recluses.

In DSM-III, many such cases would be classified as *personality disorders* (q.v.).

schizophrenia, systematic In Leonhard's classification, one of the two major subdivisions of schizophrenic disorders, comprising catatonias, hebephrenias, and paraphrenias. Systematic schizophrenias follow a progressive course. The other subdivision, with a better prognosis, he called *nonsystematic*, further divided into affect-laden paranoia, schizophasia, and periodic catatonia.

schizophrenia, toxic *Toxiphrenia* (q.v.).

schizophrenic defect state See *symptoms, negative*.

schizophreniform Resembling schizophrenia. See *psychosis, process; psychosis, reactive*.

schizophreniform disorder Any disorder with psychotic features similar to schizophrenia except that duration is less than six months and manifestations include features that are usually associated with good prognosis, such as confusion or perplexity at the height of the psychotic episode, affect not blunted or flat, premorbid social or occupational functioning good. Within six months of onset of the episode there is a complete or almost complete return to the premorbid level of functioning.

schizophrenogenic Producing or fostering the development of schizophrenia; Frieda Fromm-Reichmann was the first to discuss schizophrenogenic mothers.

schizophrenosis Southard's term for schizophrenic reactions in general.

schizotaxia Genetic predisposition to schizophrenia, whose phenotypical expression may be largely dependent on noxious or stressful environmental influences.

schizothyme (-thīm) One who has a schizoid personality.

schizothymia (-thī′mē-à) Introversion; *schizoidism* (q.v.).

schizotypal disorders See *personality disorders; psychodynamics, adaptational*.

Schmidt's syndrome (Johann F.M. Schmidt, German laryngologist, 1838–1907) A bulbar syndrome due to involvement of the vagus and spinal accessory nerves. Symptoms are homolateral paralysis of the soft palate, pharynx, and larynx; and homolateral sternocleidomastoid paralysis.

Schnauzkrampf (shnouts′krämpf) Term coined by Karl Ludwig Kahlbaum (1828–99) for protrusion of the lips such that they resemble a snout. The condition is found almost exclusively in the catatonic form of schizophrenia.

Schneider, Kurt (1887–1967) German psychiatrist, best known for his phenomenologic approach and description of the diagnostically significant symptoms in schizophrenia. See *symptoms, first-rank*.

Schneiderian first-rank symptoms See *symptoms, first-rank*.

Scholz's disease (Willibald Scholz, German neurologist, 1889–1971) See *sclerosis, diffuse*.

school-marmitis A personality type seen in some teachers, characterized by "magnified self-awareness . . . in the role of dispenser of knowledge and wisdom to children and, on occasion, to their parents; a tendency to 'lord it over' and a patronizing attitude toward others." (Kanner, L. *Child Psychiatry*, 1948) Emotional attitudes of a schoolteacher can be powerful determinants of the child's own attitude, for good or ill, as the case may be. This is especially true if the child is already emotionally insecure in his home life. Happily, there also exist teacher attitudes that reflect a healthy degree of emotional integration at a high level of personal maturity.

school, Montessori See *Montessori, Maria*.

school phobia See *phobia, school*.

school refusal syndrome See *phobia, school*.

schoolsickness An occupational neurosis in children maladjusted to their school situation, characterized by anxiety, restlessness, and irritability. See *phobia, school*.

Schreber, Schreber case In 1911, Freud published *Psycho-Analytic Notes Upon an Autobiographical Account of a Case of Paranoia (Dementia Paranoides)*. This consisted of an analysis of *Memoirs of a Neurotic*, a previously published (1903) autobiographical account by Dr. jur. Daniel Paul Schreber. Freud's analysis of these memoirs formed the basis for the psychoanalytic view of paranoid delusions which, at least in the male, are interpreted as attempts to contradict the underlying homosexual wish-phantasy of loving a man. See *paranoia.*

Schuele's sign *Omega melancholium* (q.v.).

Schüller-Christian-Hand's syndrome *Xanthomatosis* (q.v.).

sciatica (sī-a′ti-ka) See *disk, herniated lumbar intervertebral.*

scierneuropsia See *scieropia.*

scieropia (sī-êr-ō′pē-à) Visual defect in which objects appear to be in a shadow; when of emotional or psychologic origin, such defect is termed *scierneuropsia.*

sclerosis, amyotrophic lateral Progressive muscular atrophy; progressive bulbar palsy; chronic poliomyelitis; known popularly as Lou Gehrig's disease. Some authorities believe that amyotrophic lateral sclerosis is a hereditary disorder, others that it is due to a toxin with a predilection for the anterior horn cells; currently, however, most believe that it is a slow virus (see *virus infections*). It begins most often between the ages of 50 and 70 years, usually with an insidious onset. Pathological changes include progressive degeneration of the anterior horn cells of the spinal cord, the medullary motor nuclei, and the pyramidal tracts. Wasting begins in the upper limbs, first in the hands and later in the forearm and shoulder. Then it spreads to the tongue, palate, larynx, and pharnyx, resulting in slurred speech. Degeneration of both pyramidal tracts above the medulla produces pseudobulbar palsy: dysarthria, dysphagia, and spasticity of the muscles; when severe, pseudobulbar palsy results in impaired voluntary control over emotional reactions which may be exaggerated, explosive, and quite inappropriate. The disease is fatal within 1 to 4 years.

sclerosis, atrophic lobar *Little's disease* (q.v.).

sclerosis, diffuse "A group of progressive diseases usually occurring early in life and characterized pathologically by widespread demyelination of the white matter of the cerebral hemispheres, and clinically in typical cases by visual failure, mental deterioration, and spastic paralysis. Both sporadic and familial cases are encountered. The aetiology of these disorders is unknown and there is no general agreement as to their classification. At present their resemblances to one another appear to outweigh their differences and they are therefore included under a common title." (Brain, *DNS*) The various entities that Brain includes are encephalitis periaxialis diffusa (Schilder's disease), centrolobar sclerosis, encephaloleukopathia scleroticans, progressive degenerative subcortical encephalopathy, leukodystrophy, leukoencephalopathia, myeloclastica primitiva, encephalomyelomalacia chronica diffusa, *concentric demyelination* (*Baló's disease*), Krabbe's disease, Scholz's disease, and Pelizaeus-Merzbacher's disease. It has been suggested that some of this group are caused by specific biochemical defects affecting different stages in the metabolism of myelin.

The demyelination typically begins symmetrically in both occipital lobes and spreads forward. Onset is usually before the age of 14; males are more frequently affected than females. Symptoms may begin acutely or insidiously and include headache, giddiness, visual impairment progressing to blindness; diplopia, nystagmus; spastic diplegia, aphasia and/or spastic dysarthria, epileptiform attacks, and progressive dementia. Survival period is rarely longer than three years after the onset of symptoms. There is no known treatment.

sclerosis, disseminated Multiple sclerosis.

sclerosis en plaque (F. "in patches") Multiple sclerosis.

sclerosis, multiple Insular sclerosis; disseminated sclerosis. One of the demyelinating diseases of the nervous system and, at least in temperate zones, one of the most common neurological disorders. It is characterized pathologically by swelling and then demyelination of the medullary sheath, which is followed by glial proliferation. The result is an irregular scattering of well-demarcated sclerotic plaques throughout the white and gray matter of the brain and spinal cord. The lesions show a predilection for the pyramidal tracts and posterior columns of the spinal cord, the posterior longitudinal bundle and cerebellar connections of the brain stem, the white matter of the frontal lobes, and the optic tracts. The disease was first described by Cruveilhier in 1835 and Carswell in 1838. Charcot described a triad of symptoms—

nystagmus, intention tremor, and scanning speech—but this is found only in about 10% of cases and even then usually only when lesions are far advanced.

At the present time, cardinal features are the presence of symptoms of more than one central nervous system lesion at one time and a course of remissions and exacerbations.

The etiology of multiple sclerosis is unknown; both infectious (?virus ?spirochete) and autoimmune mechanisms have been implicated by some studies. The highest incidence of the disorder is in Northern Europe and Switzerland; the incidence in Great Britain is about half that in Switzerland, and the incidence in the United States is about one-quarter that in Great Britain. In the United States, incidence is considerably greater in the North than in the South. While heredity may be a contributing factor in the genesis of the disorder, evidence does not substantiate its designation as a major factor.

The disease usually begins between the ages of 20 and 40; the average age at onset is 30 years for females and 34 years for males. The age at onset tends to be lowest in those areas with the highest incidence. In 50% of cases, the initial symptom is weakness or loss of control over one or more limbs; in 29% the initial symptom involves the visual apparatus (blindness, dimness of vision, double vision, field defects, etc.); in 11% the initial symptom is numbness or similar painless paresthesia. The earliest symptoms tend to be fleeting and fluctuating, so that a misdiagnosis of hysteria is often made. The disappearance or alleviation of symptoms may last for months or years until the patient suffers another exacerbation. In general, three main types can be distinguished: an acute form, with a survival period of 1 to 2 years; a chronic, progressive form with a slowly downhill course that may last for 20 or 30 years; and a remittent form in which there is almost complete relief from symptoms during the period between acute exacerbations. The average life expectancy after the onset of the illness has been estimated to be 20 to 25 years.

"The end is distressing. . . . Ataxia, weakness, and spasticity confine the patient to bed and prevent him from carrying out the simplest actions for himself. Swallowing becomes difficult and speech almost unintelligible. Urinary or cutaneous infection or pneumonia finally releases the sufferer. In rare cases the last even is an acute exacerbation of the disease itself, taking the form of an acute myelitis or encephalomyelitis." (Brain, *DNS*)

In the mental sphere, euphoria with a sense of mental and physical well-being despite obvious handicaps is characteristic, although dejection, irritability, and emotional lability are seen in some patients. Usually there is some reduction in intellectual capacity and a few patients develop a delusional state or a terminal dementia.

There is no known treatment for the disorder.

sclerosis, posterolateral Subacute combined degeneration of the spinal cord; a deficiency disease due to lack of intrinsic factor (which combines with extrinsic factor to form the cobalt-containing complex, or vitamin B_{12}), seen in pernicious anemia, sprue, cachexia, and postgastrectomy cases. Pathological changes include irregular demyelination of the posterolateral columns and peripheral nerves. Symptoms are paresthesiae; early loss of position and vibratory sensation; later loss of touch and pain sensation, often with a glove and stocking type of anesthesia; sphincter disturbances; moderate muscular wasting; and ataxia. Symptoms usually begin in the lower limbs. Various mental changes may be seen: mild dementia, confusional psychosis, Korsakoff psychosis, or affective reactions. Associated with the neuropsychiatric changes are gastric achlorhydria, glossitis, and anemia. Duration of life in untreated cases is approximately two years. Treatment with vitamin B_{12} can restore the patient to good health indefinitely.

sclerosis, tuberous *Epiloia;* a chronic heritable disorder, transmitted as an autosomal dominant with variable penetrance. Symptoms appear in early childhood: mental retardation (often severe), epileptic convulsions, and special tumors (adenoma sebaceum) of the skin and viscera. Pathologically, there are various malformations and numerous glial tumors within the brain. The disease was originally described by Bourneville.

SCN Suprachiasmatic nucleus of the interior hypothalamus. See *clock, biological.*

SCOPE Acronym for an accepted set of diagnostic procedures that are systematic, complete, objective, practical, and empirical.

-scopia, -scopo, -scopy Combining form meaning to look at, examine, inquire, from Gr. *skopeīn.*

scopolagnia *Voyeurism; scop(t)ophilia* (qq.v.).

scopophilia Sexual pleasure derived from contemplation or looking. It is a component instinct and stands in the same relation to exhibitionism as sadism does to masochism. Freud calls them paired instincts. See *sadism, phallic; voyeur; voyeurism.*

Autoscopophilia refers to the pleasure of looking at one's own body. Active scopophilia is the pleasure derived from looking at the sexual organs of another. Passive scopophilia is the desire to be looked at by others and is thus seen to be equivalent to active exhibitionism.

"The pleasure which a person takes in his own sexual organ may become associated with scoptophilia (or sexual pleasure in looking) in its active and passive forms." (Freud, *CP*)

In Freudian literature the German *Schaulust* has been translated as scoptophilia, but scopophilia is the more correct form.

scopophobia Fear of being looked at; morbid shyness.

scoptophilia See *scopophilia.*

SCOR Skin conductance orienting response, an electrodermal response that occurs in the presence of a novel stimulus that bids for the subject's attention. Many adult schizophrenics do not produce SCORs unless the intensity of the novel stimulus is increased beyond that ordinarily required to elicit the response.

scotoma (skō-tō′ma) An abnormal blind spot in the visual field.

scotoma, mental Lack of insight; a mental "blind spot" for the problem before one's eyes.

scotomization A process of psychic depreciation, by means of which the subject attempts to deny everything which conflicts with his ego.

scotophobia Fear of darkness.

scrapie A naturally occurring spongiform encepalopathy in sheep and goats, presumed to be caused by an unconventional virus, or, perhaps, a viroid. See *virus infections.*

screen A form of concealment. When, for instance, in a dream one stands for another or others, by virtue of some common feature, the person so standing is called a screen. See *memory, screen.*

"Identification consists in giving representation in the dream-content to only one of two or more persons who are related by some common feature, while the second person or other persons appear to be suppressed as far as the dream is concerned. In the dream this one 'screening' person enters into all the relations and situations which derive from the persons whom he screens." (Freud, *ID*)

screen, dream See *hallucination, blank.*

screen memory See *memory, screen.*

screen phantasy See *phantasy, screen.*

screening See *review.*

screening, genetic Systematic search for persons in a population who possess certain genotypes that (1) are associated with existing disease or predispose to future disease (because of genetically determined susceptibilities to environmental agents, for example), (2) may lead to disease in their descendants, or (3) produce other variations of interest but not known to be associated with disease.

It is conventional to screen (1) blood of newborns (*newborn screening*) for the hyperphenylalaninemias, the tyrosinemias, the amino acidopathies, the galactosemias, and aberrations of thyroid hormone biosynthesis and (2) urine of newborns for disorders of amino acid or monosaccharide metabolism and transport.

Fetal screening permits detection of genetic disease in the fetus and thus permits selective termination of pregnancy. With the use of recombinant DNA, restriction enzymes, and oligonucleotide probes, it has become possible to detect many more diseases than previously and the methods pose fewer dangers to the fetus than earlier methods.

Carrier screening aims to identify persons heterozygous for a gene for a serious recessive disease, and it is now common to screen young adults in relevant high-risk ethnic communities to initiate genetic counseling for indications of Tay-Sachs, beta thalassemia, and sickle cell heterozygosity. Screening to identify persons with variant phenotypes, such as alpha-1 antitrypsin deficiency, has become a form of epidemiologic research to discover the natural history of the variant.

screening, periodic See *EPSDT.*

script analysis See *transactional analysis.*

scruple, defloration *Rare.* Hirschfield's term for a compulsion neurosis in young men about to marry; it implies a dread of being the first one to "injure" a woman and carries with it also the fear of castration on the part of the male.

scruple, virginity *Rare.* Doubt on the part of the man regarding his wife's virginity; delusion of infidelity.

scrupulosity Excessive meticulousness or punctiliousness, most often displayed in relation to questions of right or wrong and hence often couched in religious or moral terms. The scrupulous patient sees evil where there is no evil, serious sin where there is no serious sin, and obligation where there is no obligation. Scrupulosity may appear as part of an obsessive-compulsive pattern but if long maintained it is suggestive of an underlying schizophrenic process.

Scull's dilemma See *dilemma, Scull's.*

SDAT Senile dementia, Alzheimer's type; also known as primary degenerative dementia of senile or presenile onset. See *senile dementia.*

SDD Sporadiac (nonfamilial) depressive disease, in Winokur's classification.

SE Spongiform encephalopathy. See *virus infections.*

seasonal affective disorder See *affective disorder, seasonal.*

sebastomania *Obs.* Religious psychosis.

seclusion See *restraint.*

second messenger system See *adenyl cyclase.*

secondary defense symptom See *symptom, secondary defense.*

secondary gain See *gain, epinosic.*

secondary sleep disorder A sleep disorder associated with or caused by identifiable disease in some organ system such as central nervous system or respiratory system.

security operations Sullivan's term for feelings—such as anger, boredom, contempt, depression, or irritation—that, no matter how rational or explicable at first glance, are really defenses against the recognition or experiencing of anxiety; the term is approximately equivalent to *defense* (q.v.)

sedation A state of decreased responsivity to usual stimuli that may proceed to sleepiness, but not to drowsiness (which would be a *hypnotic* effect). In practice, the line between the sedative and the hypnotic dose of a drug is a fine one.

sedation threshold See *threshold, sedation.*

sedativism Alcohol and drug abuse.

seed psychosurgery See *tractotomy, stereotactic.*

Séglas type See *type, Séglas.*

segmentation Synonymous with *cleavage* (q.v.).

segregation In a social sense, separation or isolation.

In genetics this term refers to an essential principle in the Mendelian mechanism of inheritance, in which the gene units derived from the two parents segregate out in the hybrid, as if independent of each other. This phenomenon allows the gene units to enter into new combinations, especially in those involving more than one pair. See *Mendelism.*

Séguin, O. Edouard (1812–80) French psychiatrist; humanistic treatment and education of the mentally retarded.

Seitelberger's disease See *degeneration, neuro-axonal.*

seizure An attack, or sudden onset of a disease or of certain symptoms, such as convulsions.

seizure, audiogenic Convulsion or fit induced by prolonged exposure to intense sounds of high frequency.

seizure, automatic A type of psychomotor epilepsy. See *epilepsy.*

seizure, erotic See *epilepsy, erotic.*

seizure, gustatory A form of epilepsy in which the sensation of a definite and usually peculiar taste is a part of the seizure pattern. The seizures are often also associated with sensations of peculiar odors. See *fit, uncinate.*

seizure, psychic A type of psychomotor epilepsy. See *epilepsy; psycholepsy.*

seizure, subjective A type of psychomotor epilepsy. See *epilepsy.*

seizure, temporal lobe Psychomotor epilepsy. See *epilepsy.*

sejunction Wernicke's term for blocking and other forms of dissociation. The concept is seldom used today, because it includes forms of dissociation which are widely removed both psychologically and nosographically.

selaphobia Fear of a flash.

selection In a specific biological sense, this term applies in a mixed population to the intentional or unintentional choice of those individuals who possess a particular genetic character or a certain combination of characters. This choice may be exercised by the failure to reproduce or by the lack of an adequate partner for marriage, if preference is given to other types or if the given type is biologically incapable of reproduction.

Natural selection takes place in evolution through a variety of processes that enable types (adapted to their environment) to reproduce their kind in marked degree, so that an improvement is gradually carried on from one stage of development to the other.

In human genetics, one usually distinguishes between *positive* and *negative* factors of selection, according to (1) whether a given factor is favorable to the reproduction of healthy or tainted family stocks, or (2) whether the general life conditions of a population facilitate or hinder the reproduction of the average type.

selection, adverse In insurance terminology, accumulation of high-risk consumers within a given insurance plan; self-sorting of a population to which insurance plans are offered on the basis of how extensively they plan to use the services. Employees who use many health services, including psychiatric benefits, for example, will often gravitate toward the few carriers offering high benefit levels. As an increasingly higher percentage of the members of a plan use unusually high amounts of care, the premiums must rise to pay for it. Each premium increase to accommodate the cost of *high utilizers* results in a new wave of *low utilizers* opting out (i.e. deciding not to buy that plan), and as a result the selection process spirals higher and higher.

seleniasmus *Obs.* Lunacy.

selenogamia (L. "state of being wedded to the moon") *Obs. Somnambulism* (q.v.).

self The psychophysical total of the person at any given moment, including both conscious and unconscious attributes. Horney's term for self as thus defined is *actual self* or *empirical self*. See Jung's definition of *ego*.

self-absorption Erikson describes *generativity vs. self-absorption* as one of the eight stages of man. See *ontogeny, psychic*.

self-abuse *Obs.* A moralistic term for *masturbation* (q.v.)

self, actual In Horney's terms, the whole person—as he really exists at any point in time. The *real self* is the person's potential for further growth and development. The person the neurotic believes himself to be (the result of identification with an idealized image of what he feels he should be) is the *idealized self*.

The *neurotic process* includes all the behavior and mechanisms by which the person maintains his identification with the idealized image even though this alienates him from his real self and requires him to deny and reject his actual self.

self-actualization See *humanistic psychology*.

self-attack See *syndrome, deliberate self-harm*.

self-awareness See *image, body*.

self, bad A psychoanalytic concept referring to the tendency on the part of both analyst and patient to project on each other their guilty images of their instinct-ridden selves. Behind the shield of unconscious countertransference, an analyst may make the patient a whipping boy for his own unconscious image of his infantile instinctual self. Conversely, the analyst must frequently tolerate (and analyze) the patient's tendency to project his own instinctual urges onto the analyst and to castigate him (the analyst) for them.

Much "holier than thou" missionary zeal in the psychopathology of everyday life finds its source in this process of projection of the *bad self* upon others. E.F. Sharpe (*Collected Papers on Psychoanalysis*, 1950) says: "The analyst must be sufficiently analysed to enable him to detect, and so consciously control, any tendency to regard the patient as the 'Bad Self' who needs reforming."

self, cohesive See *autonomy, sense of*.

self-defeating personality disorder *Masochistic personality disorder;* characteristics include involvement in situations leading to disappointment or mistreatment even when other options are available; reluctance to seize opportunities for pleasure or disinterest in people who are consistently supportive and gratifying; failure to accomplish crucial tasks despite clear-cut ability to perform them; attainments bring depression or guilt feelings rather than contentment, or lead to behavior that brings about pain (such as an automobile accident or losing something of value); rejection of others's help; martyrdom and unwarranted self-sacrifice; sabotaging one's own efforts (including therapy).

Being the victim in an abusive situation does not by itself justify a diagnosis of self-defeating personality disorder, and the very existence of such an entity has been questioned. For that reason, the category has been placed in the appendix of DSM-III-R rather than within the body of the text.

self-directed exposure See *exposure, self-directed.*

self-dynamism The fabric of the motivational forces and processes that lead to the development of the *self-system*, in Sullivan's theory of interpersonal relations. The human personality is founded on a biological substrate and is the product of the interpersonal and social forces acting on the person from the time of birth. The human being is concerned with two goals: (1) the pursuit of satisfaction, which deals chiefly with biological needs; and (2) the pursuit of security, which deals primarily with cultural pressures. To maintain security and avoid anxiety, the child develops and strengthens those sides of his nature which are pleasing or acceptable to the significant adults. The resulting configuration of traits is the *self-system* (q.v.).

self-effacement Horney's term for the behavior of the type of neurotic character who idealizes compliance, dependence, and love as a result of identification with the despised self.

self-esteem A state in which narcissistic supplies emanating from the superego are maintained so that the person does not fear punishment or abandonment by the superego. In other words, self-esteem is a state of being on good terms with one's *superego* (q.v.). Pathologic loss of self-esteem is characteristic of clinical depression. See *omnipotence.*

self, ethical See *superego.*

self-extinction Horney's term for that form of neurotic behavior in which the person lives vicariously through the actions of others and has no personality that he experiences or identifies as his own. See *personality, as if.*

self-fellator See *autofellatio.*

self, hidden See *personality, multiple.*

self-hypnosis See *autohypnosis.*

self, idealized See *self, actual.*

self-identification A process in which the subject projects his own personality upon another and then proceeds to admire himself as he appears in the other person. While this is the usual process of self-identification, it is possible to include under the term the process of projecting one's undesirable traits upon another and then hating his own traits, as if they belonged to another. The latter happens in paranoid states.

Self-identification is based on narcissism and homosexuality.

self-irrumation (-ir-oo-mā′shun) Autofellatio.

self-maximation The drive (involving a part of the ego) associated with the numerous competitive situations a person encounters in the course of living, such as competitions for affection, attention, and status, at home, at school, in groups of peers, and elsewhere. There are competitions in the vocational, intellectual, and social fields, as well as for love objects. This drive is to maintain feelings of personal adequacy.

self-mutilation Maiming or injuring the self, including the willful production of any symptom, syndrome, or disease. See *factitial; morsicatio buccarum; syndrome, Munchhausen.*

Self-mutilation, in general, is nonspecific in its origin and significance and can thus be observed in a variety of settings. It is sometimes part of a suicide attempt and may then represent a discharge of aggression against the self or against parental introjections. It may represent a way of relieving guilt by expiating acts committed or phantasies entertained. It has been reported in soldiers who attempted thereby to evade their assignment to battlefield stations; many observers have noted the high frequency of schizophrenic disorders in such soldiers.

In psychiatric hospitals, probably the

two most frequent forms of self-mutilation are repetitive wrist-cutting (the "*slashers*") and cigarette burning of the forearms; both tend to be repeated in a stereotyped way, with the patient seemingly fascinated by the sight of blood oozing from the cut or by the sight and odor of burning flesh. Most such patients give little if any indication that they are suffering the pain one would anticipate from such wounds. Some authors consider wrist-cutting as distorted autoerotic activity that simultaneously defends against and gratifies the libidinal impulses; the cuttings on the skin represent the female genitalia. Other authors, while agreeing that wrist-slashing is more common among females, find it to be indicative of more serious pathology than mere neurotic distortion. It occurs most often in women with a history of physical trauma(ta) in childhood, with menstrual irregularities, with difficulty in sexual identification, and with depression. For such women, the act seems to be a way of gaining self-control and reintegration in situations of stress where they experience difficulty in thinking clearly and acting effectively. See *syndrome, Lesch-Nyhan.*

In addition to wrist-cutting and burning, the following have also been reported: abrasion, head banging, ingestion of medication and other objects, jumping from heights, hair pulling, insertion of foreign bodies into the urethra, self-enucleation of the eye, self-castration, removal of tongue.

From the point of view of psychiatric diagnosis, probably the most frequent currently reported as self-mutilators are borderline personality or schizophrenia. In these patients, the motives included relieving feelings of depersonalization, lessening inner tension, trying to solve genital conflicts, using the sight of his blood to gain assurance that he is alive, and denying the inability to control the body. See *syndrome, deliberate self-harm.*

self-observation Scrutiny of one's physical and/or mental state of functioning, one of the perceptive tasks of the *ego* (q.v.).

self-peeping, narcissistic Self-voyeurism on the basis of primary *narcissism* (q.v.). Ordinarily, the original self-voyeurism is transformed into voyeurism directed against the parents. E. Bergler considers this voyeurism to be the true basis for choosing acting as a profession. In the beginning, the child says: "I want to be a voyeur of mother and father, later of intimacies between them." But the superego reproaches the child for this wish, and the child denies having this wish by asserting the opposite: "No, I am not a voyeur, I am just the opposite—an exhibitionist." This, too, receives reproaches from the superego, and the desire is sublimated: "I am neither a voyeur nor an exhibitionist; I merely want to give other people pleasure, so I am an actor." (*Psychoanalytic Quarterly Supplement 23,* 1949)

self-pitying constellation A group of symptoms characteristic of "neurotic depression" (used in the sense of lacking endogenous symptoms such as early morning waking, weight loss, psychomotor retardation, and guilt feelings), consisting of self-pity, irritability, reactivity, and fluctuating symptoms. Neurotic depression also used to refer to related but not identical or interchangeable groups of depressed patients, meaning that their disorders were less incapacitating; nonpsychotic (= no hallucinations, delusions, confusion, memory impairment, etc.); situational or reactive to a social stressor; characterological, in a longstanding maladaptive personality pattern; due to unconscious conflicts over loss, fall in self-esteem, aggressivity, or narcissism, dependency, and ambivalence.

self psychology Object relations theory as it relates to the earliest stages of development, before the infant differentiates between self and non-self, ego and non-ego. See *object relations theory.*

self-punishment See *ego-suffering; masochism; resistance, superego.*

self-punishment, expiatory See *expiation.*

self, real See *self, actual.*

self-referential See *reference, ideas of.*

self-regulation, physiologic See *biofeedback.*

self-reporting See *psychodynamics, adaptational.*

self, secondary See *personality, multiple.*

self-sentience Awareness of self; in Sullivan's terminology, recognition of the bodily self as "me," and differentiated from the rest of the world or the "not me." See *ego, body.*

self, subconscious See *personality, multiple.*

self, subliminal See *personality, multiple.*

self-system A term used by Sullivan, in his theory of personality development, to denote final formation of self from a limited number sifted out of a greater number of potentialities, through parental influence on the developing personality of the child. Security rests on the feeling of belonging and being accepted. The child's actions or attributes that meet with disapproval tend to be blocked out of awareness and dissociated. As the child realizes that certain earlier devices for obtaining satisfaction, such as crying when hungry, bring on disapproval in the environment, the earlier pattern of behavior is inhibited: the child tends to develop and emphasize those aspects of his nature that are pleasing or acceptable to the significant adults, and the configuration of the traits that have met with approval constitutes the self-system.

After the self-system has been established, secondary anxiety appears whenever there is a possibility that the dissociated thoughts or feelings will become conscious: the dissociated impulses are not necessarily destructive, but because there is an emotional stake in maintaining the self-system, anything threatening it will nonetheless produce anxiety. It is obvious that the self-system tends to lead to a rigidity in personality and that even many positive potentialities of the person may never be realized or put into operation.

"The self-system of Sullivan has this in common with Freud's concept of character: it is formed as a result of the influence of the parents on the developing personality of the child. Freud presents this idea more mechanistically when he says character is the result of the sublimation of instincts under the influence of the Superego, the Superego being mainly the incorporated attitude of the parents and society. The self-system is different from the concept of character in that it includes more than sublimation, whereas Freud seems to conceive of character as nothing but sublimation. No true comparison of the two can be made, because the frames of reference are entirely different. Freud's system emphasizes what happens to instincts. Sullivan's system stresses what goes on between people. For Sullivan, personal-

ity does not develop mechanically. Always the emphasis is on a dynamic interaction between people. Freud's orientation is mechanistic-biological; Sullivan's dynamic-cultural (inter-personal)." (Thompson, C. *Psychoanalysis, Evolution and Development,* 1950)

self, true The sum total of a person's potentialities that might be developed under the most favorable social and cultural conditions. Fromm considers neurosis in terms of cultural pressures (which often thwart potentialities) and the interaction of people. Since some of the patient's best potentialities are repressed, therapy aims at helping the patient to become himself and discover his "true self." Neurosis stems from the new needs a person's culture creates in him and, as a secondary concomitant to cultural pressures, from the person's deprivations and the frustrations of his potentialities.

"Fromm points out that in the course of therapy one often needs to stress the essential healthiness of some of the patient's tendencies which had met with the disapproval of his environment. The goal of therapy is not primarily to make the person adjusted to his culture but to develop a sense of integrity and a respect for his true self. All adjustments to the culture which violate a person's integrity produce the feeling of guilt and shame and a loss of self-esteem. Fromm sees a real respect for oneself as essential to genuine love and respect for others." (Thompson, C. *Psychoanalysis, Evolution and Development,* 1950)

semantic dissociation See *dissociation, semantic.*

semantic memory See *memory, episodic.*

semiconscious Imperfectly conscious.

semiobsession à deux "The name 'semiobsession à deux' follows the expression *folie à deux,* by which is understood an identical and simultaneous psychosis in two members of a family group. However, while in *folie à deux* the psychosis in one individual is induced and/or influenced by the partner, we wish to call a symptom a phenomenon *à deux* when it occurs in two members of a group independently from each other." (Wilder, J. *American Journal of Psychotherapy 1,* 1947)

semiology, semeiology The study of signs, signals, symbols, or symptoms; symptomatology; the science that studies the life of signs within society.

semiopathic Relating to the organism's affective or emotionally distorted use of the symbol. The result of the impingement of the symbolic or semiotic (partitive) reaction pattern upon the organism's total pattern of behavior and the concomitant substitution of projected affects for intrinsic feeling. (Burrow, T. *The Biology of Human Conflict,* 1937)

semiotic Relating to symptoms. See *semiology.* "Every view which interprets the symbolic expression as an analogous or abbreviated expression of a known thing is semiotic. A conception which interprets the symbolic expression as the best possible formulation of a relatively unknown thing which cannot conceivably, therefore, be more clearly or characteristically represented is symbolic . . . the explanation of the Cross as a symbol of Divine Love is *semiotic,* since Divine Love describes the fact to be expressed better and more aptly than a cross, which can have many other meanings." (Jung, *PT*)

senescence See *aging.*

senile Relating to, characterized by, or manifesting old age with the implication of pathology or something more than the usual aging process.

senile chorea See *chorea, senile.*

senile dementia *Alzheimer's disease* (q.v.).

senility Old age, but almost invariably it is intended to convey the idea that the person or some part of him has undergone involution or degeneration attendant upon advanced age. The onset of senility varies considerably, though in general it begins clinically at about the age of 70. See *aging.*

senium Feebleness of old age; also, the period of old age. In general, psychoses, psychoneuroses, or behavioral reactions appearing in old age are not considered due to senility and senile brain deterioration unless the patient is 70 years or older.

W. Mayer-Gross et al. (*Clinical Psychiatry,* 1960) classify the mental diseases of old age as follows: (1) affective psychosis; (2) *senile dementia* (q.v.); (3) arteriosclerotic psychosis (see *arteriosclerosis, cerebral*); (4) delirious states (see *delirium; delirium, senile*); (5) late *paraphrenia* (q.v.); and (6) miscellaneous disorders such as paresis, epilepsy,

head injury, and organic brain syndrome associated with cardiovascular disorder.

senium praecox (L. "premature old age") Premature senility. As average senility begins, at least clinically, at about the age of 70, senile manifestations under the age of 55 may be regarded as definitely premature. In psychiatry senium praecox is associated, for example, with *Pick's disease* or *Alzheimer's disease* (qq.v.).

sensate focus In sex therapy, one of the early stages of interaction with the sexual partner in which attention is diverted from erection and orgasm to mutual, nondemanding pleasurable experiences with the body (but not genital stimulation, which is added at a later stage).

sensation, feeling See *feeling-sensation.*

sensation, kinesthetic The sensation derived from muscles, joints, and inner ear, giving the perception of body weight, position, location, and movement. P. Schilder points out that primitive perception shows in motion in the majority of the senses, and emphasizes his belief that this inner motion is an important factor for the recognition and understanding of the space in which the body moves. Kinesthetic sensation is an important element "for the final evaluation of space in our minds." Without such a knowledge, achieved through kinesthetic sensation, the individual would not have a complete perception of his own body, nor would he be able to evaluate his relationship to all other objects. (*Perception and Thought,* 1942)

sensation, proprioceptive See *proprioception.*

sensation, secondary Stoddart uses this expression as synonymous with the *synesthesias.* They are those sensations "which accompany sensations of another modality; for example, some people experience with every auditory sensation an accompanying visual sensation: the tone G is perhaps associated with the colour red or the tone D with blue. Similar sensations of color may accompany perceptions of taste, touch, pain, heat or cold: they are called 'photisms.' With some people certain words are accompanied by a sense of color, varying with different words (verbochromia). Again, there are secondary auditory sensations called 'phonisms,' secondary taste sensations called 'gustatisms,' secondary smell sensations called 'olfactisms,' and so on." (*Mind and Its Disorders*, 1926)

sensitive, volume See *volume sensitive.*

sensitiver Beziehungswahn Sensitive delusion of reference; paranoid sensitivity psychosis; a term coined by Kretschmer in 1918 to refer to a reactive psychosis described in persons with a rigid, sensitive personality who feel some action of theirs is contradictory to the high ethical or moral standards they espouse. The result is an embarrassment and self-consciousness that color the whole life of the subject, sometimes progressing to the development of self-referential delusions.

sensitivity Capacity to respond to stimulation, often with the sense that the subject is able to recognize the stimulus even when it is presented at minimal intensity. When applied to a diagnostic test, sensitivity refers to the test's ability to identify diagnostically true cases. *Specificity* refers to a test's ability to exclude false cases, and *diagnostic confidence* is a measure of a test's sensitivity and specificity, expressed as the percentage of true positive test results over the total number of index cases plus the number of false positives.

sensitivity training *T-group* (q.v.).

sensitizers See *anxiety typology.*

sensorimotor intelligence See *developmental psychology.*

sensorimotor stage In Piaget's scheme of development beginning at birth and lasting until approximately 18 months of age. In this stage, responses are first only reflexive and to a limited range of sensory stimuli. Motor responses become more coordinated and can be elicited by more complex combinations of stimuli. By the end of this stage, information can be retrieved from memory (*representation* ability) and action can be regulated through stored knowledge.

sensorium The hypothetical "seat of sensation" or "sense center," located in the brain, is usually contrasted with the *motorium*, the two constituting the so-called animal organ system, while the *nutritive* and *reproductive* apparatus make up the vegetative organ system. Occasionally this term is applied to the entire sensory apparatus of the body.

When a person is clearly aware of the nature of his surroundings, his sensorium is said to be "clear" or "intact." For example, correct orientation is a manifestation of a clear sensorium. When a person is unclear, from a sensory (not a delusional) standpoint, his sensorium is described as impaired or "cloudy."

Sensorium is interchangeable with *consciousness* (q.v.). The major disturbances of the sensorium are lowering of consciousness with reduced awareness (*cloudiness, clouding*), dreamlike states such as delirium, and narrowing of consciousness as in *twilight state* (q.v.).

sensory deprivation See *deprivation, sensory.*

sensory neglect See *neglect, sensory.*

sentience Mere sensation, apprehension, or cognition, without accompanying associations or affect.

sentiment According to McDougall, a sentiment is an organized system of emotional tendencies concerning an object or a class of objects. It is a learned form of behavior, built upon experiences and acting in the form of emotional tension. Sentiments are not pure emotions or motives because they cannot exist apart from a relationship to some person or object. The object may call forth different emotional behavior at different times, but this behavior is still consistent with the sentiment.

sentinel activity *Vigilance* (q.v.).

separation See *anxiety, separation; depression, anaclitic.*

separation anxiety Fear, anxiety, etc., occasioned by the threat or actuality of separation from mother and home. *School phobia* is a type of separation anxiety. See *anxiety disorders of childhood.*

separation-individuation A phase in the mother-child relationship during which the child begins to perceive himself as distinct from the mother and develops a sense of individual identity and an image of the self as an object. Earlier work suggested that this stage begins at the time the child can walk and thus separate himself physically from the mother, at about 18 months of age, immediately following the *symbiotic stage.* More recent studies indicate that individuation occurs earlier, at about 7 months, when the infant comes to sense self and other as both physically and mentally separate entities. It is separation that appears later because it is dependent on motor development, which will make individuation possible only at about 18 months. Margaret Mahler (*On Human Symbiosis and the Vicissitudes of Individuation,* 1968) described four subphases of the process: differentiation, practicing, rapprochement (active approach toward the mother, replacing the relative obliviousness to her that prevailed during the practicing period), and separation-individuation proper (psychologic awareness of discrete identity, separateness, and individuality). Much of the pathology of the borderline states is believed to be rooted in failure to progress satisfactorily through the separation-individuation stage. See *borderline psychosis; personality disorders.*

sequela The aftereffect of an illness and, particularly, permanent or persistent dysfunction. Mental defect, epilepsy, and spastic palsies, for example, are possible *sequelae* of viral encephalitis.

sequence, genetic Growth sequence; the genetically determined order of development of structure or functions.

sequencing disability Difficulty in abstraction. See *abstracting disabilities.*

sequestration *Isolation* or *denial* (qq.v.) of those parts of one's psyche that are unacceptable or cannot be controlled.

seriatim functions See *functions, seriatim.*

Sernyl *Phencyclidine* (q.v.).

serotonin A potent cerebral synaptic inhibitor, also known as 5-hydroxytryptamine, and identical with enteramine (which is found in the enterochromaffin system of the mammalian gastrointestinal tract). Various functions have been attributed to serotonin, but its chief interest for psychiatry lies in the evidence that serotonin is normally involved as a synaptic agent in the regulation of centers in the brain concerned with wakefulness, temperature regulation, blood-pressure regulation, and various other autonomic functions. Serotonin appears to be a major transmitter in the central parasympathetic system (the "trophotropic" system, in Hess's terminology), and *norepinephrine* (q.v.) appears to be the major transmitter in the central sympathetic ("ergotropic") system. *Monoamine oxidase* (q.v.) is involved in the metabolic breakdown of serotonin. See *ergotropic; neurotransmitter.*

servomechanism A governing or regulating device for maintaining output of a system

at the desired rate or strength or in the desired direction.

set 1. A group or series, such as a *set* of rules. 2. A readiness to respond in a certain way or to respond selectively to certain stimuli; in this sense, also called *Aufgabe; determining tendency; mental set.*

setting, social *Milieu* (q.v.).

sex The division of members of a species into two subclasses, male and female. Such division depends upon five biological factors—nuclear sex (chromosome pattern), gonadal sex (the presence of testes or ovaries), hormonal sex, internal accessory structures (the presence of uterus or prostate), and external genital morphology. Ordinarily all five are consonant and thus allow assignment of sex, initially, and rearing in a gender role on the basis of simple inspection of external genital morphology.

As *maleness* is the state associated with the production of spermatozoa, a male is an individual that is efficiently equipped for the elaboration of functional sperms and for their conveyance to the site of fertilization. *Femaleness* is associated with the elaboration of ova; in mammals, in addition to possessing the property of producing eggs, the female has equipment for the prenatal care of the embryo and fetus and for the nurture of the offspring. An individual exhibiting both maleness and femaleness is called a *hermaphrodite.*

The organs that carry on the reproductive functions are known as *primary* sex organs. Those that distinguish the sexes from each other but play no direct part in reproduction are called *secondary* sexual characters.

sex chromosome The pair of heterosomal chromosomes that differ in the male and female members of a species, in contrast to the other pairs of autosomal chromosomes that are alike in both sexes. See *chromosome.*

sex determination In biology, the genetic mechanism by which in bisexual organisms the primary difference between the sexes originates in accordance with the laws of heredity. It is a difference in the heterosomal chromosome constitution between male and female individuals that explains the generally sharp segregation of the two sexes. See *sex chromosome.*

In the female homogametic animals, sex

is determined by whether an X-bearing or Y-bearing sperm fertilizes the ovum, resulting in a female and a male offspring respectively. In male homogametic animals, sex depends on whether a sperm fertilizes an X-bearing or Y-bearing egg, resulting in male and female offspring respectively.

Before the era of physiological genetics it was dogmatically held that the fully developed sex characters in the phenotype are dependent on this simple mechanism of sex determination. Since Goldschmidt's studies of sex differentiation it has been realized, however, that it is only the *predisposition* to sex that is transmitted by heredity, and that the expression in the phenotype is furthered or inhibited by physiological and environmental conditions as well as by age factors. See *sex differentiation.*

sex differentiation Although this term sometimes embraces both sex determination and sex differentiation, it actually relates only to the developmental processes operating in the manifestation of sex differences in higher animals as expressed by Goldschmidt's "balance theory." The term thus indicates what happens during development after two sexually different types of zygotes have been formed by the chromosomal mechanism of *sex determination* (q.v.).

The conception of sex-differentiation in terms of a ratio between male-determining and female-determining elements is based upon the observation that in a number of species of animals there have appeared, in addition to normal males and females, peculiar individuals that are neither typical males nor typical females. These *intersexes* (q.v.) have some male and some female characters that "may be so intimately mixed as to give their possessors the appearance of being true intermediates between maleness and femaleness." (Sinnott, E.W., & Dunn, L.C. *Principles of Genetics,* 1939) They suggest that sex differentiation is "a competition between opposed tendencies in which the race is eventually won by the type of process (either male or female) which proceeds most rapidly, at the critical period of determination."

In normal sexual growth, the 23rd pair of chromosomes contains an XX complex in females, and the normal female pattern of cell nuclei is chromatin-positive. In males, the 23rd pair of chromosomes contains an XY complex, and the normal male pattern of cell nuclei is chromatin-negative. In true hermaphrodites (who have both ovarian and testicular functioning tissues) and in pseudohermaphrodites (where the external genitalia are the sex opposite to the genetic sex), there is often difficulty in deciding on the sex of the infant. In general, infants with anomalous sex development should be reared in accordance with their genetic sex and given appropriate hormonal treatment.

sex limitation The principle of a trait occurring in one sex only, namely, one characterized by the phenotypical development of those physiological sex characters that are the necessary anatomical basis of the trait in question.

In contrast to *sex-linked* characters produced by genes which are bound to the X or Y chromosomes, the phenomenon of sex limitation is *not* due directly to differences in the manifestation of the effects of genes located in one sex chromosome. See *sex linkage.*

sex linkage The genetic phenomenon of the coupling of a hereditary factor with an individual's sex chromosome structure responsible for the development of the respective sex. It rests upon the fact that in bisexual organisms the sex distinction is transmitted by heredity in accordance with the Mendelian law of segregation, and is not to be confused with the more common mechanism of *sex limitation.* If one of the sex chromosomes carries a gene for a certain character, the transmission of the character and the distribution of the sexes must run together. See *sex determination.*

The particular distribution of the sex chromosomes in man, having heterogametic XY males, explains why sex linkage gives different sex proportions of linked characters with respect to dominance or recessiveness. *Dominant* sex-linked characters are able to appear when only one predisposition is present. Their manifestation is therefore twice as frequent in females as in males, since the number of X chromosomes is double in females.

Recessive sex-linked anomalies can be manifested by a female only when she is a homozygote for the factor in question. As the female has two X chromosomes, one from each parent, the heterozygotic manifestation of a recessive trait, transmitted on a mother's X chromosome to her daughter, is antagonized by the effect of the X chromosome which she has from her father. In males, however, the anomaly is manifested in the heterozygotic condition, since in the case of a son who receives his single X chromosome from his mother, there is no paternal X chromosome with a dominant gene to overcome the recessive gene on the X chromosome of the mother.

Consequently, these recessive traits, of which hemophilia and color blindness are the classic examples, are usually transmitted by the female and appear in the male. They do not appear in both father and son unless the mother also possesses the gene. It is the rule that, through their daughters, who do not exhibit it, men transmit the trait to half of the daughter's sons.

sex preselection Predetermination of the sex of offspring; through sex-control technology, the parents-to-be choose whether their child will be a boy or girl.

sex reversal See *reversal, sex.*

sex role A repertoire of attitudes, behaviors, perceptions, and affection reactions more commonly associated with one sex than with the other.

sex role inversion Adoption of the sex role of, and introjection of the psychologic identity of, the opposite sex.

sex, third Bisexuality; homosexuality. Use of the term is discouraged since it seems to ignore the fact that a very considerable measure of latent or unconscious homosexuality can be detected in all heterosexuals.

sex typing That part of the process of socialization in which the child learns to adopt traits, values, and behavior that the culture deems appropriate to the child's *gender identity* (q.v.).

sexism The social system that divides life roles according to sex rather than individual abilities, assigning to women the role of housekeeper, nursemaid, playmate, etc., and to men the role of manager, ruler, scholar, scientist, etc. It is this system (i.e. patriarchy) that the feminist movement seeks to eliminate and to re-

place with a system that allows life roles to be self-assigned, independent of sex. See *racism.*

sexology The study of sexual and sex-related behaviors and their evolutionary, physiological, developmental, and sociological foundations.

sexopathy (seks-op′ȧ-thē) Sexual abnormality; sexual perversion; paraphilia. Roland Dalbiez uses this term in preference to perversion, because of the undesirable moralistic connotation of the latter. Sexopathy includes both anomalies of sexual aim and anomalies of sexual object, no matter what their etiology.

sexual Pertaining to, characterized by, springing from or endowed with sex. In biology the term *sexual,* pertaining to the property of being male or female, is used not only to characterize what is peculiar to sex or the sexes, but also to denote the method of reproduction by sexes, as distinguished from *asexual* reproduction.

sexual, contrary *Homosexual* (q.v.).

sexual deviation See *deviation, sexual.*

sexual disorders In DSM-III-R, this term replaces the *psychosexual disorders* of DSM-III, emphasizing that many of these dysfunctions are biological rather than psychological in origin. Included within this category are:

1. *Paraphilias*—known in some systems as *sexual deviations;* a group of conditions characterized by sexual urges and sexually arousing phantasies that (a) involve nonhuman objects, or the suffering or humiliation of one's self or the sexual partner, or children or other nonconsenting persons and that (b) are of sufficient intensity to cause marked distress to the person or to have led him or her to have acted them out.

2. *Sexual dysfunctions*—inhibition at one or more phases of the *sexual response cycle* (q.v.), including *sexual desire disorders* (hypoactive sexual desire disorder, sexual aversion disorder), *sexual arousal disorders* (which include conditions that are often referred to as frigidity and impotence), *orgasm disorders* (inhibited orgasm and premature ejaculation), and *sexual pain disorders* (dyspareunia and vaginismus).

Gender identity disorders, which were included in this category in DSM-III, have been moved in DSM-III-R to "Disorders

Usually First Evident in Infancy, Childhood, or Adolescence."

sexual dysfunctions In DSM-III-R, this category includes:

1. *Sexual desire disorders*—hypoactive sexual desire disorder and sexual aversion disorder.

2. *Sexual arousal disorders*—female and male, approximately equivalent to frigidity and erective impotence in other terminologies.

3. *Orgasm disorders*—inhibited female orgasm, inhibited male orgasm (approximately equivalent to ejaculatory impotence), and premature ejaculation.

4. *Sexual pain disorders*—functional dyspareunia (genital pain before, during, or after sexual intercourse) and functional vaginismus.

sexual identity See *gender identity*.

sexual orientation The preferred adult sexual behavior of a person; specifically, heterosexuality, homosexuality, or bisexuality.

sexual orientation disturbance Concern or uncertainty about, or desire to change, one's sexual preferences or behavior. The term is most often applied to ego-dystonic homosexuality; neither term has been retained as a diagnostic entity in DSM-III-R. See *homosexuality*.

sexual response cycle The complete cycle is subdivided into four phases: (1) *appetitive*—phantasies about, interest in, or desire to have sexual activity; (2) *excitement*—subjective sense of pleasant sexual arousal and accompanying physiologic changes (penile tumescence and erection in the male and vaginal lubrication and swelling of the external genitalia, labia minora, and breast in the female); (3) *orgasm*—a peaking of sexual pleasure (ejaculation in the male) and rhythmic contractions of the perineal muscles and pelvic reproductive organs in both sexes; (4) *resolution*—relaxation, a sense of well-being, and, for males, a variable period of refractoriness to further erection and orgasm. Disturbances in any part of the cycle are termed sexual dysfunctions, which form one group of *sexual disorders* (q.v.).

sexual revolution The marked change in prevalent sexual attitudes that has been particularly evident in the United States since the Kinsey reports of 1948 and 1953, which brought sexual practices "from the realm of inference and secrecy into accepted, if still private, reality." (Sadock, V. in *Psychiatry 1982*, ed. L. Greenspoon, 1982) The Presidential Commission on Pornography in the 1970s advised against sexual repression and encouraged the acceptance of frank and even sexually stimulating material. The advent of effective birth control methods and legalized abortion drew a line between pleasurable and procreative aspects of sexuality. The feminist movement attacked the double standard, challenged the previous stereotyping of male and female roles, and focused attention on rape and incest. Gerontologists shed new light on the sexual needs of the aged. Concurrent with these changes were advances in research and treatment of psychosexual dysfunctions, beginning with the Masters and Johnson work on the physiology of the sexual response in 1966 and the description of their approach in 1970.

sexualism *Rare. Sexuality* (q.v.).

sexualitas senilis Krafft-Ebing's expression for sexual potency exhibited in the senile period of life.

sexuality Freud's concept of sexuality is to be understood in a broad sense. Psychic energy connected with sensual and somatic satisfactions is said to be sexual energy, which is expressed also in the multiple forms of sublimation. "We suppose that there are two fundamentally different kinds of instincts, the sexual instincts in the widest sense of the word (*Eros*, if you prefer that name) and the aggressive instincts, whose aim is destruction." (Freud, S. *New Introductory Lectures on Psychoanalysis*, 1933)

"An attempt to formulate the general characteristics of the sexual instincts would run as follows: they are numerous, emanate from manifold organic sources, act in the first instance independently of one another and only at a later stage achieve a more or less complete synthesis. The aim which each strives to attain is 'organ-pleasure'; only when the synthesis is complete do they enter the service of the function of reproduction, becoming thereby generally recognizable as sexual instincts." (Freud, *CP*)

The meaning of *sexuality* to Freud apparently is twofold: the sexual instincts serve two major functions—those associated with self-preservation and those with race-preservation.

The race-preservative component is really not put into actual service of reproduction until some time after puberty. There seems to be no objection, indeed, there is universal agreement, to referring to the instincts, devoted to the reproductive act, as sexual.

It has been difficult, however, to accept the idea that the sexual instincts are present and operative during the so-called latency period (from the age of 5 to puberty). It is not reasonable to believe that, without any conditioning whatever, the sexual instinct is dormant somewhere for 12 or 14 years, only to put in a sudden appearance at puberty in an individual wholly unprepared for adult sexuality.

Freud holds that the preparations for adult sexuality are intensive and cover a long period. The sexual instincts, so universally acknowledged after puberty, are given definite assignments already during the latency period, for purposes of preparing the person for the severest test of all, the harmonious union of the sexes, culminating in reproduction. During the latency period, however, the sexual energies do not possess specific sexual coloring; they are sublimated or hidden under the cloak of nonreproductive forms of activities. See *altrigenderism; suigenderism*.

Freud uses the term *sexual* to refer to many activities of the infantile period (extending from birth until approximately the fifth year). There is sexuality, for instance, associated with infantile oral, anal, and genital organization. It seems true that part of the energies of the erogenous zones is destined for final adult sexual participation; moreover, that the zones themselves, particularly the oral and genital, are prepared from early life for the participation. For both Adler and Jung the meaning of sexuality more closely approximates the general opinion of scientists. "We ought to be able to recognize and to admit that much in the psyche really depends on sex, at times even everything, but that at other times little depends on sex, and nearly everything comes under the factor of self-preservation, or the

power-instinct, as Adler calls it.... At times sex is dominant, at other times self-assertion or some other instinct.... When sex prevails, everything becomes sexualized, as everything then either expresses or serves the sexual purpose." (Jung, *CAP*)

In biology the term *sexuality* relates to the state of being distinguished by sex. See *sex determination*.

sexuality index See *index of sexuality*.

sexuality, infantile See *sexuality*.

sexualization The act of sexualizing. See *sexuality*.

sexualize To endow with sexual energy or instinct. The genitals become sexualized at an early age. Other parts of the body (breasts, oral region, hands, etc.) may possess sexual qualities. Thoughts may be sexualized, as for example, when they appear in the form of sexual jokes.

shadow In Jung's analytical psychology, the unconscious.

"For the sake of understanding, it is, I think, a good thing to detach the man from his shadow, the unconscious.... One sees much in another man which does not belong to his conscious psychology, but which gleams out from his unconscious, and one is rather tempted to regard the observed quality as belonging to the conscious ego." (Jung, *PT*)

sham rage See *rage, sham*.

shaman A practitioner whose ability to heal comes from trancelike experiences and inspiration from a supernatural spirit-partner with whom he works in curing sick people. The word shaman originated in the Tungus tribe of northeastern Siberia. The Navajo draw a distinction between the "handtrembler," whose inspiration is supernatural in origin, and the "medicine man," whose knowledge comes from systematic learning in an apprenticeship. See *folk medicine*.

shame An affect that follows the revelation of one's previously hidden shortcoming(s), believed to be founded in the anal (and urethral) stages of psychosexual development.

Psychodynamically, shame is considered to be the specific force directed against urethral-eroticism, just as the fear of being eaten is the specific oral fear, and the fear of being robbed of body contents is the specific anal fear. Ambition is the fight against this shame.

Shame is also used as a defense against exhibitionism and voyeurism; "I feel a-shamed" means "I do not want to be seen."

Shame is given particular attention in self psychology and developmental psychology, where it is regarded as a master emotion that influences all the others. *Guilt* (q.v.) refers to feelings about an act, a real or imagined transgression. It does not usually bring with it self-loathing, as shame does. Shame involves one's basic sense of self and is typically experienced as embarrassment or humiliation.

Shame emerges earlier in psychological development than guilt. Signs of it can be detected in the second year of life at the time the infant's sense of self is forming. As the infant comes to recognize that he is a separate person, he begins to understand that others direct emotions toward him. Pride and shame appear—pride at pleasing others, shame at displeasing others. Pathological shame develops when parents fail to respond with empathy and attention to the infant's strivings to show his competence.

Shame can be a normal feeling, but when it colors one's most basic ideas about one's identity or worth it signals pathology. Normal shame might result from having some dark secret about the self exposed. Shame is pathological, however, when it arises with every rebuke or tiny failure, or as an undercurrent in all interpersonal relationships. Whenever shame appears, there tends to be an inhibition of other emotions with the exception of anger. Unlike other emotions, which tend to pass with time or with catharsis, shame is the most difficult emotion to admit to and the most difficult to discharge. Some clinical studies suggest that the most effective antidote to shame is a person's ability to laugh at himself.

Shame is often at the root of irrational rage outbursts in the adult; it probably plays a key role in family violence, for example. Men who for one reason or another (psychological vulnerability, limited intellectual development, physical abnormalities, etc.) are especially dependent on their spouses to function well are ashamed of that dependence and feel in-

tensely humiliated when the spouse says something they perceive as demeaning, trivializing, or critical of their competence. They react with rage and violence in an attempt to deny or overcome their feelings of disorganization and helplessness.

shaping *Method of successive approximations;* a type of operant conditioning in which the behavior that is initially reinforced is generally or approximately of the kind desired, and subsequent reinforcement becomes increasingly limited until only the specific response desired is reinforced. See *practice, reinforced.*

shared paranoid disorder See *association, psychosis of; folie à deux; paranoia.*

Sheldon, William Herbert (1899–1977) American psychologist, best known for his work in constitutional typology and description of the ectomorph, mesomorph, and endomorph somatotypes.

shell shock A general term, particularly wide in its application to psychic disorders occurring during active warfare. Many of the illnesses called shell shock, or *combat neurosis,* are encountered in civil life and are then usually regarded as traumatic neuroses. See *neurosis, traumatic; post-traumatic stress disorder.*

shift, biobehavioral A relatively sudden advance in development that occurs at around 2 or 3 months of age. It is characterized by a change in the infant's EEG patterns; more clearly social and instrumental usage of smiling, babbling, and similar behaviors; and increased tolerance for stimulation.

shinekeishitsu A syndrome described by Japanese psychiatrists consisting of obsessions, compulsive perfectionism, social withdrawal, multiple somatic complaints, and neurasthenia.

shock 1. A sudden physical or mental disturbance.

2. A state of profound mental and physical depression consequent upon severe physical injury or an emotional disturbance.

3. In Rorschach scoring, any delay or failure in responding to the blot; shock indicates ambivalence regarding the advisability of acting out the traits revealed by the blot component causing the shock. Thus *color shock* (as on plate II and/or VIII) is interpreted as ambivalence in

relation to gratifying emotional needs, and human movement shock (*M* shock or Plate III shock) reflects ambivalence over acting in accordance with one's prototypal life role. *M* shock in addition indicates conflict over insufficiently strong heterosexual tendencies.

shock, culture A type of interface shock. See *network*.

shock, future A term coined by Alvin Toffler (1970) to refer to the psychologic syndrome occurring when the subject is continuously overwhelmed by frequent, sudden, and abrupt changes in the environment.

shock, psychodramatic "A procedure which throws a patient, barely escaped from a psychosis, back into a re-experience of the psychotic attack is a psychodramatic shock treatment. The patient is asked to throw himself back into the hallucinatory experience when it is still most vivid in his mind. He is not asked to describe it; he must act.

"Acting upon a psychotic level at a time when he is extremely sensitive to the vanished mental syndrome, the patient learns to check himself. It is a training in mastering of psychotic invasions, not through analysis but through a reconstruction of the psychotic experiences from act to act, from role to role, and from delusion to delusion, until the whole sphere of the psychosis is projected upon the therapeutic stage. It is a preventative therapy. The patient is trained to develop spontaneous controls with which to ward off the sudden onset of a psychotic invasion. The procedure produces a cathartic effect. Psychodramatic procedure, as differentiated from other shock procedures which leave a patient helpless and inarticulate, insists that the patient reproduce with his own body that fantastic world in which he has been lost." (Moreno, J.L. *Sociometry 2*, 1939)

shock therapy See *therapy, shock*.

shock treatment See *therapy, shock*.

short stare epilepsy A type of petit mal epilepsy. See *epilepsy*.

short-term Brief. See *psychotherapy, brief; transient*.

short-term memory See *amnestic syndrome*.

shortening reaction See *rigidity, decerebrate*.

show, half See *"half-show"*.

ShR In Rorschach scoring, shading response. Piotrowski (*Perceptanalysis*, 1957) differentiates four categories: *c*, *Fc*, *c'*, *Fc'* (qq.v.). The *ShR* indicate the self-regulating mechanisms of control over outward manifestations of emotion; *c* responses indicate that action tendencies are inhibited or delayed, while *c'* responses indicate a readiness to do something overt and definite to alleviate anxiety. Reaction formation is characteristic of *c* types, while acting out is characteristic of *c'* types. The greater the number of *c'* responses, and the more the number of *c* responses exceeds the number of *C* responses, the greater is the amount of anxiety and/or pathological fears.

shut-in August Hoch's term for the premorbid personality which is seen in approximately 60% of schizophrenics: quiet, reserved, asocial, withdrawn, seclusive, "lone-wolf" types, those who live among but not with, etc. Bleuler's term, *schizoid*, is approximately equivalent to shut-in.

sialorrh(o)ea (sī-à-lo-rē'à) Excessive salivation.

sibling In human genetics, one of two or more children not simultaneously born of the same two parents. It thus excludes twins or other multiples as well as half-brothers and half-sisters, and stepbrothers and stepsisters. However, the definition in all leading dictionaries makes it a far less restricted term.

sibship A genetic term pertaining to one series of siblings, that is, to all the biological children of a union of two parents, excluding multiples. See *birth, multiple*.

sibship method See *method, sibship*.

sicchasia (si-kā'zē-à) Disgust for food.

sick role The use of illness or complaints about bodily functioning as a means of escaping personal failure and the expectation to succeed, or as a way of avoiding other social responsibilities. In many Western cultures, sickness automatically excuses the subject from many responsibilities and protects his assumed right to be taken care of. *Hypochondriasis* (q.v.), or escape into the sick role, is frequently encountered among the elderly population. High bodily concern is used by many older people as a defense against anxiety and a way of gaining the sympathy and help of others.

side effect Any action of a drug other than the desired therapeutic effect. No drug has a single pharmacologic action; consequently, for every wanted effect it may be necessary to accept one—or many—unwanted effects. Most side effects are extensions of a drug's known pharmacological actions. Neuroleptics and antidepressant agents, for example, affect a number of different receptor systems, and their numerous side effects are attributable to nonspecificity of pharmacological action. Allergic and idiosyncratic reactions are far less common than nonspecificity reactions, and they are generally unpredictable. To a large extent, drug response is genetically determined, particularly drug absorption and its utilization at effector sites, and the family history may provide significant information about how a patient is likely to respond to a specific drug, or even to a family of drugs.

side impulse See *impulse, side.*

siderodromophobia Fear of railroads or trains.

siderophobia Fear of the heavens and what comes from them—the elements, etc.

Sidis, Boris (1876–1923) American psychiatrist; hypnosis, multiple personality.

Siemerling, Ernst (zē'mĕr-ling) (1857–1931) German psychiatrist and neurologist.

sigmatism Difficulty in pronouncing the *S* (and *Z*) sound.

sign Signal, representation; in medicine, an objective symptom or abnormality indicating disease. For specific signs, see listings below and also those under *reflex.*

sign, Ballet's (Gilbert Ballet, French neurologist, 1853–1916) *Ophthalmoplegia externa;* loss of movements of eye and pupil with preservation of autonomic responses, often associated with exophthalmic goiter and other forms of hyperthyroidism.

sign, bonbon One form of the buccal-lingual-masticatory syndrome, consisting of pressing the tongue against the cheek. See *dyskinesia, tardive.*

sign, Bonhoeffer's (Karl Bonhoeffer, Berlin psychiatrist, 1868–1948) Loss of normal muscle tone in chorea.

sign, Brudzinski (broo-jĕn'ski) (J. Brudzinski, Polish physician, 1874–1917) The Brudzinski sign is indicative of meningitis. By passively flexing the head on the chest, a flexion of the lower limbs is produced.

sign, echo *Rare.* A speech disorder observed in epileptic patients characterized by the repetition of a word in some part of a sentence; *logoclonia* (q.v.).

sign, eyelash In a case of unconsciousness due to functional disease, such as hysteria, stroking the eyelashes will make the lids move, but no such reflex will occur in case of organic brain lesion such as apoplexy, fracture of the skull, or other severe traumatism.

sign, eye-roll An index of susceptibility to hypnosis developed by psychiatrist Herbert Spiegel; the subject is directed to roll his eyes upward as far as possible and at the same time to lower his eyelids slowly. The amount of white space showing under the corneas is scored from zero (no space or "eye-roll") to five. Low scores are not hypnotizable; they tend also to be critical, controlling personality types who favor thinking over feeling. The readily hypnotizable high scorers tend to be uncritical and gullible people who are "feelers" rather than "thinkers."

sign, Hoffmann (Johann Hoffmann, German neurologist, 1857–1919) In hemiplegia due to organic brain disease, snapping of the index or ring finger produces flexion to the thumb.

sign, Kernig's (Waldemar Kernig, Russian physician, 1840–1917) The Kernig sign is observed in meningitis. Flexing the thigh at the hip, and extending the leg at the knee, produces pain and resistance.

sign, Litten's (Moritz Litten, German physician, 1845–1907) In paralysis of the diaphragm, nonprojection of shadow by the diaphragm X-rayed during respiration.

sign, Magnan Formication; "cocaine bug," a tactile hallucination found in some cocaine abusers consisting of the feeling that small animals are moving in or under the skin. The phenomenonn was first described by Magnan and Saury in 1889. It is relatively rare and when it does appear it is usually in association with intravenous use of the drug.

sign, Marcus Gunn (Marcus Gunn, contemporary British surgeon) The raising of a ptosed lid on opening the mouth and moving the jaw to the opposite side.

sign, mirror A symptom seen frequently in schizophrenic patients, who tend to stand in front of a mirror or other shining surface for an unduly long time. The mirror sign is generally regarded as an expression of the patient's autistic withdrawal.

The same sign can also occur in advanced organic dementia (e.g. Alzheimer's disease): the patient sits for hours in front of a mirror, talking to his own reflection; because of complete loss of personal identity, the patient does not realize that the reflection is his own.

sign, palmomandibular Reflex opening of the mouth in response to pressure on the palms or forearm, present in the neonate until about the tenth day of life, when it is replaced by the palmomental reflex. See *reflex, palmomental.*

sign, Romberg (Moritz Heinrich Romberg, German physician, 1795–1873) Swaying of the body when the patient stands with the feet together and the eyes closed, suggestive of ataxia.

sign, Rosenbach's (Ottomar Rosenbach, German physician, 1851–1907) Inability of neurasthenics to close the eyes immediately and completely on command.

sign, Rumpf (Theodor Rumpf, German physician, 1862–1923) In cases of neurasthenia pressure over a painful point will accelerate the pulse from 10 to 20 beats/minute.

sign, sawtooth A type of oscillation on the flow-volume loops in spirometric evaluation that suggests the presence of *SAHS-UAO* (q.v.), and thus provides a means of detecting the disorder when the patient is awake.

sign, Schuele's (Heinrich Schuele, German psychiatrist, 1839–1916) See *omega melancholium.*

sign, sniff A diagnostic pattern of breathing observed in patients with tracheal tumors at the stage when occlusion of the trachea during expiration is almost total. In order to breathe, the patient draws in small, sharp, sniffing breaths. Many patients with such tumors are puzzling diagnostic problems in the early stages of tumor growth and are often labeled as psychiatric problems.

sign, Stiller's (Berthold Stiller, Budapest physician, 1837–1922) The presence of a floating tenth rib as indicative of a neurasthenic tendency; called also *costal stigma.*

sign, Strümpell (Adolf von Strümpell, German neurologist, 1853–1925) In organic

hemiplegia, dorsiflexion of the hand occurs on making a fist.

sign, tibialis In organic hemiplegia, dorsal flexion of the foot occurs on flexion at the knee and hip.

sign, Westphal's (vest'fålz) (Carl F.O. Westphal, German neurologist, 1833–90) Loss of the knee jerk.

sign, wobbly knee See *knee, wobbly.*

sign, Woltman's See *reflex, myxedema.*

signal anxiety See *anxiety.*

signe de Magnan (sēn'yu dû man-yan') Formication (q.v.).

signe du miroir (sēn'yu dê mē-wår') Mirror sign. See *sign, mirror.*

significance Meaning; value; importance. Statistical significance is the likelihood or probability that the value or score obtained is not due to chance but is instead meaningfully related to some specific factor or variable.

signs, soft A phrase applied to subtle signs of disability or dysfunction; used particularly to refer to the results of neurologic examination of children who are schizophrenic and/or who have minimal brain dysfunction. In both categories, it is difficult to pinpoint specific damage, but tests of patterned motor and perceptual behavior are often suggestive of subtle, slight deviations from the normal. See *impulse disorder, hyperkinetic.*

silence, insane *Obs.* T.S. Clouston's term for insanity with mutism.

silence, selective Deliberate withholding of response, information, or free association that a patient resorts to at a point of anxiety or negative transference toward the therapist or the group in order to resist the therapeutic situation.

silver cord syndrome See *syndrome, silver cord.*

Simmonds' disease (Morris Simmonds, German physician, 1855–1925) See *cachexia, hypophysial.*

Simon-Binet tests See *tests, Binet-Simon.*

simple adult MBD Minimal brain dysfunction in the absense of psychiatric diagnosis; primary or idiopathic attention deficit disorder.

simple schizophrenia See *schizophrenia, simple.*

simulant Simulator, malingerer.

simultagnosia Ability to describe the action represented in a picture; often lacking in children with generalized brain dysfunction, who may merely name the objects represented rather than being able to discuss the action of the picture. *Simultanagnosia* is the lack of, or any disability in, such simultaneous form perception, and is suggestive of a lesion in the anterior part of the left occipital lobe.

simultaneous tactile sensation See *tactile sensation, double simultaneous.*

single-major-locus model See *inheritance.*

singultus Hiccup.

sinistrad Toward the left; sinistrad writing is mirror-writing. See *strephosymbolia.*

sinistral See *dominance, cerebral.*

sinistrality See *dextrality-sinistrality.*

sinistrosis *Obs.* Shellshock (q.v.).

sitiophobia *Sitophobia* (q.v.).

sitomania *Obs.* Bulimia; a morbid, voracious appetite.

sitophobia Fear of (eating) food.

situation, danger See *anxiety.*

situation, either-or The term for a situation of doubt and vacillation in which the neurotic places himself, especially in dreams. In such situations the patient desires two different things at the same time and does not know which to choose. An example of this is the neurotic patient with a strong mother attachment who is also deeply in love with his fiancée: in his dreams he symbolizes either his mother or his fiancée, but always with a profound doubt about which of them he should love more. The patient vacillates between two principles and this vacillation may refer to persons, objects, or ideas.

situation ethics See *ethics, situation.*

situational attribution See *attribution.*

situational reaction See *transient situational disturbances.*

sixty-nine A slang expression referring to fellatio and/or cunnilinction practiced simultaneously by two persons, the head of each being near the feet of the other.

Sjobring, Henrik (1879–1956) Swedish psychiatrist; described certain personality types and reactions to stress as based on constitutional psychological variables and cerebral lesions.

skelic See *index, skelic.*

sketch, biographic Used in the field of objective psychobiology (Adolf Meyer) to refer to the life history of the patient as the latter records it. To facilitate the recording Meyer devised what he calls *The Life Chart,* consisting of topical guides for the person who is writing his biographic sketch. The life chart typically consists of three columns—one for life events, one for physical illness, one for mental illness—enabling the evaluator to highlight the time relations between episodes of physical and mental illness and potentially stressful events in the subject's life.

skew-deviation See *deviation, skew.*

skew, marital See *marital skew.*

skimming Accepting or admitting the less costly cases in a case-mix prospective payment system, but avoiding the more costly cases, so as to keep total actual cost of operations below the predicted cost. In most prospective payment systems, the agency or facility demonstrating such a "savings" is allowed to keep at least part of it as profit.

Skinner, Burrhus Frederic (1904–   ) American psychologist; operant behaviorism; *Walden Two,* 1948; *Science and Human Behavior,* 1953; *Beyond Freedom and Dignity,* 1971. See *behaviorism.*

skoptsy A Russian religious sect (a subdivision of the *raskol'nike,* the schismatics or dissenters) whose adherents practiced castration, in conformity with the passage: "And there be eunuchs, which have made themselves eunuchs for the kingdom of heaven's sake. He that is able to receive it, let him receive it." (Matt. 19:12)

Castration among the skoptsy was of two degrees: (1) *the small seal (first purity; mounting a piebald horse),* involving removal of scrotum only, with the testicles; (2) *the grand seal (second purity; mounting a white horse),* total castration, with the excision of both the scrotum and reproductive organ. Women, too, undergo castration and even remove their breasts.

slasher See *self-mutilation.*

Slater, Eliot Trevor Oakeshort (1904–1983) British psychiatrist, one of the founding fathers of 20th-century biological psychiatry, best known for his studies of the genetics of schizophrenia and manic-depressive illness. *Physical Methods of Treatment* (1944, with W. Sargant); *Clinical Psychiatry* (1954, with W. Mayer-Gross and M. Roth); *The Genetics of Mental Disorders* (1971, with V. Cowie).

slavering *Obs.* Drooling.

sleep Sleep is composed of two relatively distinct physiologic and behavioral states, non-rapid eye movement sleep (NREM), consisting of four successive stages, and rapid eye movement sleep (REM). The four stages of NREM are (1) a transition between waking and sleep, characterized by a decrease in alpha activity (12–14 Hz) in the EEG and a predominance of theta activity (4–7 Hz); (2) bursts of 12–14 Hz, or *sleep spindles;* (3) increasing concentration of delta activity (2–4 Hz), which constitutes 20–50% of the EEG tracing; (4) concentration of delta activity greater than 50%.

REM sleep occurs in episodes during the sleep period, with the first episode usually beginning about 90 minutes after sleep onset. It is characterized by the occurrence of low-voltage mixed-frequency EEG activity, a precipitous drop in electromyogram (EMG) activity and skeletal muscle paralysis, and conjugate eye movements that can be measured by the electrooculogram (EOM).

REM sleep is associated with dreaming and with considerable autonomic activation. NREM sleep, in contrast, is associated with more primitive mental content if cognitive activity can be elicited at all, with slow heart and respiratory rate and low blood pressure.

sleep, activated See *dream.*

sleep apnea See *apnea, central; sleep disorders.*

sleep, continuous See *treatment, continuous sleep.*

sleep disorders Also *sleep and arousal disorders;* somnipathy; any abnormality of the sleeping-waking cycle, divided into:

1. DIMS (disorders of initiating or maintaining sleep, the *insomnias*), or excessive daytime sleepiness (in DSM-III-R, this group is called the *dyssomnias*).

    a. Disorders primarily of insomnia include learned insomnia, childhood-onset idiopathic insomnia, and restless legs sleep disorder (in DSM-III-R, *insomnia disorder*).

    b. Disorders primarily of excessive daytime sleepiness (in some classifications, a separate category called DOES, disorders of excessive somnolence, and in DSM-III-R called *hypersomnia disorder*), including *narcolepsy* (q.v.), idiopathic hypersomnolence disorder, and the Kleine-Levin syndrome.

    c. Disorders of insomnia or excessive daytime sleepiness include *sleep apnea,* nocturnal myoclonus (see *myoclonus, nocturnal*), insomnia or excessive daytime sleepiness secondary to other physical disorder, and subjective sleep complaint without objective findings. The most common cause of sleep apnea (*sleep-induced respiratory impairment;* in DSM-III-R classified as "insomnia related to a known organic factor") is obstruction or occlusion of the airway by atonic or excessive tissue. The number and length of the apneic periods determine the extent of cardiovascular involvement and change in oxygen saturation. Apnea is associated with bradycardia and electroencephalographic and behavioral arousal; it often terminates with a loud snore, body jerks, sleep talking, or tachycardia. In addition to disturbing sleep, apnea also produces chronic fatigue and sleepiness during the day. Sleep apnea that occurs in NREM and REM sleep is associated with hypertension, right heart failure, secondary polycythemia, nocturnal cardiac arrhythmias, and possibly sudden, unexplained nocturnal death. Treatment may include surgical resection of portions of the soft palate or even tracheostomy in severe cases.

2. *Sleep-wake schedule disorders,* including *phase shift* (advanced sleep phase disorder: feeling sleepy when one should be awake and alert; delayed sleep phase disorder: feeling alert when one should be sleepy), jet lag and work shift syndromes (frequently changing sleep-wake schedule disorder), and disorganized sleep-wake pattern disorder.

3. Parasomnias, dysfunctions associated with sleep, sleep stages, or partial arousals; included here are sleepwalking disorder (somnambulism), sleep terror disorder (pavor nocturnus), nocturnal enuresis, dream anxiety disorder (nightmares), and sleep paralysis.

sleep drunkenness *Somnolentia;* a disorder of excessive somnolence (DOES) consisting of prolongation of the period between sleep and waking with protracted (as long as two hours) obnubilation and confusion following arousal, sometimes accompanied by agitation, aggressivity, and assaultiveness. In at least some cases it appears to be familial; further, it seems to occur only in males.

sleep efficiency The ratio of time spent asleep to the total polysomnograph recording period; the most "efficient" sleep is that in which sleep latency is short and no wakenings occur after sleep onset. *REM sleep efficiency* is the time in REM sleep over the time from the beginning to the end of a REM period.

sleep-induced respiratory impairment Sleep apnea. See *sleep and arousal disorders.*

sleep latency See *latency, sleep.*

sleep paralysis or numbness See *paralysis, sleep.*

sleep, paroxysmal Sleep epilepsy, *narcolepsy* (q.v.); a sudden uncontrollable disposition to sleep occurring at irregular intervals, with or without obvious predisposing or exciting cause.

sleep, telencephalic See *dream.*

sleep terror disorder *Pavor nocturnus; night terror; sleep terror;* a rare type of sleep disorder, allied to but more serious than nightmares, which occurs in children and is not seen after puberty. The child awakes abruptly, screaming with fright, may stand up in bed or run about the bedroom, may have hallucinations of animals or strange people in the room, is disoriented and does not recognize the people about him. The attack ends after several minutes; the child drops off to sleep and does not remember the epidsode.

Episodes occur usually during periods of EEG delta activity, in stages 3 and 4 of sleep, and not during REM sleep. There is no evidence of abnormal electrical activity during the sleep of affected children. See *sleep and arousal disorders.*

sleep, thrombencephalic See *dream.*

sleep time, total The amount of time actually spent in sleeping, measured by subtracting *wake time after sleep onset* (q.v.) from the duration of the period from onset to termination of sleep.

sleep-wake schedule disorders Any shift in the time of the sleep cycle, such as the *delayed sleep phase syndrome,* in which the sleep and wakefulness pattern is permanently shifted and going to sleep and

waking times are substantially later than desired. It is found more frequently in adolescents and young adults and may be partly constitutional and partly the result of intrusion of work or social activities into the normal sleep cycle.

sleep, yen (Chinese *yen,* smoke, opium) A slang expression used by morphine or heroin addicts for the somnolence that affects them when the drug is withdrawn.

sleepwalking See *somnambulism.*

sliding of meanings Making minute alterations in how facts are reported as a way to externalize blame and thereby preserve self-esteem. The phenomenon has been reported frequently in narcissistic personality disorder.

slip See *act, symptomatic; intentional unvoluntary behavior.*

slip of tongue *Lapsus linguae.* See *act, symptomatic.*

slippage, cognitive See *cognitive slippage.*

slow virus See *virus infections.*

Sluder's syndrome Sphenopalatine neuralgia; vidian neuralgia. See *headaches, cluster.*

slum An urban area characterized by physical deterioration and social disorganization so marked as to result in the personal disorganization of its residents in the form of juvenile delinquency, adult crime, vice, substance dependence, gambling, mental disorders, etc. Children of the slums are both materially and emotionally disadvantaged and underprivileged.

SML Single-major-locus; one of the models of *inheritance* (q.v.).

smother love See *love, smother.*

SMR training A biofeedback technique that teaches the subject to produce 14–16cps rhythms. Insomniacs are deficient in these rhythms even when awake, and SMR is effective in 10–20% of psychophysiologic and childhood sleep onset insomniacs who are relaxed but even so cannot fall asleep.

SNE See *encephalomyelopathy, subacute necrotizing.*

snow (From cocaine powder's resemblance to snow both in whiteness and powder consistence) Slang expression for cocaine.

snow lights A type of visual pseudohallucination in which the subject, usually a cocaine user, sees twinkling lights similar to the sparkling of cocaine crystals or frozen snow crystals.

snowbird Slang expression for a cocaine addict. See *cocainism*.

SOAP See *problem-oriented record*.

social breakdown syndrome See *syndrome, social breakdown*.

social class and mental illness See *class, social*.

social cohesion, hedonic See *hedonism*.

social control See *dilemma, Scull's; forced treatment*.

social impulse, fundamental See *impulse, fundamental social*.

social integration-disintegration model See *psychiatry, community*.

social interest See *interest, social*.

social phobia See *phobia, social*.

social policy planning Known variously as *community organization, community action, social action,* and *social engineering,* social policy planning is a deliberate, organized, and collaborative approach to the analysis and manipulation of social structures and systems. It aims to improve the quality of life in a community, which is viewed as an organism, a total biotype, an ecological entity. Emphasis is upon superordinate goals (viz. the welfare of people), rather than on institutionally defined goals (e.g. the pathology and condition of specific people who appear at the door of a mental health center). Its methods may even include such an approach as founding a new town with a sociopetal arrangement to promote participation by such means as organization, architectural structure, and other environmental factors that program behavior. The goal is to develop a process within the community—not to devise a specific prescription, but to initiate interaction and expand the spectrum of possible action in overcoming poverty, minority problems, and other urban crises, which currently are ordinarily defined in terms of jobs, housing, education, crime on the streets, drug and alcohol abuse, and suicide. See *psychiatry, community*.

social psychiatry See *ecology; psychiatry, community; psychiatry, comparative*.

social psychology See *sociology*.

social skills training (SST) A behavioral technique designed to help patients to organize or improve their ability to relate to other people and to conform with social norms, with emphasis on changing specific behaviors that are bizarre or mal-adaptive. Training and instruction may include description of particular social skills or maneuvers, modeling or demonstration by others who are competent in those skills, imitation and rehearsal by the patient, feedback from others who have witnessed or participated in practice sessions or from videotaped recordings of the sessions, and reinforcement for achieving the objectives or goals of the training approach. Such training is often a part of therapy with families of schizophrenics, whose social ineptness can predispose the family to recurrent dysfunction. See *therapy, behavior*.

social stressor See *event, life*.

social therapy Rehabilitation therapy; any form of treatment whose primary focus is on the patient's level of social functioning and whose aim is to improve the patient's ability to function in a socially approved manner. The social therapies include any number of socioenvironmental approaches that concern themselves with the patient's behavior, rather than his intrapsychic state—the therapeutic community, patient government, remotivation, attitude therapy, compensated work, etc. See *deinstitutionalization*.

social type See *type, social*.

social work, family "Family social work is a field of organized practice having to do with human relationships. Its main purpose is to help individuals deal effectively with difficulties experienced in relating themselves to others in their families and in their communities. This practice is based on a growing body of knowledge about human beings as functioning members of society and it employs the technique and art termed social case work." (*Social Work Year Book 1939*)

social work, psychiatric The adaptation and application of social psychiatry and mental hygiene to casework practice. "Psychiatric social workers are usually concerned with the social case study and treatment of children or adults whose personal and social maladjustments are primarily due to mental health problems, including nervous and mental diseases and defects, and emotional behavior, and habit disorders." (*Social Work Year Book 1939*)

socialization The processes through which the individual becomes a competent member of society. Anthropologists stress cultural transmission or enculturation; personality psychologists focus on impulse control; sociologists concentrate on role learning. Recent work using direct observation of infants suggests that socialization is an interactive process based on reciprocity. The human infant is an active participant in the socialization process and much more than a mere passive recipient of information doled out by others.

In occupational therapy this term is applied to the development (in a patient) of those tendencies that induce him to be companionable and inclined to seek and mingle easily with a group.

In psychiatry the term means the condition in which inner impulses (i.e. instincts and their derivatives) are expressed or lived out in conformity with the cultural demands of the environment. It is synonymous with *sublimation* (q.v.).

socialize 1. To *sublimate* (q.v.). 2. To mix in a group.

societal reaction theory *Labeling theory* (q.v.).

society The network of relationships between a person and every other organizational unit of mankind, ranging from the mother-child dyad or family to a league of nations.

sociobiology The study of the biological basis for social behavior and of how such behavior affects the individual's (or society's) fitness to survive. Sociobiology is also concerned with how specific traits serve as adaptations and with the identification of the evolutionarily stable strategy that enables the individual organism to adapt optimally within a social context that is determined by the behavior of others.

sociogram "The sociogram projects the results of sociometric, spontaneity and population tests into a pattern and makes visible the relationship of every individual to every other individual of the group tested. Thus, the position of every individual is defined as well as the configuration of the total structure.

"The sociogram is primarily a method for exploring the invisible structure of society. As a guide it has led to discoveries of social structures which could not have been revealed through other means. It showed, for example, the positions of emotional isolates in a group, of pair attrac-

tions and pair rejections, of triangles, of chains of interpersonal relations, the positions of leader structures and the cliques of individuals who are separated from the group as a whole." (Moreno, J.L. *Sociometry 1*, 1937)

sociology The behavior science that concerns itself with the conceptualization and study of group life, and particularly the functions, structures, and organization of institutions and communities, the interactions between them, and the changes within them. Even though systematic sociology developed in response to recognized social problems (specifically, crime, delinquency, and suicide), the sociologist is as interested in understanding "normal" social actions as in gathering knowledge of social problems and uncovering the crucial factors in their incidence. Current clinical emphasis on how social organizations may, both implicitly and explicitly, program or dictate the behavior of the people within them is more akin to *social psychology* than to sociology; but in practice the distinction between the two is not finely drawn.

sociology, clinical See *psychiatry, comparative*.

sociometry "Sociometry is the study of the actual psychological structure of human society. This structure, rarely visible on the surface of social processes, consists of complex interpersonal patterns which are studied by quantitative and qualitative procedures.

"Sociometry proceeds upon the premise that there is some sort of order in the phenomena with which it deals. The psychological situation of a community viewed as a whole has a discernible ordered pattern. It presents itself in laws and tendencies which are discoverable by means of experiment and analysis.

". . . A fundamental part of the sociometric procedure is to apply to a community an actual social situation which is confronting its people at the moment. The social situation applied is of such a nature as to make repetition possible at any time in the future without loss of spontaneous participation. In this manner, the procedure reveals the organization and evolution of groups and the position of individuals within them." (Moreno, J.L. *Sociometry 1*, 1937)

sociopath *Psychopathic personality* (q.v.).

sociopathic personality disturbance In the 1952 revision of psychiatric nomenclature, this term was used to refer to those who are ill primarily in terms of society and of conformity with social, cultural, and ethical demands. This group does *not* include those whose conduct and behavior are symptomatic of more primary personality disturbance. Included in this group were:
1. *Antisocial reaction*—approximately equivalent to the older terms constitutional psychopathy and psychopathic personality and to *antisocial personality disorder* in DSM-III.
2. *Dyssocial reaction*—disregard for and conflict with the social code as the result of having lived in an abnormal moral environment.
3. *Sexual deviation*—such as homosexuality, transvestism, pedophilia, fetishism, sexual sadism.
4. *Addiction* (q.v.).
    a. *Alcoholism* (q.v.).
    b. Drug addiction.

sociopathology The pathology of society. Society at large, or any segment of society, is composed of or comprises an aggregate of individuals, and the psychopathology of the patient as an individual or of a few or many of the group is quantitatively and qualitatively reflected ultimately as the psychopathology of the society that contains the individuals. Individual psychopathology is thus closely intermeshed with communal sociopathology.

sociopathy (sō-sē-op'á-thē) 1. Generally used to designate an abnormal or pathological mental attitude toward the environment. Thus criminality and vagabondage are regarded by some authorities as manifestations of sociopathy. In this sense the term refers to mental states that are commonly subsumed under psychopathy.
    2. Abnormality or pathology of society or social units.

sociotaxis See *network; taxis.*

sociotherapy Any type of treatment whose primary emphasis is on socioenvironmental and interpersonal factors in adjustment; it is sometimes used to refer specifically to the establishment of a therapeutic community. See *community, therapeutic.*

sodium pump See *conduction, nerve.*

sodomite One who practices sodomy; a sodomist.

sodomy Most often the term refers to anal intercourse, although in different jurisdictions and in different countries it has been defined to refer to various forms of sexual expression that are considered unnatural, perverse, or otherwise unacceptable.

soft signs Neurological signs without localizing significance, often involving stereognosis, graphesthesia, balance, and proprioception and thus suggestive of a defect in integrating sensory information.

soiling See *encopresis.*

soliloquy, sexual Hirschfeld says that many sexually timid individuals, who find difficulty in suppressing or repressing their sexual impulses, engage in long soliloquies as a means of relieving the sexual tensions.

solipsism The doctrine that *my self, alone,* is the essence of existence and that nothing counts except one's own ego, in which all else is reflected.

soluble RNA See *chromosome.*

solution, auxiliary In Horney's terminology, any partial or temporary solution of intrapsychic conflict, such as automatic control of feelings, compartmentalization, externalization, intellectualization, or self-alienation.

solution, comprehensive In Horney's terminology, an unrealistic avoidance of conflict by believing oneself to be the *idealized self* (q.v.), i.e. by actualizing the idealized image of oneself.

solution, expansive See *expansiveness.*

solution, major In Horney's terminology, a type of neurotic solution consisting of repression and denial of trends that conflict with the idealized self, or consisting of withdrawal into resignation.

soma The organic tissues of the body. Whether correctly or not, the terms *soma* and *psyche* are often employed as if they were opposites. The psyche, however, is currently considered as an organ of the total person; it is not looked upon as an antithesis of the soma, but rather as a harmonious constituent of the entire organism. See *psyche; psychosomatic.*

somatagnosia See *somatognosia.*

somatalgia Pain due to organic causes, as distinguished from psychalgia or pain due to psychical causes. See *hypochondriasis; psychalgia; somatoform disorders..*

somatic Relating to or involving the soma.

somatist Psychiatrist or scientist who regards any particular neurosis or psychosis as of organic or physical origin.

somatization Stekel's term for a type of bodily disorder arising from a deep-seated neurotic cause. It is as if the organs of the body were translating into a physiopathological language the mental troubles of the individual. The term somatization is identical with the phenomenon Freud calls *conversion*. Stekel refers to it also in terms of *organ speech* of the mind, meaning the organic expression of mental processes. Such physical expressions are also encountered in dreams, and when they occur, the oneiric phenomena or process is known as a functional dream. See *conversion*.

somatization disorder Briquet's syndrome, one of the *somatoform disorders* (q.v.); a chronic and fluctuating condition of relatively early onset (before 30 years) characterized by recurrent and multiple somatic complaints that lead to repeated medical examinations and consultations, multiple diagnoses, and in many cases multiple surgical interventions. Most commonly, symptoms are related to the gastrointestinal, cardiopulmonary, reproductive, and neurological systems, or to psychosexual functioning, or they involve pain (e.g. in back, joints, genitals).

soma, some- Combining form meaning body, from Gr. *soma*.

somatobiology The study of the biology of the body, as contrasted with psycho-biology, which is the study of the biology of the mind.

somatoform disorders A group of disorders whose symptoms resemble physical disorders but cannot be explained by any demonstrable organic findings. Included are *somatization disorder* (q.v.), conversion disorder (see *hysteria*), somatoform pain disorder (preoccupation with severe, prolonged, and disabling pain that leads often to doctor-shopping, overuse of analgesics, solicitation of surgery, and adoption of the invalid role), *hypochondriasis* (q.v.), and body-dysmorphic disorder, consisting of preoccupation with some imagined defect in physical appearance that is not warranted by objective evidence.

somatogenesis Origination in organic tissue (the soma).

somatognosia (sō-mȧ-tog-nō′sē-ȧ) The awareness of one's own body as a functioning object in space. *Macrosomatognosia* is a disturbance of the body scheme in which the body or parts of the body are experienced as abnormally large; *microsomatognosia* is a disturbance of the body scheme in which the body or parts of the body are experienced as abnormally small. Such disturbances have been reported in organic neurological lesions, epilepsy, migraine, schizophrenia, and experimental psychosis. See *ego, body; image, body.*

Note that absent or defective awareness may be expressed in two ways: as *asomatognosia* or as *somatagnosia*.

somatopathic drinking See *alcoholism*.

somatoplasm The somatic tissues of an animal body, to distinguish them, according to the *germ plasm* theory, from the reproductive tissue that produces the germ cells.

somatopsychic Relating to or originating in both body and mind.

somatopsychonoologia *Obs.* Psychosomatism.

somatopsychosis Southard's term for a psychosis associated with visceral disease.

somatosexual Pertaining to or characterized by organic manifestations of sexuality.

somatosexuality Somatosexual condition or state, or sexuality as it exists in the tissues or soma or organs. For example, sexuality, expressing itself through the genitals, is a form of somatosexuality.

somatotonia A personality type described by Sheldon that is correlated with the meso-morph body type and shows a predominance of vigorous assertiveness and muscular activity.

somatotopagnosia (top-ag-nō′zē-ȧ) *Autotopagnosia* (q.v.).

somatotype In some systems of constitutional medicine, the physical structure and build of a person as assessed by particular photographic techniques of *anthropometry*. Its scientific meaning thus applies only to one aspect of an *anthrotype*, which has physiological, immunological, and psychological aspects as well. See *anthrotype*.

somesthetic area See *lobe, parietal*.

somite In the development of an embryo, a mesodermic segment formed by the medial portions of the third germ layer or *mesoderm*.

Sommer, Robert (1864–1937) German psychiatrist.

somnambulism *Sleepwalking disorder*, consisting of repeated episodes of rising from bed during sleep and walking about. Episodes rarely last more than 30 minutes and once awake the subject is amnesic for his actions during the episode. See *sleep disorders.*

Somnambulism is primarily a male disorder and is rare in homosexuals of either sex; in one series a reported 35% of sleepwalkers were overtly schizophrenic, and another 28% were markedly schizoid in character. Dynamic characteristics of this series were inadequate male identification, passive-dependent strivings, and conflicting feelings over aggression. (Sours, J.A. *Archives of General Psychiatry 9,* 1963)

Somnambulism usually occurs in sleep stages 3 and 4 and not during REM sleep. Those somnambulists so far studied have given no evidence of abnormal electrical brain activity during sleep.

Somnambulism may occur as a complication of neuroleptic medication, and particularly if neuroleptics are combined with lithium.

somnambulism, cataleptic A cataleptic state occurring during somnambulism.

somnambulism, monoideic (mon-ō-ī-dē′ik) Janet's term for a single idea constituting the content of a somnambulistic episode. When the content contains many ideas he calls it polyideic somnambulism.

somnambulism, polyideic (pol-ē-ī-dē′ik) See *somnambulism, monoideic.*

somnial *Rare.* Pertaining to dreams.

somnifacient (som-ni-fā′shent) Hypnotic; sleep-inducing.

somniferous Hypnotic; somnific.

somnifugous (som-nif′ū-gus) Driving sleep away; agrypnotic.

somniloquism (som-nil′ō-kwiz′m) Talking during sleep. Somniloquism is not pathognomonic of any specific disorder and is only rarely presented as a symptom or chief complaint.

somnipathy 1. Any *sleep disorder* (q.v.). 2. *Obs.* hypnotism.

somnolence Unnatural sleepiness, drowsiness.

somnolent detachment See *detachment, somnolent.*

somnolentia *Obs.* 1. *Sleep drunkenness* (q.v.). 2. somnolence.

somnolism *Obs.* Hypnotism.

somnovigil *Obs.* Somnambulism.

sonoencephalogram (SEG) *Echoencephalogram.* See *echoencephalography.*

sonography See *NMR.*

sophomania A form of megalomania in which the patient stresses the excellence of his wisdom.

sopiet Soporific.

sopite *Rare.* Drowsy.

sopor *Obs.* A disorder of consciousness in which the subject can be aroused only by strong stimulation.

soporiferous Soporific, making drowsy.

soporific, soporifical Any sleep-inducing agent.

soporose Characterized or affected by morbid sleepiness.

sororate Marriage to a deceased wife's sister. See *levirate.*

soteria (sō-ter′ē-à) Possessions and objects that bring security and protection, as the objects that a collector admits to his collection. Collecting and soteric objects are to be distinguished from accumulation and the objects accumulated; *accumulation* is "the continued possession of unclassified, useless, meaningless, annoying objects" and, unlike true collecting, "cannot be understood in terms of its symbolic meaning, but is a by-product of the accumulator's indecision, an unwillingness to commit himself to a clear and realistic self-definition." (Phillips, R.H. *Archives of General Psychiatry 6,* 1962) See *coprophilia; mania, collecting.*

Soteria also means deliverance, and in that sense it has been used as a name for residences for schizophrenics. See *domicile.*

Soteria also refers to a nonmedical treatment systems approach that rejects medication and formal professional services in favor of peer support, with the family kept at a friendly distance.

Soteria House See *domicile.*

soul See *anima.*

soul, folk A kind of mystical group mind, the presence of which is deduced from the way each individual displays properties and modes of reaction not present when he remains outside the group. The folk soul is considered a sort of supermind that is transcendental and possesses more good than the individual minds that contribute to it. The following terms are nearly synonymous with folk soul: group mind (McDougall); general will (Rousseau); collective consciousness

(Renan); social consciousness (Espinas, Durkheim, Wundt); group consciousness (Heard). Many do not accept the presence of a folk soul or group mind and instead would explain collective reactions like communism and anarchism as racial neurosis (see *psychosis, collective*). Freud explains group psychology on the basis of individual identification with one another, secondary to the sharing of a common emotional situation.

source In psychoanalysis, "That somatic process in an organ or part of the body from which there results a stimulus represented in mental life by an instinct." (Freud, *CP*) Freud claims that "the study of the sources of instincts is outside the scope of psychology," because it probably involves physiochemical processes. "Although its source in the body is what gives the instinct its distinct and essential character, yet in mental life we know it merely by its aims." (Ibid.)

Southard, Elmer Ernest (1876–1920) American psychiatrist; social psychiatry, industrial hygiene.

space, life See *life space*.

space, personal See *proxemics*.

space, subarachnoid See *meninges*.

spacing Distancing; the distance an organism puts between itself and another member of its own group. When spacing is so close as to be nonexistent, as in the mother-infant relationship, the term *bonding* is applied; close spacing under other conditions may be termed *crowding*, with the implication that such closeness is undesirable rather than facilitating. In humans and other primates, crowding is associated with a significant increase in aggressiveness.

span, auditory The number of digits (or letters, or words) that can be repeated after one hearing; determination of auditory span is a common test of immediate memory.

span of attention See *attention; memory*.

spasm A slow, at times prolonged, patterned movement of a muscle or groups of muscles occurring anywhere in the body.

spasm, masticatory Tonic closure of the jaw; it may be part of a syndrome of hysteria, meningitis, tetanus, epilepsy; it occasionally occurs in tumors or other diseases of the pons.

spasm, nodding A stereotyped movement disorder consisting of repetitive head-shaking and sometimes accompanied by nystagmus. The syndrome is rare in adults. In children it is seen most frequently in association with mental retardation or pervasive developmental disorders, although it may occur as an isolated syndrome not associated with any recognizable mental disorder.

spasm, oculogyric An involuntary tonic contraction of the extraocular muscles characterized by fixed upward gaze (or forced conjugate movements in other directions) that lasts from several minutes to several hours. Oculogyric crises or spasms are often a sequel of encephalitis, or they may appear as an acute dystonic side effect of medication with neuroleptics.

spasm, salaam (or **salutation**) A variety of spasm seen in young children, consisting of periodic and rhythmic movements of the head and upper part of the body of about 2 seconds duration with intervals of approximately 10 seconds. They resemble the oriental form of greeting. The condition is mostly associated with neuropathologic findings.

spasm, saltatory Spasm of the muscles of the lower extremities producing jumping or skipping movements, usually of hysterical origin.

spasmophemia *Obs.* Speaking in spasms; stammering or *stuttering* (q.v.).

spasmophilia 1. A neuropsychiatric syndrome, described by Joyeux in 1958, consisting of moderate anxiety, irritability, hypermotility, insomnia, dysfunction in various organ systems (gastrointestinal, cardiovascular, genital, skin), and positive Chvostek sign. All the symptoms may be precipitated or aggravated by hyperventilation. See *syndrome, hyperventilation*.

     2. In general and constitutional medicine a syndrome characterized by undersecretion of the parathyroids and frequently associated with a generalized hypoparathyroid constitution. See *constitution, hypoparathyroid*.

spasmus nutans A rhythmic nodding or rotatory tremor of the head occurring in infants between the ages of 6 and 12 months; frequently accompanied by nystagmus. See *spasm, nodding*.

spatial nonrecognition See *nonrecognition*.

spatial summation See *summation*.

species In natural science, a group of animals or plants that rank below the genus and divisible into varieties or *subspecies*. The individuals forming a species are assumed to resemble one another in the essential features of their organization and to produce fertile offspring that vary from the general type of the group to a limited extent only.

specific *Biol.* Pertaining to a *species*.

specific developmental disorders See *developmental disorders, specific*.

specific dynamic pattern Franz Alexander's term for the specific nuclear conflict or dynamic configuration unique to a particular psychosomatic disorder or organ-neurosis. See *psychosomatic*.

specificity See *sensitivity*.

specificity, encoding See *encoding*.

specificity, individual-response The tendency of a subject to respond maximally and consistently in one particular physiological system. Such specificity is hypothesized to be a significant factor in organ choice, that is, in determining in what bodily system dysfunction will be expressed, as in psychosomatic disorders. *I-R specificity* is approximately equivalent to what used to be referred to as locus minoris resistentiae in that it is one manifestation of susceptibility of, overactivity on the part of, or damage to a particular organ system. See *compliance, somatic; inferiority, organ; psychosomatic medicine*.

specificity of research See *research, specific*.

specificity, symptom The phenomenon of heightened reactivity to stress in that organ system in which a psychosomatic patient's symptoms are localized; e.g. greater heart rate and heart rate variability in patients with cardiovascular complaints than in subjects without such complaints.

SPECT Single photon emission computed tomography, a type of imaging in which the camera rotates around the patient while the computer compiles images of transverse slices, as in CT or CAT scanning. Unlike the latter, however, which produces an anatomic image, SPECT uses radioactive tracers and provides an image of radioactivity distribution. In this aspect, it is similar to *PET* (q.v.), whose major disadvantage is that cyclotrons must be maintained on-site to develop the short-lived isotopes needed for imaging. PET's major advantage in comparison with SPECT is that short-lived isotopes enable visualization of processes that cannot be seen with longer lived isotopes. Although the SPECT image is not as clearly defined as the PET image, the cost is much lower. See NMR.

spectral photography See *BEAM*.

spectrophobia "The hysterical phobia for mirrors and the dread of catching sight of one's own face in a mirror had in one case a 'functional' and a 'material' origin. The functional one was dread of *self-knowledge;* the material, the flight from the *pleasure of looking and exhibitionism.* In the unconscious phantasies the parts of the face represented, as in so many instances, parts of the genitals." (Ferenczi, *FCT*)

spectrum, psychotherapeutic The entire range of psychotherapeutic techniques.

spectrum, schizophrenic A hypothesized range of psychopathologic states that share a genetic etiology with classic schizophrenia; the differences between the states are differences in intensity that may be due to environmental or genetic modification of the genetic diathesis necessary for development of any of the spectrum's variants. (Kety, S.S., Rosenthal, D., Wender, P.H., & Schulsinger, F. *Schizophrenia Bulletin 2,* 1976) See *psychosis, reactive; schizoidia*.

spectrum, subaffective An inexact term that varies with the diagnostic/classificatory system of the user to refer to a range of mood abnormalities that do not fulfill the criteria for major affective disorder because they are chronic and prolonged rather than acute and self-limited in duration, or because they are subtle and ill-defined rather than clear-cut and unmistakable, or because they fail to crystallize into discrete or predictable episodes. Included within the group by one or more workers at one time or another are cyclothymia, dysthymic disorder, atypical depression or mania, hysteroid dysphoria, and masked depression. See *affective disorders*.

speech, cerebellar In diseases of the cerebellum, the speech may be jerky, explosive, irregular, and scanning. This condition is also called *asynergic* or *ataxic speech*.

speech disorders Lalopathies; logopathy; all abnormalities in language production that are not due to faulty innervation of speech muscles or organs of articulation: included on the motor end are disturbances in gestures (*amimia*), voice (*aphonia*), speech (*aphasia*), and pictorial or symbolic representation (*agraphia*); and on the sensory end inability to perceive or understand gestures (*sensory amimia*), sounds (*sensory aphasia*), or writing (*alexia*). Some use the term in a very limited sense, to refer only to *stuttering* and *specific developmental disorders* (qq.v.). Others include a broader range of disorders within the term, and although there is no standard classification, a tripartite subdivision is often used: (1) central disorders, or *aphasia* (q.v.); (2) output disorders (also called production disorders), such as stuttering and cluttering; and (3) input disorders (also called reception disorders), such as auditory agnosia and pure word-deafness (see *aphasia, auditory*).

There is a confusing array of terms that refer to specific speech disorders, but many of them include generally accepted combining forms that make them more readily comprehensible:

1. *a-* or *an-* means absence or total loss, as in *aphonia* (loss of voice) or *aphasia* (q.v.).

2. *dys-* means a partial loss or one limited to a discrete function, as in *dyslexia* (q.v.), where only certain letters or words are misread or transposed.

3. *mogi-* or *moli-* means labored, effortful functioning, as in *mogilalia* (labored speech).

4. *tachy-* means rapid, as in *tachylogia* (rapid word production).

5. *brady-* means slow, as in *bradyphrenia* (slowed thinking).

6. *hyper-* means excessive in amount, as in *hyperphrasia* (garrulousness).

7. *hypo-* means reduced, inadequate, as in *hypomimia* (constricted range of gestures).

8. *para-* means a qualitative change in the faculty, as in *paraphrasia* (use of a wrong phrase, malapropism).

9. *agito-* means agitated, as in *agitolalia* (speech that is both rapid and disorganized).

10. *embolo-* means interjection of unnecessary elements, as in *embolophrasia* (speech that is filled with meaningless or irrelevant phrases).

11. *echo-* means repetition, as in *echolalia* (repetition by the subject of sounds or words that he hears).

Some articulation disorders have specific names:

1. *gammacism*—*g* is pronounced as *d*.

2. *lambdacism*—*l* is pronounced as *w* or *y*.

3. *rhotacism*—*r* is pronounced as *w* or *l*.

4. *sigmatism*—*s* is pronounced as *sh, th,* or *f*.

speech, labyrinthine See *labyrinthine.*

speech, organ Any physical symptoms that represent conscious or unconscious mental impulses; used particularly to refer to those schizophrenics who concentrate almost all their energy on complaints about a particular organ or body part (such as the nose). See *dysmorphophobia.*

speech, plateau Speech whose monotonal quality is due to loss or reduction in the pitch characteristic of each vowel sound; it occurs in epilepsy, multiple sclerosis, and other central nervous system disorders.

speech, scattered A type of speech commonly found in hebephrenic schizophrenia and marked especially by the lack of relevancy and coherence. This lack is due primarily to the patient's tendencies to condensation and the formation of neologisms. The patient condenses a whole series of allied events into a single word or phrase. See *scattering.*

spell, vacant *Absence* (q.v.).

spells of doubting and brooding See *brooding-spells.*

SPEM Smooth pursuit eye movements, reported to be disordered in 70–80% of schizophrenic patients and in 45–50% of their first-degree relatives, but only in about 6% of normal subjects. P.S. Holzman and his coworkers posited that the abnormalities may represent a failure of inhibiting, modulating, or integrating control centers in the pontine paramedian reticular formation. (*Archives of General Psychiatry 33,* 1976)

spending spree Oniomania.

sperm, spermatozoon In contradistinction to the large reproductive cells in the female, which are called *eggs* (or ova), the *spermatozoa* (or sperms) are the very small male germ cells. They are unlike any other kind of cell, but like the eggs are subject to *meiosis* (q.v.). When mature they have only half the number of chromosomes characteristic of the individual that produces the germ cells.

Before undergoing meiosis, the spermatozoa multiply by repeated cell divisions of the ordinary duplicating type and are called *spermatogonia*. When these cells cease to divide by ordinary division, they become *primary spermatocytes*, but grow considerably less than the oocytes.

The first meiotic division produces in the male two *equal* cells, both functional, which are known as *secondary spermatocytes*. Each cell produced by this first *maturation division* immediately proceeds to divide again (*equation division*). The two identical new cells are called *spermatids* and, by changing shape, produce the *mature spermatozoa*.

In the process of fertilization, a spermatozoon enters an egg either after the maturation is completed or at some earlier time during the maturation process. When an egg is fertilized, a new individual is started.

spermatid In genetics a stage in the development of a mature *spermatozoon* (q.v.).

spermatocyte In sexual reproduction, the *spermatogonium* divides into *primary* and *secondary spermatocytes*, before maturing into a *spermatozoon* (q.v.).

spermatogonium In sexual reproduction, the spermatogonium represents the first stage in the development of a male's mature reproductive cell. See *spermatozoon*.

spermatophobia Fear of semen.

spes phthisica (spās′ ftē′zē-kȧ) The feeling of hopefulness and confidence of recovery experienced by many sufferers from tuberculosis even in the later stages of the disease.

sphacelismus (sfas-ē-liz′mus) *Obs.* Phrenitis (q.v.).

spheresthesia (sfer-es-thē′zē-ȧ) *Obs.* Globus hystericus (q.v.).

sphincter morality See *morality, sphincter*

Spielmeyer-Vogt's disease (Walter Spielmeyer, German neurologist, 1879–1935, and Oskar Vogt, contemporary German neurologist) A type of *Tay-Sachs disease* (q.v.); pigmentary retinal lipoid neuronal heredodegeneration.

spike-and-wave The dart-and-dome type of electroencephalographic tracing seen in petit mal epilepsy. See *epilepsy*.

spina bifida (spē′nȧ bēf′fē-dȧ) Rachischisis; a developmental defect in the spinal col-

umn due to failure of fusion of the dorsal walls of the primitive ectodermal neural canal. Although this defect may exist anywhere along the spine, it is usually situated posteriorly in the median line in the lumbar region.

spina bifida occulta (ô-kool′tȧ) That type of spina bifida in which the bony defect is covered by skin and therefore hidden from view.

spinal gate See *gating, spinal*.

spindles, sleep See *sleep*.

spine, railway *Obs.* A general term for injuries, real or feigned, to the back or spine, sustained during a railway accident.

Spitz, René A. (1887–1974) Austrian-born psychoanalyst; developmental studies; pioneer in applying research methods to Freud's analytic concepts of child development.

splanchnic Referring to the viscera. In psychiatry, the term ordinarily has reference to Viola's system of typology. See *type, megalosplanchnic; type, microsplanchnic; type, normosplanchnic*.

splicing, gene Any of the various techniques of *recombinant DNA* experiments, in which pieces of the genetic material from different species can be combined ("spliced") and inserted into living bacterial cells. It is clear that such experiments can yield invaluable information about heredity and the ways in which genes function, but at the same time many possible hazards have been envisaged (e.g. "supergerms" of high virulence or the deliberate, malevolent manipulation of human heredity). It is generally agreed that the possible dangers warrant some regulation of recombinant DNA research; the question of how stringent and restrictive such regulation should be remains a hotly debated issue.

split-brain preparation A surgical procedure in which the corpus callosum and other fibers connecting the two cerebral hemispheres are severed.

split double-bind See *bind, double*.

splitting According to Melanie Klein, splitting is an ego mechanism that precedes, and to some extent determines the type of repression. See *position, paranoid-schizoid; personality, multiple*. The term is used in a variety of ways by different authors—as the counterpart to synthesis in psychic structure formation, as a description of pathologic coexistent suborganizations of psychic structure, as a way to organize external reality on the basis of whether the specific early experiences were "pleasurable good" or "painful bad," and as a mechanism of defense against ambivalent feelings toward an object. (Lichtenberg, J.D., & Slap, J.W. *Journal of the American Psychoanalytic Association 21*, 1973)

Splitting consists of compartmentalization of opposite and conflicting affect states; the subject may be aware of his contradictory, ambivalent attitudes but fails to recognize that they spring from his own internal conflicts. See *identity diffusion. Split object-relations unit* refers to a self-percept and self-concept of being damaged, bad, incomplete, etc. This pathologic form of internalized object relation is an outgrowth of inadequate mother-infant interaction during the process of *individuation-separation* (q.v.), particularly in the rapprochement subphase. See *fault, basic; partialism, persistent.*

In DSM-III-R, splitting is a defense mechanism in which the subject, when faced with emotional stress or conflict, views himself or others as all good or all bad, or alternately idealizing and devaluing the same object. In splitting, the subject in unable to integrate the positive and negative qualities of self or object, or both, into cohesive images.

splitting, alliance and See *alliance and splitting.*

splurge, stealing A form of behavior disorder in children: the child strives to attain status in the group either by proving itself daring and competent in acts of stealing or by using the articles or money stolen as gifts to purchase the favor of the other members of the group.

spoiled-child reaction See *reaction, spoiled-child.*

spondylitis Inflammation of one or more of the vertebrae.

spongiform encephalopathy See *virus infections.*

spontaneity See *state, spontaneity.*

spontaneous imagery See *imagery, spontaneous.*

spoon feeding Feeding of another person (e.g. an infant) by putting a spoon filled with food to his lips; by extension, the expression has come to refer to any mani-

festation of oversolicitude that prevents or obstructs the development of independence on the part of the one being "fed." Psychiatric residents, for example, who receive so much individual case supervision that they never treat a patient completely by themselves, are spoken of as being spoon-fed.

spoonerism See *cluttering.*

spot, hypnogenic In susceptible patients the body sometimes presents a spot or point, pressure upon which will throw the person into a hypnotic state. See *zone, hysterogenic.*

SRO In psychiatry, sociology, and related fields, single room occupancy, referring to buildings made up of single rooms for occupants who are drawn from the outcasts of society—alcoholics, addicts, the mentally ill, the crippled and chronically disabled, and the lonely aged. SRO buildings are the privately owned equivalents of 19th-century poorhouses and a major indicator of social disintegration. They form a closed and isolated ghetto, separated from the surrounding community because their residents have no reference groups or roles outside the physical limits of the buildings themselves. They are characterized by profound dehumanization of welfare occupants who lack primary families and live with others of their kind in close quarters under control of a landlord-manager. The occupants need outreach services and education on how to use available facilities if they are to be rescued from the cycle of poverty, sickness, and crime.

SSPE See *panencephalitis, subacute sclerosing.*

SST 1.*Social skills training* (q.v.). 2. Self-Statement Training, a cognitive approach to the treatment of agoraphobia that aims to replace self-defeating cognitions with positive self-statements in confronting and coping with the feared situation.

stable cells See *neurometrics.*

stage, biting A subdivision of the oral phase of libido development. Abraham divided this phase into two parts. One is the sucking stage and the other, in consequence of the appearance of teeth, is the biting stage. Based on the nature of the fixation, the oral character will be (1) submissive if the fixation takes place in the sucking stage, or (2) aggressive, if in the biting stage. Thus psychoanalysts speak of oral receptive and oral aggressive characters. See *character, oral*.

stage, developmental See *ontogeny, psychic.*

stage, ideoplastic Verworn's term referring to the fact that the young child draws what he knows rather than what he sees. In the ideoplastic stage the child tends to exaggerate items that seem important or interesting and to minimize or omit the other parts.

stage, physioplastic Verworn's term for the ability to draw what is seen, in contrast to the ideoplastic stage, in which the child draws what he knows. See *stage, idioplastic.*

stage, postambivalent The final stage in the development of object love in which real love of an object is possible. As infantile sexuality develops, it passes through several stages associated with the various erogenous zones. The libido is organized successively around these various erogenous zones. The final stage in the development of sexuality is the genital stage and it occurs when all sexual excitations can be discharged through the use of the genital apparatus. See *ontogeny, psychic.*

Development of object love is interwoven with the development of sexuality. As infantile sexuality develops, the type of relationship to objects changes, for associated with each stage and related to the particular erogenous zone around which the libido is being organized is a different type of relationship to objects. In general, the development proceeds from an objectless state associated with the early oral (sucking) stage to the final stage of real love.

The stages of object love before real love is reached are ambivalent: in these stages, the process of achieving satisfaction destroys the object. This is based chiefly on the physiological nature of oral and anal erogeneities—that is, biting, swallowing, defecating, etc.—which are the usual models for these object relationships. The personality of the object itself does not matter, as the object is important only insofar as it can give satisfaction to the individual. When satisfaction has been achieved, the object itself may disappear—as far as the infant is concerned.

The final stage of object relationship, real love, is termed the postambivalent stage. No traces of hateful or destructive feelings toward the object remain. Instead, "consideration of the object goes so far that one's own satisfaction is impossible without satisfying the object, too." The prerequisite for real love is genital primacy, the ability to attain full satisfaction through genital orgasm. This emerges only in the final genital stage of libidinal organization. (Fenichel, *PTN*)

stagefright A type of anxiety hysteria in which the patient, an actor, fears to go onto the stage, or if he goes on, forgets his lines and/or begins to stutter. Stagefright is often based upon a need to ward off heightened exhibitionism and scopophilia, which if indulged in might provoke castration, and at the same time to gain reassurance from the audience that the dreaded castration has not occurred. See *pseudoaggression.*

stagnant anoxia See *anoxia, cerebral.*

stalemate, analytic See *resistance, id.*

staleness See *neurasthenia, aviator's.*

stammering A speech disorder characterized by spasmodic, halting, or hesitating utterance. The term is used by many authorities interchangeably with *stuttering* (q.v.).

standard deviation See *deviation, standard.*

standing mute *Rare.* Refusing to plead or say anything when arraigned; in such cases, the court may order a plea of not guilty to be entered for the accused and the trial or hearing may then continue.

Stanford-Binet Intelligence Scale See *tests, Binet-Simon.*

STAPP Short-term anxiety-provoking psychotherapy. See *psychotherapy, short-term anxiety-provoking.*

stasibasiphobia Fear of standing or walking. See *astasia-abasia.*

stasiphobia Fear of standing (up), delusion of inability to stand. See *astasia.*

stasis, libido Accumulation of libidinous excitations or tensions consequent upon blockage of their motor discharge. When the free flow of libido has been thus dammed, a stasis results, giving rise to the feeling of anxiety.

According to Kardiner, "Freud made an early attempt to describe the *Aktualneurosen*, and in this category were anxiety neurosis and neurasthenia. In connection with these neuroses Freud noted irritability, a diminished ability to tolerate accumulations of excitation, auditory hyperesthesia, anxious expectation, hypochondria, paresthesias, vasomotor disturbances, and so on. The essential pathology Freud considered an 'accumulation of tensions which were prevented from motor discharge.' "

The physiological accompaniments of anxiety are mediated by way of the autonomic nervous system. Kardiner points out that stasis phenomena resulting from overactivity of this system do not necessarily produce anxiety. "The autonomic phenomena need to be explained as regards their role in the failure reaction which is traumatic neurosis. . . . These phenomena may be considered 'discharge' manifestations. One may say that [the inhibitions of a traumatic neurosis] produce stasis phenomena, on the principle that since the demands of the external world continue to be the same as those before the neurosis was established, and the executive apparatus cannot carry out the necessary adaptive manipulations, stasis of some kind will accumulate. In other words it is as if the internal environment were geared for action, and the executive apparatus not. Hence autonomic activity that is shunted from its proper function continues unaccompanied by the activity of which it was originally an integral part.

"In the traumatic neurosis the place of the autonomic system in the action system is quite clear. It stands in direct relation to activity that is inhibited and in this neurosis is a part of the disorganization phenomena. The relations of autonomic disturbances in other neuroses are more difficult to disentangle. . . .

"The disorders of this autonomic system can be classified roughly by their correspondence to the normal physiologic accompaniments of anxiety. Such a picture is found in the usual autonomic imbalance of what is called by Lewis 'the soldier's heart' or 'effort-syndrome.' This autonomic picture may or may not be accompanied by the affect of anxiety or terror in the chronic forms of the disturbance. The affect of anxiety may completely disappear and in proportion as it disappears the more obtrusive these autonomic disturbances may become. In place of the anxiety or terror there remains a residual irritability. In the chronic cases the affect

is generally not present nor are there any displacement phobias. But there is one constant in the traumatic neurosis, the fact that the motility is blocked or guarded while the need tensions which can only be released by activity continue unabated. Hence one can regard these autonomic phenomena as evidence of stasis, since the autonomic system is not susceptible to inhibition—at least not by the same quantities of stimuli that are effective in inhibiting the skeletal system." (Kardiner, A., & Spiegel, H. *War Stress and Neurotic Illness*, 1947) See *neurosis, traumatic.*

stasobasophobia *Stasibasiphobia* (q.v.).

stasophobia *Stasiphobia* (q.v.).

stataesthesia (stat-es-thē′zē-à) Perception of constancy of pressure, as in maintaining pressure in a balloon by hand compression.

state, alpha See *alpha wave training.*

state, anxiety See *anxiety.*

state, central excitatory See *summation.*

state, clouded See *sensorium.*

state dependence Behavior that is a reflection to or a reaction of the state under which it occurs, rather than being primarily determined by the subject; reactive rather than constitutionally determined behavior.

state-dependent learning Acquisition of a skill during a drug state and subsequent best performance when the subject is in the same drug state, with worst performance when the subject is free of drug; also known as *dissociated learning.*

state, dreamy A state of arrested consciousness, akin to epileptiform seizures, but unaccompanied by convulsions. The patient suddenly passes off into a dream world, often with olfactory, auditory, and/or visual hallucinations, and usually recovers within a few minutes. Such states are most commonly associated with temporal lobe lesions. See *lobe, temporal.*

state, fatigue See *hypoglycemia.*

state, lacunar See *lacuna.*

state, paraphonic See *action, automatic.*

state, spontaneity "Spontaneity state is the condition which a subject has to attain in order to produce an emotion or role at will. The state is usually felt by the subject as a novel experience and frequently without a concrete precedent in his life history. Ordinarily, emotions like anger and jealousy are determined by the influence of common tensions and stresses. The emotions produced during the spontaneity state are voluntary. The subject must make an effort to reach the state or to warm up to it. Getting angry or jealous may be enforced upon the subject in life situations by determinants he cannot control, but getting angry or jealous in a spontaneity state is exactly the opposite. The subject voluntarily realizes a state which he usually experiences as something coming up against his will. In the spontaneity state he develops a relative distance from the states or roles which he ordinarily embodies. Spontaneity and spontaneity state are operational terms and cannot be fully understood by intellectual definition." (Moreno, J.L. *Das Stegreif Theater,* 1926)

state, twilight In Bleuler's classification, one of the acute syndromes in *schizophrenia* (q.v.). The twilight states appear as waking dreams that portray desires, wishes, or fears in a direct or symbolic way as being already fulfilled. They often persist for long periods; duration of six months is not uncommon.

stationing, interface See *network.*

statistical trend See *trend, statistical.*

statistics The branch of mathematics dealing with data that vary relatively as a result of the interaction of many causes; a body of data, numerical facts, or enumerations that must be analyzed in accordance with the statistical method.

status The relative position or rank of a person in a group, or of a group in reference to some larger grouping.

In medicine this term implies the presence of some abnormal state or pathological condition and requires further qualification by an adjective for the particular type of condition.

status, deemed See *deemed status.*

status degenerativus Bauer describes this as an accumulation, in a given person, of extreme variants of certain constitutional characteristics that, taken alone, may have little, if any, pathological significance such as a scaphoid shoulderblade, a supernumerary breast, a deformed earlobe, or an anomalous distribution of hair. However, any combination of these anomalies in the same person may be taken to indicate a type of general constitution that deviates too much from the average type and therefore is to be regarded as "biologically inferior."

This definition shows that from the constitutional standpoint *degeneration* simply implies a marked deviation from the type of a species, without regard to the clinical value of the deviation itself.

status dysraphicus (dēs-rä'fē-koos) A variety of developmental anomalies resulting from faulty closure of the neural groove at an early embryological stage. It seems to be hereditary and is believed to be the basis of such neurological diseases as hereditary ataxia and spinal gliosis (syringomyelia).

status epilepticus The recurrence without interruption of grand mal seizures in an epileptic.

Status epilepticus is the most common cause of death in epileptics. It occurs more frequently in symptomatic than in idiopathic epilepsy, and it often appears to be precipitated by withdrawal or change of anticonvulsant medication, or by intercurrent infection (where pyrexia may produce a state of internal withdrawal from medication). Other causes include occlusive cerebrovascular disease, hypertensive and metabolic encephalopathies, neoplasm, head trauma, degenerative diseases of the brain, and, sometimes, collagen disorders and similar systemic diseases.

status hypoplasticus Bartel and Wiesel use this term for a constitutional type characterized by generalized hypoevolutism, fibrous diathesis, hyperplasia of the lymphatic tissue, and the ready aging of the differentiated elements. This general hypoplastic condition is bound to lead to a poor functional capacity of the natural defense mechanisms and to a tendency on the part of the connective tissue to replace the elements constituting the parenchyma, which easily undergoes atrophy.

status hystericus *Obs.* Frequently recurring attacks of hysterical conversion symptoms extending over a period of hours or days.

status lymphaticus A constitutional type characterized by hyperplasia of the lymphatic tissue system and poor development of the blood vessels. Slight injuries to a person in this state may prove fatal.

status marmoratus See *dystonia, torsion.*

status, mental See *mental status.*

status offender See *offender, status.*

status raptus *Ecstasy* (q.v.).

status, social See *class, social.*

status, thymicolymphaticus Those cases of status lymphaticus in which an enlargement of the thymus is conspicuous. The condition may be *primary* and congenital or acquired *secondarily* in extrauterine life, especially through changes in other endocrine glands, occurring before the period of physiological involution of the thymus.

The symptomatology of both forms chiefly consists of enlarged thymus, general hyperplasia of the glands, dissemination of hyperplastic lymphatic tissue throughout the body, hyperthyroidism, sclerosis of ovaries and testes, and hypoplasia of the circulatory system. This condition attains its significance for constitutional medicine from the fact that the persons affected by it are under constant threat of infection and even of sudden death from minor psychical or physical traumata.

statuvolence *Obs.* Statuvolent state; self-induced hypnotism.

Stauder's lethal catatonia See *paralysis, catatonic cerebral.*

steady state In pharmacokinetics, the period during which daily elimination of drug equals the amount of drug ingested. Once the steady state is reached, plasma levels of the drug reflect the amount of drug available for biologic action.

steal, subclavian See *syndrome, subclavian steal.*

steatopygia, steatopygy (stē-à-tō-pī′jēà, stē-à-top′i-jē) Excessive fatness of the buttocks, a biological peculiarity observed among Hottentot and Bushman women.

Stedman, Charles H. (1805–66) American psychiatrist; one of "original thirteen" founders of Association of Medical Superintendents of America (forerunner of American Psychiatric Association).

Stekel, Wilhelm (1868–1940) German sexologist and psychoanalyst; advocated activity as a means to shorten the duration of treatment. Through sympathy and imaginative or intuitive insight the therapist alerts himself to the patient's repressed complexes and then is expected to intervene actively to make the patient aware of them.

stem, brain This refers to the *pons* (q.v.) and *medulla oblongata* (q.v.).

stema (stē′mà) *Obs.* Penis.

steppingstone theory The assumption that use of *gateway drugs* (such as alcohol and marihuana) predisposes to use and abuse of other classes of ("harder") drugs.

stereoencephalotomy Production of cortical or subcortical lesions through the use of the stereotaxic apparatus, which permits carefully controlled penetration of brain matter by the needle.

stereognosis The ability to judge the shape and form of an object by means of touch.

stereopsyche The primitive part of the mind that has to do with primitive types of motility. Storch applied this term to certain motor manifestations seen in schizophrenia: the catatonic postures and movements that seem to be isolated from the personality and to have a meaning independent of the rest of the psychic structure. These archaic types of motility arise from the deeper layers of the motor apparatus after the ego has disintegrated. They indicate an indistinct apperception of objects, indistinct ego boundaries, and a deep ambivalence toward reality objects in general. An example is the fetal position assumed by catatonics: this position suggests that at least certain motor manifestations in the catatonic are carryovers from the intrauterine period of existence.

stereotactic tractotomy See *tractotomy, stereotactic.*

stereotype An individual motor pattern that was originally meaningful to the subject and/or carried some private, autistic meaning for him. Stereotypes are thus to be distinguished from *primitive motor patterns* that are meaningless, inborn, or acquired very early in life, and that consist of simple movements or groups of simple movements.

stereotype, dynamic A term used mainly by Russian neurophysiologists to refer to the end result of cortical analysis and synthesis of all stimuli arising from both the external and the internal world. The dynamic stereotype represents a balanced, classified, and homogeneous arrangement of all the conditioned and unconditioned processes reflected in the cortex.

stereotyped movement disorders In DSM-III, a group of childhood disorders, about three times more frequent in boys than in girls, whose central feature is gross disturbance in motility manifested as recurrent, involuntary, rapid, purposeless movements (tics). Included are (1) *transient tic disorder*—typically, an eye blink or facial tic, exacerbated by stress but attenuated by absorption in some task and absent during sleep, persists less than 12 months; (2) *chronic motor tic disorder*—tics involving no more than three muscle groups at any one time; lasting more than 12 months (and usually for life); (3) *Tourette's disorder*—see *syndrome, Gilles de la Tourette; (4)* a miscellaneous group including head-banging and rocking.

In DSM-III-R, stereotypy/habit disorder is included among "Other Disorders of Infancy, Childhood, or Adolescence" and is separate from *tic disorders* (q.v.). It refers to repetitive, nonfunctional behaviors such as head-banging and rocking.

stereotypy A repeated movement that does not appear to be goal-directed, such as incessant rubbing of some part of the body; it is more complex than a tic.

The foregoing is often called *stereotypy of motion.* There is also *stereotypy of posture*, the patients maintaining a given posture for inordinately long periods. And there is *stereotypy of place;* catatonic patients may occupy an identical place month in, month out, year in, year out.

In Rorschach testing, stereotypy of responses suggests a lack of imagination, one of whose indicators is a high animal response percentage.

sterility The state or quality of being infertile or barren. This condition may be produced either by primary genetic disturbances in the sex chromosome constitution of an individual or by secondary effects on the phenotype, both of internal pathological processes and of surgical interference for medical or eugenic purposes. See *sterilization.*

The pathological processes disturbing the physiology of normal reproduction may affect (1) the sexual center in the hypothalamus, (2) the anterior pituitary gland with the follicle-stimulating and the luteinizing hormones, (3) the ovaries with the follicle and the corpus luteum hormones, and (4) the uterus. About 50 % of sterile women are reported by Wiesbader

to show evidence of endocrine disturbance, a form of sterility usually subdivided into the pituitary, ovarian, and hyperthyroid types. The Froehlich syndrome and Cushing's pituitary basophilism are the best known instances of the pituitary type of sterility.

sterilization Any process (brought about spontaneously or by deliberate action) that causes a person to become sterile.

When performed for medical reasons, it aims at rendering conception impossible, ordinarily without affecting the ovaries or testes. Accordingly it is not an "unsexing" operation, and neither inhibits sex desires nor interferes with normal sex functioning. In men it is the simple process of cutting and tying the vas deferens, while in women it requires an abdominal incision to tie the fallopian tubes.

Stevens-Johnson See *syndrome, Stevens-Johnson.*

Stewart-Morel syndrome See *syndrome, Stewart-Morel.*

STH Somatotrophic or growth hormone; one of the anterior pituitary hormones. See *syndrome, general adaptation.*

sthenia (sthē′-nē-à) In a general medical sense, strength and vigor.

sthenic In general medicine, strong and active. It is applied especially to morbid states with excessive action of the vital processes, as in sthenic fever or sthenic mental (delusional) reaction.

In constitutional medicine, the term is applicable in a general way to all types that correspond to Kretschmer's *athletic type* or its equivalents in other systems. It is even used by Mills for one of his three types. See *type, athletic.*

In general psychology, the term indicates strength and vigor in different fields of emotional reactivity and adaptability. In accordance with this concept, the psychopathological behavior of a sthenic type has been described by Kretschmer as inclined to delusional reactions of a predominantly aggressive nature (paranoia, querulous ideas of reference), in contrast to the introspective tendency of paranoid or hypochondriac reactions in sensitive types.

sthenoplastic In constitutional medicine, a type contrasted by Bounack with the *euryplastic,* and corresponding to the *asthenic* in Kretschmer's system and the *mi-*

crosplanchnic hypovegetative constitution of Pende.

stick, fecal Fecal mass. See *phase, anal.*

stigma, costal See *sign, Stiller's.*

stigmata Marks resembling the wounds on the crucified body of Christ. Most psychoanalytic writers consider these monosymptomatic conversions, the afflicted areas unconsciously symbolizing the genitals, the hyperemia and swelling representing erection, and abnormal sensations imitating genital sensations. The first person known to have experienced stigmata was St. Francis of Assisi; since that time, more than 300 cases have been reported, most of them in women.

stigmata, external See *insufficiency, segmental.*

stigmatization The process of labeling or branding, or the process of developing the signs or traits that appear to justify being labeled or branded or singled out. *Stigmata* (q.v.) originally denoted marks resembling the bleeding wounds, on the hands, feet, or chest, of the crucified body of Christ. They were generally assumed to be signs of Divine favor. Later, stigmata referred to similar marks produced exogenously by suggestion or hypnosis or endogenously as a form of conversion hysteria. Currently the term is used to signify indicators or pathognomonic signs of a disorder or syndrome. By extension, stigmatization has come to mean the labeling or branding of any person or group as being mentally disordered or abnormal, and the use of such labels as justification for discriminating against them.

Stiller's sign See *sign, Stiller's.*

stimulation See *activation.*

stimuli, accidental Among the four general types of dream stimuli—which are (1) external sensory; (2) internal sensory (subjective); (3) internal physical (organic); (4) psychic—the group of accidental stimuli belongs to the first type, external sensory. Accidental stimuli denote those chance happenings that take place in the environment of the sleeper and seemingly precipitate dreams or become part of them. For example, the backfire of an automobile passing in the street may emerge in the dream as the firing of a gun or as the "pop" of a champagne cork. The pain of muscles cramped by an awkward position during sleep may start a dream of being

hurt in that area of the body. An alarm clock ringing may be heard by the sleeper simultaneously dreaming of that very thing.

stimulus-bound Referring to difficulty in willed, intentional control of motor behavior. In the normal person, motor behavior is stimulus-resistant and can be controlled through thinking or reasoning despite the presence of distracting visual, tactile, or other stimuli. Stimulus-bound behavior, such as echopraxia or gegenhalten, suggests frontal lobe dysfunction.

stimulus, dream See *dream stimulus.*

stimulus-tension The tension produced by a stimulus. "But we have unquestioningly identified the pleasure-pain-principle with this Nirvana-principle. From this it would follow that every 'pain' coincides with a heightening, every pleasure with a lowering, of the stimulus-tension existing in the mind." (Freud, *CP*)

stimulus word The word used in association tests to provoke a response. See *association.*

stir fever See *psychosis, prison.*

stirps, stirpes Stem; stock; the person from whom a family is descended. In genetics, all the genes that are present in, and determine the development of, the fertilized egg.

STM Short-term *memory* (q.v.), often defined as recall of material presented to the subject up to 20 minutes prior to assessment. Recent reesearch suggests that short-term memory does not exceed three minutes.

STP A hallucinogenic drug that appears to be identical with DOM (2,5-dimethoxy-4-methylamphetamine); in low dosage (less than 3 mg), DOM produces mild euphoria, but in higher dosage it produces hallucinogenic effects that last for about 8 hours. Black market preparations of STP usually contain about 10 mg of DOM. The name is derived from a commercial gasoline additive (although some maintain it is an abbreviation for serenity-tranquility-peace).

STR The scientific-technical revolution, generally described as being based on the belief that science can be applied to all areas of life.

strabismus (stra-biz′mus) Squint; heterotropia; deviation of one or both eyes from the normal axis. See *nerve, oculomotor.*

straitjacket See *camisole.*

straitjacket, chemical *Rare.* The arresting of psychomotor overactivity by chemical means, specifically by the hypodermic injection of morphine sulfate, ¼ grain, and hyoscine hydrobromide, $^{1/50}$ grain.

Stransky, Erwin (1877–1962) Viennese neuropsychiatrist, pupil of Wagner von Jauregg; first to publish textbook in Germany on mental health; concept of intrapsychic ataxia, the dissociation of the thymopsyche from the noopsyche, as the essential characteristic of schizophrenia.

strategic compliance See *compliance, strategic.*

strategic family therapy See *family therapy, strategic.*

strategic intervention See *therapy, paradoxical.*

strategic planning Planning based on specified goals; planning geared to defining the tasks to be accomplished and assessing the need to continue those already being done. Strategic planning is opposed to *operational planning,* which is a control system geared to making sure that what is done is being done right; altering the resource commitment to programs that support the major goals of an organization in a planned way. See *budgeting, functional.*

Strauss syndrome See *impulse disorder, hyperkinetic.*

"street people" The homeless who live on the streets of mainly metropolitan centers. Many of them—but by no means all—give ample evidence of psychopathology, and a significant number of these are products of *deinstitutionalization* (q.v.). The group includes *bag ladies* (so called because they often carry all their worldly possessions in one or more paper shoppingbags) and *vent ment* (so called because in cold weather they typically sit on or sleep over vents or grates that might be sources of warmth).

strength, ego See *ego strength.*

strephosymbolia The perception of objects or graphic symbols reversed as if in a mirror. A term coined by Orton for the specific reading disability due, he believes, to poorly established hemisphere dominance, so that visual impressions coming to both hemispheres are not clearly differentiated, and symmetrical engrams oriented in opposite directions are confused, as *b* and *d*, *p* and *q*. See *impulse disorder, hyperkinetic.*

stress "Any interference which disturbs the functioning of the organism at any level, and which produces a situation which is natural for the organism to avoid." (Howard, L. *British Journal of Medical Psychology* 33, 1960) Definitions of stress fall into two groups, those emphasizing the noxious or aversive nature of the stimulus originating in the person's environment, and those emphasizing the physiologic responses of the subject to the noxious stimuli. Reactions to stress are typically manifested as disturbed psychologic and/or physiologic functioning; in psychiatry, they are seen most commonly when strong, involuntary, often unconscious internal impulses press for action that conflicts with the subject's conscious, reality-oriented behavior. See *holistic healing; syndrome, general adaptation.*

stress disorder See *post-traumatic stress disorder.*

stress, ego Broadly speaking, anything requiring adaptation maneuvers on the part of the ego, although usually the term implies that the strain is such as to require unusual defensive reactions. The stress itself may arise from the external world (the demands of reality), or from within (the pressure of the id for discharge and gratification of drives or superego demands). As stress increases so will defenses increase until there may result distortion or even alteration of the ego. Responses may vary from normal emergency reactions (phantasy, reaction-formation, etc.), to exaggerations of normal function (somatization), to partial withdrawal (depersonalization, dissociation), to transitory ego rupture (panic, oneiric episodes), to retreat with phantasies (psychoses), to complete disintegration (suicide).

stress interview A type of interview in which the patient is intentionally pressured, and the usual ways of reducing anxiety during the session are deliberately avoided. Such interviews may be useful in diagnosis, but their repeated use is generally contraindicated in the course of psychotherapy.

stressor, social See *event, life.*

Stribling, Francis T. (1810–74) American psychiatrist; advocated training of psychiatric attendants, occupational therapy.

stridor dentium *Obs.* Grinding of teeth. See *bruxism; bruxomania.*

striving, conative appetitive Striving in one particular direction, toward the particular goal appropriate for the gratification of the appetite involved. "The distinguishing feature of Freud's instinct theory is that it is based on a conative-appetitive-striving, rather than on a structural principle like sensation or reflex." (Kardiner, A., & Spiegel, H. *War Stress and Neurotic Illness*, 1947)

stroking See *transactional analysis*.

structural Pertaining to organization or arrangement. The *structural hypothesis* pertains to the description of the mental apparatus in terms of ego, superego, and *id* (q.v.). O. Kernberg emphasizes the importance of stability and continuity of the intrapsychic organization over time, particularly as reflected in the quality of object relations (identity integration vs. identity diffusion), defensive operations (advanced vs. primitive), and reality testing (presence vs. absence) in making a *structural diagnosis. Structural interviewing* uses elements of the traditional mental status examination combined with a focus on the here-and-now aspects of the patient-therapist interaction and on the patient's interpersonal functioning in general to arrive at an assessment of his intrapsychic organization.

structural imbalance See *imbalance, structural*.

structural integration *Rolfing* (q.v.).

structural profile In multimodal behavior therapy, the patient's self-rating of proclivities in each of the seven areas of the *BASIC-ID* (q.v.). The patient is asked to what extent he perceives himself as doing, feeling, sensing, imagining, thinking, and relating, and also to what extent he observes and practices health-promoting habits.

structure, character A relatively permanent constellation of habitual ways of reacting to the world, connoting only habitual attitudes developed as reactions to life situations; not to be confused with *temperament*.

"Character structure, as Freud saw it, is the result of sublimation or reaction formation. That is, it is formed unconsciously through the efforts of the Super-ego to bind the forces of the Id in such a way that the Ego accepts them, and its relation to the outside world is not jeopardized. It is, in effect, a defensive mechanism. Al-

though the result, sublimation, seems to be a positive attitude of the Ego, it is formed primarily as a defense against instincts. Freud's philosophy of character makes it the result of the transformation of instinctual drives." (Thompson, C. *Psychoanalysis, Evolution and Development*, 1950) See *character; defense, character*.

structure, mental The organization of the *psyche* (q.v.).

strychnomania See *poisoning, deadly nightshade*.

study groups See *Conferences, A.K. Rice Group Relations*.

study, Midtown See *Midtown study*.

study, natural Also known as *study in nature*, an investigation in which the researcher is a passive observer of the course of some natural process, such as disease. See *follow-through*.

stupemania Manic stupor. See *mania*.

stupor An imprecise term for (1) organically determined unconsciousness; (2) unresponsiveness with immobility and mutism but retention of consciousness, and often with open eyes that follow external objects; (3) mutism only.

stupor, affective See *stupor, emotional*.

stupor, akinetic *Cairns stupor* (q.v.).

stupor, anergic Stupor with immobility. As a rule patients showing the psychogenic stuporous reaction are inactive, immobile, anergic.

According to older concepts, *anergic stupor* was synonymous with *primary dementia* and *stuporous insanity*.

stupor, benign Depressive stupor, usually described as the most severe form of manic-depressive disorder, depressed type; termed benign in that it was believed to share the generally favorable prognosis of manic-depressive psychoses. Most such cases are in fact schizophrenic and in time show a more classical deteriorative course; they thus more appropriately should be termed *malignant stupors*.

stupor, Cairns See *Cairns stupor*.

stupor, catatonic See *schizophrenia, catatonic*.

stupor, depressive See *stupor, benign*.

stupor, diencephalic *Cairns stupor* (q.v.).

stupor, emotional Affective stupor; characterized by mutism and intense anxiety or depression.

stupor, examination When the affects are so strong as to bring thoughts and actions to a standstill, Bleuler speaks of *examination* or *emotional stupor*. See *anxiety, examination*.

stupor, exhaustive Stupor or coma as a result of infection or intoxication. See *psychosis, infective-exhaustive*.

stupor, malignant See *stupor, benign*.

stupor, manic See *mania*.

stupor vigilans *Obs.* Catalepsy (q.v.).

stuporous Relating to or under the influence of stupor; comatose or semicomatose.

Sturge-Weber-Dimitri's disease See *angiomatosis, trigeminal cerebral*.

stuttering A *speech disorder* (q.v.) of childhood, consisting of a spasmodic utterance with involuntary halts, breaks, and repetitions, usually characterized (in more severe cases) externally by sputtering due to violent expulsion of breath following a halt or stop. For the sake of convenience, stuttering denotes a visually more violent or explosive form of stammering.

Other terms by which stuttering has been known are ischnophonia, ischophonia, psellism, and psallismus hesitans.

Any sound, in any position, any part of a word and any word may be the obstacle in stuttering, varying with the individual stutter or the severity of the symptom.

Some authorities hold that stuttering is the result of an organic brain disease or physiological defect, but that is still a moot question. The first hesitations and halts in a child's speech are as normal as the missteps, stumbles, and falls in the child's earliest attempts in walking, due to lack of coordination and control of the walking mechanism, which in comparison with the speech mechanism is as simple as that of a wheelbarrow by the side of a delicate watch movement. The staggering burden on the child's powers to reproduce the movements of speech organs (many of them concealed from his view within the other people's mouths) can be surmised from the exertions adults have to make in learning the sounds of a new language even from a teacher with aid of diagrams, illustrations, and mirrors.

Whether originating in a physiological disorder or not, in its subsequent stages, the symptom is predominantly a psychic condition that causes shrinking from speaking through fear of not succeeding; the remedy of *relaxation* (to reduce or entirely do away with the nervous and muscular tension) has worked nearly always in the various institutions for curing stuttering.

"Of the initial stage of speech development, the mental process is in advance of the powers of muscular control, and the resulting lack of muscular coordination often produces a *temporary stammer [stutter]*. If the child is worried and nervous during this period of adjustment, he will become conscious of his speech and of the difficulties surrounding its acquisition, and at once the second stage is reached—that of fear or dread of speech—unconscious probably, but none the less potent." (Boome, E.J., Baines, H.M.S., & Harries, D.G. *Abnormal Speech*, 1939)

Stuttering is seen in about 1% of the population and usually appears between the ages of 2 and 6 years. It occurs more frequently in males, in twins, and in those who are left-handed. It is rarely seen among diabetics and it is most uncommon among primitive peoples.

From the psychoanalytic point of view, stuttering is regarded as due in most instances to displacement of anal libido onto the throat and mouth and onto the act of word-forming. The anal-sadistic stutterer equates words with feces, and the expulsion or retention of words means the expulsion or retention of feces. Further, words acquire the same omnipotence they had in the infantile stage; "words can kill" and the stutterer is constantly anxious about using so dangerous a weapon. While anal sadism forms the core of the problem, other component instincts typically contribute to the symptom. Phallic impulses, for example, often lead to an equation of speaking ability with potency and of disability with castration.

stygiophobia Fear of hell; hadephobia.

style, cognitive *Cognitive control;* the characteristic way in which a person organizes environmental stimuli, relates such information to other perceptions, ideas, and memories, and translates that information into a potential response. *Cognitive psychology* and in particular *cognitive personality theory* are concerned with how different cognitive styles develop in different people, and with how the different models of reality that people have affect their behavior. One of the major differences between Piaget's theories and Freudian theories of personality is the former's emphasis on formal thinking and cognitive maturation (rather than instinctual needs or affective states) as determinants of identity formation and the development of autonomy. See *therapy, cognitive.*

Information processing approaches view the person as a complex information processing system and use computer technology (such as artificial intelligence) to build models of human cognitive processes. Such *cognitive science* seeks to understand how symbols are recognized, how memories are retrieved, how learning develops, how problems are solved, etc. See *intelligence, artificial.*

style, life See *constancy.*

style, perceptual The way in which a person attends to, alters, and shapes the sensory stimuli that bombard him. Some workers have found that schizophrenics have an altered, unusual, or abnormal perceptual function.

stylistics See *psycholinguistics.*

subacute combined degeneration of the spinal cord See *sclerosis, posterolateral.*

subacute delirious state See *delirium, subacute; subdelirious state.*

subaffective spectrum See *spectrum, subaffective.*

subception Autonomic response to a stimulus, which is not consciously recognized by the subject.

subclavian steal See *syndrome, subclavian steal.*

subconsciousness 1. Partial unconsciousness. 2. The state in which mental processes take place without conscious perception on the subject's part.

subcortical dementia See *dementia, subcortical; dysmentia, tardive.*

subcortical encephalopathy (en-sef-a-lop′ă-thē) See *sclerosis, diffuse.*

subdelirious state, subdelirium The prodromata of a full-blown delirium: restlessness, headache, oversensitiveness to auditory and visual stimuli, irritability, lability of emotions.

The term *subacute delirious state* is applied to "a syndrome in which incoherence of thought, speech and movement appear together with perplexity, in a setting of clouding of consciousness, fluctuating in degree. The state may follow a typical delirium or appear independently. It may

persist over a considerable period, weeks or months, outlasting the signs of the underlying physical illness, but always ending in recovery." (Mayer-Gross, W., et al. *Clinical Psychiatry,* 1960)

subject homoerotic See *homosexuality, male.*

subject-ill The subject-ill patient uses his own body to symbolize his emotions. This is achieved through somatization, which constitutes an organic language of the mind. See *somatization.*

In opposition to this type, Stekel calls object-ill the patient who is the victim of compulsions and expresses his emotions through symbolization of objects outside his body—usually a close member of the family.

"The 'subject-ill' makes efforts to extravert himself in order to adjust himself to the world; the 'object-ill,' however, is introverted and makes no attempts at extraversion." (Stekel, *CD*)

subject system See *complex, systematized.*

subjective mentation *Autism* (q.v.).

sublimate To externalize or objectivate instinctual impulses in ways that meet the situation. To sublimate is to refine, to purify instinctual manifestations. The instincts are not changed; their mode of expression is altered.

sublimation In psychoanalytic psychology, the process of modifying an instinctual impulse in such a way as to conform to the demands of society. Sublimation is a substitute activity that gives some measure of gratification to the infantile impulse that has been repudiated in its original form. Sublimation is an unconscious process and is a function of the normal ego. It is not technically a defense mechanism, for unlike the latter it does not lead to any restriction or inhibition or ego functioning by requiring a constant countercathexis; rather, the impulse or wish is modified in such a way that gratification can be achieved without disapprobation or disapproval. Unlike the usual defenses, in sublimation the ego is not acting in opposition to the id; on the contrary, it is helping the id to gain external expression. Sublimation, in other words, does not involve repression. It is to be noted that the original impulse is never conscious in sublimation.

To put it another way, sublimation is a

form of *desexualization* (q.v.) in which the instinctive impulses, instead of requiring control by constant countercathexis, are deflected (by means of identification, displacement, and substitution) into acceptable channels. The aim or object (or both) of the drive is changed without blocking an adequate discharge. It seems likely that sublimation is intimately related to *identification* (q.v.), for both depend upon the presence of models and upon incentives supplied directly or indirectly by the environment.

subliminal fringe See *summation.*

submania Hypomania. See *mania.*

submissiveness, submission Passivity, acceptance, especially as contrasted with *ascendance* (q.v.) or dominance.

subpsyche A term introduced by Bumke as synonymous with unconscious life.

subshock See *treatment, ambulatory insulin.*

substance abuse and dependence disorders See *psychoactive substance dependence.*

substance-induced syndromes See *psychoactive substance-induced organic mental disorders.*

substance P See *peptide, brain.*

substantia nigra See *midbrain.*

substantial comorbidity See *comorbidity.*

substitute See *surrogate.*

substitute, displacement The affect, idea, object, etc., onto which the original affect or impulse is displaced. See *displacement.*

substitute formation Symptom-formation; the tendency of repressed impulses to use any opportunity for indirect discharge. The energy of the warded-off instinct is displaced to any other impulse that is associatively connected with the repressed one, and the intensity of this substitute impulse is increased and often, in addition, the affect connected with it is changed in quality. Such substitute impulses are known as *derivatives;* most neurotic symptoms are derivatives.

substitute, regressive Displacing the unconscious sexual aim or object in the course of psychosexual development to a chronologically earlier one from which pleasure was derived.

In describing a patient with a phantasy of being beaten by the father, Freud states that "it is not only the punishment for the forbidden genital relation [*incest*], but also the *regressive substitute* for it." (*CP*)

substitution neurosis *Obs. Obsessive-compulsive psychoneurosis* (q.v.).

subthalamus That portion of the brain bounded by the dorsal thalamus anteriorly, the tegmentum of the midbrain posteriorly, the hypothalamus medially, and the internal capsule laterally. The subthalamus contains the rostral extensions of the red nucleus and substantia nigra from the midbrain, the fields of Forel (which are probably a rostral extension of reticular nuclei), and the subthalamic nucleus (*body of Luys*). The last is functionally connected with the globus pallidus.

subwaking Being or held in a state intermediate between sleeping and waking; hypnoidal.

success, failure through A term used by Freud to describe the self-injuring conduct of those who, on the verge of achieving a long-desired aim, renounce it, obtaining gratification through its renunciation. Examples are "the clinical assistant who for so long desired to become professor and renounced the position on his predecessor's sudden death," or "the girl who withdrew from the beloved man at the sudden death of his wife, her rival." It is a moral veto. The fact is that at such a moment the force of conscience prevents the enjoyment, and even the acceptance, of success. The moral veto can enforce itself in different ways. "A young man who has been dependent on an uncommonly thrifty, rich father, is suddenly notified that his father had died from apoplexy. He is the only heir. A few hours later he is so clumsy when driving his car that he perishes in an accident." In a less spectacular reaction, this young man could have wasted his heritage, or he could have acquired a severe neurosis. It seems that this moral veto, with its reaction of renunciation, occurs only when it is preceded by a period of phantasy that anticipates the misfortune or the death of the rival. (Reik, T. *Masochism in Modern Man,* 1941) See *destiny, neurosis of; masochism; obedience, deferred.*

successive approximations See *practice, reinforced.*

succinylcholine A muscle relaxant, usually administered intravenously; in psychiatry, used in association with electroconvulsive treatment to prevent or minimize the occurrence of bone fractures.

succubus (suk'u-bus) Demon or witch; specifically, a female demon who has sexual intercourse with men during their sleep. See *incubus*.

sucking, thumb The earliest and one of the most common manipulations of the body found in young children. In some children, it is observed at birth, to continue on through infancy and early childhood, when it becomes an undesirable habit and is classified as a neurotic trait. During the first months of life, thumb sucking is a physiological and common, but not universal, characteristic of the infant. With the waning of the hand-to-mouth reaction phase, which takes place at about 12 months of age, according to Gesell, the habit ceases. Even past the age of 12 months and on through 3 and 4 years (2 years according to Kanner) it is considered normal when recurring before nap, sleep, or at times of fatigue or emotional stress. Thumb sucking is accompanied by movements and positions of the free hand, as well as the remaining fingers of the sucked thumb hand, which are characteristic of and constant for the individual child, the so-called accessory movements. (Levy, D.M. *American Journal of Psychiatry 7,* 1928) According to Levy, thumb sucking occurs in children with insufficient lip movements or incompleteness of the sucking phase of earlier feeding, breast or other type.

The psychoanalytic school considers thumb sucking an autoerotic gratification, as an expression of infantile sexual cravings, the oral erogenic zone being in this case the level of stimulation and gratification.

suckling, eternal Freud's term for that type of person who throughout life feels he or she should be cared for, protected, and supported by someone else.

suffocatio hysterica Hysterical suffocation; hysterical spasm of the muscles of the throat; often seen as part of the symptom picture in *globus hystericus* (q.v.). Like the latter, suffocatio hysterica is often based on the unconscious rejection of incorporation phantasies of a sexual and/or aggressive nature.

suggestibility The state, quality, or ability of being influenced by *suggestion* (q.v.). *Negative suggestibility* is doing the opposite of

what is suggested to the patient. See *schizophrenia, catatonic*.

suggestion The process of influencing a person to the point of uncritical acceptance of an idea, belief, or other cognitive process. Some would differentiate between heterosuggestion (when the source of the idea is someone outside the person) and autosuggestion (when the source of the idea is the subject himself, as when he keeps saying to himself that he is getting better and better every day, perhaps in hopes that he will one day come to believe his own statement).

While suggestion does not afford a complete explanation of hypnosis, it is obvious that it plays a large part in it, in that the subject comes to accept the hypnotist's repeated suggestions that he is becoming drowsy and soon finds that this is so. This is even more clear with posthypnotic suggestion, when the subject will carry out some action that has been proposed to him during the trance state.

The psychoanalytic method is a modification of hypnosis, and, like the latter, depends upon suggestion in the force of influencing "a person through and by means of the transference-manifestations of which he is capable." (Freud, *CP*) See *conditioning, operant*.

Prestige suggestion is another form of psychotherapy; unlike psychoanalysis, however, it does not attempt to uncover or deal with the unconscious determinants of behavior. Its efficacy is chiefly dependent upon gratification of the patient's security needs; the patient submits to and identifies with the omnipotent authority (the therapist) and gives up his symptoms as part of his obedience to the therapist.

suggestion, affective See *hypotaxia*.

suggestion, posthypnotic Suggestion given during the hypnotic stage to be acted upon after the hypnotic phase has passed.

suggestion, prestige A form of supportive psychotherapy in which the therapist, because he occupies a position of omnipotence in the eyes of the patient, is able to dictate the disappearance of symptoms. "The motivation to comply is usually conditioned by a wish to gratify important security needs through archaic mechanisms of submission to and identification with an omnipotent authority." (Wolberg, L.R. *The Technique of Psychotherapy*, 1954) Prestige suggestion is probably the least successful of all treatment methods.

suggestion, verbal See *ideoplasty*.

suggestive In psychiatry this usually relates to hypnotic suggestion; thus one speaks of hypnotic or suggestive therapeutics.

suicide The act of killing oneself. Suicide is the tenth leading cause of death in the United States, accounting for at least 1% of all deaths (in numbers, somewhere between 30,000 and 100,000 per year). For every death from suicide ("successful suicide") there are eight other attempts. More people die from suicide each year than from homicide.

The official rate has remained at 10 to 12 per 100,000 per year since 1945, but statistics on suicide are notoriously unreliable. Some researchers believe that a high rate reflects a high rate of autopsies and toxicological examination; whether it is recorded as suicide may also depend on age, sex, race, social class, and other factors.

The highest rates of suicide occur in German-speaking countries. Austria, which has the highest official rate in the world, is followed by Switzerland, the Scandinavian countries, eastern Europe, and Japan. There is a relatively low rate in Spain, Italy, and the Netherlands. The official rate in the United States is about average for industrialized countries.

In 1980 in the United States, white males accounted for 70% of all suicides. That year, the median age of suicides dropped from 47 years to under 40 years. Even so, it is still true that incidence of suicide is highest in old age. Among the elderly, males may account for as many as 90% of suicides. Persons over 60 years of age constitute 20% of the population but contribute 40% of the suicides. Among people 75 years of age and older, the annual rate is three times the average.

Suicide is rising in the younger population. In the age range of 15 to 25 years, suicide is the third leading cause of death. In 1961, the rate in this age group was 5 per 100,000; the incidence peaked in 1977 at 13.3 per 100,000, and in 1984 it was 12.5 per 100,000 (a total of 5,026 suicides).

As in previous years, females remain more likely than males to attempt suicide, but males are more likely to succeed.

As compared with the 150% increase in suicides in the 15- to 25-year-old group as a whole, the suicide rate in the 15- to 19-year-old subgroup has tripled since 1950. Every day, 18 teenagers kill themselves; every hour, 57 children and teenagers attempt suicide.

In the 25- to 35-year-old age group, there has been an overall increase of 30% in the same period (although among females in this cohort the rate dropped by 20%).

Overall, blacks have a lower suicide rate than whites. Even so, young black men (20 to 35 years of age) have a rate double that of young white men. Native Americans have a higher suicide rate than whites at all ages.

In at least 90% of suicides, there is an associated mental or emotional disorder: depression (although this is not the leading factor in the mounting number of suicides in young white males), alcoholism, drug abuse (a significant factor in over half of suicides in the young, where the pattern is typically one of chronic use of multiple drugs), and schizophrenia.

Depression accounts for suicide in approximately 30 to 70% of cases (suicide accounts for 15% of all deaths among patients with mood disorders), alcoholism for 15 to 25% (the lifetime prevalence of suicide among alcoholics is about 10%, ten times the average). Suicide rate among drug abusers is at least five times the average. Schizophrenics also have a high suicide rate: over 20% attempt it, and 10% eventually succeed.

It is a common misconception that the patient who threatens suicide is not likely to commit suicide. The reverse is probably closer to the truth, for about 75% of successful suicides had previously threatened or attempted it. Typically, the genuinely suicidal patient departs with a surge of hatred for the world and pejorative accusations of the self, leaving definite instructions and restrictions for those he has purposely deserted. Among the clinical depressions, those with prominent anxiety features, a feeling of losing ground, and/or a marked hypochondriacal trend are the most likely to make a suicide attempt.

Among schizophrenics, suicide is most likely in the young, unemployed male with no family who has had many relapses requiring repeated hospitalization. The greatest danger is during a relapse, in the first six months of hospital stay, when he is let out of hospital on a pass, and just after discharge.

People who have never married are twice as likely to commit suicide; the divorced and widowed have the highest rates of all. High unemployment increases suicide rates. Physicians have a higher than average rate, and the rate in psychiatrists is higher than other physicians. Among physicians, women have a higher rate than men.

Psychodynamically, suicide or a suicide attempt is seen most frequently to be an aggressive attack directed against a loved one or against society in general; in others, it may be a misguided bid for attention or it may be conceived of as a means of effecting reunion with the ideal love object or mother. That suicide is in one sense a means of release for aggressive impulses is supported by the change of wartime suicide rates. In World War II, for example, rates among the participating nations fell, sometimes by as much as 30%; but in neutral countries, the rates remained the same.

In depressions, the following dynamic elements are often clearly operative: the depressed patient loses the object that he depends upon for narcissistic supplies; in an attempt to force the object's return, he regresses to the oral stage and incorporates (swallows up) the object, thus regressively identifying with the object: the sadism originally directed against the deserting object is taken up by the patient's superego and is directed against the incorporated object, which now lodges within the ego; suicide occurs, not so much as an attempt on the ego's part to escape the inexorable demands of the superego, but rather as an enraged attack on the incorporated object in retaliation for its having deserted the patient in the first place.

suicide, anomic See *anomie.*

suicide, attempted Uncompleted suicide, survival following an apparently suicidal act. Some writers prefer the terms *deliberate self-poisoning, deliberate self-injury, deliberate self-harm,* or *parasuicide* to indicate that the behavior was not accidental while making no assumption about the presence of a desire for death. See *syndrome, deliberate self-harm.*

suicide, focal See *syndrome, deliberate self-harm.*

suicide pact An agreement or pledge of two (rarely more) people to take their own lives at the same time. It is estimated that suicide pacts account for 1 in 300 completed suicides, and that there are twice as many uncompleted suicide pacts as completed ones.

suicide, psychic The killing of one's self without resorting to any physical agency; used in reference to those who make up their minds to die and actually do so. It is presumed that the same forces that lead a person to commit physical suicide are active in psychic suicide cases, but that, instead of operating overtly, these forces work endopsychically.

suicidogenic Pertaining to suicidogenesis; causing suicide.

suigenderism (sū-i-jen'dĕr-iz'm) The natural drift on a child's part to associate or group with others of his own *gender.* During latency the activities of boys are largely confined to boys, while those of girls are mainly limited to girls. For the manifestation of these natural, unerotic relationships between members of one's own gender, the term *suigenderism* is recommended. When sex feelings begin to crop up in suigenderism, it may become *homoerotism, homosexuality,* or *homogenitality* (qq.v.).

Sullivan, Harry Stack (1892–1949) The chief proponent of the so-called dynamic-cultural school of psychoanalysis, which emphasizes sociologic rather than biologic events, present-day contacts with people rather than past experiences, current interpersonal relationships rather than infantile sexuality. Orthodox Freudians consider this a superficial approach that is limited to a single facet of experience, the cultural.

summation An accumulation of elements that individually produce no discernible effects, but whose aggregation results in pathologic changes and/or an overreaction to minor stimuli. According to Freud, "Persons who tolerate coitus interruptus apparently without harmful results are in reality becoming thereby disposed to the disorder of anxiety neurosis, which may break out either at any time spontaneously or after an ordinary and otherwise insufficient trauma." (*CP*)

In neurophysiology, summation refers to a response obtained when two stimuli are applied, neither of which by itself is of sufficient intensity to elicit a response. In this sense, there are two types of summation, temporal and spatial. *Temporal summation* is seen when two successive stimuli, each of them too weak to elicit a response, are applied to the same nerve trunk within 0.1 to 0.5 msec of each other, in which case a response will be evoked because of the enduring character of the local excitatory process. *Spatial summation* is seen when two different afferent nerves, which play upon the same reflex center, are stimulated either simultaneously or within a short interval (not more than 15 msec); a response is evolved even though neither stimulus alone will elicit a response. Spatial summation is believed to be a result of additive excitatory alterations in the neurons involved. Sherrington and his associates refer to this excitatory alteration as the central excitatory state, which is often abbreviated as c.e.s. The nerves affected are said to be in the *subliminal fringe* of excitation.

summation, spatial See *summation.*

summation, temporal See *summation.*

sundowner The older person whose mental functioning is adequate during the day but at night is impaired by confusion and agitation; also known as deliriant *confusion*. See *syndrome, organic.*

superego In psychoanalytic psychology, there are three functional divisions of the psyche: the id, the ego, and the superego. The superego is the last of these to be differentiated. It is the representative of society within the psyche (i.e. *conscience* or morality) and also includes the ideal aspirations (*ego-ideal*). The superego is mainly unconscious; its functions include (1) approval or disapproval of the ego's actions, i.e. judgment that an act is "right" or "wrong"; (2) critical self-observation; (3) self-punishment; (4) demands that the ego repent or make reparation for wrongdoing; (5) self-love or *self-esteem* as the ego reward for having done right.

In general, the superego may be regarded as a split-off portion of the ego that arises on the basis of identification with certain aspects of the introjected parents. Since introjection and identification are among the earliest defense mechanisms to appear, it is obvious that the precursors of the superego are in evidence early in life, in the prephallic or preoedipal phase. Such precursors consist mainly of the various effects that the demands and prohibitions of the parents (and their surrogates) have on the child, and these are particularly evident in regard to bowel training (and thus Ferenczi's term, *sphincter morality*). Yet until the oedipal phase, the superego does not make itself felt as a disturbance of the harmonious accord between the strivings of the ego and the strivings of the id. Morality in the young child, such as it is, is more a response to immediate external demands of the environment than obedience to an inner authority. It is only with the oedipal phase that the superego begins to take its final form as an internal authority that stands between ego and id, compelling the child on his own to renounce certain pleasures, and imposing punishment (loss of self-esteem, guilt feelings, etc.) for violations of its orders. The superego develops as a reaction to the Oedipus complex; as is often said, it is the *heir of the Oedipus complex*. It is a solution to the impulses of this period that have no prospect of succeeding in reality and that, if allowed to continue unchanged, would have been dangerous. These impulses, deriving from the id, are allowed access to the ego; the forbidden impulses (love for the mother, hatred of the father) are withdrawn from their objects and deposited in the ego, which thus becomes changed. The changed portion of the ego is the superego, and it contains the sadism originally directed against the father; so also does it contain the love originally felt for the mother, but the very process of introjecting the mother and changing the libido attached to the maternal object into ego libido has resulted in desexualization. Thus the love portion of the superego (the ego-ideal) is a nonsensual love.

What has happened, in short, is that the frustrations of the Oedipus complex have caused the ego to resort to primitive methods of defense: introjection and identification. As a result, the oedipal objects are regressively replaced by identifications, and sexual longing for the maternal object has been replaced by an asexual alteration within the organization of the ego. These newly introjected objects, which replace the sexual and hostile impulses toward the parents, combine with the parental introjects from the prephallic period (internalized parental prohibitions), and the superego is formed.

In practice it is difficult to differentiate sharply between the superego, which is an image of the hated and feared objects, and the ego-ideal, which is an image of the loved objects in the libido. "The ego ideal seems to contain more maternal libido, the superego, more of the paternal; in reality both are fused. Furthermore, just as there are some destructive elements to be found within the ego ideal because the libido is desexualized, there are also libidinal forces at work in the formation of the superego, since it develops through identification with the ambivalently loved father. The predominantly maternal ego ideal starts to develop as early as the pregenital stages, but the predominantly paternal superego is observed first in the genital stage. The impetus for the formation of the superego is the danger of castration, a danger that threatens the entire ego in consequence of its identification with the genitals. By taking the father into his ego, the boy not only escapes the danger of castration but also gains a protector in the image of the father absorbed by the ego." (Nunberg, H. *Principles of Psychoanalysis*, 1955)

Melanie Klein and her followers believe that the superego begins to function much earlier than Freud (and most psychoanalysts since him) believed. "Where I differ is in placing at birth the processes of introjection which are the basis of the superego. The superego precedes by some months the beginning of the Oedipus complex, a beginning which I date, together with that of the depressive position, in the second quarter of the first year. Thus the early introjection of the good and bad breast is the foundation of the superego and influences the development of the Oedipus complex. This conception of superego formation is in contrast to Freud's explicit statements that the identifications with the parents are the heir of the Oedipus complex and only succeed if the Oedipus complex is successfully overcome." (*International Journal of Psychoanalysis 39*, 1958)

superego, autonomous The normal superego, which demands that the ego behave in a "good" way, in contrast to a heteronomous superego, which demands that the ego behave in accordance with what is expected. The heteronomous superego is a possible outcome of inconsistent handling of a child by his parents. The inconsistency makes it impossible for him to foresee what particular conduct might ensure continued affection from the parents; the child consequently renounces attempts to differentiate between good and bad, and instead responds only to the demand of the moment.

superego, double The double conscience sometimes seen in *psychic dualism*. The two consciences, or superegos, are usually antagonistic and regard each other vigilantly and belligerently. One conscience is usually considered masculine, the other feminine. Oberndorf cites the case of a male physician as an illustration of double superego. The patient's courtesy, conscientiousness, and consideration for others was often exaggerated to the point of masochistic subservience. The patient complained of depression secondary to the constant criticism which he underwent at the hands of his second superego. This second conscience, which never agreed with his masculine conscience, was traced to the story of the Dybbuk he had heard from his mother. In the story, the Dybbuk is the disembodied spirit of a wicked person which can reach heaven only after purification by entering the body of a young, virtuous girl. Thus the second conscience, which required almost absolute goodness, was viewed as feminine, and the patient's goodness became almost synonymous with femininity.

superego, group S.R. Slavson differentiates between the group superego and the infantile superego. (*IGT*) He considers that this superego is an outcome of the adaptations to and experiences with various groups of people beyond the relationship with parents.

superego, heteronomous See *autonomy-heteronomy*. A special type of superego which demands of the ego that it behave according to what is expected at the moment. A person with such a superego is irresolute and weak, for his behavior at any given moment is controlled by the desire to secure the approval of those about him; and he is likewise in constant fear of being criticized or punished—i.e. he has "social anxiety." This is in contrast to the normal type of superego, which demands only that the ego behave in a "good" way, according to a certain set of standards or ideals. Here the person goes by rule of thumb and is thus free of constant fear of criticism; he can come to decisions and carry out behavior independently of the approval or disapproval at the moment.

The heteronomous superego arose, for example, "when the parents had shown so inconsistent a behavior that it became impossible for the child to foresee what conduct on his part would be most likely to ensure the continuance of their affection; whereupon, renouncing all attempts to distinguish between good and bad, he would take his bearings according to the demand of the moment." (Fenichel, *PTN*)

superego, parasites of the Ideals and values absorbed by the person "which usurp the functions of the super-ego." After one has entered the latency period, ideals usually continue to undergo modification. As the emotional ties to the family begin to loosen, becoming less intense, one's standards become more independent of the infantile models based upon the parents. Other persons or ideas begin to serve as models. These become part of the original superego which was formed at an earlier age from the parents' attitudes and activities. When the new ideals are only "a slight modification of old ideals, the situation is not difficult . . . Sometimes, however, internal or external situations may create parasites of the superego which usurp the functions of the superego for a varying length of time." Even though the later identifications with authorities other than the parent are usually superficial, they may be very influential. An example of a parasitic superego is the influence of mass suggestion. A person with a normal superego may, under mass suggestion, yield to impulses which would normally be suppressed and yet show no guilt-feelings: "Individuals acting as a group . . . (or mob) . . . are capable of instinctual outbreaks that would be entirely impossible for them as individuals."

Another example of a parasitic superego occurs under hypnosis, when the hypnotist takes over the functions of the patient's superego. In the patient's psyche the hypnotist acts as a parasitic superego. "As such he tries to undo the previous work of the super-ego that gave rise to the defensive struggle." (Fenichel, *PTN*)

superego, parasitic A temporarily coexisting body of commands that conflict with the subject's own superego standards, such as internalizations of the leader's exhortation to kill during wartime.

superego, primitive A superego that exists apart from the parental superego and is older in origin than the force established by parents and teachers. The primitive superego is assumed to be hereditary and susceptible to the influence of hereditary factors in contrast to the parental superego, which reflects tradition.

superfemale Metafemale; a female with a sex chromosome pattern of XXX (instead of the normal XX). Rather than being more "female" than the normal, however, such women are amenorrheic, sterile, and have underdeveloped female sexual characteristics. See *chromosome*.

supergene A type of variation of hereditary traits caused by chromosomal rearrangement; such a mutation affects an entire section of a chromosome but simulates the single factor type of inheritance (which is produced by one major mutant gene).

superior paraplegia See *paraplegia*.

superiority strivings See *psychology, individual*.

supermoron A person slightly subnormal mentally, but in a grade above that of a moron.

superordinated See *ego* (Jung's definition).

supersex A sexually abnormal type of sterile organism, first observed by Bridges, which shows intersexual features owing to the disturbed ratio of autosomes to heterosomes.

Supersexual individuals are either *"superfemales"* characterized by three X chromosomes and two sets of autosomes or *"supermales"* with one X chromosome and three sets of autosomes.

superstition An irrational belief in magic, chance, etc., or an exaggerated fear of the unknown. See *delusion.*

supervalent Referring to the excessive intensity of an idea that the subject cannot rid himself of; the intensity results from the multiple unconscious determinants of the idea, and/or from the need to keep the idea as a screen for a reverse or contrary thought. See *reaction formation.*

supervision In psychiatry, the critical evaluation by an experienced therapist of the clinical work of a therapist in training.

support See *psychotherapy.*

suppression The act of consciously inhibiting an impulse, affect, or idea, as in the deliberate attempt to forget something and think no more about it. Suppression is thus to be differentiated from *repression* (q.v.), which is an unconscious process. It is probable that there is no sharp line of demarcation between suppression and repression, and it seems also likely that on occasion the unconscious defense of repression may be directed against material which the individual consciously suppresses. Nonetheless, it seems advisable in most instances to regard suppression and repression as distinctly different mechanisms.

suppression neurosis See *neurosis, suppression.*

supraindividuals See *collective unconscious.*

supramarginal gyrus See *lobe, parietal.*

supramolecular receptor complex See *receptor complex, supramolecular.*

supranuclear palsy *Steele-Richardson-Olszewski syndrome;* a subcortical dementia characterized by progressive supranuclear paralysis of extraocular movements, dysarthria, pseudobulbar palsy, and dystonic rigidity of the neck and trunk. Underlying the clinical dementia is an impaired ability to manipulate acquired knowledge, even though if given enough time the patient may show that he retains verbal and perceptual motor capacities. The pathological changes include cell loss, neurofibrillary alterations, gliosis, and demyelination in the basal ganglia, brain stem, and cerebellum. The cortex is usually normal.

suprarenalism (su-pra-ren'al-iz'm) Overactivity of the suprarenal glands.

surface-ego "Freud conceives the ego as essentially a 'surface-ego,' that is to say, one which in its principal function is directed toward the outside world whose stimuli it receives or wards off. It is therefore more readily able to assimilate a piece of knowledge presented to it from without than one which proceeds from within the psychic apparatus." (Sachs, H. *International Journal of Psychoanalysis VI,* 1925)

surface imaging See *NMR.*

surrender, schizophrenic A term used by C. MacFie Campbell to characterize the type of schizophrenia in which the mechanism is one of passive repression without initial anxiety or any conspicuous restitutional attempts.

The symptoms of schizophrenia can be divided into two major groups: (1) the regressive symptoms and (2) the restitutional symptoms. The first category comprises those symptoms that are a direct expression of the regressive breakdown of the ego and an undoing of differentiations acquired through mental development. Some examples are phantasies of world destruction, feelings of depersonalization, delusions of grandeur, and physical sensations. In the second category are those symptoms that express the schizophrenic's attempt to regain the lost objective world; hallucinations, delusions of persecution, and some catatonic symptoms are in this category.

Hebephrenia is the purely regressive type of schizophrenia in which there are no restitutional or defensive attempts. The ego takes refuge in successively older types of adaptation, finally arriving at a vegetative existence and perhaps even intrauterine attitudes. The loss of the objective world and of any interest in it has become complete. The patient has undergone a "schizophrenic surrender." (Fenichel, *PTN*)

surrender, will to The psychic process through which the neurotic patient comes to the point of giving up his neurosis: a renunciating mental attitude through which the patient expresses his desire to submit to the analyst's aim of curing the illness. At the beginning of his psychotherapy, the patient's only aim seems to be a desire to protect and cherish his illness in defiance of the doctor's therapeutical endeavor. It is only through the development of the will to surrender that the patient is ready to renounce his neurosis.

According to Stekel, a positive transference during analysis is a manifestation of this will to surrender. This desire is the opposite of the patient's "will to power," which is the expression of the patient's wish to master the analyst by love and attention, and defend his neurosis by so doing. (ID)

surrogate One who takes the place of another is a surrogate or substitute. From the standpoint of instinctual psychology, during growth, affective states originally expressed toward the parents are normally transferred from them to others who stand for them. Thus a sister may be the first mother surrogate, later a teacher, still later the mother of a friend, and finally a lover. With each new surrogate there is normally less and less resemblance to the original (mother). See *surrogate, mother.*

surrogate, father See *surrogate, mother.*

surrogate, human Euphemism for corpse or for a portion of a dead body.

surrogate, mother 1. *Mother substitute;* one who takes the place of the mother. The female schoolteacher, for instance, takes over part of the care of the child; she becomes a mother surrogate.

The same concepts hold true with regard to the father: hence the expressions *father surrogate* and *father substitute.*

2. Surrogate mother or *host mother* also refers to the woman who agrees to be inseminated artificially with the sperm of the husband of an infertile woman, to carry the fetus so conceived to term, and to relinquish all parental rights to that child once it is born, typically by giving it back to the couple for adoption. (The phrase "new reproductive technology" is currently preferred to "surrogate motherhood.")

survival skills workshop See *psychoeducation.*

survivor syndrome See *syndrome, survivor.*

suspenopsia Suspension of sight. A tendency for the image arising in either eye to be entirely disregarded for a short period of time so that the subject is using one eye only for the time being.

sustaining cause, distinct Any recognizable or discrete determiner, of particular relevance in differentiating between an environmental condition that causes discomfort and an illness or malady that causes discomfort. Profuse sweating on a hot and humid day is not an illness, although the same discomfort and observable signs would constitute a malady or illness or disorder in the absence of such a distinct sustaining cause as high environmental temperature. See *disease.*

susto *Fallen fontanel syndrome;* an acute anxiety state seen in Peruvian children and adolescents, usually precipitated by an experience of violent fright. Susto, or magic fright, is characterized by anxiety, excitability, dejection with considerable weight loss, and a belief that the patient's soul has been stolen from his body. See *curanderismo.*

Sweetser, William (1797–1875) American psychiatrist who wrote the first American treatise on mental hygiene (1843).

swindler, epileptic See *epilepsy, affective.*

swindler, pathological See *impostor; liar, pathological.*

swinging Slang for uninhibited sexual activity, often manifested in frequent casual sexual encounters, group sex, and combinations of heterosexual and homosexual acts.

Sydenham's chorea See *chorea, Sydenham's.*

syllable-stumbling A form of stuttering or stammering: the patient halts on syllables that he finds difficult to enunciate.

symbiontic Symbiotic; used to refer to psychosis of association, *folie à deux* (q.v.).

symbiosis Intimate living together in a mutually beneficial relationship; technically, the term refers to an interdependent relationship between dissimilar organisms (i.e. members of two different species). In psychiatry and psychology, the term is used in a less restrictive sense to refer to any degree of mutual cooperation or interdependence, as between mother and child. It includes any of the following: *commensalism,* when one member in a dependent relationship benefits and the other is relatively unaffected; *parasitism,* when one member's benefit is achieved at the expense of the other, who is disadvantaged by the relationship; and *mutualism;* when both members benefit. See *mutualism; symbiotic stage.*

symbiotic infantile psychosis See *psychosis, symbiotic infantile.*

symbiotic stage A phase in the mother-child relationship during which the child dimly recognizes the mother as a need-satisfying object and functions as though he and the mother formed a single omnipotent system. At this period, the mother must function as the child's auxiliary ego, performing functions he cannot yet perform for himself (e.g. control of frustration tolerance, setting ego boundaries, impulse control). This phase extends from the age of 3 months to 18 months, when it is succeeded by the stage of *separation-individuation* (q.v.).

symbol An object that stands for or represents something else. E. Jones (*Papers on Psycho-Analysis,* 1948) has pointed out that a symbol (1) is a representative or substitute of some other idea; (2) represents the primary element through having something in common with it; (3) is typically sensorial and concrete, whereas the idea represented may be relatively abstract and complex; (4) utilizes modes of thought that are more primitive, both ontogenetically and phylogenetically; (5) is a manifest expression of an idea that is more or less hidden, secret, or kept in reserve; and (6) is made spontaneously, automatically, and, in the broad sense of the word, unconsciously.

In psychoanalytic psychology, the symbol is a conscious representation or perception that replaces, and is a substitute for, unconscious mental content. The unconscious mental content is not recognized and its repression is maintained by the countercathexis of ego defenses; by the very fact that its meaning is unknown to the subject, the repressed psychic energy can, through the symbol, attain primary-process discharge, which would not be possible if the unconscious mental content were recognized as such. Symbols are the building stones for various other forms of indirect representation of unconscious content, viz. dreams, phantasies, hallucinations, symptoms, and even language.

Jones has this to say in regard to the extraordinary predominance of sexual symbols: "A Swedish philologist, Sperber, has in a remarkable essay elaborated the theory, which has been several times suggested on other grounds by biologists, that sexual impulses have played the most important part in both the origin and later development of speech. According to this theory, which is supported by very weighty considerations, the earliest speech sounds were those that served the purpose of calling the mate (hence the sexual importance of the voice to this day), while the further development of speech roots accompanied the performance of work. . . . Words used during these common tasks thus had two meanings, denoting the sexual act and the equivalent work done respectively. In time the former meaning became detached and the word, now applying only to the work, thus 'desexualized.' . . . The symbolic association is the relic of the old verbal identity; things that once had the same name as a genital organ can now appear in dreams, etc., as a symbol for it. Freud aptly likens symbolism to an ancient speech that has almost vanished, but of which relics still remain here and there." (Ibid.)

As psychiatric symptoms, symbols may be expressed in any one or all of these general categories: (1) affects alone; thus in anxiety hysteria the symbol is intense anxiety without any relevant ideas; other symptoms (rapid pulse and breathing, feelings of impending collapse, etc.) are generally secondary symptoms; (2) affects with ideas, the latter being looked upon as thoroughly foreign and painful to the conscious ego (For example, a patient was "tormented to death with the idea that I am slowly but certainly killing my children; that thought is furthest removed from my mind. I love them too dearly."); or (3) organic symptoms: the patients whose mental symptoms take an organic route of expression usually complain of a disease and not of symptoms; a woman, 35 years old, inordinately attached to her mother since early childhood, developed a deep sense of guilt when she left her invalid mother, who had a hemiplegia at the time. She repressed the guilt, replacing it with good intellectual reasoning, that is, with rationalization. The daughter later developed symptoms identical with those of her mother, and although these were not organically determined, the repressed guilt and its associated impulses returned to consciousness in the guise of a physical ailment.

Symbols may appear as delusions, hallucinations, morbid affects, compulsions, obsessions, conversions (i.e. hysterical), hypochondriasis, personalization of organs or organ systems, etc. Dreams form a special class of symbols.

symbol, memory A memory or idea that stands for, i.e. is substituted for, some other idea.

symbol, phallic Anything that represents the penis. Many phallic symbols have been described: knife, spear, gun, and other similar weapons; tree, column, pillar, skyscraper, automobile, airplane, bird, snake, wild animals, cigar, cigarette, pen, pencil, key, screw, hammer, and any number of other objects that go up and down, go in and out, or extend and retreat.

symbolamblyopia, congenital (sim-bol-am-blē-ō′pē-ȧ) Claiborne's term (1906) for a type of *reading disability* (q.v.).

symbolic categorization See *categorization, symbolic*.

symbolic computation See *cognitive science*.

symbolic wounding See *syndrome, deliberate self-harm*.

symbolism The act or process of representing an object or idea by a substitute object, sign, or signal. In psychiatry, symbolism is of particular importance since it can serve as a defense mechanism of the ego, as where unconscious (and forbidden) aggressive or sexual impulses come to expression through symbolic representation and thus are able to avoid censorship. The symbolic expression of the unconscious impulse may then appear as the patient's symptom. In one of Freud's cases, for example, Dora's cough was a hysterical symptom that symbolized her unconscious phantasy of oral intercourse between her father and another woman, and this phantasy in turn covered her own erotic feelings for the other woman's husband. See *symbol*.

symbolism, anagogic (an-ȧ-goj′ik) Pertaining to or arising from the striving of the inner psychic forms toward progressive ideals; pertaining to the interpretation and psychotherapy of dreams, symptoms,

etc., with emphasis on such striving: as, *anagogic methods*.

Silberer takes the symbol "to be the expression of a striving for a high ethical ideal, one which fails to reach this ideal and halts at the symbol instead; the ultimate ideal, however, is supposed to be implicit in the symbol and to be symbolized by it." (Jones, E.J. *Papers on Psycho-Analysis,* 1949)

Therapists who embrace this concept of anagogic symbolism regularly make use of it in their treatment of patients. Recognition and understanding of anagogic symbols is stressed and the striving for the achievement of the ideals expressed therein is encouraged.

symbolism, cryptogenic Silberer's term for any form of pictorial representation or image formed in mental functioning. In other words, all functions of the mind, save the ideational, are represented by cryptogenic symbolism.

symbolism, cryptophoric See *symbolism, metaphoric*.

symbolism, functional Silberer subdivides symbolism into the first and second types; his first is called by Jones the *material* type; his second, the *functional* type. "The first type is that which arises on the basis of an apperceptive insufficiency of purely intellectual origin, where the symbolized idea is not hindered by the influence of any affective complex; the second type arises, on the other hand, on the basis of an apperceptive insufficiency of affective origin." (Jones, E. *Papers on Psycho-Analysis,* 1938)

Formerly Silberer used the expression *functional symbolism* with reference to the speed with which the mind was working, whether it was fast, slow, etc.

symbolism, material See *symbolism, functional*.

symbolism, metaphoric According to Jones, a form of indirect representation. It seems that he prefers the expression *indirect pictorial representation* to *symbolism* or *metaphoric symbolism*. The latter may be defined, then, as a pictorial representation based on a metaphor.

symbolism, threshold Silberer's term for symbolism occurring during the transition from one state of consciousness to, i.e. on the threshold of, another, for example, from sleep to wakefulness or vice versa. The term is the equivalent of *hypnagogic hallucination*. It is a subdivision of what Silberer calls *functional symbolism*.

symbolism, true "The typical attributes of *true symbolism*, as modified from the description given by Rank and Sachs, are: (1) representation of unconscious material; (2) constant meaning, or very limited scope for variation in meaning; (3) non-dependence on individual factors only; (4) evolutionary basis, as regards both the individual and the race; (5) linguistic connections between the symbol and the idea symbolized; (6) phylogenetic parallels with the symbolism as found in the individual existing in myths, cults, religions, etc." (Jones, E. *Papers on Psycho-Analysis*, 1938)

symbolization "Symbolization according to psychoanalytic usage is an unconscious process built up on association and similarity whereby one object comes to represent or stand for (symbolize) another object, through some part, quality, or aspect which the two have in common. The resemblance is generally so slight or superficial that the conscious mind would overlook it." (Healy et al., *SMP*)

symbolophobia Fear of symbolism, i.e. of having a symbolical meaning attached to one's acts or words.

symmetrical See *complementary*.

sympathetic nervous system See *autonomic nervous system*.

sympathicotonia Eppinger and Hess's term for a clinical syndrome in which there is increased tonus of the sympathetic nervous system with a marked tendency to vascular spasm and high blood pressure, excessive functioning of the adrenals, and a hypersensitivity to adrenalin.

sympathin (sim′pa-thin) See *epinephrine*.

sympathism Suggestibility.

sympathize To experience a feeling similar to that possessed by another. Usually reciprocal motivation is implied.

sympathomimetic See *mydriasis*.

sympathy In general, the existence of feeling identical with or resembling that which another experiences. According to Freud, identification may arise when there is no emotional attachment with the person imitated: for example, one person may copy the feelings and actions of another, because the imitator has an unconscious impulse set free upon hearing about or looking at the one copied. In sympathy the feelings of the imitator remain essentially within him. When one or both share similar feelings, based upon some common unconscious quality, the term *identification* is used. See *empathize*.

symptom 1. Any sign, physical or mental, that stands for something else. 2. In a medical sense, pathology, although in its broader meaning a symptom may reflect physiological action (as in hunger).

Before the advent of modern psychiatric knowledge, when almost all psychic manifestations were traced directly to cells of the body, the term symptom denoted a sign relating to mental and physical phenomena, that is to say, by tradition it carried with it thoughts of the soma or tissues. With the expansion of psychiatric understanding, *symbol* has become identified with the realm of the psyche, i.e. a symptom of the psyche is a symbol. However, in this transitional period, many psychiatrists prefer symptom to symbol, particularly when there is any doubt concerning the origin of the symptom. But there is general agreement when a signal from the psyche is called a symbol. See *symbolism*.

symptom, accessory Bleuler differentiates between fundamental symptoms and accessory symptoms of the schizophrenias. The accessory, secondary symptoms include hallucinations, illusions, delusions, certain memory disturbances (e.g. déjà vu, déjà fait), some of the disturbances of the person (e.g. speaking of one's self in the second or third person and other pronominal reversals), speech and writing disturbances (e.g. coprolalia, verbigeration, neologisms, metonymy, asyndesis, interpenetration), and physical symptoms such as headache, paresthesiae, "will-o'-the-wisp" gait, weight loss, and general signs of metabolic asthenia. See *symptom, fundamental*.

symptom, Anton's Anosognosia (q.v.).

symptom, biphasic A compulsive symptom or action that has two component parts, the second of which is the direct reverse of the first: e.g. the patient has the compulsion first to open the water tap and then to close it again. Obsessive thoughts or impulses may likewise have two parts, the second directly contradicting the first.

The first phase of the symptom represents an instinctual demand, whereas the second phase represents the *anti-instinctual force* or threat of the superego. "The patient behaves alternately, as though he were a naughty child and a strict punitive disciplinarian." (Fenichel, *PTN*) See *anticathexis*.

symptom, fundamental Bleuler differentiates between fundamental symptoms and accessory symptoms of the schizophrenias. The fundamental, primary, or principal symptoms are those that are characteristic of and pathognomonic of *schizophrenia* (q.v.). The accessory symptoms, on the other hand, while they may overshadow the fundamental symptoms in their intensity, are not the essential or basic elements of the schizophrenias since they are seen also in other diseases, particularly in the organic brain syndromes. The fundamental symptoms include disturbances in the associations, in the affect, in the person, in the will, in attention, in activity and behavior, and also ambivalence (of affect, intellect, and/or will), autism, and schizophrenic dementia.

symptom, gramophone Mayer-Gross's term for a symptom seen often in *Pick's disease* (q.v.): the patient repeats "with correct expression and diction an elaborate anecdote, seeming himself to be highly amused by it, and could not be stopped until he had told the whole story. After a short interval he would repeat his anecdote as something quite new." (Mayer-Gross, W., et al. *Clinical Psychiatry,* 1960)

symptom, primary See *symptom, fundamental.*

symptom, primary defense A term used by Freud in describing the early development of obsessional neurosis. At the onset of sexual maturity, self-reproach for the memories of pleasurable sexual activities in childhood is avoided by primary defense symptoms, such as conscientiousness, shame, and self-distrust. These introduce the period of "apparent health or better—that successful defense." (Freud, *CP*)

symptom, principal See *symptom, fundamental.*

symptom, secondary See *symptom, accessory.*

symptom, secondary defense The protective measures to which the ego resorts in obsessional neurosis, when the primary defense (against repressed memories and self-reproach) has failed. The secondary defense symptoms include obsessive actions, obsessive speculating, obsessive thinking, the compulsion to test everything, *folie du doute;* "secondary defense against the obsessional affects calls into being a still wider series of protective measures, which may be transformed into obsessive acts. These may be grouped according to their tendencies: *Penitential* measures (burdensome ceremonials, the observation of numbers), *precautionary* measures (all kinds of phobias, superstitions, pedantry, exaggeration of the primary symptom of conscientiousness), *dread of betrayal* (collecting paper, misanthropia), *hebetude* (dipsomania)." (Freud, *CP*)

symptom specificity See *specificity, symptom.*

symptomatic Having the nature or quality of a *symptom* (q.v.); indicative of underlying (organic) pathology. Thus the symptomatic psychoses are secondary disturbances of psychic function dependent upon primary alterations in brain tissue function. Some reserve the term symptomatic psychoses for *acute brain disorders* (q.v.); the chronic brain disorders are then referred to as organic psychoses.

symptomatize In psychiatric usage, equivalent to symbolize. See *symbolization.*

symptoms, compulsive The orderly and systematic behavior exhibited by the obsessive-compulsive in order to protect himself against dangerous anal-erotic instinctual demands. The obsessive-compulsive feels threatened by unconscious anal-sadistic drives. He is protecting himself against a rebellion of sensual and hostile demands (such as murder and incest), which through regression have become anal-erotic in nature. He accomplishes this by doing things in a compulsive systematic way, according to a prearranged plan, a routine. This protects him against the danger associated with spontaneity. He can be sure he is not committing a sin of which he is both unconscious and afraid. He knows beforehand what he will do and how he will do it and thus he overcomes his fear that his own excitement may induce him to do things he is afraid of. The systematization is especially noticeable with respect to money and time. "Many compulsion neurotics have an exaggerated interest in all kinds of timetables."

The unconscious anal-sadistic drives, however, "usually sabotage orderliness and clinging to a 'system.' They may reappear in the form of disorder or events that disturb the system." Furthermore, the obsessive-compulsive never can feel that he has provided enough rules to govern all possibilities, that he knows all the rules sufficiently well, or that he is safe because the unconscious drives have actually permeated the systems themselves.

Frequently, people around the obsessive-compulsive are bidden to follow his systems in an effort to ensure the validity of the systems. The others' refusal to submit increases the patient's hostility as well as his attempts to compel those around him to conform, with the end result that the fear engendered by this show of hostility increases the patient's systematizing needs.

The systematization of the obsessive-compulsive often leads him to make false generalizations. All ideas are classified into certain mutually exclusive categories. Thus the likelihood of an unforeseen new event is excluded. The attitude is that the phenomenon or idea is already known—that is, has been classified—for unforeseen events are dangerous and are interpreted as temptations. (Fenichel, *PTN*) See *compulsion; obsession; obsessive-compulsive psychoneurosis.*

symptoms, deficit In schizophrenia, emotional blunting, withdrawal, and anhedonia. See *symptoms, productive.*

symptoms, first-rank A group of symptoms described by Kurt Schneider, and used by him and his followers as a basis for making a diagnosis of *schizophrenia* (q.v.). The signs include:

A. Hallucinations
 1. *audible thoughts*
 2. hearing voices arguing
 3. hearing voices commenting on the subject's behavior

B. Changes in thought process
 4. *thought insertion*—the experience that the subject's thoughts belong to others who have intruded their thoughts upon the subject
 5. *thought withdrawal* or *thought interruption* by some outside person or force (castrophrenia; nooklopia)
 6. thought broadcasting so that the

subject's private thoughts are known to others

C. Delusional perceptions
 7. attributing highly personal meaning to perception(s) without any comprehensible justification

D. Somatic passivity
 8. body sensations that the subject attributes to outside forces, such as X-rays or hypnosis

E. Other external impositions
 9. "forced" or "made" impulses—the subject is being forced to do things that he does not want to do
 10. made volition—the subject is being forced to want things he does not really want
 11. made feelings—the subject is being made to feel emotions or sensations (often sexual) that are not his own

Schneider worked in Munich in the 1930s and during the period 1945–55 occupied Kraepelin's chair in Heidelberg. Even though he accepted the wider post-Kraepelinian concept of schizophrenia that had begun with Bleuler, he and his followers held to a more narrow delineation than was upheld by most American psychiatrists.

In the International Pilot Study of Schizophrenia (IPSS, 1973), 57% of the patients diagnosed schizophrenic by the nine participating countries demonstrated first-rank symptoms.

symptoms, negative In schizophrenia, symptoms of the chronic phase such as apathy, lack of drive or will, underactivity, slowness, and social withdrawal; also called *deficit symptoms*, which together constitute the *schizophrenic defect state.* See *symptoms, positive.*

Negative thought disorder includes poverty of speech, poverty of content, and alogia; *positive thought disorder* includes derailment, incoherence, illogicality, tangentiality, and pressured speech. Negative thought disorder occurs mainly in schizophrenia, whereas positive thought disorder occurs at least as frequently in mania as it does in schizophrenia.

symptoms, phylogenetic See *schizophrenia, hebephrenic.*

symptoms, positive In schizophrenia, symptoms of the acute phase such as hallucination, delusions, and disturbances in thinking. See *symptoms, negative; symptoms, productive.*

symptoms, productive In schizophrenia, hallucinations, delusions, and in some descriptions autism. See *symptoms, deficit.*

symptoms, withdrawal A general term for abstinence syndrome (see *addiction*), or used more specifically to refer to the symptoms (restlessness, yawning, chills, characteristic pilomotor activity, excessive nasal secretion, lacrimation, sneezing, cramps in abdomen and lower extremities, vomiting and diarrhea, excessive perspiration, muscular twitching) experienced by addicts to morphine and heroin when the drug is suddenly withdrawn, that is, no longer taken.

synapse A specialized structure at which the *bouton* (q.v.) makes contact with the receptor elements of the adjacent neuron. Mitochondria in the bouton contain the elements that generate cellular energy through metabolism of glucose, enzymes involved in the synthesis and degradation of neurotransmitter, and storage vesicles for the neurotransmitter itself.

When a neuron is stimulated, the nerve impulse or electrical action potential causes neurotransmitter to be released into the *synaptic cleft* (the space between the neurons), where it interacts briefly with the adjacent neuron's dendritic membrane. That interaction results either in electrical stimulation, which heightens the likelihood that an action potential or nerve impulse will be generated in the postsynaptic neuron, or in electrical inhibition, which decreases the likelihood of such an impulse. See *conduction, nerve; neuron; neurotransmitter.*

Receptors concentrated on the dendritic membrane are of two types: *recognition site,* which allows the "right" neurotransmitter, i.e. one that fits the site, to be bound to it; and *transducer,* which is activated by the binding of neurotransmitter to recognition site. It is activation of the transducer that produces the physiologic effects.

Transducers themselves are of two types: ion channels, which regulate passage of ions through the neuronal membrane; and transducers, which are linked to enzymatic processes within the neuron.

synaptic cleft See *neurotransmitter.*

synaptic delay See *facilitation.*

synchiria (sin-kī′rē-à) Perception of a stimulus to one side of the body as having been applied to both sides of the body.

synchronism The simultaneous occurrence of several developmental faults. In Down's syndrome, for example, all organ systems of ectodermal, mesodermal, and entodermal origin that undergo specific development during the neofetal period are impaired; the particular synchronism of such symptoms points to the period between the sixth and twelfth weeks of fetal life as the time when the etiologic factors exert their greatest effect.

syncope (sing′kō-pē) Fainting; a swoon.

syncretism See *thinking, physiognomonic.*

syndrome A collection or grouping of disjunctive, variable signs and symptoms whose frequency of occurrence together suggests the existence of a single pathologic process or disorder that will explain them. "A syndrome is fundamentally a statistical notion based on covariation; it seems obvious that its derivation will be placed on more secure grounds when it is carried out (i) on the basis of a properly formulated model, (ii) with awareness of the statistical requirements and difficulties involved, (iii) on the firm foundation of quantitative measurement of objective test performance, (iv) in relation to properly selected samples of the population in question, (v) in accordance with the rules of significance widely accepted in biological statistics. It is not implied that the syndromes isolated by psychiatrists in the last hundred years or so are inevitably imaginary and to be discarded; it seems more likely that such consensus as there is points to important and fruitful dimensions which could be validated by proper statistical research, and perhaps improved and sharpened." (Eysenck, H.J. *Handbook of Abnormal Psychology,* 1960)

In general, three levels of categorization can be differentiated in medicine: (1) an isolated sign or symptom, without reference to associated features or cause, and with little predictive value; headache, stuttering, constipation, etc., are examples; (2) a clinical picture formed by a grouping of signs or symptoms into a distinctive syndrome, such as a combination of diarrhea, dementia, and dermatitis (suggestive of pellagra); (3) a distinctive clinical picture that is accounted for by an identifiable pathophysiologic process or etiologic agent, such as intellectual deterioration occurring in irregular spurts over a period of several years in a 67-year-old hypertensive man who also demonstrates dysarthria, small-step gait, and fundoscopic changes indicating arteriosclerosis (multi-infarct dementia). See *abnormality; disease.*

For descriptions of specific syndromes, see listings below and see also listings under *disease* and *disorder.* Some disorders have so long been known by their eponymic name that they are described under that name rather than in this section (e.g., *Alzheimer's disease, Guillain-Barré syndrome, Tay-Sachs disease*).

syndrome, acquired immune deficiency (AIDS) A cluster of disorders such as Kaposi's sarcoma (KS) and opportunistic infections to which the subject is abnormally vulnerable because of the collapse of his immune defense system. The cause is a retrovirus, identified in different laboratories and given different names: human T-lymphocytic virus type III (HTLV-III), lymphadenopathy-associated virus (LAV), and AIDS-associated retrovirus (ARV). Because it seems possible that all those organisms are the same, the International Committee on the Taxonomy of Viruses proposed (1986) the term *HIV (human immunodeficiency virus)* to include all of them.

The virus specifically infects and suppresses the T-4 lymphocyte or helper-inducer cell, the focal cell of the immune system. The virus not only reduces the number of T-4 cells; it also impairs their ability to propagate and synthesize immunoglobulins. In addition, the virus directly attacks specific types of cells in the central nervous system and lungs (and perhaps in other tissues as well).

Approximately 70% of reported cases in the United States have occurred in homosexual and bisexual males, and about 25% in male and female intravenous drug users. There is no known cure and mortality rate is high. Concern about the possibility of developing the disorder has led to severe anxiety reactions and somatic overconcern in many homosexual men.

AIDS is frequently complicated by central nervous system dysfunction because the AIDS retrovirus directly infects the brain. The dual tissue tropism of the virus may reflect similarities in surface membrane determinants of T lymphocytes and certain brain cells. Over 40% of AIDS patients develop neurologic complications at some point in their illness. The most common CNS dysfunction is a generalized encephalopathy or *progressive multifocal leukoencephalopathy (PML)* that includes dementia as a dominant feature. Less commonly, the dysfunction is due to well-defined focal lesions, including opportunistic infection by *Toxoplasma gondii*, which may invade nervous tissue and give rise to seizures or more subtle alterations in mentation and behavior. Myelopathy and peripheral neuropathy are other neurologic complications.

Of all the AIDS patients who develop neurological problems, about 10% have neurological symptoms first, before any signs of AIDS-related complex (ARC); 40% develop neurological symptoms after signs of ARC appear; 50% manifest symptoms after AIDS is diagnosed.

AIDS dementia characteristically begins with impaired concentration and mild memory loss and progresses to severe global cognitive impairment. Motor signs, including generalized hyperreflexia and increased tone, may accompany the dementia and some patients develop a spastic-ataxic gait or frank paraparesis. The neurological symptoms and signs usually progress over a course of several weeks to months.

The brain of an AIDS patient typically is shrunken, with dilated ventricles—changes that can be detected in a living patient by CAT scan. On microscopic examination, abnormalities are seen in the white matter and the subcortical and limbic areas rather than in the cortex. The white matter does not stain as darkly as normal (for unknown reasons), and in the spinal cord the white matter shows *vacuolar myelopathy*—a bubbly change in myelin tracts. The AIDS virus infects macrophages, monocytes, and endothelial cells that line brain capillaries (but not endothelial cells elsewhere in the body). Neurons and glia are minimally affected and there is poor correlation between the severity of neurological symptoms and the degree to which the brain appears abnormal on histological examination.

Many of those infected also become apathetic, withdrawn, agitated, or depressed. Mood disturbances have been observed in about 80% of subjects with ARC or AIDS. A chronic depression begins with mild symptoms and steadily worsens over time; although "reactive depression" on a psychological basis is frequent, the chronic type of depression is believed to be organic because it begins long before AIDS or ARC is diagnosed. Cases in which the presenting picture was one of acute psychosis without dementia have also been described.

syndrome, Addisonian (Thomas Addison, English physician, 1793–1860) Addison's disease; melasma suprarenale; adrenocortical insufficiency, due usually to atrophy or destructive inflammatory lesions. Symptoms include weakness, anorexia, hypotension, cutaneous pigmentary changes (bronzed skin), hyponatremia, hyperkalemia, vomiting, diarrhea, irritability, periodic hypoglycemia, and decreased or absent secretion of α-ketosteriods and 11-oxysteriods. In some cases, paranoid reactions are seen. Treatment consists of replacement therapy with desoxycorticosterone acetate and supplementary sodium chloride or aldosterone.

syndrome, Adie's A syndrome of unknown etiology characterized by enlarged pupil that shows the tonic pupillary reaction (when the patient is directed to gaze at a near object, the affected pupil slowly contracts to a size even smaller than the normal pupil) and by diminution or loss of tendon reflexes. The disorder occurs almost exclusively in females and usually has its onset in the third decade. It is a benign condition and unrelated to syphilis; also known as pseudo-Argyll Robertson pupil and pupillotonic pseudotabes.

syndrome, air pollution Symptoms associated with exposure to air pollutants, such as headache, fatigue, irritability, depression, and impaired judgment.

syndrome, akinetic-abulic A group of symptoms that frequently appear in the course of treatment with neuroleptics: pseudoparkinsonism (tremor), bradykinesia, hypertonia, decreased mental drive, and lack of interest.

syndrome, Alajouanine's (Theophile Alajouanine, French neurologist, 1890–1980) A congenital neurological disorder with lesions of cranial nerves VI and VII, double facial paralysis, convergent strabismus, and double clubfoot.

syndrome, amotivational Passivity, lack of interest, loss of drive; "dropping out," and difficulties in attention and concentration, described by some as the usual effect of long-term marihuana use. See *residual*.

Some use the phrase *amotivational states* to refer to deficit symptoms in schizophrenia. See *symptoms, deficit; symptoms, negative*.

syndrome, angry woman A personality disorder described in housewives consisting of a morbidly critical attitude to others, perfectionism, obsessive neatness and punctuality, marital maladjustment, proneness to alcohol or drug abuse, periodic outbursts of unprovoked anger, and serious suicide attempts. (Rickles, N.K. *Archives of General Psychiatry 24*, 1971)

syndrome, angular gyrus A symptom complex associated with focal lesions of the dominant posterior hemisphere consisting of alexia with agraphia or Gerstmann's syndrome (acalculia, agraphia, difficulty in differentiating left from right, finger agnosia, and constructional disturbances), in addition to fluent aphasia. Unlike *Alzheimer's disease*, with which it is often confused, the angular gyrus syndrome begins abruptly, memory and topographic orientation are relatively well maintained, and affected subjects are aware of their language deficits and can be engaged in conversation. Neurologic examination may reveal right-sided defects, and both electroencephalography and CT scan may show left-sided abnormalities. Positron emission tomography typically shows a left posterior deficit, whereas bilateral hypometabolism is characteristic in Alzheimer's.

syndrome, aniridia-ataxia A combination of absence of the iris in both eyes, cerebellar ataxia, and mental retardation. Because of the aniridia, visual acuity ranges between 20/100 and 20/200.

syndrome, Anton's See *hemiasomatognosia*.

syndrome, apallic Kretschmer's term for a prolonged state of disturbed consciousness, generally following closed head trauma, characterized by mutism, akinesia, primitive mass reflex, oral reflex, contractions, and extrapyramidal disturbances.

syndrome, Asperger's See *psychopathy, autistic.*

syndrome, atropine See *syndrome, central anticholinergic.*

syndrome, Babinski's See *hemiasomatognosia.*

syndrome, Balint's (Rezsoe Balint, Hungarian physician, 1874–1929) Spatial agnosia due to opticomotor disturbances of cortical origin.

syndrome, Bärtschi-Rochaix See *migraine, cervical.*

syndrome, battered child Term coined by pediatrician C.H. Kempe in the 1960s denoting physical injuries to children secondary to intentional acts of omission or to repeated, volitional, excessive beatings, by a parent or caretaker. Other than the obvious immediate dangers to the child's life and adequate physical growth, it is possible that such cruelty and abuse may constitute a long-term hazard in that it predisposes to a psychic development along the lines of delinquency and violence. See *psychopathic personality.*

The parents of abused or battered children show as wide a variation in character and personality makeup as do people in general; a small percentage of them can be classified as borderline psychotic, while only a few are overtly psychotic. Many, however, have poor self-esteem and a lack of self-confidence, difficulty in extracting pleasure from daily living, social isolation, a past history of abuse within their own families, and a lack of empathy with their child's needs. Such factors are often expressed in problem drinking, repeated job loss, unwanted and early pregnancies, unrealistic expectations of their children, and an inability to maintain children on various behavior and school schedules. (Coltoff, P., & Luks, A. *Preventing Child Maltreatment: Begin with the Parent,* 1978)

Sexual abuse of children—including incest, rape, and sexual relations between adults and children—appears to be rooted in defective family functioning. To describe it only in terms of violence by an adult against an innocent victim is an oversimplification. *Incest,* for example, involves at least three people—the incestuous pair and the nonparticipating parent—and

each of them plays an essential role in sustaining the situation. (Rosenfeld, A.A. *Journal of the American Medical Association 240,* 1978)

syndrome, Behçet's A syndrome that may be allergic in nature consisting of recurrent iritis, aphthous lesions of the mouth, and ulcerations of the genitalia, all of which run a benign course. Some cases show neuropsychiatric complications in addition, and these indicate a much more serious prognosis; they include episodic or progressive brain stem syndromes, meningoencephalitic syndrome, and organic confusional syndrome.

R.N. De Jong (*Neurologia 9,* 1964) suggested that Behçet's syndrome is one of a group of related symptom complexes (rather than disease entities) and that multiple and diverse etiologies, such as virus or allergy, may be involved. The other syndromes that he includes in the grouping are:

1. *Harada's syndrome*—uveitis, retinochoroidal detachment, cataract, and meningoencephalitis.

2. *Vogt-Koyanagi syndrome*—bilateral uveitis, vitiligo, alopecia, poliosis, dysacousia, often accompanied by meningoencephalitis.

3. *Fuch's syndrome*—headache, fever, cyanosis, swelling of the face, ulceration of the mucous membranes, and conjunctivitis.

4. *Klauder's syndrome*—fever, vesicular eruption of hands and feet, and eruption of the mucous membranes and orifices.

5. *Stevens-Johnson syndrome*—fever, severe and generalized maculopapular or vesicular or erythema multiformelike eruptions of the orificial mucosa.

6. *Reiter's syndrome*—arthritis, nonspecific urethritis, and conjunctivitis.

syndrome, Behr's (Carl Behr, German physician, b. 1876) A familial disorder beginning in infancy and involving temporal nerve and optic atrophy, ataxia, loss of coordination, and mental retardation.

syndrome, Bianchi's Hemiplegia, hemianesthesia, agraphia, apraxia, and alexia due to a lesion of the left parietal lobe.

syndrome, Bing-Neel See *macroglobulinemia, Waldenstrom's.*

syndrome, binge-eating See *syndrome, night-eating.*

syndrome, body-packer Drug overdose as a result of the ingestion of multiple small packages of contraband drugs (most commonly cocaine) in order to transport them. Rupture of the package or leaking from semipermeable wrappings (such as condoms) results in acute drug intoxication and, often, death.

syndrome, Bogorad's *Crocodile tears syndrome;* profuse tearing during eating or drinking, due to a seventh nerve lesion and subsequent misdirection of regenerating nerve fibers. Nerves that formerly supplied the salivary gland are diverted to the lacrimal glands. Affected subjects usually also show some degree of residual facial paralysis.

syndrome, Briquet's (brē-kāz′) *Hysteria* (q.v.) , so-named because P. Briquet was the first to describe hysteria systematically, in 1859. Some use the eponym to refer specifically to the polysymptomatic form of hysteria with many visits to different physicians, excessive medications, excessive hospitalizations, and excessive surgery. (Bibb, R., & Guze, S. *American Journal of Psychiatry 129,* 1972) Criteria for the diagnosis of Briquet's syndrome include (1) vague or dramatic medical history beginning before the age of 35 years; (2) a history of multiple symptoms (usually not less than 20) severe enough to interfere significantly with the patient's life and/or require medication or a visit to a physician; and (3) a lack of any medical explanation for the symptoms. See *hypochondriasis.*

syndrome, broad thumb-hallux See *syndrome, Rubenstein-Taybi.*

syndrome, Brown-Sequard (Charles Edouard Brown-Sequard, French physiologist, 1818–94) This syndrome, which follows hemisection of the spinal cord, consists of lower motor neuron type paralysis and loss of touch sensation at the level of the lesion; ipsilateral upper motor neuron type paralysis and loss of proprioception and vibratory sense below the level of the lesion; and contralateral loss of pain and temperature sense below the level of the lesion.

syndrome, Brueghel's See *syndrome, Meige.*

syndrome, buccal-lingual-masticatory See *dyskinesia, tardive.*

syndrome, buffoonery "The *buffoonery syndrome* is not always easily separated from catatonic states. In this syndrome the entire picture is taken up with playing de-

monstrative striking tricks, and with giving wrong answers; like the Ganser twilight state it probably only occurs as a reaction to a situation from which unconsciously one wants to escape through insanity." (Bleuler, *TP*)

syndrome, bulbar See *medulla oblongata.*

syndrome, Capgras's The delusional belief in the existence of identical doubles of significant others or of oneself or both, such as the delusion that one's spouse has been replaced by one or more imposters. The syndrome was first described in 1923 by J. Capgras and J. Reboul-Lachaux and is also known as *illusions of doubles* or *illusions of false recognition.* It is to be distinguished from autoscopy, defects of memory, perception, or recognition, hallucination, illusion, and prosopagnosia.

The syndrome occurs most frequently following a change in significant interpersonal relationships, which leads to negative feelings so different and alien to the subject that he rejects the idea that they could be attributable to the previously loved person. They must, instead, be due to an imposter or double. Such delusions occur most frequently as part of a paranoid schizophrenic picture, but they have also been reported in organic disorders and affective psychoses. The preconditions are a psychotic state, a paranoid tendency, and pathologic splitting of internalized object representations. (Berson, R.B. *American Journal of Psychiatry 140,* 1983)

The Capgras delusion is a negative misidentification that denies the genuineness of a known person (though admitting of a resemblance). In contrast, *Frégoli's phenomenon* (the *illusion de Frégoli,* the *illusion of a negative double*) is a positive misidentification, consisting of a belief that a persecutor has assumed the guise of various people whom the subject encounters in his daily life. (Frégoli was an actor famed for his ability to alter his appearance.) See *syndrome, intermetamorphosis.*

syndrome, carpal tunnel Numbness, tingling, and other painful paresthesiae in the hands and fingers (especially the middle three), frequently worst at night. It is often misdiagnosed as somatization, but it is due to compression of the median nerve in the carpal tunnel (as in fracture or arthritis of the wrist) or to pyridoxine (vitamin B$_6$) deficiency. The latter may occur as a side effect of treatment with monoamine oxidase inhibitors.

syndrome, cat cry A cytogenetic abnormality consisting of deletion of the distal portion of the short arm of chromosome number 5; manifestations include a high, piercing, catlike cry due to laryngomalacia *(cri-du-chat);* mental retardation, microcephaly, moonlike facies, hypertelorism, bilateral epicanthus, low-set ears, tiny external genitalia, laryngeal abnormalities, and abnormal palmar dermatoglyphs. The syndrome was first described in 1963 by L. Lejeune.

syndrome, central anticholinergic Atropine syndrome; symptoms include hallucinations, anxiety, short-term memory loss, disorientation, and agitation; seen frequently in patients receiving combinations of psychotropic drugs because of the additive anticholinergic effects of tricyclic antidepressants, the weaker phenothiazines and antiparkinson agents. The syndrome will often respond to simple reduction of anticholinergic drug, but in life-threatening situations (as in massive overdosage with tricyclic antidepressant) intramuscular physostigmine can be used as a specific antidote. See *therapy, atropine coma.*

syndrome, cervical vertigo See migraine, cervical.

syndrome, Chubby Puffer Sleep apnea in an obese child with large tonsils and adenoids, which occlude the air passages during sleep. There is some evidence that sudden infant death syndrome may be due to sleep apnea.

snydrome, Cinderella Simulation of neglect, or false accusation of neglect by a child, such as an adopted child's allegation (unfounded) that her stepmother made her do all the household chores and then left her unclothed in a snowdrift while the stepmother went off to the movies with her other children.

syndrome, clinical poverty Consisting of slowness, underactivity, reduced emotional responsivity, and impaired ability to communicate (as manifested, for example, in a wooden expression, monotonous voice, lack of gesturing, poverty of speech content). The clinical poverty syndrome is

a type of long-term impairment or disability that tends to persist in many schizophrenics even after acute symptoms have subsided.

syndrome, Cockayne's Mental retardation associated with dwarfism, wizened countenance, photosensitive skin, and cerebellar and ocular involvement ("salt and pepper"-like abnormalities of the retina).

syndrome, convexity Symptoms produced by a lesion of or near the lateral surface of the frontal lobe, most frequently *negative symptoms* such as apathy, indifference to the environment, loss of drive and ambition, or deterioration of social behavior often manifested as disheveled and dirty appearance. Motor inertia, catalepsy, and posturing are frequent. If the pathology is in the dominant hemisphere, there are also deficits in language and verbal thinking (which is impoverished, vague, and without detail), impaired verbal fluency, stereotyped speech with verbigerative and perseverative utterances, dyspraxia, and, sometimes, Broca's or transcortical aphasia.

syndrome, Cotard's (Jules Cotard, French neurologist, 1840–87) *Délire de négation(s);* the nihilistic delusion(s) found in severe depression, when the patient feels his head or bowels have been destroyed, his family has been exterminated, he is penniless, etc.

sydrome, cri-du-chat See *syndrome, cat cry.*

syndrome, Dandy-Walker's Congenital atresia of the foramen of Magendie.

syndrome, de Clérambault *Erotomania* (q.v.).

syndrome, de Lange A type of mental retardation with associated and highly variable minor physical manifestations, including low stature, mild microcephaly, low forehead, heavy confluent eyebrows, depressed bridge of the nose, flaring nostrils, small mandible, low-placed ears, micromelia and/or phocomelia, limitation of extension at the elbow joints, clinodactyly of the little fingers, low-placed thumb, webbing of the second and third toe, and hypertrichosis. Cause is unknown; the syndrome was first described by Cornelia de Lange in 1933 and is sometimes known as the Amsterdam type of retardation because it was described in subjects in that area.

Some authorities differentiate two types:

(1) the Brachman-de Lange type, or Amsterdam dwarf disease, with retarded bone maturation, short arms and fingers, and prominent features; and (2) the Bruck-de Lange type, with broad neck and shoulders, muscular hypertrophy, and a wrestlerlike appearance.

syndrome, delayed sleep phase See *sleep-wake schedule disorders*.

syndrome, delayed stress *Post-traumatic stress disorder* (q.v.).

syndrome, deliberate self-harm Conscious and willful inflicting of painful, destructive, or injurious acts on one's own body without intent to kill. Typically, the subject feels mounting tension and an impelling impulse to act, followed by a feeling of relief after the injury has been inflicted on the self. The most frequent self-destructive behavior is wrist cutting; other reported acts include abrasion, amputation (e.g. tongue or ear), biting, burning, enucleation of the eye, genital mutilation including castration, removal of the tongue, head banging, ingestion of medication and other objects, jumping from heights, hair pulling, and insertion of foreign bodies into the urethra.

The syndrome most commonly begins in late adolescence and continues for many years. It probably occurs most often in borderline or schizophrenic patients, in order to (1) relieve feelings of depersonalization; (2) lessen inner tension; (3) solve genital conflicts; (4) reassure the subject that he or she is alive by seeing his own blood; (5) deny inability to control the body by planning its destruction. Also called *autoaggression, focal suicide, parasuicide, self-attack, self-mutilation, symbolic wounding*. See *suicide, attempted*.

syndrome, Delilah Promiscuity in a woman for whom seduction of the partner is equated with rendering him weak or helpless, something she would like to have achieved with her dominating and exploitative father.

syndrome, dietary chaos See *restricters*.

syndrome, Diogenes *Hoarding* (q.v.).

syndrome, displaced child A form of separation phenomenon, often precipitated in a child by the birth of a sibling. Symptoms include a mixture of irritability, discouragement, jealousy of siblings, and feelings of rejection by other children.

syndrome, Down's Mongolian idiocy. Preferable terms are *Down syndrome, trisomy-21, autosomal trisomy of Group G, Langdon-Down disease* or *syndrome*, and *congenital acromicria*.

Trisomy-21 is an autosomal anomaly, due most frequently to nondisjunction of the 21st chromosome, this resulting in 3, rather than 2, G chromosomes (number 21 or 22), or a total of 47 chromosomes rather than the normal total of 46. The first report of an extra chromosome in this syndrome was made by the French workers Le Jeune, Gautier, and Turpin in 1959, and numerous studies since have confirmed that report. In the usual nondisjunction type of trisomy-21, the 21st (or 22nd) pair of chromosomes (for reasons not yet known) fails to separate during meiosis; this produces a germ cell with 24 instead of 23 chromosomes. When such a germ cell is united with a normal germ cell during fertilization, the resulting organism contains 47 rather than 46 chromosomes.

Pathologically, the brain is small, and there are widespread defects in the cortical cell layers and in the number of ganglion cells. Whole gyri may be faulty in development. The process apparently is stationary, for regressive changes are not seen. There are many signs characteristic of trisomy 21, but not all are seen in each case. In one reported series, the signs appeared with the following frequencies; slanting of the palpebral fissures (88%), hyperextensible joints (88%), flabby hands (84%), brachycephalic skull with flat occiput (82%), ear anomalies or small lobules (80%), diastasis recti (76%), high-arched palate (74%), irregular alignment of teeth (68%), flat nipples (56%), epicanthus (50%), speckling of the iris (30%), heart murmurs (28%), double-zoned iris (22%), and pathologically open fontanels (16%). (Levinson, A., Freidman, A., & Stamps, F. *Pediatrics 16*, 1955)

Mentally, the patient is usually docile and tractable and may give an appearance of higher mental capacity than is really present because of imitativeness. The majority have a mental age of 4 to 7 years, although there are variations from moronity to pronounced idiocy. A few are hyperactive and sometimes destructive.

Because of associated defects, probably less than 60% live more than five years.

In a less frequent type of Down's syndrome, extra genetic material does not remain in position 21 as an extra chromosome, but instead attaches itself to one of the other chromosomes—usually to a chromosome in the 13–14–15 group, and thus the process is termed *15/21 translocation*. In such cases, the normal chromosome count of 46 is retained, but the chromosome receiving the excess of genetic material is abnormally elongated.

Inherited Down's syndrome is rare, and obvious familial aggregation of cases would be expected only in the translocation type. It has been reported in both monozygotic twins and in both dizygotic twins (but not in twins of different sex). The conditions that generate excess genetic material from chromosome 21 are undetermined; ionizing radiations, viruses, and senescence have been suggested as possible factors, and it has long been known that increased frequency of the syndrome is positively correlated with advanced parental age.

The syndrome was first described by J. Langdon-Down in 1866. Data accumulated since that time suggest that the general frequency of the disorder is about 1 in 600 births. Probably not more than 10% of these are of the translocation type, although in young mothers (who contribute only a small proportion of cases to the total group) translocation may be the responsible mechanism in as many as 25%.

syndrome, Dyke Davidoff Hemiatrophy of the brain, manifested by mental retardation, seizures, facial asymmetry, and contralateral hemiplegia. (Gorlin, R.J., et al. *Modern Medicine 38,* 1970)

syndrome, effort Neurocirculatory asthenia.

syndrome, Ekbom's 1. *Restless legs syndrome* (q.v.); when it occurs spontaneously it is often associated with low serum iron. Akathisia as a side effect of neuroleptic administration is similar in appearance and may also be associated with iron deficiency. Even though not anemic, such patients show low serum iron and percentage saturation, and high total iron-binding capacity. Further, the lower the serum iron the more severe the akathisia.

2. Dermatozoic delusions. See *dermatozoic.*

syndrome, episodic dyscontrol See *dyscontrol, episodic.*

syndrome, Fahr's See *Fahr's disease.*

syndrome, fetal alcohol A pattern of retarded physical and mental growth, with associated cranial, facial, limb, and cardiovascular anomalies, that is found in 30 to 50% of the offspring of severely alcoholic mothers. Damage to the fetus by maternal alcoholism is one of the most common recognizable causes of mental retardation. The affected children do not typically "catch up" in their growth patterns, even when given a nutritionally adequate diet. The basis for the syndrome is believed to be a direct toxic effect of alcohol and/or one of its intermediate breakdown products on the fetal brain.

syndrome, fetal hydantoin See *epilepsy, gestational.*

syndrome, fetal trimethadone See *epilepsy, gestational.*

syndrome, Foster Kennedy (Foster Kennedy, American neurologist, 1884–1955) See *nerve, olfactory.*

syndrome, fragile X A chromosomal disorder consisting of a gap or constriction at the distal end of the long arm of the X chromosome at Xq28, resulting in the appearance of an X chromosome with a satellite and a tendency to break easily. The fragile X chromosome is definitely associated with mental retardation in males. Macroorchidism is a strong phenotypic indicator of the presence of a fragile X and of retardation.

The disorder is believed to occur in 1 of every 2,000 to 3,000 male births, making it second only to Down's syndrome as a cause of retardation, even though relatively few females are affected. A male born to a mother with fragile X chromosome has a 50% chance of manifesting the disorder.

There may be an association between fragile X chromosome and dyslexia (primary learning disability), but contrary to earlier claims there is little evidence for an association between fragile X and autism.

syndrome, Freud's P. Janet coined this expression: "The mania for repression . . . is still an interesting symptom; and it explains certain remarkable phenomena, such as monstrous and sacrilegious longings. It will continue to form a part of mental pathology under the name of 'Freud's syndrome.' " (*PH*)

syndrome, Fuch's See *syndrome, Behçet's.*

syndrome, Ganser (Sigbert J.M. Ganser, German psychiatrist, 1853–1931) One of the *factitious disorders* (q.v.); the Ganser twilight syndrome is factitious disorder with psychological symptoms, while the Munchhausen syndrome is factitious disorder (chronic) with physical symptoms. The Ganser syndrome is also known as "the nonsense syndrome" or syndrome of deviously relevant answers; it is often observed among prisoners, who, it is held, hope to be treated leniently by the court in virtue of their malady. It is described by many investigators as a hysterical reaction. The patient seldom does anything correctly. When shown a watch reading 3:30, the patient may say it reads 5:00; when shown a glove he says it is a hand; he designates a 50-cent piece as a dollar bill; calls a key a lock. But in addition to such approximate answers, which may be seen also in hysterical pseudodementia, behavior is bizarre, with episodes of excitement or stupor, as though the subject were acting out an artificial psychosis (neuromimesis).

syndrome, Gardner-Diamond *Painful bruising syndrome,* or *autoerythrocyte sensitization,* first described by F.H. Gardner and L.K. Diamond. (*Blood 10,* 1955) Tingling, burning, or stinging sensations often develop in the areas that will be involved in the painful swelling and erythema that later evolve into ecchymoses. The lesions may occur alone or in clusters, they vary in size from several centimeters to encompass the whole limb, and typically they arise close to a recent trauma (including surgery). A period of emotional distress preceding the development of the syndrome is so common that it is sometimes referred to as *psychogenic purpura.* Unpredictable remissions and disabling recurrences are the rule, and no fully effective therapy is known. Immunopathogenic mechanisms are believed by some workers to be of etiologic significance, but others find no evidence for such a theory. The syndrome has been observed much more frequently in women than in men.

syndrome, general adaptation The various changes in the body in response to and/or as defense against stress. Selye distinguishes three stages in this syndrome: the *alarm reaction,* in which adaptation is not yet acquired; the *stage of resistance,* in which adaptation is optimal; and the *stage of exhaustion,* in which the acquired adaptation is lost again. The hypophysis-adrenal interrelationships, which largely determine the various elements of the syndrome, are as follows: the stress agent, or stressor, acts not only upon the cells of the *target organ* but also acts (humoral or neural route?) upon the anterior pituitary and stimulates the latter to produce ACTH; in certain circumstances it may also induce a release of somatotrophic hormone (STH). ACTH, in turn, induces the adrenal cortex to produce glucocorticoids (such as cortisone). The latter exert primarily an inhibitory effect upon the various target organs—catabolism, diminution of granuloma formation and of allergic responses, etc. STH, on the other hand, by stimulating connective tissue, enhances defensive reactions in the target organs—anabolism, augmentation of granuloma formation and of allergic responses, etc. This action occurs by means of direct sensitization of the connective tissue elements to mineralocorticoids (such as desoxycorticosterone) and also by stimulating the adrenal cortex to produce mineralocorticoids. This latter corticotrophic effect, however, depends upon the simultaneous availability of ACTH. Thus the target organ response to stressors depends largely upon the balance between STH and the mineralocorticoids on the one hand, and ACTH and glucocorticoids on the other.

syndrome, Gerstmann (Josef Gerstmann, American neurologist, 1888–1969) A symptom complex described by Gerstmann in 1940 consisting of finger agnosia, right-left disorientation, acalculia, and agraphia. There may be various additional features, such as constructive apraxia, amnestic reduction of word finding, disturbed ability to read, impaired color perception, absence of optokinetic nystagmus, and disturbance of equilibrium. The agraphia often takes the form of dissociated dysgraphia.

Presence of the Gerstmann syndrome implies definite parietal lobe pathology, usually in the neighborhood of the angular gyrus.

Most present-day neurologists question the validity and usefulness of the concept, in that the deficits forming the syndrome are no more closely linked together than are a score of other combinations of behavioral deficits.

syndrome, Gilles de la Tourette (Georges Gilles de la Tourette [jēl du là toor-et'], Paris physician, 1857–1904) *Tourette's disorder; maladie des tics;* one of the *stereotyped movement disorders* of childhood, first described in 1885. It begins between 2 and 15 years of age with facial movements (motor tics) and throat noises (vocal tics); the involuntary, rapid, purposeless movements become more generalized and progressive, and phrases or sentences may be ejaculated. Coprolalia and echolalia occur in more than half the cases; also frequent are palilalia, obsessive doubting, and compulsive touching. The lifetime prevalence rate of the disorder has been estimated as between 0.1 and 0.5 per 1,000; it is three times more common in boys than in girls. It is usually of lifelong duration, but marked relief has been obtained in many cases with high doses of butyrophenones (haloperidol).

The most frequently used treatments for the disorder are neuroleptics (particularly haloperidol) and pimozide. The latter was approved for use in the United States in 1984, the eleventh product to be approved under the *orphan drug* (q.v.) law. (There are only about 100,000 persons in the United States with Tourette syndrome.)

syndrome, Gjessing's (jes'ing) Recurrent episodes of catatonic stupor or excitement occurring in schizophrenics and associated with phasic variations in the nitrogen metabolism; first described by R. Gjessing in 1938. The syndrome is related to inadequate metabolism of dietary protein, leading to periods of nitrogen retention that are concurrent with hyper- or hypokinetic episodes. Dietary regulation is sometimes enough to control such patients; in others, thyroid administration increases nitrogen output with corresponding improvement in mental state.

syndrome, Gunn's See *synkinesia.*

syndrome, Hallervorden Spatz Familial, progressive, juvenile striatopallidal degeneration. It usually begins early in the second decade; symptoms include bilateral rigidity, speech difficulties, dementia, and sometimes also optic atrophy and hyperkinesias.

syndrome, Happy Puppet A form of mental retardation characterized by protruding jaw and tongue, flat occiput, ataxic gait, epilepsy, a smiling but otherwise expressionless face, paroxysms of laughter, hypotonia, absent speech, abnormal EEG, and a variety of other congenital malformations. Etiology is unknown although it is presumed to be of genetic origin.

syndrome, Harada's See *syndrome, Behçet's.*

syndrome, holiday Sadness, anxiety, or other emotional pain—reflected in increased rates of suicide, hospital admissions, and deaths in automobile accidents—occurring during the period between Thanksgiving and New Year's Day. The syndrome appears to be an expression of unmet dependency needs triggered by the reminiscing and loving aspects of the holiday season.

syndrome, Horner's (Johann Friedrich Horner, Swiss ophthalmologist, 1831–86) Caused by paralysis of the cervical sympathetic nerve, this condition has the following signs and symptoms: (1) miosis, (2) enophthalmos, (3) pseudoptosis, (4) occasionally ipsilateral vasodilatation and anhydrosis on the side of the face and neck.

syndrome, Horton's (Bayard T. Horton, contemporary American physician) See *histamine.*

syndrome, Hunt's Dyssynergia cerebellaris myoclonica, a syndrome characterized by myoclonic crises, cerebellar ataxia and dysarthria, and, usually, epileptic seizures.

syndrome, Hurler's *Mucopolysaccharidosis* (q.v.).

syndrome, Hutchinson-Gilford progeria Premature aging and senility in children, manifested in midline facial cyanosis, sclerodermalike skin, and a grooved nasal tip. There is no evidence that this rare syndrome predisposes to emotional disturbances.

syndrome, hyperventilation Formerly termed DaCosta's syndrome, effort syndrome, irritable heart, neurocirculatory asthenia, soldier's heart, war neurasthenia;

subjective symptoms (especially breathlessness, palpitation, dizziness or faintness, paresthesiae and excessive sweating) are due to the progressive hypocapnia produced by overbreathing. The overbreathing is itself a form of reaction to anxiety or fear, but the importance of recognizing the syndrome lies in the fact that the subjective symptoms secondarily produced are of physiologic origin rather than specific symbolic representatives of the underlying neurotic conflict. See *spasmophilia.*

syndrome, imidazole *Bessman-Baldwin syndrome;* a familial disorder of imidazole metabolism, described by Samuel Bessman (American biochemist, b. 1921) and Ruth Baldwin (American pediatrician, b. 1915). It consists of cerebromacular degeneration with convulsions, retinitis pigmentosa, mental retardation, and excessive urinary excretion of carnosine, anserine, and histidine.

syndrome, intensive care Psychosis appearing in patients in postoperative recovery units or in intensive care units. Significant factors contributing to the development of such a complication include the following: (1) the physical conditions of the unit itself—often impersonal, highly mechanized, unfamiliar, isolated, windowless, and in certain ways a type of sensory deprivation experience; (2) the physical condition of the patient within the unit—he is usually immobilized to a severe degree and in considerable discomfort; (3) the nature of the underlying pathology, including the medical-surgical complications and the age of the patient, and the effects these have on brain function; (4) the effects of medication and operative procedures on brain function; and (5) the premorbid level of functioning, including personality structure and genetic-constitutional factors.

syndrome, intermetamorphosis Delusional conviction that various people in one's environment have been transformed physically and psychologically into other people. Intermetamorphosis differs from Frégoli's phenomenon, which also involves false identification, in that it includes false physical resemblance in addition to false recognition. See *syndrome, Capgras's.*

syndrome, irritable bowel Symptoms include abdominal pain, usually over the descending colon, with diarrhea or alternating diarrhea and constipation. Psychological factors are often implicated as precipitants but are not believed to be the sole cause.

syndrome, kinky hair A neurodegenerative disease of male infants characterized by coarse and kinky hair, grand mal seizures, psychomotor retardation, failure to grow, cerebrocerebellar atrophy, and early death.

syndrome, Kleine-Levin A syndrome consisting of episodes of hypersomnia, bulimia, and abnormal mental states such as clouded sensorium, partial or total amnesia for certain periods of the attack, and psychomotor retardation. The syndrome is distinct from narcolepsy, although it may be related to the latter. The Kleine-Levin syndrome appears to be a result of disturbance of function of the frontal lobe and/or the hypothalamus. Amphetamine drugs are often useful in treatment of the disorder. See *eating disorders; syndrome, pickwickian.*

syndrome, Klinefelter's A disease due to gross chromosome abnormality, consisting of 47 chromosomes (instead of the normal 46, there is an extra sex chromosome, giving an XXY pattern instead of the usual XX or XY). Affected subjects appear phenotypically to be males (indicating that the Y chromosome, far from being inert, is strongly determinant of maleness), but they show dysgenesis of the seminiferous tubules, gynecomastia, and eunuchoidism. The sex chromatin test is positive, as in the normal female. Known also as *primary microorchidism.*

syndrome, Klippel-Feil (klē-pel' fāl') (Maurice Klippel, French neurologist, 1858–1942; André Feil, contemporary French physician) A congenital anomaly characterized by absence and fusion of portions of the cervical spine, producing a shortness and stiffness of the neck. Compression of the cord may occur with motor and sensory changes. Mirror writing may occur in association with the syndrome.

syndrome, Klumpke-Déjérine (Auguste Klumpke-Déjérine, French neurologist, 1859–1927) A combination of paralysis of the cervical sympathetic nerve with paralysis and atrophy of the small muscles of the hand.

syndrome, Klüver-Bucy A syndrome, described originally by Klüver and Bucy, in monkeys that had been subjected to bilateral removal of the temporal lobes. In the human, symptoms include (1) loss of recognition of people; (2) loss of fear and rage reactions; (3) increased sexual activity (especially masturbation and homosexuality); (4) bulimia; (5) hypermetamorphosis; and (6) memory defect.

syndrome, Lauder's See *syndrome, Behçet's.*

syndrome, Laurence-Moon-Biedl (J.Z. Laurence, British ophthalmologist, 1830–74; Robert C. Moon, American ophthalmologist, 1844–1914; and A. Biedl, German physician, 1868–1933) An autosomal recessive disorder consisting of six cardinal signs in the following order of frequency: obesity, retinitis pigmentosa, mental deficiency, genital dystrophy, familial occurrence, polydactyly. Also known as *retinodiencephalic degeneration.*

syndrome, Lesch-Nyhan A heritable disorder of purine metabolism, inherited as a recessive trait, consisting of hyperuricosuria, mental retardation, choreoathetosis, spasticity, and a compulsive tendency to self-mutilation (typically, the lips and distal fingers are bitten away). Affected children usually die before puberty. There is no known treatment, but the characteristic deficiency of hypoxanthine-guanine-phosphoribosyltransferase (HGPRT enzyme, which normally catalyzes phosphoribosylpyrophosphate) can be detected in amniotic cells in time to allow termination of pregnancy before the affected fetus is viable. The original descriptions of the syndrome were by J.D. Riley in 1960 and by M. Lesch and W.L. Nyhan. (*American Journal of Medicine 36,* 1964)

Manifestations of HGPRT enzyme deficiency depend on the remaining degree of enzyme activity. In Lesch-Nyhan syndrome, the enzyme is present at only a 0.005% level of normal activity. In some members of the families of affected subjects, the HGPRT enzyme is also deficient, but not to the same degree. In those in whom the level is between 0.01 and 0.5% of normal, spinocerebellar syndromes of variable severity will develop; but if the enzyme level is as high as 1% of normal, the resultant syndrome is gout.

syndrome, Loeffler's An allergic reaction by sensitized lung tissue to various allergens, and especially drugs, consisting of pulmonary infiltration and eosinophilia. Loeffler's syndrome has been described in association with various psychotropic and psychedelic drugs.

syndrome, Louis-Bar's *Ataxia telangectasia* (q.v.).

syndrome, Lowe's See *syndrome, oculocerebrorenal.*

syndrome, Main's The ability of a patient (usually a female psychotic who is a nurse or is otherwise closely related to the field of medicine, and part of whose productions include recounting long-continued incestuous relationships) to extort "frantic sympathy and remarkable therapeutic privilege" from her attendants, and to imbue "doctor or nurse with a vivid sense of private significance for the patient, of being peculiarly attuned to her." (Bourne, H. *Archives of General Psychiatry 2,* 1960) The syndrome was first described by T.F. Main in 1957.

syndrome, Malin See *syndrome, neuroleptic malignant.*

syndrome, Marfan's (Antoine Bernard Jean Marfan, French pediatrician, 1858–1942) An autosomal dominant disorder manifested in bilateral congenital ectopia lentis, vascular defects such as dissecting aneurysm of the aorta, and skeletal system deformities such as arachnodactyly and pectus carinatum (pigeon breast or chicken breast).

syndrome, Marin Amat A syndrome described in 1918 consisting of closing of the eyelid on chewing or opening the mouth. Paralysis or spasm of the ipsilateral facial nerve usually precedes the appearance of the syndrome, which is probably due to a disturbance of intrinsic nuclear functions.

syndrome, Marinesco-Sjogren A hereditary disorder, transmitted through a polyphenous autosomal gene, consisting of congenital dementia, congenital cataract, and cerebellar ataxia.

syndrome, Mast A recessively inherited form of presenile dementia, named after the family in which it was first detected. The disorder begins in the late teens with intellectual deterioration, spasticity, and dysarthria; it progresses to complete incapacitation of the affected in their thirties or forties. Early symptoms are blank facies, an unblinking stare, loss of initiative, short attention span, loss of remote memory, failure to understand verbal orders, difficulty in walking because of spasticity, and dysarthria. Extrapyramidal and cerebellar signs, if present at all, appear late in the course of the disorder. No specific treatment is applicable, and although no underlying metabolic disorder has been identified, a specific enzyme defect, probably limited to the metabolism of nervous tissue, is suspected. (Cross, H., & McKusick, V. *Archives of Neurology 16,* 1967)

syndrome, maternal deprivation The psychobiologic response to withdrawal or withholding of the emotional, affectional, cognitive, or other supplies needed for proper development that ordinarily are provided by the mother. Most typically, it appears in children without mothers who are reared in institutions, in children who for one reason or another are separated from the mother at an early age, and in children whose mothers are incapable of providing consistently suitable emotional support for their children. See *depression, anaclitic; deprivation, emotional.*

syndrome, Meige *Brueghel's syndrome;* an idiopathic disorder of movement consisting of blepharospasm and oromandibular dystonia, first described by Henri Meige. (*Revue Neurologie* [Paris] *10,* 1910) It is easily confused with tardive dyskinesia.

syndrome, Melkersson-Rosenthal Recurrent, gradual, persistent swelling of the lips, clefts or folds in the tongue, and facial paresis; the syndrome occurs in subjects with an unstable vegetative nervous system and is usually precipitated by stress or other psychic factors.

syndrome, Ménière's (Prosper Ménière, French physician, 1799–1862) Dilatation of the endolymph system of the internal ear of unknown etiology, leading to episodic vertigo associated with tinnitus and increasing deafness. It occurs more often in males, typically in late middle age.

syndrome, Munchhausen A name suggested by Asher in 1951 to refer to patients who wander from hospital to hospital ("hospital hoboes"), feigning acute medical or surgical illness and giving false and fanciful information about their medi-

cal and social background. The diagnostic triad of symptoms comprises *pseudologia fantastica* (q.v.), peregrination, and disease simulation. The underlying motivation for such behavior (pathomimicry) is not clearly understood, but apparently it does not include attempts to obtain drugs, avoid police, etc. Such patients would seem to be a particular form of *impostor* (q.v.). See *factitial; factitious disorders.*

syndrome, neuroleptic malignant (NMS) *Malin syndrome;* a rare and sometimes fatal complication of therapy with high-potency neuroleptics, consisting of hyperthermia, neuromuscular rigidity, abnormal blood pressure (low or high or labile), sweating, and usually some disturbance of consciousness. In many cases, concurrent medical disorders and complications (such as dehydration, infection, renal failure, or pulmonary congestion) suggest that the neuroleptics may not be the direct cause, and that at least some cases develop on the basis of untreated severe or prolonged rigidity and other extrapyramidal symptoms. Malin syndrome was first described by Delay and Deniker in 1968. See *Bell's mania.*

syndrome, night-eating A type of *eating disorder* (q.v.) that occurs in some obese patients consisting of nocturnal hyperphagia, insomnia, and morning anorexia. The syndrome tends to appear episodically, and during such periods weight control is especially difficult or even impossible for the patient.

A second type of eating pattern found in obese patients is *binge eating*—consumption at irregular intervals of large quantities of food in an orgiastic manner. A third pattern is *eating without saturation,* seen most frequently in patients with central nervous system disturbances, and characterized by overeating without relationship to stress situations and without regular periodicity.

syndrome, nonsense Popular synonym for *Ganser syndrome* (q.v.).

syndrome, oculocerebrorenal One of the diffuse demyelinating scleroses of genetic origin; also known as *Lowe's syndrome.* Symptoms include congenital cataract, progressive mental impairment, hypotonia, hyporeflexia, proteinuria, hyperaminoaciduria, and hyperchloremic acidosis. So far, the syndrome has been reported only in males; those affected usually die during childhood.

syndrome of approximate answers See *answers, syndrome of approximate; syndrome, Ganser.*

syndrome, OFD I *Oral-facial-digital syndrome,* characterized by frenular hypertrophy, clefts of the palate, lips, or tongue, hypoplasia of the nasal cartilages, brachydactyly, syndactyly, and, in many cases, mental retardation. OFD I is believed to be transmitted as an X-linked dominant trait; OFD II, on the other hand, is transmitted as an autosomal recessive trait.

syndrome, orbitomedial A frontal lobe syndrome whose manifestations may include (1) asthenia, fatiguability, blandness, akinesia, aphonia, withdrawal, and fearfulness; (2) diminished wakefulness, or an oneiroid or stuporous state; or (3) *Witzelsucht,* with euphoria, lability, and rapid mood shifts; such patients are uninhibited, reckless, impulsive, intrusive, importunate, frenetic, and strongly stimulus-bound.

syndrome, organic The group of symptoms characteristic of the *organic mental disorders* (q.v.) . In any specific case, one or more of the characteristic symptoms may predominate. The signs of organicity include (1) disturbances in orientation; (2) impairment of memory; (3) impairment in the maintenance of the level of consciousness and attention; (4) impairment of all intellectual functions (comprehension, calculation, knowledge, learning, etc.); (5) defective judgment; (6) lability, shallowness, and similar instabilities of the affect; and (7) overall changes in the personality, with the appearance of conduct foreign to the patient's natural or usual behavior. In the acute brain disorders, alteration in consciousness (with preoccupation, stupor, or coma) and defects in orientation and memory tend to predominate; the acute organic syndrome is sometimes called the *delirious reaction.* In the chronic brain disorders (e.g. the Korsakoff psychosis), intellectual defects are prominent (loss of general efficiency, inability to plan, judgment defects, disturbances in orientation and memory, confabulation), and disturbed affect and personality changes are also frequent. The term *dementia* is often used to refer to the irreversible intellectual defects of the patient with chronic brain disorder. See

abstract attitude; behavior, catastrophic; drivenness, organic.

syndrome, Othello See *jealousy, morbid.*

syndrome, pedunculopontile Weber's syndrome. See *hemiplegia alternans.*

syndrome, persecution Described in war refugees with concentration camp experience or those who were persecuted in flight; consists of pervasive anxiety, overreactivity, irritability, chronic depression, psychosomatic disturbances, and defense by means of dehumanization and unconscious identification with the aggressor. The social contacts and marriages of those with the syndrome are likely to be confined to others who have had similar experiences. See *neurosis, traumatic; posttraumatic stress disorder.*

syndrome, phantom lover *Erotomania* (q.v.).

syndrome, pickwickian Alveolar hyperventilation syndrome; obesity associated with hypersomnolence (especially, daytime sleepiness), hypoventilation, and polycythemia, and often also with twitching movements, cyanosis, periodic respirations, congestive heart failure, arterial hypoxia and hypercapnia, and rightward axis deviation on electrocardiogram. The syndrome may sometimes be reversed by weight loss. Although the pathophysiology of the syndrome is poorly understood, the drowsiness, sleep, and muscular twitching appear to be related to hypercapnia, while polycythemia and cyanosis appear to be related to arterial hypoxia. See *eating disorders; syndrome, Kleine-Levin.*

syndrome, Pierre Robin Also known as the *Robin triad,* this syndrome, presumably of genetic origin, consists of glossoptosis (which leads to severe respiratory disorders), microcephaly, and mental retardation.

syndrome, Pisa *Pleurothotonus* (q.v.).

syndrome, pontocerebellar angle A group of symptoms caused by acoustic neuromas. Involvement of the acoustic nerve produces persistent tinnitus, progressive deafness, and vertigo. Involvement of the facial nerve produces homolateral facial anesthesia with loss of corneal and sneeze reflexes. Cerebellar involvement produces homolateral ataxia with staggering, and pontine involvement results in contralateral hemiplegia and slight hemianesthesia.

In addition, there are general symptoms of brain tumor and increased intracranial pressure.

syndrome, post-torture A Dutch study of refugees from nine countries examined symptoms immediately following torture. Complaints at the time were widely divergent. Psychic problems were particularly pronounced. There is not enough evidence to justify the term post-torture syndrome, on analogy with post-concentration camp syndrome. The question remains if a clearly developed syndrome will appear with passage of time.

syndrome, Potzl's Pure alexia (i.e. symbol agnosia for written characters, although the writing is seen, and without any intrinsic disturbance of speech), combined with disturbances of color sense and defects of the visual field. Potzl's syndrome is generally seen in the presence of foci in the medullary layer of the lingual gyrus of the dominant hemisphere with damage of the corpus callosum.

syndrome, Prader-Labhart-Willi A syndrome consisting of myotonia early in life, obesity and growth retardation in childhood, diabetes mellitus in early adulthood, and mental retardation, hypogonadism, acromicria, and dolichocephaly; sometimes referred to as HHHO (hypotonia, hypomentia, hypogonadism, obesity). Basis of the disorder is presumed to be an abnormal fat metabolism leading to inadequate insulin action.

syndrome, premenstrual (PMS) Changes in mood, behavior, cognition, and somatic functioning seen in some women in relation to the menstrual cycle. Symptoms usually begin a few days before the onset and end shortly after the onset of a menstrual period; most frequently reported symptoms are anxiety, irritability, depressed mood, breast tenderness, abdominal discomfort, and a feeling of distention. It is generally assumed that endocrine abnormalities are a major factor in producing the syndrome, but evidence for the assumption is no stronger than the evidence implicating psychological factors as the major cause. See *late luteal phase dysphoric disorder.*

syndrome, prisoner of war (POW) Psychopathologic manifestations occurring in prisoners of war, presumbly a reaction to capture and imprisonment. Various types of reaction have been described, among them a syndrome of withdrawal, apathy, and sometimes death, which has been likened to the anaclitic depression reported by Spitz in hospitalized or otherwise deprived children.

syndrome, psychomimic Symptoms without organic basis that resemble the illness of another; typically, the latter illness has been fatal to an ambivalently related person, and the psychomimic syndrome often occurs on or near the anniversary of the other's death.

syndrome, Puerto Rican *Fighting sickness; male de pelea;* a culture-specific syndrome consisting of an initial brooding period followed by agitation and striking out against anyone the subject encounters.

syndrome, rabbit A perioral extrapyramidal movement disturbance associated with prolonged use of neuroleptics, consisting of quickly alternating, regulator movements of the oral and masticatory musculature (except for the tongue) along a vertical axis. Often an associated poppinglike sound is produced by the rapid separation of the lips. The movements are more rapid and regular than the chewing movements that may occur in tardive dyskinesia, and the rabbit syndrome ordinarily responds to anitparkinson agents (which may intensify symptoms of tardive dyskinesia).

syndrome, radiation somnolence A transient syndrome that develops in some children exposed to radiation (for the treatment of leukemia, for instance). It is caused by radiation-induced demyelinization and appears several weeks after radiation in the form of impaired attention, concentration, and memory, and clouding of consciousness with inability to maintain wakefulness.

syndrome, Refsum's *Heredopathia atactica polyneuritiformis;* first described by the Norwegian neurologist Sigvald Refsum in 1946. Principal symptoms are pigmentary retinitis, chronic polyneuritis, ataxia and other cerebellar disturbances, and albuminocytologic dissociation in cerebrospinal fluid. Other symptoms and signs are pupillary and skeletal anomalies, anosmia, deafness, ichthyosis, and changes in the electrocardiogram.

Onset is usually in childhood, although

the disease may not appear until the third decade; most commonly the course is one of gradual progression. The disease is probably transmitted by an autosomal recessive gene that affects lipid metabolism.

syndrome, Reiter's See *syndrome, Behçet's.*

syndrome, Renpenning's A type of mental retardation that is inherited as an X-linked recessive and characterized by a lack of associated physical abnormality.

syndrome, restless legs *Tachyathetosis* (q.v.)

syndrome, Roussy Levy See *ataxia, Friedreich's.*

syndrome, Rubenstein-Taybi *Broad thumb hallux syndrome;* a type of mental retardation, first described in 1963, characterized by broad thumbs and great toes, facial abnormalities, and a cluster of congenital malformations. Etiology is unknown but is presumed to be genetic.

syndrome, Sanfilippo's Type III *mucopolysaccharidosis* (q.v.).

syndrome, savant A rare disorder in which severe developmental or psychiatric handicap is combined with islands of remarkable ability, usually artistic or memory-related, that stand out in sharp contrast to the otherwise permeating disability.

syndrome, Seitelberger's Familial, progressive, juvenile neuroaxonal dystrophy; similar to (and possibly identical with) Hallervorden Spatz syndrome.

syndrome, silver cord A family constellation consisting of a passive or absent father and a dominating mother, believed by some to be significantly related to the subsequent development of schizophrenia. See *mother, schizophrenogenic.*

syndrome, Sjogren-Larsson Hereditary disorder first described in 1957 in Sweden by Sjogren and Larsson consisting of ichthyosis, mental retardation, and spastic paralysis. Degenerative retinitis and speech disorders may occur in addition to the diagnostic triad of symptoms. Transmission of the disorder is of the autosomal recessive type.

syndrome, social breakdown The deterioration in social abilities, interpersonal relationships, and general behavior that frequently accompanies organic and functional psychoses (and especially the schizophrenias). The term emphasizes the belief that such personality distortions, rather than being an inherent part of the psychotic process, are instead a reaction to

the patient's environment; the male patient who is isolated from women will no longer make attempts to be attractive to the opposite sex, the person who is deprived of all purposeful activity or removed from any meaningful occupation will have no reason to keep track of time, etc. The social breakdown syndrome occurs in many situations—mental hospitals, prisons, concentration camps, etc. See *psychiatry, community.*

syndrome, Steele-Richardson-Olszewski See *supranuclear palsy.*

syndrome, Stevens-Johnson *Erythema multiforme major; erythema multiforme bullosum;* an acute, inflammatory, system disease characterized by lesions of skin and mucous membranes (macules, papules, wheals, vesicles, bullae) and systemic manifestations (fever, malaise, dehydration, muscle and joint pains, toxemia, prostration, and sometimes death). Etiology is unknown, although the majority of evidence points to the condition as secondary to any number of other disorders, among them infections, drug reactions (including barbiturates and tranquilizers), vaccination, malignancy, deep X-ray therapy, contact dermatitis, and collagen disease. See *syndrome, Behçet's.*

syndrome, Stewart-Morel Internal frontal hyperostosis with adiposity and mental disturbances.

syndrome, stiff-man A poorly understood syndrome, related to abnormal phosphorus metabolism, consisting of painful, ironlike spasms of muscle groups in various parts of the body. The spasms can be so severe as to cause fractures of the long bones, and most patients show secondary hypertrophy of affected muscles as well as varus deformity of the feet. Course is prolonged, and death may occur after a number of years during or shortly after a severe spasm.

syndrome, Strauss See *impulse disorder, hyperkinetic.*

syndrome, striatal Disease of the striatum or striopallidal system, characterized, in general, by the following: (1) rigidity (a general increase of muscle tonus); (2) tremor (abnormal involuntary movements); (3) hypokinesia (poverty of voluntary, especially spontaneous movements); (4) impairment of associated movements; (5) absence of sensory disturbances; (6) absence of "true" paralysis, that is, absence of signs of involvement of pyramidal tracts.

syndrome, subclavian steal Symptoms of cerebral vascular insufficiency secondary to central stenosis or occlusion of the subclavian artery; blood is shunted past the occluded artery by reversal of blood flow in the vertebral artery, and blood is thereby "stolen" from the cerebral circulation. Symptoms can sometimes be removed by reconstructive vascular surgery.

syndrome, survivor Any number of symptoms, including depression, insomnia, anxiety, psychosomatic illnesses, nightmares, etc., that are believed to be based upon guilt feelings over being a sole—or nearly sole—survivor of a disaster in which others perished who were emotionally close, such as parents, siblings, spouse, or friends. The survivor syndrome is a type of *post-traumatic stress disorder* (q.v.). See *neurosis, traumatic*.

syndrome, Tapia's See *Tapia's syndrome*.

syndrome, tea and toast A phenomenon described in older people who develop nutritional deficiencies on the basis of inadequate diet. It is difficult, and expensive, to cook for one, and depression is characterized by a loss of pleasure in eating as well as diminution in energy. Since older people often are both poor and depressed, they are likely to nibble rather than take the time to prepare nutritious meals, and in time they often develop one or more severe deficiency disorders, the first sign of which may be an acute confusional state that is mistaken as an early sign of dementia.

syndrome, temporal lobe A constellation of characteristic interictal personality changes observed in many patients with temporal lobe epilepsy, consisting of changes in sexual behavior, religiosity, a tendency toward extensive or compulsive drawing and writing, preoccupation with detail and clarity, and a profound sense of righteousness.

syndrome, thalamic See *thalamus*.

syndrome, triple X Mild mental retardation associated with trisomy of the X chromosome.

syndrome, Vogt-Koyanagi See *syndrome, Behçet's*.

syndrome, vulnerable child Symptoms often noted in a child who, though he has survived an acute episode of severe illness, continues to be treated by his parents as if his life were still in considerable danger.

syndrome, Weber's A type of *hemiplegia alternans* (q.v.).

syndrome, Werner's Premature senility with general retardation of growth, skin atrophy, and endocrine disturbances.

syndrome, Wernicke-Korsakoff (Karl Wernicke, German neurologist, 1848–1905 and Sergei Korsakoff, Russian neurologist, 1853–1900) *Alcohol amnestic syndrome; amnesic confabulatory syndrome*. Although Wernicke's syndrome and Korsakoff's syndrome (or psychosis) have classically been considered separate entities, neuropathological studies have demonstrated that the pathological changes in each are identical but differences in localization of lesions have produced different clinical pictures. The basis is generally believed to be a thiamine deficiency, which produces lesions in the 3rd and 6th nerve nuclei and adjacent tegmentum (giving rise to palsies of ocular muscles and of gaze); in the vestibular nuclei (giving rise to nystagmus and disturbances in equilibrium), in the cerebellar cortex (producing ataxia), and in the diencephalon (giving rise to the characteristic severe anterograde amnesia, with inability to retain memory for events for more than a short time even though immediate memory is unimpaired and remote memory is only mildly impaired; confabulation is frequently associated with the amnesia).

Wernicke described polioencephalitis hemorrhagica superior in 1881; the clinical picture consisted of confusion, apathy, dullness, a dreamy delirium, oculomotor palsies, ptosis, pupillary changes (such as the Argyll Robertson pupil), nystagmus, vomiting, and ataxia.

Korsakoff's psychosis was accompanied by polyneuritis in about half of the cases described. It was characterized by the severe anterograde amnesia described above and, often, *confabulation* (q.v.). See *amnestic syndrome*.

syndrome, Zieve's Transient hyperlipaemia, jaundice, and hemolytic anemia associated with alcoholic fatty liver and cirrhosis, probably due to specific damage to the alpha cells of the islets of Langerhans and to the liver; in most cases, upper abdominal pain is so severe that an operable condition is suspected. (Kessel, L. *American Journal of Medicine* 32, 1962)

syndromes, acute Bleuler differentiated between the acute and chronic forms of schizophrenia. The acute syndromes are transitory states of various kinds that may occur as simple exacerbations of the chronic state or as reactive episodes, in response to emotionally charged experiences. The acute syndromes occur more frequently in the early years of the disease process; they may last for hours only, or they may persist for years. Subsequent memory for these episodes varies, but complete amnesia for them is unusual. Bleuler listed the following acute syndromes: melancholic conditions, manic conditions, catatonic states, delusions (amentia in the terms of the Viennese school), twilight states, Benommenheit, confusional states, fits of anger, anniversary excitements, stupor, deliria, fugue states, and dipsomania. See *schizophrenia.*

syndromes, culture-specific Behavior disorders that appear to be limited to certain societies and have no counterpart in current Western nosology. Among such syndromes are *amok, amurakh,* Arctic hysteria, *bangungut,* berserk, copying mania, *delahara, echul, falling out,* fighting sickness, *grisi siknis, Hsieh-Ping, imu,* jumpers, *juramentado, kimilue, koro, lata,* mal de pelea, menerik, *miryachit,* olonism, Oriental nightmare-death syndrome, piblokto, pseudoamok syndrome, Puerto Rican syndrome, *susto,* Tropenkoller, voodoo death, wihtigo psychosis, and *windigo psychosis* (qq.v.).

syneidesis (sīn-ī-dē'sis) *Rare.* This Greek word was proposed by Monakow to replace the English *conscience.* Monakow suggests that conscience is not a specifically human phenomenon and does not belong to the sphere of consciousness, but is a characteristic of all living beings in any stage of development. This concept is at variance with prevailing psychiatric opinion, which believes that conscience is a product of the interaction of the child with frustration-producing elements in the child's environment. See *conscience.*

synergism, sexual A sexual excitation that arises from a combination of various stimuli acting simultaneously. The manifold aspects of this combination range from pleasurable stimulation of the surface of the body to unpleasant, or even painful, processes within the organism. Freud considered that perhaps every important physical process contributes to the genesis of sexual excitement. Even the combination of the two opposed instinctual tendencies—love and hate—may arouse sexual excitement: sexual synergism can be aroused provided the intensity of discomfort and pain does not pass a certain limit. According to the individual sexual constitution, this synergism manifests itself in different ways. Reik asserts that sexual synergism "constitutes the physiological basis for the psychic superstructure of masochism." This peculiar sexual excitement is independent of the attitude of the subject toward the object: in many children mechanical concussions may produce this kind of sexual excitement, and, similarly, certain affective processes such as fright or horror may act as sexual stimuli, even in adults. In this respect one may cite the patients who distinguish between "disagreeable" and "interesting" pain. (Reik, T. *Masochism in Modern Man,* 1941)

synergy 1. Coordination of muscular movements. 2. Cooperation in action, primarily a function of the cerebellum.

synesthesia See *sensation, secondary.*

syngamy (sing'gà-mē) *Fertilization,* the biological phenomenon that brings about the intermingling of paternal and maternal hereditary material.

"It is accomplished by a great variety of means in animals and plants. In the lowest groups the gametes may be equal in size and similar in structure (an *isogamous* condition), but in the great majority of all animals and plants they are unequal *(heterogamous),* the male gamete being relatively small and consisting of little but a nucleus, and the female gamete (egg) being very much larger and possessing a considerable amount of cytoplasm in addition to its nucleus." (Sinnott, E.W., & Dunn, L.C. *Principles of Genetics,* 1939)

syngignoscism (sin-jig'nos-iz'm) *Obs.* Hypnotism; suggestion.

synkinesia, synkinesis An involuntary movement accompanying a voluntary one; such as the movement (occurring in a paralyzed muscle) accompanying motion in another part; any abnormal associated movement(s), indicative of neural injury or maldevelopment; they are brought out when the subject voluntarily contracts one muscle or muscle group, for then other unintended and unneeded movements appear. Such associated movements, also termed *adventitious motor overflow*, suggest frontal lobe dysfunction.

Various forms of synkinesis have been described; Gunn, for example, described a palpebromandibular synkinesia, consisting of elevation of the upper lid during any movement of the lower jaw.

synnoetics (sin-oi-e'tiks) A term suggested by Fein for the science "treating of the properties of composite systems . . . whose main attribute is that its ability to invent, to create, and to reason—its 'mental' power of its components." Another term for synnoetics would be "the computer-related sciences," which would include such subjects as cybernetics, computer science, and bionics. (*American Scientist* 49, 1961)

synthesis The combination or grouping of parts or elements so as to form an integrated whole; the integration of the various factors making up the personality and thus the opposite of analysis. This term has been used with various shades of meaning by different writers. Prince used it to refer to the ability to keep the component parts of the psyche together in close association; any weakening of synthesis tends to produce dissociation and hence neurosis. Synthesis has also been used to refer to maintenance of intactness of personality; in this sense, synthesis is the opposite of *splitting* in Bleuler's sense. Gestalt psychologists use the term synthesis to refer to the tendency to perceive and appreciate situations as a whole. In psychoanalytic psychology, synthesis is considered to be a complex ego function, probably a derivative of libido, which impels the person to harmonious unification and creativity in the broadest sense of the term. Synthesis includes a tendency to simplify, to generalize, and ultimately to understand—by assimilating external and internal elements, by reconciling conflicting ideas, by uniting contrasts, and by seeking for causality. See *constructive; ego; ego strength; object relations theory; psychology, gestalt; psychosynthesis.*

synthesis, distributive In objective psychobiology, the "synthesis of the various factors and strivings which will offer the patient security. . . . The material for such a synthesis is obtained by analysis of all the factors and situations which are of importance in the study of the human personality and more specifically in the pathologic reactions which bring a patient to the physician. . . . Every analysis should lead to synthesis and after each consultation physician and patient should be able to formulate what has been obtained from the analysis and how it can be used constructively." (Diethelm, O. *Treatment in Psychiatry,* 1936)

synthesis, syllabic The combination of syllables of several words to form a new word or neologism. The process is common in the productions of schizophrenic patients and in dreams.

"The condensation-work of dreams becomes most palpable when it takes words and names as its objects. Generally speaking, words are often treated in dreams as things, and therefore undergo the same combinations as the ideas of things. The results of such dreams are comical and bizarre word-formations." (Freud, *ID*) See *condensation; neologism.*

syntone One whose personality is in harmony with the environment. The term implies emotional rapport, in particular. Bleuler at times uses the expression interchangeably with *cyclothyme.*

"According to a more recent theory of these two groups of psychoses one observes *even in normal people* a syntonic ('cyclothymic') reaction type, in which the whole personality uniformly participates in a definite and relatively vivid affect, suitable for the situation of the moment, and the train of ideas follows substantially quite logical laws." (Bleuler, *TP*)

The term *syntone* implies normality, while usually *cyclothyme* describes a personality that is an exaggeration of the syntonic but is less intense than that observed in the manic-depressive reaction.

syntropy (sin'trō-pē) The state of wholesome association with others.

syphilis An infectious venereal disease caused by *Treponema pallidum;* lues.

syphilis, cerebral Meningovascular syphilis; interstitial syphilis. The term includes syphilitic leptomeningitis, vascular neurosyphilis or luetic endarteritis, and the gummatous subtype. The essential lesion in cerebral syphilis is vascular and parivascular inflammation of varying degrees. Symptoms, which typically appear about three years after the primary infection, depend upon the site and extent of involvement. Thus there may be primarily a picture of acute or chronic leptomeningitis with signs of increased intracranial pressure and involvement of the cranial nerves (especially III, IV, and VII); or luetic endarteritis may lead to occlusion and thus to hemiplegia or convulsions; or development of a gumma may simulate the appearance of intracranial neoplasm. Superimposed on these neurological signs are mental symptoms such as intellectual dulling, emotional lability, stupor, fearful delirium, and/or multiple somatic complaints. Cerebral syphilis often responds favorably to penicillin treatment.

syphilis, congenital See *neurosyphilis, congenital.*

syphilis, mesodermogenic Meningovascular syphilis. See *syphilis, cerebral.*

syphilomania *Rare.* Insanity resulting from syphilophobia.

syphilophobia Fear of syphilis.

syphilopsychosis Southard's term for psychosis associated with central nervous system syphilis.

syringobulbia See *syringomyelia.*

syringomyelia *Status dysraphicus;* a chronic disease, probably due to a developmental defect, consisting of central cavitation of the spinal cord or ventricle in the medulla (*syringobulbia*). Symptoms begin in the second and third decades; 70% of those affected are male. Enlargement of the cavity affects, in order, the following structures: the anterior commissure, the anterior horn cells, and the pyramidal tracts. Pain and temperature sensation are impaired, but touch and proprioception are intact; hand and finger movements become weak and awkward, and a claw hand develops. Trophic disturbances are prominent, with thickened skin and various arthropathies (some would call this form *Morvan's disease*). In the bulbar form, symptoms referable to disturbances of the tenth, eighth, and fifth cranial nerves and of the medial lemniscus are seen. Affected patients usu-

ally live many years. Palliative X-ray irradiation of the affected region of the spinal cord or medulla is sometimes beneficial.

system In psychoanalytic psychology, any of the organizational units of the psychic apparatus; the ψ-systems (psychic apparatus) include the *P-system* (perception), the *mem-system* (memory), the *Pcs* (preconscious), and the *Ucs* (unconscious).

system, Aberdeen Day industrial feeding schools, used in the 19th century and associated with a social movement, spearheaded by Sheriff Watson, that gave priority to family ties, emphasized the rights of children, and advocated a day-care system (rather than residential placement) to meet the needs of the whole child in his family and community setting.

system, action A bodily system that enables the organism to take action in response to a desire: a desire to keep one's feet dry will cause one to walk around and not through a puddle. The means by which this action is taken is produced by the integration of receptor, coordinative, effector systems into a functioning unit or action system.

The term action system was introduced by Kardiner in connection with his studies of the traumatic neuroses. He maintains that the traumatic neuroses present a symptomatology and a psychodynamic structure that cannot be fully understood or adequately explained on the basis of instinct as an operational concept. Instead of using instinct as an operational concept in studying the traumatic neuroses, he takes as his operational concept the various action systems of the body by which instinct is put into action. The damaging of these action systems, with consequent impairment of their function, explains the traumatic neuroses and, indeed, *is* traumatic neuroses. (Kardiner, A., & Spiegel, L. *War Stress and Neurotic Illness,* 1947)

system, adviser An educational program for supervisory personnel (e.g. sergeants) used in the U.S. Armed Forces in World War II; by alerting such personnel to the emotional, domestic, and physical problems of trainees (inductees, draftees), and the ways in which they were likely to be expressed within their units, the program was able to reduce psychoneurotic reactions as well as behavior subject to disciplinary action.

system, anabolic In constitutional medicine two large systems are described—the anabolic and the catabolic, corresponding with the megalosplanchnic (pyknic) and the microsplanchnic (asthenic) habitus, respectively.

system, boarding-out A system under which psychotic patients are taken care of as boarders in private homes. See *domicile; Gheel Colony.*

system, centrencephalic Penfield's term for a hypothesized central structure of neurons in the brain stem that is conceived of as the anatomical basis for the coherent unity of mental processes. In many respects, the centrencephalic system would appear to be identical with the reticular activating system. See *formation, reticular.*

system, chronological See *complex, subject.*

system, graphogenic See *mechanism, homogenic.*

system, graphonomic See *mechanism, homogenic.*

system, intralaminar Morison and Dempsey's term for a diffuse, bilateral, nonspecific projection system of neurons in the thalamus. Also known as the *recruiting system,* the intralaminar system is associated with consciousness, sleep, and wakefulness and thus would appear to be identical with the *reticular activating system* in many respects. See *formation, reticular.*

system, perceptual-conscious The part of the mental apparatus that absorbs perceptions from both the external world and the interior of the mind (the id). Early in the development of the human mind, one part of it becomes the recipient of stimuli. In this part of the mind the feeling of consciousness originates and, for this reason, it is named the perceptual-conscious system.

As the mind develops, its new task is to protect the organism from the stimuli that are dangerous to the organism. The mind learns to retain a true picture of the external world by its memory of the perceptions that, through reality-testing, it keeps from being contaminated by instinctual demands. With this later function, anticipation, reason, and judgment become possible and take over the control of motility or action. The part of the mental apparatus that has developed the faculties of memory, reality testing, reason, and judgment

toward the end of controlling the instincts and thus protecting the organism is called the ego. But the earliest function that is decisive for the ego must be the perception of stimuli, since without this perception none of its more complex functions can be carried out. The ego thus originates in the perceptual-conscious system, "the most superficial portion of the mental apparatus." (Freud, S. *New Introductory Lectures on Psychoanalysis,* 1933)

system, pride Horney's term for the sum total of the neurotically (over-)valued and the neurotically (over-)hated attributes of the self.

system, psychodynamic cerebral See *psychodynamics, adaptational.*

system, recruiting See *system, intralaminar.*

system, reticular See *formation, reticular.*

system, rotation The method some group psychotherapists employ of treating individual patients in sequence in the presence of the group.

system, sign Schilder's term for the use of language as the main tool, or instrument, of psychotherapy. Through words, the psychiatrist gains access to and unveils the patient's hidden problems and inner personality. Words in the sign system are to the psychiatrist what knives and other instruments are to the surgeon. "The psychotherapist has no immediate access to the body of the patient and to his gratifications. The influence he has on the patient is merely due to the words he speaks." In a broader sense, every social relation between two persons speaking to each other includes the erotic. Man needs not only actual but also future gratification, "and humanity has elaborated a system for such gratification," language constituting the main, though by no means the only, element of this system. In the relationship between the sexes, words and sentences in themselves may become signs through which the individuals obtain their social and erotic gratifications. (Schilder, P. *Psychotherapy,* 1938)

system, stereogenic See *constant, central; mechanism, orthogenic.*

system, stereonomic See *constant, central; mechanism, orthogenic.*

system, villa Boarding-out system. See *domicile.*

systematic desensitization See *desensitization.*

systematic schizophrenia See *schizophrenia, systematic.*

systematic family therapy See *family therapy, systemic.*

systems interview, family See *family systems interview.*

systems theory See *general systems theory.*

T

T-group Sensitivity training group. An educational-psychotherapeutic technique in which a group of people meets regularly, usually with a specified leader, in order to learn about themselves, about interpersonal relationships, about group process, and about larger social systems. The T-group is experience-based learning (rather than a type of therapy for recognized emotional disturbance), and its major aims include increasing relatedness and opening communication channels between the group member and others within his social system. The T-group is reality-oriented and focuses on connections between current reactions and universal psychologic concepts rather than on individual genetic antecedents of those reactions. Used in industrial organizations, for example, the T-group tries to get its members to own up to their own feelings (including their feelings about each other), to become open to new ideas and experiment with new solutions to problems (i.e. to replace automaton conformity with a capacity for risk-taking), and thereby to generate effective decision making within the organization. T-groups are sometimes also called human relations groups.

TA *Transactional analysis* (q.v.).

tabes (tā′bez) (L. "a wasting, emaciation") *Tabes dorsalis, locomotor ataxia;* a chronic, progressive disease of the nervous system occurring rather late in a comparatively small percentage of persons affected with syphilis. The main pathological process involves the posterior spinal ganglia in a mild inflammation. The roots between the ganglia and the spinal cord, and, to some extent, the meninges are also involved. There is a degeneration of the nerve fibers with a selective degeneration of the posterior columns of the cord. The cranial nerves, especially the optic and those supplying the ocular muscles, are particularly involved. The symptoms are ataxia, or muscular incoordination, neuralgia, anesthesia, visceral crises, lancinating pains, and muscular atrophy. Trophic disorders of the joints (arthropathies) are frequent, atrophy of the optic nerve occurs, and paralysis may be a late symptom. Mental symptoms are not usually prominent, although a severe depression may occur.

tabes, congenital See *neurosyphilis, congenital.*

tabes, juvenile Juvenile tabes presents an essentially identical pathologic process and clinical course as in the adult. The symptoms appear from the age of 10 onward in children who have congenital syphilis or who acquired the disease in infancy or early childhood. Ataxia is rather infrequent while optic atrophy is very common in juvenile tabes. Mental symptoms and taboparesis occur frequently. The Wasserman blood reaction is often negative. The course is much more rapid than in the adult form, and the disease terminates fatally comparatively early.

tabetic curve See *Lange's colloidal gold reaction.*

table, frequency The number of subjects with a given character may be arrayed in order of size with respect to the amount of the character possessed by each individual in the series. If the entire range is divided into intervals, and if to each interval is assigned the number of cases falling within the limits of the class, the resulting distribution is called a frequency table.

Age Distribution of Admissions to Private Mental Hospitals, United States, 1975

Age (years)	No.	%
Under 15	19,178	11.6
15–24	23,972	14.5
25–34	30,586	18.5
35–44	28,271	17.1
45–54	28,767	17.4
55–64	17,359	10.5
65+	17,194	10.4

table, life An instrument for determining the number of years that any person may, on the average, be expected to live after reaching a specified age. It also enables one to determine the chance of an individual dying within any specified number of years after reaching a given age.

Expectation of Life in Years by Race, Age, and Sex, United States, 1977

Age (years)	Total	White Male	White Female	Black and Other Male	Black and Other Female
At birth	73.2	70.0	77.7	64.6	73.1
15	59.6	56.5	63.9	51.8	60.0
25	50.3	47.3	54.3	42.8	50.5
35	40.9	38.0	44.6	34.3	41.2
45	31.8	29.0	35.2	26.3	32.4
55	23.5	20.8	26.4	19.4	24.5
65	16.3	13.9	18.4	14.0	17.8
75	10.4	8.6	11.5	9.7	12.5
85+	6.4	5.3	6.8	7.3	9.6

table, statistical A summary of numerical data in accordance with logical criteria, showing the manner in which the variables included in the table are distributed with respect to their relative frequencies.

taboo, tabu "For us the meaning of taboo branches off into two opposite directions. On the one hand it means to us, sacred, consecrated: but on the other hand it means uncanny, dangerous, forbidden and unclean. The opposite for taboo is designated in Polynesian by the word *noa* and signifies something ordinary and generally accessible. Thus something like the concept of reserve inheres in taboo; taboo expresses itself essentially in prohibitions and restrictions. Our combination of 'hold dread' would often express the meaning of taboo." (Freud, *BW*)

taboparesis A disease of the nervous system that combines the features of general paresis and tabes dorsalis. The mental and physical symptoms of general paresis are present together with spinal cord changes producing absent knee or ankle jerks, the Romberg sign, and bladder disturbances.

tabula rasa (L. "erased or blank tablet") Clean slate, or, by extension, the mind at birth. The tabula rasa idea finds its modern expression in Pavlovian psychology, an environmentalist view that the nature of the response is determined by the stimulus. Such a position is much more subject than the biological to whatever ideology is defined by the political or cultural values of the moment as the fit, normal, or desirable way of life.

tachy- (tak-ē-) Combining form meaning quick, swift, fleet, from Gr. *tachýs*. Opposite of *brady-*.

tachyathetosis *Restless legs syndrome* (q.v.).

tachycardia, orthostatic Rapidity of pulse rate beyond the normal range occurring when one changes from the reclining to the standing position.

tachyglossa See *tachylogia*.

tachyglossal Pertaining to or characterized by tachyglossa, or rapidity of speech.

tachylalia See *cluttering*; *tachylogia*.

tachylogia *Hyperlogia; hyperphrasia; lallorhea; logodiarrhea; logomania; logorrhea; polylogia; polyphrasia; tachylalia; tachyphrasia; verbomania;* rapid, pressured, voluble speech. Tachylogia is characteristic of the manic phase of manic-depressive (bipolar) disorder.

tachyphagia Food-grabbing; extreme rapidity of eating. Tachyphagia is commonly seen in regressed, deteriorated schizophrenics, and often such patients will grab any object, edible or not, put it into the mouth, and swallow it.

tachyphemia See *tachylogia*.

tachyphrasia See *tachylogia*.

tachypnea, tachypnoea (tak-ip′nē-à) See *polypnoea*.

tachypragia *Rare.* Psychomotor acceleration, as in the manic phase of manic-depressive disorder.

tachytrophism Rapid or increased metabolism.

tactical research See *research, strategic*.

tactile sensation, double simultaneous The ability of the subject to perceive that he has been touched in two places at the same time. This is usually acquired by the age of 6 years and is considered an index of biological sentiency, level of organization, and discrimination of environmental changes. It is often late in developing or otherwise defective in childhood schizophrenics and in children with minimal brain dysfunction; it is also often impaired in patients with diffuse brain damage (e.g. cerebral arteriosclerosis). The *face-hand test* (of Fink-Green-Bender) is designed to measure such impairment. The patient is touched simultaneously on the cheek and the dorsum of the hand, and is asked to indicate where he was touched. Ten trials are given: eight face-hand (divided between four contralateral and four ipsilateral), and two interspersed combinations of face-face and hand-hand stimulation.

taeniphobia Fear of tapeworms.

taint In genetics, the genotypical affection of an individual by a morbid factor inherited from, and manifested by, his ancestors, whether or not this factor is exhibited by the subject himself.

taint carrier In a family survey, this genetic term is limited to the members who carry a particular genetic factor in their genotypes, but do not manifest it phenotypically. See *trait carrier.*

talion Retaliation. See *dread, talion.*

tangentiality A type of association disturbance in which thought and speech diverge or digress from the topic of the moment so that they appear unrelated or irrelevant; if often repeated (and especially if the speaker does not return spontaneously to the topic), tangentiality is labeled loosening or diffuseness of speech, and its end result is to destroy the value of speech as an effective means of communicating with others.

Tantra A group of Hindu or Buddhist sacred scriptures containing instructions for various kinds of meditation and worship with the aim of achieving unity between the worshiper and the deity. Tantric rituals include sexual intercourse (divine intercourse between god and goddess, rather than bestial or lustful human sexuality); *mantras* (sacred sounds with a magical power to gain the desired unity); visual images, including mental representation of the deity and *mandalas* or *yantras*, external diagrams representing the abode of the worshiped deity (Jung viewed them as a way to develop harmony between the conscious and unconscious); and breathing techniques, used in Tantric Yoga to achieve identity with the infinite.

tantrum A child's dramatic outburst of crying, kicking, screaming, etc., in response to frustration. Such temper-tantrums are natural to the child of 2 or 3 and are an expression of aggression, anger, rage, and defiance. The child works himself rapidly, or gradually, into a rage—yells out, stamps his feet, throws his arms about, rolls on the floor, strikes everyone, throws every object within reach against the walls, curses, bites, or even bangs his head against the wall. The tantrum thus assumes uncontrolled and sweeping proportions in contrast to normal expressions of anger and rage.

Tantrums are seen almost routinely in the children of overindulgent, oversolicitous, and overprotective parents. Though originating in physical discomforts which increase the child's irritability, tantrums either are motivated by an attempt to obtain gratifications and dominate a family that allows itself to be controlled by these outbursts, or are a result of imitation of a parent or some other member of the household.

Persistence or reappearance of tantrums after the age of 3 years indicates pathology and is classified within the *oppositional disorders* (q.v.).

taoism Chinese philosophy founded by Lao Tsu in the 6th century B.C. The *Tao te Ching* expresses this simple philosophy of life: "Empty and be full; wear out and be new; have little and gain; have much and be confused." Taoist practices include effortless, yet effective action that proceeds gently, without force; modesty and sincerity in social relationships; an awareness of one's own energetic processes (*t'ai chi*); and a transcendence of the dualizing limitations of percepts and concepts. The last allows the participant to merge with and be guided by the Tao (the ultimate source and unifying principle of all that exists or is in process). The fundamental intent is toward the experience of the unification of all opposites, falsely dichotomized by the seduction of reason, toward the gradual attainment of clarity and openness in a creative balance.

taphephobia Fear of being buried (alive).

taphophilia Morbid attraction to graves and cemeteries. A patient spent all his spare time either in cemeteries or in thoughts connected with them. Though highly intelligent, he was emotionally immature, having never resolved his childhood relationships with his parents. He was vividly anal-erotic, expressing among other things a strong coprophagic tendency. Another patient often carried out his impulse to defecate on graves, though, as he maintained, a grave was sacred to him. He endowed graves with unlimited magic power, to which he added his own power (feces). Still another patient saved most of his excrement, burying it from time to time in a neighboring cemetery. See *necrophilia*.

Tapia's syndrome (Antonio Garcia Tapia, Spanish otolaryngologist, 1875–1950) A bulbar syndrome due to involvement of the vagus and hypoglossal nerves, with homolateral paralysis and atrophy of the tongue, and homolateral paralysis of the pharynx and larynx.

tarantism *Obs.* Dancing mania; specifically, what appears to have been a culture-specific syndrome in Italy in the 16th and 17th centuries, consisting of compulsive dancing as a way to undo the bite of the tarantula.

taraxein (tar-ak′sān) See *ceruloplasmin*.

tardive As used currently in psychiatry, tardy in the sense of being (or appearing) late rather than in the more proper sense of being slow. See *dyskinesia, tardive*.

tardive dysmentia See *dysmentia, tardive*.

target multiplicity See *multiplicity, target*.

target organ See *syndrome, general adaptation*.

task, primary In group process theory, any task that a system must carry out in order to survive.

TAT Thematic apperception test. See *test, thematic apperception*.

taxis Tropism; movement toward or away from some source of stimulation. Used loosely in social psychiatry to refer to the stimulus itself, in which case *taxis* refers to inanimate stimulation, *biotaxis* to animal or human stimulation, *sociotaxis* to social stimulation. See *network*.

Tay-Sachs disease (Warren Tay, English physician, 1843–1927; and Bernard Sachs, American neurologist, 1858–1944) *Amaurotic family idiocy; cerebromacular degeneration;* first described by Tay (1881), who referred principally to the ocular changes. In 1887, Sachs described the brain changes in a paper, "Arrested Cerebral Develop-

ment." A familial disorder of lipoid metabolism, caused by a single recessive autosomal gene. A progressive deposition of lipids, mainly GM2 gangliosides, in the ganglion cells of the brain and retina, leads to blindness, muscular wasting and enfeeblement, and mental retardation.

Four forms are recognized: (1) *infantile form,* originally found mainly among Polish Jews, the symptoms appearing as early as the third month; (2) *late infantile form,* appearing between the second and fifth years; (3) *juvenile form,* appearing in older children between the sixth and twelfth years, was described by Spielmeyer. It resembles the infantile type, shows gradual mental impairment and terminates in blindness and death within two years. Although optic atrophy occurs, there are no changes in the macula lutea; (4) *adult form,* occurring after puberty, though usually not beyond the third decade. Some writers refer to the infantile form only as Tay-Sachs disease, to the late infantile form as Bielschowsky's disease, to the juvenile form as Vogt-Spielmeyer's disease, and to the adult or tardive form as Kuf's disease.

The underlying biochemical defect, a deficiency of β-hexosaminidase-A, results in accumulation of its major substrate, GM2 ganglioside. Carriers of the mutant gene can now be detected, and the enzyme deficiency can be detected in the fetus through amniocentesis. The mutation responsible for the defect is believed to have arisen during the Middle Ages in certain regions of eastern Europe. Incidence is highest among Ashkenazic Jews and their descendants; 1 in 30 Jews carries the gene, but only 1 in 300 non-Jews carries it.

TC *Therapeutic community* (q.v.).

TCA Tricyclic antidepressant drugs. See *antidepressant; psychotropics*.

tea and toast syndrome See *syndrome, tea and toast*.

technique, classical See *parameter*.

technique, play A psychotherapeutic method devised by Melanie Klein for special use in the treatment of children. By allowing a child to play with almost anything he wants, the therapist is, through this play, able to analyze and clarify the child's emotional problem. This technique is, in effect, a very useful substitute for the free-association method, in view of the child's usual lack of verbal self-expression. Adult patients will, sooner or later, translate into words not only their problems but also the actions that may take place during the analysis. With children such verbalizations are next to impossible and the play technique is of paramount importance. Toys of all kinds can be used but it is usually better to use toys that do not move by themselves. Frequently the child accompanies his play with short remarks that elucidate the situation. See *therapy, play.*

TEFRA Tax Equity and Fiscal Responsibility Act of 1982 (PL 97-248), intended to reduce Medicaid and Medicare expenditures. It is the most significant health care financing legislation since Medicaid and Medicare were created in 1965 and directly affects all hospitals, insurers, pension plans, and major corporate purchasers of health insurance.

tegmentum See *midbrain.*

tele (tel′ē) (Gr. "at a distance, far away, far off") In Moreno's system of sociometry, the intuitive reaction of liking or disliking another person based upon something real in that other person; the opposite of *transference* (q.v.), in which the reaction is an expression of the subject's needs rather than an appropriate response to the object's behavior or attitude.

telemnemonike (tel-em-nē-mon′i-kē) Acquiring consciousness of matters held in the memory of another person.

telencephalon That part of the *forebrain* (q.v.) or prosencephalon which forms the cerebral cortex, the striate bodies, the rhinencephalon, the lateral ventricles, and the anterior portion of the 3rd ventricle.

teleoanalysis See *teleological.*

teleologic regression Purposeful regression. See *regression, progressive teleologic.*

teleological Goal-directed, purposive; used particularly to refer to Adler's insistence on the holistic approach to personality and his belief that a person can best be understood by the goals he sets for himself, and not by any analysis or dissection of partial functions such as sexuality. The understanding of goals and the helping of patients to change their goals are so basic to Adlerian psychotherapy that individual psychology has sometimes been called *teleoanalysis.*

teleology The belief that natural processes are purposefully directed toward some end or goal. In psychiatry, the term is particularly used in reference to the psychologies of Jung and of Adler. Adler, for example, considers the present activity of the person as a preparation for his final state, for what he is going to be. Jung's analytical psychology is also teleological. Jung considers the mind as something much more than the result of past experiences: "It is Becoming as well as Has Been, and therefore any analysis of it must include reference to its aims and to that which it is trying to realize within itself. In this connection the dream must therefore be regarded as partly determined by the future." (Nicole, J. *Psychotherapy,* 1948) Jung treats the symbols from the collective unconscious "not only reductively as an expression of the past of the race, but synthetically also, as a sign that the unconscious is trying to exert a directive influence upon the individual's life-line. These symbols should be interpreted teleologically, as indicative of fundamental strivings that are aiming at guiding the personality along certain lines, certain necessary paths of development and fulfilment. It is only by thus giving these symbols a 'final' or purposive value as well as a 'casual' one, that we can adjust the unconscious to the conscious, the collective to the individual, the non-rational to the rational, without either principle doing violence to the other. This means that the physician's explanations must, of necessity, become educational and morally conditioned, thus performing a task that psycho-analysts refuse to undertake." (Ibid.)

teleophrenia *Obs.* Term coined by M. Nippe for a morbid mental condition that stands between traumatic neurosis and malingering; compensation neurosis. See *neurosis, compensation.*

telepathic Pertaining to telepathy or characterized or communicated by thought transference.

telepathy See *perception, extrasensory.*

telephone scatalogia A paraphilia in which the person gains sexual arousal from making lewd calls. See *psychosexual disorders; scatology.*

telesthesia Telepathy.

telodendria See *neuron.*

telophase In genetics, the final phase or stage of mitosis.

temper tantrum See *tantrum.*

temperament A constitutional tendency to react to one's environment in a certain way. Some people are more placid than others, some more vigorous, some more high-strung; it is likely that such differences are genetically based and recognizable from the moment of birth. Temperament is not identical with character, though often confused with it, especially in popular language. Temperament is probably instrumental in determining the particular type of character structure developed by a person in that it limits the potentialities for character development: it is unlikely that a constitutionally phlegmatic person would develop an anxious, rigid, and compulsive character structure. Character, on the other hand, is something in addition to temperament, as a component within the framework of the possibilities encompassed by the given temperament.

Recent studies have identified ten indicators of temperament in children: approach, withdrawal, rhythmicity (regularity), quality of mood, intensity of reaction, adaptability, activity level, threshold, distractibility, and attention span.

temperament, manic *Obs.* Kraepelin's designation for what is today known as one of the phases of *cyclothymia.* "The intellectual endowment of the patients is for the most part mediocre, sometimes even fairly good, in isolated cases excellent. They acquire, however, as a rule, only scanty, and, in particular, very imperfect and unequal knowledge, because they show no perseverance in learning, do not like exerting themselves, are extraordinarily distractible, and seek to escape in every way from the constraint of a systematic mental training, and in place of that they pursue all possible side occupations in variegated alternation." (*Manic-Depressive Insanity and Paranoia,* 1921) He adds that the mood is "permanently exalted, careless, confident" and that conduct is unsteady and restless.

temporal lobe seizure Psychomotor epilepsy. See *epilepsy.*

temporal orientation Awareness of the relationship of sounds, ability to remember sounds and rhythms, and actual knowledge of time. Disorganization in the temporospatial sphere is often manifested in motor defects, because if the subject is defectively oriented he is compromised in his ability to translate perceptions into the motor activity or reactivity that would be expected.

temporal summation See *summation.*

temptation, horrific One of Rado's subdivisions of obsessive attacks: an idea or urge of compelling intensity to kill or harm someone (usually a close relative), an idea from which the patient shrinks back in horror.

tendency, anagogic See *tendency, katogogic.*

tendency, final The ultimate goal or aim of the neurosis. Adler was the first to point out "the presence of a final tendency in the structure of every neurosis." In this respect he was guided by both Janet's theory of the *idée fixe* and Wernicke's concept of over-charged idea. See *idea, overcharged.*

"The neurotic goals are not sheer strivings for power and recognition: they betoken a secret tendency toward future triumphs expressed in many forms that might even be antagonistic to each other. Nevertheless, it may be stated that every neurosis has a central idea around which the various *lay motives* group themselves." The task of the analyst is to uncover as early as possible this central idea (the final tendency and ultimate goal of the neurosis) if success is to be expected in treatment. (Stekel, *CD*)

tendency, katagogic The "downward-leading" restrictive psychic impulses that strive to prevent the person from achieving his positive and constructive aim in life. In fact, the katagogic tendency constitutes an inhibitory mechanism in opposition to what Stekel calls *anagogic tendency,* or "upward-leading" impulses, which are of a constructive nature. (Stekel, *ID*)

tendency of action In objective psychobiology the inclinations associated with action. "One should always study the general behavior of a person while talking to him. Much can be learned from his way of entering the room, shaking hands, talking, and from his facial expression, gestures and posture . . . emotions are the regulative functions of our personality and are therefore closely related to the behavior of the person in action." (Diethelm, O. *Treatment in Psychiatry,* 1936) See *body language.*

tender years presumption See *custody.*

tenesmus penis (te-nes′moos pā′nēs) (L. "straining of the penis") *Priapism* (q.v.).

tension, instinctual The psychic and somatic manifestations of the need to gratify a primal trend or urge.

tension, mental The emotional charge with which components of the psyche are infused; *psychentonia*. See *cathexis*.

tension, need A tension that develops within the organism in connection with various needs essential for survival, which demands contact with the outer world for its relief. "Being born may be said to have already interfered with the equilibrium of the intrauterine state, because stimuli are now registered upon the organism from within (hunger) and without (cold). To relieve these *need tensions* the infant must direct itself to the outer world, or show signs of the unpleasant effects created by these tensions." (Kardiner, A., & Spiegel, H. *War Stress and Neurotic Illness,* 1947)

tension, premenstrual See *syndrome, premenstrual.*

tentigo venerea *Obs.* (L. "venereal, sexual lust") *Nymphomania* (q.v.) .

tentigo vereti *Obs.* (L. "tensions or lust of the private parts") *Satyriasis* (q.v.).

tentorium cerebelli See *meninges.*

TEPP See *psychotomimetic.*

teratology The study of birth defects and their causes; *congenital malformations* (any structural defects present at birth) account for approximately 15% of all deaths in the first year of life. Their overall incidence is in the range of 1–10% of all births, but the most severe developmental defects are not compatible with survival of the fetus so they are reported as spontaneous abortions rather than as congenital malformations.

teratophobia Fear of bearing a monster.

territoriality The characteristic behavior by which an organism lays claim to and defends an area against the encroachment of members of its own species.

terror, night or sleep *Sleep terror disorder* (q.v.).

test A systematic procedure to measure or assess some characteristic, ability, or skill of a subject, such as intelligence or personality traits. A *normative-referenced* test is one that compares the performance of the individual subject with a group whose performance on the test is used as a standard.

A *criterion-referenced* test is one in which the standard is a specified set of performances or actions; the subject is evaluated as to whether he does or does not meet the criteria, without comparing his performance to that of a group (e.g. can the patient dress himself, or can he not?). See *reliability; validity.*

test, ability Any evaluation of presently existing potentiality or capacity to function; a test of maximal performance in any area.

test, ACE The American Council on Education intelligence test, designed for use with secondary school and college students.

test, achievement Any evaluation of what gains the subject has made in an area following training and instruction.

test, Adrenalin-Mecholyl Funkenstein test; first described by Funkenstein, Greenblatt, and Solomon in 1952 as a test of prognostic significance in relation to electroshock treatment (EST). The test consists of the administration, on two successive days and under comparable basal conditions, of intravenous epinephrine hydrochloride and intramuscular Mecholyl chloride. The blood pressure response to each drug is then recorded. Response to Mecholyl appears to be the more significant of the two measures, and it has been observed that patients with a hypotensive response (1) are benefited by EST; (2) also show a high rate of improvement when psychotherapy is the sole method of treatment; (3) have good abstraction ability and good personality organization; and (4) appear clinically to maintain an appropriate and adequate level of affect. In general, patients with a hypertensive response to Mecholyl are not benefited by EST, show a relatively lower improvement rate with psychotherapy, have poor abstraction and inadequate or inappropriate affect, and give other evidence of personality disorganization.

test, Akerfeldt See *ceruloplasmin.*

test, analogies A test of ability to comprehend relationships, usually by asking the subject to name the fourth term that bears the same relation to the third as the second does to the first. Example: Ship is to water as automobile is to what?

test, aptitude A test of the probable level of future performance that will be reached following further maturation and/or training.

Test, Army General Classification See *AGCT*.

test, Arthur Point Scale A nonverbal performance measure of intellectual ability, consisting of 10 subtests, mainly of the form-board variety. The test is most reliable within the 7- to 13-year age range and is of particular value when the subject's verbal capacity is compromised by foreign language handicap, speech or hearing defect, or personal and cultural factors.

test, Bender Visual-Motor Gestalt A projective technique consisting of nine geometrical figures that are copied by the subject; devised by Lauretta Bender and first described by her in 1938. Its chief applications are to determine retardation, loss of function, and organic brain defects in children and adults, and in the study of personality deviations that show regressive phenomena. It is of limited usefulness in the study of psychoneuroses and psychosomatic disorders.

test, Bero (bā′rō) Behn-Rorschach test; a set of plates prepared by Behn with the assistance of Rorschach. Zullinger provided the norms for the Bero test.

test, beta A set of mental tests used in the U.S. Army in 1917–18, designed for illiterates. Instructions are given in signs and the material is pictorial in character, in contrast to alpha tests, which are carried out verbally.

test, block design A performance test in which the subject tries to match standard designs using colored blocks; used as a measure of intelligence and as an indicator of deterioration in brain damage and in the schizophrenias.

test, cancellation Any test in which the subject is instructed to strike out one or more specified symbols that are distributed irregularly within the test material. The symbols may be particular letters, numbers, words, or geometrical figures.

test, chi-square A statistical test, developed originally by Karl Pearson, that measures the significance of differences occurring between groups. In a group of 500 cases of lobar pneumonia treated with penicillin, for example, the overall cure rate was 94%. But not all cases were treated with the same batch of penicillin: 100 cases were treated with batch A pencillin and 98% were cured; 100 cases were treated

with batch B and 89% were cured; 100 cases with batch C and 95% were cured; 100 cases with batch D and 92% were cured; and 100 cases with batch E and 96% were cured. In this imaginary example, the chi-square test could be applied to ascertain whether the different cure rates in different groups are due only to chance or whether, all other relevant factors being equal, the different results are due to different effectiveness of the individual batches of penicillin.

test, coin A test of tactile gnosis (recognition) in which the subject is required to estimate the size of coins touched; an underestimation of the size has been believed to be indicative of a lesion of the pyramidal system, but mass examination of normal subjects reveals that approximately 70% of normals are unable to estimate coin size accurately, and that 90% underestimated the size.

test, comprehension See *comprehension*.

test, Cornell Word Form (CWF) A modification of the word-association technique devised to distinguish "normals" from subjects with neuropsychiatric and psychosomatic disorders in a way not apparent to the subject. The test is used primarily in industrial psychology. It consists of a list of stimulus words, each of which is followed by two response words. The subject is asked to encircle whichever of the two words seems to him to be the most related to the stimulus word; e.g. mother—mine, woman.

test, draw-a-person A method of personality analysis based upon the interpretation of drawings of the human figure. Although figure drawings had been used by many workers in the field, it was Karen Machover who in 1949 outlined a system of interpretation that was correlated with clinical diagnostic categories.

test, drawing-of-a-man See *test, Goodenough*.

test, face-hand A test of diffuse cerebral dysfunction devised by Bender. The subject, whose eyes are closed, is touched simultaneously on the cheek and the dorsum of the hand; retesting is done with the eyes open. Results are considered positive if the subject fails consistently to identify both stimuli within 10 trials. By the age of 7, normal children respond with a negative test. Positive results are seen not only in cases of cerebral dysfunction in children and adults, but also in schizophrenic children. See *tactile sensation, double simultaneous.*

test, Fink-Green-Bender See *tactile sensation, double simultaneous.*

test, Funkenstein See *test, Adrenalin-Mecholyl.*

test, Gesell developmental "The Gesell Schedules consist of a series of 27 age-level recorded observations and reactions to standardized situations from birth through the first five years of life. At each age level an inventory of activities is divided into four categories of behavior: (1) Motor; (2) Adaptive; (3) Language; and (4) Personal-Social. Each of these categories of behavior is evaluated by observing the infant or child in a number of standardized situations." (Masserman, J.H. *The Practice of Dynamic Psychiatry,* 1955)

test, good and evil See *responsibility, criminal.*

test, Goodenough A test of a child's intellectual level of development based upon the subject's drawing of a human figure. The test was introduced in 1926 by Florence Goodenough, who standardized the children's drawings and thereby produced a simple and satisfactory test of intelligence.

test, heel-to-knee A test of ataxia; the patient in a recumbent position, with the eyes open or closed, is requested to raise the foot high, touch the knee with the opposite heel, and carry the heel along the shin.

test, Holmgren (Alarik Fritniof Holmgren, Swedish physiologist, 1831–97) A test for color blindness, which requires the subject to match skeins of different-colored yarn with standard skeins.

test, House-Tree-Person (HTP) A type of projective test in which the subject is asked to draw a house, a tree, and a person.

test, Janet's (Pierre Janet, French physician, 1859–1947) A test for the determination of tactile sensibility; the patient answers "yes" or "no" when touched by the examiner's finger.

test, Kent EGY A series of 10 questions used for a quick estimate of intelligence.

test, Knox cube A performance test, of particular value when the subject suffers from a language handicap or barrier, in which the subject taps a series of four cubes in various prescribed sequences.

test, Kohnstamm The Kohnstamm maneuver is often used to demonstrate suggestibility to a subject being prepared for hypnotic trance induction. It is a normal neurophysiologic reaction, elicited by having the subject press his extended arm as strenuously as possible against a wall for approximately two minutes, after which the arm will rise automatically with or without a suggestion to that effect.

test, Kohs block-design An intelligence test in which the subject copies a design using small, multicolored cubes.

test, Lange See *Lange's colloidal gold reaction.*

test, Lichtheim's A means of determining the retention of inner languages in patients with expressive aphasia or other severe speech disturbances; the patient is asked to indicate the number of syllables in words he cannot utter.

test, Lowenfeld See *test, mosaic.*

test, Machover See *test, draw-a-person.*

test, Minnesota Multiphasic Personality Inventory (MMPI) A personality questionnaire consisting of 550 statements concerning behavior, feelings, social attitudes, and frank symptoms of psychopathology. To each question, the subject must answer T (true), F (false), or ? (cannot say), and his answer sheet is then scored by various keys that have been standardized on different diagnostic groups and personality types. The MMPI was originally constructed by a psychiatrist, J.C. McKinley, and a psychologist, Starke Hathaway.

test, Mooney See *Mooney Problem Check List.*

test, mosaic A projective technique, introduced by M. Lowenfeld and further developed by F. Wertham, which employs a set of 300 colored pieces (black, blue, red, green, yellow, and off-white) in six shapes (squares, diamonds, oblongs, and three different-sized triangles). The subject is presented with the test objects on a tray and is asked to make anything he wants on the board. The designs made by adults and children have been correlated with diagnostic categories, and individual designs can be interpreted on the basis of these correlations.

test, myokinetic psychodiagnosis A test devised by Mira that consists of drawings of patterns with both the right and the left hands. The left-hand drawings are believed to reveal genotypic reactions and the right-hand drawings are said to express more superficial phenotypic reactions. Comparison of the drawings is made to diagnose various conditions and character traits.

test, organic integrity (OIT) A modification of the Casgrandie test for color-dominance and form-dominance perception, described by H.C. Tien. The OIT is said to be a rapid test for organic brain disease; it is based on the theory that central nervous system damage will interfere with ability to perceive form.

test, Pándy (Kálmán Pándy, Hungarian neurologist, 1868–1945) A qualitative and quantitative test for protein (esp. globulin) in the cerebrospinal fluid. The fluid to be examined is mixed with carbolic acid and the degree of precipitation indicates the degree of protein content.

test-person The subject who is examined by the association method.

test, PMA A test of seven traits believed by Thurstone and Thurstone to account for most of the variance in primary mental abilities (PMA). These traits are: V (verbal comprehension), W (word fluency), N (number), S (space), M (associative memory), P (perceptual speed), and R (reasoning) or I (induction).

test, progressive matrices An intelligence test in which the subject is asked to choose, from several alternatives, the one part that will complete the abstract design presented to him. The test is made up of 60 such designs.

test, projective A type of psychologic test in which the test material presented to the subject is such that any response will necessarily be determined by his own prevailing mood or underlying psychopathology. See *method, projective.*

test, psycholinguistic See *Illinois Test of Psycholinguistic Abilities.*

test, psychopenetration A psychodynamic test devised by Wilcox in the 1940s used in conjunction with carbon dioxide coma to serve as a guide for therapeutic procedures in different types of cases. See *therapy, carbon dioxide inhalation.* It sorts reactions into five general classes, according to the degree of emotional flexibility or rigidity. The test consists of five questions, especially worded to elicit evidence of the degree of unconscious resistance to the concepts of attention, sex, killing, showing all feeling, and deceiving.

"Class I (flexibility plus mild CO_2 reac-

tion) calls for electroconvulsive therapy in the presence of depression. Otherwise, Class I is the essentially normal pattern. Class II (flexibility plus tension CO_2 reactions) yields remarkably well to carbon dioxide comas and intensive psychotherapy. Improvement coincides with a shift to Class I. Class III (rigidity plus mild CO_2 reaction) in the presence of paranoid symptoms calls for subconvulsive electrocoma treatments with the development of flexibility and ultimately a Class I reaction. Class IV (rigidity plus tension CO_2 reactions) is a mixed group which requires trials of various types of shock-therapy to find the most effective one. Improvement is likely to be slow and the patient may follow a varying course of reactions until Class I pattern is achieved. Class V (rigidity plus paradoxical CO_2 reaction) is the profound catatonic and requires electroconvulsive therapy, spaced by periodic psychodynamic tests. As soon as the CO_2 reaction reverses, considerable gains occur by adding CO_2 comas to the treatment. Patients who have previously been considered to be schizophrenic, but who clearly react as Class II have quite different psychodynamic mechanisms than other schizophrenics." (Spiegel, E.A. *Progress in Neurology and Psychiatry,* 1949)

test, right and wrong See *responsibility, criminal.*

test, Rorschach (Hermann Rorschach, Swiss psychiatrist, 1884–1922) A projective test consisting of ten inkblots of varying designs and colors, which are shown to the subject one at a time with the request to interpret them. Its purpose is to furnish a description of the dynamic forces of personality through an analysis of the formal aspects of the subject's interpretations. The test yields information as to the intellectual and emotional processes, the degree of personality integration, variability in mental functioning, and the degree to which the subject responds to environmental influences and to his inner promptings. The test not only is used to obtain a picture of the subject's personality, but also serves as an aid in problems of differential psychiatric diagnosis and prognosis.

test, Ross-Jones (Hugh Campbell Ross, English pathologist, 1875–1926, and Ernest Jones, English medical journalist, neurological researcher, and psychoanalyst, 1879–1958) A test for excess of globulin in cerebrospinal fluid. Fluid is floated on top of an ammonium sulfate solution; excess globulin forms a grayish-white ring at the junction of the two fluids, and the width of the ring is a crude measure of the amount of globulin.

test, SHP The *Strongin-Hinsie-Peck test* for measurement of salivary secretion, average rate of which is decreased in depressions and increased in schizophrenias.

test, sociometric "The sociometric test is an instrument with which to measure the amount of the organization shown by social groups. It requires an individual to choose associates for any group of which he is or might become a member. The test reveals that the underlying attraction-repulsion pattern of a group differs widely from its visible structure and that groups tested upon the basis of different criteria tend toward diversity of structures. These structures have been revealed when the criteria of the test have been applied to home groups, work groups, and school groups.

"The test is constructed in such a manner that it is in itself a motive, an incentive, or a purpose, primarily for the subject rather than for the tester. It is part of the procedure to put some of the choices of the subject into operation. The test can be repeated at any time without significant loss of interest to the subject." (Moreno, J.L. *Who Shall Survive?* 1934)

test, spider's web A test of the biological effects of various body fluids (urine, serum, etc.) on the pattern of a spider's web. It has been found, for example, that schizophrenic urine gives different and more marked pattern changes than does non-schizophrenic urine.

test, spontaneity "The spontaneity test proceeds by throwing the subject into standard life situations in which he improvises freely while acting opposite members of the group to whom he has been found emotionally related as revealed by the sociometric test, either through attraction or repulsion. The situations may express such emotions like anger, fear, sympathy, dominance or any other emotions. They may express roles such as father, mother, employer, or any other roles.

"The spontaneity test can be considered an intensification of the sociometric test, which does not reveal any factor beyond the attraction-repulsion pattern. The spontaneity test gives an additional insight into inter-personal relationships. In the course of the situations activated it reveals the specific emotions binding persons together, the disturbances which they may have in the course of spontaneous performance, the range of words spoken and gestures shown during the acts themselves." (Moreno, J.L. *Who Shall Survive?* 1934)

test, Stanford-Binet "The revised Stanford-Binet Intelligence Scale is the test most frequently used in the individual examination of children. It consists of 120 items, plus several alternative tests that are applicable to the age range between two years and adulthood. The tests have a variety of activities of graded difficulty, both verbal and performance, designed to tap a variety of intellectual functions such as memory, free association, orientation in time, language comprehension, knowledge of common objects, comparison of concepts, perception of contradictions, understanding of abstract terms, the ability to meet novel situations and the use of practical judgment. In addition to many other varieties of function, there are also tests of visual-motor coordination." (Masserman, J.H. *The Practice of Dynamic Psychiatry,* 1955) The score is expressed in months of mental age, which is divided by the chronological age (in months) and then multiplied by 100 to give the intelligence quotient.

test, Szondi A projective test, developed by Szondi in Switzerland in the 1940s, which consists of six sets of pictures, each set containing eight photographs. These eight photographs are of eight different psychobiologic conditions—homosexual, sadist, epileptic, hysteric, catatonic schizophrenic, paranoid schizophrenic, manic-depressive depressed, manic-depressive manic. The subject chooses from each set the two pictures he likes most and the two he dislikes the most. The eight different conditions portrayed are presumed to be extreme pathologic representatives of the eight basic emotional needs. The test is interpreted in terms of the degree of tension, and the subject's attitude to this tension, in each of these eight need-systems. The need-systems are as follows: the need for tender, feminine love (h factor); the need for aggression and masculinity (s factor); the mode of dealing with crude, aggressive emotions (e factor); the need to exhibit emotions (hy factor); narcissistic ego-needs (k factor); the expansive tendencies of the ego (p factor); the need for acquiring and mastering objects (d factor); and the need to cling to objects for enjoyment (m factor). Although the Szondi test can be used clinically, as a projective technique, without reference to the viewpoint that led to its development, the basis of the test is Szondi's theory of *genotropism* (q.v.).

test, Taschen's A test for nystagmus in which the subject is directed to turn five times around his axis within 10 seconds and must then fix his eyes on the upheld index finger of the examiner. Duration of nystagmus so provoked beyond 9 seconds is considered abnormal.

test, thematic apperception (TAT) A projective technique, originally described by Morgan and Murray in 1935, which focuses primarily on the dynamics of interpersonal relationships. In its present form (the third set to be used since 1935), it consists of a series of 31 pictures that depict a number of social situations and interpersonal relations. In clinical practice, 10 or 12 of the pictures are usually selected by the examiner on the basis of which of the total 31 are most likely to elicit information on the subject's problems. The selected pictures are then presented to the subject, who is asked to tell a story about what is going on in each picture. The stories are interpreted in terms of the subject's relationship to authority figures, to contemporaries of both sexes, and in terms of the compromises between and the needs of the id, the ego, and the superego. There are various methods of interpreting results; the one advocated by Murray is the need-press method (see *method, need-press*). L. Bellak recommends interpretation in terms of the following 14 categories: main theme, main hero, attitudes to parental figures, figures introduced, objects introduced, objects omitted, attribution of blame, significant conflicts, punishment for crime, attitude to

hero, signs of inhibition (in aggression, sex, etc.), outcome, pattern of need gratification, and plot.

It is to be noted that the TAT is only incidentally a diagnostic tool and is not primarily designed for nosologic classification.

test, TPI Treponema pallidum immobilization test for syphilis. This test, developed ca. 1954, depends on an antibody that develops as early as the reagin detected by serologic tests but is much more specific, dependable, and persistent. It is of particular value in differentiating false serologic positives (which are often seen in the collagen diseases) from true positives due to latent syphilis.

test, visual distortion A test of a subject's reaction to the visual distortion produced by fitting the subject with a set of +6.00 sphD or −6.00 sphD lenses for a period of 3–4 minutes; described by J. Ehrenwald (*Archives of General Psychiatry 7*, 1962), who theorizes that it is a measure of ego strength in that it "causes a temporary breakdown of the synthetic and integrative functions of the ego touched off by the dissociation of the visual and postural components of the patient's experiences of the body image and of the outside world."

test, Wada dominance A method for determining the side of cerebral dominance by intracarotid injection of amobarbital, introduced by J. Wada in 1949.

test, Wassermann (văs′air-măn) (August von Wassermann, German bacteriologist, 1866–1925) A diagnostic test for syphilis, based upon complement fixation. The development and refinement of this test, in the years 1901 to 1907, made it possible to identify positively as syphilitic many neuropsychiatric conditions whose etiology had previously been only a matter of speculation. In general, it may be said that the blood Wasserman is positive in approximately 70% of cases with cerebral syphilis, 70% of tabetics, and almost 100% of paretics. The cerebrospinal fluid Wasserman is positive in approximately 60% with secondary syphilis, 100% with tertiary syphilis, and 100% with congenital syphilis.

test, Wechsler-Bellevue An intelligence test, the most widely used test in the average adult, consisting of five verbal tests, five performance tests, and an additional vocabulary test. The 11 subtests are as follows: general information, general comprehension, arithmetic, digit span, similarities, vocabulary, picture arrangement, picture completion, block design, object assembly, and digit symbol. The subtests are scored on the basis of speed and accuracy, and results can be translated into standard scores that give the verbal IQ, the performance IQ, and the full-scale IQ.

test, Word-in-Context A test of capacity for verbal reasoning in which the subject is asked to determine the meaning of a given word by reading selected passages of prose.

test, Z See *test, Zulliger.*

test, Zulliger A brief Rorschach-type test of particular value for rapid screening of a group of patients; administration time averages ten minutes.

testing, reality See *reality testing.*

tests, alpha A series of mental tests, first used in the United States military service (1917) to determine the relative mental ability of recruits. There are eight different types of test: for directions, arithmetical ability, practical judgment, synonyms and antonyms, correct arrangement of sentences, completion of series of digits, analogies, and information. The tests are designed particularly for group application and for rapid mechanical scoring.

tests, army mental Tests devised during the World War I to determine the intellectual status of recruits examined for the United States Army.

tests, Binet-Simon (bē-nā′ sēmawN′) (Alfred Binet, French psychologist, 1857–1911, and Theodore Simon, French physician, 1873–1961) Tests of intellectual capacity, which is expressed as the intelligence quotient (IQ), introduced in France in 1905 as a result of studies made to determine whether children could be educated as the new laws required. The Stanford revision of the tests for use with American children was made in 1916, although they had already been introduced into the United States by Goddard in 1910.

tests, Brunet (broo-nā′) A developmental scale designed for use with infants as young as 1 month.

tests, Buhler A developmental scale designed for use with infants from birth up to school age.

tests, sorting A method of psychological testing in which the subject is required to place objects into groups on the basis of similarity or some other abstract relationship. Such sorting or *Zuordnung* tests are particularly associated with Kurt Goldstein, Vigotsky, Hanfmann, and Kaanin. Patients with cortical lesions, particularly, show impairment of abstract behavior as measured by these tests. Schizophrenics, too, do poorly on these tests; but performance is more varied than in ordinary brain damage cases, for the schizophrenic tends to project himself into the test objects and animate and embellish them.

tetanization *Obs.* Extreme fixation of the attention, often accompanied by exaltation or ecstasy and a lack of responsiveness to painful stimuli.

tetraethylpyrophosphate (te-tra-e-thil-pī-rō-fos′fāt) See *psychotomimetic.*

tetraethylthiuram disulfide (te-tra-e-thil-thī′ū-ram dī-sul′fīd) See *Antabuse.*

tetrahydrocannabinol (te-tra-hī-drō-kan-nab′in-ol) See *psychotomimetic.*

tetraplegia Quadriplegia; paralysis of the four extremities.

tetrasomy The "fourfoldness" in Jung's system of psychology. See *quaternity.*

TGA See *amnesia, transient global.*

thaassophobia (thȧ-as-ō-) Fear of sitting.

thalamotomy (thal-ȧ-mot′ō-mē) A psychosurgical procedure that produces a lesion in the thalamus by means of thermocoagulation. A stereotaxic apparatus is employed to position a wire or cannula into the desired subcortical area. Such a method results in minimal injury to superimposed cortex or white matter, and is a much less drastic procedure than are other methods, e.g. frontal lobectomy. The thalamotomy operation was devised by Spiegel and his coworkers, whose early reports indicate that small lesions of the dorsomedial nucleus of the thalamus (medial thalamotomy) relieve anxiety, emotional reactivity, and allied symptoms in psychoses and obsessive-compulsive states. This technique is obviously applicable to the production of lesions elsewhere in the brain.

thalamus An ovoid-shaped constellation of nuclei lying between the mesencephalon and corpora striata, forming the lateral wall of the 3rd ventricle, and completely covered by the cerebral hemisphere. The prominent posterior portion is the pulvinar, lateral to which is the lateral geniculate body. The medial surface of the thalamus is connected to the thalamus of the opposite side by the *massa intermedia.*

Anatomically, six major nuclear masses are recognized (Walker's terminology): midline, anterior, medial, lateral, ventral, and posterior nuclei. The posterior nuclei include the pulvinar and the medial and lateral geniculate bodies.

The thalamus has somatic, special sense, and associative sensory functions. The ventral nuclei are concerned with somatic sensory functions, the lateroventral portion with unconscious proprioception, the posteroventral portion with conscious exteroception and proprioception, the posteroventral portion with conscious exteroception and proprioception, the lateral geniculate body with vision, the medial geniculate body with audition (? and equilibrium), and the pulvinar with auditory and visual association.

Thalamic lesions are commonly followed by various paresthesiae and hyperesthesiae believed to be due to release from intradiencephalic and corticothalamic projections. The *thalamic syndrome* consists of a raising of the threshold (i.e. diminished sensitivity) to pinprick, heat, and cold, but when sensation is felt it is disagreeable and unpleasant (thalamic hyperpathia). See *dementia, thalamic.*

thalassophobia Fear of the sea.

thanatomania *Obs.* Suicidal mania.

thanatophobia Fear of death.

Thanatos According to Freud there are two sets of instincts. He terms one the life instinct or Eros, the other the death instinct or Thanatos. "For the sake of clearness I will repeat in a sentence the three stages in the development of Freud's ideas concerning the duality of instincts. The first was the contrast between sexual and ego instincts; the second the contrast between object-love or allo-erotic libido, and self-love, narcissistic libido; and the third is the contrast between life and death instincts, between Eros and Thanatos."

(Jones, E. *Papers on Psycho-Analysis,* 1938) See *instinct, death.*

thanatotic Pertaining to or manifesting the death instinct.

thank you theory See *theory, thank you.*

theater, therapeutic "An objective setting in which the subject and patient can act free from the anxieties and pressures of the outside world. In order to accomplish this, the total situation of the patient in the outside world has to be duplicated on a spontaneous level in the therapeutic theater, and even more than this, the invisible roles and invisible inter-personal relations he may have experienced must find a visible expression. This means that certain functions—a stage, lights, recording system, assistants, and psychiatrist or director—have to be introduced into its operation." (Moreno, J.L. *Sociometry 1,* 1937)

thelygonia (thē-li-gȯ′nē-à) *Obs.* 1. Procreation of female offspring. 2. *Nymphomania* (q.v.).

theme interference An emotionally toned cognitive constellation or conflict operating preconsciously in the consultee to distort his professional objectivity with his client. Usually the conflict is an outgrowth of actual life experience or phantasies in the consultee that have not been satisfactorily resolved. One of the consultant's tasks is to identify such themes and reduce or eliminate them (*theme interference reduction*). See *consultation-liaison.*

theme, mythological "The collective unconscious—so far as we can venture a judgment upon it—seems to consist of something of the nature of mythological themes or images. For this reason the myths of peoples are the real exponents of the collective unconscious. The whole of mythology could be taken as a kind of projection of the collective unconscious." (Jung, *CAP*)

theomania *Obs.* Delusion that one is God.

theophobia Fear of God.

theory A body of *principles* or *rules* (qq.v.), generally referring to the same subject, with each rule systematically related to the others.

theory, arousal The hypothesis that diminution in personal space increases arousal, and that when personal space becomes inadequate arousal may be expressed in aggression.

theory, Cannon's See *Cannon hypothalamic theory of emotion.*

theory, catastrophe The belief that the act of sexual intercourse is destructive to the penis. "In the normal coitus of individuals who are not neurotic, the inner tension seeking for discharge finally overcomes anxiety, although, as suggested in my ontogenetic and phylogenetic 'catastrophe'-theory of coitus, some traces of anxiety may still persist." (Ferenczi, *FCT*)

theory, disengagement The hypothesis that the older person most likely to achieve satisfaction and contentment is the one who can accept the inevitability of reduced social and personal interactions with advancing age.

theory, gating See *gating; gating, spinal.*

theory, immanence The closed circle hypothesis of life that describes the function of each organ in terms of what it accomplishes for the rest of the organism. According to such a view, the life process would have the pattern of a logical vicious cycle. The part processes have the function of sustaining life; and life is an aggregation of these part processes. This theory is the opposite of *holism* (q.v.).

theory, James-Lange-Sutherland "The bodily changes follow directly the perception of the exciting fact, and our feeling of the same changes as they occur is the emotion. . . . The elements . . . of physiological processes, which comprise the emotion . . . are all organic changes, and each of them is the reflex effect of the exciting object." (Lange, C.G., & James, W. *The Emotions,* 1922) This theory admits of no special brain centers for emotion and has been largely replaced by Papez's modification of the *Cannon hypothalamic theory of emotion* (q.v.).

theory, libido Technically, the psychoanalytic hypothesis concerning the development and vicissitudes of the sexual drive or instinct. Often, however, libido theory is used to refer to all of the psychoanalytic hypotheses about the instincts in man. The confusion arises from the fact that until 1920 Freud did not fully develop his dual-instinct theory; before that time, all instinctual manifestations were considered to be a part of the sexual drive. Nowadays, however, the existence of two drives is assumed: sexual (libido)

and aggressive. See *instinct; instinct, death; libido.*

theory, object relations See *object relations theory.*

theory, thank you *Ratification theory;* a test that is often proposed as a way to justify paternalistic behavior, especially in civil commitment deliberations: one may act paternalistically if one is certain that the object of one's actions will later be thankful that those actions were taken.

therapeiology (ther-à-pā-ol'ō-jē) *Obs.* Therapeutics.

therapeutic Pertaining to or consisting of medical treatment; healing, curative.

therapeutic community (TC) Although originally associated with the name of Maxwell Jones, who advocated use of every aspect of the hospital environment as a therapeutic tool (see *therapy, milieu*), the therapeutic community has become associated more specifically with nonhospital residential programs for the treatment of substance use disorders. Like Alcoholics Anonymous, therapeutic communities stress self-help, are abstinence-oriented, and reinforce drug-free behavior through intense interaction with others who have had experience with drug abuse. That interaction is heightened by reason of the fact that the members of the community are living together, and firm rules of conduct are stringently enforced within the residence through punishment for infractions by group confrontation.

therapeutic dose dependence See *dose dependence, therapeutic.*

therapeutic reaction, negative See *resistance, superego.*

therapeutic window See *window, therapeutic.*

therapeutics, differential The matching of therapies available with the patient's or family's needs; tailoring therapy to the patient or group to be treated; the process of choosing the therapy to be recommended.

therapist, auxiliary See *ego, auxiliary; psychotherapy, multiple.*

therapist, parent See *parent therapist program.*

therapy Treatment of disease; therapeutics. See listings under *psychotherapy.*

therapy, active The psychoanalytical method in which the psychiatrist does not confine himself to the interpretation of psychic material, but goes further to force the patient to actions that are hindered by his neurosis. The patient has to be forced precisely into the situations he fears, in order to accustom him to these situations and consequently to enable him to overcome his fear. According to psychoanalytical theory, such actions bring forward and make available for interpretation the psychic material that otherwise might remain hidden. "By the repetition of the act which he fears the patient will gain a better insight into his situation which, until then, he considered dangerous." Through this forced action the patient is taught that there are no insurmountable difficulties in the situation. It is very important that the psychiatrist find out just what actions he can demand of a patient, in order to avoid asking too much and thereby throwing the individual into a panic. In cases of simple anxiety neurosis, like that of a "patient who does not dare to be far away from his home, he is ordered, at first, to walk two or three blocks." After doing this three or four times, he is ordered to walk four or five blocks, and in this manner the therapy proceeds progressively. The only thing that should be asked of the patient is action; he should never be asked to exercise will-power, or suppress his thoughts: "Such demands are useless and increase the sense of failure in the patient." Very often it is difficult to find actions that are appropriate to the symptoms of the patient. According to Schilder, the principle of active therapy is "probably also valid when thoughts which seem to be unacceptable to the patient are formulated again and again": the mere formulation of words seems to have an effect similar to the repetition of the act. (Schilder, P. *Psychotherapy*, 1938)

therapy, activity group A special technique of applying psychotherapy through group activity. "So that these [very shy] children might not feel threatened, a program of picnics and trips was arranged for them, and after some months of such therapy it was found that not only did they evidence gain in their social behavior, but that they had made general improvement in their personalities. From this inauspicious practice grew Slavson's activity group therapy." (Klapman, J.W. *Group Psychotherapy*, 1946) See *psychotherapy, group.*

therapy, adjuvant Subsidiary therapy or curative means in the treatment of the psychoneuroses, in addition to psychotherapy, which they aid or assist. Adjuvant therapies consist primarily of drugs, suggestion, and hypnosis.

therapy, administrative Institutional treatment of psychologically disturbed people such as is employed in the therapeutic community, in contrast to mere custodial care. See *therapeutic community.*

therapy, analytical Therapeutic application of the principles of *analytic psychology* (q.v.). According to Jung the contents of consciousness are antithetic to those of the unconscious. One compensates for the others. "In the normal condition the compensation is unconscious, i.e., it performs an unconscious regulation of conscious activity. In the neurotic state the unconscious appears in such strong contrast to the conscious that compensation is disturbed. The aim of analytical therapy, therefore, is to make the unconscious contents conscious in order that compensation may be established." (Jung, *CAP*) See *constructive; reductive.*

therapy, assignment In Moreno's system of sociometry, placement of the individual into a group in accord with his sociometric position in the community. It tries to give the individual the best opportunity for adjustment in the group in accordance with his abilities.

therapy, atropine coma (ACT) The use of atropine sulfate to induce coma in the treatment of psychoses, first reported by Forrer in 1950. Greatest benefit has been reported in tense, anxious, and agitated psychotics. See *syndrome, central anticholinergic.*

therapy, attitude Originally, a process of treating children by working with the disturbed attitudes of their parents. Nowadays, a type of reeducative psychotherapy that focuses on the current attitudes of the patient, their distortions, their origins, and their present purpose. In this type of therapy, the patient is helped to adopt attitudes that make for harmonious relationships as substitutes for his maladaptive attitudes.

therapy, aversion Negative conditioning, consisting of pairing the unwanted symptom or behavior (e.g. alcoholism, fetishism, homosexuality, enuresis, and psychopathic behavior) with painful or unpleasant stimuli until the undesirable behavior is suppressed. See *behavior theory*.

therapy, behavior *Behavior modification:* application of the methods and findings of experimental psychology to the alteration of maladaptive behavior. The origins of behavior therapy are mainly to be found in two reports: (1) *Psychotherapy by Reciprocal Inhibition* (1958), in which Joseph Wolpe describes his work on experimental neurosis, leading to the technique of systematic desensitization; and (2) *Science and Human Behavior* (1953), in which B.F. Skinner describes how the effects on learning of the consequences of behavior could be applied therapeutically. See *behavior theory*.

Behavior therapy tends to concentrate on behavior itself rather than on any putative cause. It begins with a detailed analysis not only of the patient's behavior but also of the factors associated with them. Specific, concrete goals are set and a treatment plan is developed that is tailored to the patient's specific needs. Objective evaluation of the results of treatment is an inherent part of the process.

Many different techniques have been developed within the framework of behavior theory, including assertiveness and social skills training, cognitive therapy, contingency management procedures, exposure methods, and self-control procedures.

Assertiveness and *social skills training* help the patient to express positive or negative emotions clearly. *Behavioral rehearsal* (one or more practice sessions in expressing appropriate reactions to situations that are difficult for the patient), *modeling* (q.v.), and *information feedback* (in which patient and therapist act out troublesome situations and the therapist comments on the patient's behavior) are specific techniques that may be used. See *social skills training*.

Cognitive behavior therapy: sometimes called *cognitive restructuring;* among the many variants are Ellis's rational-emotive therapy (see *psychotherapy, rational*), Meichenbaum's *self-instructional training* (SET), and Beck's *cognitive therapy*. SET typically focuses on specific irrational beliefs the patient holds, making the patient aware of them and then helping the patient counter them by making appropriate comments while the patient is performing the behavior that has posed difficulties in the past. Beck focuses on the cognitive distortions of depressed patients and ways of guiding them to consider their problems in alternative, solvable terms. See *therapy, cognitive*.

Contingency management: the central tenet of operant conditioning is that behavior is maintained by its consequences. The approach is to determine the consequences of disturbed behavior and to ensure that such behavior is not followed by positive consequences and that desired behavior does receive positive reinforcement. See *conditionalism; conditioning, operant*.

Exposure methods: their aim is to extinguish anxiety and other symptoms by repeated, controlled exposure of the patient to the feared situation. At one level, modeling may be used to allay the patient's anxiety by having him observe the desired reaction being performed by someone else. At another level, systematic *desensitization* (q.v.) may be used to reduce anxiety by gradual increments in the fear level of trial situations. At still another level, exposure may be rapid and fear-inducing as in flooding or *implosion* (q.v.). *In vivo exposure*, exposure to the real situation, appears to be the most effective approach in the treatment of obsessional behavior.

Self-control: the best-known procedure in this category is *biofeedback* (q.v.).

therapy, brief stimulus (BST) A type of electroconvulsive therapy in which the current is modified so that the average electrical energy needed to produce a seizure is much less than with the usual method. It is claimed that BST gives as satisfactory clinical results as classical ECT, with the added advantage of reducing or even eliminating confusion. A disadvantage of BST is that patients are more fearful than with the classical method; this can be overcome by using pretreatment barbiturates.

therapy, carbon dioxide inhalation A form of somatic treatment introduced in 1945 by von Meduna (who also introduced Metrazol convulsive treatment for schizophrenia); rarely used nowadays. In CO_2 inhalation therapy, the patient breathes from a cylinder containing a mixture of 30% CO_2 and 70% O_2 to the point of unconsciousness. Treatments are given two or three times a week, sometimes to as many as 100 treatments. The method is of limited usefulness in the treatment of various psychoneuroses, and many workers feel that it may even retard or prevent recovery. Those who find it of some value feel that it is best suited to traumatic hysteria with dissociation, to conversion symptoms of recent origin, and to anxiety hysteria.

therapy, child-guidance The treatment of emotional problems of children by the simultaneous therapy of the child and its parents, especially the mother.

therapy, client-centered *Nondirective therapy;* a type of therapeutic counseling associated with Carl Rogers. Client-centered therapy is predicated on the belief that the subject possesses inherent potentialities for growth that need only to be released by the therapist. The subject is responsible for his own destiny and has the right of choice in the solution of his problems, and instead of imposing values on him the therapist must promote the free expression of feelings in the counseling relationship.

therapy, cognitive Also known as cognitive behavior therapy; an active, structured, time-limited, and directive form of therapy, based on the belief that the way a person perceives and structures the world determines his feelings and behavior. Depression, for example, is an outgrowth of a tendency to view oneself in a negative way, and treatment is aimed at altering that cognitive schema by helping the patient gather evidence for and against his distorted self-view.

Cognitive therapy emphasizes how the patient came to think in certain ways about himself, the future, and the world. It was developed by Aaron T. Beck and is rooted in the work of Alfred Adler, George Kelly, and Karen Horney, with a number of its tactics derived from behavior modification. The cognitive view assumes that one *assigns* meaning and value to one's perceptions and experiences. Cognitive schemata are organized representations of prior experience that help a person to screen, encode, and categorize perceptions. They may be reactivated, however, by stimuli that are only remotely similar to the historically etiologic context and in relation to present-day reality are distorted, maladaptive, and exaggerated. The goal of therapy is to identify and correct the subject's distorted negative cognitions, to elucidate and challenge the underlying cognitive schemata, and to increase the patient's adaptive problem-solving repertoire. See *holistic healing; therapy, behavior.*

therapy, continuation See *preventive therapy, long-term.*

therapy, contract Also known as *behavioral contracting* and *contingency contracting;* a form of behavior therapy in which a systematic way of scheduling the mutual exchange of reinforcements between the patient and his family or friends is established for the purpose of modifying reinforcement contingencies that maintain the undesirable behavior. During the initial interview the therapist may suggest to the patient and his family that if each of the family members learns to accommodate to the requests of the others, each might in turn be able to enjoy the fulfillment of more of his own desires and privileges. Then specific statements of privileges (reinforcements), responsibilities (responses), sanctions for contract violations, and bonuses for contract compliance are drawn up and negotiated. A type of *microsocial engineering,* behavioral contracting may not only change family conflict into positive interaction, but it may also train the family in a pattern of conflict resolution that can be used indefinitely. (Stuart, R.B. *Journal of Behavior Therapy and Experimental Psychiatry 2,* 1971)

therapy, delay A behavioral management technique, said to be particularly useful in obsessive-compulsive syndromes, in which the patient is placed in situations that ordinarily provoke compulsive rituals but is prevented from carrying out the ritualistic behavior. Also called *response prevention.*

therapy, directed group See *psychotherapy, group.*

therapy, diversional In occupational therapy, tasks given primarily for the amusement and distraction of the patient.

therapy, divorce See *divorce therapy.*

therapy, dual transference Treatment of the same patient by two therapists, sometimes advantageous when the patient needs both support and confrontation with reality issues but is unable to accept both from the same therapist. It is theorized that providing two therapists enables a fragile ego to differentiate more clearly between good and bad mother images as a step toward ultimate fusion and integration of those images.

therapy, electroconvulsive (ECT) Electroshock therapy; a form of somatic treatment for certain psychiatric conditions in which electrical current is applied to the brain through two electrodes placed on the temporal areas of the skull. Current is applied through a specially constructed machine, whose main features are a stop for time regulation to fractions of a second and a voltometer that regulates the voltage to be applied. The desired generalized convulsion is ordinarily obtained with voltage varying between 70 and 130 volts applied for 0.1 to 0.5 seconds. The convulsion usually occurs immediately with an initial tonic phase lasting about 10 seconds. The tonic phase slowly goes over into the clonic phase, which fades out after a total of 30 or 40 seconds for the whole seizure. The convulsion is accompanied by apnea. The seizure is followed by coma lasting from 5 to 30 or more minutes.

Complications are rare, the most frequent one being bone fractures due to muscular contraction. Intravenous muscle relaxants, such as succinylcholine, are often used to prevent this complication. Respiratory and cardiovascular complications may occur; neurological complications are extremely rare. The probability of fatal incidents does not exceed 0.06% of cases.

Electroconvulsive therapy, is indicated in mania, depressions, and certain cases of schizophrenia. Results are unsatisfactory in the psychoneuroses, except in psychoneurotic depression. All types of depression react favorably to ECT after some four treatments. ECT gives an 80 to 100% remission rate in the depressive phase of manic-depressive psychosis, in involutional melancholia, and in agitated depressions, but it does not ward off episodic recurrences. The manic phase must usually be treated more intensively, with as many as two or three treatments a day. With such treatment the remission rate approaches that in depressed phase. The paranoid type of involutional psychosis usually requires 20 treatments, in contrast to the ordinary maximum of 10 treatments in the aforementioned groups, but even so, the remission rate is less than 50%. Schizophrenics also require a minimum of 20 treatments. About 65% of schizophrenic cases of less than six months' duration respond favorably, some 40% among those ill from six months to two years, and less than 10% of those ill more than two years. In all cases, temporary remissions may be prolonged with ECT maintenance therapy at weekly, fortnightly, even monthly intervals. (Kalinowsky, L.B., & Hoch, P.H. *Shock Treatments,* 1950)

Electroconvulsive therapy was often used in combination with insulin therapy, particularly in schizophrenia. In these cases, ECT was used to relieve the anxiety and apprehension components, insulin to clear the underlying thought disorder. Because ECT does not afford insight to the patient, psychotherapy, in addition to somatic therapy, is usually indicated in order to bring more lasting benefit.

therapy, expressive A method of treatment in which the therapist's dominant aim is to encourage and help the patient to bring out, talk about, act out, or emotionally express all ideas and feelings so that both the patient and the therapist come to know the dynamic emotional roots of the patient's symptoms and illness. Through encouragement and by bringing about a reversal of the *covering up* (or normal) defensive mechanism, expressive therapy endeavors to *uncover* the roots of mental emotional illness. As epitomized in psychoanalysis, the main purpose of expressive therapy is, through a reversal of the repressive defensive mechanisms, to shift the material from the unconscious realm into the realm of conscious thought.

On the other hand, *suppressive therapy* tends to cover up, to keep down, and to strengthen the repressive, defensive forces of the personality. As such, suppressive therapy tries to build up the forces of concealment of the self toward hidden portions of itself, while expressive therapy brings about painful but valuable self-revelation. Suppressive therapy tends to maintain and continue the individual's comfortable and peaceful illusion of himself, while expressive therapy becomes painfully disillusioning and thus aims in the direction of self-realization and reality.

therapy, family See *family therapy.*

therapy, family group Treatment of the family as a unit rather than individual treatment of one or more members of the family. Among the first to undertake treatment of the family unit were John Bell and Nathan Ackerman. This type of treatment is an outgrowth of a shifting emphasis in recent years, from the view of the child as a victim of his family to a field-force concept, in which the family is viewed as a social unit whose operations can be understood only in terms of the reciprocal expectations of the family members.

therapy, family member A form of individual psychotherapy that pays special attention to how the patient's family contributes to his condition and how it can assist in his management.

therapy, family unit A type of psychotherapy in which all family members, rather than any one "patient," are considered together as a psychosocial system requiring intervention. The focus is on interpersonal relationships rather than on intrapsychic processes. The family itself is viewed as a rule-governed, change-resistant transactional system sustained by the conformity of the family members to the operational objectives of the system. The dysfunctional family fails to support children in their movement away from the family and hampers their individuation and social maturation. Family treatment attempts to improve the social functioning of the whole family so that no generation will inhibit the individuation and separation of an adjacent generation.

therapy, Gestalt A holistic form of psychotherapy that emphasizes heightened emotionality, understanding the autonomic and musculoskeletal messages transmitted by the body, and helping the subject get in touch with the primitive wisdom of the body. The person acts out a variety of roles in life and during therapy learns to recognize what is symbolized by those patterns of activity and to take responsibility for conflicts within himself and attitudes toward others that contribute to his problems. During the treatment session, the therapist considers not only what the patient says but how he is saying it—his voice inflection, posture, gestures, breathing patterns, etc. Change is viewed as a subintel-

lectual process and the here-and-now is all important. Gestalt therapy employs role-playing and other techniques to promote the subject's growth process and to develop his full potential.

Developed by Fritz Perls, Gestalt therapy is used in both individual and group therapy. It draws from many sources, including psychoanalysis, Jung's ego psychology, Reich's character armoring, existentialism, phenomenology, and behavior theory.

therapy, interpersonal From the standpoint of psychodramatics, "Inter-personal therapy is a technique which is applied in such problems and mental disorders in which the treatment interrelates dynamically all the persons involved. An illustration of a situation demanding this approach is a 'triangular neurosis' i.e. an inter-personal neurosis affecting three persons, for example, a husband, wife, and another individual.

"Inter-personal therapy is carried out in alternating sessions with each of the persons involved until the psychiatrist, the auxiliary ego, has returned to the subject with whom he began. The cycle can be repeated as often as necessary until catharsis is reached." (Moreno, J.L. *Sociometry 1,* 1937)

therapy, ludo Play therapy.

therapy, maintenance See *preventive therapy, long-term.*

therapy, major role Vocational rehabilitation counseling. See *rehabilitation.*

therapy, marriage A type of family therapy involving husband and wife, concerned primarily with their marital relationship. See *counseling, marriage; therapy, family group.*

therapy, mass A psychotherapeutic term that embraces various group techniques, particularly the didactic, recreational, and class methods used for large groups.

therapy, milieu Socioenvironmental therapy, usually in a hospital setting. See *community, therapeutic; social therapy; "total-push" treatment of schizophrenia.*

In addition to emphasizing the simple humanistic approach advocated by Tuke and Pinel in 18th-century "moral treatment" (which emphasized that treating patients as responsible human beings is effective in getting them to act that way), milieu therapy utilizes techniques that are specifically designed to promote behavioral modification within a stable social organization so that every social experience and treatment experience of the patient will be synergistically applied toward realistic and specific therapeutic goals. Among the techniques that may be used are somatic treatments (psychopharmacologic agents, ECT, etc.), behavior therapies, individual psychotherapy, group process (sensitivity training, family therapy, psychodrama, etc.), hypnosis and suggestion, communications analysis, and role-playing.

Milieu therapy is a means of providing an integrated, stable, and coherent context in which the optimal combination of specific treatments can be given to the patient. Its aim is "to make certain that the patient's every social contact and his every treatment experience are synergistically applied towards realistic, specific therapeutic goals." (Abrams, G.M. *Archives of General Psychiatry 21,* 1969) The goals may be to limit, reduce, or otherwise control pathologic behavior and/or to develop basic psychosocial skills. Group meetings that encourage participation in information sharing, decision making, conflict resolution, etc., are a prominent feature of milieu therapy, not as ends in themselves but as a way of achieving the therapeutic goals.

therapy, multimodal See *BASIC-ID.*

therapy, multiple monitored electroconvulsive (MMECT) A modification of classical ECT in which several EEG-monitored convulsions are induced in a single session in an attempt to achieve results over a shorter period of time.

therapy, network A form of group therapy, used generally with schizophrenic patients, that includes not only family members but also other relatives, neighbors, and friends who make up the patient's *social network* and provide a potential source of support, encouragement, and employment, which may reduce the likelihood of rehospitalization.

therapy, nondirective See *therapy, client-centered.*

therapy, occupational A method of treatment for the sick or injured by means of purposeful occupation, whose goals are to arouse interest, courage, and confidence; to exercise mind and body in healthy activity; to overcome disability; and to reestablish capacity for industrial and social usefulness.

therapy, old-age See *geriatrics.*

therapy, paradoxical *Strategic intervention;* tactics or techniques that on the surface appear contrary to the goals of treatment but are in fact designed to achieve them by overcoming resistance, fostering change, or otherwise hastening improvement. Strategic therapy is associated particularly with Jay Haley and Richard Rabkin. It is based on the assumption that symptoms represent an attempt to solve a problem in a way that only makes the problem worse. Therapy focuses on isolating and defining the problem, analyzing the attempts already made to solve it, and negotiating mutually acceptable and workable goals to develop a series of "strategies" or more effective ways to handle the problem.

Many theorists assume that some, if not all therapy is by definition manipulative. Paradoxical therapy consists of a deliberate use of influencing techniques that focus on the patient's symptoms, often by altering their meaning for the patient. The strategic use of paradoxical interventions is applicable to groups as well as individuals. It is an active, direct, focused, and usually short-term approach.

One of the earliest forms of strategic intervention to be described is *negative practice,* in which the patient is directed to practice repetitively the very habit he wants to eliminate. Another form is *paradoxical restraining therapy,* in which the therapist discourages the patient from attempts to change. The therapist may suggest that it might not be possible for the patient to change, or he may adopt a position that is an exaggeration of the patient's pathologic attitude. In the *anti-expectation technique,* also called *paradoxical positioning,* the therapist expresses an attitude about the patient's symptoms that appears to encourage and reinforce them rather than urging the patient to join forces with the therapist in resisting or ignoring them. Another technique, *defiance-based strategy,* is based on the expectation that the patient will resist the therapist and rebel against any directives he might issue. In the *therapeutic double-bind,* the patient is enjoined to change by remaining unchanged; if he complies and remains unchanged, he demonstrates that he can in fact control the situation, whereas if he defies by changing he has accomplished the purpose of therapy.

therapy, physical Physiotherapy; the branch of physical medicine that makes use of physical and other effective properties of light, heat, cold, water, electricity, mechanical agents, and kinesitherapy (massage, manipulation, therapeutic exercise, mechanical devices).

therapy, pineal Treatment with extracts of beef-pineal substance advocated in the 1950s for treatment of chronic schizophrenia.

therapy, play In child psychiatry, a method of treatment that in general corresponds to the method of psychoanalysis in adult psychiatry, the difference being that the child expresses himself and reveals unconscious material to the therapist by means of play rather than by verbalization of thoughts, as the adult does in psychoanalysis. See *technique, play.*

The play of children, an essential part of their life, is self-expressive in its nature. If a playroom containing all manner of toys and games is set up for the child, much can be learned about the child by observing what game he chooses to play and the manner in which he plays it. For example, during a session in the play-therapy room, a 9-year-old boy took chalk of various colors and drew on the blackboard a charming picture of a house in the countryside. When the drawing had been finished the therapist warmly complimented the boy on his work, and then asked him to make up a story about the people living in that house. It was known that he was a child from a broken, poverty-stricken home in a tenement section of the city; he would not obey his mother, and allegedly had pushed his baby sister from a fire escape to her death. In play therapy he had created what he lacked, an attractive home in the country. In telling the story of the people who lived in it, his feelings about his own home and his own family were drawn out. The therapist was able to help him face his insecurity, anxiety, and hostility and to learn better ways of dealing with them. Before this release through

play therapy, the boy had been uncommunicative and inaccessible in several interviews with the therapist.

therapy, preventive See *preventive therapy, long-term.*

therapy, reconstructive See *psychotherapy.*

therapy, recreation See *recreation.*

therapy, reeducative See *psychotherapy.*

therapy, regressive electroshock (REST) A form of electroconvulsive therapy in which several daily grand mal convulsions are produced for a number of days until the patient is out of contact and incontinent of urine and feces. In one study, four treatments were given each day for seven days; at the end of this time, in addition to the above symptoms, patients were underactive, did not talk spontaneously, lost their appetite and had to be spoon-fed, and movements were uncertain, slow, and clumsy. These symptoms last for one or two weeks; recovery from the superimposed organic brain syndrome is gradual.

Regressive EST is ordinarily used only when the more usual methods fail and prognosis is poor, as in some forms of the schizophrenias.

therapy, relationship Therapy that emerges out of the totality of the relationship between patient and therapist during the entire course of treatment. Although Allen is a pioneer in relationship therapy with children, he considers the term misleading: "It [relationship therapy] seems to imply a special brand of psychological therapy. All therapy involves a relationship between patient and therapist." However, "here the therapeutic relationship is conceived as an immediate experience. The therapist begins where the patient is and seeks to help him draw on his own capacities toward a more creative acceptance and use of the self he has. While maintaining an interest in understanding what has been wrong, the therapeutic focus is on what the individual can begin to do about what was and, more important, still is wrong. Therapy emerges, then, from an experience in living, not in isolation but within a relationship with another from whom the patient can eventually differentiate himself as he comes to perceive and accept his own self as separate and distinct." (Kanner, L. *Child Psychiatry,* 1948)

therapy, release See *release.*

therapy, rhythmic sensory bombardment A form of treatment consisting of sonic, photic, or tactile stimulation applied intermittently and rhythmically usually for a period of one hour. The affective psychoses, psychoneuroses, psychopathic personalities, and paranoid forms of schizophrenia are said to show favorable response.

therapy, shock A general term indicating the use of various somatic treatments that produce a *shock* to the central nervous system, thus favorably influencing the course of a mental disease. The shock therapies include electroshock (EST)—also called electroconvulsive therapy (ECT)—insulin coma therapy, ambulatory insulin treatment (also called subshock or subcoma insulin therapy), Metrazol convulsive treatment, brief stimulus electrotherapy, electrostimulation, electronarcosis, Indoclon inhalation therapy, atropine coma therapy.

therapy, situational A term introduced by S.R. Slavson, in connection with his activity group psychotherapy, in which the social relationship and the physical environment themselves (i.e. the situation) have a therapeutic effect.

therapy, sleep-electroshock Electroshock treatment preceded by the administration of sufficient sedative or hypnotic drug to produce sleep. The method is of particular value in patients who develop a fear of electric shock and are unwilling to continue receiving such therapy. Sodium pentothal is commonly employed, administered intravenously as a 2.5% solution. The electrodes are applied after sleep is induced. Many psychiatrists apply the current as soon as the patient spontaneously moves a limb during the waking process. The same amount of current is given as without the sleep-inducing drug. Other psychiatrists apply the current at a deeper stage of narcosis, as judged by the absence of spontaneous movements and the presence of a corneal reflex. With the latter method a nonconvulsive or minor reaction is obtained, but the clinical effects as measured by the maintenance of the improved state are equally satisfactory.

therapy, social Use and manipulation of the social setting as a major element in treatment, as in the *therapeutic community* (q.v.). Social therapy provides a model social group, which encourages use of appropriate forms of behavior, as well as immediate feedback on the effects of the patient's behavior on the people he encounters (*reality confrontation*).

therapy, supportive See *psychotherapy.*

therapy, suppressive See *therapy, expressive.*

therapy, will A form of psychotherapy associated with Otto Rank and based upon his belief that birth trauma (the separation of the child from the mother at the moment of birth) is the central element in neurosis. The trauma of birth is believed to lead to two sets of strivings: (1) to return to the womb or (2) to reenact separation and achieve independence. In will-therapy, separation reactions are studied as well as the struggle of will manifested in the patient's desire to continue it (and become independent). The patient is actively encouraged to assert himself so as to develop and strengthen his will.

thermanesthesia, thermoanesthesia Loss of the ability to distinguish between heat and cold.

thermo- Combining form meaning hot, heat, from Gr. *thermós.*

thermohyperesthesia Extreme sensitiveness to heat stimuli.

thermohypesthesia Diminished sensibility to heat stimuli.

thermoneurosis *Obs.* An elevation of the temperature of the body due to neurosis as seen sometimes in hysteria.

theta EEG activity See *sleep.*

theta rhythm or wave See *electroencephalogram.*

thinking, abstract See *thinking, physiognomonic.*

thinking, allusive Bleuler's term for loosening of the associations. It may be a normal mode of abstract thinking, found in a high percentage of schizophrenics but also in a significant percentage of normals; there is some evidence that this type of thinking is inherited. See *loosening.*

thinking, archaic-paralogical E. von Domarus (1924) classified thinking into (1) *prearchaic;* (2) *archaic-paralogical;* and (3) *paralogical-logical.* The latter two he considered to be typical of primitive savages, and common in schizophrenia, and the first as typical of man's anthropoid progenitors and of schizophrenic stupor. In 1940, Osborne recommended changing the name of schizophrenia to palaeophrenia to emphasize the importance of regression to primitive subrational forms of thinking in the schizophrenic disorders.

Primitive thinking, primordial thinking, anthropoid thinking are all synonyms for archaic-paralogical thinking. They are all characterized by impairment or deficiency of abstraction and generalization, with a tendency toward concrete rather than abstract thinking.

thinking-aside A disorder of associations seen in schizophrenic patients in which the patient loses himself in insignificant side association with the result that no unitary train of thought develops. Because of the paucity of genuinely causal links in such conversation or writing, thinking-aside would be considered a type of *asyndesis*.

thinking, associative Verbal catharsis that deals with immediate problems of patients in their everyday life rather than with traumatic problems originating in infancy. The latter sort of catharsis occurs through *free association*. Free association is regressive in its nature, which is not the case with associative thinking. Associative thinking is lateral in direction, whereas free association is vertical. (Slavson, S.R. *Analytic Group Psychotherapy*, 1950) See *presentation*.

thinking, autistic See *autism*.

thinking, categorical See *thinking, physiognomonic*.

thinking compulsion See *brooding*.

thinking, concrete See *thinking, physiognomonic*.

thinking, concretistic See *concretism*.

thinking, directed See *intellect*.

thinking disorder *Thought disorder*, including abnormalities in form (*formal thought disorder, association disturbance*), in possession (feeling that one's thoughts are not one's own), in content (delusions and similar ideas), and in quantity or stream of thought (abnormal speed or amount of thinking). See *associations, disturbances of; symptoms, negative; thought disorder*.

thinking, double An infrequently used term with unclear definition; some authorities use the term synonymously with *thought-hearing*. See *symptoms, first-rank*.

thinking, fragmentation of A disturbance in association, pathognomonic of schizophrenia, in which even such basic concepts as "father" and "mother" become vague and obscure and the thinking processes become so confused that they cannot result in a complete idea or action, but merely in vague movements. Bleuler calls this a primary symptom of schizophrenia and believes that it is due to associations no longer following the logical pathways indicated by past experience. Instead, associations easily take new and seemingly illogical pathways, and thinking becomes bizarre. Thus two ideas, fortuitously encountered, are combined into one thought. Associations lack the concept of purpose. When the symptom is of mild degree, it may be noticed only that the patient gives generalized rather than precise answers. Thus one patient, asked to give the location of London, said "Europe" rather than "England." (*Dementia Praecox or the Group of Schizophrenias*, 1950)

thinking, Janusian See *Janusian thinking*.

thinking, magical Archaic, primitive, prelogical thinking, such as is seen in the unconscious of neurotics, in small children, in normal persons under conditions of fatigue, as antecedents of thought in primitive man, and in schizophrenic thinking. The speech and thinking of the schizophrenic are frequently more concrete and active than normal, not yet capable of realistic abstractions, and more a symbolic equivalent of action. See *paleologic; process, primary psychic*.

thinking, physiognomonic (fiz-i-og-nom'ō-nik) According to Kasanin, the first stage in the development of thought in the child. In this stage, the child animates objects and projects his ego into them, as when he plays with a stick and calls it a horse. Piaget calls this *syncretic thinking*.

The second stage is concrete thinking, characterized by literalness and lack of generalizations. In this stage, for example, the word "table" refers not to tables in general but to the particular table in the subject's house.

The third stage is abstract or categorized thinking, characterized by use of abstractions and generalizations. This type of thinking appears relatively late, usually after adolescence and probably only after some degree of education.

thinking, prearchaic See *thinking, archaic-paralogical*.

thinking, preconscious One of the terms used by Fenichel to describe the preverbal, prelogical, pictorial phantasy thinking that precedes the development of logical thinking in small children.

Preconscious thinking is not in accordance with reality. All of its features are primitive and archaic. First, since it is ruled by the emotions and strives for the discharge of tensions, it is full of wishful or fear-laden misconceptions. Second, it is carried out through concrete pictorial images. Third, it is a magical type of thinking. "The object and the idea of the object, the object and a picture or model of the object, the object and a part of the object are equated: similarities are not distinguished from identities; ego and nonego are not yet separated. What happens to objects might (by identification) be experienced as happening to the ego, and what happens to the ego causes the same thing to happen to the object." Last the thinking is symbolic and thus vague, for the world is experienced and apperceived in symbolic forms. Stimuli that provoke the same emotional reactions are looked upon as identical. Thus if penis and snake provoke the same emotions they are apprehended by a common conception: they are one and the same thing. Although illogical and ineffective, this preconscious phantasy thinking is an attempt to master reality. It does postpone immediate discharge reactions and attempts to anticipate reality and bring about a more adequate discharge of tensions.

With the acquisition of words and the development of the faculty of speech, thinking becomes logical and organized. Words can be linked to ideas. This is the decisive step in the final differentiation of conscious and unconscious and in the development of reality testing. Now there can be precise anticipation of action through thinking, and instinctual excitations as well as the external world can be handled in a better way.

Preconscious thinking, however, recurs in the adult in several different ways. Before acquiring verbal formulation, all thoughts run through initial phases that resemble preconscious thinking. In dreams and in fatigue, words are retranslated into pictures. Conscious ideas may be symbols

hiding objectionable unconscious ideas and in dreams symbols appear not only in order to distort, but also as a characteristic of, archaic pictorial thinking visualizing abstract thoughts. In this way the fact that the symbol and the symbolized were once the same thing is utilized. Preconscious thinking may also appear as a substitute for unpleasant reality or a reality that cannot be influenced. This occurs, for example, in the magical daydreaming phantasies of the hysterical patient. In the obsessive-compulsive the magic power of concepts can be observed. Finally, psychotic thinking is identical with the preconscious thinking of small children, described above. (Fenichel, *PTN*)

thinking, syncretic See *thinking, physiognomonic*.

thinking, undirected See *intellect*.

third nervous system A system differentiated by Burrow on the basis of its specialization of function, not on the basis of anatomical demarcation. It involves the neural processes that govern man's symbolic interchange, and through its misuse is considered responsible for man's disordered behavior.

thirteen, original The original thirteen were the founders (in 1844) of the Association of Medical Superintendents of America: William Awl, Luther Bell, Amariah Brigham, John Butler, Nehenich Cutter, Pliny Earle, John Galt, Thomas Kirkbride, Isaac Ray, Charles Stedman, Francis Stribling, Samuel White, and Samuel Woodward. In 1893 the name of the society was changed to the American Medicopsychological Association, which became the American Psychiatric Association in 1922.

thlasis depressio *Obs.* Melancholia.

Thomism The philosophicotheological system of Thomas Aquinas, an ideological system that some assert is based on the unrecognized premise that "father is always right" or "it is right because father said so." It would consequently be incompatible with reconstruction or insight psychotherapy but consonant with supportive, persuasion, or exhortative therapy. See *psychotherapy*.

Thompson, Clara (1893–1958) American psychoanalyst; associated with Harry Sullivan and his modifications of psychoanalysis (interpersonal relationships).

thought, archaic "Schizophrenic thinking shows startling analogies to the thinking of primitive man. In other words it is *archaic* in character. A reasonably adequate discussion of schizophrenic thinking would require that it be correlated with the principal historic features of the development of thought wherein it would be shown that it throws back to historically earlier ways of thinking in which feeling, perception and concreteness dominate, while reasoning, differentiation, and abstraction are little in evidence." (White, W.A. *Outline of Psychiatry,* 1929)

thought, audible A type of auditory hallucination in which the voice is projected into the patient himself, as though he could hear his own thoughts. Such hallucinations with almost no sensory components are commonly designated as *inner voices.* Baillarger referred to them as *psychic hallucinations.* These are *hallucinations of conception* rather than of perception. Patients may use the term "soundless voices" to refer to essentially the same phenomenon. See *symptoms, first-rank.*

thought blocking See *blocking.*

thought broadcasting See *symptoms, first-rank.*

thought constraint See *constraint of thought.*

thought deprivation *Blocking* (q.v.).

thought derailment See *derailment, thought.*

thought disorder *Thinking disorder* (q.v.); sometimes used in a more limited way to refer specifically to schizophrenic disturbances of the associations such as thought blocking, thought deprivation, poverty of thought, or haphazard, seemingly purposeless, illogical, confused, incorrect, abrupt, or bizarre associations. See *associations, disturbances of; symptoms, negative.*

thought disorder, primary The type of schizophrenia in which there is striking involvement of intellectual functions with marked incoherence and irrelevance, tendency to *neologisms, word salads,* and peculiar syntactical speech formation.

thought echoing An auditory hallucination consisting of hearing one's own thoughts expressed in whispered or unbearably loud tones; *écho des pensées* (q.v.); audible thoughts. See *symptoms, first-rank.*

thought, emotional See *psychodynamics, adaptational.*

thought hearing Some patients, notably those with schizophrenia, maintain that they hear their own thoughts; they may also believe that their thoughts are heard by others too. Similar to thought echoing except that in the latter the thoughts are typically heard coming from the outside, while in thought hearing the thoughts are heard as coming from within the patient himself. See *symptoms, first-rank.*

thought, imageless A thought completely devoid of optic pictures or representations.

thought, inelasticity of Reduction of the normal flow of thought, often observed in people of old age, when thoughts become more rigid, more static than in the years of youth.

thought insertion *Thought pressure* (q.v.).

thought, latent See *cerebration, unconscious.*

thought, multifocal Arieti's term for *asyndesis* (q.v.) and similar association disturbances, which he explains as being due to the fact that the patient's thought simultaneously focuses on many different planes and on different meanings with their different objective situations.

thought omnipotence See *thinking, magical.*

thought pressure Thoughts, as patients described it, that are forced into their minds; thought insertion. The patients assume little or no responsibility for developing the thoughts. This is particularly true in patients with schizophrenia, who may ascribe all their mental processes to the alleged pressure brought upon them by others. See *symptoms, first-rank.*

The same phenomenon of thought pressure may also appear in manic-depressive disorders, as well as in certain psychoneurotic states. In these diagnostic groups no external pressure is alleged; rather, the patients assert that the irresistible force arises within their own minds.

Also known as *pressure of ideas.*

thought, reactive See *reinforcement, reactive.*

thought, reenforced See *thought, supervalent.*

thought rehearsal See *rehearsal, obsessional.*

thought, supervalent "A train of thought such as this may be described as exaggerated, or better *reenforced,* or 'supervalent' in Wernicke's sense of the word. It shows its pathological character, in spite of its apparently reasonable content, by the single peculiarity that no amount of conscious and voluntary effort or thought on the patient's part is able to dissipate or remove it." (Freud, *CP*)

thought transference See *perception, extrasensory.*

thought unemotional See *psychodynamics, adaptational*

three-cornered therapy See *psychotherapy, multiple.*

threshold, sedation The amount of sodium amytal required, by intravenous injection, to produce slurring of speech and a concomitant inflection point in the 15–30 cps amplitude curve of the electroencephalogram. The EEG change occurs within 80 seconds of the time when slur is noted. Shagass had used this test to differentiate between psychotic and neurotic depressions; according to him, thresholds are low in psychotic depressions and high in neurotic depressions.

thromboangiitis obliterans, cerebral (throm-bō-an-jē-ī′tis) Thromboangiitis obliterans is far less common in the cerebral vessels than in the peripheral vessels, but when it does occur peripheral disease is often absent. The cerebral form is more common in males and usually begins in the fifth decade; heavy smoking may be of etiologic importance. Symptoms are very similar to those found with cerebral arteriosclerosis: a focal, neurological form or a generalized mental form. See *arteriosclerosis, cerebral.*

thrombosis, cerebral See *accident, cerebrovascular.*

thumb sucking See *sucking, thumb.*

thymergasia (thīm-ēr-gas′ē-à) Adolf Meyer's term for the psychiatric syndromes commonly known as affective psychoses or reaction types. For example, the manic-depressive psychosis is a form of thymergasia.

-thymia (-thī′mē-à, -thim′ē-à), **thymo-** (thī′mō-) Combining form meaning state of mind and will, soul, spirit, temper, from Gr. *thymós.*

thymogenic drinking See *alcoholism.*

thymoleptic Influencing or changing mood; this term is used to refer to drugs that ameliorate pathologic depressive states but, in the absence of depression, do not act as central nervous system stimulants. See *psychotropics.*

thymopathic Referring to any disturbance in affect or mood tone; dysthmic; dysphoric. Bleuler used *thymopathic personality* to refer to the premorbid personality of the manic-depressive (bipolar) subject, characterized by lack of emotional poise, distractibility, feelings of inadequacy and frustration, irascibility, and periods of dejection. He believed those personality traits were evidence of an inherited predisposition to bipolar disorder.

thymopathy (thī-mop′à-thē) A general term for morbidity of the affects.

thymopsyche See *noopsyche.*

thyroidism Excessive functioning of the thyroid gland.

thyrotoxicosis Grave's disease; exophthalmic goiter. The usual personality pattern of patients with thyrotoxicosis is said to be a pseudo-self-reliance to overcome security threats combined with an unconscious longing for dependence. Neurotic-like symptoms are frequent and often lead to a misdiagnosis of anxiety state or phobic reaction; if a psychosis develops, it is usually of the affective type, often with prominent manic symptoms.

TIA Transient ischemic attack; occlusion of the internal carotid artery (usually just above the bifurcation of the common carotid artery) leading to an attack of paresis in one or both limbs on the opposite side of the body, weakness of the side of the face, visual defects such as blurring or blindness, and vertigo. Characteristic are complete recovery following each episode, repeated attacks of short duration (rarely longer than 18 hours), but eventually a hemiplegia.

tic A brief, sudden, rapid, recurrent, non-rhythmic, stereotyped, irresistible movement or vocalization. Although tics may be psychogenic (in which case they are sometimes called *habit spasm* or *habit contraction*), they may also be due to a variety of neurologic disorders. Both types are exacerbated by stress and diminished during sleep or engrossing activities. See *stereotyped movement disorders.*

Simple motor tics are blinking, shrugging the shoulders, facial twitches, or grimaces. Complex motor tics include grooming behavior (such as hair combing motions), jumping, hitting or biting oneself, smelling an object, echokinesis, and echopraxis.

Simple vocal tics include coughing, grunting, snorting, and clearing the throat.

Complex vocal tics include echolalia, palilalia, coprolalia, and repeating words or phrases out of context.

The French term *tic de pensée* refers to the involuntary habit of giving expression to any idea that happens to be present in the mind.

Abraham considered the tic a conversion symptom at the anal-sadistic level, and most psychoanalytic writers have emphasized the well-defined anal character and, in addition, the markedly narcissistic makeup of the tiqueur.

"The repressed situations, whose motor intentions return in tic, are highly emotional ones representing again either instinctual temptations or punishments for warded-off impulses. In tics, a movement that was once the concomitant sign of an affect (sexual excitement, rage, anxiety, grief, triumph, embarrassment) has become an equivalent of this affect, and appears instead of the warded-off affect.

"This may occur in different ways: (1) The tic represents a part of the original affective syndrome, whose mental significance remains unconscious; (2) the tic represents a movement whose unconscious meaning is a defense against the intended affect; (3) the tic does not directly represent affect or defense against affect but, rather, other movements or motor impulses that once occurred during a repressed emotional excitement, either in the patient or in another person with whom the patient has made a hysterical identification." (Fenichel, *PTN*)

tic, attitude Tonic rigidity in particular attitudes of the head or a limb, such as torticollis.

tic convulsif See *tic*.

tic disorders In DSM-III-R, this category includes Tourette's disorder, chronic motor or vocal tic disorder, and transient tic disorder. In DSM-III, those conditions were subsumed under the category *stereotyped movement disorders* (q.v.).

tic douloureux (tēk'dōō-lōō-rē) (F. "painful tic; facial neuralgia") Also known as trifacial neuralgia, prosopalgia, Fothergill's neuralgia, chronic paroxysmal trigeminal neuralgia; a chronic trigeminal neuralgia characterized by excruciating paroxysmal pain of short duration, flushing of the face, watering eyes, and rhinorrhea. The condition may affect either the second or the third division of the fifth cranial nerve, or both. The first division is rarely affected. The intermissions between paroxysms vary from weeks to as long as a year. With each succeeding attack seizures become more frequent and more severe. Many cases exhibit dolorogenetic or trigger zones on the face or mucous membranes, stimulation of which will evoke attacks. Tic douloureux is usually unilateral, is more common in adults over 40, and is more frequent among females. The cause is unknown, although the disease may be associated with dental or sinus pathology. There is probably some hereditary factor.

Treatment is directed first toward remedying possible local causes. Carbamazepine is often effective in controlling the pain, but permanent relief is possible only by blocking the pain fibers, either by alcohol injection of the trigeminal ganglion or by surgical division of the sensory root.

tic non-douloureux (nôN-dōō-lōō-rē) (F. "nonpainful tic") Charcot's term for a hysterical disorder of the face, usually unilateral, characterized by paroxysmal twitching of the facial muscles and anesthesia of the skin on the affected side of the face.

tic, psychic A gesture or ejaculation made under the influence of an irresistible morbid impulse.

tic scriptorius Writer's tic; fast, short, stereotyped, involuntary movements of the writing arm and hand that result in adventitious inclusions of varying size in handwriting. Such movements have been reported in patients with *Tourette's disorder*. See *syndrome, Gilles de la Tourette*.

Tilney, Frederick (1876–1938) American neurologist; comparative anatomy.

time agnosia A condition in which the meaning of time is not comprehended, even though the patient may speak of time. There is disorientation in immediate time, the patient is unable to estimate short time intervals, and long intervals of time are frequently shortened. Thus one patient with time agnosia stated that World War I had ended four years before, whereas actually it had ended ten years earlier. Patients with time agnosia are able to relate events of the distant past and their interconnection with location, but cannot give the element of time of the event or time relations. Accompanying the time agnosia, and probably a result of it, is an indifference to the past and future and a lack of concern about the condition itself. Time agnosia follows trauma, such as head injury, especially of the temporal area, cerebrovascular accident, and alcoholic coma.

The trauma usually results in a mentally confused state of short duration. Then the patient regains orientation in space, but remains disoriented in time for the immediate present as well as for past events, to a varying degree. Time agnosia often disappears gradually, depending on the extent and degree of permanency of the original lesion.

Davidson has described a syndrome of time agnosia which includes post-traumatic muscular hypertonicity, vascular eye-ground changes (congested discs), and diminution of the acuity of sensibility in a generalized way. The prepsychotic personality of such patients includes a certain simplicity of makeup and a weakness of the sexual impulse. They have ordinarily led a colorless, drifting life wherein time has had no particular meaning to them. (*Journal of Nervous and Mental Disease 94,* 1941)

time, evaluated A description of phrases or periods of life with an assessment by the subject of the feeling tone aroused by them. According to D. Chiriboga (*Journal of Gerontology 33,* 1978), 60% of subjects aged 16 to 67 years rate the teens and twenties as the best time of life, and another 18% rate the thirties as best. No one chose the later years as best.

time, reaction See *reaction time.*

time, sleep See *sleep time, total.*

time, wake See *wake time after sleep onset.*

timetable, individuation-separation See *separation-individuation.*

tiqueur (tē-kĕr′) One who suffers from a tic.

TLP Time-limited psychotherapy. See *psychotherapy, time-limited.*

TM *Transcendental meditation* (q.v.).

tobacco dependence This diagnostic group is defined as using tobacco continuously for one month or longer and, in addition, failure of attempts to stop or reduce intake on a permanent basis, or appearance of withdrawal syndrome upon attempting to stop, or continuation of use despite life-threatening physical disorder(s) known to be exacerbated by tobacco use.

tocomania Puerperal mania.

Todd's paralysis (Robert Bentley Todd, English physician, 1809–60) The temporary increase, following each convulsion, in the severity and extent of the weakness associated with Jacksonian convulsions. Permanent weakness of the part of the body that is the focus of the fit is common in Jacksonian epilepsy.

toe-walking Walking on the toes rather than on the whole foot; toe-walking has been reported in approximately 20% of childhood schizophrenics.

togetherness Ackerman's term for the earliest stage in personality development, when the infant is in a state of primary psychic union with the mother, with little or no recognition of the self.

toilet training The process of teaching a child bowel and urine control. See *morality, sphincter; phase, anal; superego.*

token economy A type of group treatment program, based upon the operant conditioning technique of positive reinforcement, in which elements in the patient's environment are arranged in such a way that reinforcing aspects of the environment are made contingent on the patient's behavior. When the desired "target behavior" occurs, a token (such as a poker chip or plastic card) is given and may be exchanged for a reinforcing agent (any desired goods or services).

tolerance Increasing resistance to the effects of a drug. Tolerance is an outstanding characteristic of the opiates and the amphetamines, and only somewhat less marked with the barbiturates. Although tolerance is not an essential for the development of drug dependence—the cocaine addict, for example, does not develop tolerance for his drug—it is an important consideration in any instance of drug dependence. For linked to tolerance is the need for increasing dosage to maintain or recapture the desired drug effect; and in general, the more saturated body cells become with any substance, the longer will be the period required to rid them of all traces of the drug. Tolerance of any marked degree also creates serious problems for the drug user in ensuring an adequate supply.

Closely allied to tolerance is *physical dependence*, the need to have some quantum of drug present within the body—or at least within some of its cellular elements or organ systems. The *abstinence* (or *withdrawal*) *syndrome* is the symptomatic expression of physical dependence—cells that have become accustomed to functioning under a mantle of drugs tend to fire or discharge or otherwise function in chaotic disorder when that mantle is suddenly removed. See *addiction; alcoholism; dependency, drug.*

tolerance, frustration The maximal point of tolerance of frustration at which the defenses of a person give way to the conflict and resentment that frustration sets up in him.

tolerance, social Public acceptance of personal variation or idiosyncrasy in matters of appearance, lifestyle, personality, or belief. Tolerance is thus differentiated from approval, in that a society may tolerate diversity of lifestyle even when a majority of its members do not approve of the variant behavior.

tomography Sectional roentgenography; during exposure, the X-ray tube is moved in a curve synchronous with the recording plate but in the opposite direction. As a result, the shadow of the selected plane remains stationary while all others are displaced and thus blurred or obliterated. *CT* (computerized tomography) scan is used in visualizing cerebral structures, including ventricles and cortical sulci. Because it is a noninvasive procedure, it is used often as a basic screening device for suspected neurological disorders such as brain tumor, infarction, hemorrhage, cerebral atrophy, and hydrocephalus. See *NMR.*

tomomania A morbid desire to be operated upon.

-tonia (-tō′nē-à) Combining form meaning stretching, tension, tone, from Gr. *tónos.*

tonicity State or condition of tone or tension, mental or physical. See *tension, mental.*

tonitrophobia Fear of thunder; astrapophobia.

tonogenic Giving rise to increased tension or tonus.

tonogeny (tō-noj′ē-ni) Tonogeny refers to any factor giving rise to increased tension or tonus. The vagus nerve is regarded

as the tone-giving nerve of the stomach and intestines. The psyche may be the origin of tone-producing stimuli; for example, anxiety may be expressed in part through states of tension or tenseness. Extreme states of tension of long duration are common in the catatonic form of schizophrenia.

tonus Tonicity.

TOP The association areas of the temporal, occipital, and parietal lobes of the cerebral hemisphere. The functions of TOP are imperfectly understood, but presumably many of the highest psychic functions are dependent upon intactness of these regions. The TOP area and the prefrontal area are the last to develop phylogenetically.

topalgia Pain localized to one spot; the presence of a painful point or spot; a symptom occurring in hysteria or neurasthenia.

topectomy A surgical operation for the excision (removal) of selected areas of the cerebral cortex (brain surface) in certain cases of mental illness; also known as the Columbia-Greystone operation since it was devised by that group. See *lobotomy, prefrontal.*

"The following types of cases show the most favorable results: (1) Schizophrenic patients who, in spite of every kind of shock treatment, continue to manifest violent behavior, suicidal tendencies, homicidal tendencies, and destructiveness. . . (2) refractory obsessive-compulsive psychoneurotics who remain uninfluenced by prolonged psycho-analysis, direct interview psychotherapy, and electroshock treatment. . .(3) involutional melancholia which has failed to respond to shock therapy. . .(4) manic-depressive psychosis, with either a chronic depressed state or a chronic mania. . . (5) chronic depressions of old age, in patients over sixty who have failed to improve after electroshock treatment." (Polatin, P. *How Psychiatry Helps,* 1949)

topical flight Cameron's term for *flight of ideas* (q.v.).

topographical hypothesis See *id.*

topography, mental The mapping out of psychic structures, a static representation of the components of the psyche, denoting their location. For example, the superego in the adult psyche is located in the realm of the unconscious; Jung's archetypes occupy one of the deeper layers of the unconscious.

"Psychoanalysis differed from academic (descriptive) psychology mainly by reason of its dynamic conception of mental processes; now we have to add that it professes to consider mental topography also, and to indicate in respect of any given mental operation within what system or between what systems it runs its course. This attempt, too, has given it the name of 'depth-psychology.' " (Freud, *CP*)

toponeurosis A localized neurosis.

topophobia A general term meaning fear of place. For each patient the nature of the place is specific, although the word has come to be used as a synonym of agyiphobia, or fear of streets.

torpedoing The application of intense electrical currents to the bodily region involved in hysterical conversions.

torpillage (tor-pē-yàzh′) (F. "act of torpedoing") A form of treating cases of hysteria, particularly in wartime, by applying electric currents to a shocking degree of pain—thus "fighting fire with fire," as it were; a type of aversion therapy.

torpor A disorder of consciousness in which the subject is drowsy, slow in thinking, and shows a narrowed range of perception.

torsion dystonia See *dystonia, torsion.*

torsion spasm A constant and irregular twisting and turning of the body, especially of the pelvis and neck muscles, with bizarre posturing of the body and limbs.

torticollis Wry neck; characterized by spasmodic contractions of the muscles of the neck, particularly those supplied by the spinal accessory nerve; the head is usually drawn to one side and rotated so that the chin points to the opposite side.

Torticollis is sometimes psychological in origin; Ferenczi regarded it as an attitude tic.

"total-push" treatment of schizophrenia A method of treatment suggested by Myerson that includes physiotherapy, irradiation, exercise and games, diets, praise, blame, reward, punishment, regard for clothing and personal care.

totem "An animal, either edible or harmless, or dangerous and feared; more rarely the totem is a plant or a force of nature (rain, water) which stands in a peculiar relation to the whole clan. The totem is first of all the tribal ancestor of the clan, as well as its tutelary spirit and protector; it sends oracles and, though otherwise dangerous, the totem knows and spares its children. The members of a totem are therefore under a sacred obligation not to kill (destroy) their totem, to abstain from eating its meat or from any other enjoyment of it." (Freud, *BW*)

totemism The selection of animals, plants, and inanimate objects as representatives for the (primitive) individual and tribes.

Freud says that he divides "the accepted theories of the derivation of totemism into three groups, (a) nominalistic, (b) sociological, (c) psychological."

Nominalistic totemism refers to that form of totemism that differentiates tribes by names. Freud, quoting from E. Durkheim, says that, "as regards sociorepresentative of the social religion of these [i.e. Australian] races, it embodies the community, which is the real object of veneration." Psychological totemism, according to Frazer, was based upon the belief in an "outward soul." The totem was meant to represent a safe place of refuge where the soul is deposited in order to avoid the dangers which threaten it. (Freud, *BW*)

toucherism A paraphilia in which arousal is dependent upon touching the sexual object.

touching A disturbance in association, peculiar to schizophrenia, in which the only recognizable association to external stimuli consists of feeling with the hands the contours of objects within reach. This process is similar to *naming* (q.v.) except that a different motor activity is involved.

Tourette disorder, Tourette syndrome See *syndrome, Gilles de la Tourette.*

tower-head *Oxycephaly* (q.v.).

toxicomania A craving for poison; drug dependency.

toxicophobia, toxiphobia Fear of poison.

toxiphrenia *Obs.* Schizophrenia associated with toxic, delirious reaction.

toxoplasmosis, congenital In utero infection with toxoplasma, a protozoanlike organism, which may produce mental retardation. Diagnosis is by serological testing of mother and infant.

TPI *Treponema pallidum* immobilization. See *test, TPI.*

TPN Total parenteral nutrition, usually implemented with an indwelling intravenous catheter and used in patients who have lost most or all of the small bowel. About 20% of such patients develop delirium or other serious psychiatric complications in the first year.

tracking In multimodal behavior therapy, analysis of the patient's usual response to a situation or experience in terms of the order in which the different modalities of the *BASIC-ID* (q.v.) are predominant. Some patients, for example, typically respond first in the sensation modality, whereas others respond first in the cognitions area. It has been found that interventions are likely to be most effective if they follow the order of the patient's response pattern. With a patient whose first-order response is sensation (e.g. "butterflies in the stomach"), the best therapeutic results are likely to be obtained if predominantly sensory techniques (e.g. relaxation and biofeedback) are used as initial treatments.

tracking, eye See *eye movements, pursuit.*

tract, pyramidal "The pyramidal tracts are the means by which the nervous impulses which excite voluntary movements pass from the cerebral cortex to the lower motor neurones which arise in the brainstem and spinal cord. The pyramidal fibres or upper motor neurones are the axones of cells of the precentral convolution. Electrical excitation of these cells causes movements of the opposite side of the body. The movements thus excited are not simply contractions of isolated muscles, but always involve groups of muscles contracting harmoniously, so that an orderly movement results. The upper motor neurones therefore are organized in terms of movements, in contrast to the lower motor neurones, which are distributed to groups of muscle-fibres in individual muscles." (Brain, *DNS*)

tractotomy, stereotactic A modification of psychosurgery consisting of implantation of radioactive yttrium-90 seeds in the substantia innominata below the head of the caudate nucleus. Sometimes called *seed psychosurgery,* the procedure has been reported to be of benefit in intractable depression, anxiety, and obsessional states.

training, alpha wave See *alpha wave training.*

training, assertiveness See *therapy, behavior.*

training, autogenic Relaxation exercises; gradual, progressive relaxation of the voluntary musculature, typically starting with the toes and feet and sweeping upwards to involve the whole body. Often used in conjunction with reciprocal inhibition psychotherapy and other forms of behavior therapy. See *behavior theory.*

training, control See *control training.*

training, habit The acquisition (by the young child) of specific behavior patterns mainly related to the functions of eating, elimination, sleep, and dress. To the behaviorist, training is in the nature of conditioning. To the psychoanalyst, habit and habit training have a different meaning: "A particular habit is for the child a defence against a particular unconscious fantasy or wish. His clinging to habit may be one of his main defences against the anxiety connected with aggressive impulses and fantasies in general." (Isaacs, S. in *On the Bringing Up of Children,* ed. J. Rickman, 1936)

training, self-instructional See *therapy, behavior.*

training, social skills See *social skills training.*

training, spontaneity "Just as the spontaneity test is an intensification of the sociometric test, so the spontaneity training process is an intensification of the assignment technique. New situations and new roles demand from some individuals spontaneous elements which are lacking. It is through graduated training of the personality in constructed situations and roles that such individuals learn how to act on the spur of the moment and how to integrate these roles into their personality without loss of spontaneity." (Moreno, J.L., & Jennings, H. *Sociometric Review 17,* 1936)

trait In genetics, the characteristic symptomatology of a hereditary factor as it appears in the phenotypes of those who have inherited the predisposition to the given attribute.

A trait is any physical or psychological characteristic that varies from one subject to another; it is a relatively stable and enduring attribute, in contrast to a *state,* which is a transient reactive condition or behavioral predisposition. Some authorities, for instance, consider hypoboulia and affective blunting as trait variables in schizophrenia, and hallucinations, delusions, and periods of agitation or excitement to be state variables.

trait anxiety See *anxiety*.

trait carrier In genetic family studies this means a tainted family member actually exhibiting the hereditary character under observation. These trait carriers are distinguished from the *taint carriers*.

traits, feminine, in male According to Adler, the following are feminine traits that the male neurotic perceives in himself either consciously or unconsciously: passive attitude, obedience, softness, cowardice, memory of defeat, ignorance, lack of capacity, and tenderness. The person attempts to overcome these characteristics by developing hatred, defiance, cruelty, and egoism.

traits, neuropathic Classically, the following are included in the term: enuresis, nail-biting, finger-sucking, sleepwalking, anxiety, nightmares, and fear of darkness. See *behavior disorders*.

traits, neurotic See *behavior disorders*.

trance A sleeplike state with markedly diminished responsivity to environmental stimuli; a daze, stupor, or coma. Trances are most commonly observed as a part of *catalepsy, ecstasy,* or *hypnotism* (qq.v.).

trance coma The deep sleep following hypnotism.

trance, ecstatic See *ecstasy*.

trance/possession disorder See *possession/trance disorder*.

tranquilizer Ataractic; neuroleptic; currently used to refer to a group of phrenotropic compounds whose effects are exerted primarily at a subcortical level so that consciousness is not interfered with, in contrast to hypnotic and sedative drugs, which also have a calming effect. See *ergotropic; psychotropics*.

Benjamin Rush in the 1790s referred to an invention of his designed to reduce blood flow to the head of the mental patient as a "tranquillizing chair." It consisted of a chair to which the patient's hands and arms were strapped, stocks for the feet, and a box for the patient's head, so that he could not move.

transactional Relating to negotiating, conducting, performing, or carrying on, as an act or process; pertaining to an interplay or interaction. R. Grinker's transac-

tional approach is an attempt to understand the interplay between therapist and patient—and ultimately between the patient and external reality—in terms of role theory.

"Activities within a transactional process, although they deal with current reality and start with well-defined explicit roles, expose the repetitive nature of the patient's unadaptive behavior and stimulate his recall of past experiences ... this transactional approach evokes implicit expressive or emotional roles and incites repetition of old transactions and illuminates the genetic source of the current behavior." (In *Contemporary Psychotherapies*, ed. M.I. Stein 1961) See *role*.

Both transactional and interactional refer to cross-communication and cross-influencing of each member in a relationship by the other member(s). In psychiatry, the terms are generally used to refer to the dynamic, two-way interaction between therapist and patient. The earlier assumption that the psychoanalyst is totally objective and reflects none of his own values to his patient has undergone gradual modification in recent years. It is now recognized that in the psychoanalytic process, "The therapist's personality, his value system, and his techniques of interaction, nonverbal as well as verbal, are ... at least as important, and in many instances even more important than the uncovering of repressed content which has been the cornerstone of the traditional model of the psychoanalytic process. The increasing awareness of this among psychoanalysts has been reflected in recent years in the growing literature on the subject of 'countertransference' attitudes in the analyst and their effect upon the analytic process." (Marmor, J. *Archives of General Psychiatry 3*, 1960)

transactional analysis (TA) A type of psychotherapy developed by Eric Berne that emphasizes the influence of the ego states of Parent, Adult, and Child on a person's interactions with others. The Parent ego state relates to limit-setting and nurturing; it is based on the subject's perception of his own parents. The Adult ego state is concerned with reality testing and estimating probabilities in transactions with the outside world. The Child ego state comprises the feelings, wishes, and adaptations actually experienced in childhood.

Most outcomes of an exchange are decided by *ulterior transactions,* psychological responses that are outside the awareness of the participants. People play *games,* adopting the role of Persecutor, Rescuer, or Victim and using ulterior transactions in such a way that everyone loses. Treatment focuses on *feelings analysis, script analysis,* and *stroking* (stimulating and recognizing other human beings). Feelings may be reactions (appropriate responses in the here and now); they may also be *rubber bands* (feelings from the past reactivated by a stimulus in the present) or *rackets* (indulgences or displaced feelings that are a backdrop in today's scene of living). The script refers to plans decided upon in early life when the subject was under parental influence; they are based on myths about the self and the world and are perpetuated by games and rackets. The major scripts are *winner, nonwinner* (tolerable but unsatisfying), and *loser.*

transcendental meditation (TM) A psychophysiologic technique, usually associated with the name of the Indian guru (teacher) Maharishi Mahesh Yogi. Maharishi began teaching the technique throughout India in 1955 and in 1958 initiated a worldwide movement to train others who wished to learn it. TM is neither a religion nor a philosophy even though in the past it may have been related to both. It appears to be a natural process, perhaps a fourth physiologically and biochemically definable state of consciousness (the others being sleeping, dreaming, and waking), that does not require any mental or physical control, any change in lifestyle or belief system, nor does it involve hypnosis or suggestion. TM is associated with a hypometabolic state, during which there is a reduced activity of the adrenergic component of the autonomic nervous system. The physiologic and psychosomatic accompaniments of the state lead to a lowering of tension and anxiety and an increase in contentment and tolerance of frustration.

transcultural psychiatry See *psychiatry, comparative.*

transducer See *synapse.*

transduction, sensory Conversion of sensory stimuli into the electrochemical activity of neurons, accomplished through specialized sensory receptors for exteroception, proprioception, and interoception.

transfer In connection with institutional statistics, a transfer is a shift from one institution directly to another institution of the same class.

transfer RNA See *chromosome.*

transference In psychoanalytic therapy, the phenomenon of projection of feelings, thoughts, and wishes onto the analyst, who has come to represent an object from the patient's past. The analyst is reacted to as though he were someone from the patient's past; such reactions, while they may have been appropriate to the conditions that prevailed in the patient's previous life, are inappropriate and anachronistic when applied to an object (the analyst) in the present.

"During psychoanalytic treatment, the repressed unconscious material is revived, and since this material contains many infantile elements, the infantile strivings are reactivated and seek gratification in the transference. As the most important relationship of the child is that with his parents, the relationship between patient and analyst established in the transference becomes analogous to, or, at times, even similar to the patient's relationship with his parents in childhood. The patient endows the analyst with the same magic powers and omniscience which, in childhood, he attributed to his parents. The traits of submissiveness and rebellion, in transference, likewise reflect the attitude of the child to his parents. The patient behaves irrationally in the psychoanalytic situation; it often takes a long time to make him see the irrationality of his behavior, which is deeply rooted in his unconscious infantile life." (Nunberg, H. *Principles of Psychoanalysis,* 1955)

Transference may be positive, as when the patient unrealistically overvalues or loves the analyst; or it may be negative, as when the patient dislikes or hates the analyst without due cause in reality. See *distortion, parataxic.*

It is to be noted that the term transference does not refer to reactions of the patient to the analyst that are based on reality factors in the therapeutic relationship; thus a patient may be angry with his therapist if the latter misses an appointment, but to call such a reaction a manifestation of transference is incorrect. It should also be recognized that transference can exist outside the analytic situation in relation to other people in the person's environment.

E. Krapf (*Psychoanalytic Quarterly 26*, 1957) considers positive transference to be predominantly libidinal and negative transference as predominantly aggressive. He notes that there is a third type of transference, the transference of anxiety, which always serves as a defense, while libidinal and aggressive transference are defensive in many instances but not in all. "Thus we may list five types of transference: 1, libidinal; 2, aggressive; 3, libidinal-defensive; 4, aggressive-defensive; and 5, anxious-defensive."

Jung stresses the question of transference, which he calls psychological rapport. He calls it "the intensified tie to the physician which is a compensation symptom for the defective relationship to present reality." He holds that "the phenomenon of transference is inevitable in every fundamental analysis. . . . The patient must find a relationship to an object in the living present, for without it he can never adequately fulfill the demands that adaptation makes upon him." (Jung, *CAP*)

transference cure See *flight into health.*

transference, floating Also known as the floating positive; those generally positive and spontaneous attitudes and feelings that the patient has for the analyst and the analytic situation in the beginning of treatment. The floating transference is a preliminary sort of relationship and usually merges imperceptibly into the specific transference of affect brought about by the analytic situation and the fundamental rule.

transference, identification A term employed by S.R. Slavson to differentiate between *libidinal* transference and *sibling* transference, which occur in analytic group psychotherapy. It refers to the attitude and relations derived from identifying with other members of a therapy group and the desire to emulate or be like them. See *transference, libidinal; transference, sibling.*

transference, institutional Emotional dependence upon hospital, clinic, or similar establishment, rather than on a particular therapist or person within the institution; observed frequently in latent schizophrenics.

transference, libidinal The transference derived from and charged with libidinal and other drives that the patient had felt toward his parents and now is redirecting upon the therapist. See *transference, identification; transference, sibling.*

transference, negative See *transference resistance.*

transference neurosis See *neurosis, transference.*

transference, positive See *transference.*

transference resistance Positive libidinal transference that occurs when the patient harmoniously transfers repressed material upon the physician. The material, however, may be rejected by the ego or superego, that is, there is resistance offered to the appearance of the material in consciousness, as a consequence of which it may be held in the unconscious; the patient gives an indirect clue by remaining silent on the topic in question. Or the material may be projected upon the physician, then appearing as something undesirable allegedly possessed by the physician. The repressed material may return to consciousness in one of the many known forms, but it is only when it constitutes a conflict between the patient and the physician that it is known as transference resistance. The resistance gives rise to negative transference, an animosity or opposition to the physician. See *resistance, ego.*

transference, sibling Attitudes and feelings similar to those a patient has heretofore entertained toward the siblings of the family and now has toward other members of the group.

transformation See *affect, transformation of in dreams.*

transformation, affective "There is a psychological law of 'affective transformation,' which says that emotionally toned and affectively emphasized values constantly strive to increase their dimensions. . . . This inclination to transformation on the part of the affects seems to play a very important role in primitive man. In drawings by children and primitives, the parts which are affectively toned are much enlarged." (Storch, A. *The Primitive Archaic Forms in Schizophrenia*, 1924) Affective transformation may be observed in all forms of psychiatric conditions; it is particularly noticeable in schizophrenia.

transformation of affect See *affect, transformation of in dreams.*

transfusion, exchange Total replacement of blood by transfusion. See *icterus gravis neonatorum.*

transient Lasting for a short period of time, quickly passing through, time-limited. The differences between transient, transitory, time-limited, short-term, etc., are more a matter of usage than of precise definition, and different groups employ the terms in different ways. In descriptions of sleep disorders, for example, transient insomnia indicates DIMS (disorder of initiating and maintaining sleep) of one to several days, whereas *short-term* insomnia indicates DIMS of up to three weeks, and *persistent* insomnia indicates a duration of at least two months and usually of many months or years.

transient situational disturbances In the 1968 revision of psychiatric nomenclature (DSM-II), adjustment reactions of acute symptom formation to an overwhelming situation; crisis reaction. Recession of symptoms occurs when the stress stimulus diminishes or disappears; persistence of symptoms indicates a more severe underlying disturbance. Included in the group are adjustment reactions of (1) infancy; (2) childhood; (3) adolescence; (4) adult life; (5) late life. See *adjustment disorders.*

transinstitutionalization Moving people or populations from one segment or sector to another, used particularly in regard to "depopulation" of state mental hospitals and "deinstitutionalization," where follow-up studies suggested that the criminal justice system had often been substituted for the mental health system. What seemed to be an advance in care of the chronically mentally ill seemed to be no more than a statistical ploy: patients were put into jails and prisons for disturbing the peace, rather than into the medical facilities they needed, but because they had been shifted out of the health care system they no longer appeared on the rolls of that system. See *chronic mentally ill.*

transitional object See *object, transitional.*

transitivism (tran'si-ti-viz'm) One of the accessory or secondary changes in the person of the schizophrenic, consisting of detachment of a part of the personality from the patient with subsequent displacement of this part onto another person. In such cases, whatever the patient hallucinates or does is believed to be an experience of that other person.

transitivity The character of passing over into something, a term applied principally to patients with schizophrenia. "Transitivistic manifestations are nowhere so frequent as in schizophrenia. Very commonly, patients are convinced that those about them also hear their voices, sometimes even that they undergo the physical persecutions with them. A patient has holes in her hands and maintains that the nurse also has holes in her hands." (Bleuler, *TP*)

transketolase A thiamine-dependent enzyme of central nervous system cells that has been reported to be deficient in Korsakoff psychosis.

translocation A chromosomal abnormality in which part or all of one member of a chromosome pair, instead of maintaining its proper position and joining with its counterpart from the other gamete in fertilization, drifts or migrates to another chromosome pair. In some cases of Down's syndrome, for example, the defect is due to translocation of the long arm of an extra chromosome 21 to chromosome 15; the resulting chromosome is called a 15/21 translocation chromosome.

transmethylation A biochemical step in which one or more methyl groups are added to the structure of a compound. The *transmethylation hypothesis*, based on the observation that one of the major differences between naturally occurring amines (e.g. indoles, such as tryptamine and serotonin, or phenethylamines, such as dopamine and norepinephrine) and hallucinogenic indoles or phenethylamines is the increased number of methyl (CH_3) groups in the latter compounds, suggests that an alteration in the biochemical transmethylation of naturally occurring amines might result in the endogenous synthesis of methylated amines that function as hallucinogens and produce some of the symptoms of schizophrenia.

transmissible Can be transmitted; formerly used synonymously with *inheritable*.

transmission Practically synonymous with *inheritance* (q.v.).

transmission, vertical Transplacental infection, as contrasted with *horizontal* (host-to-host) *transmission*.

transmitter See *neurotransmitter*.

transpersonal psychology An extension of the field of psychology to include the study of optimal psychological health and well-being. It recognizes the potential for experiencing a broad range of states of consciousness, in some of which identity may extend beyond the usual limits of the ego and personality. Transpersonal psychotherapy adds to traditional areas and concerns an interest in facilitating growth and awareness beyond traditionally recognized limits of health. The importance of modifying consciousness and the validity of transcendental experience and identity are affirmed. (Walsh, R., & Vaughan, F. *Beyond Ego: Transpersonal Dimensions in Psychology*, 1980)

Transpersonal psychology is distinguished from religion and theology by its basis in empirical, scientific study of the experiences that people actually have. Topics of particular interest include ultimate values, unitive consciousness, peak experiences, ecstasy, mystical experience, self-actualization, essence, bliss, wonder, ultimate meaning, transcendence of the self, oneness, cosmic awareness, individual and species-wide synergy, maximal interpersonal encounter, cosmic self-humor and playfulness, maximal sensory awareness, responsiveness, and expression.

transplantation Removal from one place to another; most commonly used to refer to removal of a body organ from a donor to a recipient. Also used to refer to transfer of a person from familiar to alien surroundings (as in admission of an elderly person to a nursing home). The concomitant anxiety, depression, or other manifestations of distress are sometimes termed transplantation shock.

transposition of affect See *affect, transposition of*.

transposon A naturally occurring genetic element that specifically inserts itself at various points in recipient genetic material and thereby controls the synthesis of specific nucleotide sequences.

transsexualism The condition in which the gender role and sexual identity of the subject are of the sex opposite to the subject's anatomic sex, usually with an overwhelming feeling of "being in the wrong body" and a desire for a sex conversion operation (*sex reassignment*). The desire for sex change starts early in life, from which time the male transsexual behaves, phantasizes, and talks as if he were a girl. The male transsexual does not prize his penis nor does he consider it primarily an organ for the expression of erotic desire; the few transsexuals who do experience orgasm typically phantasize that the sensations are being felt in an imagined vagina. Transsexualism has also been termed eonism, psychic hermaphroditism, metatropism, and severe intersexuality. See *transvestitism*.

Origin of the condition is unknown. Some authorities emphasize the symbiotic relationship with a mother whose own sexual identity is confused; others hypothesize that constitutional and endocrinologic factors, such as abnormal development of the hypothalamus during gestation, might be responsible.

In DSM-III-R, *nontranssexual cross-gender disorder* refers to similar discomfort with and feelings of inappropriateness about one's assigned sex, with recurrent cross-dressing or phantasies about cross-dressing but lacking the preoccupation with sex reassignment.

transvestitism *Transvestic fetishism* (in DSM-III-R); transvestism; *cross-dressing;* a type of sexual deviation characterized behaviorally by donning garments of the opposite sex. As R.J. Stoller (*Archives of General Psychiatry 24,* 1971) points out, cross-dressing by itself is a symptom, not a syndrome or diagnostic entity, and it may be manifested in several different ways.

1. *Fetishistic cross-dressing*—limited to males, who consider themselves to be heterosexual, whose behavior and appearance when not cross-dressing are masculine rather than feminine; such men derive genital excitement by donning women's clothes, and the excitement usually leads to masturbation and orgasm. See *girl, phallus*.

2. *Transsexualism*—the patient's cross-dressing is not a means to induce genital excitement, but only one of the means used to transform himself into the opposite sex, and to deny his own masculinity. The transsexual has no interest in his penis as an executive organ of erotic desire, and far from wanting to preserve his penis the transsexual from his early years has a strong desire for transformation anatomically into a female. In some, the desire is so strong that they seek castration (*castrophilia*) or prefer suicide to living as a man.

3. *Effeminate homosexuality*—the overt homosexual may put on women's clothes as part of a performance or act in which he both identifies with women and mocks them through mimicry and caricature; the wearing of women's clothes is not in itself sexually exciting, however.

Transsylvania effect Correlation of abnormal behavior with moon phases (and thus the term "lunacy'). Despite the frequent and persistent belief that such a correlation exists, there is little evidence to support the notion.

trauma Injury, damage, wound, shock. As originally described, psychic trauma referred to a sudden intense surge of anxiety, secondary to some external event, that exceeds the subject's ability to cope and to defend. The concept was subsequently extended to include overwhelming anxiety related to intrapsychic events, then to include later intrapsychic elaboration of external events that had originally seemed benign (as when cognitive development allowed a different interpretation or clearer understanding of the significance of an earlier event, or when psychosexual development rendered the subject susceptible or reactive to an event to which he or she had earlier been unresponsive), then to a summation or accumulation over time of events that individually had been inadequate to provoke overwhelming excitation. *Screen trauma* referred to a memory occurring after a trauma that concealed and stood for a deeply repressed memory of a traumatic experience; *constructive trauma* suggested that at least some traumata might benefit the child and constitute a positive learning experience.

Because such diffusion and overexten-sion of meanings threatened to reduce or even negate the usefulness of the term, the tendency since the 1970s has been to return to the original and more restricted meaning. See *adjustment disorders; anxiety disorders; neurosis, traumatic.*

trauma, birth The trauma of birth is a topic extensively considered in psychiatry, particularly by psychoanalysts. The concept is described comprehensively by Otto Rank, who maintains that the circumstances of birth are deeply imprinted upon the psyche of the infant and often reappear in symbolic form in psychiatric patients.

It is said that intrauterine existence is blissful, free from all conflicts of a psychical nature. The act of being born is believed to mark a radical upheaval from both the psychical and physical points of view; it produces a psychic shock of great consequence, a trauma with which the person is never reconciled. Rank holds that certain people are always attempting to reconstruct the conditions of intrauterine existence. In its most vivid and literal form intrauterine life is reproduced by the patient showing the catatonic form of schizophrenia.

Freud says: "The act of birth, moreover, is the first experience attended by anxiety, and is thus the source and model of the affect of anxiety." (*BW*) He believes that Rank overestimates the importance of birth upon the psyche of the infant. Freud says that "we certainly may not presuppose that the fetus has any kind of knowledge that it is in danger of annihilation"; the fetus can only sense "a wholesale disturbance in the economy of its narcistic libido."

As an example of the symbolic representation of the birth act Rank refers to the phobia concerning animals entering and leaving holes.

Ferenczi states: "The more I observe, the more I realize that none of the developments and changes which life brings finds the individual so well prepared as for birth." (*FCT*) He believes that birth is an agreeable and triumphant transition for the infant. What Rank calls birth phantasies Ferenczi says are coital phantasies.

Referring to the analysis of a dream, Jones says: "Emergence, after great difficulty, from a dark chamber containing water, is a very usual way for unconscious thoughts about the birth act to be expressed. . . . In mythology the situation is often reversed by the hero being placed in an enclosing chamber and put *into*, or *onto*, water, such as with Moses in the bulrushes, Noah in the Ark, and so on." (*Papers on Psycho-Analysis*, 1938)

trauma, head See *compression, cerebral; concussion; contusion, brain.*

trauma, infantile The occurrence in infancy or childhood of a situation in which the psyche is bombarded by stimulation of such intensity that it cannot be mastered or discharged. In such situations, anxiety develops automatically.

trauma, primal The original, supremely important, and most painful situation to which the person has been exposed early in life. Such a basic situation is necessarily of paramount importance and often constitutes the nucleus of the neurosis.

trauma, puberty The painful, disagreeable, or unacceptable experiences that occur during puberty. Acording to Stekel, such traumatic experiences during puberty are as important for the development of neurosis as the traumas suffered in childhood (see *trauma, infantile*), especially among girls, whose unpleasant sexual experiences can have fateful effects in their later lives. (Stekel, *ID*) See *trauma, primal.*

traumasthenia Nervous exhaustion following an injury; traumatic neurasthenia. See *neurosis, traumatic.*

traumatic defect state See *neurosis, traumatic; psychosis, traumatic.*

traumatic neurosis Post-traumatic stress disorder (q.v.).

traumatization See *libido, traumatization of the.*

traumatophilia Love of injury or the unconscious desire to be injured. See *diathesis, traumatophilic.*

traumatophobia Fear of injury.

treatment Any measure designed to ameliorate or cure an abnormal or undesirable condition.

For specific treatments, see also listings under *therapy.*

treatment, ambulatory Therapeutic measures carried out while the patient is up and about or is not hospitalized.

treatment, ambulatory insulin A modification of insulin coma treatment consisting of intramuscular injection of relatively

small doses of insulin, until hypoglycemia is reached. It has been observed that such subcoma treatment often relieves severe anxiety, tension, and anorexia; the mechanism of action is unknown. Also called *subshock* or *subcoma insulin treatment.*

treatment, continuous sleep A symptomatic method of treatment in which the patient is sedated with any of a variety of drugs; the aim of treatment is to provide 20 hours of sleep per day, for periods up to 3 weeks in more agitated patients. Klaesi, in 1922, introduced continuous sleep treatment with barbiturates. The method has been superseded in large part by insulin coma, ambulatory insulin, electroconvulsive therapy, and treatment with the tranquilizing drugs; its chief uses at the present time are in manic excitements, agitated depressions, and acute anxiety neuroses.

treatment, forced See *forced treatment.*

treatment, insuiin A form of treatment introduced into psychiatry by Sakel and used in certain psychiatric conditions. It consists of the production of coma, with or without convulsions, through the intramuscular administration of insulin.

treatment, malarial A form of treatment introduced by Wagner-Jauregg for syphilis of the central nervous system, especially general paralysis; blood containing tertian or quartan malaria parasites is injected into the patient, as a result of which he develops malarial fever.

treatment, Metrazol A form of treatment, introduced by von Meduna in 1934 in certain psychiatric conditions. It consists of the production of coma with or without convulsions, through the intravenous administration of Metrazol (cardiazol).

treatment, milieu Treatment effected through the medium of the patient's surroundings and immediate environment, and specifically through the medium of the psychiatric hospital. See *community, therapeutic; therapy, milieu.*

treatment, prolonged sleep See *treatment, continuous sleep.*

treatment, psychiatric social The supervision of the patient in the community in such a way as to bring about a better social adjustment for him. In some cases all that is possible may be the modification of the environment so that a fairly satisfactory social adaptation may be made for him in

spite of his mental handicap. Wherever the outlook for improvement is at all favorable, however, the aim of both the social and psychiatric treatment is to bring about a change in the attitude of the patient himself, to replace undesirable mental habits by wholesome ones, to modify his conduct by a training of his emotions, and to give him insight into his difficulties, so that he may eventually overcome his disabilities and be able to make a satisfactory adjustment in any environment.

treatment, psychoprophylactic Mental hygiene.

treatment, shock A form of treating certain psychotic conditions by inducing coma (or convulsions) usually by electrical or chemical means, such as Metrazol, insulin, camphor. See *therapy, shock.*

treatment, subcoma insulin See *treatment, ambulatory insulin.*

treble safeguard, principle of See *principle, treble safeguard.*

tremophobia Fear of trembling.

tremor Shaking or trembling; *hyperponesis.* A disorder of muscular tone in which the usual, normal unappreciable tonic contractions of a muscle become exaggerated to the point of awareness.

In general, tremors can be classified into:

1. Coarse tremors, usually indicative of organic disease; included are—

a. *passive tremor* or *rest tremor,* a tremor that occurs while the affected area is at rest, as the pill-rolling tremor of parkinsonism;

b. *action tremor* or *intention tremor,* which may be absent while the affected area is at rest and which is exaggerated by voluntary movement of the area, as the intention tremor of multiple sclerosis;

2. Fine tremors, often psychogenic although they may also be on a toxic basis (alcoholism, drug poisoning, hyperthyroidism, etc.);

3. *Fasciculation,* involuntary twitchings of a portion of a muscle; seen in fatigue, also in brain stem or anterior horn cell damage.

tremor, flapping *Asterixis* (q.v.). Rapid burst of flexion and extension in the wrist and metacarpophalangeal joints similar to the flapping of a bird's wings; such a tremor is indicative of hepatic failure.

tremor, hovering
kinson's disease t
full-blown conditi
consisting of a fin
and fingers with 3
pears when the subj
without resting his
temple.

trend, death See *suicide.*

trend, malignant The pr
nents that ordinarily poi

trend, pernicious *Trend, m*

trend, statistical Uniform
direction as shown by su
long period of time natu
phenomena tend to increa
in a regular manner.

TRH Protirelin, or thyroid-r
mone, which normally ind
(thyroid-stimulating hormon
that may be blunted or inadequ
types of depression.

triad, anal The group of three
outstanding traits of the so-ca
character: (1) obstinacy; (2) parsin
pedantic orderliness. In every
guage the connection between mi
and the retention of stool, both ha
common the tendency to hold on to
thing, or holding something back, is
clearly manifested. The folk saying
so tight he couldn't pass a raspberry se
is an example of this. (Sterba, R. *Intro*
tion to the Psychoanalytic Theory of the Lil
1942) See *phase, anal.*

triad, Charcot (Jean Martin Charcot, Fren
neurologist, 1825–93) See *sclerosis, multipl*

triad, interdependent See *psychotherapy*
family.

triad, oral Lewin's term for the desires of the
infant in the early oral phase—the wish to
devour, the wish to be devoured, and the
wish to go to sleep.

triad, Robin See *syndrome, Pierre Robin.*

triad, Sandler's See *Sandler's triad.*

triage (trē-àzh′, trī′àj) The process of choosing, selecting, sorting, or weeding out; in medicine, the immediate sorting out and classification of medical casualties (as in disasters and crises) so that patients may be routed to and referred to appropriate treatment services.

trial, clinical A prospective study involving human subjects designed to provide evaluation of preventive, diagnostic, or thera-

ic practice, such as the use of a certain ?, medical device, or procedure.

randomized See *randomized clinical*

ulation See *scapegoating*.

e (trib'ad) A woman with an abnor-lly large clitoris, who plays the part of a le in homosexual practices. See *lesbian-;*; *sapphism*.

alin The molecule in normal human rine believed to be both an inhibitor of onoamine oxidase receptor binding and n inhibitor of benzodiazepine receptor inding.

chologia *Carphology* (q.v.).

chopathophobia Fear of hair.

chophagy (tri-kof'ă-jē) The tic of biting the hair.

ichophobia *Trichopathophobia* (q.v.).

ichotillomania *Hair pulling* (q.v.); in DSM-III-R classified as an impulse control disorder.

rifacial neuralgia See *tic douloureux.*

trigeminal cerebral angiomatosis See *angiomatosis, trigeminal cerebral.*

trigeminal neuralgia See *tic douloureux.*

trihybrid Hybrid that differs in three hereditary characters. See *hybrid.*

triolist In a triangular sex relationship the person whose opposite-sex partner has a same-sex partner; the triolist typically derives as much sexual satisfaction from watching the other two indulge in homosexual activity as from engaging in heterosexual activity with either or both of them. Example: Alice has sex with Ted, whose male lover is Gordon; much as she enjoys intercourse with Ted, she finds even more satisfaction in watching Ted and Gordon having sex together.

triplet One of three children born at the same birth. See *birth, multiple.*

trisexuality The symbolic representation, especially in dreams, of the three currents or aspects—man, woman, and child—in which sexuality may be studied in a psychoanalytical sense. In other words, trisexuality may be considered as a kind of tripartition of the mind by which the subject may have at the same time the impulses of the three trends of sexuality. The patient will have simultaneously the desire to be a man, a woman, and a child, playing, at least symbolically, the three roles. (Stekel, *ID*)

triskaidekaphobia Morbid fear of (the number) thirteen. Thirteen at table is viewed by many as an ill omen, and one more person is usually invited to join in the meal. The thirteenth day of the month is looked upon with dismay by those swayed by the superstition and, if it falls on a Friday, with double dismay—for Friday, long referred to as "hangman's day," was the usual day for hanging a criminal in the England of old. To prevent the possible loss of such fearsome clients (who would not live in a house No. 13) many office buildings, and particularly hotels, have no thirteenth floor or rooms No. 13, or multifigured numbers ending with 13. Apparently the "baker's dozen" (adding one roll for good measure, to avoid the severe penalties for short-counting) is an exception to this common fear of thirteen.

trisomy A type of chromosomal abnormality in which three chromosomes appear in a position that normally is occupied by a chromosome pair. The most important known trisomy in psychiatry is 21-trisomy, or *Down's syndrome.* See *chromosome; syndrome, Down's.*

tristemania *Obs.* Melancholia.

tristitia (trē-stē'tē-ă) *Obs.* Melancholy.

tromomania *Obs.* Delirium tremens.

trophicity, neural The concept, emphasized particularly by Russian neurophysiologists, that is an outgrowth of Pavlov's views of trophic functions of the nervous system. Pavlov believed the nervous impulses arising from one group of neurons do not only stimulate other neurons but also act upon the entire trophicity of those neurons: oxygen and nutrient supply, and assimilation and metabolism of these substances within those cells.

trophodermatoneurosis *Acrodynia* (q.v.).

trophoneurosis A nutritive disturbance, organically determined. It is believed that each organ of the body is supplied with nerves whose functions are definitely identified with nutrition or trophism. When such nerves are disordered, nutrition of the organ suffers.

trophotropic See *ergotropic.*

-trophy (-trō-fē) Combining form meaning nutritive, from Gr. *trophē,* nourishment, food.

tropism *Taxis* (q.v.).

-tropy (-trō-pē) Combining form meaning turn(ing), from Gr. *trope.*

trust, basic See *relatedness.*

trust vs. mistrust One of Erikson's eight stages of man. See *ontogeny, psychic.*

truth serum See *narcotherapy.*

TTR Type token ratio. See *ratio, type token.*

TSD *Tay-Sachs disease* (q.v.).

TSH Thyroid-stimulating hormone; see *TRH.*

tube, neural See *cephalogenesis.*

tubectomy See *salpingectomy.*

tuberculomania An unfounded but unalterable conviction that one is suffering from tuberculosis; phthisiomania.

tuberculophobia Fear of tuberculosis or of associating in any way with a sufferer from that disease; phthisiophobia.

tuberous sclerosis See *sclerosis, tuberous.*

Tuke, Daniel Hack (1827–95) British psychiatrist; editor of *Dictionary of Psychological Medicine.*

tumescence Swelling, engorgement; used particularly to refer to the swelling of genital tissues associated with sexual excitement.

tumescence, penile Erection of the penis. *Nocturnal penile tumescence (NPT)* is associated with over 90% of REM sleep episodes and is thus a useful aid in differentiating between psychogenic impotence (where NPT is ordinarily preserved) and impotence due to organic impairment (where NPT is typically reduced or absent). Before the use of comprehensive polysomnographic studies of various physiologic processes, almost 90% of cases of male impotence were believed to be psychogenic in nature. Now that physiologic studies can be performed it is realized that approximately 65% of patients are organically impaired.

tumor, intracranial Any localized intracranial lesion, whether of neoplastic or of chronic inflammatory origin, which by occupying space within the skull tends to cause a rise in intracranial pressure. According to W.R. Brain (*DNS*): "Over 1 percent of all deaths are due to intracranial tumors which form about 17 per cent of all malignant neoplasms in man."

Primary brain tumors account for approximately 10% of nontraumatic neurologic disease. Even more frequent are metastatic cerebral neoplasms, secondary to tumors of the lung, breast, stomach, thyroid, or kidney.

Gliomas, the most common primary brain tumors, include (1) astrocytomas, which arise in both cerebral and cerebellar tissue, at any age; (2) glioblastoma multiforme, a highly malignant tumor of the cerebral hemispheres which appears in middle age; (3) medulloblastoma, a rapidly growing tumor most often of the cerebellum, and frequently in children; and (4) oligodendrogliomas and ependymomas, rare and slowly growing.

Meningiomas are extracerebral tumors of the meninges which often invade the overlying bone of the skull. Other brain tumors are angioblastomas and angiomas (which arise from the cerebral blood vessels); chromophil and chromophobe adenomas and craniopharyngioma (all from the pituitary); pineal tumors; colloid cysts from the choroid plexus of the third ventricle; and acoustic neuroma, from the eighth cranial nerve.

Symptoms of intracranial tumors are of two types: general symptoms, due to increased intracranial pressure, and focal symptoms, due to the local effects of the growth. The general symptoms of increased intracranial pressure include the classical triad of headache, papilledema, and vomiting. Other general symptoms are epileptiform convulsions, aphasia, vertigo, disturbances of pulse rate and blood pressure, and mental symptoms such as coma, confusion, disorientation, and progressive dementia.

tumultus sermonis *Obs.* Tumultuous speech.

turbid Muddled, mentally confused. "Naturally we often observe very mild twilight states and deliria, in which the thought process is only more or less unclear. These mild forms together with deliria and twilight states may provisionally be called *turbid states.*" (Bleuler, *TP*)

Turkish-bath method See *method, Turkish-bath.*

turmoil, adolescent An inexact term describing what some observers believed to be an expected, normal phase of adolescence, consisting of rebelliousness, concern about identity and role, instability of mood, and changeable and unpredictable behavior. Studies of nonpatient adolescents do not support this concept of significant disruption in psychological equilibrium as being a typical phase of normal adolescence.

Turner's syndrome A chromosomal abnormality characterized by 45 chromosomes, rather than the usual number of 46; it is presumed that a Y chromosome is lacking. Symptoms and signs include retardation in physical growth, ovarian dysgenesis, and phenotypically the appearance of mainly female sex characteristics even though the sex chromatin test is negative (XO).

turpitude, moral Sexual misconduct or other kinds of misbehavior on the part of the physician toward his patient, such as alcoholism or dishonesty.

turrecephaly *Oxycephaly* (q.v.).

TVD Transmissible virus dementia. See *virus infections.*

twilight state Absence, a transitory disturbance of consciousness during which many acts, sometimes very complicated, may be performed without the subject's conscious volition and without retaining any remembrance of them.

Responsive as a rule only to some given complex, the subject acts in accordance with the demands of the complex, the rest of the personality being subordinated to or, as a rule, more or less completely submerged during the period of the twilight state. For example, an epileptic patient, entirely unmindful of his natural surroundings, believed that he was walking around in Heaven; during the phase he was utterly unable to recall any part of his real life.

"During this period, if they [i.e. such patients] can be observed, they usually strike one as being abnormal; at times, however, they can use correctly ordinary means of intercourse, can associate with fellow travelers, and can even visit relatives, without betraying their condition." (Bleuler, *TP*) See *fugue.*

The term twilight state is also applied to one of the variations of delirium in which the patient passes abruptly into a state of severe clouding of consciousness combined with generally slow, monotonous movements but occasionally outbursts of rage and fear.

twilight state, alcoholic A type of pathological drunkenness, characterized by "sudden excitations or twilight states set free by alcohol, usually with mistaking of the situation, often also with illusions and hallucinations, and excessive affects, most of anxiety and rage. In individual cases the entire morbid process can transpire in hardly a minute, but it usually lasts longer, up to several hours." (Bleuler, *TP*) See *intoxication, alcoholic.*

twilight state, clear See *equivalent, epileptic.*

twilight state, postepileptic Sometimes after an epileptic attack, a so-called twilight state exists for a variable period of time. During the twilight state the patient may carry out acts for which he is later amnesic.

twin One of two organisms born from a female that ordinarily brings forth only one offspring at a time.

In human beings there are two distinct types of twins, the *monozygotic* or *identical* twins, developed from a single egg, and the *dizygotic* or *fraternal* twins, developed from two eggs. Dizygotic twins are held to be as separate in their origin and biological development as are siblings in general. Monozygotic twins are like the right and the left halves of *one* organism; accordingly, they not only have the same genotypical structure, but also exhibit frequently the phenomenon of *reversed asymmetry* (mirror-imaging) in handedness, hair whorl, dentition, palm patterns, and other asymmetrical characters, i.e. characters that are asymmetrical in one person. The presence of mirror-imaging is confirmatory evidence of monozygosity, but its absence does not refute it.

Of the two methods used for diagnosing twins with respect to their zygotic origin, the *similarity* method is now generally preferred to the *fetal-membrane* method, since it has been discovered that one-egg twins often have separate chorions and even separate placentae.

Twin studies are of great scientific significance in human genetics, because they throw light upon many fundamental aspects of the *nature-nurture* problem as well as of the *developmental* mechanism of the human organism throughout its life from the fertilization of the ovum to death. For these purposes a twin survey is usually based upon the particular technique of comparing the likenesses or differences between identical twins with the likenesses and differences between fraternal twins.

twin-study See *method, twin-study.*

twinned Born as a twin.

twinning The attribute of producing or state of being twins.

twins, Siamese (Chinese twins [Eng and Chang, born in Siam, 1811, died in North Carolina, 1874] whose bodies were joined by a band extending from umbilicus to the xiphoid cartilage) Among various kinds of freak twins, the variety of *Siamese twins* is characterized by an incomplete separation of the halves of the originally single embryo, from which the given set of monozygotic twins is developed. The division may be almost complete, so that the remaining link between the twins can be severed by operation, or it may be so incomplete as to result in twins with one body and two heads, or with one body and four legs and arms. See *birth, multiple.*

type See *type, constitutional.*

type A A behavior pattern characterized by anger, impatience, irritation, and aggravation. The personality syndrome was first formulated by cardiologists Meyer Friedman and Ray Rosenman, who in 1959 reported their finding that men with such a behavior pattern were seven times more likely than others to have evidence of heart disease and two to three times more likely than men with the more easygoing *type B* behavior to have heart attacks. Type A subjects are also at higher risk for accidents, suicide, and murder than are type B subjects.

Characteristics of type A behavior include a sense of urgency; competitiveness; easily aroused hostility and aggressivity, often manifested in obvious facial tension or muscular set; a ticlike drawing back of the corners of the mouth; a hostile, jarring laugh; an explosive, staccato speech pattern; frequent use of obscenities; periodic "bulging" of the eyes to show white above and below the pupils. The syndrome is often identified through a questionnaire, which discloses such behavior as often trying to do two things at once; walking fast, eating fast, and leaving the table immediately after eating; taking pride in always being on time, having difficulty sitting and doing nothing, and often being told by a spouse to slow down. He is a workaholic and a Don Juan of achievement. When speaking, he typically blinks or moves his eyes rapidly, jiggles a knee, taps his fingers, licks his lips, nods his head, and rapidly sucks in air. He hurries or interrupts the speech of others, sits on the edge of his chair as if poised to leap out of it, talks with his hands, pounds his fist for emphasis, and sighs deeply, especially when discussing an annoying or frustrating event. He moves rapidly and often trips over things, is annoyed if kept waiting, distrusts others' motives; even in games with children he plays to win and is ravenous for success and accomplishment. See *character, exploitative; choleric; type, hypercompensatory.*

Most studies suggest that type A behavior is only a secondary risk factor in cardiac disease, less important than the major risk factors such as smoking, high blood pressure, high blood cholesterol, and diabetes. Some investigators believe it more important than that, however; they report that type A behavior can be modified through counseling, and that the risk of heart attack is significantly lower in those whose type A characteristics are reduced or eliminated.

type, adenoid In constitutional medicine, a type in which the hypertrophy of the pharyngeal tonsil is believed to be a sign of serious general constitutional anomaly. The more marked cases of this type are associated with such degenerative states as oxycephaly, deaf-mutism, cretinism, status thymicus, and facial asymmetry.

type, apoplectic See *habitus apoplecticus.*

type, asthenic Within the system of constitutional types described by Kretschmer, this term designates the type characterized by the general impression of a deficiency in volume combined with an average unlessened length, so that the subject appears taller than he really is (see *type, constitutional*).

The head of the asthenic rises like a bud upon a lean, long neck. In profile, the curve of the head is interrupted by sharp irregularities. The nose is a prominent feature and juts out from the long face, thus throwing back the forehead and chin. The line connecting the upper forehead, tip of nose, and chin tends to be angular on account of this disproportion between the long, sharp nose and the small mandible. In frontal outline the face is of short egg form. The middle face is long in proportion to the rest and the upper lip is short. The primary hair is strongly developed and has a tendency to grow down the neck and into the face, producing a fur cap appearance. When baldness occurs, it has an irregular outline.

The chest of the asthenic is long, narrow, and flat. The upper ribs fall inward and the xiphoid angle is acute. The prominence given to the clavicle is accentuated by the stooping attitude characteristic of the asthenic. The cavity of the abdomen is poorly developed, while the limbs appear long and thin, with lean muscles. The hips in the male are usually wider than the chest measurement, accentuating the waist. The skin tends to be pale, dry, and cold with scant subjacent fat.

As a *psychological* type, the asthenic is thought to be basically *schizothyme* (q.v.), thus constituting the bulk of the schizothymic group, although the athletic and dysplastic types also contribute to it. According to Kretschmer's theories, the asthenics may fall into any one of the three divisions accepted by him: namely, the *healthy schizothymes* (polite, sensitive types; world-hostile idealists; cold-hearted egoists); the *schizoids* (the predominantly hyperesthetic temperaments including despotic or passionate types and unsteady loafers); and the *schizophrenics*.

When no attention is paid to particular modifications, it is appropriate to say that the asthenic type thus described corresponds fairly closely to the following types in other systems: the *habitus phthisicus* of Hippocrates, the *sensory, pneumatic, chlorotic, phthisic,* and *lymphatic* type with a disposition to tuberculosis of Rokitansky-Benecke, the *first combination* of De Giovanni, the *macroskelic* type of Viola, the *hypovegetative (dolichomorphic)* biotype of Pende, part of the *hypotonic* group of Tandler, the *asthenic habitus* of Bauer and Mills, the *narrow-chested* type of Brugsch, the *slender* biotype of Stockard, the *T type* of Jaensch, the *regressive* type of Lewis, the *ectomorphic* type of Sheldon, the *sthenoplastic* type of Bounak, and the *hyperontomorphic* type of Beau.

type, athletic Robust, strong, vigorous, sthenic, possessing a well-developed muscular system with resultant physical activity and prowess. Kretschmer's athletic type is characterized by a strong development of the locomotor apparatus, so that the bones and muscles stand out in plastic relief. The head shares in the overdevelopment of the skeleton, as is usually demonstrated by prognathous jaws and marked occipital protuberance. A line connecting the upper forehead, tip of nose, and chin forms a gentle curve. The frontal facial outline is steep egg-shaped. The head hair is abundant and tends to grow in a peak in the center of the forehead, receding in a baylike manner on either side toward the temples.

The neck is strong and the shoulders are large. The trunk tapers down from the broad shoulder girdle, so that the trunk outline from the front appears inverted trapezoid. The limbs are relatively long, the hands and feet are large, and the fingers are often blunt, thick, and acromegaloid in character. The skin is thick, of good turgor, moderately tinted, and medium as to sweat secretion.

As a psychological type, the athletics, too, are assumed by Kretschmer to be basically *schizothymic,* like the asthenics and the majority of the dysplastics. According to his theories, they constitute a considerable proportion of the total group of schizothyme, although a decidedly smaller one than do the asthenics, and they may also fall into any one of his three divisions of the schizothymes group, that is, the healthy schizothymes, the schizoids, and the schizophrenics (see *type, asthenic*).

The athletic type thus described corresponds approximately to the following types in other systems: the *muscular* type of Rostan, the *second (plethoric) combination* of De Giovanni, the *normosplanchnic* type of Viola, the *hypertonic* type of Tandler, the *sthenic* type of Mills, the *medium* biotype of Davenport, the *normal* type of Aschner, the *mesoskelic* type of Pende, part of the *hypercompensatory* type of Lewis, and the *mesomorphic* type of Sheldon.

type, attitudinal One or the other of two types of introvert and extravert attitudes toward the world and oneself, in the Jungian system of psychology.

"The introvert turns in upon himself, is absorbed in his inner world, while the extravert turns outward to the world, and is much more concerned with what goes on there than with his own private experiences. Both of these types he [Jung] subdivides into thinking, feeling, intuition, and sensation types. That is, there may be a thinking introvert, a thinking extravert, a feeling introvert or extravert and so on." (Thompson, C. *Psychoanalysis: Evolution and Development,* 1950) Introversion and extraversion are *attitudinal types;* thinking, feeling, intuition, and sensation are *functional types.* Jung believes that—probably by constitutional determination—every person is a combination of one or the other attitudinal type plus one functional type of the four. "Whereas the functional type describes the way in which the empirical material is specifically grasped and formed, the attitudinal type introversion-extraversion characterizes the general psychological orientation, i.e. the direction of that general psychological energy which Jung conceives the libido to be. . . . The functional type to which he belongs would be in itself an index to a man's psychological character. It alone, however, would not suffice. In addition, his general psychological attitude, i.e. his way of reacting to what meets him from without or within, must be determined. Jung distinguishes two such attitudes: extraversion and introversion. They represent orientations that essentially condition all psychic process—the reaction habitus, namely, through which one's way of behaving, of subjectively experiencing, and even of compensating through the unconscious is given." (Jacobi, J. *The Psychology of C.G. Jung,* 1942)

type B See *type A.*

type, B See *imagery, eidetic.*

type, belief Ferenczi holds that there are two fundamental types of personality from the standpoint of belief. There are those who have a tendency to "blind beliefs"; they accept statements without any question. He believes the tendency is derived at the time when the child is disillusioned about his own omnipotence upon others, originally upon his parents, later upon anyone in authority. There is the second type, constituting "blind disbelief"; it is said also to stem from associations with the parents. It is a phase of disillusionment in the power of the parents or other superior people.

type, broad See *type, pyknic.*

type, C See *type, M.*

type, cerebral In the system of constitutional types described by Rostan and Sigaud, this type is distinguished from the *muscular, digestive,* and *respiratory* types (qq.v.) by a predominance of the brain and nervous system over the other body systems. See *type, asthenic.*

type, choleric In constitutional medicine, this is one of the four classical temperamental and constitutional types of antiquity. Galen attributed the irritability of this type to the predominance of the yellow bile over the other three humors (or fluids) of the human organism. See *type, pyknic.*

type, constitutional The constellations of traits, morphological, physiological, and psychological, that are assumed to be associated with tendencies to certain diseases, physical and mental. Often used in a wider sense to include types of body and mind, even where no relations to any particular tendency to disease is postulated. See *constitution.*

The first typological system was developed by Hippocrates, who described a tendency to apoplexy, the *habitus apoplecticus* (q.v.), in persons of thick-set, rounded appearance, and a tendency to pulmonary tuberculosis, the *habitus phthisicus* (q.v.), in persons of slender, angular appearance. This dichotomizing system was extended by Galen to four human types that were related to the four fluids or humors assumed to form the basis of the body. The *sanguine* type was thought to owe his enthusiasm to the "strength of the blood," the *melancholic* type was said to be sad because of the overproduction of the "black bile," the *choleric* type was irritable owing to the predominance of the "yellow bile," and the *phlegmatic* type was sluggish because of the abundance of "phlegm." These four classical humors lived on as the explanation of temperamental and constitutional types for centuries, until Harvey's discovery of the circulation of the blood had the twofold effect of focusing attention on the blood as the important humor, and of emphasizing the role of the blood vessels. It was Haller who demonstrated the loose connection between the blood and the temperaments, and thereby paved the way for the modern typologists to describe their types in terms of anatomical systems instead of humors.

The discovery of the internal secretions and their effect on the morphology of body and mind led in all countries to a new humoral doctrine and thus to a classification of types on the basis of altered secretion of one of these glands. The prefixes *hyper-*, *hypo-*, and *dys-* were employed to indicate oversecretion, undersecretion, or qualitatively altered secretion. The main typological systems developed on the basis of these concepts were those of the modern French, Italian, German, and American typologists.

The ordinary system of the *French* school has consisted, from the time of Rostan (1828), of the *digestive, respiratory, cerebral,* and *muscular* types (qq.v.). Other types accepted by Rostan's successors are the *reproductive* and the *atonic* types, corresponding to the old hypergenital and lymphatic types, and also the *round* and the *flat* types, explained by MacAuliffe in terms of colloidal chemistry.

The system of the *Italian* school dates from the work of De Giovanni (about 1890), who formulated the *law of underdeformation* and described three types of body build: the *first combination* or phthisic type, the *second combination* or plethoric type, and the *third combination*. Other tritypal classifications are based either on the form of the viscera, distinguishing *microsplanchnic, megalosplanchnic,* and *normosplanchnic* types (Viola), or on the total external characteristics, distinguishing *dolichomorphic, brachymorphic,* and *eumorphic* types. Pende modified this system by distinguishing a *hypervegetative* and a *hypovegetative* biotype, in addition to a number of *dysplastic* types.

The typological work of the modern *German* school was initiated by the phrenologist Gall at the end of the 18th century and continued by Beneke (*asthenic* or *hypoplastic* type, *apoplectic* or *hyperplastic* type, *normal* type); Carus (*athletic, phlegmatic, phthisic, cerebral, sterile* constitutions); Bauer (*status degenerativus, arthritic habitus, asthenic* type); and by E.R. and W. Jaensch (*integrated* and *disintegrated* types). In the field of psychiatry, the typological system of Kretschmer has certainly become the most

influential one (*pyknic, asthenic, athletic,* and *dysplastic* types on the physical side: and *cyclothymic* and *schizothymic* temperaments).

In the modern *American* school, the most systematic and effective work has been done by Draper (*panels of personality*), Davenport (*fleshy, slender,* and *medium* biotypes), Stockard (*lateral* and *linear* types), Lewis (*regressive, hypercompensatory,* and *normally compensating* types), and Sheldon (*ectomorphic, mesomorphic,* and *endomorphic* types).

Well-known *English* typologists are E. Miller, Spearman, and Cohen, and in the modern *Dutch* school Hymans and Wiersma are the outstanding workers.

type, degenerative See *status degenerativus.*

type, delicate See *type, cerebral.*

type, digestive In the system of constitutional types described by Rostan and Sigaud, this term is distinguished from the *muscular, respiratory,* and *cerebral* types by a predominance of the alimentary system of the body over the other systems. Persons of this type correspond to Kretschmer's *pyknic* type. See *type, pyknic.*

type, disintegrated In the system of constitutional types described by E.R. and W. Jaensch, this term refers to persons with a *disintegrated* psychological state, which is indicated by the *T type* of *eidetic imagery* and is further associated with particular physiological, biochemical, and clinical characteristics. See *imagery, eidetic.*

type, dysplastic In Kretschmer's system of constitutional types a form of physique that varies markedly from the average form of one of the main types called *asthenic, pyknic,* and *athletic* (qq.v.). Most dysplastic subjects are said to fall either into the category of elongated *eunuchoidism* with tower skull and, in the female, with masculinism, or into the groups of polyglandular *fat abnormalities* and *infantilism;* their psychological makeup is held by Kretschmer to be basically *schizothymic* (q.v.).

The anomalies of the dysplastic type seem to be comparable to the *sterile, atrophic constitutions* described by Carus and to Bauer's *status degenerativus* (q.v.).

type, eidetic Constitutional type characterized by a particular kind of *eidetic imagery* and by associated differences in other psychological qualities as well as in certain physiological, biochemical, and clinical features. There are two eidetic types, the *integrated* and the *disintegrated*. See *imagery, eidetic.*

type, extraverted When "the state of extraversion becomes habitual," Jung speaks of the person as possessing the extraverted type of personality. When introversion is habitual, the personality is of the introverted type.

"Thus in both *general attitude* groups (the *extravert* and *introvert*) individuals with regard to *function* (i.e., reaction to a stimulus or event) may be either (1) *rational* (a) thinking, (b) feeling, or (2) *irrational* (c) intuitive, or (d) sensational." (Jung, *PT*) See *type, general attitude.*

type, feeling The second of the four functional types of personality described by Jung. With his first (*thinking* type) it constitutes the *rational* class of *functional* types.

"When the total attitude of the individual is orientated by the function of feeling, we speak of a *feeling-type.*" (Jung, *PT*)

type, flaccid See *atonic.*

type, flat MacAuliffe's name for one of his two fundamental constitutional types evolved from considerations of colloidal chemistry. The flat type is believed to result from a slight craving of the tissues for water and is characterized by little surface tension, rapid metabolic processes, quick general reactions, economical energy expenditure, and, on the psychological side, by an inherent general sobriety. It is distinguished from the *round* type by its marked cellular irritability and should not be confused with the type of a merely thin person. See *type, round.*

type, fleshy See *type, pyknic.*

type, function Same as *type, functional* (q.v.).

type, functional Jung uses this term to designate personality types from the standpoint of function. He postulates four functional classes, viz., thinking, feeling, intuitive, and sensational. "In so far as such an attitude is *habitual,* thus lending a certain stamp to the character of the individual, I speak of a psychological type. These types, which are based upon the root-functions and which one can term the thinking, the feeling, the intuitive, and the sensational types, may be divided into two classes according to the quality of the respective basic function:

viz., the *rational* and the *irrational.* The thinking and feeling types belong to the former. The intuitive and sensational to the latter." (*PT*)

But since *functioning* presupposes a static state or general attitude as the basis for the functioning, any one of the four functional types may occur in either of the two *general attitude* groups—the *extravert* or the *introvert;* i.e. there are: (1) thinking, (2) feeling, (3) intuitive, (4) sensational *extraverts,* and *introverts,* or *eight* varieties of psychological types in all.

type, general attitude Jung's expression for the total mental cast or psychic makeup that statically determines a person's general attitude independently of or in advance of the external stimulus. This conception aggregates all human beings into two groups of *extraverts* and *introverts.* See *introvert; type, extraverted.*

With regard to the person's dynamic reaction to a life stimulus, Jung classifies all mankind into *functional types* (see *type, functional*) and also in two classes: (1) *rational* and (2) *irrational.*

type, heavy See *diathesis, arthritic.*

type, hyperaffective In the system of constitutional types described by Pende, a psychological type characterized by an abundance of emotional reactivity and roughly corresponding to the *cyclothymic* type.

type, hypercompensatory In the system of constitutional types described by Lewis, the type that on the physical side is characterized by *hyperplasia* of blood and lymph vessels, intestines, and ductless glands, and on the psychological side is inclined to *hypercompensatory* reactions taking the form of manic-depressive psychosis or paranoid reactions.

type, hypergenital In constitutional medicine, a type distinguished by Pende as a subgroup of the *dolichomorphic* type and, in general, corresponding roughly to the *reproductive* type of Rostan.

The *male* type is characterized not only by an exaggerated and premature development of primary, secondary, and tertiary sexual characteristics, but also by a dolichomorphic form of trunk with a noticeable excess of thorax over abdomen, relative shortness of the extremities, large skull and heart, marked development of the skeletal muscles, and definite parasympathicotonia, and, on the psychological side, by a calm, stable, and energetic character and a strong development of artistic impulses.

In addition to an exuberant and premature development of the sexual system, especially of the pelvis, the female type is characterized by early menarche, a tendency to leucorrhoea in the intermenstrual periods, exaggerated local sensitiveness of the genital organs and breasts, megalosplanchnic proportions, great fecundity, and a stature which is somewhat below the average. "When hypergenitalism is secondary or is combined with anomalies of the other endocrine glands, we observe as a rule marked dissociations in the sexual development or a tendency to assume the characteristics of the opposite sex. Thus, women with hyperpituitary or hyperadrenal constitutions may present masculine characteristics, homosexual inclinations and an exaggerated libido." (Pende, N. *Constitutional Inadequacies*, 1928)

type, hypertonic In the system of constitutional types described by Pende this term is used in connection with the *hypersthenic* type to designate a subgroup of both the *megalosplanchnic hypervegetative* constitution, where it stands in contrast to the *atonic* and *flaccid* subgroup, and of the *microsplanchnic hypovegetative* constitution, where it stands in contrast to the *atonic* and *hyposthenic* subgroup.

The term hypertonic is also used in the constitutional system of Tandler to indicate a type characterized by a high degree of tonus of the voluntary muscles. This corresponds roughly to Kretschmer's *athletic* type.

type, hypervegetative The hypervegetative biotype is contrasted with the hypovegetative biotype and corresponds exactly to the megalosplanchnic and brachymorphic types, and approximately to the equivalents of the pyknic type. See *hypovegetative.*

type, hypoaffective In Pende's system of constitutional types, a psychological type that in contrast to the *hyperaffective* type is characterized by a deficiency in emotional reactivity, corresponding roughly to the *schizothymic* type.

type, hypogenital The *primary* hypogenital type is usually called *eunuchoid* and is characterized by exaggerated length of the

lower extremities, a relatively hypoplastic state of trunk and head, and a deficient development of the genital organs and sexual characteristics. Various recent observations have suggested that this eunuchoid condition is inheritable as a sex-linked genetic factor. It seems to occur in women, too, although in a milder and less recognizable form.

In addition to the complete form of primary hypogenitalism, there is an attenuated type distinguished by Pende as the *hypogenital temperament.*

type, integrated In their system of constitutional types E.R. and W. Jaensch denote by this term subjects with an *integrated* psychological state, of which the *B type* of *eidetic imagery* is an indicator.

type, introverted See *extraversion; type, extraverted.*

type, intuitive The third of Jung's four functional types of personality. With his fourth (*sensational* type) it constitutes the *irrational* class of *functional types.*

One who "adapts himself by means of unconscious indications, which he receives through an especially fine and sharpened perception and interpretation of faintly conscious stimuli. How such a function appears is naturally hard to describe, on account of its irrational, and, so to speak, unconscious character." The intuitive type "raises unconscious perception to the level of a differentiated function, by which he also becomes adapted to the world." (Jung, *PT*)

type, irrational See *type, rational.*

type, lateral See *type, pyknic.*

type, linear See *type, asthenic.*

type, lymphatic In the system of Carus, this corresponds to the asthenic type (Kretschmer) and the habitus phthisicus (Hippocrates). See *type, asthenic.*

type, M Rorschach differentiated two types of personality on the basis of the ratio between human movement (*M*) responses and color (*C*) responses. In the M type, M responses are more numerous than C responses; in the C type, the reverse is true. The M type shows a more imaginative and discriminating intelligence, more stability of emotions, and a more awkward and clumsy motility than the C type. In a general way, the M type corresponds to the obsessional type in Reich's description of character types, while the C type corresponds to the hysterical character.

type, medium See *type, athletic.*

type, megalosplanchnic In Viola's system, this corresponds to *type, pyknic* (q.v.).

type, microsplanchnic In Viola's system, this corresponds to *type, asthenic* (q.v.).

type, muscular This type was first described in 1828 by Rostan of the French school. In contradistinction to the *digestive, respiratory,* and *cerebral* (qq.v.), this type is characterized by the predominance of the muscular and locomotor system over the other systems of the body and corresponds to Kretschmer's athletic type. See *type, athletic.*

type, normal See *type, athletic.*

type, normally compensating In the system of constitutional types described by Lewis, this type is intermediate between his *hypercompensatory* and *regressive* types (qq.v.) and is characterized by an average intermediate degree of development of the viscera and, on the psychological side, by its capacity for compensatory reactions that are moderate and reversible and therefore usually of a temporary nature.

type, normosplanchnic In Viola's system, this corresponds to *type, athletic* (q.v.).

Type I schizophrenia See *Crow Type I schizophrenia.*

type, organic reaction See *syndrome, organic.*

type, phlegmatic One of the four classical temperamental and constitutional types of antiquity. Galen attributed the torpor and apathy of this type to the predominance of the *phlegma* (mucus secreted in the air passages of the throat) over the other three humors (fluids) of the human body. See *type, pyknic.*

type, phthisic See *habitus phthisicus.*

type, plethoric See *type, athletic; type, pyknic.*

type, pneumatic See *type, asthenic.*

type, pyknic In Kretschmer's system of constitutional types, this is the type characterized by roundness of contour, amplitude of body cavities, and a plentiful endowment of fat.

The head of a pyknic is usually circular and smooth in profile, without any sharply prominent parts. The frontal facial outline is pentagonal or shield-shaped. The face is definitely broad and fleshy, particularly the nose. The neck is short and thick, with the head set a little forward on smoothly rounded shoulders. The line from the tip of the chin to the suprasternal notch is characteristic: it tends to be a smoothly sloping or even a straight line, but not an angle. The hairline borders the forehead in a regular, unindented curve. There is a tendency to baldness, the areas of which are regular in outline and have a smooth shiny surface.

The typically pyknic trunk is thick-set and barrel-shaped, with the chest broadening to the lower part of the body. The abdomen is protruding and the xiphoid angle is wide. The limbs are well developed in thickness rather than in length, and the lower extremities, while not actually short, tend to appear short relative to the rest of the body because of their massiveness. The feet are broad and well covered, while the hands are square or broad, with pudgy, fusiform fingers. The skin is warm and moist, with a well-developed fatty layer beneath it.

Pyknics may fall into any one of the three divisions of the *cyclothymes* as distinguished by Kretschmer: (1) the *healthy* cyclothymes (the gay chatterbox, the quiet humorist, the silent good-tempered man, the happy enjoyer of life, the energetic practical man); (2) the *cycloids* (the cheery hypomanic type, the quiet contented type, the melancholic type); and (3) the *manic-depressives.*

The pyknic type corresponds approximately to the following types in other leading systems: the *habitus apoplecticus* of Hippocrates, the *abdominal* and *digestive* types of the French school, the *phlegmatic, boeotic, plethoric venous, choleric* constitutions of Carus, the *hyperplastic* type with a disposition to carcinoma of Rokitansky-Benecke, the *third combination* of De Giovanni, the *brachyskelic (mikroskelic)* type of Manouvier, the *megalosplanchnic* of Viola, the *hypervegetative (brachymorphic)* biotype of Pende, the *arthritic habitus* of Bauer, part of the *hypotonic* group of Tandler, the *hypersthenic* type of Mills, the *wide-chested* type of Brugsch, the *fleshy* type of Davenport, the *mesontomorph* of Beau, the *lateral* type of Stockard, the *broad* type of Aschner, the *B* type of Jaensch, the *euryplastic* type of Bounak, the *endomorphic* type of Sheldon, and part of the *hypercompensatory* type of Lewis.

type, rational According to Jung there are four basic psychological types—the thinking, feeling, intuitive, and sensational. He calls the first two *rational* types "because they are characterized by the supremacy of the reasoning and the judging functions. It is a general distinguishing mark of both types that their life is, to a large extent, subordinate to reasoning judgement." The second two (intuitive, sensational) are termed *irrational* "because their commissions and omissions are based not upon reasoned judgment but upon the absolute intensity of perception. Their perception is concerned with simple happenings, where no selection has been exercised by the judgment." (Jung, *PT*)

type, reaction See *reaction type.*

type, regressive In the system of constitutional types described by Lewis, this type is characterized on the physical side by *hypoplasia* of blood and lymph vessels, intestines, and ductless glands and by its tendency to *tuberculosis.* Since on the psychological side this type is distinguished by its disposition to *schizophrenia,* the most severe of all regressive changes, persons of this type are comparable to the *asthenic* type in Kretschmer's system and its equivalents in other systems.

type, reproductive In Rostan's system of constitutional types this type was characterized by a predominance of the reproductive system over the other systems of the body. Although no major type of other systems is based on the degree of development of the reproductive system, this type of Rostan is comparable to the *hypergenital* type, which is a subgroup of the *dolichomorphic* type in the system of Pende, and may best be contrasted with the sterile *atrophic* constitution in the system of Carus.

type, respiratory In the system of Rostan and Sigaud, this type is distinguished from the *muscular, digestive,* and *cerebral* types by predominance of the circulatory and respiratory systems over the others. Many typologists classify such persons in the *asthenic* type, although they seem to be at the pole opposite to the asthenic with his flat, underdeveloped chest, hypoplastic blood vessels, and poorly expanding lungs. See *type, asthenic.*

type, reversal Abraham and Jones use this expression for persons with a tendency to act in a way contrary to normal. They may express contrary opinions, though they know them to be illogical; they may dress "out of style"; they may enumerate irrelevant items, etc.

type, round One of the two fundamental constitutional types evolved by MacAuliffe from considerations of colloidal chemistry. In contradistinction to the *flat type,* this type is characterized by an extremely *hydrophilic* tendency of the colloidal cells, great surface tension, increased osmotic pressure, and a considerable expenditure of energy with a corresponding dynamic sweep. See *type, flat.*

type, sanguine One of the four classical temperamental and constitutional types distinguished by Galen. He attributed the good humor and enthusiasm of this type to the predominance of the blood over the other three humors.

type, Séglas (sā-glå′) (Jules Séglas, French physician, 1856–1939) The so-called psychomotor type of paranoia.

type, sensational The last of Jung's four functional types.

"Sensation, or sensing, is that psychological function which transmits a physical stimulus to perception. It is, therefore, identical with perception. . . . Primarily sensation is a *sense-perception,* i.e. perception transmitted *via* the sense organs and 'bodily senses' (kinaesthetic, vasomotor, sensation, etc.)." Sensation "always predominates over thinking and feeling, though not necessarily over intuition." It is a conscious function or conscious perception.

The sensational type of person shows "little tendency either for reflection or commanding purpose. To sense the object, to have and if possible to enjoy sensations, is his constant motive. He is by no means unlovable; on the contrary, he frequently has a charming and lively capacity for enjoyment; he is sometimes a jolly fellow and often a refined aesthete." (Jung, *PT*)

type, sensory See *type, asthenic.*

type, slender See *type, asthenic.*

type, social The role which a person assumes and to which he is assigned by society. See *gender role.*

type, sthenic (sthen′ik) In constitutional medicine, this corresponds to Kretschmer's athletic type and its equivalents in other systems. See *type, athletic*.

In general psychology, the term sthenic indicates strength and vigor in different fields of emotional reactivity and adaptability. In accordance with this concept, the psychopathological behavior of the sthenic type has been described by Kretschmer as inclined to delusional reactions of a predominantly aggressive nature (paranoia, querulous ideas of reference), in contrast to the introspective tendency in paranoid or hypochondriac reactions in sensitive types.

type, T See *imagery, eidetic*.

type, Tartar See *syndrome, Down's*.

type, "the exceptions" A character type first described by Freud; such persons, because of early frustrations, arrogate unto themselves the right to demand lifelong reimbursement from fate. This behavior is intensified if they are required to contradict a deep inner doubt as to their right to compensation. See *entitlement*.

type, thinking The first of the four functional types of personality described by Jung. With Jung's second (*feeling* type) it constitutes the *rational* class of *functional* types.

"It is a fact of experience that all the basic psychological functions seldom or never have the same strength or grade of development in one and the same individual. As a rule, one or another function predominates, in both strength and development. When *supremacy* among the psychological functions is given to thinking, i.e., when the life of an individual is mainly ruled by reflective thinking so that every important action proceeds from intellectually considered motives, or when there is at least a tendency to conform to such motives, we may fairly call this a *thinking type*. Such a type can be either introverted or extraverted." (Jung, *PT*)

type token ratio See *ratio, type token*.

type, vital See *biotype*.

type, wide-chested See *type, pyknic*.

types, family See *family types*.

types, personality See *personality types*.

typhlomegaly (tif-lō-meg'á-lē) An unusually large size of the caecum. In Pende's system of constitutional types, this condition is frequently characteristic of the *ptotic habitus*.

typholexia, congenital (tēf-ō-lek'sē-à) A term used by Variot and Lecomte (1906) to refer to a type of *reading disability* (q.v.).

typical Pertaining to, or serving as, a type.

typing, sex See *sex typing*.

typology Study of types.

typology, anxiety See *anxiety typology*.

U

Ucs Abbreviation for *unconscious*.

UDDA Uniform Determination of Death Act, advocated for use in defining death by the President's Commission for the Study of Ethical Problems in Medicine and Biomedical and Behavioral Research (1981): "An individual who has sustained either (1) irreversible cessation of circulatory and respiratory functions, or (2) irreversible cessation of all functions of the entire brain, including the brainstem, is dead. A determination of death must be made in accordance with accepted medical standards."

ulcer, peptic A psychophysiologic disorder of the digestive tract consisting of circumscribed erosion of any of those areas exposed to acid-pepsin gastric juice, most commonly the lesser curvature of the stomach and the duodenal bulb. Etiology is uncertain, but even the most psychologically oriented theories assume the coexistence of somatic as well as emotional factors. Among the latter, Alexander has stressed conflict between repressed passive-receptive, oral-dependency needs and conscious desires for independence; oral needs are frustrated and the patient regresses to a desire to be fed. Gastric activity responds appropriately and the mucosa secretes as if preparing for actual feeding.

ulterior transactions See *transactional analysis*.

ultradian See *rhythms, biologic*.

ultrasonic irradiation See *irradiation, ultrasonic*.

ultrasound probe See *NMR*.

ululation The inarticulate crying of hysterical or psychotic persons.

Umwelt Whatever is subjectively meaningful in the subject's environment; the environmentally significant as contrasted with hereditary factors.

uncanny emotions See *not-me*.

uncertainty In information theory, *incongruity* (q.v.).

uncinate seizure (un'si-nāt) See *fit, uncinate*.

unconditioned response See *conditioning*.

unconscious (Ucs) Used as a noun or an adjective. In psychiatry it is used with two different and separate meanings.

1. The absence of participation of the conscious ego or the so-called perceptive-self. When the conscious part of the mind is not functioning, the subject is said to be unconscious. Unconsciousness is usually associated with absence of orientation and perception, particularly in its extreme expression.

2. A division of the psyche, *the unconscious* or *unconsciousness*. In general it may be stated that all psychic material not in the immediate field of awareness is in the unconscious. When it is near enough to the former to be more or less easily accessible to it, it is said to be in the foreconscious or preconscious. See *ego; id*.

"Modern psychopathology has in its possession a wealth of observations regarding mental activities that are entirely analogous to conscious functions, and yet are unconscious. One can perceive, think, feel, remember, decide, and act, unconsciously. . . . How this is possible can best be seen if one imagines the mental functions and contents as resembling a night landscape over which the beam of a searchlight is playing. Whatever appears in this light of perception is conscious; what lies in the darkness beyond is unconscious, although none the less living and effective." (Jung, *CAP*)

"An appropriate and descriptive term to characterize that which is devoid of the attributes of consciousness. . . . Unfortu-

790

nately, however, the term has been also employed to characterize another and distinct class of facts, namely *Co-* [or *Sub-*] *conscious Ideas. . . .* It is sufficient to say here, that as conceived of, and as we have seen, there are very *definite states of coconsciousness—a coexisting dissociated consciousness or coconsciousness of which the personal consciousness is not aware,* i.e., of which it is 'unconscious.' Hence they have been called 'unconscious ideas.' . . . But this is plainly using the term in a different sense—using it as a synonym for the longer phrase, 'ideas we are unaware of,' and not as a characterization of that which is physiological and nonpsychological.

" 'Unconscious ideas' in this sense (the equivalent of conscious ideas) would include conscious states that we are not aware of simply because not in the focus of attention but in the fringe of the content of consciousness. The term would also include pathologically split-off and independently acting conscious ideas or systems of ideas such as occur in hysteria, reaching their apogee in coconscious personalities and in automatic writings." (Prince, M. *The Unconscious,* 1916)

unconscious, absolute Collective unconscious. See *collective unconscious.*

unconscious, collective See *collective unconscious.*

unconscious, impersonal See *collective unconscious.*

unconscious, personal See *collective unconscious.*

unconscious, superpersonal See *collective unconscious.*

unconsciousness See *unconscious.*

unconventional virus See *virus infections.*

uncus See *lobe, temporal.*

underachievement See *academic underachievement disorder.*

underachiever A person who fails to produce or perform at the level for which he is qualified and capable; specifically, a student whose academic performance is below his known potential.

underclass A permanent, irreversibly impoverished social stratum in which maladaptive treatment of children engenders psychological unpreparedness for self-improvement. Families in this stratum often appear clinically as multiproblem welfare families. Although there are ex-

ceptions, the general tendency of underclass families to reproduce hopelessness, alienation, and antisocial behavior in each subsequent generation has been noted by many observers.

undercutting, cortical See *lobotomy, prefrontal.*

underload, informational See *deprivation, sensory.*

undinism *Urolagnia; urophilia* (qq.v.).

undoing One of the unconscious defense mechanisms, consisting of a positive action that, actually or magically, is the opposite of something against which the ego must defend itself. Expiatory acts, countercompulsions, and some forms of compulsive ceremonials and counting compulsions are among the more frequent expressions of undoing, which is characteristic of the obsessive-compulsive psychoneurosis.

unfocused delirium See *délire chronique.*

unforthcomingness Impairment of motivation, and particularly that type of poor or disorganized motivation that has been observed in some children born of a stressful or complicated pregnancy. Some workers believe that minimal brain damage associated with stressful pregnancy may express itself behaviorally as unforthcomingness, and that the child so affected may be predisposed to delinquent breakdown.

unipolar See *depression, unipolar.*

unipolar double-bind See *bind, double.*

unit character A single-gene trait transmitted independently of other unit characters, such as pigmentation vs. albinism.

unit, least publishable *LPU* (q.v.).

unitization Administrative organization of a large hospital into several units, each with its own chief, staff, and carefully delineated responsibilities. The several autonomous units form a confederation that is supervised by the hospital director or superintendent. Hospitals may be unitized on the basis of function (e.g. adolescent units, geriatric units, alcoholism units), or on the basis of geography, with each unit serving a specified region of the larger area from which the hospital draws its patients.

unlust (un-lust') A German psychoanalytic term synonymous with the English terms *ego pain, unpleasure,* or *anxiety.*

Unpleasure, or unlust, refers to the sensation of mild discomfort or frustration tension that is felt in consciousness (by the ego) when instinctual trends, seeking gratification, are totally or partly opposed or blocked by the ego. This feeling of discomfort stands in marked contrast to the expected feeling of pleasurable relief from tension that usually follows full gratification of the instinct.

The feeling of pain, unpleasure, frustration, tension, or discomfort is frequently mixed with, or associated with, anxiety. Unlust, or unpleasure, represents ego suffering as an antithesis to pleasurable instinct satisfaction. It is this state of affairs that embodies the catalogue of all neurotic symptoms. (Sterba, R. *Introduction to the Psycho-analytic Theory of the Libido,* 1942)

unnatural Contrary to nature, abnormal, atypical, unusual; most often applied to sexual behavior that the user of the term judges to be repugnant or otherwise unacceptable.

"Especially when difficulties beset a population already inclined to value conformity for its own sake, those who are perceived as willfully different are apt to be viewed not only as mistaken (or 'unnatural') but as potentially dangerous." (Boswell, J. *Christianity, Social Tolerance, and Homosexuality,* 1980)

unpleasure See *unlust.*

unreality, feelings of See *depersonalization.*

unveiling Fritz Wittels's term for the uncovering or revelation of psychic components.

unvoluntary behavior See *intentional involuntary behavior.*

up-regulation Receptor supersensitivity, characteristic of postsynaptic receptors when the endogenous ligand (their normal innervation) is removed. Degeneration of the nigrostriatal pathway in Parkinson's disease, for example, results in up-regulation of dopamine receptors. It is because of that supersensitivity that L-dopa is effective in alleviating symptoms of the disorder. If treatment continues for a long time, however, the result is a *down-regulation* (q.v.) of the originally up-regulated receptors and a refractoriness to L-dopa, sometimes referred to as the *on-off* phenomenon. In some cases, temporary cessation of L-dopa permits sensitivity to build up again so that treatment can be reinstituted with beneficial results.

upper class See *class, social.*

UR *Utilization review;* see *review.*

Ur defenses Masserman's term for what he considers the three fundamental psychological maneuvers of man—the delusion of invulnerability and immortality, the delusion of the omnipotent servant (in the form of some abstract being or gnostic principle or system), and the conviction of man's kindness to man.

uranism (ū'rà-niz'm) *Obs.* (From Uranus, most ancient of Greek gods and the first ruler of the universe) A term used by Karl Heinrich Ulrichs in 1862 for homosexuality; the female homosexual he called *urninde,* the male *urning.*

The corresponding term for heterosexuality is *dionism* (from Dione, mother of Venus Pandemos).

uranomania *Obs.* The delusion that one is of divine or celestial origin.

uranophobia Fear of heaven.

Urbach-Wiethe disease See *disease, Urbach-Wiethe.*

urban crises See *social policy planning.*

urethra The canal leading from the urinary bladder to the outside of the body, in the male by way of the penis. In psychoanalysis, the urethra is regarded as an erogenous zone, and psychoanalysts speak of urethral erotism and sadism.

urine, dirty Used in reference to substance abusers and drug addicts who are on a drug-free treatment program, when chemical analysis of their urine indicates that they have taken narcotics or other drugs.

urninde (oor-nin'dē) *Obs.* Female homosexual. See *uranism.*

urning (oor'ning) *Obs.* Male homosexual. See *uranism.*

urningism *Uranism* (q.v.).

urolagnia Pleasure connected with urine. For example, some persons drink their own urine; others gain gratification in watching others urinate, and/or in having a sexual partner urinate upon them ("golden shower").

urophilia A pathologic love for, or interest in, urine; one of the miscellaneous paraphilias within the *psychosexual disorders* (q.v.); *urolagnia* (q.v.).

urorrhea *Enuresis* (q.v.).

user A slang expression to describe a morphine or heroin addict who takes small doses daily for years to keep himself comfortable. See *hog.*

uteromania *Obs.* Insanity associated with uterine disorder.

utilitarian principle See *principle, utilitarian.*

utilitarianism The moral theory that there is only one basic principle in ethics, the principle of utility, which decrees that in all circumstances the morally right thing is to produce the greatest possible balance of value over disvalue for all persons affected or, in situations where only evils are involved, the least possible balance of disvalue.

utilitarianism, act Use of the principle of utility to decide whether a specific act is right. This is in contrast to *rule utilitarianism,* in which general rules of conduct are established as morally right in accordance with the principle of utility. A specific act can be considered right only if it conforms with the established rule, and its rightness or wrongness is not determined on an individual basis.

utilitarianism, hedonistic A type of utilitarianism (q.v.) in which value is defined in terms of happiness or pleasure. See *utilitarianism, pluralistic.*

utilitarianism, negative The ethical theory that the morally correct choice is made by comparing evils prevented with evils caused and deciding in favor of the lesser evil. Such a theory, which is often used to justify *paternalism* (q.v.), fails to take into account the consequences of universally allowing the violation of a moral rule, if that happens to seem to be the lesser evil in a particular situation. See *ethics, situation.*

utilitarianism, pluralistic A type of *utilitarianism* (q.v.) in which many kinds of intrinsic value are recognized: happiness, friendship, beauty, courage, health, etc. See *utilitarianism, hedonistic.*

utilization See *review.*

utilization behavior A form of *magnetic apraxia* or bilateral grasping response described in lesions of the frontal lobe, and particularly in those involving its orbital surface and perhaps the head of the caudate nucleus. When confronted with the tactile, visuotactile, or visual presentation of an object, the subject feels compelled to grasp or use it. (Lhermitte, F. *Brain 106,* 1983)

utilization technique Milton Erickson's term for one of his methods of handling resistance in hypnotic subjects and patients in brief psychotherapy: "Erickson first asks the subject to do what he is already doing to resist him, and so do it under his own direction. Then he begins to shift the patient's behavior into more co-operative activity until the patient is fully following his directions." (Haley, J. *Archives of General Psychology 4,* 1961)

utilizer User; most commonly, a user of insurance benefits. See *selection, adverse.*

uvula See *cerebellum.*

uxoricide (uks-or'i-sīd) Killing of a wife by her husband.

V

vaccinophobia A morbid fear or dread of being vaccinated.

vagina dentata A vagina with teeth; a phantasy, more often unconscious than conscious, in which the female genitalia are equated with a castrating, devouring mouth.

vaginismus A sexual dysfunction consisting of painful spasm of the vagina. It generally takes place at some time during coitus or it may have its onset during the stage of preparation for the sexual act. Etiology is often psychic.

Typical cases develop spasms that make insertion of the penis impossible, and such spasms are responsible for the rare cases of penis captivus. Vaginismus usually represents inhibition of sexual excitement along with positive action to ensure maintenance of inhibition; in addition, it may be a conversion symptom expressing a wish to break off the penis and keep it.

vaginismus, psychic Painful spasm of the vagina preventing coitus; caused by repugnance to the sexual act.

vagotonia Excessive excitability of the vagus nerve.

valence See *life space*.

valid consent See *consent, informed*.

validation, consensual See *distortion, parataxic*.

validity The degree to which a test measures what it is supposed to measure; a valid intelligence test, for example, is truly a measure of general intelligence and not a test of rote memory. The degree of validity of a test depends upon the magnitude of the errors present in the measures obtained from it. Some indication of the validity of a given test is gained from a study of the correlations between scores on the given test and scores from other tests designed to measure the same factor.

value That which is esteemed, prized, or deemed worthwhile and desirable by a person or a culture. See *superego*.

Values are experientially determined; unlike needs, they are not innate.

vampirism Belief in bloodsucking ghosts (vampires); performing the actions of a vampire. While in neither sense is the term often used in clinical psychiatry, when it does appear in the literature it is generally in the second sense, as the act of drawing blood from an object with accompanying sexual pleasure. The blood may be drawn by cutting, biting, or similar means, and sometimes the drinking of the drawn blood is an important part of the action. Some writers regard the "love-bite," i.e. the biting of the sexual partner during sexual activity, as a form of vampirism. Psychodynamically, vampirism is usually interpreted as expressing conflicts in any or all of the following areas: oral sadism and incorporation, fear of castration, aggressive hostile wishes (including murder), and oedipal strivings for the mother.

vampirism, parasitic H.G. Baynes uses the expression parasitic vampirism in a special sense, namely, that in a psychoneurotic patient compulsive mechanisms are present that are constantly driving the person. These drives have a demonic appetite—the more they have the more they demand. They know no reasonable bounds. Baynes believes that the neurotic symptoms, such as phobias, obsessions, and aggressions, are similar to a devouring monster that overpowers and possesses the patient in the manner of a bloodthirsty vampire. (*Mythology of the Soul*, 1940)

vandalism, sexual An inordinate impulse to destroy the sexual zones represented in pictures, statuary, etc.

vapores uterini *Obs.* It was an ancient belief that vapors, originating in the uterus, passed into the brain, thus producing mental disorders.

vapors *Obs.* Hysteria; hypochondriasis.

variant, epileptic There are many clinical phenomena of the so-called epilepsies. Among them are the varieties listed by S.A. Wilson in the *Journal of Neurology and Psychopathology*, 1928:

A. Motor Variants
   1. Myoclonic or regional epilepsy
   2. Epilepsia partialis continua
   3. Tonic epilepsy
   4. Coordinated epilepsy
   5. Inhibitory or akinetic epilepsy
B. Sensory Variants
   1. Reflex epilepsy
   2. Sensory epilepsy
   3. Affective epilepsy
C. Psychical Variants
D. Visceral Variants

variation The varying phenotypical expressivity of hereditary characters, whose individual manifestations are *modifiable.* Since in a species originating through sexual reproduction no real hereditary homogeneity among its various individuals can be expected, the offspring of higher organisms are never exactly like the parents, but vary to a certain extent, each organism inheriting the entire characteristic modifiability of its kinship.

According to genetic theories, there are three possible mechanisms that can cause an organism to become different from its parents: *modification, combination,* and *mutation* (qq.v.).

The items in any frequency distribution differ from each other with respect to the amount of a given character they all possess (e.g. height), and any frequency distribution may differ in a similar way from another frequency distribution describing the same character. Such differences constitute the phenomenon of variation.

vasectomy The *sterilizing* operation on men of cutting and tying off the seminal ducts (vasa deferentia). Usually no unfavorable effect on the secondary sexual characters follows vasectomy, in contrast with the *castrating* operation of removing the testicles. See *sterilization.*

vasopressin, arginine (AVP) A peptide synthesized in nuclei of the medial hypothalamus. It is stored in the posterior pituitary and released into the circulation to regulate water reabsorption by the distal renal tubule; hence it is also called antidiuretic hormone. It is also transported to the third ventricle and into the cerebrospinal fluid, through which it exerts its neuromodulator effects on biogenic amine activity and on the release of other peptide modulators, including the endorphins. Evidence suggests that AVP may augment memory functions in both cognitively normal and cognitively impaired subjects.

vasotocin, arginine (AVT) A peptide of the neurohypophysial unit and perhaps the prototypic neurohypophysial hormone. In function, it is more closely linked to adenohypophysis-regulating activities than to antidiuresis.

vasovagal attack of Gowers Gowers described a syndrome characterized by nausea and belching, precordial discomfort, respiratory difficulty, anxiety of impending death, and mild mental upset. The attack may last from a few minutes to an hour.

VBR Ventricle to brain ratio, often reported increased as assessed by CAT scan in some acutely psychotic subjects (as well as in subjects with various forms of brain atrophy). Increased VBR is associated with abnormal performance on a number of neuropsychological tasks.

VDRL Venereal disease research laboratory; used generally to refer to a slide test for syphilis developed in that laboratory.

VDT Visual distortion test. See *test, visual distortion.*

vecordia *Obs.* Any mental disorder.

vegative nervous system See *autonomic nervous system.*

vegetative symptoms Used particularly in referring to mood or affective disorders, the expression includes sleep and appetite disturbances, weight change, fatigue, and low energy that are a part of the clinical picture as the major depressive disorder develops.

vent men See *street people.*

ventricle puncture See *puncture, ventricle.*

ventricle to brain ratio *VBR* (q.v.).

ventriculogram An X-ray of the skull following replacement of cerebrospinal fluid with air by means of ventricular puncture. This drains the ventricular system but not the subarachnoid spaces and cisterns; the procedure is used when an expanding intracranial lesion is suspected, since ventriculography is considered safer than encephalography in such cases.

ventriculography Radiography of the brain cavity. A means of determining the presence of structural changes in the intracranial contents, which are visualized by the X-ray, after the direct injection of air into the lateral ventricles.

VEP Visual evoked potential, the brain wave response to visual stimulation such as exposure to different flash intensities. See *neurometrics*.

Veraguth, fold of (Otto Veraguth, German neurologist, 1870–1940) Contraction upward and backward of the inner third of the upper lid, thus changing the arch of the upper lid into an angle. Veraguth described this change as a characteristic sign of the depressed type of manic-depressive psychosis.

verapamil A calcium channel blocker, used in the treatment of cardiac arrhythmias, angina pectoris, and hypertension because of its action on myocardial and vascular smooth muscle cells. Because it seems also to inhibit calcium ion influx within the brain, it has been used as a substitute for lithium in the treatment of mania.

verbalization The state of being verbose or diffuse, commonly encountered in extreme degree in patients with the manic form of manic-depressive psychosis. In a more general sense, verbalization refers to the expression in words of thoughts, wishes, phantasies, or other psychic material that had previously been on a nonverbal level because of suppression or repression. "Verbalize" is often used in a pseudoerudite way when "talk about" is meant.

verbigerate (vĕr-bij'ĕr-āt) To repeat the same word, phrase, or sentence over and over again.

verbigeration A manifestation of stereotypy, consisting of the morbid repetition of words, phrases, or sentences; also called *cataphasia*. A patient with the catatonic form of schizophrenia kept repeating "muscle, muscle, muscle," in reply to all forms of questioning.

verbigeration, hallucinatory A type of *thought-echoing* (q.v.) in which the patient hears, in endless repetition or with slight changes, the same meaningless sentences.

verbochromia A type of *synesthesia* in which certain words evoke a sensation of color. See *sensation, secondary*.

verbomania *Tachylogia* (q.v.).

verbose Overproductive in speech.

vermis See *cerebellum*.

Verstehen See *Erklären*.

vertical transmission See *transmission, vertical*.

vertigo Dizziness; a feeling that the subject or the world around him is spinning or revolving.

vertigo, cervical See *migraine, cervical*.

vesania (vē-sā'nē-ä) An old term, as well as an old concept, that meant insanity in general. It was used by Sauvages in his *Nosologia Methodica*, of 1763. The group termed *vesania* embraced psychiatric disorders not known to be associated with any organic disease or disorder.

vesania anomala (ä-nō'mä-lä) *Obs*. *Mania transitoria* (q.v.).

vesania, typica circularis (tē'pē-kä kēr-koo-lä'rēs) In 1882 Kahlbaum used the term *cyclothymia* to designate the milder, recoverable forms of manic-depressive psychosis, and the expression *vesania typica circularis* for the chronic forms.

vestibular nerve See *nerve, acoustic*.

VF See *vigil, fatiguing*.

vice allemand (vēs'äl'mäN) Used by Hirschfeld synonymously with homosexuality. In the 18th century the French called homosexuality "the German vice"; at an earlier period Europeans referred to homosexuality as "the Oriental disease." It seems that every nation disowns responsibility for originating homosexuality, and would like to shift it upon another's shoulders. But, as a matter of fact, homosexuality is recorded in classical literature.

vicissitudes, instinctual See *libido, plasticity of*.

Victim See *transactional analysis*.

victim recidivism See *recidivism*.

victimology The study of the victim(s) of kidnaping, rape, assault, or other crime—how they came to be the object of the crime, what physical and mental injuries they were forced to endure, what kind of assistance they might require in returning to their usual pattern of daily living, what type of restitution or compensation they might merit, etc. Observations that some persons appeared to be "accident prone" or more likely than most to be the victims of assaults fostered a tendency to look upon victims as *agents provocateurs*. On another front, civil libertarians became so successful in protecting the rights of persons accused of crimes that it became exceedingly difficult for their victims to establish that any wrong had been done. Then came an emphasis on entitlement, and the idea that victims should somehow, by someone, be compensated for the pain and anguish to which they had been subjected. Finally, the spotlight has turned back on the perpetrator of the action. In the case of rape, spousal abuse, and other forms of domestic violence, for instance, the social attitude is changing from one of blaming the victims of abuse to one of holding the abusers accountable.

The myth of provocation by an abused spouse has become increasingly suspect, and attention is now focused on the behavior of the abuser, and also on social norms that have sanctioned and encouraged such behavior under the guise of protecting privacy and preserving the sanctity of the home. See *diathesis, traumatophilic*.

view, Equus-Laingian See *Equus-Laingian view*.

vigil, fatiguing A type of sleep deprivation in which the experimental subject is required to perform mental work while he remains awake.

vigilambulism *Fugue* (q.v.). A condition of unconsciousness regarding one's surroundings, with automatism, resembling somnambulism, but occurring in the waking state.

vigilance The general alerting function or sentinel activity of the nervous system; in conditioned reflex experiments, each positive or negative conditioned stimulus causes a sharp spike of sudden alertness, termed stimulus-vigilance. Stimulus-vigilance is considered to be an emergency reaction to a stress stimulus in a stressful situation. "When an animal un-

dergoing a regimen of difficult conditioning succumbs to an experimental neurosis we may suppose that its final traumatic reaction to the repeated stress situations of the conditioning laboratory was due to a gradual heightening of the vigilance level from day to day in consequence of the summation of the after-effects of stimulus-vigilance enduring for days, weeks, or months. Finally, an end point or breaking point is reached beyond which the animal's management of its emergency function becomes faulty as indicated by its neurotic manifestations. The intensity of the vigilance level of the day depends then not only upon the total stimulus load, i.e., upon the number, intensity, duration, and temporal spacing of the specific vigilance reactions aroused by the positive and negative conditioned stimuli of the experimental day, but also upon the lingering traces of stimulus-vigilance from previous conditioning sessions." (H.S. Liddell, in *The Biology of Mental Health and Disease*, 1952)

In 19th-century writings, vigilance was equivalent to *insomnia* and *agrypnia*.

vigilant See *anxiety typology*.

villa system See *system, villa*.

villus biopsy See *biopsy, chorion*.

violence Physical aggression; willful physical harm inflicted by a persop or group on itself or on another person or group. Violence represents the extreme pole of the aggressive spectrum of behavior, characterized by an explosive, sudden quality and the use of force to injure or destroy an object, a person, or an organization. Aggression, in contrast, refers to the use of force (not necessarily physical) to overcome resistance by an object, person, or organization to the will of one of the participants in a struggle or conflict so that the outcome will conform to the intention of one of the adversaries. Anger, hate, and rage are frequent internal, emotional concomitants of aggression, but not universally so, since simple assertion is also aggression. How much aggression and violence are biologically inherent, and how much are a consequence of social learning, are moot questions. Ethology, for example, views man as a killer ape, while genetic anthropologists see him as a noble savage characterized by cooperation with other men. The absolute negative position says that violence is always bad, and with this view is correlated the negative therapeutic position that considers any excessive display of violence as sick. The absolute positive position states that violence is good, in that those who feel free to display it constitute an elite who are fit to lead and able to resist corruption; the correlated positive therapeutic position considers the display of violence under conditions of injustice to be therapeutic in itself. In recent times, there has tended to be a move away from either of the absolutes to a relative or conditional position, which considers violence acceptable under certain conditions, as in self-defense or the "just" war.

violence, domestic *Family violence;* included are child and spouse homicide, spouse abuse, wife battering, child abuse, child sexual abuse, severe child neglect, adolescent abuse, sibling abuse, parental abuse, and abuse of the elderly. The family is the most frequent single locus for all violence, including homicide. Violence is estimated to occur in at least 50% of American families. See *syndrome, battered child; wife battering.*

VIP Abbreviation for very important person, and in clinical psychiatry applied to any patient who is able through personal influence or professional status to exert unusual pressure on the staff of a psychiatric hospital. A staff usually reacts adversely to such pressure with fear, anger, and withdrawal from the patient, and a vicious circle of increased patient pressure and further staff withdrawal is created. This has been termed the *VIP syndrome* and is of particular importance in that it generally ends in therapeutic failure, often in the form of suicide or discharge against medical advice.

viraginity (vir-à-jin′i-tē) The adoption by women of male characteristics. It is an expression of homosexuality.

virium lapsus *Obs.* Lypothymia; melancholy.

viroids The smallest RNA viruses, whose small size renders them highly resistant to ultraviolet inactivation. See *virus infections.*

virus infections Rabies, Japanese B encephalitis, and St. Louis encephalitis, among others, have long been recognized as viral encephalitides. More recently, evidence has accumulated to suggest that viruses can sometimes persist in host cells for long periods—even years—without producing symptoms. Such infections, called *conventional slow virus infections,* comprise a wide spectrum of chronic and degenerative diseases, including subacute postmeasles leukoencephalitis and subacute sclerosing panencephalitis (SSPE) due to paramyxovirus of measles; subacute herpetovirus encephalitis of herpes simplex; progressive congenital rubella togavirus; cytomegalovirus brain infection; epilepsia partialis continua or Kozhevnikov's epilepsy; chronic meningoencephalitis in immunodeficient patients. It is suspected that many other chronic diseases may fall into this group, and slow virus has been proposed as a causative agent of multiple sclerosis, Parkinson's disease, amyotrophic lateral sclerosis, tuberous sclerosis, disseminated lupus, ulcerative colitis, and some forms of schizophrenic dementia. To date, however, no virus has been identified from in vitro tissue cultures and attempts to transmit the disorders to other species have not succeeded.

During the 1970s, interest has grown in still another group, the *unconventional viruses* or *spongiform encephalopathies (SE),* which differ from other viruses in several ways: they do not evoke a virus-associated inflammatory response in brain or a pleocytosis or rise in CSF protein; there is no demonstrable immune response to the causative virus; they show unusual resistance to various chemical and physical agents that destroy conventional viruses. Some have speculated that the unconventional viruses may be *viroids*—very small DNA or RNA molecules about one-tenth the size of the nucleic acids in conventional viruses and without the protein coat that normally covers viral nucleic acids.

Included within the unconventional virus infections are (1) in man—*kuru* (q.v.) and transmissible virus dementia (TVD), including the sporadic familial forms of Creutzfeldt-Jakob's disease (CJD; see *degeneration, cortico-striato-spinal*), and familial *Alzheimer's disease* (q.v.); (2) in animals—scrapie and transmissible mink encephalopathy (TME). The work of D. Carleton Gajdusek and his colleagues at the National Institute of Neurological Communicative Diseases and Stroke suggests that scrapie-infected sheep tissue might be the source of TME (mink are often fed sheep scraps), of CJD by means of kitchen or butchery accidents (and secondarily from those so affected by means of neurosurgical or ophthalmologic surgical procedures performed on them), and of kuru through cannibalism.

visceral epilepsy See *epilepsy, visceral.*

visceral learning See *biofeedback.*

viscerotonia A personality type described by Sheldon correlated with the endomorph body type which shows a love of food, comfort, and conviviality and a tendency to general relaxation.

viscosity of libido See *libido, viscosity of.*

vision See *lobe, occipital.*

vision, tubular See *field defect.*

visionism *Obs.* Voyeurism (q.v.).

visions, hypnagogic The optic perceptions present in a state midway between sleep and waking. They are a phase of dream phenomena.

visitor, health Any person who goes to the family as a way to provide linkage to health services; it has been suggested that a visiting nurse or, perhaps even better, a mature and supportive mother who is recognized as such by the community, can provide health supervision to the young family whose child might otherwise fall victim to abuse or neglect. See *syndrome, battered child.*

visual field See *field defect.*

visual-spatial agnosia. See *agnosia, visual-spatial.*

VLSIC Very large scale integrated circuits, necessary to render a computer system *friendly* (q.v.).

VNA Visiting Nurse Association.

vocational counseling See *counseling; rehabilitation.*

Vogt, Oskar (fôKt) (1870–1959) German neuropathologist; Tay-Sachs disease.

Vogt-Spielmeyer's disease See *Tay-Sachs disease; Spielmeyer-Vogt's disease.*

voice, soundless See *thought, audible.*

volition Will, motivation, desire. To have volitional ability, one must be able both to will and do, and also to refrain from willing and doing when there are appropriate reasons for so willing. The compulsive handwasher, for example, acts intentionally but not voluntarily, for he can will and perform the act of handwashing, but he cannot refrain from doing it even though he has good reasons for not washing his hands.

volition, derailment of See *derailment of volition.*

volition, made See *symptoms, first-rank.*

volubility Overproductivity in speech.

volume sensitive Affected or determined by amount or quantity. A special operation that requires highly polished technical skills, for instance, is likely to be better performed in an institution where it is performed frequently than in an institution where it is only rarely performed. Thus part of valid consent includes informing a patient about to undergo a volume-sensitive operation in a low-volume hospital that he is at somewhat greater risk than if the same operation were to be performed in a high-volume hospital. See *consent, informed.*

voluntary See *volition.*

voluntary euthanasia See *euthanasia.*

vomiting, cyclic A disorder of children characterized by attacks of vomiting. The attacks begin suddenly, last several days, cease abruptly, and then recur in intervals or cycles of several weeks or months.

vomiting, nervous Functional vomiting of psychogenic, emotional, or neurotic origin, occurring most frequently in young women between the ages of 20 and 40. It usually expresses, in organ-language, symbolically and physically, the desire to reject a hated idea, or person, concerning whom there exist conscious and unconscious conflicts of an emotional nature; this is the only way out of the conflict left to these patients, because, in consciousness, they cannot stand their hostility and yet cannot express it verbally.

E. Weiss and O.S. English report the following case: "A young white woman, with markedly repressed sexuality, developed frequent vomiting attacks after a marriage to which she had consented, in the main, because of her mother's urging. Her passive and dependent nature did not allow her to express hostility openly but instead her unconscious mental forces caused her to vomit as though to say: 'I cannot stomach this situation.' " (*Psychosomatic Medicine*, 1949)

von Gierke's disease *Glucogenosis* (q.v.).

von Graefe's sign (Albrecht von Graefe, German ophthalmologist, 1828–70) Lag of the upper lid in following the downward movement of the eye, due to retraction of the upper lid such as occurs in exophthalmic goiter and in lesions in the upper part of the midbrain.

von Recklinghausen's disease (Friedrich Daniel von Recklinghausen, German pathologist, 1833–1910) *Neurofibromatosis* (q.v.).

Vorbeireden (fōr-bī-rā'den) One who is at cross purposes with another; applied to the person with Ganser syndrome who seems to miss the point of questions put to him by talking around or past them and giving nonsensical or approximate answers. See *factitious disorders; syndrome, Ganser.*

voyeur Peeping Tom; scopophiliac; one who obtains sexual gratification by looking at the genitals of another. See *voyeurism.*

voyeurism Peeping; obtaining sexual pleasure from watching an unsuspecting person who is nude, in the act of disrobing, or engaging in sexual intercourse. It is the watching or the later recall of it in phantasy that gives sexual excitement and is an end in itself (although often accompanied by masturbation to effect orgasm). Further sex contact between the observed and the voyeur does not occur. Voyeurism as defined has not been reported in females. It is one of the paraphilias within the group of *psychosexual* (q.v.) disorders. "Sublimation of the looking impulse can be brought about if the interest is turned from the genitals to the form of the body. This, Freud thinks, normally occurs as an intermediary sexual aim and makes possible the directing of a certain amount of the libido in artistic channels." (Healy et al., *SMP*)

vulnerability factor Any condition that renders the subject more susceptible than the average or normal population to stress, stimulation, disease, or any other factor under study.

Many depressions are observed to be triggered by life events that ordinarily would not be sufficient to provoke such a reaction. Such events appear to be acting as the "last straw" in a series of adverse circumstances that render the subject less able to cope, and those predisposing or sensitizing adverse circumstances have been called vulnerability factors. While not all studies have been confirmatory, some investigators have suggested that depressions are most likely to be triggered by life events in those who are caring for young children, who have no work outside the home, who have no one to confide in, or who have lost the mother by death or separation before they were 11 years of age. See *risk factor.*

vulnerability, genetic Inherited predisposition to developing an illness, either because of a heavy loading of those factors that contribute to the development of the illness or because of inadequate resistance or defenses against the illness. The concept implies that the vulnerability is an actual or measurable variation in structure or function, that it is continuous and chronic, and that the affected person carries the constitutional susceptibility even during periods of health. This is in contrast to the stress concept of psychiatric illness, which implies that in the well state a person is equivalent to a normal control and it is only when stress appears that he deviates from the normal. See *risk; risk factor.*

vulnerable child See *syndrome, vulnerable child.*

vulvismus *Vaginismus* (q.v.).

W

W In Rorschach scoring, a whole response; i.e. a percept determined by the entire inkblot. According to Piotrowski, the *W* is primarily a measure of the tendency to organize and plan in the pursuit of external goals.

Wada test See *test, Wada dominance.*

Wagner von Jauregg, Julius (väg'nēr fôn you'reg) (1857–1940) Austrian psychiatrist and neurologist; fever treatment of general paresis.

Wahnstimmung (vahn'shtim-ung) *Delusional mood,* consisting of a change in general mood that precedes the appearance of the delusional idea itself, such as a feeling of foreboding that some sinister event is about to occur.

WAIS Wechsler Adult Intelligence Scale.

wake time after sleep onset The duration of the intervals of time the subject is awake between onset of sleep and the end of the sleep period.

wakefulness *Arousal* (q.v.), attentiveness; sleeplessness, insomnia.

Wallenberg's syndrome (Adolf Wallenberg, German physician, 1862–1949) The symptoms following occlusion of the posterior inferior cerebellar artery (which is known as "the artery of thrombosis"): ipsilateral facial analgesia, ipsilateral Horner's syndrome, ipsilateral ataxia, and contralateral analgesia.

wandering Straying, wandering, roaming, traveling without a fixed course or particular destination in mind; also known as drapetomania, dromomania, ecdemomania, wanderlust, and many other nonspecific terms. Sometimes wandering refers to fugue states, but the current trend is to use it in a more specific way to denote episodes of sudden confusion (disorientation) in senile dementia or other organic disorders. See *deterioration, simple senile.*

wanderlust Morbid impulse to roam or wander, believed to be associated with the Oedipus situation in the sense that the wanderer is incessantly seeking to establish affiliation with one or both parents as he had experienced it, or longed to experience it, when he was a young child.

war neurosis See *neurosis, traumatic; shell shock.*

warn, duty to The responsibility of a psychiatrist to notify the possible victims of a patient's assault when the psychiatrist has sufficient evidence that such dangerous acts are likely to occur.

Wassermann reaction See *test, Wassermann.*

watchfulness, frozen See *frozen watchfulness.*

watchspring theory See *aging, theories of.*

Watson, John Broadus (1878–1958) American psychologist; behaviorism.

Watson-Crick model See *chromosome.*

waxy flexibility *Cerea flexibilitas.* See *catalepsy.*

weak-mindedness, hallucinatory *Obs.* Kraepelin's term for one of the terminal states of schizophrenia.

Weber's syndrome (Sir Herman Weber, English physician, 1823–1918) Pedunculopontile syndrome. See *hemiplegia alternans.*

weighted harm principle See *principle, weighted harm.*

Weltmerism (After Sidney A. Weltmer, founder of the method and the Weltmer Institute at Nevada, Mo.) A system of therapeutics based on suggestion.

Wernicke, Carl (vâr'ni-kē) (1848–1905) German neurologist; aphasia.

Wernicke's aphasia See *aphasia, Wernicke's.*

Wernicke's encephalopathy (en-sef-a-lop'-a-thē) *Polioencephalitis hemorrhagica superior,* described by Wernicke in 1881; a very severe disorder consisting of degeneration of nervous tissue especially marked in the midbrain. The syndrome occurs in a small percentage of alcoholics and is probably due to a combination of nutritional deficiencies, especially a vitamin B deficiency. Onset is insidious, with vomiting, oculomotor palsies, ptosis, pupillary changes (such as Argyll Robertson pupil), ataxia, insomnia, and a mental state consisting of an acute hallucinatory picture similar to delirium tremens except that there is no tremor and the delirium is dreamy and confused. Impaired consciousness may progress to stupor. The encephalopathy may terminate fatally, or there may be progression to a Korsakoff syndrome. Thiamine chloride has been used successfully to reverse the ophthalmoplegia and has sometimes been of help in the mental state. See *syndrome, Wernicke-Korsakoff*.

Westphal-Strümpell's pseudosclerosis See *degeneration, hepatolenticular*.

Westphal's sign See *sign, Westphal's*.

wet dream Popular term for seminal ejaculation during sleep; oneirogonorrhea.

whiplash A syndrome following sudden hyperextension or hyperflexion of the neck consisting of rapid loss of memory of life experiences without loss of intellectually learned facts. The syndrome is based on bilateral vascular disturbances in the hippocampal gyri, consisting of thrombosis and embolism in the hippocampal branches of the posterior cerebral arteries.

whipping See *flagellation*.

whirling See *schizophrenia, childhood*.

White, Samuel (1777–1845) American psychiatrist; one of the "original thirteen" founders of the Association of Medical Superintendents of America (forerunner of American Psychiatric Association).

White, William A. (1870–1937) American psychiatrist; psychodynamics, psychotherapy, forensic psychiatry.

wife battering Wife beating, probably the most unreported type of violence and the leading form of *domestic violence;* other terms sometimes include *intraspousal assault, interspousal violence,* and *intramarital assault.* "Wife-battering behavior" is sometimes quantitatively defined as deliberate, severe, and repeated (more than three times) physical assault resulting in demonstrable injury, such as severe bruising. It has been estimated that in the United States almost 1.8 million wives are battered at least once by their husbands.

The social attitude toward wife beating is slowly changing from one of blaming the victim of abuse to one of holding the man who perpetrates such abuse accountable. As with rape, attention is turning away from the myth of provocation by the woman to the abuse behavior of the man and the social norms that sanction and encourage such behavior under the guise of protecting the privacy and the sanctity of the home.

Wife battering is frequently accompanied by child abuse, both physical and sexual. Battering, as well as sexual abuse and incest, frequently occur hand-in-hand with alcohol or other substance abuse. Wife batterers are typically men with aggressive personalities or, less often, depression; in either case, they are often pathologically jealous or heavy drinkers, or both. See *violence, domestic*.

Wihtiko See *windigo psychosis*.

Wilbur, Hervey Backus (1820–83) American pioneer educator in the field of mental deficiency.

will, disturbances of the One of Bleuler's fundamental symptoms of the schizophrenias. Usually, the disturbance is in the direction of deficiency (hypobulia, hypoboulia) or lack (abulia, aboulia); such patients appear lazy, negligent of their duties, purposeless, and with no aims, ambitions, or desires. *Platonization* (q.v.) is often seen and patients appear apathetic toward their environment and uninterested in the reality about them. At other times, because they have no real goals, they appear flighty, capricious, and undependable, adopting momentarily any goal that is thrust upon them. Or they may appear stubborn, robotlike, and wedded in a perseverative way to a particular activity, which they cling to rather than have to make any decision or move toward purposeful change.

A few patients are hyperbulic and show a bizarre or inappropriate application and assiduity to unimportant and trivial occupations; these are the faddists, the shifters, persons who are forever brewing storms in teapots.

will therapy See *therapy, will*.

will to be above Adler borrowed this term from Nietzsche to indicate the tendency of the neurotic female to identify herself with the male.

will to be up Adler borrowed this term from Nietzsche to denote the neurotic's striving toward masculine aggression.

will to power This term, borrowed by Adler from Nietzsche, denotes the strivings of the neurotic toward masculinity, in order to escape the feeling of uncertainty and inferiority that connotes femininity.

Willowbrook consent See *consumerism.*

Wilson's disease (Samuel A.K. Wilson, English neurologist, 1878–1936) See *degeneration, hepatolenticular.*

windigo psychosis A culture-specific disorder of some Indian tribes of northern Canada, consisting of a fear or delusion that one will be transformed into a *wihtigo,* a giant monster that eats human flesh. No such psychosis has ever been witnessed by a psychiatrist or anthropologist, and the existence of such an entity seems doubtful.

window, therapeutic The range of plasma levels of a drug within which optimal therapeutic effects occur; levels outside that range, be they higher or lower, are associated with absent, minimal, or otherwise unsatisfactory response. A therapeutic window may exist for many psychotropic drugs, but it has been most convincingly demonstrated for some tricyclic antidepressants. It is worthy of emphasis that the phrase refers to plasma levels and not dosage levels, since the same dosage level may produce widely varying plasma levels in different patients, depending upon multiple factors including the recipient's age, sex, race, genetic makeup, underlying disorder, and concurrent medications.

Winner See *transactional analysis.*

wird A secret or holy sound or prayer that is repeated in conjunction with rhythmic exercises and breathing control as part of the ritual to induce *relaxation response* (q.v.).

WISC Wechsler Intelligence Scale for Children.

Wise Old Man See *analytic psychology.*

wish An impulse, a purpose, a desire, a tendency, an urge, a striving, "a course of action which some mechanism of the body is set to carry out, whether it actually does so or does not." (Holt, E.B. *The Freudian Wish and Its Place in Ethics,* 1915)

wish, child-penis In psychoanalytic psychology, the wish for a child with which, in her

psychosexual development, the little girl replaces her wish for a penis.

The little girl's first love object is the mother, since it was she who provided the first satisfactions of life, nourishment, warmth, etc. The little girl's libidinal impulses to her first object, her mother, are manifold and express themselves through oral, anal, and phallic wishes, both active and passive. They are also completely ambivalent, being both tender and hostile. The phallic wishes are expressed by "the desire to get the mother with child as well as the corresponding one, to have a child by the mother." The mother contributed to these wishes in reality, since she aroused "pleasurable sensations in the child's genitals in the ordinary course of attending to its bodily needs." As the child develops, her strong attachment to her mother is replaced by an attachment to her father. This takes place in an atmosphere of hatred for the mother. Although there are many obvious sources for this hatred of the mother—the unavoidable necessity in the child's development of frustrating her insatiable desire for the breast; the birth of a sibling who deprives the little girl of the mother's exclusive attention; the frustration (with threat and disapproval from the mother) of the child's masturbatory activities, which the mother herself had unwittingly stimulated; the other necessary restrictions associated with education; and finally the strong ambivalence of the child's impulses toward her mother— Freud feels that in the girl's turning from her mother to her father the main and specific factor is her penis envy, her wish for a penis. For when the girl first notices that the boy has something she has not— his male genitals—she feels at a great disadvantage. Now the little girl no longer enjoys her phallic sexuality. Her self-love is wounded "by the unfavourable comparison with the boy who is so much better equipped," and therefore she "gives up the masturbatory satisfaction which she obtained from her clitoris . . . and . . . repudiates her love towards her mother." See *envy, penis.*

Having given up her love for her mother, who, too, is found to be castrated and therefore cannot satisfy her daughter's desire for a penis or the sexual phantasies associated with her masturbation, the little girl turns her love toward her father. She has not, however, relinquished her wish for a penis, which, in effect, her mother has refused her, and which she now expects from her father. Also, her passive instinctual impulses have gained the upper hand, since a certain amount of activity was surrendered along with the clitoric masturbation. Thus a symbolic equation, child = penis, can come into effect and the wish for a penis is replaced by the wish for a child. The girl's strongest wish now is for a child by her father. "With the transference of the child-penis-wish onto her father, the girl enters into the situation of the Oedipus complex."

At an earlier age, before the development of her penis envy, the little girl had expressed a wish for a child by playing with dolls. This wish for a child, however, was an expression of her active identification with her mother: she could do to the doll all that her mother used to do with her. It was not, however, associated with a wish for a penis. "Only with the onset of the desire for a penis does the doll-child become a child by the father." (Freud, S. *New Introductory Lectures on Psychoanalysis,* 1933)

wish dream, masochistic A dream that has to do with injury to the dreamer himself. According to Freud, even dreams with a painful content are to be analyzed as wish fulfillments.

wish fulfillment, asymptotic Gratification of an impulse or desire in a substitute or "almost but not quite" way.

wish, id Instinctual urges having their source in the realm of the repressed, unconscious, primitive, and infantile regions of the personality (psyche or mind).

Id wishes, or instinctual urges, emanating from the unconscious are thought of in conflict with, and in juxtaposition to, wishes having their origin in the ego, on the one hand, and in the conscience, or superego, on the other. Wishes having their origin in the ego make for reality adjustment and control; those having their origin in the conscience, or superego, make for the attainment of "goodness" and "approval."

Id wishes are characterized by a driving urgency representative of their infantile

and primordial biologic nature. They are mainly of a crudely aggressive and erotic nature.

wish, penis See *envy, penis; wish, child-penis.*

wishes, fundamental Basic wishes have been subdivided into (1) the desire for new experience; (2) the desire for security; (3) the desire for response; and (4) the desire for recognition.

wit The background of wit is fundamentally the same as the background of many other psychic phenomena, but wit is usually not a manifestation of morbidity, any more than are slips of the tongue or pen. There are no nosological disorders, or syndromes, in which wit occupies the position of abnormality in the general sense of that term. To be sure, wit appears in certain clinical conditions, but its import to the total clinical picture is usually insignificant.

Freud regards wit "as the most social of all those psychic functions whose aim is to gain pleasure. It often requires three persons, and the psychic process which it incites requires the participation of at least one other person. It must, therefore, bind itself to the condition of intelligibleness; it may employ distortion made practicable in the unconscious through condensation and displacement, to no greater extent than can be deciphered by the intelligence of the third person."

Freud defines wit as a "developed play" that "seeks to draw a small amount of pleasure from the free and unencumbered activities of our psychic apparatus, and later to seize this pleasure as an incidental gain."

The pleasure of wit originates "from an *economy of expenditure in inhibition;* the comic arises from an *economy of expenditure in thought;* while humor originates from an *economy of expenditure in feeling." (BW)*

wit, tendency There are two major classifications of witty productions. "Word- and thought-wit on the one hand, and abstract and tendency-wit on the other hand, bear no relation of dependence to each other; they are two entirely independent classifications of witty productions."

When "wit is wit for its own sake and serves no other particular purpose," it is called *abstract* or *harmless wit.* Freud cites an example from Lichtenberg: "They sent a small octavo to the University of Göttingen; and received back in body and soul a quarto" (a fourth-form boy).

Wit may serve some purpose; it may have deep meaning; it may be tendential; when such is the case, Freud speaks of *tendency-wit.* "It makes possible the gratification of a craving (lewd or hostile) despite a hindrance which stands in the way; it eludes the hindrance and so derives pleasure from a source that has been inaccessible on account of the hindrance." (*BW*)

wit work In this expression Freud uses the component element work in the same sense as he does in *dream work,* namely, to denote the psychic processes operating to produce the witticism.

withdrawal The act of retracting, retiring, retreating, or going away from. Withdrawal is used in psychiatry to refer to (1) voluntary removal of the penis from the vagina in coitus interruptus; (2) abstaining from a drug on which the patient is dependent, and/or the symptoms associated with such abstinence (see *addiction; alcoholism; dependency, drug; tolerance*); (3) the turning away from objective, external reality that is seen so often as an expression of schizophrenic autism. In this third sense, withdrawal refers to the patient's retreat from society and interpersonal relationships into a world of his own. External stimuli are reduced, and if internal stimuli predominate one speaks of preoccupation that may progress to stupor or even to coma. The withdrawn person appears aloof, detached, uninterested, removed, and apart; he has difficulty in spontaneously initiating or planning with other people. He is unable to mingle freely and communication with others is an effort. He cannot share his experiences with others and even in a group appears to work independently rather than cooperatively. In its more extreme forms, withdrawal appears to be a regressive phenomenon in which the subject relinquishes his higher symbolic and social functions and falls back to the infantile level of shutting off the perceptive system in order to avoid the anxiety aroused by interpersonal relationships.

withdrawal, thought See *symptoms, first-rank.*

Wittkower, Eric D. (1899–1983) Berlin-born psychoanalyst whose earliest work in psychosomatic medicine began in 1929.

He moved to London in 1933, and to Canada (McGill University) in 1951. He founded the Section for Transcultural Psychiatric Studies and was a cofounder of the Canadian Psychoanalytic Society.

Witzelsucht (vit'sel-zookt) Facetiousness; seen in lesions of the frontal lobe. See *lobe, frontal.*

Wolf-Man The patient reported on by Freud in his 1918 paper "From the History of an Infantile Neurosis." The patient is so called because of a dream he had had at the age of 4 concerning six or seven white wolves sitting on a tree in front of a dreamer's window; he woke in terror, evidently of being eaten by the wolves. The interpretation of the dream extended over several years. Although the Wolf-Man responded well to psychoanalytic therapy, he suffered several relapses during which he showed increasingly severe paranoid symptoms.

Woltman's sign See *reflex, myxedema.*

womb phantasy See *phantasy, womb.*

women with penis See *penis, women with.*

Woodward, Samuel B. (1787–1850) First president of Association of Medical Superintendents of America (the forerunner of the American Psychiatric Association); treatment of alcoholism.

word blindness Kussmaul's term (1877) for a type of *reading disability* (q.v.).

word cathexis See *cathexis.*

word deafness Auditory aphasia. See *aphasia, auditory.*

word dumbness See *aphasia, motor.*

word salad This is the type of speech, heard most frequently in advanced states of schizophrenia, characterized by a mixture of phrases that are meaningless to the listener and, as a rule, also to the patient producing them; also known as *jargon* or *paraphrasia.* A word salad is a group of neologisms. They are meaningless until the patient discusses the neologisms at length, thus revealing their underlying significance. It is, so to speak, a coded language, not unlike dreams in principle; the patient holds the table to the code and only he can provide meanings to the otherwise incomprehensible dialect.

words, microcosm of "Words and worded concepts are shadows of things, constructed for the purpose of bringing order through trial acting into the chaos of real things." Thus words create a replica of the real world, a model or microcosm of the world. "The macrocosm of real things outside is reflected in the microcosm of things representative within." The normal person uses this microcosm for calculating and acting out in advance, before real action is taken. To him, then, words will have the characteristics of the things that they represent, but they will not have the reality or "seriousness" that the things have. The normal person has mastered the words and, by using his words, will master the real things.

Such mastery of the real world through words is markedly disturbed in the obsessive-compulsive. Being afraid of emotions, he is afraid of things that cause emotions. He therefore retreats from the macrocosm of things to the microcosm of words. He tries to repeat the process by which as an infant he learned to use words to master frightening aspects of the real world. However, "under the pressure of his warded-off impulses" words have now acquired "that emotional value which things have for other persons." They have regained the magical quality they first had in infancy, when there was no clear differentiation between the microcosm and the macrocosm. That is, the words themselves now have the values and meanings they express. Unconsciously, words and thoughts are believed to have real effects. Therefore, the obsessive-compulsive handles words and thoughts very cautiously. This is the origin of compulsive thinking. (Fenichel, *PTN*)

work, case See *casework, social.*

work cure Treatment by occupation. See *therapy, occupational.*

work decrement Decrease in amount of work performed per unit time during a period of continuous practice; this phenomenon is probably a function of muscular (peripheral) and central fatigue induced by continuous work. In most studies of the work curve, schizophrenics have been found to show more rapid work decrement than normals.

work, group See *group-work, social.*

work inhibition See *academic (work) inhibition.*

work, social See *social work, psychiatric.*

worker, aftercare Social worker.

worker, indigenous See *caregiver.*

worker, mental health Staff other than the core mental health professionals (clinical psychologists, psychiatric social workers, psychiatric nurses, psychiatrists) who have had special training to help them develop the skills in helping patients and clients deal with social and psychological problems. In general, such workers perform either a therapeutic role or an advocate/ombudsman/expediter role. See *advocacy; expediter; psychiatry, community.*

working class See *class, social.*

working-over In psychoanalysis, an internal process of rearranging, adjusting, reconstituting, and remolding the excitations produced in the psyche and thereupon being able to prevent their harmful effect because of the impossibility or undesirability of discharging them outward.

"We have recognized our mental apparatus above all as a device for mastering excitations which would otherwise be felt as unpleasant or would have pathogenic effects. The 'working-over' of stimuli in the mind accomplishes wonders for the internal discharge of excitations which are incapable of direct discharge is for the moment, undesirable." (Freud, *CP*)

working-through An ill-defined psychoanalytic concept no single definition of which has achieved general acceptance. Freud considered it a spontaneous psychic process that was the only effective means of countering id resistance (see *resistance, id*). On a descriptive level, working-through usually refers to a doldrum period, that is, a phase of relative inactivity on the part of the patient in psychoanalytic treatment, a period when the analyst's interpretations, no matter how extensive or intensive, seem to have no effect. Such a period is generally assumed to be due to an inability (perhaps constitutional) of the patient to be hurried through his analysis, and/or as due to the persistence of deep transference attitudes (such as hurt, suspicion, or ambivalence) that require prolonged periods of ventilation. "It is easy to observe that after any crisis either in analysis or in ordinary life most individuals tend to 'draw in their horns' until the situation has been stabilized. This process of spontaneous recuperation is best illustrated in the phenomena of normal grief; and it is of interest that this may vary in duration from a few weeks to a few years, indicating that the degree of 'working through' varies normally within wide limits." (Glover, E. *The Technique of Psycho-Analysis,* 1955)

Looked at in another way, working-through may be interpreted as the intrapsychic processes that must take place if insight in one area is to be amalgamated with other areas of the personality, if the patient is to be enabled to experience new perceptions and conflict-free affects appropriate to those perceptions. Working-through involves the recognition and assimilation of newly learned truths, an alteration of balance among the defenses, neutralization of resistance, formation of new identifications, and reconstruction of the ego ideal. To a large extent, successful working-through depends upon the analyst, who is not only a mirror for the patient but must also be a teacher, a definer of reality, a nonjudgmental object of drive-motivated behavior, a representative of the superego who influences by suggestion and even authority, and an idealized object who influences by example. Identification of the patient with the analyst is the basis for expansion and reconstruction of the ego ideal, which stimulates future attainment and is the source of realistic self-esteem. (Karush, A. *Psychoanalytic Quarterly 36,* 1967)

It must also be recognized that the concept of working-through is sometimes used as a rationalization by the therapist for his failure to understand the origins of the patient's resistance at some point during psychoanalytic treatment.

working type See *assimilation.*

workshop, survival skills See *psychoeducation.*

wound See *disease.*

wounding, symbolic See *syndrome, deliberate self-harm.*

wrist-cutting See *self-mutilation.*

writing, automatic Writing without conscious volition, while in hypnotic trance. "Automatic writing is a splendid means of gaining access to unconscious material that lies beyond the grasp of conscious recall. The portion of the cerebrum that controls the automatic writing seems to have access to material unavailable to centers that control speech. Consequently hypnotic verbalization of feelings and impulses may not yield information as vital as that brought up through automatic writing." (Wolberg, L.R. *Hypnoanalysis,* 1945)

writing disorder, expressive An academic skills disorder consisting of impaired performance in spelling, grammar, and other writing skills.

writing, mirror See *strephosymbolia.*

wryneck See *torticollis.*

WS In Rorschach scoring, a whole response (see *W*) that includes some white spaces as well as the entire blot.

Wyatt v. Stickney See *consumerism; forced treatment.*

X

X chromosome See *chromosome*.

xanthomatosis (zan-thō-ma-tō'sis) Schüller-Christian-Hand's syndrome; diabetic exophthalmic dysostosis. A rare disturbance of lipoid metabolism in which tissues are infiltrated by xanthomatous masses rich in cholesterol, this leading to diabetes insipidus, exophthalmos, and progressive erosion of the bones. Infiltration of the reticuloendothelial cells with the lipoid material results in the characteristic foam cell. Retardation of growth and mental development occurs in about half of the cases. The disorder begins in childhood; males are three times as frequently affected as females.

xenoglossia Speaking in a foreign tongue, with the implication that the use of a foreign language is inappropriate to the situation (i.e. the foreign tongue is chosen to avoid rather than enhance communication) and/or that the words are a pseudolanguage or a collection of private metaphors that only the subject understands. Less commonly, the term is used to indicate a person's aversion to any situation in which a language that is not his native tongue is spoken.

xenophobia Fear of strangers.

xerostomia Dryness of the mouth, due to reduced or absent salivary secretion; seen in states of fear, anxiety, or depression, and also as a side effect of many psychopharmacologic agents.

XYY A chromosomal abnormality in which an extra Y (male) chromosome is present, bringing the total chromosomes to 47 (instead of the usual 46, with XY chromosomes in the normal male, and XX chromosomes in the normal female). The XYY pattern is uncommon in the general population; it is estimated to occur in from 1 in every 300 to 1 in every 2,000 men. But the pattern occurs much more frequently (perhaps in as many as 4%) in delinquents and criminals. Some of the adult XYY men studied to date showed a tendency toward tallness, thinness, myopia, disfiguring acne, mental dullness, and behavioral problems, including aggressive, sometimes even violent behavior.

Y

Y chromosome See *chromosome*.

yantra See *Tantra*.

yen sleep See *sleep, yen*.

Yerkes, Robert Mearns (1876–1956) U.S. psychobiologist; behavior of primates.

ylophobia (ī-lō-fō′bē-à) Less correct form of *hylophobia*. Fear of the forest.

yoga psychology A system for the cultivation of self-control. In ordinary life the mind is distracted by real and ideal objects and restlessly in flux. Yoga is designed to overcome infestation of the self by objects. By distancing himself from immediate experience, the yogin achieves both passionlessness and mastery. This requires passing through a sequence of deletions of the contents of consciousness. From *vitarka*, deliberation on ordinary sense experience, delete direct experience (*abhoga*). From reflection, the state thus achieved, delete deliberation; from the resulting stage, joy, delete reflection; and from the last stage delete joy and one has *samvid*, pure "sense of personality" without content.

The essence of the technique is concentration, facilitated by the repetition of a mystic syllable to attain singleness of intent. (Woods, J.H. *The Yoga-System of Patanjali*, 1914)

yohimbine An α_2-antagonist that binds to the α-adrenergic autoreceptor and increases the amount of neurotransmitter secreted by the presynaptic neuron, producing an anxiety syndrome.

young adult chronic patient See *chronic mentally ill*.

Z

Zeitgeber See *rhythms, biologic*.

zelophobia Fear of jealousy.

zelotypia Zealotry; excessive zeal, carried to the verge of insanity, in the advocacy of any cause. Zelotypia is sometimes an expression of *schizoidia* (q.v.).

Zieve's syndrome See *syndrome, Zieve's*.

Zilboorg, Gregory (1890–1959) Russian-born psychoanalyst; criminology, history of psychiatry, ambulatory schizophrenia.

zoanthropy *Lycanthropy* (q.v.).

zoara (zō-ä'rà) *Obs.* Insomnia.

zone, erogenous An organ or organ system that is invested with libidinal energy. Of the many erogenous zones, three are particularly important in psychoanalytic psychology: the oral, the anal, and the genital. See *anal-erotism; genitality; ontogeny, psychic; orality*.

zone, hypnogenic Hypnogenic spot. See *spot, hypnogenic*.

zone, hysterogenic Any area of the body that precipitates a hysterical reaction when stimulated. See *spot, hypnogenic*.

zone, primacy Any dominating erotogenic area, by means of which more subordinated areas find instinctual discharge through displacement. The fashion in which the weaker or residual instinct sources are subordinate to the primacy zone has been termed *libido organization*.

In the development of the libido, one primacy zone tends to succeed another in a typical and characteristic chronological order: (1) the oral; (2) the anal; (3) the phallic; (4) the genital. See *ontogeny, psychic*.

zones, ultramarginal "Some of these marginal elements [see *fringe*] may be so distinctly within the field of awareness that we are conscious of them, but dimly so. Others, in particular cases at least may be so far outside and hidden in the twilight obscurity that the subject is not even dimly aware of them. In more technical parlance, we may say, they are so far dissociated that they belong to *an ultra-marginal zone and are really subconscious*." (Prince, M. *The Unconscious*, 1916)

zoo- (zō'ō-) Combining form meaning animal, from Gr. *zöion*, living being, animal.

zooerasty (zō-ō'ēr-as-tē) Krafft-Ebing's term for the paraphilia consisting of sexual intercourse with an animal. It is usually considered to be synonymous with *sodomy;* many psychiatrists prefer zooerasty, since etymologically it has a more definite meaning than sodomy.

zoolagnia (zō-ō-lag'nē-a) Sexual attraction to animals; a paraphilia.

zoophilia Sexual excitement caused by the stroking and fondling of animals; *zoolagnia* (q.v.). It does not refer to sexual intercourse with animals, which Krafft-Ebing termed *zooerasty* (q.v.).

zoophilism, erotic (zō-of'i-liz'm) Erotic impulse to pat or stroke animals for sexual pleasure; a paraphilia.

zoophobia Fear of animals.

zoopsia (zō-op'sē-à) Act of "seeing" insects or any animal, as in the visual hallucinations of patients with delirium tremens.

zoosadism (zō-ō-) The act of injuring animals for the morbid (as a rule ultimately sexual) pleasure derived from it; a paraphilia.

Zuordnungs (tsoo-ord'nungs) Sorting tests. See *tests, sorting*.

Zwischenstufe (tsvish'en-shtoo-fē) (Ger. "intermediary stage") Magnus Hirschfeld's term for a homosexual.

zygote A fertilized egg produced by the union of two cells to form one single cell in sexual reproduction. By an extension of meaning, however, the organisms themselves that develop from fertilized eggs are also called zygotes, in order to distinguish them from their germ cells, which are called *gametes*.

Zygotes are *diploid* with respect to their chromosomes and have two genes of each pair, whereas gametes are *haploid* and have only one gene of each pair. See *chromosome*.

zygotic Pertaining to a zygote. Referring either to a single cell produced by the union of two cells in reproduction or to the individual developing from such a fertilized egg.